Register Now for Ces to Your Book

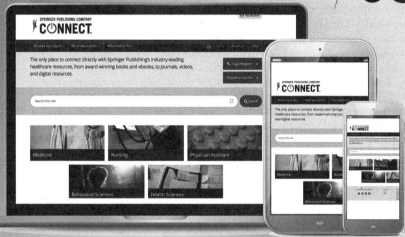

SPRINGER PUBLISHING COMPANY
CONNECT™

Your print purchase of *AACN Core Curriculum For Pediatric High Acuity, Progressive, And Critical Care Nursing, Third Edition,* **includes online access to the contents of your book**—increasing accessibility, portability, and searchability!

Access today at:

http://connect.springerpub.com/content/book/978-0-8261-3303-8 or scan the QR code at the right with your smartphone and enter the access code below.

C2BMU6J1

Scan here for quick access.

SPRINGER PUBLISHING COMPANY
View all our products at springerpub.com

Margaret C. (Peggy) Slota, DNP, RN, FAAN, is an associate professor and director of DNP Graduate Studies at Georgetown University. Her experience includes professional positions as a critical care clinical nurse specialist, flight nurse, staff development educator, university faculty, and healthcare administrator for pediatric critical care services. She was responsible for operations in multiple critical care units and respiratory care, palliative care, critical care transport, and extracorporeal membrane oxygenation (ECMO) services. She initiated a collaborative research program for bedside nurses, led professional development and peer recognition programs, initiated a hospital-based cardiopulmonary nursing fellowship program, and implemented an inpatient and outpatient palliative care program. She has presented frequently and published many peer-reviewed articles, chapters, and three books. Dr. Slota was a member of the national steering committee of the Pediatric Special Interest Group for the American Association of Critical-Care Nurses, an Editorial Board member for *Critical Care Nurse*, first department editor for pediatric critical care in *Critical Care Nurse*, and editor of the first and second editions of the *Core Curriculum for Pediatric Critical Care Nursing* in 1998 and 2006.

AACN CORE CURRICULUM FOR PEDIATRIC HIGH ACUITY, PROGRESSIVE, AND CRITICAL CARE NURSING

Third Edition

Margaret C. Slota, DNP, RN, FAAN

Editor

CO-PUBLISHED WITH THE AMERICAN ASSOCIATION
OF CRITICAL-CARE NURSES (AACN)

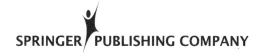

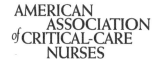

Springer Publishing Company, LLC
11 West 42nd Street
New York, NY 10036
www.springerpub.com

Acquisitions Editor: Elizabeth Nieginski
Compositor: diacriTech, Chennai

ISBN: 978-0-8261-3302-1
ebook ISBN: 978-0-8261-3303-8

18 19 20 21 22 / 5 4 3 2

The author and the publisher of this Work have made every effort to use sources believed to be reliable to provide information that is accurate and compatible with the standards generally accepted at the time of publication. Because medical science is continually advancing, our knowledge base continues to expand. Therefore, as new information becomes available, changes in procedures become necessary. We recommend that the reader always consult current research and specific institutional policies before performing any clinical procedure. The author and publisher shall not be liable for any special, consequential, or exemplary damages resulting, in whole or in part, from the readers' use of, or reliance on, the information contained in this book. The publisher has no responsibility for the persistence or accuracy of URLs for external or third-party Internet websites referred to in this publication and does not guarantee that any content on such websites is, or will remain, accurate or appropriate.

Library of Congress Cataloging-in-Publication Data
Names: Slota, Margaret C., editor. | American Association of Critical-Care
   Nurses, publisher.
Title: AACN core curriculum for pediatric high acuity, progressive, and
   critical care nursing / [edited by] Margaret C. Slota.
Other titles: Core curriculum for pediatric critical care nursing. | Core
   curriculum for pediatric high acuity, progressive, and critical care
   nursing
Description: Third edition. | New York, NY : Springer Publishing Company, LLC;
   [Aliso Viejo, CA] : co-published with the American Association of
   Critical-Care Nurses, [2018] | Preceded by Core curriculum for pediatric
   critical care nursing / edited by Margaret C. Slota. 2nd ed. c2006. |
   Includes bibliographical references and index.
Identifiers: LCCN 2018000371 | ISBN 9780826133021 | ISBN 9780826133038 (ebook)
Subjects: | MESH: Critical Care Nursing—methods | Pediatric Nursing—methods |
   Infant | Child | Outlines
Classification: LCC RJ370 | NLM WY 18.2 | DDC 618.92/00231—dc23
LC record available at https://lccn.loc.gov/2018000371

Contact us to receive discount rates on bulk purchases.
We can also customize our books to meet your needs.
For more information please contact: sales@springerpub.com

Printed in the United States of America.

Dedicated with love to the current and future generations of children,
the hope for our world . . .

Especially my very loved grandchildren, Jackson, Wyatt, and Finlay Hayes

CONTENTS

Contributors   ix
Reviewers   xi
Foreword   Mary Fran Hazinski, MSN, RN,
    FAAN, FAHA   xiii
Preface   xv
Acknowledgments   xvii
Introduction   Mary Frances D. Pate   xix

1. **Caring for Critically Ill Children and Their Families**   *1*
   Jodi E. Mullen and Mary Frances D. Pate

2. **Pulmonary System**   *35*
   Elizabeth Flasch, Nicole Brueck, Justin Lynn, and Jennifer Henningfeld

3. **Cardiovascular System**   *147*
   Louise Callow and Alissa Scheffer

4. **Neurologic System**   *349*
   Paula Vernon-Levett

5. **Renal System**   *445*
   Michelle A. Dokas

6. **Endocrine System**   *479*
   Jennifer LaMie Joiner

7. **Gastrointestinal System**   *531*
   Sarah A. Martin

8. **Hematology and Immunology Systems**   *585*
   Jessica L. Spruit

9. **Multisystem Issues**   *667*
   Section I.   Multiple Trauma
   Frances Blayney and Colleene Young
   Section II.   Toxicology
   Maureen A. Madden
   Section III.   Sepsis and Septic Shock
   Larissa Hutchins and Megan D. Snyder
   Section IV.   Burns
   Amanda Bettencourt and Melissa Gorman
   Section V.   Disaster Preparedness and Response
   Nancy Blake
   Section VI.   Initial Stabilization and Transport
   Bradley A. Kuch and Michael McSteen

10. **Professional Issues—Quality, Safety, Work Environment, and Wellness**   *883*
   Brandis Thornton and Jaime Manley

Index   927

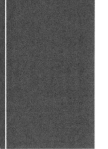

CONTRIBUTORS

Amanda Bettencourt, MSN, RN, CNS, CCRN-K, ACCNS-P
Predoctoral Fellow
Center for Health Outcomes and Policy Research
University of Pennsylvania School of Nursing
Philadelphia, Pennsylvania

Nancy Blake, PhD, RN, CCRN-K, NEA-BC, NHDP- BC, FAAN
Assistant Adjunct Professor
University of California, Los Angeles
Los Angeles, California

Frances Blayney, MS, RN-BC, CCRN
Clinical Educator Patient Care Services
Children's Hospital Los Angeles
Los Angeles, California

Nicole Brueck, MSN, APNP, FNP-BC
Pediatric Pulmonary Nurse Practitioner
Cystic Fibrosis Program Coordinator
Children's Hospital of Wisconsin
Medical College of Wisconsin
Milwaukee, Wisconsin

Louise Callow, MSN, CPNP-PC
Pediatric Cardiac Surgery Nurse Practitioner
C. S. Mott Children's Hospital
Michigan Medicine
Congenital Heart Center
Ann Arbor, Michigan

Michelle A. Dokas, MSN, RN, CPNP-AC
Pediatric Nurse Practitioner
Children's Hospital of Michigan
Detroit, Michigan

Elizabeth Flasch, MSN, APNP, PNP-PC
Pediatric Pulmonary Nurse Practitioner
Children's Hospital of Wisconsin
Medical College of Wisconsin
Milwaukee, Wisconsin

Melissa Gorman, MSN, RN-BC, CCRN-K
Clinical Education Coordinator
Shriner's Hospital for Children—Boston
Boston, Massachusetts

Jennifer Henningfeld, MD
Assistant Professor of Pediatrics
Director of the Pediatric Tracheostomy and Home
  Ventilator Program
Department of Pulmonary and Sleep Medicine
Children's Hospital of Wisconsin
Medical College of Wisconsin
Milwaukee, Wisconsin

Larissa Hutchins, MSN, RN, CCRN-K, CCNS
Director of Nursing, Professional Development
  Simulation Center, and Emergency Care Programs
Children's Hospital of Philadelphia
Philadelphia, Pennsylvania

Jennifer LaMie Joiner, MSN, RN, CPNP-AC/PC
Lead Nurse Practitioner
Pediatric Intensive Care Unit
The Children's Hospital of San Antonio
Baylor College of Medicine
San Antonio, Texas

Bradley A. Kuch, MHA, RRT-NPS, FAARC
Director, Respiratory Care Services and Transport Team
Clinical Research Associate
Department of Pediatric Critical Care Medicine
Children's Hospital of Pittsburgh of UPMC
Pittsburgh, Pennsylvania

Justin Lynn, BS, RRT-NPS
Lead RCP, Tracheostomy/Ventilator Program
Children's Hospital of Wisconsin
Adjunct Faculty
Milwaukee Area Technical College
Milwaukee, Wisconsin

Maureen A. Madden, MSN, RN, CPNP-AC, CCRN, FCCM
Associate Professor of Pediatrics
Rutgers Robert Wood Johnson Medical School
New Brunswick, New Jersey

Jaime Manley, MSN, RN, CPN
H4B/CTICU Program Coordinator
Heart Center Float Pool Manager
Nationwide Children's Hospital
Columbus, Ohio

Sarah A. Martin, MS, CPNP-AC/PC, CCRN
Advanced Practice Nurse—Pediatric Surgery
Ann & Robert H. Lurie Children's Hospital
Chicago, Illinois

**Michael McSteen, BSN, RN, MBA,
CCRN, CNPT**
Transport Nurse
Children's Hospital of Pittsburgh of UPMC
Pittsburgh, Pennsylvania

**Jodi E. Mullen, MS, RN-BC, CCRN,
CCNS, ACCNS-P**
Clinical Leader
Pediatric Intensive Care Unit
UF Health Shands Children's Hospital
Gainesville, Florida

Mary Frances D. Pate, PhD, RN
Assistant Professor
Capstone College of Nursing
University of Alabama
Tuscaloosa, Alabama

Alissa Scheffer, MS, CPNP-PC
Pediatric Cardiac Surgery Nurse Practitioner
C. S. Mott Children's Hospital
Michigan Medicine
Ann Arbor, Michigan

Megan D. Snyder, MSN, RN, ACCNS-P, CCRN
Clinical Nurse Specialist
Pediatric Intensive Care Unit
Children's Hospital of Philadelphia
Philadelphia, Pennsylvania

Jessica L. Spruit, DNP, RN, CPNP-AC
Pediatric Acute Care Nurse Practitioner Program
Coordinator
College of Nursing
Wayne State University
Detroit, Michigan

Brandis Thornton, MS, RD, CSP
Senior Service Line QI Coordinator
Nationwide Children's Hospital
Columbus, Ohio

Paula Vernon-Levett, MS, RN, CCRN-K
Nursing Practice Leader PICU/PCICU
University of Iowa Stead Family Children's
Hospital
Iowa City, Iowa

Colleene Young, BSN, RN, NE-BC, CCRN
Lead/Clinical Nurse IV
Children's Hospital Los Angeles
Los Angeles, California

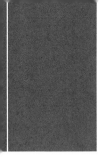

REVIEWERS

Cardiopulmonary Section Reviewer/ Editor

Kathryn E. Roberts, MSN, RN, CNS, CCRN, CCNS, FCCM
Associate Chief Nursing Officer–Innovation and Advancement
Children's Hospital of Philadelphia
Philadelphia, Pennsylvania

Elumalai Appachi, MD MRCP(UK)
Associate Professor of Pediatrics
Baylor College of Medicine
Chief, Pediatric Critical Care Medicine
The Children's Hospital of San Antonio
San Antonio, Texas

Cheryl Bartke, MSN, ARNP, PNP-BC, CPNP-AC
Supervisor
Pediatric Advanced Practice Provider Team
Department of Pediatrics
Division of Critical Care
Seattle Children's Hospital
Seattle, Washington

Kathleen M. Brown, DNP, MSHA, BSN
Executive Vice President and Chief Clinical Officer
Post Acute Medical, LLC
Enola, Pennsylvania

Joseph Carillo, MD
Professor, CCM and Pediatrics
Children's Hospital of Pittsburgh of UPMC
Pittsburgh, Pennsylvania

Kathryn Carpenter, MSN, RN
Pediatric and Neonatal Transport Clinical Lead RN
OHSU Doernbecher Children's Hospital
Portland, Oregon

Roland Chu, MD
Assistant Professor of Pediatrics
Fellowship Director, Pediatric Hematology/Oncology
Division of Hematology/Oncology/BMT Medical Director of Informatics
Children's Hospital of Michigan
Detroit, Michigan

Diana DeArment, PA-C
Supervisor, Advanced Practice Providers
Division of Endocrinology
Children's Hospital of Pittsburgh of UPMC
Pittsburgh, Pennsylvania

Michele Dunstan, MSN, RN, CCRN
Pediatric Trauma Coordinator
Lehigh Valley Health Network
Allentown, Pennsylvania

Julie C. Fitzgerald, MD, PhD
Assistant Professor of Anesthesiology and Critical Care Medicine
University of Pennsylvania
Perelman School of Medicine
The Children's Hospital of Philadelphia
Philadelphia, Pennsylvania

Patricia Harris, DNP, NP-C, PNP-AC, CCRN, CWOCN, CCTN, CCTC
Department of Pediatric Abdominal Transplant Surgery
Thomas E. Starzl Transport Institute
Children's Hospital of Pittsburgh
Pittsburgh, Pennsylvania

Amy J. Howells, PhD, CPNP-AC/PC
Assistant Professor
Department of Family Child Nursing
University of Washington
School of Nursing
Seattle, Washington

Jessica Huber, MSN, CCRN
Senior Professional Staff Nurse
Children's Hospital of Pittsburgh
Instructor/Course Coordinator for Pediatrics
Carlow University
Pittsburgh, Pennsylvania

Aimee Jennings, MSN, ARNP
Supervisor, Pediatric Advanced Practice Provider
Team Department of Pediatrics
Division of Critical Care Medicine
Seattle Children's Hospital
Seattle, Washington

Vanessa Kalis, DNP, ACNP-BC, CPNP-AC, CNS, RN
Associate Professor
Director, Acute Care DNP Programs: Pediatric and
    Adult–Gerontologic
Marybelle and S. Paul Musco School of Nursing and
    Health Professions
Brandman University
Irvine, California

**Serena Phromsivarak Kelly, MSN, FNP-BC,
    CPNP-AC, CCRN, CPEN**
Pediatric Intensive Care Unit Nurse Practitioner
Assistant Professor of Pediatrics
Pediatric Critical Care Medicine
OHSU Doernbecher Children's Hospital
Portland, Oregon

**Michael A. Maymi, DNP, ARNP, CPNP-AC,
    CCRN**
Lead Nurse Practitioner Cardiac Critical Care, Orlando
Cardiac Intensive Care Unit
Nemours Children's Hospital
Orlando, Florida

William J. Mohr, MD
Medical Director, Burn Program
Regions Hospital
St. Paul, Minnesota

Radhika Muzumdar, MD
Chief, Pediatric Endocrinology
Associate Professor of Pediatrics and Cell Biology
Children's Hospital of Pittsburgh
Pittsburgh, Pennsylvania

Lisa Remaley, MPAS, PA-C
Physician Assistant
Department of Pediatric Abdominal Transplant Surgery
Thomas E. Starzl Transport Institute
Children's Hospital of Pittsburgh
Pittsburgh, Pennsylvania

Melissa Reynolds, MSN, RN, NE-BC, CCRN-K
Nurse Manager, Pediatric Intensive Care Unit
University of Florida Health Shands Children's Hospital
Gainesville,Florida

Lindsay Wilson Shah, MSN, RN, CPNP-AC
Nurse Practitioner
Instructor, Critical Care Medicine
Baylor College of Medicine
Texas Children's Hospital
Houston, Texas

Robert Sheridan, MD, FAAP, FACS
Medical Director, Burn Service
Shriners Hospital for Children—Boston
Boston, Massachusetts

Kyle A. Soltys, MD
Associate Professor of Surgery
Thomas E. Starzl Transport Institute
Children's Hospital of Pittsburgh
Pittsburgh, Pennsylvania

James E. Squires, MD, MS
Division of Gastroenterology
Hepatology and Nutrition
Children's Hospital of Pittsburgh of the University of
    Pittsburgh Medical Center
Pittsburgh, Pennsylvania

Kathleen Stevenson, RN, BSN
Senior Project Manager
Healthcare Technical Services Inc
Pasadena, California

Roberto R. Trevizo, MPH, MSN, RN, FNP-BC
Nurse Practitioner
University Medical Center of El Paso
El Paso, Texas

Danielle Van Damme, MSN, CPNP-AC, CPHON
Pediatric Nurse Practitioner
Pediatric Critical Care Medicine
C. S. Mott Children's Hospital
University of Michigan Health System
Ann Arbor, Michigan

Lee Ann Wallace, MBA, BSN, RN, NEA-BC
Vice President
Neonatal Services and Critical Care Transport Services
Nationwide Children's Hospital
Columbus, Ohio

Tracey Weifenbaugh, MSN, MBA, RNC-NIC, CCM
Associate Director, Medical and Clinical Operations
United Healthcare
Pittsburgh, Pennsylvania

Martha Yee, MSN, RN, PNP-C, AC&PC
Instructor in Clinical Nursing, PNP-AC&PC Programs
University of Texas at Arlington
Arlington, Texas

L. Caulette Young, BSN, RN, CCRN, CHSE
Education Manager
CHLA Simulation Center
Children's Hospital Los Angeles
Los Angeles, California

Ahmar Urooj Zaidi, MD
Assistant Professor, Pediatrics
Division of Pediatric Hematology/Oncology
Children's Hospital of Michigan
Wayne State University School of Medicine
Detroit, Michigan

FOREWORD

This is the third edition of the previously published *Pediatric Critical Care Core Curriculum*. All three books have been edited by Margaret C. (Peggy) Slota. The title of this third edition, *AACN Core Curriculum for Pediatric High Acuity, Progressive, and Critical Care Nursing*, has been changed to reflect the expansion of the practice of pediatric critical care beyond the bounds of critical care units and beyond the acute phase of illness or injury. As in the first two editions, this edition contains detailed information regarding pediatric critical care physiology, pathophysiology, clinical evaluation, and management presented in a narrative outline style for quick reference and later study. All parts of this text convey Peggy's respect for both the science and the art of nursing care of children and their families. They also reflect Peggy's keen insights about approaches to the challenges faced by pediatric critical care nurses today.

The subspecialty of pediatric critical care nursing is a relatively new one. Pediatric critical care units initially evolved as postoperative care units for children. However, in the 1960s and 1970s, during the first wave of the subspecialty's evolution, several simultaneous developments contributed to the rapid expansion of the pediatric critical care patient population and the technology they needed. First, successful mechanical ventilation of premature newborns engendered development of commercially available newborn ventilators and successful arterial blood gas and other laboratory analysis with smaller and smaller specimen volumes. Neonatal ventilators soon populated pediatric critical care units, often used to support older infants with lung disease. In fact, for several years, the options for pediatric mechanical ventilators were the neonatal ventilators (the "baby Byrd" or the Bournes), ventilators borrowed from the operating suite, or Bennet "adult" (MA-1) ventilators. Simultaneous advances in prehospital emergency and trauma care and successful closed-chest cardiopulmonary resuscitation enabled at least short-term survival of children with what had been immediately fatal illnesses and injuries, adding more facets to pediatric critical care. Open-heart cardiovascular surgery was becoming more successful in infants and young children, and prostaglandin E1 enabled better preoperative stabilization of infants with ductal-dependent congenital heart defects; this resulted in a substantial rise in perioperative survival. Although these factors contributed to the expansion of the pediatric critical care population, technology, and the types of care provided, Reye's syndrome was the first disease that was unique to children and it was one that necessitated continuous and meticulous care by all members of the healthcare team. This disease, probably more than any others, demanded that all aspects of pediatric critical care move beyond techniques and technologies modified from experience with newborn or adult patients. It also required the critical care providers to function as a cohesive team.

The 1980s and 1990s saw the second wave in the development of the pediatric critical care nursing subspecialty. In the early 1980s, pediatric nurse members of the American Association of Critical-Care Nurses (AACN) initially organized within a special interest group, and pediatric content at the National Teaching Institute (NTI) was limited. However, pediatric critical care units were growing in size and scope, and the number of pediatric critical care nurses was increasing rapidly. Several seminal journal publications documented specific physiologic differences between children and adults and how those differences influenced the pathophysiology, clinical presentation, and management of common critical care conditions, but much of our understanding of these aspects still had to be derived and modified from neonatal and adult published literature. At this time, a substantial portion of the equipment used in pediatric critical care units came from newborn or adult ICUs. By the 1990s, there was sufficient demand for pediatric content at the AACN NTI that pediatric "tracts" were offered, and pediatric nurses successfully lobbied for the establishment of a pediatric critical care certification process, because it was now clear that pediatric critical care nursing required unique knowledge and skills. In the late 1990s, AACN invited Peggy Slota to edit the first edition of the *Pediatric Critical Care Core Curriculum*. Peggy was a recognized pediatric critical care author, researcher, teacher, and leader who helped define the subspecialty. The first edition of the *Pediatric Critical Care Core Curriculum*, published in 1998, explained many of the reasons that critically ill or injured children and the care they require are unique, and this edition focused on those skills, assessments, and interventions that were unique or essential to pediatric critical care nursing, and that differed from the practice of physicians and other members of the critical care team.

By the time the second edition of the *Core Curriculum* was published in 2006, pediatric critical care had a stronger evidence base, and this was reflected in more detailed content with greater emphasis on pathophysiology, clinical assessment and pharmacology, and evidence-based management. The patient population in pediatric critical care units had much higher acuity, with patients much more dependent on technology. As a result, more content was added about the function and troubleshooting of equipment, while still emphasizing the crucial role of the critical care nurse in supporting the child and family.

This third edition addresses complex patient problems and solutions, with the core content reflecting the greater independence of the nursing role. The additional emphasis on evidence-based practice and professionalism is apparent throughout the text. A new chapter (Chapter 10) has been added at the request of the nurses who use the *AACN Core Curriculum*. This chapter includes information about the professional role of the nurse, and the nurse's contributions to processes of continuous quality improvement. Any consideration of issues of quality of care and safety must address the importance of supporting the caregivers, acknowledging the challenges inherent in a profession that addresses life-threatening emergencies on a daily basis.

As the challenges of pediatric critical care evolve, so must the knowledge, skills, and preparation of pediatric critical care nurses. In three editions of this important book published over a 20-year period, Peggy Slota has contributed substantially to the generation, synthesis, and dissemination of the knowledge and skills that pediatric critical care nurses require to care for their patients and families . . . and themselves.

Mary Fran Hazinski, MSN, RN, FAAN, FAHA
Professor, Division of Trauma & Surgical Critical Care
Vanderbilt University School of Nursing
Nashville, Tennessee

PREFACE

Infants and children cared for in critical care units leave a legacy. Beyond the lessons learned from the phenomenal resilience of children and their amazing will to survive, the collaborative experience of working together as a team to support children in their battle for recovery provides knowledge that we cannot provide in a text. The art and science of pediatric critical care nursing has grown exponentially over my career and it has been exciting to witness, from our very early hybridization of the adult critical care model and "downsized" adult interventions to the development of an independent evidence-based, family-centered, specialty discipline. Our patient population is challenging, requiring the knowledge and contributions of multiple disciplines and a cohesive team of care providers. Although skilled and technically competent nursing care has made significant contributions to patient outcomes, much more is required: Compassion—an affirmation to families that although we cannot fully know their pain, we will always be there for them; persistence balanced by realism so that we know when it is time to let go; caring focused not only on the children, but on their parents, siblings, and extended family, all of whom are impacted; evidence-based practice and monitoring of quality to ensure best practices; and a sense of humor and acceptance to find the sun in the clouds and the path to tomorrow.

The *Core Curriculum for Pediatric Critical Care Nursing*, last published in 2006, has always been a resource for nurses caring for acutely ill or injured children. This third edition has been retitled: *AACN Core Curriculum for Pediatric High Acuity, Progressive, and Critical Care Nursing*, which reflects the increasing acuity in all inpatient departments and the fact that these children are cared for in a variety of settings, including many specialty units in hospitals and in the emergency department, cath lab, diagnostic testing, and more. Experienced contributing authors representing diverse geographic regions have created a thorough and relevant source of information, providing a review of a wide variety of conditions. Using a systems approach and narrative outline for easy reference, each chapter reviews developmental anatomy and physiology, pathophysiology and defining characteristics of neonatal and pediatric disorders, clinical assessment, pharmacology, monitoring, diagnostic testing, pain and palliative care management, and a multidisciplinary approach to the plan of care. Each health problem is discussed along the continuum of the American Association of Critical-Care Nurses (AACN) Synergy Model for Patient Care and family-centered care with integration of ethical, legal, and environmental issues. Application of the principles of care is exemplified in the embedded case studies. This third edition builds on and updates the information provided in the first two editions, with expansion to the acute and progressive phase of care. The content is based on the most current standards of care, scope of practice, national guidelines, key AACN initiatives, and the AACN Certification Corporation Pediatric CCRN Test Plan (AACN, 2017). In addition, based on focus group feedback from critical care nurses, we have added a chapter on professional issues. This new chapter includes content on quality, safety, communication, teamwork, work environment, and personal wellness. In 2008, Berwick, Nolan, and Whittington's Triple Aim framework was introduced to influence quality and ensure high-value care in the United States, focusing on *improving the individual experience of care, improving the health of populations*, and *reducing the per capita cost* of healthcare. More recently, the Quadruple Aim added the aim of *improving the experience of providing care* (Sikka, Morath, & Leape, 2015). Workforce engagement and safety are significant in this. Achieving the metrics of this goal would ensure that we remember what motivated us to choose this career in the first place and allow us to find joy and meaning in our work. Our work as pediatric critical care nurses is dedicated to the memory of the children and families we have cared for; those for whom our best technology, knowledge, effort, and compassion were not enough for survival; and those children who have recovered from critical illness and injury, able to smile and play again . . . this gives us strength.

As critical care nurses, you make a difference in someone's life in ways you cannot imagine *every single day* that you work. I cannot imagine a greater gift from a profession.

Margaret C. (Peggy) Slota

REFERENCES

American Association of Critical-Care Nurses. (2017). *CCRN exam handbook.* Aliso Vieja, CA: AACN Certification Corporation.

Berwick, D. M., Nolan T. W., & Whittington, J. (2008). The Triple Aim: Care, health and cost. *Health Affairs, 27*, 759–769.

Sikka, R., Morath, J. M., & Leape, L. (2015). The quadruple aim: Care, health, cost and meaning in work. *BMJ Quality & Safety, 24*, 608–610. doi:10.1136/bmjqs-2015-004160

ACKNOWLEDGMENTS

Without a team, this book would not have been possible.

Caring for children in eight different ICUs over the course of my career in neonatal and pediatric critical care, emergency department, and transport team nursing practice, I met and worked with more caring and dedicated healthcare professionals than I can count—nurses, physicians, respiratory therapists, pharmacists, and those in many other disciplines. I have witnessed an unparalleled devotion to this career path, especially among nurses. As a previous administrator, I continuously heard and read the praise and gratitude of families that will never forget the team's efforts to save the life of their child. Thank you, pediatric healthcare professionals, for all that you taught me.

I have learned so much from the many children and families we cared for over the years. I admire and respect the strength and courage of children and families in the face of devastating and unexpected illness and injury.

I am grateful to the contributing authors for their extensive commitment of time and for sharing their expertise so readily and for the thoughtful critiques given by our many reviewers.

Over the years, critical care nurses who used the text provided valued feedback and suggestions. I especially appreciate the critical care nurses who completed the American Association of Critical-Care Nurses (AACN) survey in anticipation of the revision and those who participated in the focus groups, which assisted immensely in setting direction for the third edition.

Thank you to the AACN publishing staff, especially Michael Muscat, and the production staff and administrative support at Springer Publishing, especially Rachel Landes, Elizabeth Nieginski, and Lindsay Claire. Your support and patience was critical to the success of this project.

Mary Frances D. Pate, a contributing author for both the 2006 edition and this one, was invaluable in reviewing all the chapters for AACN, ensuring that the content included all of the AACN key initiatives, guidelines, and standards. I appreciate the introduction she wrote to provide an overview of the critical role of professional oversight played by AACN. I appreciate Kathryn Roberts's support in coordinating the development of the key cardiac and pulmonary chapters.

I have been an active member of many professional organizations, but the most valuable to me has been AACN. As a member for more than 37 years, I am so appreciative of the goldmine of education and support offered through the journals, newsletters, evidence-based resources, and professional colleagues. As a critical care nurse, educator, clinical nurse specialist, and manager, I always knew that AACN had my back.

Special thanks to Mary Fran Hazinski, who has been an influential part of my career from the beginning. We met as members of AACN's first Pediatric Critical Care Special Interest Group, which she led. In those times, there was no map—we were creating our own directions as we paved the way for pediatric critical care to emerge as a nursing specialty. I am grateful for our collegial and supportive friendship.

I feel so very privileged to have been a pediatric critical care nurse.

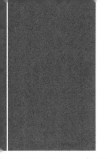

INTRODUCTION

Mary Frances D. Pate

AACN Core Curriculum for Pediatric High Acuity, Progressive, and Critical Care Nursing provides the essential knowledge needed by those caring for pediatric patients receiving high acuity and intensive nursing care. Nursing students involved in their first pediatric clinical experiences and those studying for certification exams may find the book useful as a reference. Although the clinical placement of critically ill children may vary from a Level 1 pediatric intensive care unit (PICU) to a unit that cares primarily for adult patients, the care young patients receive must remain consistent across all contexts and care models. Critical care is not a place, but rather it describes care requiring a high level of vigilance and intervention. Nationally recognized guidelines standardize admission and discharge criteria for children in such units, and pediatric-specific, evidence-based standards need to be integrated into the care of all young patients.

The American Association of Critical-Care Nurses (AACN) Synergy Model for Patient Care instructs us that the needs or characteristics of patients and families influence and drive the characteristics or competencies of the nurse. Synergy results when the needs and characteristics of a patient, clinical unit, or system are matched with the nurse's competencies (AACN, 2017a). Those caring for acutely and critically ill children must demonstrate initial and ongoing professional competencies related to the care of this population. Nursing is a dynamic field, so it is the responsibility of the professional to apply the most current, evidence-based literature during care planning. For example, when working with pharmacologic agents, professional nurses are required to be familiar with manufacturers' information, appropriateness of the agents for children, and dosing and administration guidelines.

As the largest specialty nursing organization in the world, AACN is the standard setter for leading-edge clinical resources for pediatric acute and critical care nurses that empower them to make their optimal contribution to patients and families. Healthcare organizations can use the following resources to assist in the evidence-based care of our youngest patients. AACN's online course, Essentials of Pediatric Critical Care Orientation (EPCCO), uses an online learning format to orient nurses to the care of critically ill children, and

is available from AACN. The AACN Pediatric Critical Care Pocket Reference Card (2016) provides a succinct, readily accessible resource for the bedside nurse. Professionals interested in gaining a broader view of pediatric critical care, learning from pediatric experts, and having an opportunity to network with others caring for children may consider attending AACN's National Teaching Institute & Critical Care Exposition. This annual educational event provides attendees with several venues and activities developed to connect professionals experiencing similar clinical and work-related situations. In addition, AACN's impact grant programs have supported—and will continue to support—researchers and clinicians working with pediatric populations.

Nurses caring for critically ill children are often required to complete the American Heart Association's Pediatric Advanced Life Support (PALS) course, which is co-branded with AACN and provides detailed algorithms to assist healthcare providers in the care of children who are deteriorating physiologically. Emergency simulations related to pediatric assessment and resuscitation are used to reinforce learning.

Specialty certification is a hallmark of excellence, demonstrating a commitment to quality and patient safety. Nurses interested in validating pediatric critical care knowledge and becoming recognized for additional learning can register for the CCRN (Pediatric) and/or CCRN-K (Pediatric) professional examinations for the registered nurse. (The CCRN-K is a specialty certification for nurses who influence the care delivered to patients but do not primarily or exclusively direct care.) Similarly, the ACCNS-P (Pediatric) certification reflects the clinical nurse specialist's dedication to excellence in the care of pediatric critical care patients. AACN offers study materials and practice exam questions to help prospective certificants prepare for the exam. The association also offers a CCRN (Pediatric) review course, and both online and in-person review courses are available at various sites from other organizations across the country (AACN, 2017b).

Children and families admitted to pediatric critical care units benefit from a healthy environment in which healing is facilitated. Annually, an award co-sponsored by AACN, the Society of Critical Care Medicine (SCCM), and the Committee on Architecture for Health of the American Institute of Architects, recognizes units that combine functional design with humanitarian delivery of care (SCCM, 2017). These elements are critical for children and families recovering from serious illness or injury.

Nurses and intraprofessional teams benefit from work environments that are healthy. Unfortunately, the results of the 2013 AACN Critical Care Nurse Work Environment Survey revealed that the health of critical care nurse work environments has declined since 2008 (Ulrich, Lavandero, Woods, & Early, 2014). This finding is important as toxic work situations impact both nurses and patient outcomes. Healthcare providers should experience a work life that is conducive to stimulating, satisfying employment. The *AACN Standards for Establishing and Sustaining Healthy Work Environments* (AACN, 2017c), now in its second edition, was developed to provide evidence-based guidance to those interested in fostering such workplaces. The AACN Healthy Work Environment Assessment Tool is available for those who wish to examine the baseline health of their workplace. Using the assessment tool, caregivers can measure performance improvement following implementation of the standards.

Much has changed since 1967 when the first multidisciplinary PICU opened in the United States at the Children's Hospital of Philadelphia (CHOP; Foglia & Milonovich, 2011). The need for healthy work environments for nurses and intraprofessional teams, synergy between the competencies of the nurse and the needs of patients and families, and the need for patients to be seen as persons (Koloroutis & Trout, 2012) hasn't changed. This is especially important for children, who may be viewed as human *becomings* versus human beings. When true collaboration occurs, children and families will be viewed as full partners in healthcare with the intraprofessional team.

Pediatric critical care technology, pharmacology, research, and patient care management are fields that are rapidly changing and growing. Although we have made every effort to provide current information and data, it is not possible to provide an up-to-the-minute resource in a print publication. As licensed professionals, nurses are responsible for using current resources to evaluate treatment approaches, especially with medications and other products as well as checking their employers' policies and procedures, as well as manufacturers' product information; and verifying dosages, administration guidelines, and contraindications. AACN, the publisher, editor, and contributing authors assume no liability for injuries or damages arising from this publication.

The editor, contributors, and reviewers of the *AACN Core Curriculum for Pediatric High Acuity, Progressive, and Critical Care Nursing* hope this new edition will assist pediatric acute and critical care nurses along their professional journey.

REFERENCES

American Association of Critical-Care Nurses. (2017a). AACN synergy model. Retrieved from https://www.aacn.org/nursing-excellence/aacn-standards/synergy-model

American Association of Critical-Care Nurses. (2017b). *AACN Certification Corporation*. Retrieved from https://www.aacn.org/certification?tab=First-Time%20Certification

American Association of Critical-Care Nurses. (2017c). AACN Standards for Establishing and Sustaining Healthy Work Environments: A Journey to Excellence. Retrieved from https://www.aacn.org/nursing-excellence/healthy-work-environments

Foglia, D. C., & Milonovich, L. M. (2011). The evolution of pediatric critical care nursing: Past, present, and future. *Critical Care Nursing Clinics of North America, 23*(2), 239–253. doi:10.1016/j.ccell.2011.02.003

Koloroutis, M., & Trout, M. (2012). *See me as a person: Creating therapeutic relationships with patients and their families*. Minneapolis, MN: Creative Healthcare Management.

Society of Critical Care Medicine. (2017). *ICU design citation*. Retrieved from http://www.sccm.org/Member-Center/Awards/Pages/ICU-Design-Citation.aspx

Ulrich, B. T., Lavandero, R., Woods, D., & Early, S. (2014). Critical care nurse work environments 2013: A status report. *Critical Care Nurse, 34*(4), 64–79. doi:10.4037/ccn2014731

1 CARING FOR CRITICALLY ILL CHILDREN AND THEIR FAMILIES

Jodi E. Mullen and Mary Frances D. Pate

AJ was almost 2 years old and had never been in the hospital. In the weeks before admission, his parents noticed that he was holding his head to one side and resisting efforts to straighten it. AJ was also becoming ataxic. A few days before admission, he experienced emesis and became lethargic. His parents were frightened when they were told that AJ had a malignant brain tumor. He was admitted to the pediatric intensive care unit (PICU) after craniotomy for removal of the tumor, was medically stable, and required routine postoperative care. The morning after surgery, AJ was awake and looked around but avoided eye contact. He refused to smile or to pay attention to books or toys. He held his special blanket close to his face. His eyes were huge under the gigantic turban of gauze and tape. With pain medication, he relaxed somewhat but still refused to interact with his nurse.

AJ initially brightened when his mother arrived but showed little interest in her efforts to beguile him. Because AJ was preverbal, it was impossible for him to tell us why he was so unhappy. As his mother talked, she stated that AJ was one of four boys. His oldest brother was almost 5 years old, the next boy was 3 years old, and AJ had a twin brother, NJ. The boys' father was at home with them until grandparents arrived from another state to help with their care.

AJ's mother was assured that the children were welcome to visit and that the certified child-life specialist would help them understand what to expect before coming into the unit. When the rest of the family arrived, AJ was observed closely. The sight of his father and older brothers elicited a response similar to that of his mother's arrival, but when AJ saw his twin brother, a metamorphosis occurred. When twin NJ saw AJ, he broke loose from his father's hand and ran to the bed. It was suggested that his mother pick up NJ and place him on the bed next to AJ, at which time AJ became a "new man." He sat up straight, looked around the room, and smiled with his nurse and his entire family. AJ's twin had brought Mylar balloons, and within minutes both AJ and NJ were hitting the balloons and laughing out loud. AJ's mother later expressed her feelings about the encounter. When she and AJ's father had seen the change in their son, they were able to remain hopeful

about their ability to face the future. Their need, at that time, was for their family to be together. AJ's special need was to be with his twin brother.

Regardless of the anticipated outcome, admission of a child to the PICU is a highly stressful event for families. Effective pediatric critical care nurses see the child and family as an integral unit that is central to the healthcare system and are perceptive to the needs of the entire family as they move through the crisis. Nurses who view patients and families as partners in care acknowledge both the psychosocial and physical needs of the developing child and family. When guided by the American Association of Critical-Care Nurses (AACN) Synergy Model for Patient Care, nursing practice places the patient's and the family's needs as its central or driving force. When nursing competencies are based on these needs, optimal patient outcomes result (Curley, 2001). By practicing within the Synergy Model for Patient Care, the pediatric critical care nurse can articulate how he or she contributed to the patient's outcomes.

THE SYNERGY MODEL FOR PATIENT CARE

The AACN Synergy Model for Patient Care was initially developed by the AACN Certification Corporation to serve as the foundation for certifying critical care nursing practice (AACN Certification Corporation, 2015; Hardin & Kaplow, 2017).

A. Core Concepts

The following are core concepts of the Synergy Model for Patient Care:

   1. The needs and characteristics of patients and their families influence and drive the competencies of the nurse.

   2. Synergy occurs when individuals work together in ways that move them toward a common goal.

   3. An active partnership between the patient and the nurse will result in optimal outcomes.

B. Patient and Family Characteristics

Every patient and his or her family bring a unique set of characteristics to the care situation. Each characteristic exists along a continuum, and the patient can fluctuate along that continuum as his or her needs evolve over time.

1. *Stability.* The ability to maintain a steady state

2. *Complexity.* The intricate entanglement of two or more systems (body, family, therapies)

3. *Predictability.* A collective characteristic that allows the nurse to anticipate the patient moving along a certain illness trajectory

4. *Resiliency.* The capacity to return to a previous level of functioning

5. *Vulnerability.* Susceptibility to stressors that may affect outcomes

6. *Participation in Decision Making.* The extent to which the patient and family participate in decision making

7. *Participation in Care.* The extent to which the patient and family can participate in care

8. *Resource Availability.* Resources (e.g., personal, financial, social) the family brings to the care situation

C. Nurse Competencies

Nurse competencies are driven by the needs of the patient and family. These competencies reflect the integration of nursing knowledge, skills, and experiences that are required to meet the patient's and family's needs and to optimize their outcomes. Each competency has different levels of experience ranging along a continuum from novice to competent to expert practitioner. Although the competencies, as a whole, reflect the entirety of nursing practice, each competency becomes more or less important depending on the patient's needs at the time.

1. *Clinical Judgment.* Clinical reasoning and critical thinking skills

2. *Caring Practices.* Creating a therapeutic environment based on the unique needs of the patient and family

3. *Advocacy/Moral Agency.* Working on another's behalf; resolving ethical concerns

4. *Collaboration.* Working with others in a way that encourages each person's contribution toward the patient's goals

5. *Systems Thinking.* Recognizing the interrelationship within and across healthcare systems

6. *Response to Diversity.* Recognizing and incorporating differences into care

7. *Clinical Inquiry.* Ongoing questioning and evaluation of practice

8. *Facilitator of Learning.* Facilitating patient and family learning

D. Outcomes

Optimal outcomes result when the patient characteristics and nursing competencies are matched. Because the Synergy Model for Patient Care views the patient and family as active participants in the model, the outcomes measured should be patient and family driven. The following are examples of potential outcomes to be measured (Curley, 2001).

1. Outcomes from a patient perspective
   a. Functional change
   b. Behavioral change
   c. Trust
   d. Satisfaction
   e. Comfort
   f. Quality of life

2. Outcomes from a nursing perspective
   a. Physiologic changes
   b. Presence or absence of complications
   c. Extent to which treatment objectives are obtained

3. Outcomes from a system perspective
   a. Costs
   b. Rehospitalization
   c. Resource utilization

The following case study illustrates the use of the Synergy Model for Patient Care in practice:

DK, a 9-year-old male, was diagnosed with asthma at the age of 4. He presented at the emergency department with a 24-hour history of increasing difficulty breathing, wheezing, and coughing. DK has been hospitalized once or twice a year since diagnosis and has been in the PICU on three occasions. He was placed on continuous oxygen and nebulized aerosol therapy and was admitted to the PICU for further observation and care. DK was admitted within the past hour and a physical assessment had been completed. In addition, he was evaluated from a nursing perspective using the Synergy Model for Patient Care. According to the patient characteristics of the model, he could be described as follows.

Stability

DK was moderately stable. He was currently able to maintain a steady state but had the potential of deteriorating. He was receiving oxygen, aerosol treatments, and intravenous (IV) fluids. He was tachypneic and tachycardic and had moderate work of breathing.

Complexity

DK's case was mildly complex. Currently, only one body system was affected. His family system was relatively uncomplicated; his mother was a single parent and DK had two younger siblings, aged 7 and 4 years.

Predictability

DK's condition was moderately predictable. He was moving along the expected course of his illness. Although he has been in the PICU on three previous occasions, he had not required mechanical ventilation and had always improved as expected once therapies were initiated.

Resiliency

DK was highly resilient. He had no other underlying conditions that would complicate his situation and had demonstrated previously that he could return to his usual level of functioning.

Vulnerability

DK had a low level of vulnerability. He was only mildly susceptible to stressors that might affect his outcome. This susceptibility was influenced by his history of asthma, previous medication regimen, and young and relatively healthy physique.

Participation in Decision Making

DK and his mother both had a high level of participation. He was alert and asking questions and had a fairly good understanding of his condition and what would help him get better. His mother was present and asking appropriate questions.

Participation in Care

DK and his mother both had a high level of participation in care. His mother had made care arrangements for her other children so as to allow her to remain at the hospital with DK. She was informed about our unit's family-centered care philosophy and invited to participate as a partner with staff in DK's care.

Resource Availability

DK and his mother had moderate resource availability. His mother expressed some financial concerns related to recently changing jobs and not yet having health insurance for her family. In addition, the family car had broken down and they were relying on public transportation. She did have an extended family that was supportive of her situation and her son's medical needs.

By having a holistic picture of DK and his family's characteristics, nurses were able to think about what nursing competencies would be an important match for improved patient outcomes. Although all the competencies are important, some would be more valuable in this situation. Nurses would need to rely on strong *clinical judgment* skills to monitor DK for improvement or worsening of his condition. Nurses would use *caring practices* to create a therapeutic environment for this family, and nurses would be vigilant to prevent complications from DK's therapies and the hospitalization itself. Nurses would use *collaboration* skills when working with him and his mother and also in determining whom to consult to help with the family's financial and transportation needs. Finally, nurses would be a *facilitator of learning* by ensuring that DK and his mother received additional asthma education.

Outcome goals were discussed with DK and his mother, and we agreed that satisfaction with care, absence of complications, and progressive improvement with discharge from the PICU and, eventually the hospital, were important.

CHILDHOOD DEVELOPMENT: PSYCHOSOCIAL, EMOTIONAL, AND COGNITIVE FACTORS

Knowledge of normal growth and development and the ability to assess the child's developmental level are crucial to working effectively with children and parents in any healthcare setting. Historically, children used to be viewed as small adults. Pediatric nurses now understand that using a developmental perspective is the ideal norm. Those who experience children as individuals at a particular level of development find caring for children a rich and rewarding adventure.

The following section describes general childhood developmental concepts. Individual differences exist, and these stages serve as a general guide for the nurse. Erikson's stages of psychosocial development,

Freud's theory of personality development, and Piaget's stages of cognitive development are summarized.

A. Developmental Stages in Infancy (0–12 Months)

1. *Psychosocial Development: Trust Versus Mistrust.* Infants develop a sense of trust when their basic needs for affection, security, and survival are satisfied. Older infants may fear an unfamiliar person and may not want to be held or approached by a stranger.

2. *Personality Development: Oral Stage.* Sucking provides the major source of enjoyment.

3. *Cognitive Development: Sensorimotor Stage.* Reflexes are gradually replaced with voluntary behaviors. Infants learn to differentiate themselves from others. Infants begin to develop object permanence at 4 to 8 months. Security objects may alleviate anxiety responses in older infants. For instance, infants use their parents as a social reference; that is, by looking at their mother or father, infants determine how to react to new and unfamiliar situations.

B. Developmental Stages of Toddlers (1–3 Years)

1. *Psychosocial Development: Autonomy Versus Shame and Doubt.* Toddlers gradually develop the ability to control their bodies and begin to seek independence. When frustrated or when their need for independence is thwarted, toddlers can express themselves through negativism, temper tantrums, and physical resistance. At times, older toddlers are eager to please adults. Toddlers learn through sensorimotor experiences.

2. *Personality Development: Anal Stage.* Toddlers learn bladder and bowel control. They have an egocentric view of life.

3. *Cognitive Development: Sensorimotor Stage Matures to Preoperational Stage.* Toddlers exhibit egocentric development and increased use of language. In addition to early memory development, toddlers develop a sense of time as it relates to their daily routine of meals, naps, and playtime.

4. *Concept of Death.* Toddlers view death as a temporary event and may continue to act as though the dead person is still alive.

C. Developmental Stages of Preschoolers (3–5 Years)

1. *Psychosocial Development: Initiative Versus Guilt.* Preschoolers begin to develop the superego and learn right from wrong. They have a strong need to explore the environment. Preschoolers may feel guilt or fear in response to inappropriate thoughts or actions. Many preschoolers are eager to conform to adult expectations.

2. *Personality Development: Phallic Stage.* Preschoolers develop a beginning gender awareness and identify with the parent of the same sex.

3. *Cognitive Development: Preoperational Stage (2–7 Years).* The preschooler's vocabulary increases, and magical thinking is used. Preschoolers communicate through play and have vivid imaginations. They are unable to see anyone else's point of view at this stage of development.

4. *Concept of Death.* Death is viewed as temporary. Preschoolers may say that someone is "dead" without any understanding of the finality of death. Preschoolers may fear death as a separation from someone they love, as being injured, or as a punishment for misbehavior.

D. Developmental Stages of School-Age Children (6–12 Years)

1. *Psychosocial Development: Industry Versus Inferiority.* School-age children have a need to develop a sense of achievement and competence and are usually willing and eager to cooperate.

2. *Personality Development: Latency Period.* Development of the superego continues, and school-age children gain a greater understanding about what is right and wrong.

3. *Cognitive Development: Concrete Operational Stage (7–11 Years).* School-age children begin to use logic in thought and can consider another person's point of view. Language and problem-solving abilities improve. Rules, rituals, and conformity are important to school-age children because they provide order to their world. They expect others, including parents, to obey the rules and will complain if something seems "unfair" to them.

4. *Concept of Death.* Early-school-age children still believe death is temporary and may view it as scary or violent. Older school-age children understand death as permanent and inevitable.

E. Developmental Stages of Adolescents (12–18 Years)

1. *Psychosocial Development: Identity Versus Role Confusion.* Teens are often preoccupied and frequently are dissatisfied with their physical appearance. The adolescent years are a time of emotional

---

struggle for independence as the teen searches for a personal identity.

2. *Personality Development: Genital Stage.* This stage begins at puberty with the development of secondary sex characteristics and sex hormones. Teens display frequent mood swings with emotional lability. Teens often fluctuate between wanting to be with their family and avoiding their family.

3. *Cognitive Development: Formal Operational Stage.* The ability to use abstract thinking begins in the early teens. Logical thinking becomes more developed, although teens may retain some magical thinking as well. For example, they may feel that an illness is a punishment for something they did. Use of verbal communication increases.

4. *Concept of Death.* Teens understand death as permanent and inevitable but as something that will occur only in the distant future.

DEVELOPMENTALLY APPROPRIATE ASSESSMENT OF CHILDREN

Children usually respond well to honesty, gentleness, and respect. Most children want to please their parents and other adults as well.

A. General Principles for Working With Children

1. *Introduce Yourself to the Child and Family.* Include the child in conversation even if the child does not seem to be responding. Children may not respond verbally but will listen to everything that is said and decide how much comfort or danger the situation holds for them. Assure the child that it is all right to talk or not to talk.

2. *Honesty Is Vital to Establishing a Trusting Relationship With Children.* Be honest with the child if the procedure will hurt. To deny that something will hurt and then do something that causes the child pain could destroy the possibility of establishing a trusting, cooperative relationship with that child. Admit that you do not know the answer if the child asks a question you cannot answer. Promise to try to find the answer.

3. *Make Eye Contact and Address the Child by Name.* The child may not return eye contact, but can still be listening intently.

4. *Stoop or Bend to Communicate at the Child's Eye Level When Possible.*

5. *Allow the Child to See Your Hands and Any Instruments You Will Use.* If possible, allow the child to touch and examine the instruments because this will tap into his or her curiosity. Most children are cooperative if they know you are not planning a painful procedure.

6. *Allow the Child to Make Choices Whenever Possible, But Avoid Giving the Child Artificial Choices.* For example, do not ask permission to measure the child's blood pressure unless you are prepared to respect his or her choice if the child refuses. Simply state what you need to do in a gentle but matter-of-fact manner and do it. Examples of realistic choices include desired Popsicle flavor and choice of video game to play.

7. *Allow the Parents to Participate in the Child's Care Whenever Possible.* Some procedures can be accomplished with the child sitting on a parent's lap or in a position of comfort, such as a hug.

8. *Use a Calm, Soothing Voice.*

9. *Encourage the Family to Bring the Child's Favorite Articles From Home.*

B. Principles for Working With Infants

1. Before touching the infant, assess affect, color, level of consciousness, and respiratory rate and effort because changes can occur in these parameters when the infant is touched. Infants express their distress in physiologic and behavioral ways.

2. When possible, perform the assessment while a parent is holding the infant.

3. Warm the stethoscope and other appropriate instruments before use.

4. Smile and speak softly to the infant before touching and during the examination.

5. Bright objects may be useful as a distraction.

6. Start the examination with the least invasive process, such as listening to breath sounds, and end with more invasive processes, such as examining the ears.

C. Principles for Working With Toddlers

1. Assess affect, color, level of consciousness, and respiratory rate and effort before touching the toddler.

2. Name each body part for the toddler as you examine it.

3. Make the experience fun by drawing faces on tongue blades.

4. The toddler will feel more in control if allowed to sit up and to hold a security item.

5. Allow the toddler to inspect and touch the equipment.

6. Before approaching the toddler, demonstrate the equipment on a doll, a stuffed toy, or the toddler's parent.

D. Principles for Working With Preschoolers

1. In simple terms, explain what you are doing as you progress through the assessment.

2. Praise the preschooler frequently, and make the experience fun.

3. Allow the preschooler to inspect and touch the equipment.

4. Demonstrate the equipment on a doll, a stuffed toy, or the preschooler's parent.

5. Avoid holding your hands behind your back because preschoolers may wonder what you are hiding.

6. Avoid using words or phrases like "cut," "take," "broken," or "put you to sleep."

E. Principles for Working With School-Age Children

1. Speak directly to the school-age child, explaining what you are doing and why.

2. Take time to listen to the school-age child.

3. Allow the child to ask questions. The school-age child can understand simple bodily functions, so incorporate this knowledge into the answers.

4. Accord the child respect, privacy, and dignity.

5. Encourage as much mobility as possible to help reduce stress.

6. As appropriate, allow the child to help with the examination.

F. Principles for Working With Adolescents

1. Respect the adolescent's desire for privacy, and avoid unnecessary physical exposure.

2. Give adolescents the choice of whether or not they want their parents to be present.

3. Explain what you are doing and why.

4. Encourage teens to discuss their concerns, and include them in decision making regarding their health and illness.

5. Teach the adolescent about normal physical and sexual development.

6. Facilitate visits with peers when possible.

G. Principles for Working With Adolescents as Parents

1. Affirm the role of an adolescent parent as "mom" or "dad."

2. Discourage grandparents or other relatives from usurping the parent's control.

3. Teach the adolescent parent about normal child development, nutrition, discipline, and care.

4. Assess the parent's level of understanding, and teach without condescension.

5. Direct questions and explanations to the parent even when older relatives are present.

STRESS RESPONSES AND COPING BEHAVIORS

Critical illness and hospitalization in the PICU are stressful experiences for all children. This stress arises not only from the underlying medical condition, but also from the PICU environment and experience itself.

A. Physiologic Response to Stress

When a human body is faced with a stressful stimulus, the autonomic nervous system is activated, releasing hormones that control physiologic defense mechanisms. The following are signs of this nervous system activation:

1. Tachycardia, tachypnea, and increased blood pressure

2. Peripheral vasoconstriction with cool extremities

3. Inhibition of the digestive system

4. Inhibition of the immune system

5. Hyperglycemia in older infants or children, hypoglycemia in young infants

6. Dilated pupils

7. Increased level of alertness

B. Response to Psychological Stress and Hospitalization

An important part of the human stress response is what the child thinks or feels about what is happening. As children mature, their perception of stress becomes more important to their overall stress response.

1. *Infants.* Infants respond to stress with crying and increased motor activity. The infant may be experiencing pain or fear or may feel the need to be comforted. Infants may suck on fingers, pacifiers, blankets, or endotracheal tubes to calm themselves and cope with stress. Older infants may avert their gaze or attempt to turn away from an unpleasant experience. In an attempt to calm themselves, older infants may rock their bodies or use their arms or legs to make rhythmic movements.

CM is an 11-month-old female who was riding in a car with her 12-year-old brother and her mother. Another car ran a stop sign and collided with the car in which they were riding. CM and her brother are now hospitalized in the PICU with stable injuries while their mother is being evaluated at another hospital. CM's father is spending his time going back and forth between both his children's hospital rooms. As CM's PICU nurse, you notice that every time her father leaves, she screams loudly and cries "Daddy, Daddy" over and over. She reaches her arms toward his direction and searches for him constantly with her eyes. Your attempts to comfort the infant are unsuccessful until she is reunited with her father.

2. *Toddlers.* Toddlers may react to stress with increased physical activity, loud crying, or screaming that may continue to the point of exhaustion. The mobile toddler may try to resist a frightening situation physically. This age group is particularly susceptible to distress when separated from parents. Toddlers tend to experience regression when hospitalized. For example, previously toilet-trained toddlers may lose bladder control or revert to thumb sucking. Toddlers are frequently attached to security items and often hold them close to the face.

Twenty-two-month-old TS is admitted to the PICU with pneumonia. He is receiving oxygen by face mask, has a pulse-oximeter probe taped to his right index finger, electrocardiographic electrodes on his chest, and an IV catheter in his left hand while his hand is secured to an arm board. TS is extremely restless in his crib and keeps getting tangled in the wires and tubing. In addition, he is left-handed and unable to feed himself because his hand is secured to the arm board. As his mother tries to comfort TS, he hits at her with the arm board and cries loudly. The PICU nurse recognizes that this toddler is showing frustration as he tries to maintain his independence despite the medical interventions.

3. *Preschoolers.* Hospitalization of preschoolers interrupts and challenges children at a time when they are learning to control their own bodies and environment. To gain control in at least some area, preschoolers may refuse food and not cooperate with caregivers. Preschoolers continue to hold on to security items. Regression to the toddler stage is common. Preschoolers may project feelings of sadness, anger, or guilt onto others or onto toys and frequently express their feelings about illness through dramatic play. Preschoolers may withdraw from interaction with others if they are angry, sad, or in pain.

Four-year-old MB needs to have a percutaneously inserted central catheter (PICC) placed for ongoing antibiotic delivery. Recognizing that a child this age has a strong imagination and communicates well through play, the IV therapy nurse brings a doll for MB to play with. This doll has a PICC taped to her arm, and the nurse guides MB as she plays with the doll so that she can gain some understanding about the PICC and what it will be like to have the PICC in her own arm.

4. *School-Age Children.* A child of this age will ask questions and try to understand the experience. Fear of a loss of control may lead school-age children to deny fears and act "grown up" even when frightened. School-age children may regress to earlier stages of development and fear bodily mutilation and intrusion. If feeling out of control, school-age children may withdraw from caregivers, refuse to communicate, or use television or sleep as a means of escape. He or she finds comfort in familiar routines, the presence of parents, and contact with siblings.

BG, who is 8 years old, is recovering in the PICU after having brain surgery to remove a tumor. He is awake and alert. His mother has stated that he likes to put together puzzles. BG and his mother work on an intricate puzzle all afternoon, and when the puzzle has been completed, he shows everyone who comes into the room his "awesome puzzle." The nurse smiles and tells BG what a great job he has done. In doing so, the nurse is recognizing that a child of this age is developing a sense of achievement and competence.

5. *Adolescents.* Teens may deny obvious pain and discomfort, especially if peers are present. If feeling out of control, teens may withdraw and refuse to communicate or cooperate. Teens may regress to an earlier stage and become demanding and clinging with caregivers or parents. The hospitalized teen may experience labile and conflicting emotions, especially about the hospitalization itself and any disruption to body or body image.

Sixteen-year-old RM was recently transferred to the PICU because of hemodynamic instability following the administration of several chemotherapeutic agents needed to treat her newly diagnosed leukemia. When she is more stable, RM spends time on the telephone with one of her friends. The nurse overhears her crying and talking about how "terrible I'm going to look when I lose my hair! No boys will ever want to talk to me!" The nurse recognizes that adolescents are often preoccupied with their physical appearance and are developing a sense of identity.

ISSUES RELATED TO HOSPITALIZATION

A. Fear and Anxiety

Most children experience some fear and anxiety when hospitalized. Fears may be reality based, related to previous procedures or hospitalizations, or the result of magical thinking. Information given to a child by friends or relatives may be incorrect, and the child may inadvertently hear frightening comments made by others. Children in the hospital may witness fear in others and may see or hear things from other bed spaces that cause fear and anxiety.

   1. *Age-Specific Fears Related to Developmental Level*

   a. *Infants.* Separation anxiety and fear of strangers begin at 6 to 7 months of age. Crying and clinging to parents are normal behaviors and generally indicate a healthy parent–child relationship. Older infants frequently resist being separated from parents. When parents leave, infants may exhibit loud and active grief that may continue to the point of exhaustion. Over time, they may become passive and withdrawn if cries do not cause the immediate return of parents or if the separation is prolonged. Infants may accept food and comfort from the nursing staff while avoiding eye contact or other interactions.

   b. *Toddlers* may fear separation from parents, large animals, strangers, "the doctor," changes in their environment, or "shots." Temper tantrums, clinging to parents, attachment to security objects,

and regression may be used as means of coping with the fears and perceived threats to security.

   c. *Preschoolers* may fear bodily injury or mutilation, darkness, separation from parents, loss of control, the unknown, death, or "shots." They may regress and act like a toddler or become quiet and withdrawn if feeling out of control. Preschoolers may be able to express anxiety through play and drawing.

   d. *School-age children* may fear bodily injury, loss of control, failure in school, supernatural beings, rejection by others, or death. They may also fear intrusive procedures and being separated from family and friends. Incomplete information and misconceptions about illness, injury, and body function may exacerbate their fears. For example, they may believe that illness is a punishment for bad behavior. Some school-age children may be reluctant to ask questions and feel that they must act "grown up." Additional explanations may be required by this age group, even if an understanding of information is exhibited.

   e. *Adolescents'* fear may revolve around social isolation, loss of control, rejection by peers, the appearance of being different, or helplessness. Teens may use denial or regression despite a fear of appearing younger than they are. They may dramatize events or intellectualize illness or injury.

B. Pain

Children in pain frequently receive too little medication or they may receive no analgesia at all. Despite an increase in the emphasis on pain management in children over the past several years, some misconceptions about children and pain persist (Table 1.1). AACN's Essentials of Pediatric Critical Care Orientation (EPCCO) provides a broad overview of this topic, and can be used to orient nurses caring for critically ill children, and as a review to reinforce concepts.

TABLE 1.1 Misconceptions About Pain in Children

Misconceptions	Truth About Pain
Children do not experience pain the same as adults.	Pain is "an unpleasant sensory and emotional experience associated with actual or potential tissue damage, or described in terms of such damage" (International Association *for the Study of Pain*, 2015, p. 1).

(continued)

TABLE 1.1   Misconceptions About Pain in Children *(continued)*

Misconceptions	Truth About Pain
A child who is not crying is not in pain.	Children express pain in varying ways at different ages.
A child who is asleep is not experiencing any pain.	Some children sleep to try to escape pain, just as adults attempt to do.
Infant nerve pathways are not developed enough to have pain.	Infants, even preterm babies, may experience harmful physiologic and long-term behavioral development effects from stress responses related to pain.
Children will always tell you if they are in pain.	Children may interpret pain as punishment for misbehavior or believe they are supposed to have pain if nothing is done to relieve it.
Children will become addicted if given narcotics.	Physical tolerance can occur, necessitating increasing doses of medication to achieve the same effect, but psychological dependency is unusual. These drugs can be weaned just as with adults.
Children always tell the truth about pain.	Children may deny pain to avoid injections or out of concern for worrying their parents. Teens may deny pain in the presence of peers.

C. Separation From Family and Friends

Support from family and friends is important to children, and the need for support and closeness increases during times of illness. If children are separated from loved ones, long-term effects, such as impaired trust, diminished intellectual and motor functioning, and disturbed behavior, are possible. Preventing separation of the child from his or her family is the standard of care in pediatric acute and critical care units. Family-centered care practices ensure the closeness of loved ones as familiar trusted sources of security.

D. Limited Understanding

Misconceptions about illness, treatment, and caregiver motives may result from a child's limited understanding. Magical thinking may lead children to conclude that an illness is punishment for misbehavior. Words such as "cut" or "take" can be misconstrued by children

and increase levels of fear. The vivid imagination of childhood supplies answers to any unanswered questions or unexplained situations.

E. Loss of Control

Hospitalized children are rarely given choices related to their treatment regimen, which results in little sense of control. Physical restraint can increase the anxiety related to hospitalization and, when at all possible, should be reserved as a measure of last resort. Frequently restraints can be avoided with proper preparation of the child, and therapeutic holding may be used for temporary immobilization. Therapeutic holding with the child on the caregiver's lap or in a hug position allows close physical contact with a caregiver or family member during procedures and helps to decrease patient anxiety. Allowing choices, when choices are truly present, can assist the child in dealing with feelings that result from the perceived loss of control.

ISSUES RELATED TO CRITICAL CARE UNITS

FB was 5 years old and had been admitted to the PICU after she fell from a second-story window while jumping on the bed. She had experienced a traumatic brain injury from the fall and was intubated. She lay unresponsive, sedated, and in a darkened room to decrease stimuli as the rhythmic swoosh of the ventilator breaths continued. On occasion, an alarm or a conversation would break the silence. Another healthcare provider entered the room to examine her and without a word started turning her side to side as FB winced in pain. The nurse gasped, went to the bedside, and stopped any further "assessment." As the nurse whispered a soft-spoken apology to FB, a tear ran down her face.

A. Sensory Overload

Sensory overload can occur for the child in the PICU because of the around-the-clock activity.

1. Noise levels can be high from communication devices, bedrail openings and closings, in-room equipment, alarms, and voices of families and caregivers (Tripathi et al., 2014; Watson et al., 2015). Recommendations have been made by the U.S. Environmental Protection Agency stating that hospital noise levels should be no greater than 45 dB during the day and 35 dB at night (U.S. Environmental Protection Agency, 1974), which is needed for rest, although noise levels in PICUs are known to exceed recommended levels (Watson et al., 2015). Many times, the sources of noise, such as monitors and infusion pumps, are located close to the child's head. Hearing loss can result from persistent humming of equipment, especially when these noises are combined with the administration of ototoxic antibiotics (Hockenberry & Wilson, 2013). Patient annoyance, increased length of stay, delirium, and delayed wound healing also have been correlated with excess noise (Hsu, Ryherd, Waye, & Ackerman, 2012). Noise can also have an impact on nurses who care for our youngest patients. Elevated heart rates, which may negatively impact health (Watson et al., 2015), have been recorded in nurses in PICUs.

2. Constant light leads to confusion of day and night. Differentiation between day and night is difficult if no windows are available. Lights are frequently bright and are located directly over the child's head.

3. Unfamiliar tactile and olfactory stimulation over which the child has little or no control can be disturbing. Children are unfamiliar with hospital food. Medicinal smells may be powerful and unpleasant.

B. Sensory Deprivation

Although there is an excess of stimulation in most PICUs, there is a lack of the normal types of stimulation beneficial for children. Mealtimes and clothing will most likely change. Important bedtime rituals are changed, especially with unfamiliar blankets, beds, toys, and pajamas. Adults other than parents are directing the child's activities and schedule. Restricted activity leads to feelings of isolation and boredom and interferes with the child's ability to cope with the stress of hospitalization. Physical activity is a method frequently used by children to cope with stress. Sensory deprivation may lead to depression and regression and can interfere with normal development. Children who are intubated also have difficulty communicating and may fear that they might never be able to speak again.

C. Sleep Deprivation

Children in the PICU may experience sleep deprivation because of repeated caregiver interactions and environmental stimuli, and each child has a unique sleep experience (Kudchadkar, Aljohani, & Punjabi, 2014; Table 1.2). Sleep assessment is difficult as each child is an individual and differs by age, illness, medication, and type of interventions (Kudchadkar et al., 2014). Day–night orientation can be lost because children in the PICU sleep less than normal, and often any sleep that is achieved will be interrupted. The physical effects of sleep deprivation may result in immune-system vulnerability, inefficient temperature regulation, and impaired healing of cells and tissues. Anxiety, irritability, confusion, and

TABLE 1.2   Causes of Sleep Deprivation in the PICU

Noise levels
Decreased light–dark cycles
Disruption of home sleep rituals
Pain and discomfort
Isolation
Immobilization
Anxiety
Depersonalization
Restraints
Tense atmosphere
Pharmacologic paralysis
REM and NREM suppressant drugs

NREM, nonrapid eye movement (sleep); REM, rapid eye movement (sleep).

Source: Reproduced with permission from Slota, M. C. (1988). Implications of sleep deprivation in the pediatric critical care unit. *Focus on Critical Care, 15(3),* 35–43.

hallucinations are just a few of the psychological symptoms that may be seen in children experiencing sleep deprivation (Gregory & Sadeh, 2012). Nonpharmacologic interventions that can improve sleep include subdued lighting, unit quiet times, earplugs, and formalized noise-reduction protocols (Kudchadkar et al., 2014).

D. Lack of Privacy

Some PICUs are large, open units where patients and families experience "living in public." Open areas allow "strangers" (other visitors and hospital employees) to see the children and their parents. Children may also be aware of procedures and crises that occur at beds close to their own, and the need for close observation sometimes leads to physical exposure of the child.

E. Technology Dependence

The number of technology-dependent patients has increased since the development of mechanical ventilation (Rennick & Childerhose, 2015). Critically ill, unstable children are the highest priority in the PICU. Chronically ill but stable children who are technology dependent may receive less developmental and psychosocial support when the PICU is busy or understaffed. Technology may interfere with parental attachment or lead to the parents' emotional withdrawal from their child. Technology-dependent children may experience long periods of separation from home, school, and friends. Children are aware that alarms are related to them and exhibit fear when any alarm is triggered. Chronic sleep disruption can affect learning, growth, healing, and developmental progress.

F. PICU Design Considerations

Issues associated with hospitalization may be decreased through the intentional design of critical care units. AACN partners with the Society of Critical Care Medicine and the American Institute of Architects Academy of Architecture for Health to recognize such units. These care areas integrate the needed functionality of a high-acuity setting with the humanitarian needs of patients and families.

DEVELOPMENTALLY APPROPRIATE INTERVENTIONS

A. Pain Management

1. *Assessment of Pain.* An accurate assessment of the critically ill or injured child's pain is vital for appropriate pain intervention. The child who states that he or she is in pain should be believed. Family caregivers can provide input about their perception of the child's pain and can also provide a history of the child's experience with pain, what words the child uses to describe pain, and what interventions were previously successful. The pain assessment should be tailored to the child's developmental level and needs (Table 1.3). Other important considerations include the following:

a. Some hospitalized children may be too ill to display typical pain behaviors because energy is directed toward maintaining physiological stability.

b. Pain assessment scales are useful to quantify and supplement the nurse's observations.

c. It may be difficult to distinguish between pain and anxiety. Pain should be considered when the patient's behavior is associated with actual or

TABLE 1.3   Guidelines for Age-Appropriate Assessment of Pain

Age Group	Behavioral Indicators of Pain	Pain Assessment Scales
Neonate (0–28 days)	Preterm infant may show a less robust response than a term infant Cry (can be high pitched, tense, or irregular) Facial grimace (eyes tightly closed, brows lowered and drawn together, mouth square shaped) Increase or decrease in body movements Change in feeding patterns Change in vital signs Change in oxygen saturation Vagal tone Palmar sweating	CRIES (Krechel & Bildner, 1995) Neonatal Facial Coding System (Peters et al., 2003) NIPS (Lawrence et al., 1993) N-PASS (Hummel, Puchalski, Creech, & Weiss, 2008) PIPP-R (Stevens et al., 2014)
Infant (0–12 months)	Response may be blunted by state of arousal, level of consciousness, and severity of illness Cry (can be high pitched, tense, or irregular) Facial grimace (eyes tightly closed, brows lowered and drawn together, mouth square shaped) Increased or decreased level of activity, restless, irritable, inconsolable Withdrawal from stimulus (newborns show poorly localized response; older infants localize more and may attempt to pull away) Changes in vital signs Lacrimation	COMFORT-B (Boerlage et al., 2015) FLACC (Merkel, Voepel-Lewis, & Malviya, 2002) N-PASS (Hummel et al., 2008)
Toddler (1–3 years)	Cries, screams May lie still or rigid Physically attempts to avoid painful stimuli Facial grimace of pain Irritable, sad, uncooperative Touching or guarding site of pain Verbalized expressions ("ow," "ouchie," "it hurts," "stop") May verbalize where something hurts Unable to describe pain intensity May regress behaviorally	COMFORT-B (Boerlage et al., 2015) FLACC (Merkel et al., 2002)

(continued)

TABLE 1.3   Guidelines for Age-Appropriate Assessment of Pain *(continued)*

Age Group	Behavioral Indicators of Pain	Pain Assessment Scales
Preschooler (3–5 years)	Cries, screams May demonstrate aggressive behavior Irritable, difficult to comfort Easily frustrated Increasing ability to describe verbally the location and intensity of pain	Body Outline Tool (Savedra, Tesler, Holzemer, Wilkie, & Ward, 1989) Faces Pain Scale-Revised (Hicks, von Baeyer, Spafford, van Korlaar, & Goodenough, 2001) FLACC (Merkel et al., 2002) Oucher (Beyer et al., 2005) Visual analogue scale
School age (6–12 years)	May cry less than younger peers May grunt, moan, or sigh Verbalizes protest Describes pain location, intensity, and quality Restless or overly still and quiet Irritable May try to appear brave May clench teeth or fists; body stiffness	Adolescent Pediatric Pain Tool (Jacob, Mack, Savedra, Van Cleve, & Wilkie, 2014) Body Outline Tool (Savedra et al., 1989) Faces Pain Scale-Revised (Hicks et al., 2001; von Baeyer et al., 2009) FLACC (Merkel et al., 2002) Numerical Rating Scale (von Baeyer et al., 2009) Visual analogue scale
Adolescent (13+ years)	Describes pain location, intensity, quality, and duration May clench teeth or fists; body stiffness May grunt, moan, or sigh Restless or overly still and quiet Irritable, moody May be stoic in the presence of peers	Adolescent Pediatric Pain Tool (Jacob et al., 2014) Body Outline Tool (Savedra et al., 1989) Faces Pain Scale-Revised (Hicks et al., 2001; von Baeyer et al., 2009) Numerical Rating Scale (von Baeyer et al., 2009) Oucher (Beyer et al., 2005) Visual analogue scale
Children with cognitive impairment	Varies depending on child's developmental level Ask parents to describe child's typical behavioral responses to pain	r-FLACC (Dubois, Capdevila, Bringuier, & Pry, 2010) INRS (Solodiuk et al., 2010) NCCPC (Breau, McGrath, Camfield, & Finley, 2002) Paediatric Pain Profile (Hunt et al., 2004)

CRIES, Crying Requires increased oxygen administration, Increased vital signs, Expression, Sleeplessness; FLACC, Faces, Legs, Activity, Cry, and Consolability; r-FLACC, Faces, Legs, Activity, Cry, and Consolability-Revised; INRS, Individualized Numeric Rating Scale; N-PASS, Neonatal Pain Agitation Sedation Scale; NCCPC, Non-Communicating Children's Pain Checklist; NFCS, Neonatal Facial Coding System; NIPS, Neonatal Infant Pain Scale; PIPP-R, Premature Infant Pain Profile-Revised.

potential tissue damage or injury. The underlying disease and the presence of lines, tubes, and drains can contribute to the child's pain.

d. It is challenging to assess pain adequately in the nonverbal patient (e.g., young child, developmentally delayed patient, sedated or pharmacologically paralyzed patient). The nurse must rely on myriad assessment strategies in this situation.

e. Reassessment of pain should take place at appropriate intervals around nonpharmacologic and pharmacologic interventions to evaluate the adequacy of the interventions. For instance, depending on the route and dosage of a pain medication, reassessment should take place after the onset of action and then at a frequency determined by the duration of action.

2. *Nonpharmacologic Management of Pain*

a. Various types of nonpharmacologic measures are useful in the management of children's pain. These techniques work best when combined with appropriate analgesia. See Table 1.4 for a developmental perspective of nonpharmacologic pain interventions.

b. When possible, tell the child how long the pain will last, and be sure to tell the child when the procedure ends.

c. Encourage the child to express feelings of pain. Assure the child that it is all right to cry when something causes pain.

TABLE 1.4   Age-Appropriate Nonpharmacologic Pain Management Strategies

Age Group	Strategies
Neonate (0–28 days)	Swaddling Positioning Skin-to-skin/kangaroo care Developmental care Nonnutritive sucking (e.g., pacifier) Oral administration of sucrose (infants <30 days of age or <44 weeks gestation) Music or fetal heart sounds Decrease noxious environmental stimuli
Infant (0–12 months)	Bundling and rocking Presence of primary caregiver Nonnutritive sucking (e.g., pacifier) Oral administration of sucrose (infants <30 days of age or <44 weeks gestation) Familiar sounds (voices, music, etc.) Security object Distraction with visual stimuli Cutaneous stimulation
Toddler (1–3 years)	Rocking, holding, touching Presence of primary caregiver Security objects Distraction (e.g., music therapy, books) Controlled breathing (e.g., blowing bubbles) Cutaneous stimulation
Preschooler (3–5 years)	Rocking, holding, touching Presence of primary caregiver Age-appropriate explanations and reassurance Security objects Distraction (e.g., kaleidoscopes, music therapy, books) Controlled breathing (e.g., blowing bubbles) Cutaneous stimulation
School age (6–12 years)	Presence of primary caregiver Focused relaxation techniques Distraction (e.g., imagery, music therapy, watching television, use of technology-based device or smartphone) Controlled breathing Cutaneous stimulation
Adolescent (13+ years)	Presence of primary caregiver or friends, as desired Focused relaxation techniques Distraction (e.g., imagery, music therapy, watching television, use of technology-based device or smartphone) Controlled breathing Cutaneous stimulation

Note: To be combined with appropriate analgesia, as indicated.

d. Educate parents about their role in supporting the child who is in pain. Ask the parents what comfort measures they have found successful at home.

e. Distractions, such as singing, blowing bubbles, storytelling, reading to a child, music therapy, watching television, or interacting with technology-based devices, may help a child cope with pain.

f. The use of rhythmic motion is helpful. Infants often like to be patted on the back or bottom. Infants, toddlers, and preschoolers like rocking motions. Holding the child may be comforting at all ages.

g. Controlled breathing, imagery, and hypnosis can bring about relaxation. These techniques should be practiced before the painful event takes place.

h. Cutaneous stimulation by means of massage, the application of heat or cold therapy, acupuncture, or acupressure can provide low-level sensory input to reduce the transmission of painful stimuli.

i. Sucking a pacifier may comfort infants experiencing pain. Dipping the pacifier in a 24% sucrose solution 2 minutes prior to a painful stimulus may augment pain reduction in preterm and term infants (Stevens, Yamada, Lee, & Ohlsson, 2013). Some centers may have inclusion and exclusion criteria to guide the administration of sucrose analgesia. Examples of exclusion criteria might include the risk for necrotizing enterocolitis or unstable glucose levels.

j. Collaborate with child-life specialists, behavioral medicine specialists, and other members of the pain-management team to establish an individualized and comprehensive approach to pain management.

3. *Pharmacologic Pain Management*

a. *Administration.* The goal of pain-management therapy is to optimize pain relief while minimizing adverse effects. For intermittent dosing, consider the duration of action and anticipate redosing before pain returns. Continuous infusion provides a constant level of analgesia and may be preferable to bolus administration. Administer a bolus dose when the continuous infusion is started and consider repeating each time the infusion rate is increased. Patient-controlled analgesia (PCA) has been used successfully in children as young as 5 years and gives the patient a sense of control over his or her pain. In children younger than 5 years or those who cannot use the PCA system because of developmental delays or neurologic impairment, nurse- or parent-controlled analgesia may be initiated (Mondardini et al., 2014). Some patients benefit from epidural or intrapleural analgesia. Topical anesthetics can be applied prior to a painful event, such as venipuncture.

b. *Nonopioids* are useful for mild to moderate pain and can frequently be given in combination with opioids for control of more severe pain.

　　i. Acetaminophen is a mild analgesic frequently used for pain and fever in children. It works well for mild pain or when given in combination with an opioid.

　　ii. Ibuprofen has anti-inflammatory and analgesic effects with potential for gastrointestinal side effects, platelet aggregation, and bleeding.

　　iii. Ketoralac is an anti-inflammatory agent that can be administered via the parenteral route.

c. *Opioids.* A wide choice of drugs is available to provide relief of moderate to severe pain (Table 1.5). Medications can be given by several routes and may be administered intermittently (scheduled or as needed) or by continuous infusion, depending on the child's need. A common side effect of opioids is constipation, so consider giving the child a stool softener routinely.

d. *Sedative and adjuvant medications* can be helpful if the child remains agitated despite receiving appropriate analgesia. An assessment scale should be used to assess the child's sedation level and response to interventions. Examples include the State Behavioral Scale (SBS; Curley, Harris, Fraser, Johnson, & Arnold, 2006) and the COMFORT Behavioral Scale (Boerlage et al., 2015). Sedatives should not be used in isolation when there is a pain component involved but can work in combination with opioids to control pain more effectively. The benefits (decreased days of ventilation, less sedation, etc.) of a daily interruption of sedation in the critically ill child is still being debated (Vet et al., 2014).

　　i. *Benzodiazepines* (i.e., midazolam, lorazepam, and diazepam) provide muscle relaxation, amnesia, and relief of anxiety. When a patient has received a benzodiazepine for an extended period, taper the drug slowly and observe for symptoms of withdrawal such as a state of agitation, confusion, choreoathetoid movements, and ataxia.

ii. *Ketamine* provides sedation and analgesia. Ketamine raises blood pressure and should not be used in children at risk for increased intracranial pressure. It is a useful drug for children with asthma because of its bronchodilatory effect. Observe for emergence reactions such as excitement, hallucinations, or delirium. Maintain a dark, calm environment if this reaction occurs.

iii. *Barbiturates* have anticonvulsant and sedative properties. They have a longer half-life and are particularly helpful in patients with acute head injury.

iv. *Chloral hydrate* can be used to induce sleep and control agitation. Side effects can occur with long-term use because of a buildup of active metabolites.

v. *Dexmedetomidine* is an alpha$_2$-adrenergic agonist with sedative and analgesia effects. It is administered via continuous infusion and has minimal effect on respiration. The patient may need a lower opioid dose when receiving dexmedetomidine.

4. *Pharmacologic Paralysis.* The intubated patient may receive neuromuscular blocking agents to augment other therapies. These medications do not affect the child's state of consciousness or perception of pain. Every child receiving a paralytic should also receive appropriate analgesia and sedation.

TABLE 1.5   Select Medications Used to Manage Pain and Sedation in Acute and Critically Ill Children

Drug	Dose[a]	Route	Frequency
Opioids			
Morphine[b]	0.2–0.5 mg/kg/dose immediate release	PO	Every 4–6 hr
	0.3–0.6 mg/kg/dose controlled release	PO	Every 12 hr
	0.03–0.2 mg/kg/dose (usual maximum dose: 10 mg/dose)	IV, subcutaneous, IM	Every 2–4 hr
	Neonates (use preservative-free formulation) 0.01–0.02 mg/kg/hr	IV infusion	Continuous
	Infants/children 0.02–0.06 mg/kg/hr	IV infusion	Continuous
Fentanyl	0.5–3 mcg/kg/dose	IV	Every 1–3 hr
	0.5–2 mcg/kg/hr	IV infusion	Continuous
Hydromorphone	0.05–0.1 mg/kg/dose (maximum dose: 5 mg/dose)	PO	Every 6 hr
	0.015 mg/kg/dose	IV	Every 4–6 hr

(*continued*)

TABLE 1.5 Select Medications Used to Manage Pain and Sedation in Acute and Critically Ill Children *(continued)*

Drug	Dose[a]	Route	Frequency
Methadone[b]	0.1 mg/kg/dose initial (maximum dose: 10 mg/dose)	Oral, IM, subcutaneous	Every 4 hr for 2–3 doses, then every 6–12 hr
	Narcotic dependency; 0.05–0.1 mg/kg/dose increase by 0.05 mg/kg/dose until withdrawal controlled	Oral, IV	Every 6 hr; after 24–48 hr the dosing interval can be lengthened to every 12–24 hr during weaning
Nonopioids			
Acetaminophen	10–15 mg/kg/dose (maximum dose: 75 mg/kg/day infants, lesser of 100 mg/kg/day or 1,625 mg/day children)	PO, PR, IV	Every 4–6 hr
Nonsteroidal Anti-Inflammatories			
Ibuprofen[d]	5–10 mg/kg/dose for ages >6 months (maximum single dose: 400 mg/dose; maximum daily dose: 1200 mg/day)	PO	Every 6–8 hr
Ketorolac[c]	0.5 mg/kg/dose (maximum dose: 15 mg/dose)	IV	Every 6 hr
Sedatives and Adjuvants			
Lorazepam	0.025–0.05 mg/kg/dose (maximum dose: 2 mg/dose)	IV	Every 2–4 hr
	0.025–0.2 mg/kg/hr	IV infusion	Continuous
Midazolam	0.05–0.2 mg/kg/dose	IV	Every 1–2 hr
	0.06–0.12 mg/kg/hr	IV infusion	Continuous
Diazepam	0.04–0.3 mg/kg/dose (maximum of 0.6 mg/kg within an 8 hr period if needed)	IV	Every 2–4 hr
Ketamine	0.2–1 mg/kg/dose	IV	Titrate to effect
	10–15 mcg/kg/minute	IV infusion	Continuous
Dexmedetomidine	0.1–0.5 mcg/kg	IV	Titrate to effect
	0.1–0.75 mcg/kg/hr	IV infusion	Continuous

IM, intramuscular; IV, intravenous; PO, by mouth; PR, by rectum.
Drug dosages may vary based on prescribing practitioner preference, indication for use, and chronicity of the illness. Always check additional references, such as the hospital formulary or manufacturer recommendations, for dosage and administration guidelines.

[a]This table is for children weighing <50 kg; consider maximum recommended dosage in children >50 kg.
[b]Decrease dose in patients with renal impairment.
[c]Do not use in patients with renal impairment.
[d]Use caution in patients with renal impairment.

Source: Micromedex®. (2015). Retrieved from http://www.micromedexsolutions.com

B. Iatrogenic Withdrawal Syndrome

Children who receive prolonged administration of opioids and/or benzodiazepines (>5 days) are at risk for iatrogenic withdrawal syndrome, which can occur with the abrupt discontinuation or too-rapid weaning of these medications. Symptoms may include agitation, increased motor tone, dilated pupils, sweating, nasal congestion, fever, mottling, seizures, poor sleep, hallucinations, grimacing, yawning, poor feeding, vomiting, and diarrhea (Mondardini et al., 2014). An assessment tool, such as the Withdrawal Assessment Tool-1 (Franck, Scoppettuolo, Wypij, & Curley, 2012) or the Sophia Observation withdrawal Symptoms-scale (Ista, de Hoog, Tibboel, Duivenvoorden, & van Dijk, 2013), should be used to identify and monitor withdrawal symptoms. Switching to medications with a longer half-life, using the enteral route when possible, and gradually tapering medications are appropriate interventions for iatrogenic withdrawal (Mondardini et al., 2014). The family or the older child may fear medication addiction. Help them understand that tolerance and dependency are physiologic phenomenon and that the child is not psychologically addicted to the medication. This fact is often not well understood by families and may be a source of anxiety.

C. Communication

The nurse's words, tone of voice, body language, facial expressions, actions, and emotions all convey messages to patients and families. It is important to communicate in a developmentally appropriate manner. Acute and critical care nurses can use communication in a positive way to help children and families as they struggle to cope with the stress of hospitalization.

1. *Preparation for Procedures.* When given the option, most parents will choose to be present with their child during procedures. With proper preparation and guidance, parents can provide support and comfort to their child. If a parent does not feel able to remain with the child, this decision should be respected. A child-life or play specialist is invaluable in preparing and supporting children in a developmentally appropriate manner for surgery or procedures.

  a. *Infancy.* Even infants will learn quickly which cues predict painful events. Awaken infants before any painful procedure so they are not aroused from sleep by pain. Avoid repetitively playing familiar music during procedures, such as suctioning or needle sticks, so the infant will not associate the music with discomfort or learn to interpret the sounds as a cue to imminent pain.

  b. *Toddlers.* Use simple words and phrases to explain the procedure immediately before performing the procedure. Allow the child to handle the equipment when possible. Use restraints only when necessary. Use phrases like "all done" when appropriate so the toddler knows when the procedure is over.

  c. *Preschoolers.* Use pictures, puppets, dolls, or toys during explanations or demonstrations, and allow the preschooler to handle them. If time permits, preschoolers may be prepared hours in advance for minor procedures or a few days ahead of time for more serious events. Help preschoolers identify safe times and places when no procedure, vital sign measurement, or other care is planned. Allow preschoolers to keep a security item during procedures. Avoid using confusing phrases such as "put you to sleep" for anesthesia or "move you to the floor" for transfer. The child may interpret these phrases literally.

  d. *School-age children.* Use as many choices as possible. Ask the school-age child to explain what was heard to verify understanding of explanations. Allow time for and encourage questions. Depending on the nature of the procedure, school-age children may be prepared weeks before the event. When advanced planning is not possible, allow the school-age child as much time as possible between the explanation and the event. Teach and encourage the use of cognitive behavioral coping techniques, such as imagery and relaxation, before the procedure.

  e. *Adolescents.* Provide factual explanations of what will happen and encourage questions. Promote a sense of control by allowing the adolescent to make appropriate choices. Allow teens to choose whether they want to have a parent present. Teach coping techniques, such as imagery or relaxation, before the procedure. Prepare adolescents as soon as it is known that the procedure or surgery is needed.

2. *Communicating With Intubated Children.* Children who remember being intubated find the experience of not being able to communicate anxiety producing.

ET is a 10-year-old male admitted to your PICU with severe status asthmaticus. He is intubated and mechanically ventilated. His arms are restrained to prevent him from dislodging his endotracheal tube and other medical devices. He is receiving intermittent medications for pain and sedation and does not remember having the endotracheal tube placed or why he is in your PICU.

Strategies for communicating with such a child include the following:

   a. Introduce yourself, and orient the child to the place and situation. Speak to the child before and during procedures. Explain what is happening and why the child is in the PICU (e.g., "You were hurt in an accident," "You became very sick," or "You are in the hospital, and you are getting better"). As the child gains awareness, you may need to repeat these explanations.

   b. Explain why the child cannot make noise or cry out.

   c. Use frequent, gentle touching when you are with the child.

   d. Encourage parents to stay with the child, and teach them to assist with appropriate care (e.g., diaper changes, bath, oral hygiene, eye care) if they desire to do so.

   e. Allow these children to point to a picture or a word board to express their needs.

   f. Teach the child how to summon help if needed (e.g., using a call light).

   g. Ask questions that require only a "yes" or "no" answer so the child can shake or nod his or her head or give a thumbs up or down if moving the head is ill advised.

   h. Consult a speech or child-life therapist as needed for additional augmentative communication devices.

3. *Communication With Children Who Are Sedated and Pharmacologically Paralyzed.* The child receiving sedation and chemical paralysis will retain the ability to hear and may recollect the experience later.

   a. Use the child's name, and tell the child what you plan to do even if you think the child might not be able to hear you. Explain noises that the child might hear, such as the monitor alarming or the sounds of the ventilator. Describe things the child might feel, such as vital signs, turning, oral hygiene, suctioning, or bathing.

   b. Touch the child gently, and speak to the child before painful interventions.

   c. Explain to the child why he or she cannot move and that the condition is temporary until the child gets better.

   d. Tell the child that he or she will not be left alone. If the family must leave temporarily, inform the child that the family will return. Family members may record a message that can be played in their absence, such as the reading of a favorite story for the child.

   e. Encourage parents to touch, stroke, and talk to the child. Parents may tell the child about things family members are doing, read stories, or sing to the child.

   f. Ask parents what type of music the child prefers, and play this periodically. Before performing any procedures, turn off the music and then explain the procedure. In this way, the child may realize that procedures do not take place while music is playing.

   g. Place a sign in the room that reminds others that the child may hear them, even though he or she is not moving.

D. Delirium

Delirium is a common yet underrecognized problem for acutely ill hospitalized children. The delirious child experiences an onset of cerebral dysfunction with a change or fluctuation in baseline mental status, which includes inattention and either disorganized thinking or an altered level of consciousness (AACN, 2016a).

1. The condition may develop within hours or days.

2. The delirious child can be hyperactive, hypoactive, or in a mixed state. The child's behavior often fluctuates during the day and may worsen in the evening.

3. Risk factors for the development of delirium include the child's severity of illness; certain patient factors, such as infections, metabolic disorders, withdrawal from medications, restraints and sleep disturbance; and factors from the hospital environment, such as light and noise, which contribute to disturbances of circadian rhythms (Silver et al., 2015).

4. Use a valid tool to screen for pediatric delirium. Options include the Cornell Assessment of Pediatric Delirium (CAPD; Traube et al., 2014), the Pediatric Confusion Assessment Method–Intensive Care Unit (pCAM-ICU; Smith et al., 2011), and Preschool Confusion Assessment Method–Intensive Care Unit (psCAM-ICU; Smith et al., 2016).

5. The frequency of delirium screening has not been determined and will vary depending on the tool used.

6. Interventions to prevent delirium and manage the symptoms when it occurs are focused on identifying and modifying contributing factors in the child's condition; modifying the hospital environment to promote a normal sleep–wake cycle; surrounding the child with familiar people, routines, and personal belongings; as well as offering family education and support.

E. Interventions for Sleep Deprivation, Sensory Deprivation, and Sensory Overload

1. *Minimize Noise Levels.* Be aware of the noise level in the care area and attempt to eliminate unnecessary noise. Alarm volumes should be kept just to the level that will alert the nurse to a problem. Anticipate when infusion pumps are likely to complete their cycle and alarm so they can be responded to quickly. Monotonous sounds, such as the beep of the bedside monitor, can be turned off if not needed. Limit loud conversation both in and outside patients' rooms, and speak in soft, soothing tones. Use headphones or ear plugs to decrease noise exposure for the children even if they are not listening to music. Turn music or headphones off periodically so the child can have quiet periods.

2. *Maintain a Day–Night Cycle.* Determine the child's usual morning and daytime routines, such as awakening time, mealtime, and playtime. Depending on the child's condition, adhere to these routines when possible. Try to maintain the child's normal bedtime routine, which may include a bath at night, reading a story, or having a security object in bed. Dim lights as much as possible at night, and use indirect lighting around the child. Organize nursing care and that of other caregivers so the child can be undisturbed for at least 90 minutes of sleep. When awakening a child, always offer an explanation before performing any procedures. It can be beneficial to establish a schedule that enhances circadian rhythms when possible. For this schedule to be successful, everyone, including parents, needs to follow it as much as possible. Ask parents about their preferences regarding usual home routines. Incorporate this knowledge into the schedule. Initially, the child may be tired and irritable during awake periods and want to sleep. After a few days, however, the child's body will reestablish a circadian rhythm and the irritability will diminish. A sample schedule to be used as the child progresses through recovery is outlined in Table 1.6.

F. Facilitation of Play

Having an opportunity to play while in the hospital normalizes and humanizes the environment while allowing the child to release tension and express feelings.

TABLE 1.6 Sample Schedule to Enhance Circadian Rhythms During Hospitalization

Time	Activities
8:00 a.m.–1:00 p.m.	Awake Lights on Window blinds open Child out of bed, if possible TV and electronic devices (as appropriate) on Playtime
1:00–3:00 p.m.	Nap Lights off TV off Sleep or quiet time
3:00–9:00 p.m.	Awake Lights on Window blinds open Child out of bed, if possible TV on Playtime
9:00 p.m.–8:00 a.m.	Asleep Lights off TV and electronic devices off Allow 90 minutes of uninterrupted sleep when possible by grouping interventions or by delaying interventions that can wait until after the sleep period.

Note: Schedule adapted as possible during hospitalization and recovery.

Play can also provide diversion while giving children the opportunity to exercise control over their hospital experience. The child who is acutely or critically ill presents a different challenge to caregivers interested in providing play opportunities for their patients.

1. Child-life or play specialists can assist in finding appropriate play activities for children at different levels of development.

2. If so desired, parents can bring special toys from home for the child. Children appreciate being surrounded by familiar objects.

3. Caregivers or parents may play for the child who cannot play at all. In some cases, the child can verbally direct the play. Make passive forms of play, such as being read a book, available for these children.

4. Medical play with equipment and supplies can correct misconceptions about the equipment and lessen the anxiety of a procedure.

5. *Infants* enjoy mobiles, pictures of faces, and soothing music or parents' voices. Older infants enjoy toys they can grasp and manipulate. When their use is possible, equipment, such as bouncy seats and swings, may provide support and enable play.

6. *Toddlers* enjoy books, security objects, and music, stories, or recorded family voices. Immobility is difficult for the toddler, who may benefit from watching the caregiver play with puppets, cars, or other active toys.

7. *Preschoolers* like to talk and have questions answered. They enjoy water play and having stories read to them. They usually enjoy favorite television shows and will often take part in medical play if given the tools.

8. *School-age children* often enjoy medical play, coloring, books, and crafts. Most enjoy children's movies or television shows. Ask the parents what type of shows the child is allowed to watch at home to avoid conflict related to television. A child of this age may also enjoy playing video or computer games or using other technology-based devices.

9. *Adolescents* enjoy books, magazines, and television. Peer visits and the use of a smartphone, if available, can help the teenaged patient feel connected to peers and social media. Video or computer games and other technology-based devices are also an enjoyable distraction.

G. Provision of Psychosocial and Emotional Support for the Child

SM and EM were 3-year-old and 7-year-old siblings who were unrestrained during a motor-vehicle crash. Both their parents suffered extensive injuries and were being treated in the adult intensive care unit. The sisters had serious injuries but were being admitted to the PICU in stable condition. Both were awake and experiencing fear and pain.

SM cried when the nurse placed her in the bed and attached electrodes and monitoring equipment to her body. She continually tried to remove her IV catheter. Her nurse spoke in soothing tones as pain medication was administered, and she was given a toy to distract her attention away from the IV. Soon SM's grandparents arrived, and she was observed to visibly relax when she made reassuring eye contact with a familiar face.

In the next room, EM was very quiet. Because of her injuries, her eyelids were swollen shut. She would

not speak but would nod "yes" or "no" when asked a question. EM was oriented to the room around her and was told her why she was in the hospital, reminding her that nothing was her fault. She nodded "yes" when asked if she wanted to listen to cartoons on the television. Her nurse arranged for a volunteer to sit with EM when her grandparents could not be with her.

1. Recognize that hospitalized children may experience a range of emotions. Sadness, anxiety, fear, and anger may arise. These emotions may be a response to being in the hospital, having painful procedures done, having to take medicine, or any number of things that happen in the hospital. Ask about their feelings, and assure them it is all right to feel that way. Some children may be unwilling or unable to express their feelings but sometimes display them by facial expression, crying, withdrawal, or being uncooperative.

2. Arrange for care by consistent staff members to limit the number of caregivers each child and family encounter. Having a familiar nurse helps to allay parental anxiety and may make it easier for parents to leave the child's bedside for a time. The nurse who takes time to know the child will become familiar with the child's responses and psychosocial needs. Most children communicate more readily with familiar caregivers. Caregivers who are familiar with a child more easily establish predictable routines.

3. Some children do not respond verbally but are willing to nod or shake their heads in response to a "yes" or "no" question or point to a picture on a communication board.

4. Assure children that they did not get sick because of something they thought or did. This assumes that the hospitalization is not related to the child's actions or inactions, such as driving without a seatbelt or taking an overdose of medication.

5. Limit the use of restraints and remove them whenever someone is able to stay with a child or as soon as the child's condition allows for restraint removal.

6. With planned admissions, offer hospital and PICU "tours" for both the child and parents. Identify equipment that will be used with the child. Explain the purposes of the alarms. Assure the parents and the child that the nurses know which alarms require an immediate response and which do not. Introduce the child and parents to at least one nurse or staff member whom they will see when the child is admitted.

7. If the child chooses, allow him or her to wear personal clothing as soon as possible. Being able to wear clothing from home, including underwear, socks, and shoes, is comforting for most children.

8. Respect the child's "space." Speak when approaching the child. Tell the child what you plan to do before touching the bed or the child.

9. Explain equipment, medications, and procedures in terms of what the child will experience. Tell children what they can expect to feel, see, hear, smell, and taste. Allow the child to hold the electronic thermometer, remove the blood pressure cuff, and remove old tape. Give as much control to the child as is safely possible.

10. Recognize regression as a normal defense mechanism in the hospitalized child, and help others, particularly parents, understand the process.

11. Set reasonable limits that a child can understand. For example, explain that it is all right to feel angry and cry, but it is not all right to bite or kick people. Do not threaten or shame a child. Be positive when speaking; for instance, say that you are going to help the child hold still rather than that the child will be held down. If parents use threats (e.g., "If you don't hold still, that nurse is going to give you a shot"), explain in a tactful manner, but within the child's hearing, the importance of telling a child the truth and avoiding threats so that the child will trust the caregivers.

12. Offer whatever comfort the child is willing to accept. Some children may accept stroking and hugging only in the absence of their parents. Interact with children at their eye level, but do not force eye contact with a child who is avoiding it. Interact with the child in a developmentally supportive manner, which can include being physically close, speaking in a soft voice, and using an empathetic touch.

13. Suggest that the parents bring in family pictures, and place them where the child can see them.

PSYCHOSOCIAL NEEDS OF FAMILIES

A. Family Assessment

1. *Sources of Stress Related to the PICU.* The sight and sound of equipment attached to sick children cause anxiety and fear. Parents often cannot distinguish between alarms that signal life-threatening conditions and those that might indicate something as simple as a completed medication or a false alarm

(Board & Ryan-Wenger, 2003). The changes in the appearance of a child and procedures are stressful to parents, especially during the first few days of hospitalization (Jee et al., 2012). Later in hospitalization, stress related to the communication and behavior of staff increase parental stress (Curley & Meyer, 2001). Parents fear that their child is in pain and may fear that the child will die. The presence of other sick, injured, or crying children and their apprehensive parents causes additional stress. Alteration in the parental role occurs as they watch strangers care for their child. This can lead to feelings of loss of control because they do not know how to care for the child themselves. Feelings of inadequacy may result when parents perceive professionals as better able to care for their child than they can. Parents may question their self-image as protector and nurturer of their child as they adjust to a new role as parent to an ill child. Restrictions on visitation and separation from the child can cause additional stress (Jee et al., 2012).

2. *Needs of Parents of Children in the PICU* (Curley & Meyer, 2001; Jee et al., 2012)

   a. Receiving as much information as possible

   b. Assurance that their child is receiving best possible care

   c. Feeling that there is hope

   d. Vigilance

   e. Being near their child as much as possible

   f. Assistance with physical care

   g. Being recognized as important to the child's recovery

   h. Talking with other parents

   i. Prayer

   j. Resources (e.g., transportation, meals)

3. *Responses to Stress and Coping Behaviors.* Stress reactions for families increase when a child's illness is severe, unexpected, or has an uncertain outcome.

   a. *Reactions*

     i. A shock reaction may occur when parents first see their child in the PICU.

     ii. Parents might be unable to remember information and might repeat the same question several times.

     iii. The initial response of parents may be to focus on the equipment and monitors and to be afraid to approach the bed or their child. Parents might want caregiver's "permission" and encouragement to approach the bed and touch their child.

iv. Some parents blame themselves or other family members for the child's illness and may show hostility toward caregivers.

v. Parents may assist in their child's care with repetitive tasks such as suctioning their child's mouth or draining urine from the tubing into the bag.

vi. Parents may focus on a detail and repeatedly complain if they feel it is not addressed adequately.

vii. There may be a delay in approaching the patient's bedside while visually scanning the environment for purposes of orientation to the situation (Soulvie, Desai, White, & Sullivan, 2012).

viii. Parents may display signs of withdrawal or passive behaviors, or they may intellectualize the illness (Soulvie et al., 2012).

b. *Support systems*

i. Family members are anyone who is considered important in the child's life (Meert, Clark, & Eggly, 2013).

ii. Family members close to the child may provide emotional support for parents, or they may be an additional source of stress if they are unable to cope with the child's illness or injury.

iii. Parents are often more willing to leave the hospital temporarily if a member of their support system remains with their child or if they have grown comfortable with a staff member caring for their child.

iv. Parents sometimes ask family members of another child in the PICU to "keep an eye on" their child while they leave the hospital for a rest even if a familiar caregiver is providing care for their child.

v. Parents may miss and worry about children at home or left in the care of others.

c. *Physical needs*

i. If a child's admission to the PICU was unexpected, parents may need assistance with finding a place to rest (if rooming-in accommodations are unavailable), bathe, find clothing, and obtain food.

ii. If the parents live near the PICU, they may want to go home to rest.

iii. Some parents are not able to cope with leaving the hospital and will need a place to lie down in the PICU or in a place as close as possible to the PICU.

iv. Assistance from social services should be obtained if parents do not have enough money for food.

v. Parents of critically ill children may forget or decline to eat. Encouraging them to eat and rest will help them to maintain their strength so that they will be able to support and care for their child.

d. *Cultural implications.* The cultural and spiritual identity and perspective of families may influence their understanding, roles, and expectations regarding illness, healthcare interventions, and end-of-life care. Diversity is respected and supported by acute and critical care nurses (Bell, 2015).

i. Some parents whose first language is not English may be able to speak English but have difficulty understanding what is being said because of the stress of the situation and the unfamiliar medical language. Obtain the assistance of an interpreter when the family is having difficulty understanding the professionals. It might be easier for them to ask questions in their own language.

ii. Be aware that wrist bracelets, ankle bracelets, or objects pinned to the child's clothing may have cultural or spiritual significance for the family. Treat these objects with respect. Do not remove such objects without parental permission unless absolutely necessary. Consider adding the patient identification bracelet. If objects are pinned to linens, be sure they do not get lost when linens are changed.

iii. Avoid categorizing or stereotyping members of a cultural group.

e. *Spiritual considerations*

i. Many parents experience guilt and helplessness when a child is ill or injured because they feel they must protect their children from harm of any kind. The illness of a child sometimes causes parents spiritual distress.

ii. Some parents express feelings that God caused the child's illness because of a parent's personal sin or fault.

iii. If the parents are religious, offer to contact a minister, priest, rabbi, or other religious leader. Offer the assistance of hospital chaplains if they are available.

iv. Ensure privacy by closing a door or curtain when parents wish to pray or participate in other religious and spiritual rituals. Some parents believe prayer is more effective when several faith-community members are gathered together and lay their hands on the child. Allowances in visiting policies should be made for this type of visit.

v. Assess dietary or treatment restrictions related to religion or culture. These may include rules about some foods or a prohibition against certain treatments, such as a ban on the use of blood products.

f. *Financial concerns.* Critical illness usually causes financial stress. Even parents who have insurance may have additional expenses related to hospitalization, which may include the cost of food, travel, babysitting for other children, or loss of pay. Parents may have to return to jobs earlier than desired. It may be necessary for family, friends, neighbors, and faith communities to assist with financial stressors.

B. Interventions With Families

Multiple studies have been done to identify family needs when a child is critically ill. Families want reassurance, access to the ill child, and information. Nurses caring for the child and family unit ensure that interventions take into account concepts of family-centered care, which allow for family involvement (as much as desired by the family) in the planning and implementation of care. Family-centered care has been shown to be beneficial to the child and family unit—and healthcare providers—through intentional planning, implementation of family-centered care policies, education, and ongoing family-centered competency building by the entire healthcare team (Coats et al., 2018 ; see Chapter 10 for more information on family-centered care).

1. *Supporting Families.* Full partnerships should be developed between family members and healthcare providers that share mutual interdependence and equal status. Implementation of the Nursing Mutual Participation Model of Care (Curley & Meyer, 2001) reduces parental stress (Table 1.7). Providing structured education and support to parents has also demonstrated improved outcomes in both mothers and young children.

2. *Communicating With Parents*

a. Make an effort to know the parents' first names, so they are not always addressed as "Mom" or "Dad." Ask permission before calling them by their first names.

b. Make an effort to learn how the parents are coping. Asking whether they were able to sleep or have been able to eat or drink anything demonstrates an interest in their well-being.

TABLE 1.7   Nursing Mutual Participation Model of Care

Admission
Extend care to include parents Acknowledge their importance
Daily Bedside Contact
Enable strategies that provide the parent with system savvy • Information: teach and clarify • Anticipatory guidance–illness trajectory • Provide instrumental resources Facilitate transition to *"parent-to-a-critically-ill-child"* • Enhance parent–child unique connectedness • Role-model interactions • Invite participation in nurturing activity • Provide options during procedures Communication pattern • Establish a caring relationship with the parent How are you doing today? • Assess parental perception of the child's illness How does he or she look to you today? • Determine parental goals, objectives, and expectations What troubles you most? • Seek informed suggestions and preferences, and invite participation in care How can I help you today?

Source: Reproduced with permission from Curley, M. A. Q., & Meyer, E. C. (2001). Caring practices: The impact of the critical care experience on the family. In M. A. Q. Curley & P. A. Moloney-Harmon (Eds.), *Critical care nursing of infants and children* (2nd ed.). Philadelphia, PA: W. B. Saunders.

c. Engage the parents as partners in care by asking them how they think the child is doing. Parents often detect subtle changes. Such questions also help the parents feel they are important in the child's care.

d. Ask about the parents' understanding of their child's condition and whether they have any outstanding questions, worries, or suggestions. After you have answered any questions, explore the information you shared with them to ensure that they understood the answers and whether your responses were adequate.

e. Consider forming a parent support group for the families. Groups can be facilitated by clinical-nurse specialists, nurses from the PICU, or social workers. Personally invite each parent of every child in the PICU to the group and keep all discussions confidential.

f. Assist the parents with physician contact. Let them know that they may request a joint meeting between the family and staff at any time, or offer to arrange a standing meeting for children anticipated to have a lengthy stay.

3. *Building a Relationship of Trust.* Parents need to trust the caregivers to feel comfortable enough to leave the bedside. Ask the parents to let you know where they are when they are not in the PICU and how they can be contacted. Agree about when they want to be called. Some parents prefer to be called if any change at all occurs, whether positive or negative. If you have agreed to call the parents when their child asks for them, do so. This will enhance a trusting relationship between the nurse and the parents as well as between the nurse and the child. Determine whether the parents have access to a cellular phone and consider loaning them a pager if needed so they will know you can easily contact them wherever they are.

4. *Mutual Care Planning With Parents*

a. Help the family understand which things are safe to touch and which must remain the caregivers' responsibility. Some parents turn off alarms to be helpful. Their point of view may be that they are doing the same thing as the nurse who walks into the room, touches a button, and walks away. Take time to explain the unseen assessment that is performed by the nurse as the alarm is silenced.

b. Collaborate with the multidisciplinary team (which includes the family) regarding the daily plan for the child. Daily rounds with family members provide a time for information gathering, clarification of understanding, questioning, and participation in decision making. Encourage the family to share their observations about the child, especially any changes they notice. If the plan is to observe the child and not make any changes, let them know that also so that they are not disappointed by a perceived lack of progress. Rounds with family members also improve trust with the healthcare team and increase transparency of intention (Meert et al., 2013).

c. Assist the parents in gaining as much control as possible by maintaining the parental role. Offer choices as much as possible. For example, when possible, let the parents decide when to give a bath or perform oral hygiene.

d. Offer to be a gatekeeper for the parents. If parents are being stressed by too many visitors who stay too long, let parents know that the staff is willing to place limits on visiting so they do not need to do so.

5. *Caring for Parents of Chronically Ill Children*

a. Children with a chronic illness may experience multiple PICU admissions. When possible, assign nurses who are familiar to the child and family from previous admissions.

b. Parents may be accustomed to performing many procedures at home and have developed their own ways of doing them. Ask how they perform care at home, and be open to the possibility that the staff can learn from experienced parents. Their expertise and contributions to care should be recognized. Parents will also have the ability to assess their child and provide input into clinical management.

c. Nurses caring for chronically ill children in the PICU should maintain the child's home routine as much as possible and provide developmentally supportive care.

d. To ensure the continuity of care, the multidisciplinary team should convene a discharge-planning session with the family before the child returns home or to another facility.

6. *Working With Siblings of a Child in the PICU*

a. Siblings of critically ill children have special needs. The PICU nurse can help to ensure that family-centered visiting policies are in place and that the PICU environment is such that children feel welcome.

b. Certified child-life specialists provide excellent preparation for siblings and help them to know what to expect before they visit in the PICU. Siblings may imagine that a brother or sister is far more seriously ill or injured when they are not allowed to see for themselves. The child-life therapist can assist siblings to communicate feelings they might have difficulty expressing. Formal programs for siblings may also be developed and can decrease behavioral and emotional problems following visitation (Meert et al., 2013).

c. Siblings may fear that they caused the illness or injury by something they said or did. Siblings may also experience signs of stress such as sleep disturbances or changes in behavior.

d. Parents may need assistance in making decisions regarding care of the child's siblings and whether and when siblings should visit.

e. Best friends and other close family members of the child in the PICU, such as cousins, may have concerns and needs similar to those of the child's siblings.

7. *Facilitating Transfer From the PICU.* Although transfer from the PICU signals the child's improvement and stability, it can engender anxiety and worry about future care, and may cause as much stress as the initial PICU admission (Berube, Fothergill-Bourbonnais, Thomas, & Moreau, 2014).

a. When their child is transferred, parents may experience anxiety related to the following changes:

   i. Being placed on an unfamiliar unit after becoming accustomed to the PICU

   ii. Unfamiliar staff members caring for the child

   iii. Changes in how frequently the child is assessed

   iv. Discontinuation of frequent monitoring

   v. The lack of the continuous presence of a nurse at the bedside

   vi. Concerns that the child is not well enough to be transferred

b. Family should be prepared for transfer plans before the event and told of any changes to expect. The nurse should assist in understanding that a transfer means the child is now doing better and no longer needs ICU care. If possible, offer a visit to the new unit before the transfer, emphasizing the positive aspects of the transfer, such as a more private and quiet environment.

c. A tour of the new unit and introductions to the staff can decrease stress. Care conferences with the family and new-unit staff before the transfer and follow-up visits by PICU nurses can facilitate transition. A critical care outreach team that is available following transfer to a new unit can provide families a bridge back to the PICU providers if any concerns arise (Berube et al., 2014).

8. *"Visiting Privileges" in the PICU.* To suggest that parents need our permission to be with their child is the antithesis of a system of healthcare that is driven by the needs of the patient. The primary need of the parents is to be with their child.

a. Parents should have 24-hour access to their child (Meert et al., 2013).

b. Parents should be given the option of staying with their child during procedures and tests; studies suggest that families would like to be given the option of and may actually benefit from being present during resuscitation events (AACN, 2016b; Guzzetta, 2016).

c. Extended family and individuals who are significant to the child by providing care and support should be included in educational and informational processes as desired by the child and family (Meert et al., 2013).

d. Privacy and confidentiality are important in the PICU but are not barriers to family presence.

e. Meeting the needs of the children

   i. Encourage an open, supportive atmosphere where family members can come and go around the clock to meet their own needs and those of the child.

   ii. Make exceptions to unit policies based on the child and family's individual needs, especially if a child is dying.

INTERVENTIONS FOR DYING CHILDREN

NK, a previously healthy 9-month-old, had been admitted to the PICU overnight and diagnosed with bacterial meningitis. His condition had quickly deteriorated, and he required intubation and placement on a mechanical ventilator. Medications were being used to improve his blood pressure, and an arterial catheter and a central venous catheter had been placed. NK was not responsive and did not seem to be aware of anything taking place around him.

As the shift began, the nurse quickly surveyed the situation in NK's room. It would be challenging to keep up with the multiple care priorities this patient needed, including ongoing assessments, administration of blood products, antibiotics, and placement of a device to monitor pressure in the brain. In addition, two devastated parents clung to each other in the corner of the room, unable to fathom what unspeakable things were happening to their precious child. His nurse established communication with NK's parents by introductions. Using simple words, his nurse explained what the nurses were doing for NK and answered what questions his parents could bring themselves to ask. Although not aware of it at that moment, his nurse was soon to become the catalyst that would help this family start transitioning from being the "parents of a healthy boy" to the "parents grieving for a lost child."

The extremely high pressure in NK's brain then confirmed the worst: A child who had been eating Cheerios and playing with his 2-year-old brother just yesterday was now neurologically devastated to the point that he would not survive. The critical care team's outcome goals for NK changed from curing his illness to orchestrating his peaceful and dignified death experience.

The nurse facilitated communication between the pediatric intensivist and the parents and talked about how the parents would say good-bye to their son. The PICU has a strong bereavement philosophy, and the program has many interventions that we offer families during this devastating time. NK's parents were assisted in deciding what options would be right for themselves and their son. Supported by the research-based policy of family-centered care, loving grandparents, aunts and uncles, a godfather, and the family priest encircled the parents when, for the last time, the child was placed in his mother's arms. At the parents' request, the intensivist and the nurse joined this intimate circle. All eyes were overflowing with tears when the child's godfather said a prayer for the parents and then prayed blessings on the critical care team.

A. Pain Management in the Terminally Ill

1. When a child is dying, the focus of care becomes pain relief and comfort of the child and family. Parents want their child to die peacefully and this desire influences how long they are willing to maintain life support (Hoover, Bratton, Roach, & Olson, 2014). Most parents are keenly sensitive to their child's pain and do not want their child to suffer (de Vos et al., 2015). In addition, there is a moral imperative to relieve the pain and suffering of dying children.

2. As the child develops a tolerance toward the analgesic used, higher doses of opioids may be required to provide adequate pain relief. High doses of opioids carry the risk of respiratory depression. According to the "principle of double effect," when the intended goal is to relieve pain, it is ethically correct to give whatever dose of analgesic is necessary to relieve pain, even with the potential for life to be shortened as a secondary effect (Reynolds, Drew, & Dunwoody, 2013). It is not legal, however, to administer more than is necessary to manage pain or to attempt to hasten death.

3. Nonpharmacologic means of pain relief are useful in the dying child but should never be used to the exclusion of medications.

4. To provide better control of pain, give analgesics around the clock rather than on an as-needed basis.

5. Fear of tolerance or addiction should not be a consideration in the dying child.

6. Neuromuscular blocking agents do not provide sedation or analgesia for the patient, thereby providing no comfort. Administration of these agents during withdrawal of life support provides no benefit to patients and may unethically hasten death (Sprung et al., 2014).

B. Forgoing Life-Sustaining Medical Treatment

1. Forgoing life-sustaining medical treatment includes decisions to withhold, withdraw, or limit medical treatment. AACN's online course, Promoting Excellence in Palliative and End-of-Life Care, is a resource that covers this topic across the life span.

2. Most ethicists believe there is no difference between withholding medical treatment and withdrawing treatment that has already been in use if the treatment is not beneficial to the patient (American Academy of Pediatrics Committee on Child Abuse and Neglect and Committee on Bioethics, 2000).

3. When considering the value of medical treatment in children, the benefits of treatment must be continually weighed against the burdens of treatment placed on the child. For instance, mechanical ventilation may be viewed as life prolonging, whereas noninvasive positive-pressure ventilation may relieve dyspnea and improve the child's time left (American Academy of Pediatrics Section on Hospice and Palliative Medicine and Committee on Hospital Care, 2013).

4. In most cases, parents are the appropriate decision makers for children. Ideally, parents and caregivers collaborate in making decisions about limiting or withdrawing treatment. The wishes and desires of conscious, coherent children should be given serious consideration (American Academy of Pediatrics Committee on Bioethics, 1994). Parents want to receive understandable explanations of their child's condition and need to feel that everything possible was done to help their child (Brooten et al., 2013). Parents consider many factors when deciding whether to withdraw life support for their child, including the quality of life, the likelihood that the child might get better (different from survival), and the amount of pain and suffering, in addition to chances for survival. This is more complex and somewhat different from what the ICU staff may consider. For instance, they may view survivability as the most important factor.

5. A decision to withhold or withdraw any medical treatment applies only to that specific treatment and should not be generalized to other treatments or care.

6. A do-not-resuscitate (DNR) order means only that no life-saving measures will be instituted in the event of a cardiac or respiratory arrest unless other measures have been discussed as well. It does not mean that the child should receive any less or different care compared with the care given to another child. It does not necessarily mean that the child is expected to die soon. A care-and-comfort-only policy is written in positive terms and describes the care that will be given to the child, such as supportive care and pain management. Limitation of treatment may include the decision not to institute any new therapies or to stop specific therapies already in use or both.

7. Any decision to forgo life-sustaining treatment for a child who has been abused should be made using the same process or deliberation criteria used for other critically ill children. Parents or guardians may have a conflict of interest because the perpetrator of the abuse risks having legal charges changed from assault to manslaughter or homicide (American Academy of Pediatrics Committee on Child Abuse and Neglect and Committee on Bioethics, 2000).

8. *Withdrawal of Treatment.* Consult parents when planning the time of withdrawal of treatment. There is no urgent need to withdraw support immediately simply because a decision was made. Allow time for parents to gather whatever family members they wish to be with them. Consult multidisciplinary team members, such as a chaplain, child-life therapist, interpreter, and social worker, for assistance as appropriate to family needs. Families may want the clergy from their community to be contacted in addition to or instead of the hospital chaplain, or they may not desire either. They may also want the family pediatrician to be involved (Wender & Committee on Psychosocial Aspects of Child and Family Health, 2012).

9. Acknowledge that parents may be in a stronger agreement with healthcare providers concerning treatment discontinuation than with family members and friends. This may occur because the healthcare providers are knowledgeable concerning end-of-life issues and may have been more involved in the decision-making processes (de Vos et al., 2015).

10. Provide anticipatory guidance to family members related to how treatment will be discontinued and how the child might respond. Allow parents all the time they need to say their good-byes to the child both before and after treatment is withdrawn. Parents may wish to hold the child before and after treatment is withdrawn, especially if death is expected to follow quickly after withdrawal of support. Parents may wish to play specific music for the child, have certain toys or security objects available, or carry out other rituals that have had meaning for them as a family, especially if the child is likely to die when support is withdrawn.

11. *Consider Discontinuation of Monitoring.* If the unit has central-monitoring capability, consider turning off the monitor in the child's room and continuing monitoring at the central station. Avoid having alarms go off in the child's room if no response to the alarms is planned.

12. Neuromuscular blocking agents should be stopped and allowed to wear off prior to withdrawal of life support. These agents can hasten death and impede assessment of the child (Delaney & Downar, 2016).

13. Privacy is essential for a family when treatment is withdrawn from a child. Transfer the patient to a private room with less traffic flow, or provide a curtain if no private room is available. Ask parents who, if anyone, they want to have in attendance when life support is withdrawn. Many parents, but not all, wish to be alone, whereas some fear being alone. Assure parents that if they choose to be alone, assistance will be close by.

C. Caring for the Potential Organ and Tissue Donor

1. Organ donation may occur after a child is diagnosed as brain dead or as a donation after circulatory determination of death (DCDD).

2. *Brain death* is defined as the irreversible cessation of function of the whole brain, including the brainstem. If organ donation ensues following brain death determination, the child's body is supported and mechanical ventilation continues until organ recovery can take place in the operating room.

3. The process for DCDD starts with end-of-life decision making prior to the child's death. In this situation, the child does not meet criteria for brain death, but cardiac cessation is expected quickly once mechanical ventilation and other therapies are removed (Nakagawa & Bratton, 2016). Once the child experiences asystole and is pronounced dead, organ recovery proceeds.

4. Critical care staff members are required by law to identify potential organ and tissue donors. Early referral to an organ procurement organization affords the best opportunity for skilled professionals to help both caregivers and parents through the process of organ donation.

5. Some families see organ donation as a chance to have "something good" come from the death of their child (Hoover et al., 2014).

6. Uncouple the child's death from the idea of organ donation. Allow the family time to be with the child. Assess the family to determine whether they are acknowledging the child's death to themselves. Note that acknowledgment is not acceptance. If the family is still asking whether there is any chance that the child will recover, they have not acknowledged that the child is dead. Avoid raising the issue of organ donation at the same time the parents are told of the child's death. Allow at least a brief period between these events. If possible, allow time between raising the idea of organ donation and asking for a decision.

7. It may be difficult for parents to believe a child is dead when the child's chest is still moving and a heart rate is visible on the monitor.

8. Parents may need to ask the same questions repeatedly before they are able to hear and remember what they have been told.

9. Assure the parents that organ donation will not disfigure the child's body, preclude an open casket, or delay funeral arrangements (Hoover et al., 2014).

10. Offer parents the opportunity to hold the child before the organs are removed.

11. Some parents may want to leave the hospital before the child's organs are removed, whereas others may need to see the child again following the recovery procedure (Hoover et al., 2014).

12. Be careful to treat the child who is going to be an organ donor with the same respect and dignity afforded to any child who is still living.

13. In cases of child abuse, federal and state regulations may require permission of the parent or guardian for organ donation. If organs are to be donated, the medical examiner or district attorney should be notified so that valuable evidence is not altered or lost during donation (American Academy of Pediatrics Committee on Child Abuse and Neglect and Committee on Bioethics, 2000).

D. Caring for the Conscious, Dying Child

The conscious, dying child may benefit from the opportunity to communicate about his or her own personal dying process. The use of an age-appropriate, advance-planning guide can provide a framework for guiding this dialogue (Mullen, Reynolds, & Larson, 2015). Occasionally, families insist that children not be told about their impending death. Whether and how impending death is disclosed to a child can be influenced by the family's religious and cultural heritage, previous experience with death, and other influences. It is important to help the parents realize that the child

probably already knows or suspects and may not talk about it simply because he or she senses the parents' avoidance.

1. Ask the family about the child's understanding of death. Explore their thoughts concerning death to help you understand and support them.

2. Encourage parents to discuss the subject with the child and answer the child's questions.

3. Obtain support from clinical nurse specialists, child-life therapists, psychologists, social services, or chaplains as needed for the family and child.

4. Answer the child's questions openly and honestly.

5. Assure the child that he or she will not be left alone.

6. Allow whatever visitors the child wishes to see.

7. Provide opportunity for a child or adolescent to obtain spiritual guidance and to continue peer relationships.

E. Caring for Bereaved Families

Grief is the cognitive, emotional, physical, psychological, and spiritual response to an overwhelming loss. Grief is frequently described in terms of stages, phases, or symptoms. Although these references are helpful in understanding grief, grief is not a linear process. The bereaved person moves in and out of the phases at various times in the grief process. Symptoms of one phase may overlap with another, and time limits should not be imposed on the individual for completion of this painful process. When a child dies, parental grief is the subjective, individualized response to a hideous loss. The impact is long lasting and life altering.

1. Lindemann (1944) described symptomatology that was pathognomonic for grief:

a. *Somatic distress.* Feelings of tightness in throat or chest, sighing, weakness, shortness of breath

b. *Preoccupation with the image of the deceased.* Hearing or seeing the person who has died, inability to focus on anything other than loved one who died, emotional distance from others

c. *Feelings of guilt.* Feeling responsible for the loved one's death, searching for things that could have been done differently, thinking in terms of "if only"

d. *Hostile reactions.* Feelings and expressions of anger

e. *Loss of patterns of conduct.* Restlessness and an inability to complete things started

2. Kübler-Ross (1969) described the stages of death and dying. As with grief, a person may move in and out of various stages at different times before reaching acceptance:

   a. *Denial.* Shock and disbelief

   b. *Anger.* Angry and hostile reactions expressed

   c. *Bargaining.* Attempts to delay the death

   d. *Depression or despair*

   e. *Acceptance*

3. Miles and Perry (1985) identified three phases of parental grief: (a) a state of numbness and shock, (b) a period of intense grief, and (c) a period of reorganization. During the early phase of numbness and shock, parents may use a variety of coping behaviors and display a wide range of emotions.

   a. Some parents may seem to be in a trance and display no emotion at all. They may show concern for others and even try to comfort other family members while expressing little emotion themselves.

   b. Parents can display a wide range of emotions. Many parents will cry. Some express grief loudly with keening and wailing, whereas others cry quietly. Some parents exhibit inappropriate silliness or euphoria. It is a mistake to judge a parent as unaffected or uncaring because of emotional reactions at the time of a death.

   c. Although parents are in emotional shock and forget much of what is said to them, paradoxically they often remember verbatim the things that were said to them at the time of their child's death.

   d. Psychic numbness protects the person from feeling the full impact of their loss. It protects the mind from a grief that is too horrible to be faced at one time.

4. *Interventions With the Family at the Time of Death*

   a. *Be a calm, nonanxious presence.* If you are unable to think of something to say, with family permission, be a silent presence (Mullen et al., 2015). Being with a family may assist the parents in several ways. Feelings of isolation experienced by the parents may be reduced. Being with the family helps them to know that nothing is being hidden from them. One of the reasons for malpractice suits is that families sometimes feel they are not being told the truth or that information is being hidden. A receptive, nonverbal posture lets people know you are willing to listen if they need to talk. Bereaved family members have described caring people as those who were able to show that they cared by just "being there."

   b. *Consider the use of a gentle touch to express caring and concern.* Be sensitive to those who are not comfortable with being touched. This can usually be discerned by stiffening in the person who was touched. Those who respond to touch will frequently grasp your hand or lean toward you as you touch them.

   c. *Keep the focus on the family.* Caregivers who feel compelled to share their own losses may be attempting to meet their own needs rather than those of the family.

   d. *Provide opportunity to be with the child.* Go into the room with family members. Prepare them for what they will see if they were not there at the time of death. Ask the parents if they prefer some time alone with the child. Remain close by and available to them. Offer parents the chance to hold their child. If death is imminent, be sure they understand their child could die while being held. Offer more than once if they seem to be having difficulty processing information given to them. In some circumstances, the parents may ask the nurse to hold their child as he or she dies. Parents may wish to help care for the child's body. Offer the chance to bathe and dress the child or brush the child's hair. Provide a rocking chair if possible for parents to rock their child one last time. Siblings may benefit from being able to say good-bye and need to be reassured that they did not cause the illness and death.

   e. *Assist parents in telling siblings of the child's death.* The information given to siblings should be truthful and in terms appropriate to their developmental age. Child-life therapists can be helpful with this process. Surviving siblings have had issues with feeling alone or guilty, or feeling that they did not have enough time to say good-bye to their brother or sister (Youngblut & Brooten, 2013). Many excellent written resources are available for children to assist them in the grieving process.

   f. *Encourage families to seek professional psychosocial support as needed.* It would be impossible to judge who in the family may need professional help following the death of a child. Parents, understandably, might be sensitive if they are deemed to be "coping poorly." Bereavement support groups may also be helpful to families in the aftermath of childhood death.

g. *Call the child by name.* Parents need to know that their child was special to others as well as to them.

h. *Avoid platitudes* such as "time heals all wounds," "you wouldn't want him or her to live like that," or "you're lucky, it could have been worse." These phrases, although meant to comfort, tend to minimize a person's loss.

i. *Things you can say that are helpful.*

    i. "I'm sorry."

    ii. "This must be terribly hard for you."

    iii. "Is there anyone I can call for you?"

    iv. "Would you like me to stay with you for a while?"

j. *Avoid delaying the onset of grief* by offering the parents tranquilizers or sedatives on a routine basis. Medications may ease the situation for caregivers but only delay the inevitable for the parents. Parents may feel they are being told that their grief is not acceptable.

k. *Offer a remembrance packet to the family.* Keep a camera on the unit and offer to take a picture of the child if the parents wish either before or after the child's death. This may be especially important when an infant dies if the parents have few (if any) pictures. Handprints or footprints can be made easily on a card for the family. Parents may wish to have a lock of hair from the back of the child's head. Ask their permission before cutting the hair. Baptismal certificates or candles can be provided. Hand or foot molds can be made and placed in a memory box to provide a special keepsake (Mullen et al., 2015).

l. *Provide factual information, but do not dwell on details that the family has not requested.* Be prepared to answer the same questions more than once.

m. *Allow the family to talk about the child.* Ask questions about the child and listen to the family's answers. Do not be afraid of their tears or your own. Crying is a normal expression of grief for both family and caregivers. There is no need to say, "I didn't mean to remind you"; the parents have not forgotten.

n. *Develop a resource file on the unit* that includes information about grief for families and caregivers, materials to develop a remembrance packet, sympathy cards to be mailed to families, and a list of effective local self-help groups.

o. *A follow-up program is helpful to families.* An index card file system or electronic database is useful to keep a record of the children who have died. Sympathy cards and letters may be sent to bereaved parents a few weeks following the child's death and again on the first anniversary of the child's death, at Christmas, or any time chosen by the unit staff (Mullen et al., 2015). Follow-up telephone calls give parents the chance to ask questions and to relate how they are doing. An offer to return to the hospital to visit with physicians or nurses may be helpful for some parents. If an autopsy was done, allow parents to ask questions and review the autopsy report if they so desire (Eggly et al., 2011).

p. *Consider developing a checklist* to guide caregivers at the time of a child's death. Include those things your unit considers most important for parents.

5. *Staff Support.* (Please see Chapter 10 for additional information.)

    a. Offer emotional support and assistance to the multidisciplinary team members caring for a child who dies. Allow the healthcare providers to "get out of the unit" for a break as necessary.

    b. Consider support sessions following a death in the unit. Debriefing sessions may be facilitated by a clinical-nurse specialist, child-life therapist, social worker, psychologist, or chaplain.

        i. Some healthcare providers may attend the funerals or memorial services for children for whom they cared. This ritual may assist the caregivers and offer support to the family as well.

        ii. If a child is expected to die, provide a resource person for the nurse who has never cared for a child at the time of death.

Pediatric critical care nurses play a special role and have myriad opportunities to help children and their families cope with hospitalization, the intensive care unit environment, and the stressors that accompany this disruption to their daily lives. Children should be approached in a manner consistent with their developmental level and interventions tailored to their unique needs. Hospitalized children require assistance to help them cope with fear, anxiety, and pain. Nursing interventions will focus on facilitating communication, sleep, play, and providing for the emotional needs of the child and family. Finally, when children and their families must face the end of life, pediatric nurses will rely on important strategies to support bereavement needs.

REFERENCES

American Academy of Pediatrics Committee on Bioethics. (1994). Guidelines on forgoing life-sustaining medical treatment [Reaffirmed 2008]. *Pediatrics, 93*(3), 532–536. Retrieved from http://pediatrics.aappublications.org/content/pediatrics/93/3/532.full.pdf

American Academy of Pediatrics Committee on Child Abuse and Neglect and Committee on Bioethics.(2000). Forgoing life-sustaining medical treatment in abused children [Reaffirmed 2007]. *Pediatrics, 106*, 1151–1153. doi:10.1542/peds.106.5.1151

American Academy of Pediatrics Section on Hospice and Palliative Medicine and Committee on Hospital Care. (2013). Pediatric palliative care and hospice care commitments, guidelines, and recommendations. *Pediatrics, 132*(5), 966–972. doi:doi:10.1542/peds.2013-2731

American Association of Critical-Care Nurses. (2015). The AACN synergy model for patient care. Retrieved from https://www.aacn.org/nursing-excellence/aacn-standards/synergy-model

American Association of Critical-Care Nurses. (2016a). AACN practice alert: Assessment and management of delirium across the life span. Retrieved from https://www.aacn.org/clinical-resources/practice-alerts/delirium-assessment-and-management

American Association of Critical-Care Nurses. (2016b). AACN practice alert: Family presence during resuscitation and invasive procedures. Retrieved from https://www.aacn.org/clinical-resources/practice-alerts/family-presence-during-resuscitation-and-invasive-procedures

Bell, L. E. (Ed.). (2015). *AACN scope and standard for acute and critical care nursing practice*. Aliso Viejo, CA: American Association of Critical-Care Nurses.

Berube, K. M., Fothergill-Bourbonnais, F., Thomas, M., & Moreau, D. (2014). Parents' experience of the transition with their child from a pediatric intensive care unit (PICU) to the hospital ward: Searching for comfort across transitions. *Journal of Pediatric Nursing, 29*(6), 586–595. doi:10.1016/j.pedn.2014.06.001

Beyer, J. E., Turner, S. B., Jones, L., Young, L., Onikul, R., & Bohaty, B. (2005). The alternate forms reliability of the Oucher pain scale. *Pain Management Nursing, 6*(1), 10–17. doi:10.1016/j.pmn.2004.11.001

Board, R., & Ryan-Wenger, N. (2003). Stressors and stress symptoms of mothers with children in the PICU. *Journal of Pediatric Nursing, 18*(3), 195–202. doi:10.1053/jpdn.2003.38

Boerlage, A., Ista, E., Duivenvoorden, H., Wildt, S., Tibboel, D., & van Dijk, M. (2015). The COMFORT behaviour scale detects clinically meaningful effects of analgesic and sedative treatment. *European Journal of Pain, 19*(4), 473–479. doi:10.1002/ejp.569

Breau, L. M., McGrath, P. J., Camfield, C. S., & Finley, G. A. (2002). Psychometric properties of the non-communicating children's pain checklist-revised. *Pain, 99*(1), 349–357. doi:10.1016/S0304-3959(02)00179-3

Brooten, D., Youngblut, J. M., Seagrave, L., Caicedo, C., Hawthorne, D., Hidalgo, I., & Roche, R. (2013). Parent's perceptions of health care providers actions around child ICU death: What helped, what did not. *American Journal of Hospice & Palliative Care, 30*(1), 40–49. doi:10.1177/1049909112444301

Coats, H., Bourget, E., Starks, H., Lindhorst, T., Saiki-Craighill, S., Curtis, J. R., . . . Doorenbos, A. (2018). Nurses' reflections on benefits and challenges of implementing family-centered care in pediatric intensive care units. *American Journal of Critical Care, 27*(1), 52–58. doi:10.4037/ajcc2018353

Curley, M. A. Q. (2001). The essence of pediatric critical care nursing. In M. A. Q. Curley & P. A. Moloney-Harmon (Eds.), *Critical care nursing of infants and children* (2nd ed., pp. 3–16). Philadelphia, PA: W. B. Saunders.

Curley, M. A. Q., Harris, S. K., Fraser, K. A., Johnson, R. A., & Arnold, J. H. (2006). State behavioral scale: A sedation assessment instrument for infants and young children supported on mechanical ventilation. *Pediatric Critical Care Medicine: 7*(2), 107–114. doi:10.1097/01.PCC.0000200955.40962.38

Curley, M. A. Q., & Meyer, E. C. (2001). Caring practices: The impact of the critical care experience on the family. In M. A. Q. Curley & P. A. Moloney-Harmon (Eds.), *Critical care nursing of infants and children* (2nd ed., pp. 47–67). Philadelphia, PA: W. B. Saunders.

Delaney, J. W., & Downar, J. (2016). How is life support withdrawn in intensive care units: A narrative review. *Journal of Critical Care, 35*, 12–18. doi:10.1016/j.jcrc.2016.04.006

de Vos, M. A., Bos, A. P., Plotz, F. B., van Heerde, M., de Graaff, B. M., Tates, K., ... Willems, D. L. (2015). Talking with parents about end-of-life decisions for their children. *Pediatrics, 135*(2), e465–e476. doi:10.1542/peds.2014-1903

Dubois, A., Capdevila, X., Bringuier, S., & Pry, R. (2010). Pain expression in children with an intellectual disability. *European Journal of Pain, 14*(6), 654–660. doi:10.1016/j.ejpain.2009.10.013

Eggly, S., Meert, K. L., Berger, J., Zimmerman, J., Anand, K. J., Newth, C. J., ... Nicholson, C. (2011). A framework for conducting follow-up meetings with parents after a child's death in the pediatric intensive care unit. *Pediatric Critical Care Medicine, 12*(2), 147–152. doi:10.1097/PCC.0b013e3181e8b40c

Franck, L. S., Scoppettuolo, L. A., Wypij, D., & Curley, M. A. (2012). Validity and generalizability of the withdrawal assessment tool-1 (WAT-1) for monitoring iatrogenic withdrawal syndrome in pediatric patients. *Pain, 153*(1), 142–148. doi:10.1016/j.pain.2011.10.003

Gregory, A. M., & Sadeh, A. (2012). Sleep, emotional and behavioral difficulties in children and adolescents. *Sleep Medicine Reviews, 16*(2), 129–136. doi:10.1016/j.smrv.2011.03.007

Guzzetta, C. (2016). Family presence during resuscitation and invasive procedures. *Critical Care Nurse, 36*, e11–e14. doi:10.4037/ccn2016980

Hardin, S. R., & Kaplow, R. (Eds.). (2017). *Synergy for clinical excellence: The AACN synergy model for patient care* (2nd ed.). Burlington, MA: Jones & Bartlett.

Hicks, C. L., von Baeyer, C. L., Spafford, P. A., van Korlaar, I., & Goodenough, B. (2001). The Faces Pain Scale–Revised: Toward a common metric in pediatric pain measurement. *Pain, 93*(2), 173–183. doi:10.1016/S0304-3959(01)00314-1

Hockenberry, M., & Wilson, D. (Eds.). (2013). *Wong's essentials of pediatric nursing* (9th ed.). St. Louis, MO: Mosby.

Hoover, S. M., Bratton, S. L., Roach, E., & Olson, L. M. (2014). Parental experiences and recommendations in donation after circulatory determination of death. *Pediatric Critical Care Medicine, 15*(2), 105–111. doi:10.1097/PCC.0000000000000035

Hsu, T., Ryherd, E., Waye, K. P., & Ackerman, J. (2012). Noise pollution in hospitals: Impact on patients. *Journal of Clinical Outcomes Management, 19*(7), 301–309. Retrieved from https://pdfs.semanticscholar.org/27db/5536c0a580983f3efd1b30374f64cacacd65.pdf

Hummel, P., Puchalski, M., Creech, S., & Weiss, M. (2008). Clinical reliability and validity of the N-PASS: Neonatal pain, agitation and sedation scale with prolonged pain. *Journal of Perinatology, 28*(1), 55–60. doi:10.1038/sj.jp.7211861

Hunt, A., Goldman, A., Seers, K., Crichton, N., Mastroyannopoulou, K., Moffat, V., ... Brady, M. (2004). Clinical validation of the paediatric pain profile. *Developmental Medicine & Child Neurology, 46*(1), 9–18. Retrieved from https://onlinelibrary.wiley.com/doi/pdf/10.1111/j.1469-8749.2004.tb00428.x

International Association for the Study of Pain. (2015). *IASP terminology*. Retrieved from https://www.iasp-pain.org/terminology?navItemNumber=576#Pain

Ista, E., de Hoog, M., Tibboel, D., Duivenvoorden, H. J., & van Dijk, M. (2013). Psychometric evaluation of the Sophia observation withdrawal symptoms scale in critically ill children. *Pediatric Critical Care Medicine*, 14(8), 761–769. doi:10.1097/PCC.0b013e31829f5be1

Jacob, E., Mack, A. K., Savedra, M., Van Cleve, L., & Wilkie, D. J. (2014). Adolescent pediatric pain tool for multidimensional measurement of pain in children and adolescents. *Pain Management Nursing*, 15(3), 694–706. doi:10.1016/j.pmn.2013.03.002

Jee, R. A., Shepherd, J. R., Boyles, C. E., Marsh, M. J., Thomas, P. W., & Ross, O. C. (2012). Evaluation and comparison of parental needs, stressors, and coping strategies in a pediatric intensive care unit. *Pediatric Critical Care Medicine*, 13(3), e166–e172. doi:10.1097/PCC.0b013e31823893ad

Krechel, S. W., & Bildner, J. (1995). CRIES: A new neonatal postoperative pain measurement score. Initial testing of validity and reliability. *Pediatric Anesthesia*, 5(1), 53–61. doi:10.1111/j.1460-9592.1995.tb00242.x

Kübler-Ross, E. (1969). *On death and dying*. New York, NY: Macmillan.

Kudchadkar, S. R., Aljohani, O. A., & Punjabi, N. M. (2014). Sleep of critically ill children in the pediatric intensive care unit: A systematic review. *Sleep Medicine Reviews*, 18(2), 103–110. doi:10.1016/j.smrv.2013.02.002

Lawrence, J., Alcock, D., McGrath, P., Kay, J., MacMurray, S. B., & Dulberg, C. (1993). The development of a tool to assess neonatal pain (NIPS). *Neonatal Network*, 12(6), 59–66. doi:10.1016/0885-3924(91)91127-U

Lindemann, E. (1944). Symptomatology and management of acute grief. In J. J. Parad (Ed.), *Crisis intervention: Selected readings* (pp. 141–148). New York, NY: Family Service Association of America.

Meert, K. L., Clark, J., & Eggly, S. (2013). Family-centered care in the pediatric intensive care unit. *Pediatric Clinics of North America*, 60(3), 761–772. doi:10.1016/j.pcl.2013.02.011

Merkel, S., Voepel-Lewis, T., & Malviya, S. (2002). Pain assessment in infants and young children: The FLACC scale: A behavioral tool to measure pain in young children. *American Journal of Nursing*, 102(10), 55–58. Retrieved from http://www.jstor.org/stable/3522977

Micromedex. (2015). Retrieved from http://www.micromedexsolutions.com

Miles, M. S., & Perry, K. (1985). Parental responses to sudden accidental death of a child. *Critical Care Quarterly*, 8(1), 73–84.

Mondardini, M. C., Vasile, B., Amigoni, A., Baroncini, S., Conio, A., Mantovani, A., ... L'Erario, M. (2014). Update of recommendations for analgosedation in pediatric intensive care unit. *Minerva Anestesiologica*, 80(9), 1018–1029. Retrieved from https://www.minervamedica.it/en/journals/minerva-anestesiologica/article.php?cod=R02Y2014N09A1018

Mullen, J. E., Reynolds, M. R., & Larson, J. S. (2015). Caring for pediatric patients' families at the child's end of life. *Critical Care Nurse*, 35(6), 46–55; quiz 56. doi:10.4037/ccn2015614

Nakagawa, T. A., & Bratton, S. L. (2016). Pediatric donation after circulatory determination of death: Past, present, and hopeful future changes. *Pediatric Critical Care Medicine*, 17(3), 270–271. doi:10.1097/PCC.0000000000000605

Peters, J. W., Koot, H. M., Grunau, R. E., de Boer, J., van Druenen, M. J., Tibboel, D., & Duivenvoorden, H. J. (2003). Neonatal facial coding system for assessing postoperative pain in infants: Item reduction is valid and feasible. *Clinical Journal of Pain*, 19(6), 353–363.

Rennick, J. E., & Childerhose, J. E. (2015). Redefining success in the PICU: New patient populations shift targets of care. *Pediatrics*, 135(2), e289–e291. doi:10.1542/peds.2014-2174

Reynolds, J., Drew, D., & Dunwoody, C. (2013). American Society for Pain Management Nursing position statement: Pain management at the end of life. *Pain Management Nursing*, 14(3), 172–175. Retrieved from http://www.aspmn.org/documents/PainManagementattheEndofLife_August2013.pdf

Savedra, M. C., Tesler, M. D., Holzemer, W. L., Wilkie, D. J., & Ward, J. A. (1989). Pain location: Validity and reliability of body outline markings by hospitalized children and adolescents. *Research in Nursing & Health*, 12(5), 307–314. doi:10.1002/nur.4770120506

Silver, G., Traube, C., Gerber, L. M., Sun, X., Kearney, J., Patel, A., & Greenwald, B. (2015). Pediatric delirium and associated risk factors: A single-center prospective observational study. *Pediatric Critical Care Medicine*, 16(4), 303–309. doi:10.1097/PCC.0000000000000356

Slota, M. C. (1988). Implications of sleep deprivation in the pediatric critical care unit. *Focus on Critical Care*, 15(3), 35–43.

Smith, H. A., Boyd, J., Fuchs, D. C., Melvin, K., Berry, P., Shintani, A., ... Ely, E. W. (2011). Diagnosing delirium in critically ill children: Validity and reliability of the pediatric confusion assessment method for the intensive care unit. *Critical Care Medicine*, 39(1), 150–157. doi:10.1097/CCM.0b013e3181feb489

Smith, H. A., Gangopadhyay, M., Goben, C. M., Jacobowski, N. L., Chestnut, M. H., Savage, S., ... Pandharipande, P. P. (2016). The preschool confusion assessment method for the ICU: Valid and reliable delirium monitoring for critically ill infants and children. *Critical Care Medicine*, 44(3), 592–600. doi:10.1097/CCM.0000000000001428

Solodiuk, J. C., Scott-Sutherland, J., Meyers, M., Myette, B., Shusterman, C., Karian, V. E., ... Curley, M. A. (2010). Validation of the individualized numeric rating scale (INRS): A pain assessment tool for nonverbal children with intellectual disability. *Pain*, 150(2), 231–236. doi:10.1016/j.pain.2010.03.016

Soulvie, M. A., Desai, P. P., White, C. P., & Sullivan, B. N. (2012). Psychological distress experienced by parents of young children with congenital heart defects: A comprehensive review of literature. *Journal of Social Service Research*, 38(4), 484–502. doi:10.1080/01488376.2012.696410

Sprung, C. L., Truog, R. D., Curtis, J. R., Joynt, G. M., Baras, M., Michalsen, A., ... Avidan, A. (2014). Seeking worldwide professional consensus on the principles of end-of-life care for the critically ill. The consensus for worldwide end-of-life practice for patients in intensive care units (WELPICUS) study. *American Journal of Respiratory and Critical Care Medicine*, 190(8), 855–866. doi:10.1164/rccm.201403-0593CC

Stevens, B. J., Gibbins, S., Yamada, J., Dionne, K., Lee, G., Johnston, C., & Taddio, A. (2014). The premature infant pain profile-revised (PIPP-R): Initial validation and feasibility. *Clinical Journal of Pain*, 30(3), 238–243. doi:10.1097/AJP.0b013e3182906aed

Stevens, B. J., Yamada, J., Lee, G. Y., & Ohlsson, A. (2013). Sucrose for analgesia in newborn infants undergoing painful procedures. *Cochrane Database of Systematic Reviews*, 2013(1). doi:10.1002/14651858.CD001069.pub4

Traube, C., Silver, G., Kearney, J., Patel, A., Atkinson, T. M., Yoon, M. J., ... Greenwald, B. (2014). Cornell assessment of pediatric delirium: A valid, rapid, observational tool for screening delirium in the PICU. *Critical Care Medicine*, 42(3), 656–663. doi:10.1097/CCM.0b013e3182a66b76

Tripathi, S., Andring, C., Beadling, A., Klarr, E., McNamara, M., Duncan, J., … Nemergut, M. (2014). 804: Noise levels in the PICU and staff perception regarding effect of noise exposure on sleep quality. *Critical Care Medicine, 42*(12), A1553–A1554. doi:10.1097/01.ccm.0000458301.54861.01

U.S. Environmental Protection Agency. (1974). *Protective noise levels: Condensed version of EPA levels document*. Washington, DC: Author Retrieved from http://www.nonoise.org/library/levels/levels.htm

Vet, N. J., de Wildt, S. N., Verlaat, C. W., Knibbe, C. A., Mooij, M. G., Hop, W. C., … de Hoog, M. (2014). Daily interruption of sedation in critically ill children: Study protocol for a randomized controlled trial. *Trials, 15*(1), 55. doi:10.1186/1745-6215-15-55

von Baeyer, C. L., Spagrud, L. J., McCormick, J. C., Choo, E., Neville, K., & Connelly, M. A. (2009). Three new datasets supporting use of the numerical rating scale (NRS-11) for children's self-reports of pain intensity. *Pain, 143*(3), 223–227. doi:10.1016/j.pain.2009.03.002

Watson, J., Kinstler, A., Vidonish, W. P., 3rd, Wagner, M., Lin, L., Davis, K. G., … Daraiseh, N. M. (2015). Impact of noise on nurses in pediatric intensive care units. *American Journal of Critical Care, 24*(5), 377–384. doi:10.4037/ajcc2015260

Wender, E., & Committee on Psychosocial Aspects of Child and Family Health. (2012). Supporting the family after the death of a child. *Pediatrics, 130*(6), 1164–1169. doi:10.1542/peds.2012-2772

Youngblut, J. M., & Brooten, D. (2013). Parents' report of child's response to sibling's death in a neonatal or pediatric intensive care unit. *American Journal of Critical Care, 22*(6), 474–481. doi:10.4037/ajcc2013790

2 PULMONARY SYSTEM

Elizabeth Flasch, Nicole Brueck, Justin Lynn, and Jennifer Henningfeld

DEVELOPMENTAL ANATOMY OF THE PULMONARY SYSTEM

A. Embryology of the Lung

In humans, there are five well-recognized stages of lung development: embryonic, pseudoglandular, canalicular, saccular, and alveolar (Figure 2.1).

1. *Embryonic Stage. Day 26 to 52*—In primitive development, the foregut forms a lung bud from the pharynx 26 days after conception. This lung bud elongates and forms the trachea and two bronchial buds, which then separate from the esophagus. By the end of the embryonic period, the larger airways, including the trachea, main stem, and segmental and subsegmental bronchi are developed. During this phase, the respiratory endothelium and diaphragm develop (Schnapf & Kirley, 2010).

2. *Pseudoglandular Stage. Day 52 to week 16*— During this stage, branching morphogenesis continues, leading to the formation of subsegmental bronchi, bronchioles, and primitive acinar tubules. Cilia appear on the surface of the epithelium of the trachea and the main stem bronchi at 10 weeks of gestation and are present on peripheral airways by 13 weeks gestation. Lymphatics appear in the lung itself by week 10. Goblet cells appear in the bronchial epithelium at 13 to 14 weeks gestation (Schnapf & Kirley, 2010).

3. *Canalicular Stage. Week 17 to 26*—This stage is so named because of the appearance of vascular channels, or capillaries, which begin to grow by forming a capillary network around the air passages. By the end of this period, pulmonary acinar units are formed, consisting of a respiratory bronchiole, alveolar ducts, and alveolar sacs. By 20 to 22 weeks of gestation, type I and type II epithelial cells can be differentiated. By the end of this period, the development of the air–blood barrier is thin enough to support gas exchange. These developments, along with increasing synthesis of surfactant, are critical to the extrauterine survival of the fetus. At 22 to 24 weeks gestation, the survival of the fetus becomes possible during this stage (Schnapf & Kirley, 2010).

4. *Saccular Stage. Week 26 to 36*—During this period, there is a marked increase in the potential gas-exchanging surface area due to thinning of the epithelium and mesenchyme and further formation of the capillary net. The terminal structures are referred to as *saccules* and are relatively smooth-walled cylindrical structures. They then become subdivided by ridges known as *secondary crests*. As the crests protrude into the saccules, part of the capillary net is drawn with them, forming a double capillary layer. Further septation between the crests results in smaller spaces termed *subsaccules* (Schnapf & Kirley, 2010).

5. *Alveolar Stage. Week 36 and beyond*— Alveolarization is rapidly progressing during this period. Alveologenesis is characterized by a complex interaction of epithelial, fibroblast, and vascular growth factors with extracellular matrix components (Schnapf & Kirley, 2010).

6. *The First Breath*. The thorax is compressed as it passes through the birth canal, forcing out some of the fetal lung fluid. Chest recoil after the thorax is delivered results in air entry into the lungs. The first inspiratory effort must be large enough to overcome the viscous resistance to movement of the intrapulmonary liquid and overcome the tissue and surface tension. For the first several minutes to 2 hours, expiration is often incomplete, resulting in progressively increasing functional residual capacity (FRC). For infants born by cesarean section, it takes longer to establish FRC (Schnapf & Kirley, 2010).

B. Postnatal Lung Development

Normal lung growth is a continuous process that begins early in gestation and extends through infancy and childhood. Estimates of alveolar number at birth vary greatly but the general accepted number is 50 million. Eventually 300 million alveolar will form after birth. Lung volume will increase 23-fold, alveolar number will increase sixfold, alveolar surface area will increase 21-fold, and lung weight will increase 20-fold. Alveolar development is thought to continue through early childhood with implications for recovery of lung function after certain childhood insults (Schnapf & Kirley, 2010).

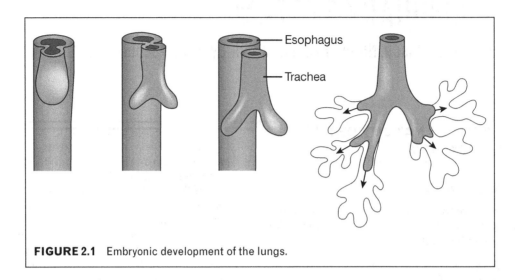

FIGURE 2.1 Embryonic development of the lungs.

C. Upper Airway Development

The upper airway is responsible for warming, humidifying, and filtering air before it reaches the trachea. There are notable differences between pediatric and adult airways (Table 2.1).

1. *Nose*

a. *Embryology.* Nasal cavities begin as widely separated pits on the face of the 4-week-old embryo. The ethmoid and the maxillary sinuses form in the third to fourth gestational month and, accordingly, are present at birth. The sphenoid *sinuses* are generally pneumatized by 5 years of age; the frontal sinuses appear at age 7 to 8 years but are not completely developed until late adolescence. The ethmoid cells are present and increase in size throughout life. Frontal and sphenoid sinuses do not begin to invade the frontal or sphenoid bones until several years after birth (Walsh & Vehse, 2010).

b. Until the age of 6 months, infants are obligatory nose breathers because the elongated epiglottis, positioned high in the pharynx, almost meets the soft palate. However, they are still able to mouth breathe because blocked nares do not lead to complete upper airway obstruction. By the sixth month, growth and descent of the larynx reduce the amount of obstruction. Nasal breathing doubles the resistance to airflow and proportionately increases the work of breathing (WOB; Walsh & Vehse, 2010).

2. *Pharynx*

a. *Embryology.* The oropharyngeal membrane between the foregut and the stomodeum begins

TABLE 2.1 Anatomic Differences Between Pediatric and Adult Airways

Pediatric Anatomic Difference	Clinical Significance
Proportionally larger head	Increases neck flexion and obstruction
Smaller nostrils	Increases airway resistance
Larger tongue	Increases airway resistance
Decreased muscle tone	Increases airway obstruction
Longer and more horizontal epiglottis	Increases airway obstruction
More anterior larynx	Difficult to perform blind intubation
Cricoid ring is the narrowest portion	Inflated cuffed tubes not recommended for routine intubation in children younger than 8 years of age
Shorter trachea	Increases risk of right main stem intubation
Narrower airways	Increases airway resistance

to disintegrate to establish continuity between the oral cavity and the pharynx in the 4-week-old embryo (Walsh & Vehse, 2010).

b. The *pharynx* is a musculomembranous tube that extends from the base of the skull to the esophageal and laryngeal inlets. The pharynx is the conduit for inhalation and exhalation and is vital to the production of speech. The *nasopharynx* is located above the soft palate. The *oropharynx* extends from the soft palate to the level of the hyoid bone. The *hypopharynx* extends from the level of the hyoid bone to the esophageal inlet (Walsh & Vehse, 2010).

3. *Larynx*

a. *Embryology.* During the fourth week of embryologic life, the laryngotracheal groove begins as a ridge on the ventral portion of the pharynx. Vocal cords begin to appear in the eighth week. In the newborn infant, the larynx is approximately at the level of the second cervical vertebra. In the adult, the larynx is opposite the fifth and sixth cervical vertebrae (Walsh & Vehse, 2010).

b. The *larynx* is a funnel-shaped structure that connects the pharynx and trachea. It includes the thyroid cartilage, vocal cords, epiglottis, and the cricoid cartilage. It is important in the production of the cough and protects the airway from aspiration of food during deglutition (Walsh & Vehse, 2010).

c. Compared with the adult epiglottis, the child's *epiglottis* is longer and more flaccid. The epiglottis in a newborn extends over the larynx at approximately a 45-degree angle. This more anterior and cephalad epiglottis may make intubation of the airway more difficult in the small infant (Walsh & Vehse, 2010).

d. The *cricoid cartilage ring* is the only point in the larynx in which the walls are completely enclosed in a circumferential ring of cartilage. In the rest of the trachea, the incomplete C-shaped cartilaginous rings are located anteriorly and laterally and the posterior wall is membranous. Resistance to airflow is inversely proportional to the fourth power of the radius. Thus, swelling from trauma or infection can produce large increases in airway resistance (Walsh & Vehse, 2010).

e. *Vocal cords* must abduct to allow inhalation and exhalation and adduct to prevent aspiration (Walsh & Vehse, 2010).

4. *Trachea*

a. *Embryology.* The trachea begins to develop in the 24-day-old embryo. At 26 to 28 days, a series

of asymmetric branchings of the primitive lung bud initiate the development of the bronchial tree (Walsh & Vehse, 2010).

b. The *trachea* is a thin-walled rigid tube flattened posteriorly that is characterized by a framework of 16 to 20 cartilages that encircle the trachea, except in its posterior aspect, which is membranous and contains smooth muscle.

c. The trachea's nervous, vascular, and lymphatic supplies are independent of those in the lungs.

D. Lower Airway Development (Figures 2.2 and 2.3)

1. *Lung*

a. At birth, the lungs weigh about 40 g and double in weight by 6 months. By age 2 years, they weigh about 170 g. Normal adult lungs weigh approximately 1,000 g.

b. The right lung has three lobes, and the left has two lobes separated by divisions called *fissures*, each further subdivided into bronchopulmonary segments. The surface of the lung is covered with the visceral pleura.

2. *Conducting Zone*

a. *Intrapulmonary airways* are divided into three major groups: cartilaginous bronchi, membranous bronchioles, and gas exchange units.

    i. *Cartilaginous bronchi* are the large airways that include nine to 12 divisions terminating in bronchi having a diameter of approximately 1 mm.

    ii. *Membranous bronchioles* comprise an additional 12 divisions before ending as

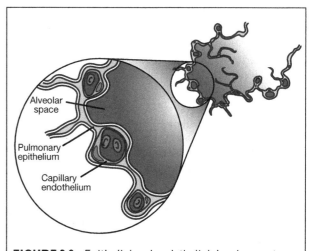

Alveolar space

Pulmonary epithelium

Capillary endothelium

FIGURE 2.2 Epithelial and endothelial development.

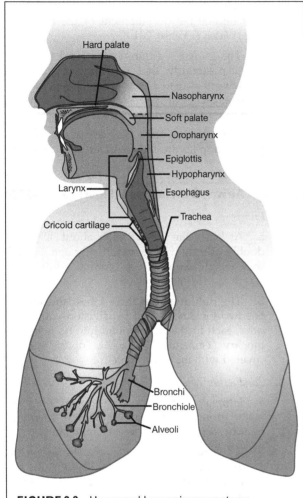

FIGURE 2.3 Upper and lower airway anatomy.

terminal bronchioles, the last conducting structure in the lung.

b. The airways are lined with an epithelial membrane, which gradually changes from ciliated pseudostratified columnar epithelium in the bronchi to a ciliated cuboidal epithelium near the gas exchange units.

c. In the largest airways, a smooth muscle bundle connects the two ends of the C-shaped cartilage. As the amount of cartilage decreases, the smooth muscle assumes a helical orientation and gradually becomes thinner.

3. *Gas Exchange Units (Alveoli)*

a. *Alveoli* are complex networks in which gas exchange takes place. Alveoli are lined with two epithelial cell types. Type I cells cover about 90% of the total alveolar surface. These cells are adapted to allow for the rapid exchange of gases.

Type II cells constitute the other 10% and secrete surfactant material that lowers surface tension and maintains the patency of alveoli during respiration. *Alveoli patency* refers to the alveoli's ability to maintain a spherical shape, preventing collapse, which is necessary for efficient gas exchange.

b. Two types of *intercommunicating channels* provide collateral ventilation for the gas exchange units. *Alveolar pores of Kohn* are holes in the alveolar wall that provide channels for gas movement between alveoli. These pores are not present until 6 to 8 years of age. While the pores of Kohn connect alveoli to adjacent alveoli, the canals of Lambert are accessory channels in the lungs connecting some terminal bronchioles to adjacent alveoli.

c. *Gas exchange* involves the movement of gas between the atmosphere and the alveoli and the pulmonary capillary blood. This movement occurs via simple passive diffusion whereby the gases travel from an area of high pressure to an area of low partial pressure.

E. Thoracic Cavity

1. *Diaphragm*

a. The diaphragm is the principal muscle of inspiration. If the chest wall is stiff, contraction of the diaphragm during inspiration decreases the pressure within the thoracic cavity and increases thoracic volume. This negative intrathoracic pressure in the chest cavity is discussed in detail later in this chapter. The diaphragm is innervated by the phrenic nerve (third, fourth, and fifth cervical spinal nerves).

b. The diaphragm sits more horizontally in the infant than in the older child or adult.

2. *The Chest Wall.* The infant's chest wall is very compliant compared with the rigid chest wall of the older child and adult. In the presence of lung disease, contraction of the diaphragm results in intercostal and sternal retractions rather than in inflation of the lungs. These retractions occur because the intercostal muscles are not strong enough to stabilize the chest against the stronger diaphragm contraction.

F. Pulmonary Circulation

The development of pulmonary circulation closely follows the development of the airways and alveoli.

1. *Embryology.* Preacinar arteries, which branch along the airways, develop in utero. Muscular arteries end at the level of the terminal bronchiole in the fetus and newborn but gradually extend to the alveolar level during childhood. Prematurely born infants have less well-developed vascular smooth muscle.

2. *Pulmonary Blood Volume.* The lungs receive the entire cardiac output from the right ventricle (RV) if no intracardiac right-to-left shunts are present.

3. *Pulmonary Lymphatics.* The lymphatic system is composed of a superficial network found in the pleura and the deep network around the bronchi and pulmonary arteries and veins. An increase in the hydrostatic pressure of the pulmonary and systemic circulation can result in effusions by decreasing the rate of pleural fluid absorption. Lymphatics may be disrupted by thoracic surgery or trauma, leading to lymphatic effusions.

DEVELOPMENTAL PHYSIOLOGY OF THE PULMONARY SYSTEM

A. Physiologic Function

The primary function of the lung is gas exchange. Its prime function is to allow oxygen to move from the air into the venous blood and for carbon dioxide to move out. Other functions include metabolizing certain compounds, filtering the blood, and acting as a reservoir for blood. During inspiration, the diaphragm contracts, the chest wall expands, and the volume of the lungs increases. Gas flows from the atmosphere into the lungs and oxygen diffuses into the blood at the alveolar–capillary interface. During expiration, the diaphragm and the chest wall relax, thoracic volume decreases, intrathoracic pressure increases, and gas flows out of the lungs. This process is affected by pulmonary compliance and resistance and by pulmonary vascular pressures and resistance (West, 2012).

1. *Pulmonary Compliance and Resistance*

   a. *Compliance* (CL) is the measure of the distensibility of the lungs, influenced by surfactant and elasticity of lung tissue. The compliance of a lung depends on its size (Figure 2.4; West, 2012).

      i. Volume change is produced by a transpulmonary pressure change (CL = $\Delta V / \Delta P$). For example, if the volume change produced by a given pressure change is small, the lungs must be stiff or have decreased compliance (West, 2012).

      ii. Compliance of the infant chest wall (especially in premature infants) is considerably greater than that of the adult. There is less opposition to lung collapse. Compliance

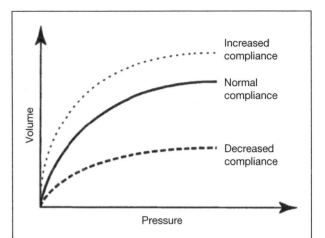

FIGURE 2.4 Compliance curve. Compliance reflects the amount of pressure required to deliver a given volume of air into an enclosed space such as the lung. Increased compliance of a lung unit indicates that less pressure is needed to distend the lung with a given volume. Decreased compliance indicates that more pressure is required to deliver the same volume of air.

is decreased by pulmonary edema, pneumothorax, pulmonary fibrosis, and atelectasis. Compliance is increased by asthma, lobar emphysema, and in the normal aging lung (West, 2012).

   b. *Airway resistance* is the driving pressure of air divided by the airflow rate determined by airway diameter. It is directly proportional to flow rate, the length of the airway, and the viscosity of the gas and is inversely proportional to the fourth power of the airway radius (Poiseuille's law; West, 2012).

      i. The upper airway contributes 70% of the total airway resistance in adults and 50% of total airway resistance in infants. In infants, the small peripheral airways may contribute as much as 50% of the total airway resistance compared with less than 20% airway resistance for the adult (West, 2012).

      ii. Resistance is increased by asthma, cystic fibrosis (CF), bronchopulmonary dysplasia (BPD), bronchiolitis, tracheal stenosis, and increased respiratory secretions. High resistance increases the WOB and creates respiratory distress.

2. *Pulmonary Vascular Pressures and Resistance*

   a. *Changes in pulmonary circulation at birth.* The fetus has low pulmonary blood flow related to high pulmonary vascular resistance (PVR).

This high PVR is due to hypoxic vasoconstriction, thicker pulmonary musculature, relatively low lung volumes, and smaller surface area. At birth, there is a decrease in PVR associated with ventilation and the effect of oxygen. This drop in PVR after birth increases blood flow to the lungs, thus facilitating the transition from fetal circulation. In the 6 to 8 weeks following birth, there is a further progressive fall in resistance associated with thinning of the smooth muscle layer (West, 2012).

b. *Intravascular pulmonary pressure* is measured by placing a catheter in the pulmonary artery and measuring systolic, diastolic, and mean arterial pressures (MAPs). The pressures in the pulmonary circulation are remarkably low. The mean pressure in the main pulmonary artery is about 15 mmHg; the systolic and diastolic pressures are about 25 and 8 mmHg, respectively (West, 2012).

c. *Ventilation–perfusion matching.* Regional differences in lung perfusion exist. Blood flow is lightest at the apex and increases at the base of the lung in an upright position (Figure 2.5; West, 2012).

  i. Zone I is located in the apexes of the lungs of an upright adult. Mean pulmonary arterial pressure is less than alveolar pressure (West, 2012).

  ii. Zone II is located in the midlung field. Here pulmonary artery pressure is greater than alveolar pressure, which is greater than pulmonary venous pressure (West, 2012).

  iii. Zone III is found in the base of the lung of an upright adult. Here the pulmonary artery and venous pressures are greater than alveolar pressure (West, 2012).

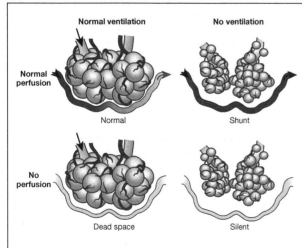

FIGURE 2.5 Ventilation–perfusion relationships.

d. *PVR* can be calculated by dividing the pressure across the lungs by the pulmonary blood flow. A decrease in resistance to blood flow can occur only through an increase in the blood vessels' diameters or an increase in the number of perfused vessels, that is, an increase in the cross-sectional diameter of the pulmonary vascular bed. An increase in cardiac output decreases the calculated PVR. The interrelationship between lung volume and PVR is complex and is influenced by pulmonary blood volume, cardiac output, and initial lung volume. Active changes in PVR can be mediated by neurogenic stimuli, vasoactive compounds, or chemical mediators (West, 2012). The pulmonary vascular resistance can be calculated as

$$\frac{80 \times (\text{mean pulmonary arterial pressure} - \text{mean pulmonary artery wedge pressure})}{\text{cardiac output}}$$

This equation is conceptually equivalent to the following:

$$R = \Delta P / Q$$

where R is the PVR, ΔP is the pressure difference across the pulmonary circuit, and Q is the rate of blood flow through it.

3. *Control of Breathing*

a. *Central respiratory centers.* The medullary respiratory center is essential for the generation of the respiratory rhythm. In addition, the medulla is associated with inspiration and expiration. The pons contains the apneustic center and pneumotaxic center responsible for "fine tuning" the respiratory rhythm.

b. *Cortex.* Within limits, the cortex can override the function of the brainstem.

c. *Other parts of the brain.* The limbic system and hypothalamus can alter the pattern of breathing during emotional states (including rage and fear).

d. *Peripheral neural reflexes.* Respiratory mechanoreceptors that can affect respiration are located within the upper airways, trachea, and lungs. Impulses are transmitted to the brainstem respiratory centers via the vagus nerve.

e. *Chemical control of respiration* (Figure 2.6)

  i. Central chemoreceptors: The central chemoreceptors are surrounded by brain extracellular fluid and respond to changes in its H^+ ion concentration. An increase in H^+ concentration stimulates ventilation, whereas a decrease inhibits it. The composition of the extracellular fluid around the receptors is governed by the cerebrospinal fluid (CSF), local

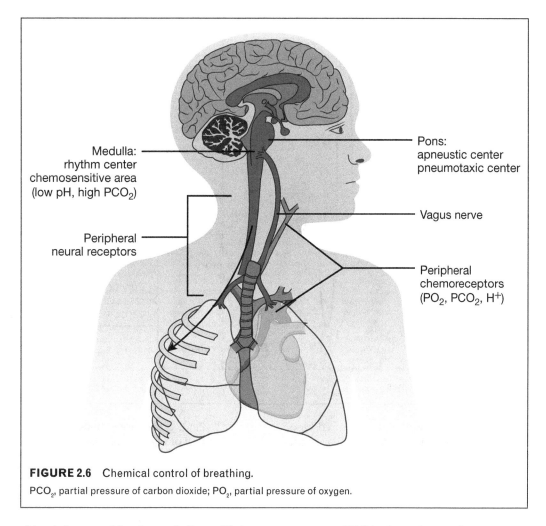

FIGURE 2.6 Chemical control of breathing.

PCO_2, partial pressure of carbon dioxide; PO_2, partial pressure of oxygen.

blood flow, and local metabolism. Of these, the CSF is the most important.

ii. Peripheral chemoreceptors: These are located in the carotid bodies at the bifurcation of the common carotid arteries and in the aortic bodies above and below the aortic arch. The carotid bodies are the most important in humans.

4. *Mechanics of Breathing.* Elastic properties of the lung come from the elastic tissue and collagen that support the lungs' internal structures. Lung compliance changes with age. The thorax of the infant is much more compliant than that of an adult.

5. *Lung Volumes* (Figure 2.7; West, 2012)

a. *Total lung capacity* is the total volume of the gas contained in the lung at maximum inspiration.

b. *Vital capacity* (VC) is the maximum volume expired from the total lung capacity with maximal expiration.

c. *FRC* is the volume of gas remaining in the lung after a normal expiration.

d. *Residual volume* is the volume of gas remaining in the lung following a maximal respiratory effort.

B. Gas Exchange and Transport

Respiratory gas exchange involves the movement of gas from the atmosphere to the alveoli to the pulmonary capillary blood. The alveolar capillary membrane permits the transfer of oxygen and carbon dioxide while restricting the movement of fluid from the pulmonary vasculature to the alveoli.

1. *Diffusion*

a. Oxygen diffuses from the alveolus through the alveolar epithelial lining, basement membrane, capillary endothelial lining, plasma, and red blood cell. Blood passing through the lung resides in a pulmonary capillary for only 0.75 second. Diffusion of oxygen depends on the difference (gradient) between alveolar and oxygen tension (West, 2012).

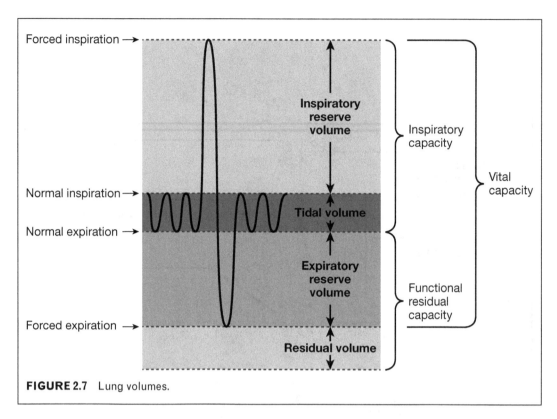

FIGURE 2.7 Lung volumes.

b. Carbon dioxide diffuses from the red blood cell to the plasma, through the capillary endothelial lining, basement membrane, and alveolar epithelial lining. The pulmonary capillary mean alveolar carbon dioxide gradient is smaller than that of oxygen (i.e., CO_2 diffuses more readily than O_2; West, 2012).

2. *Oxygen Transport*

a. Oxygen is carried in the blood in two forms: in combination with hemoglobin (Hgb) and dissolved in plasma. The arterial oxygen content (CaO_2) describes the total amount of oxygen carried by arterial blood. Parameters are defined and other oxygen values are calculated in a similar fashion as in Table 2.2. CaO_2 is represented in the following equation (West, 2013):

$$(\text{Hgb} \times 1.34 \times SaO_2) + (0.003 \times PaO_2)$$

b. *Oxyhemoglobin dissociation curve* (Figure 2.8)

   i. The oxyhemoglobin dissociation curve is an S-shaped curve with Hgb on the y-axis and PaO_2 on the x-axis. The release of oxygen to the tissues is directly related to Hgb concentration and the affinity of oxygen for Hgb. Thus, on the steep portion of the dissociation curve, relatively small changes in

PaO_2 cause large changes in oxygen saturation of Hgb (West, 2012).

   ii. A shift to the right, which facilitates the unloading of oxygen from Hgb, is caused by a decrease in pH, an increase in $PaCO_2$, elevated temperature, or an increase in 2,3-diphosphoglycerate (2,3-DPG). 2,3-DPG decreases the affinity of Hgb for oxygen. During hypoxia or anemia, oxygen availability is increased within a matter of hours by an increase in 2,3-DPG (West, 2012).

   iii. A shift to the left, which increases the binding of oxygen to Hgb, is caused by an increase in pH, a decrease in $PaCO_2$, a decrease in temperature, or a decrease in 2,3-DPG. Fetal Hgb has decreased 2,3-DPG, shifting the curve to the left of the adult Hgb curve. Thus, at a given PaO_2 and hematocrit, fetal Hgb is more readily saturated than adult blood is. Fetal Hgb also releases oxygen less readily to the tissues than adult Hgb. Fetal Hgb is replaced by adult Hgb within 4 to 6 weeks after birth (West, 2012).

3. *Cellular Respiration.* All cells depend on a continuous supply of oxygen to support aerobic metabolism. Oxygen delivery data do not provide information about the adequacy of tissue oxygenation. In septic

TABLE 2.2   Normal Oxygenation Profile Values

Parameter	Calculation	Norms
CaO_2	$CaO_2 = (Hgb \times 3.4 \times SaO_2) + (PaO_2 \times 0.003)$	20 mL/dL
CvO_2	$CvO_2 = (Hgb \times 3.4 \times SvO_2) + (PvO_2 \times 0.003)$	15 mL/dL
a-vDO_2	$CaO_2 = CvO_2$	3.5–5 mL/dL
DO_2	$DO_2 = CaO_2 \times CI \times 10$	620 ± 50 mL/min/m²
VO_2	$VO_2 = (CaO_2 - CvO_2) \times CI \times 10$	120–200 mL/min/m²
O_2ER	$(CaO_2 - CvO_2)/CaO_2 \times 100$	25% ± 2%
SvO_2		75% (60%–80%)

a-vDO_2, arteriovenous oxygen difference; CaO_2, arterial oxygen content; CI, cardiac index; CvO_2, venous oxygen content; DO_2, oxygen delivery; Hgb, hemoglobin; O_2ER, oxygen extraction ratio; PaO_2, arterial oxygen partial pressure; PvO_2, venous partial pressure of oxygen; SaO_2, arterial oxygen saturation; SvO_2, venous oxygen saturation; VO_2, oxygen consumption.

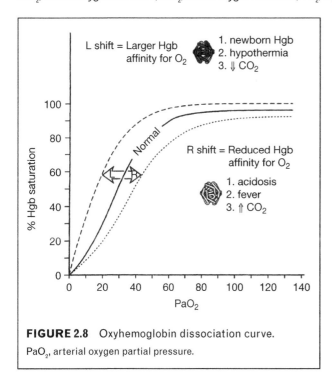

FIGURE 2.8   Oxyhemoglobin dissociation curve.

PaO_2, arterial oxygen partial pressure.

shock, tissue oxygen extraction is altered. To assess tissue oxygen extraction, a true mixed venous blood sample should be obtained from the pulmonary artery.

CLINICAL ASSESSMENT OF PULMONARY FUNCTION

A. History

1. *Prenatal and Delivery*

   a.   Birth weight

   b.   Gestational age

   c.   Apgar scores

   d.   Respiratory distress in the neonatal period, including oxygen requirements and ventilatory assistance

   e.   Length of hospital stay

2. *Childhood*

   a.   Verify immunization history and tuberculosis (TB) tests

   b.   Family history of asthma, allergies, eczema, respiratory illnesses

   c.   Episodes of wheezing with previous illness

   d.   Frequency of colds and upper respiratory tract infections

   e.   Has the child every been intubated

   f.   Environmental exposure to smoke, molds, or pets

   g.   Supervise child, especially younger than 5 years, to evaluate risk of foreign-body aspiration

   h.   Recent illnesses of child or family members

   i.   Recent emergency room visits and/or hospitalizations

   j.   Use of medications, medications to treat respiratory symptoms, and nonprescription and alternative medications

   k.   Recent international travel

3. *Other Significant Information*

   a.   Chest pain (rarely of cardiac origin) is described in quality, timing with respiratory phase, duration (continuous or intermittent), and precipitating factors.

b. *Growth and development.* Failure to gain weight is often the first sign of chronic pulmonary disease. Activity level or milestones may be delayed with chronic pulmonary dysfunction.

c. *Gastrointestinal (GI) symptoms*

    i. Pneumonic processes frequently manifest as generalized abdominal pain in young children.

    ii. Acute or chronic infection may cause anorexia and occasional vomiting.

    iii. Upper airway mucus may impede swallowing and cause gagging, vomiting, or diarrhea in infants and toddlers.

    iv. Bulky, foul-smelling stools may indicate CF.

    v. Gastroesophageal reflux may cause chronic pulmonary aspiration.

d. *Sleeping habits*

    i. Evaluate duration of sleep at night and causes of interruptions.

    ii. Nighttime coughing is a frequent symptom of asthma or other lower respiratory tract diseases.

    iii. Note positioning for sleep, such as head flat or requiring head elevation.

    iv. If a humidifier is used, note care and maintenance of the humidifier.

    v. Note signs of obstructive sleep apnea, such as sleeping propped up on pillows, apnea, orthopnea, and snoring.

B. Physical Examination

1. *Inspection*

Anatomic landmarks of the thorax provide a method for describing physical examination findings (Figure 2.9).

    a. *Thoracic inspection*

    i. Note thoracic contour: A neonate's chest is round with the anteroposterior diameter equal to the transverse diameter. Chest contour is more oval by 2 to 3 years of age. Disproportionate size may be detected by comparing head circumference (occipitofrontal circumference [OFC]) to chest circumference. From birth to 2 years, the head and chest circumferences are generally equal. During childhood, chest size

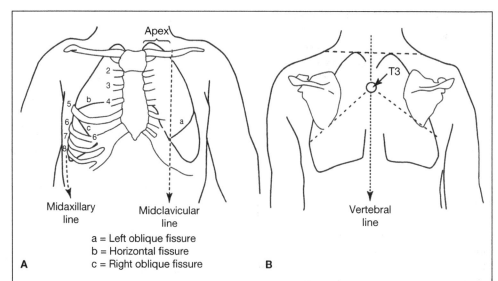

FIGURE 2.9 Anatomic landmarks of the thorax. The lower lobes of both lungs have only small projections on the anterior plane on the x-ray film and can be better visualized on a lateral or posterior x-ray film. The midaxillary line, midclavicular line, vertebral line, and intercostal spaces are frequently used landmarks in describing the location of pulmonary findings. (A) Anterior view: Left lung is divided into two lobes by the left oblique fissure. The right lung is divided into three lobes by the horizontal fissure with landmarks between the fourth rib medially and the fifth rib laterally. The right oblique fissure is found from the inferior margin (midclavicular line) to the fifth lateral rib. (B) Posterior view: Fissures dividing upper and lower lobes begin at T3, medially, extending in a line inferiorly below the inferior tips of the scapula.

is 5 to 7 cm greater than the OFC. Chronic disease may cause enlarged anteroposterior diameter or "barreled chest" which is similar to the neonate's chest contour (Figure 2.10).

ii. Note any skeletal deformities: Anomalies, such as sternal depression (pectus excavatum) or protrusion (pectus carinatum), may cause or be associated with respiratory abnormalities by altering pulmonary mechanics. Inspect posterior thoracic structures and the spine. Kyphosis and scoliosis can impair pulmonary mechanics.

iii. Note symmetry of excursion (depth of respiration).

b. *Respiratory effort*

i. Rate and rhythm are age related: Respiratory rate is about one fourth of the pulse rate in the normal infant at rest.

ii. Evaluate the adequacy of thoracic excursion.

iii. Note the effort of breathing: Infants and young children breathe principally with the diaphragm because of immature intercostal muscles. Infants in respiratory distress may exhibit nasal flaring, head bobbing, expiratory grunting, or head extension.

iv. Note the use of accessory muscles: Signs of respiratory insufficiency include suprasternal, substernal, intercostal, and subcostal retractions.

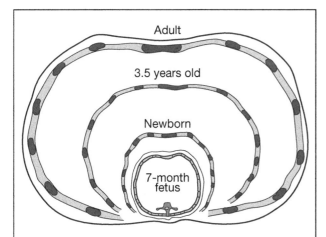

FIGURE 2.10 Thoracic contours by age. Illustrates the comparison of the anteroposterior diameter and contour of the chest wall according to age.

v. Variations in respiratory patterns are also observed with various neurologic abnormalities (Figure 2.11).

vi. *Note the quality of the voice and breathing;* pay particular attention to a muffled voice; stridor; expiratory/inspiratory wheezing; and a barky, loose, congested, or paroxysmal cough.

c. *Skin color and appearance*

i. Cyanosis is observed when 3 to 5 g of Hgb becomes desaturated. Conditions that can mask or mimic cyanosis include hypothermia, anemia, or polycythemia. If cyanosis persists with oxygen administration, this may indicate the presence of an intracardiac shunt.

ii. Clubbing of fingertips is an indication of chronic hypoxia. The distal phalanx is flat and broad, causing a "club" appearance.

iii. Cyanosis is not related to increased $PaCO_2$ (hypercarbia). A patient may be well oxygenated with a supplemental flow of oxygen diffusing through the airway but still be significantly hypercarbic and without a cyanotic appearance.

2. *Palpation*

a. This is a limited technique in infants, but can be useful in older children.

b. Expand the hands bilaterally and symmetrically across the anterior chest wall and then across the posterior chest wall to evaluate the following:

i. What is the expansion of the thoracic cage?

ii. Fremitus is conduction of the child's voice while the child says, for example, "99." Vibrations should be noted at the trachea and upper airway. Decreased sensation is normally observed centrally near large airways, otherwise it is associated with occlusions. Increased sensation is associated with solid masses (consolidations). In infants, palpation during crying allows a similar evaluation.

c. Palpation of fine vibrations may indicate underlying pleural friction rub.

d. Palpate the entire thoracic cage for crepitus, a coarse, crackly feeling (and sound) of air in the subcutaneous tissue.

e. With a history of trauma, evaluate the skeletal structure, especially the clavicles.

f. Palpate the tracheal position (midline); if it is shifted, locate the position of maximal impulse

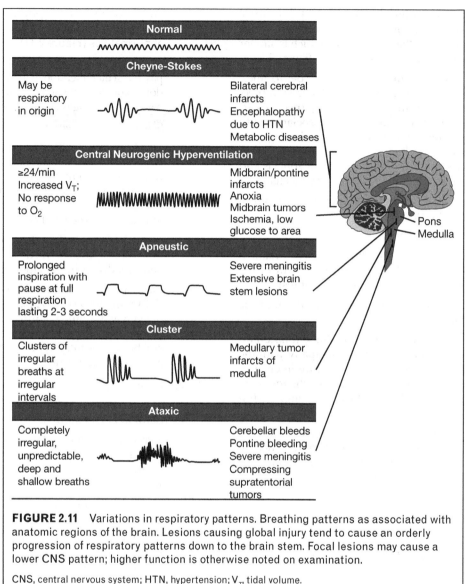

FIGURE 2.11 Variations in respiratory patterns. Breathing patterns as associated with anatomic regions of the brain. Lesions causing global injury tend to cause an orderly progression of respiratory patterns down to the brain stem. Focal lesions may cause a lower CNS pattern; higher function is otherwise noted on examination.

CNS, central nervous system; HTN, hypertension; V_T, tidal volume.

of the heart. A shift in either or both may indicate fluid or air collection or a collapsed lung.

3. *Percussion*

a. Technique used to determine the presence of air, fluid, or masses in the underlying lung and to determine anatomic landmarks (such as the upper margin of the liver; Figure 2.12).

b. Percuss using the middle finger of one hand flush against the chest wall in interspaces, noting the quality of sound produced by striking this finger with the middle finger of the other hand.

i. Right side of the anterior chest: Percussion sounds should be resonant in each intercostal space down to the fifth to sixth intercostal space, where the superior liver margin begins. There the sound changes and has a dull quality. Farther down where the lung field ends and the liver border continues, the percussion note goes flat.

ii. Left side of the anterior chest: Percussion of the heart borders can be determined. The superior border is often percussed between the second and third intercostal spaces. The inferior border is at the fourth to sixth intercostal spaces, and the left border is just lateral to the midclavicular line. At the sixth intercostal space and below, tympany may be observed because of an air-filled stomach.

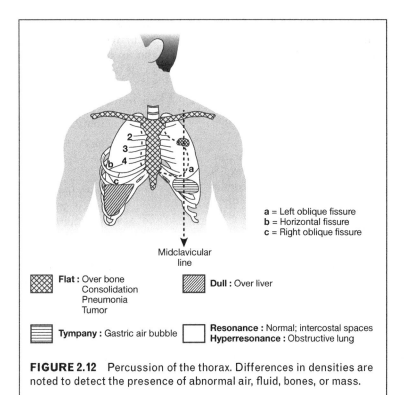

a = Left oblique fissure
b = Horizontal fissure
c = Right oblique fissure

Midclavicular line

Flat : Over bone
Consolidation
Pneumonia
Tumor

Dull : Over liver

Tympany : Gastric air bubble

Resonance : Normal; intercostal spaces
Hyperresonance : Obstructive lung

FIGURE 2.12 Percussion of the thorax. Differences in densities are noted to detect the presence of abnormal air, fluid, bones, or mass.

iii. Posterior chest: Percuss side to side to identify abnormal densities.

c. *Variations in sounds* define the density of structures:

i. Flat: Short, soft; heard over bone

ii. Dull: Medium pitch; duration heard over the liver, spleen, and mass densities

iii. Resonance: Low, loud, and long; heard over an air-filled lung

iv. Hyperresonance: Deep pitched, loud, and prolonged; heard over an overinflated lung or air collections such as pneumothorax

v. Tympany: High, musical quality, loud; heard over gas-filled organs such as the stomach

4. *Auscultation*

a. Evaluate the pitch, intensity, quality, and duration of each phase using the diaphragm of the stethoscope. For small infants, using either a small diaphragm or the bell of a stethoscope may enable localization of sounds.

b. Compare side to side, starting at the apex and proceeding methodically to the bases. The thin-walled chests of infants create transmitted breath sounds throughout the lung fields. Listen for discreet changes from one location to the next. For emergent situations, a quick check under each axilla (rather than the upper lobes of the lungs) allows gross determination of the presence of bilateral aeration.

c. Quality of pitch. *Vesicular breath sounds* (inspiratory [I] >expiratory [E]) are of long inspiration, low pitch, and soft intensity and are heard over most of the lungs. *Bronchial breath sounds* (I <E) have an equal or longer expiratory phase; are high pitched, loud, and blowing; and are heard over the large airways. Bronchial breath sounds are abnormal when heard over the peripheral lung tissue. Bronchovesicular breath sounds (I = E) are high-pitched tubular sounds.

d. Adventitious sounds are abnormal sounds superimposed on normal breath sounds. Abnormal sounds have classically been defined as rales, rhonchi, and wheezes. However, confusion over definitions has prompted a focus on describing the *quality* and *location* of these sounds to associate them with common causes. Attention should be given to pitch, timing (I or E), location, and whether they clear with cough.

e. Fine, high-pitched crackling noises (similar to the sound of rolling hair between fingers) may be heard at end inspiration over peripheral lung fields in pneumonia and pulmonary edema. Medium-pitched crackles are heard in early to midinspiration with pulmonary edema and diffuse secretions in the bronchioles. These may partially clear with coughing. Upper airway secretions may cause coarse, bubbling (rhonchi) sounds that clear with cough.

f. Inflamed pleural surfaces may result in a very fine, low-pitched crackle over the focal areas of the chest during both I and E phases. With cessation of breathing, the crackles are not heard.

g. Wheezing results from narrowed airway lumina. Inspiratory wheezing usually results from high obstruction, such as laryngeal edema or foreign bodies. Expiratory wheezing often results from lower obstruction, such as with bronchiolitis, severe asthma, or chronic obstructive lung disease.

h. Diminished or absent breath sounds are noted as the focal absence of sounds with occasional crackling, or as an abnormal quality or abnormal location of normal sounds. This may occur with severe asthma, atelectasis, pneumothorax, or pleural fluid accumulation. This finding is usually an ominous sign.

C. Abnormal Physical Examination Findings

1. *Stridor* (Table 2.3)

a. *Description*. Stridor is noisy breathing caused by increased turbulence of airflow through a lumen.

i. Inspiratory stridor is related to the inward collapse of structures during inspiration. It is most common with supraglottic or glottic lesions because of the negative pressure generated during inspiration. Inspiratory stridor is common in laryngotracheomalacia and viral croup. Postextubation endotracheal tube (ETT) trauma is another possible source of stridor.

TABLE 2.3 Evaluation of Stridor

Description of Stridor	Supraglottic	Subglottic	Tracheal
Phase of respiration	Inspiratory	Inspiratory or biphasic	Expiratory
Phonation	Muffled	Weak or breathy	Absent or high pitched
Pitch of stridor	Coarse, low pitch	High-pitched, barking, or rough cough	
Etiology of Stridor		**Differential Diagnosis for Upper Airway Stridor**	
Intrinsic lesions		Subglottic stenosis Web laryngocele Tumors such as papillomas Laryngomalacia Tracheomalacia Tracheoesophageal fistula	
Extrinsic lesions		Vascular ring Cyst hygroma Neurologic lesions such as lymphomas	
Infections		Epiglottitis Laryngotracheobronchitis Peritonsillar abscess Bacterial tracheitis Infectious mononucleosis	
Other		Craniofacial abnormalities Trauma Foreign body aspiration Hypertrophic tonsils or adenoids Allergic reactions Corrosive ingestions	

ii. Expiratory stridor is most commonly observed with subglottic lesions.

iii. Fixed lesions (e.g., subglottic stenosis) may cause both inspiratory and expiratory stridor.

b. Evaluation of the child with stridor includes checking nasal patency, the size of tongue and mandible, the quantity of oropharyngeal secretions, the presence of drooling, the quality of phonation, head and neck range of motion, evidence of tooth evulsion or oral trauma, presence of fever or infectious symptoms, neurologic status, and the rate of progression of symptoms.

i. Note the position of preference. Infants with laryngomalacia, micrognathia, or macroglossia often have less distress when placed in a prone position. Children with epiglottitis or croup (laryngotracheobronchitis) often position themselves upright; children with moderate obstruction may exhibit forward extension of the head.

2. *Cyanosis*

a. *Description.* Central or peripheral blue discoloration of skin tissue caused by desaturated Hgb. Cyanosis is usually not appreciated until 3 to 5 g Hgb per deciliter of serum is desaturated, corresponding to an SaO_2 of 80% to 85% in a normal child. Cyanosis is *not* caused by an elevated $PaCO_2$. Cyanosis can be caused by other nonpulmonary conditions (Figure 2.13).

b. Cyanosis may be masked by anemia, causing a more pallid color; or polycythemia, which may create a more "ruddy" color.

c. *Evaluation of the cyanotic child*

i. Oxygen should be administered before proceeding with the evaluation. Note the response to oxygen and the general degree of distress. If distress is moderate or severe, emergency management should be given before proceeding with further evaluation.

ii. Note whether cyanosis is peripheral (nail beds), central (lip and tongue color), or both.

iii. Assess pulmonary function to identify upper or lower airway causes, including the presence or absence of stridor, phonation, use of accessory muscles, and general state of alertness and activity level.

iv. Obtain historical information such as the evolution of the cyanosis (sudden or gradual onset) and associated factors such as illness or decreased environmental temperature.

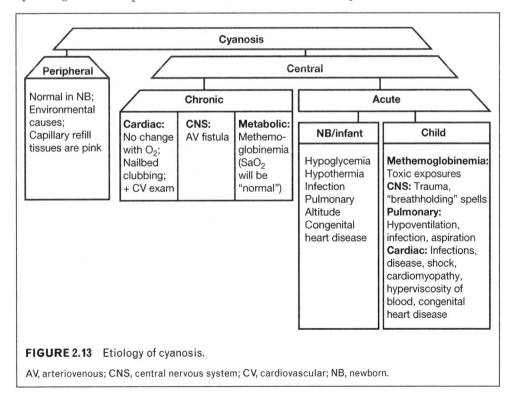

FIGURE 2.13 Etiology of cyanosis.

AV, arteriovenous; CNS, central nervous system; CV, cardiovascular; NB, newborn.

3. *Cough*

a. *Description.* A cough is an attempt to clear the airway of particulate matter or may result from general tissue irritation. It is produced by a reflex response in cough receptors, found in ciliated epithelium, or it may be initiated in higher cortical centers.

b. *Evaluation*

i. Many causes of cough are age specific (Table 2.4).

ii. Note historical information such as the presence or absence of infectious disease or exposures.

iii. Characteristics of the cough may suggest the cause:

1) Loose and productive. CF, bronchiectasis, asthma

2) Croupy. Viral laryngotracheobronchitis

3) Paroxysmal. Pertussis, mycoplasma, foreign body, chlamydia

4) Brassy. Tracheitis, upper airway drainage, psychogenic

5) Nocturnal. Asthma, sinusitis, gastroesophageal reflux, upper respiratory tract disease

6) During exercise. Asthma, CF, bronchiectasis

7) Loud honking that disappears with sleep: Psychogenic

iv. Other associated symptoms. Examine sputum samples for white blood cells (WBCs) or eosinophils. Note hemoptysis. Poor weight gain, steatorrhea, and cough are strongly suggestive of CF.

v. A cough that persists longer than 2 weeks or a cough that causes immediate respiratory distress warrants investigation.

INVASIVE AND NONINVASIVE DIAGNOSTIC STUDIES

A. Diagnostic Approach

1. *Individualization of Evaluation.* All sick children are at higher risk for respiratory insufficiency or failure than adults because of the age-related anatomic differences described previously. Monitoring of pulmonary function can be individualized according to the acuity of illness and the age of the child. For a patient with the lowest acuity, clinical examination and serial observations are adequate, but with increasing severity of illness, other monitoring devices should be used. The options for monitoring include continuous observation and clinical examination, oxygen monitoring, CO_2 monitoring, monitoring of pulmonary function, and laboratory and roentgenographic studies.

2. *Immediate Assessment and Care.* A brief estimation of the severity of distress should be made to determine whether oxygen or airway assistance is needed.

B. Baseline Respiratory Monitoring

1. *Physical Examination.* All children suspected of having respiratory distress should have their clothing removed for maximum observation, ensuring that ambient temperature is controlled. Refer to the clinical assessment section in this chapter for details on physical examination techniques. A quick-look observation should be done with all patients for early recognition of respiratory distress requiring emergency management. This 20-second appraisal should include level of consciousness, color, and respiratory effort.

2. *Diagnostic Studies for Children in Respiratory Distress From Any Cause*

a. Complete history and physical examination

b. Chest x-ray examination

TABLE 2.4 Common Causes of Cough by Age Groups

Neonates	Infections Chlamydia Viral: cytomegalovirus, rubella, pertussis Congenital malformations TEF Vascular rings Airway malformations
Infants	Causes mentioned for neonates plus Viral bronchiolitis Diffuse interstitial pneumonia Gastroesophageal reflux CF
Preschoolers	Infections in suppurative disease (e.g., CF) Viral infections with or without reactive airway disease Foreign body aspiration Environmental pollutants Gastroesophageal reflux Reactive airway disease
School age/adolescents	Reactive airway disease *Mycoplasma pneumoniae* infection CF Cigarette smoking Psychogenic cough tic Pulmonary hemosiderosis

CF, cystic fibrosis; TEF, tracheoesophageal fistula.

c. Sinus x-ray examinations (depending on age)

d. Simple oxygen saturation monitoring

e. Nasal cannula end-tidal CO_2 monitoring

f. Complete blood count (CBC)

g. Tuberculin skin test (TST)

h. Nasopharyngeal swab for respiratory syncytial virus (RSV) and viral panel and pertussis, if applicable

i. Diagnostic studies to consider for children in respiratory distress according to symptoms:

    i. Bronchoscopy with alveolar lavage (BAL)

    ii. Laboratory testing as indicated

    iii. pH probe testing for suspected gastroesophageal reflux disease (GERD)

    iv. Pulmonary function testing (PFT)

C. Laboratory Studies (Table 2.5)

D. Blood Gas Analysis

1. Arterial, venous, or capillary blood gas (CBG) analysis can assist in the respiratory assessment (Table 2.6). Typically, interpretation of blood gas values involves acid–base interpretation to evaluate the pH and PCO_2 values and evaluation of oxygenation, or PO_2, separately. An arterial blood gas (ABG) analysis is the traditional method of estimating the systemic carbon dioxide tension and pH, usually for the purpose of assessing ventilation and/or acid–base status. However, an ABG analysis requires a sample of arterial blood, which can be difficult to obtain. A venous blood gas (VBG) analysis is an alternative method of estimating systemic carbon dioxide and pH that does not require arterial blood sampling. A VBG analysis can be performed using a peripheral venous sample (obtained by venipuncture), central venous sample (obtained from a central venous catheter), or mixed venous sample (obtained from the distal port of a pulmonary artery catheter). CBG samples may be used in place of samples from arterial punctures or indwelling arterial catheters to estimate acid–base balance (pH) and adequacy of ventilation ($PaCO_2$). Capillary PO_2 measurements are of little value in estimating arterial oxygenation.

2. $PaCO_2$ directly reflects the adequacy of alveolar ventilation (V_A). Hypercarbia is $PaCO_2$ greater than 55 mmHg.

3. Oxygenation is evaluated using the PaO_2 value. Hypoxemia is an arterial PaO_2 less than 60 mmHg.

TABLE 2.5 Summary of Diagnostic Laboratory Evaluation of Pulmonary Function

Test	Significant Associations With Altered Levels
Immunoglobulins	
Norms are age-related assays.	Decreased levels of any immunoglobulin are usually associated with congenital deficiencies and patterns of infections beginning early in life. Altered levels are associated with specific causes as follows
IgA: Deficiency is associated with an increased incidence of mucosal bacterial infections	
IgG: Found in blood, lymph, CSF, pleural fluid, peritoneal fluid, and breast milk; slow response (appears 1 wk after stimulus)	Myeloma Bacterial infections Collagen disorders
IgM: Intravascular; predominant first response to bacterial or viral infection; activates the complement system	Appears early in infectious course but may persist with chronic infection
IgD: Predominant activity on the surface of B cells (involving antibody formation)	Increased with chronic infections
IgE: Found in the serum and triggers release of histamine	Increased with allogenic stimulation (e.g., asthma, associated with allergenic stimulus)

(continued)

TABLE 2.5 Summary of Diagnostic Laboratory Evaluation of Pulmonary Function *(continued)*

Test	Significant Associations With Altered Levels
Differential WBC Count	
Total WBC <1 y: maximum = 20,000 1–12 y: maximum = 15,000	Infections may cause an elevated or remarkably low (<4,000/mm³) WBC count
Segmented neutrophils (PMNs) <12 y = 25%–40% ≥12 y = >50%	
Band neutrophils <10%	Increase in bands associated with bacterial infections
Lymphocytes <12 y = >50% ≥12 y = <40%	Increased with specific infections such as pertussis, Epstein–Barr virus, hepatitis
Monocytes 4%–6% Eosinophils 2%–3% Basophils 0.5%	
Pilocarpine Lontophoresis (Sweat Chloride Test)	

Sodium <70 mEq/L
   Chloride <60 mEq/L
   Potassium <60 mEq/L
	Higher levels suggest CF

Sputum or Tracheal Aspirate Cultures	
Normally should have few if any PMNs and mixed flora	PMNs: 3–4+ with dominant organism is more likely to be valid indicator of infection than one with <2+ PMNs and multiple organisms
Deep tracheal secretions preferred; protected brush specimen technique	
Evaluate Gram stain for presence of PMNs	
Endotracheal tubes and tracheostomy tubes become quickly colonized with existing flora, which may be misleading if microbiology results are interpreted independent of other clinical indicators	

CF, cystic fibrosis; CSF, cerebrospinal fluid; IgA, immunoglobulin A; IgD, immunoglobulin D; IgE, immunoglobulin E; IgG, immunoglobulin G; IgM, immunoglobulin M; PMNs, polymorphonuclear neutrophils; WBC, white blood cell.

TABLE 2.6 Normal Blood Gas Values

Parameter	Arterial	Mixed Venous	Capillary
pH	7.35–7.45	7.31–7.41	7.35–7.45
PO_2	80–100 mmHg	35–40 mmHg	Less than arterial[a]
O_2 saturation	95%–97%	70%–75%	Less than arterial
PCO_2	35–45 mmHg	40–50 mmHg	35–45 mmHg
HCO_3	22–26 mEq/L	22–26 mEq/L	22–26 mEq/L
Total CO_2 content	20–27 mEq/L	20–27 mEq/L	20–27 mEq/L
Base excess	+2 to −2	+2 to −2	+2 to −2

PO_2, partial pressure of oxygen.

[a]Capillary PO_2 is approximately 10 mmHg less than arterial PO_2 except when decreased tissue perfusion is present, that is, during cardiovascular collapse or hypothermia. In these states, capillary samples will not accurately reflect arterial PO_2.

4. Acid–base balance is indicated by the pH. Acidosis is an arterial pH less than 7.35, and alkalosis is an arterial pH greater than 7.45.

E. Radiologic Procedures for Pulmonary Evaluation

A variety of imaging techniques allow visualization of anatomy, motion dynamics, and identification of abnormalities. Frequently, a patient may require more than one imaging procedure to detail a specific anatomic site.

1. *Chest roentgenography* permits visualization of lung parenchyma (tissue), pulmonary vascular markings, heart silhouette, and bone densities.

2. *Fluoroscopy* provides evaluation of thoracic motion, particularly diaphragm movement, which is essential to the infant, and is especially useful in the evaluation of a paralyzed diaphragm.

3. *CT scan* is the visualization of very thin slices of tissue in a predetermined plane of dimension, enabling identification of masses, fluid accumulation, and anatomic definition. A spiral CT may provide better definition. A spiral CT is especially useful in the evaluation of a pulmonary embolus.

4. *MRI* uses an external magnetic field around the patient to cause rotation of cell nuclei. Imaging provides well-defined visualization of soft tissues. No radiation is involved in this procedure.

5. *Ventilation–perfusion scan (V/Q scan)* is obtained by injecting a radioisotope into a peripheral vein and imaging its flow through the pulmonary vessels. The V/Q scan is made following the inhalation of a radioactive gas, which distributes to aerated alveoli. Comparison between *ventilated* areas with *perfused* areas of the lung can be made, looking for "matched" segments. Although many disorders may cause a ventilation–perfusion mismatch, a complete segmental mismatch is a useful clue to the diagnosis of pulmonary embolism (PE).

6. *Pulmonary angiography* involves the introduction of a catheter into a peripheral vein; the catheter is guided to the right side of the heart and to the pulmonary artery trunk. Injection of contrast media with serial radiographic examinations of the pulmonary vascular bed allows definitive recognition of vascular obstruction.

7. *Echocardiography* utilizes ultrasound waves to detect the structures and function of the heart and its surrounding vasculature. This method serves as a standard noninvasive diagnostic screening tool for pulmonary hypertension (PH). Abnormal findings obtained through this exam may be confirmed via a more invasive heart catheterization.

RESPIRATORY MONITORING

A. Oxygen Monitoring

1. *Pulse Oximetry*

  a. *Principles of operation.* The device consists of a probe that contains an infrared light source and a photodetector. Both are housed in a wraparound strip so that the light source is aligned to emit light through tissue (such as a nail bed) to the photodetector. Saturated Hgb absorbs little light, whereas desaturated Hgb absorbs a large amount of light. The photodetector measures the amount of light that crosses the tissue and with a microprocessor computes the percentage of saturated Hgb.

  b. *Uses.* The pulse oximeter requires pulsatile tissue to provide accurate measurements. Fingers, palmar wrap (in small infants), toes, and ear clips are used. The microprocessor unit measures pulse rate and most units have a mechanism to provide a "poor signal" alert or perfusion indicator if the tissue has an inadequate pulse. It provides a stable, accurate measurement over a wide variety of physiologic conditions.

  c. *Limitations*

    i. Poor perfusion (low cardiac output states) may interfere with a stable signal.

    ii. A major source of error in children is motion artifact, which causes poor tracking of the pulse. New oximeters feature an algorithm to identify both motion artifact and poor perfusion (Fouzas, Prifitis, & Anthracopoulos, 2011).

    iii. With elevated carboxyhemoglobin or methemoglobin levels, the true oxygenated Hgb values are inflated because the pulse oximeter does not distinguish between Hgb saturated with oxygen and other bound molecules.

    iv. When retinopathy is a concern in the neonatal population, SaO_2 may not provide any margin of safety because the PaO_2 can vary widely when oxygen saturations are greater than 90% as the result of factors that alter the oxygen dissociation curve.

    v. Newborns and children with uncorrected congenital heart disease may have variance in measurements depending on the placement of the oximeter. In cardiac lesions with right-to-left shunting, the right hand or foot is used for preductal measurement and the left hand or foot is used for postductal measurement.

2. *Transcutaneous Oxygen Monitoring*

 a. *Principles of operation.* A small, heated probe is placed on the skin surface. Localized heating increases capillary blood flow to the site. Oxygen diffuses across the skin and is measured by a thermistor in the probe.

 b. *Uses.* Transcutaneous oxygen monitoring ($PtcO_2$) functions well in infants and has shown good correlation with PaO_2 measurements. It can reduce the quantity of invasive blood gas measurements and provide continuous data for patients who are either being weaned or are otherwise labile. In the past, $PtcO_2$ demonstrated utility in detecting hyperoxia in neonates; however, this has been demonstrated to be more readily monitored through maintaining SpO_2 between 85% and 93% (Kacmarek, Stoller, Chatburn, & Kallet, 2017).

 c. *Limitations.* With increasing skin thickness, the accuracy of measurements diminishes. Poor perfusion and local skin hypoxia can interfere with measurements. The probe requires site change every 4 to 6 hours with a 10- to 15-minute warm-up time (and a blood gas analysis to verify measurement accuracy). Note that the heated probe may cause blisters in some infants.

3. *Mixed Venous Oxygen Saturation Monitoring*

 a. On occasion, pediatric patients are monitored with pulmonary artery catheters for hemodynamic measurements. One type of catheter includes a fiberoptic tip that measures reflected wavelengths of light from saturated Hgb in the local (pulmonary artery) blood flow (Kacmarek et al., 2017).

 b. The mixed venous oxygen saturation (SvO_2) measurement, which is usually between 65% and 80%, is a global indicator of total oxygen consumption (VO_2).

 c. Either a change in oxygen supply (arterial oxygen saturation) or in oxygen demand (VO_2) will alter this measurement (see Chapter 3 for further information).

B. Carbon Dioxide Monitoring

1. *Transcutaneous Carbon Dioxide Monitoring*

 a. *Principles.* A CO_2 sensor, housed in a small probe, is mounted on the skin surface to measure diffused carbon dioxide with an electrode similar to that found in standard blood gas machines. Although in the past $PtcO_2$ electrodes used local heat to "arterialize" the site, recent studies showed that a predictable linear relationship can be obtained with nonheated electrodes. Typically, the $PtcO_2$ is higher than the $PaCO_2$, but the gradient should remain stable.

 b. *Uses.* In the past, consistent correlations have been documented in neonates particularly; however, recent advances in technology have expanded this technology for use in older children and adults (Kacmarek et al., 2017). After the probe is positioned and the warm-up period has passed, the monitor measurement should be compared with a simultaneous blood gas measurement to establish the gradient. After this point, blood gas measurements can be reduced until the next site rotation (usually every 4 hours).

 c. *Limitations*

  i. The sensors appear to be somewhat fragile and prone to discreet alterations, such as inadequate fluid in the sensor. If the gradient between $PtcO_2$ and $PaCO_2$ is unstable, a site change is warranted.

  ii. Calibration procedures must be exact, necessitating the presence of personnel who are well trained in the operation of these monitors.

2. *End-Tidal Carbon Dioxide Monitoring.* The measurement of exhaled carbon dioxide gas provides direct evidence of ventilatory function. An increased carbon dioxide level is an objective parameter for the identification of respiratory failure. This can be measured with or without a waveform.

 a. *Principles of operation.* A small device placed in the respiratory circuit (may be on a ventilator circuit, a port on an oxygen mask/bilevel positive airway pressure [BiPAP]/continuous positive airway pressure [CPAP] mask) at the proximal airway, measures expired carbon dioxide by mass spectrometry or infrared absorption. Exhaled gas passes through this device, which emits infrared light. A detector measures the light absorption in this sample. The carbon dioxide level is *inversely* proportional to the light absorption.

 b. *Uses.* In the normal subject, $PtcO_2$ is theoretically within 2 mm of $PaCO_2$.

  i. Alveolar hypoventilation will lead to an increase in arterial and end-tidal carbon dioxide monitoring ($ETCO_2$), which can be used in patients who are being weaned from mechanical ventilation. $ETCO_2$ detection—whether qualitative, quantitative, or continuous—is the most accurate and easily available method to monitor correct ETT position in patients who have adequate tissue perfusion (Kacmarek et al., 2017).

ii. An estimation of dead space ventilation can be inferred when $PaCO_2$ measurements and $ETCO_2$ are compared serially. When the dead space (V_d/V_t) increases, the gradient between $PaCO_2$ and $ETCO_2$ increases. Conversely, as ventilator adjustments are made in an attempt to improve V_A, the gradient should diminish.

iii. Carbon dioxide monitoring can be useful in patients with increased intracranial pressure (ICP) or PH in which the patient's $PaCO_2$ needs to be regulated.

c. *Limitations*

i. The choice of sensor used for a child must be guided by its sensitivity for smaller exhaled volumes. Clinically, infants weighing less than 5 kg may not be good candidates for this device, but the final decision should be based on comparative measurements with a blood gas analysis.

ii. Additional considerations are the warm-up time required and the calibration process, which requires operator competence.

iii. During a cardiac arrest or extubation, the $ETCO_2$ measurement acutely disappears. However, this lack of measurement can be an indicator of quality cardiopulmonary resuscitation (CPR) and cardiac output during chest compressions. High-quality CPR is associated with improved outcomes after cardiac arrest. Animal data support a direct association between $ETCO_2$ and cardiac output. Capnography is used during pediatric cardiac arrest to monitor for return of spontaneous circulation as well as CPR quality. There is no pediatric evidence that $ETCO_2$ monitoring improves outcomes from cardiac arrest. Studies in adults suggest that $ETCO_2$ values generated during CPR were significantly associated with chest compression depth and ventilation rate. $ETCO_2$ monitoring may be considered to evaluate the quality of chest compressions, but specific values to guide therapy have not been established in children (de Caen et al., 2015).

C. Diagnostic PFTs

Critically ill children require continuous surveillance of pulmonary function. For those who are not in frank respiratory failure, clinical assessment, including respiratory rate, observation of chest expansion, and use of accessory muscles, provides an estimation of adequacy of minute ventilation (V_E). For those in distress, further measurements may be warranted. With children, standard measurements of pulmonary function may not be possible because of lack of patient cooperation.

1. *Spirometry* (Figure 2.14). In the cooperative child, lung volumes can be estimated with simple flow spirometers. Flow spirometers, which measure exhaled V_T, can provide an *estimation* of V_C and can be used for trending. In general, 80% of the V_C can be exhaled in 1 second and is called the forced expiratory volume, or FEV_1.

a. In *obstructive* disease, the patient is unable to breathe out fully and has both decreased V_C and FEV_1.

b. In *restrictive* disease, in which the lung cannot fully expand, the V_C is low, but FEV_1 is still proportionally normal (i.e., ≥80% of V_C).

c. In the *weakened patient*, lower volumes may be observed with a faster respiratory rate (see Figure 2.1).

2. *Pressure Manometers.* Both negative and inspiratory pressure (effort) can be quantified by using a manometer to provide an estimation of muscle condition. A normal school-age child should be able to generate a minimum of about 30 cm H_2O on *inspiration* (called *negative inspiratory force [NIF]*). An infant may generate an NIF of about 20 cm H_2O, although infant effort is difficult to capture; "crying effort" measurement is sometimes used, however. On *expiration*, a school-age child should be able to generate a pressure of at least +30 cm H_2O.

3. *Measurement of Compliance*

a. *Lung compliance* (C_L) is the measure of the distensibility of the lung and thoracic wall. It is defined as the volume change per unit of pressure change across the lung. This is expressed as $\Delta V/\Delta P$ (see Figure 2.4).

b. *Dynamic compliance* is the relationship of the delivered (tidal) volume to the total pressure required to deliver that volume. Dynamic compliance includes both elastic recoil and airway resistance factors.

c. *Static compliance.* At the end of a breath, gas flow delivery is paused. The friction created by that flow disappears, causing the inspiratory pressure to drop slightly (airway plateau pressure). The $\Delta V/\Delta P$ (*static* pressure) reflects the elastic properties of the lung (or

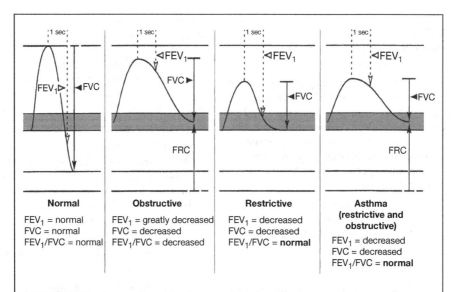

FIGURE 2.14 Comparison of pulmonary function measurements in the person with obstructive and restrictive pulmonary disease. The ratio of FEV_1/FVC is greater than 80%. Note that in restrictive disease the ratio is normal, but the separate measurements of FEV_1 and **FVC** are abnormally low.

FEV_1, forced expiratory volume in the first second of exhalation; FRC, functional residual capacity; FVC, forced vital capacity.

average distensibility of all participating alveoli). Normal range is the same in an infant as in an adult: 60 to 100 mL per centimeter of H_2O. Static compliance decreases with restrictive disease and increases with obstructive disease. Serial monitoring of *static* compliance may facilitate identification of optimal tidal volumes (V_T), optimal positive end-expiratory pressure (PEEP), and prediction of weaning readiness.

PULMONARY PHARMACOLOGY

A. General Principles

1. Pharmacologic management of pulmonary diseases in children requires understanding of both the pharmacokinetics of the various drugs and the disease conditions for which the drugs are prescribed. Most medications have been studied in adult populations and application to children has often occurred by extrapolation of data.

2. *Physiologic Differences.* Infants and young children have a greater percentage of total body water, predominately extracellular fluid. The total volume of distribution of a drug, depending on solubility, occurs within intracellular, extracellular, and interstitial fluid compartments. In general, drug doses are higher per kilogram of body weight in the infant than in the adolescent or adult.

3. *Underlying Pathophysiology.* Decreased blood flow to major organs influences absorption, delivery of the drug to the targeted site, and elimination. Inflammation can cause an increase in regionalized blood flow with altered capillary permeability, which can result in abnormally high drug delivery to these regions. Extravascular fluid collections may provide a protein-rich reservoir for drugs, diverting them from their intended distribution site.

4. *Dosing of Medications.* The dosing of medication is frequently based on one of two strategies:

a. *Target concentration.* The basis for following this strategy is that serum concentrations for a given drug have defined both therapeutic and toxic ranges. These assays are guidelines and are not specific to an individual patient. Knowledge of pharmacokinetics is important to the successful use of this strategy.

b. *Target effect.* A drug is selected with a therapeutic endpoint clearly defined before administration. Dosing is titrated to achieve this effect or until toxic effects are observed. Discontinuation of the drug may be necessary if toxicity occurs or if no therapeutic effect is achieved. Many of the medications used in a critical care setting are prescribed in this manner.

5. *Protein Binding.* Binding of drugs to plasma proteins determines the amount of free drug available for body distribution. Although plasma albumin levels reach adult levels soon after birth, differences in the binding properties of infant albumin can influence the dosing of selected medications.

B. Routes of Drug Delivery

1. *Inhaled Administration.* Inhaled administration bypasses the need for absorption as with enterally administered medications. Often smaller doses are required and a more rapid onset of action can be obtained. As infants and young children have smaller lungs and airways, the delivery of medications via inhalation can be considered more difficult. In very severe cases, this route alone may not be appropriate because the drug cannot reach the affected area (Lexicomp Online, 2016; Spahn & Szefler, 2008).

2. *Enteral Administration/Absorption.* The enteral route of administration requires absorption from the GI tract as an initial step (Lexicomp Online, 2016; Spahn & Szefler, 2008).

    a. Gastric acid secretion and motility appear to be developmentally regulated. Intestinal transit is more rapid in the infant than in the adult. Many medications might not be absorbed as completely as in the older child or adult because of the following factors:

        i. **Bioavailability.** A drug given enterally must be bioavailable from the GI tract.

        ii. An acidic pH favors absorption of acidic medications; likewise, an alkaline pH improves absorption of alkaline compounds.

        iii. The rate of gastric emptying and intestinal transit affects absorption of medications. Delayed gastric emptying or rapid intestinal motility will decrease absorption. Conditions that can decrease absorption include gastroesophageal reflux, respiratory distress syndrome (RDS), and congenital heart disease.

        iv. Gastric, jejunal, or duodenal feedings may alter bioavailability. Drugs administered through these tubes may bind with proteins in the feedings. Feedings may need to be stopped for a while before and after administration. Adjustment of drug doses (based on serum assay) is reliable only with consistency in the administration of the drugs and when steady-state concentrations have been achieved.

3. *Parenteral Administration.* Parenteral routes of administration include the subcutaneous, intramuscular, and intravenous (IV) routes. For those routes to be viable, a medication must be water soluble or in suspension. The IV route bypasses the absorption step resulting in 100% bioavailability. There is a rapid onset of action (Lexicomp Online, 2016).

C. Neuromuscular Blocking Agents

1. *Description* (Table 2.7). Muscle relaxants are used in the pediatric ICU (PICU) to facilitate assisted ventilation by intervening within the neuromuscular junction in one of two ways:

    a. Depolarizing agents cause a continuous release and subsequent depletion of acetylcholine.

    b. Nondepolarizing agents bind the receptor sites of acetylcholine so that synaptic transmission is blocked. (Lexicomp Online, 2016; Weiner, Halfaer, & Allen, 2008)

2. *Indications for Use* (Weiner, Halfaer, & Allen, 2008)

    a. Placement of an ETT requires administration of a neuromuscular blocking (NMB) agent in many instances.

    b. Control of ventilation is often needed in patients with severe respiratory disease, increased ICP, or cardiac failure.

    c. Reduction of VO_2 from muscle movement can be achieved with the use of an NMB.

3. *Nursing Considerations* (Lexicomp Online, 2016)

    a. The choice of an NMB agent depends on the purpose and intended duration of pharmacologic paralysis. All patients who will receive a paralytic drug should be given adequate sedation and analgesia.

    b. Monitoring of all children who are given an NMB agent should include ECG monitoring and pulse oximetry (see the discussion in the "Respiratory Monitoring" section). Increased heart rate (increases from baseline) may be caused by pain, fear, or seizures; increased systolic blood pressure may indicate pain or anxiety; and pupil size (dilation) may indicate earlier in the chapter fear, pain, or other causes of sympathetic stimulation such as seizures.

    c. An assessment of level of NMB is required on a regular basis. Intermittent peripheral nerve stimulation and drug holidays are two techniques that can be utilized.

    d. Long-term use of muscle relaxants may mask pain, anxiety, and seizures. Whenever possible, scheduled withholding of paralytic medications should be done to enable adequate

TABLE 2.7 Neuromuscular Blocking Agents

Drug	Dose/Onset/Duration	Contraindications	Comments
Pancuronium (IV)	Dose: 0.05–0.15 mg/kg Onset: 2–5 min Duration: 24 min	Renal failure 60%–90% renal elimination	Vagolytic: Increased heart rate and blood pressure
Vecuronium (IV)	Dose: 0.08–0.1 mg/kg Onset: 2.5–3 min Duration: 45–60 min	Liver failure	Renal elimination <25%
Atracurium (IV)	Dose: 0.3–0.5 mg/kg Onset: 2–3 min Duration: 20–70 min	Hypotension Need for rapid onset	Hoffman elimination makes it ideal for kidney or liver failure Very slow onset
Succinylcholine (IV or IM)	IV dose: 1–2 mg/kg/dose IM dose: 1–3 mg/kg/dose Onset: 30–60 sec Duration: 3–10 min	Myasthenia gravis Malignant hyperthermia Avoid in patients with hyperkalemia Guillain–Barré syndrome Skeletal muscle myopathies Crush, burn, electrical injuries Open-globe injury Increased intracranial pressure	Dysrhythmias Use a defasciculating dose Potassium efflux Muscle rigidity
Rocuronium (IV)	Dose: 0.5–1.2 mg/kg Onset: 30–60 sec Duration: 30–60 min	None	Short duration

IM, intramuscular; IV, intravenous.

Sources: Lexicomp Online. (2016). Pediatric & neonatal Lexi-Drugs. Retrieved from http://webstore.lexi.com/Pediatric-Lexi-Drugs; Weiner, D., Halfaer, M., & Allen, J. (2008). Respiratory effects of anesthesia and sedation. In L. Taussig (Ed.), *Pediatric respiratory medicine* (2nd ed., pp. 347–357). St. Louis, MO: Mosby.

assessment of the patient's awareness and condition. Prolonged use of muscle relaxants has been associated with myopathy, particularly if steroids are given concurrently.

D. Sedatives and Analgesics

1. *Benzodiazepines*

a. *Description.* Benzodiazepines are believed to cause anterograde amnesia through the inhibition of the neurotransmitter gamma-aminobutyric acid (GABA) in the limbic system. They have little or no effect on retrograde memory and have no analgesic properties. However, there is an increase in delirium with the use of benzodiazepines (Table 2.8) (Kost & Roy, 2010; Lexicomp Online, 2016; Weiner et al., 2008).

b. *Indications* include short-term general sedation and amnesia for procedures, long-term use for facilitating compliance with assisted ventilation, and acute therapy for seizure management.

c. *Nursing considerations* include the following:

i. Benzodiazepines do not provide pain relief. In many situations, use of an analgesic

in conjunction with sedation should be considered.

ii. To avoid hypotension, patients should be euvolemic (well hydrated) before administration of a benzodiazepine to avoid hypotension.

iii. Prolonged administration may result in physical dependence. Withdrawal symptoms, such as anxiety, sweating, agitation, or hallucinations, may occur with abrupt withdrawal.

iv. Some patients may exhibit a paradoxical response to benzodiazepines, which worsens with escalating doses. If an agitated child is given additional doses and the agitation worsens, consideration of a paradoxical response might prompt discontinuation of the benzodiazepine.

2. *Chloral Hydrate* (Kost & Roy, 2010; Lexicomp Online, 2016)

a. *Description.* An alcohol-based sedative–hypnotic that is safe and effective in children younger than 3 years of age (not recommended in children older than 4 years or in children with

TABLE 2.8 Sedatives and Analgesics

Drug	IV Dose/Onset/Duration	Contraindications	Comments
Other Sedatives and Analgesics			
Chloral hydrate	Oral dosing: Infants and children 25–50 mg/kg/d divided every 6–8 hr, maximum dose 500 mg/dose Onset: 15–30 min Duration: 1–2 hr	Hypersensitivity to chloral hydrate or any component of the formulation Marked hepatic or renal impairment	Very limited use in the United States Respiratory obstruction may occur in children with tonsillar and adenoidal hypertrophy, obstructive sleep apnea, and Leigh's encephalopathy
Dexmedetomidine (IV)	Loading dose: 0.5–1 mcg/kg (over 10 min) followed by a maintenance infusion of 0.2–0.7 mcg/kg/hr (although higher doses are being used at 1 mcg/kg/hr) Onset: 30 min Duration: 4 hr	None listed in the U.S. manufacturer's labeling	Administer using a controlled infusion device Infuse loading dose over 10 min; dexmedetomidine may adhere to natural rubber
Propofol (IV)	Dose: 0.5–2 mg/kg IV push 50 µg/kg/min infusion Onset: 1–2 min Duration: 5–10 min	Hypersensitivity to propofol or any component of the formulation Hypersensitivity to eggs, egg products, soybeans, or soy products When general anesthesia or sedation is contraindicated	Helpful with refractory bronchospasm Caution with hypovolemia or congestive heart failure May ↓ ICP May produces green urine (rare) Does not provide analgesia
Ketamine (IV/IM)	IV dose: 1–2mg/kg over 30 to 60 sec; may administer additional doses of 0.5–1 mg/kg every 5–15 min as needed IM dose: 4–5 mg/kg as a single dose; may give a repeat dose (2–5 mg/kg) if additional doses are required Onset: <30 sec Duration: 10–15 min	Hypersensitivity to ketamine Conditions in which an increase in blood pressure would be hazardous Infants younger than 3 months Known or suspected schizophrenia	Analgesic, amnestic, hallucinogen Monitor for emergence delirium and nightmares Bronchodilator used for patients with asthma Prevent emergence reaction with benzodiazepines at the end of the procedure
Benzodiazepines			
Midazolam (IV/IM)	IV dose (children 6 mo–5 y): 0.05–0.1 mg/kg IV dose (children 6–12 y): 0.025–0.05 mg/kg. IV dose (12–16 y): 0.02–0.04 mg/kg titrate up to desired effect or up to 0.1–0.2 mg/kg IM dose (preprocedure): 0.1–0.15 mg/kg 30–60 min before procedure Onset: 2–4 min Duration: 20–30 min Maximum dose: 0.6 mg/kg	Severe hypotension CNS depression	Sedative-anxiolytic, anticonvulsant Alternate routes of delivery, including oral, rectal, and transmucosal (nasal)

(continued)

TABLE 2.8 Sedatives and Analgesics *(continued)*

Drug	IV Dose/Onset/Duration	Contraindications	Comments
Lorazepam (IV; IM give preprocedure in adults)	Dose: 0.05–0.1 mg/kg Onset: 2–4 min Duration: 20–30 min	Severe hypotension CNS depression	4–12-hr half-life may be used by intermittent bolus No active metabolite
Diazepam (IV)	Dose: 0.05–0.1 mg/kg Onset: 2–4 min Duration: 20–30 min Maximum dose: 0.6 mg/kg in an 8-hr period	Not recommended for use by continuous infusion Severe hypotension CNS depression	Prolonged effect because of long half-life and presence of active metabolites
Opiates and Analgesic Agents			
Fentanyl (IV/IM)	IV/IM dose: 1–2 mcg/kg Onset: 3–5 min Duration: 0.5–1 hr	Severe respiratory depression	Analgesic, mildly sedating
Hydromorphone (IV; IM use may result in various absorption rates and is not recommended for use)	Dose for children <50 kg: 0.015mg/kg/dose Dose for children >50 kg: 0.2–0.6 mg/dose Onset: 15 min Peak effect: 30–60 min Duration: 5 hr	Hypersensitivity to hydromorphone or any component of the formulation Acute or severe asthma Respiratory depression	
Methadone (IV/IM)	IV dose: 0.1 mg/kg IM dose: 0.1 mg/kg/dose every 4 hr for 2–3 doses, then every 6–12 hr as needed Onset: 10–20 min Peak effect: 1–2 hr Maximum dose: 10 mg per dose		Half-life 15–29 hr Used for managing opiate dependence
Morphine (IV/IM)	IV/IM dose: 0.1–0.2 mg/kg (variable depending on age and condition) Onset: (patient dependent; dosing must be individualized) Oral (immediate release): ~30 min IV: 5–10 min Duration: Immediate-release formulations (tablet, oral solution, injection): 3 to 5 hr	Respiratory depression Metabolite accumulation in renal failure	May cause histamine release
Remifentanil (IV)	Peak: 20 min Duration: 4–5 hr	Not for intrathecal or epidural administration	Monitor respiratory and cardiovascular status
Alfentanil (IV)	Children <12 years: Limited dosing data available	Hypersensitivity	Monitor respiratory, cardiovascular, and neurological status for degree of analgesia/anesthesia

(continued)

TABLE 2.8 Sedatives and Analgesics *(continued)*

Drug	IV Dose/Onset/Duration	Contraindications	Comments
	Children >12 years*: Incremental injection: Anesthesia <30 min Induction: 8-20 mcg/kg IV Maintenance: 3-5 mcg/kg IV increments every 5-20 min, or 0.25-1 mcg/kg/min IV Total dose: 8-40 mcg/kg IV		

CNS, central nervous system; ICP, intracranial pressure; IM, intramuscular; IV, intravenous.

*Dose varies depending on duration of procedure.

Sources: Kost, S., & Roy, A. (2010). Procedural sedation and analgesia in the pediatric emergency department: A review of sedative pharmacology. *Clinical Pediatric Emergency Medicine, 11*(4), 233–243. doi:10.1016/j.cpem.2010.08.002; Lexicomp Online. (2016). Pediatric & neonatal Lexi-Drugs. Retrieved from http://webstore.lexi.com/Pediatric-Lexi-Drugs; Weiner, D., Halfaer, M., & Allen, J. (2008). Respiratory effects of anesthesia and sedation. In L. Taussig (Ed.), *Pediatric respiratory medicine* (2nd ed., pp. 347–357). St. Louis, MO: Mosby.

neurodevelopmental disorders due to lack of efficacy). It has very limited availability in the United States, although it is still available in other countries.

b. *A central nervous system (CNS) depressant.* Effects are due to its active metabolite trichloroethanol, mechanism unknown.

c. *Indications* include use as a sedative/hypnotic prior to nonpainful therapeutic or diagnostic procedures (EEG, CT, MRI, ophthalmic exam, dental procedure, infant PFT, echocardiogram).

d. *Nursing considerations.* Nurses should monitor level of sedation, vital signs, and oxygen saturation prior to and during the procedure. The taste is very bitter (disadvantage).

E. Dexmedetomidine

a. *Description.* Selective alpha2-adrenoceptor agonist with anesthetic and sedative properties thought to be due to activation of G-proteins by alpha2a-adrenoceptors in the brain stem resulting in inhibition of norepinephrine release; peripheral alpha2b-adrenoceptors are activated at high doses or with rapid IV administration resulting in vasoconstriction. Patients continue to breathe while on dexmedetomidine and therefore it is a good choice for patients who are not mechanically ventilated (Kost & Roy, 2010; Lexicomp Online, 2016).

b. *Indications.* Sedation of initially intubated and mechanically ventilated patients during treatment in an intensive care setting; sedation prior to and/or during surgical or other procedures of nonintubated patients; duration of infusion should not exceed 24 hours per the manufacturers recommendations; however, many studies exist regarding its longer term usage.

c. *Nursing considerations*

  i. Episodes of bradycardia, hypotension, and sinus arrest have been associated with rapid IV administration.

  ii. Use of a loading dose is optional.

  iii. Transient hypertension: This has been primarily observed during loading-dose administration and is associated with the initial peripheral vasoconstrictive effects of dexmedetomidine. Treatment is generally unnecessary; however, a reduction in infusion rate may be required.

  iv. Use of infusions for more than 24 hours has been associated with tolerance and tachyphylaxis and a dose-related increase in adverse reactions.

  v. When withdrawn abruptly in patients who have received more than 24 hours of therapy, withdrawal symptoms similar to clonidine withdrawal may result (e.g., hypertension, tachycardia, nervousness, nausea, vomiting, agitation, headaches).

  vi. Recovery times for sedation are somewhat longer than propofol and ketamine but shorter than pentobarbital and chloral hydrate.

  vii. Patients require continuous monitoring with level of sedation, heart rate, respiration, ECG, blood pressure, and pain control.

2. *Morphine and Morphine-Like Opioids* (Kost & Roy, 2010; Lexicomp Online, 2016)

a. *Description.* Opioid receptors are found in the brain and spinal cord. Five receptors have been described, but three—the mu (M), kappa (K), and sigma (S)—are the most clinically recognized targets for opiate binding:

    i. M: Supraspinal anesthesia; euphoria, respiratory depression, physical dependence

    ii. K: Spinal anesthesia; sedation, miosis, and respiratory depression

    iii. S: CNS stimulant; dysphoria, hallucinations, respiratory, and vasomotor stimulation

    iv. Most morphine-like narcotics are described as M and K agonists. Other agents work at different receptor sites, such as nalbuphine (Nubain). Nalbuphine is a K and S receptor agonist and M receptor antagonist. Administration of nalbuphine after morphine may "antagonize" or reverse some of the morphine effects because of its antagonistic effects on the M receptor.

b. Indications for analgesic medications include procedures, relief of pain from underlying disease, and continuous analgesia for facilitating assisted mechanical ventilation. Opioids are not a substitute for an anxiolytic and amnestic agents. Although sedation occurs with opioid administration, the mechanisms do not duplicate those found in conventional sedatives such as benzodiazepines.

c. *Nursing considerations*

    i. Some opioids, such as morphine, can cause vasodilatory effects from histamine release. Histamine release is minimal with the synthetic narcotics such as fentanyl. Most opioids, except meperidine, induce a central parasympathetic stimulation and direct depression of the sinoatrial node. All opioids also cause dose-dependent respiratory depression.

    ii. Routes of delivery should be individualized with the goal of using the lowest possible dosing to provide continuous relief without side effects.

    iii. Fentanyl is a synthetic opioid with approximately 100 times the analgesic potency of morphine. This concentrated solution (unless adequately diluted) may increase the risk for chest-wall rigidity especially with rapid, high-dose IV administration, and decreased seizure threshold. These side effects can be seen with all opioids and are not necessarily contraindications for their use. Slower administration and lower dosing can attenuate or prevent these side effects.

    iv. Prolonged use of hydromorphone during pregnancy can result in neonatal opioid withdrawal syndrome, which may be life threatening if not recognized and treated.

    v. Remifentanil and alfentanil are being utilized with increasing frequency in pediatrics.

        1) Remifentanil is an approved medication for maintenance of general anesthesia in ages 0 to 2 months, 1 to 12 years, and adults. It binds with stereospecific mu-opioid receptors at many sites in the CNS, increasing pain threshold, altering pain reception, and inhibiting ascending pain pathways. In pediatric patients, pharmacokinetic data showed variable age-related changes with distribution and clearance; however, no age-related changes occur with half-life.

        2) Alfentanil is an analgesic adjunct for the maintenance of anesthesia with barbiturate/nitrous oxide/oxygen, analgesic with nitrous oxide/oxygen in the maintenance of general anesthesia, analgesic component for monitored anesthesia care, primary anesthetic for induction of anesthesia in general surgery when endotracheal intubation and mechanical ventilation are required (Food and Drug Administration [FDA] approved in ages older than 12 years and adults).

    vi. Current research suggests that implementation of a nurse-driven sedation protocol in a PICU is feasible. Outcomes suggest that evaluation of sedation and analgesia were better after a protocol implementation; duration of mechanical ventilation and occurrence of withdrawal symptoms tended to be reduced (Dreyfus, Javouhey, Denis, Touzet, & Bordet, 2017; Neunhoeffer, et al., 2015).

3. *Barbiturates* (Kost & Roy, 2010; Lexicomp Online, 2016)

a. *Description.* Barbiturates are one of the oldest classes of sedative agents in use today.

They provide good sedation but are not analgesic or amnestic agents. The cardiopulmonary effects are dose dependent and well defined. Several drugs are available and classified according to the duration of activity. In addition to their sedative effect, barbiturates have potent anticonvulsant properties and can decrease cerebral metabolism, thus affecting ICP.

b. *Indications.* Include short-term sedation for procedures and long-term sedation for ongoing management of assisted ventilation (rarely), increased ICP, and continuous procedures such as with use of the intra-aortic balloon pump (IABP). Barbiturates are not a substitute for analgesic medications unless the dosing is high enough to produce complete anesthesia.

c. *Nursing considerations*

 i. Cardiovascular effects are dose related. With higher doses, venodilation and depressed myocardial function can occur.

 ii. Pulmonary effects are also dose related, with apnea occurring in the mid dose ranges. Bag, mask, and oxygen should always be at the bedside.

 iii. Most barbiturates are in an alkaline solution and therefore must be administered separately from other medications and IV solutions.

4. *Ketamine* (Kost & Roy, 2010; Lexicomp Online, 2016)

a. *Description.* Ketamine is both an analgesic and an amnestic medication. The mechanism of this drug, including S receptor stimulation, is mediated through the sympathetic nervous system causing a brief, immediate release of endogenous catecholamines. A brief increase in heart rate, blood pressure, and general stimulation are observed with administration of lower doses (0.5–2 mg/kg). It produces dissociative anesthesia in which the eyes may be open and nystagmus may be noted; even at lower doses, however, it provides intense analgesia and amnesia. Higher doses provide good anesthesia and respiratory depression, but as the patient recovers, the stimulation and dysphoria can reappear.

b. *Indications.* Ketamine has a minimal effect on cardiopulmonary stability at doses less than 2 mg/kg and is a good choice for unstable patients. Bronchodilation occurs (through the release of endogenous catecholamines), which makes ketamine a good agent for patients with bronchospasm. However, ketamine may increase cerebral blood flow and ICP and therefore may not be a good agent for patients with altered intracranial compliance.

c. *Nursing considerations*

 i. Emergence phenomena are observed more often in older children and adults than in younger children. Previously, it was believed that administration of a benzodiazepine at the end of the procedure could decrease or prevent this occurrence. However, more recent data refute this belief; in fact, some children exhibit paradoxical response to benzodiazepines, causing them to be more agitated and dysphoric (Weiner et al., 2008).

 ii. Although respiratory depression is dose dependent with ketamine administration, even with normal respiratory function, it is unclear whether airway reflexes are completely intact. Therefore, bag, mask, oxygen, and suction should be available at the bedside, particularly if any other sedative agents have been given with ketamine.

5. *Propofol* (Kost & Roy, 2010; Lexicomp Online, 2016; Weiner et al., 2008)

a. *Description.* Propofol is an anesthetic agent administered intravenously, with rapid onset and short duration of action. The effects are dose dependent. Propofol is provided in a lipid emulsion of soybean oil, glycerol, and egg phosphates. It has multiple properties, including bronchodilation and rapid recovery (with minimal posthypnotic obtundation), which makes it an attractive agent for deep sedation or anesthetic induction. The drug is unrelated to any of the currently used barbiturate, opioid, benzodiazepine, arylcyclohexylamine, or imidazole IV anesthetic agents. Propofol causes global CNS depression, presumably through agonism of type A gamma-aminobutyric acid (GABAA) receptors and perhaps reduced glutamatergic activity through NMDA receptor blockade.

b. *Indications.* In pediatrics, use is limited to procedural sedation only.

c. *Nursing considerations*

 i. Propofol may produce hypotension by direct vasodilation.

ii. The Academy of Allergy, Asthma, and Immunology has issued a statement that soy- and egg-allergic patients can safely receive propofol (Lexicomp Online, 2016).

iii. Anaphylactic reactions to propofol appear not to be related to soy or egg allergy.

iv. Prolonged infusions are not recommended in pediatrics.

F. Remedial Agents

1. In providing sedation, analgesia, or pharmacologic paralysis for a child, some agents exhibit predictable but unwanted effects that can be prevented or remediated pharmacologically. The following medications may be used to manage the side effects (Table 2.9).

2. *Anticholinergic Agents* (Atropine and Atropine-Like Medications)

a. *Description.* Anticholinergic agents antagonize the actions of acetylcholine, producing a central vagal blockade (tachycardia, increased blood pressure, mitosis) and specific sympathetic effects in target organs.

i. Atropine crosses the blood–brain barrier and is known to cause CNS stimulation, whereas synthetic agents, such as ipratropium, do not cross into brain tissue.

ii. In addition, the lungs have both cholinergic and adrenergic receptors that regulate bronchomotor tone. An anticholinergic agent may be considered in the management of a patient with asthma.

b. *Indications.* Include premedication for procedures or medications known to potentiate bradycardia, reduction of salivary secretions, bronchodilation (not as a first-line agent but as an adjunct), and symptom control while using a beta-blocker agent.

c. *Nursing considerations*

i. Pupil size and responsiveness are altered with atropine administration. This is important to note when a neurologic condition is being monitored. Fixed dilated pupils should not occur.

ii. Side effects may be bothersome to patients who are awake, including a fast heart rate, dry mouth, and CNS effects (delirium, agitation).

iii. Atropine crosses the blood–brain barrier and will cause CNS effects such as agitation.

3. *Naloxone (Narcan)*

a. *Description.* Naloxone is an opioid antagonist that has an affinity for opiate receptors, blocking them from binding to narcotics. Narcotics attached to the receptor are displaced. Naloxone is used to reverse the effects of morphine-like

TABLE 2.9 Remedial Agents

Side Effects Treated	Drug	IV-Dose Duration	Comments
Bradycardia or bronchospasm	Atropine	Bradycardia Dose: 0.01–0.02 mg/kg Minimum: 0.1 mg Maximum: 1 mg Bronchospasm Dose: 0.05 mg/kg in 2.5 mL NS q6h MDI or aerosol	Monitor for muscarinic effect: bradycardia, salivation, bronchospasm
Pruritus (epidural/IV opioids)	Naloxone (Narcan) Nalbuphine (Nubain)	Continuous infusion 0.001 mg/kg/hr 0.01 mg/kg IV every 2–3 min	This dose should not significantly reverse analgesia May improve analgesia May cause increased sedation
Pruritus (systemic opioids)	Diphenhydramine (Benadryl)	0.5–1 mg/kg IV q6h	Significant sedation may be observed

(continued)

TABLE 2.9 Remedial Agents *(continued)*

Side Effects Treated	Drug	IV-Dose Duration	Comments
Respiratory depression (benzodiazepines)	Flumazenil (Romazicon)	<20 kg: 0.01 mg/kg (maximum 0.2 mg) Repeat: 0.005 mg/kg (maximum 0.2 mg) 20–40 kg: 0.2 mg (maximum 1 mg) Repeat 0.005 mg/kg	Caution in patients with seizure history Does not consistently reverse amnesia Used for reversal of conscious sedation May produce convulsions in patients physically dependent on benzodiazepines
Respiratory depression (opioids)	Naloxone (Narcan)	Mild oversedation 0.01 mg/kg; repeat 2–3 min Opiate intoxication <20 kg: 0.1 mg/kg >20 kg: 2 mg/dose Repeat 2–3 min until response noted May require repeat doses q20–60 min	May cause abrupt cessation of pain control; sudden awakening with agitation, nausea and vomiting, and headache
Nausea	Metoclopramide (Reglan)	0.1 mg/kg IV q6h	Low incidence of side effects but extrapyramidal symptoms may occur
	Droperidol (Inapsine)	2–12 y: 0.05–0.06 mg/kg/dose q4–6hr >12 y: 2.5–5 mg/dose q4hr	Can cause dysphoria, severe hypotension, extrapyramidal reaction
	Ondansetron (Zofran)	0.15 mg/kg IV × three doses at 4-hr intervals	No sedation; best used prior to anticipated stimulus (e.g., operating room) Low incidence of bronchospasm, seizures, headaches

MDI, metered dose inhaler; NS, normal saline; q, every.

Source: Lexicomp Online. (2016). Pediatric & neonatal Lexi-Drugs. Retrieved from http://webstore.lexi.com/Pediatric-Lexi-Drugs.

drugs. When given intravenously, the duration is 2 to 3 minutes.

b. *Indications.* Used for complete or partial reversal of opioid drug effects, including respiratory depression induced by natural or synthetic opioids, diagnosis and management of known or suspected acute opioid overdose, and for the prevention and treatment of opioid-induced pruritus.

c. *Nursing considerations*

i. Because of the quick onset of effect with naloxone, the patient may awaken abruptly and may be in pain or exhibit nausea and vomiting.

ii. Because of the short duration of effect with naloxone, there may be a recurrence of the narcotized state, necessitating repeated

dosing or continuous infusion. Therefore, the patient requires constant monitoring because the effects of the morphine-like narcotics may last longer than the effects of naloxone.

4. *Flumazenil (Romazicon)*

a. *Description.* Romazicon is a reversal agent used for the benzodiazepines with a central mechanism of action.

b. *Indications.* Used for the reversal of benzodiazepine-related side effects, especially respiratory depression.

c. *Nursing considerations*

i. Patients should be monitored continuously with airway equipment at the bedside.

ii. Use flumazenil with caution in patients with a history of seizures, massive overdoses, or concurrent use of tricyclic agents.

5. *Other Agents.* Nausea and pruritis frequently occur with many of the medications discussed in this section. See Table 2.9 for drug recommendations and dosing to manage these problems.

G. Agents That Affect Ventilation–Perfusion Matching

1. *Nitric Oxide*

   a. *Description.* The underlying principle of inhaled nitric oxide (iNO) is its selectivity as a pulmonary vasodilator. iNO will relax only pulmonary smooth muscle adjacent to functioning alveoli. Atelectatic or fluid-filled units will not participate in iNO uptake. Therefore, if the pulmonary vasculature is constricted in atelectatic regions of the lung, pulmonary blood flow will remain minimal in these regions, reducing intrapulmonary shunt. This is in contrast to IV vasodilators such as nitroprusside or prostacycline. These drugs will relax pulmonary vasculature globally reducing PVR, but also increasing intrapulmonary right-to-left shunt (Lexicomp Online, 2016).

   b. *Indications.* Approved for the treatment of hypoxic respiratory failure associated with clinical or echocardiographic evidence of PH used in conjunction with ventilator support and other agents to improve oxygenation and reduce the need for extracorporeal membrane oxygenation (ECMO; FDA approved for term and near-term [>34 weeks gestational age] neonates; Lexicomp Online, 2017).

   c. *Nursing considerations*

   i. Nitric oxide (NO) is an inhalational gas delivered through the ventilator circuitry at a flow of 10 to 80 parts per million (ppm). Doses above 20 ppm should not be used or be used with caution (off-label; Lexicomp Online, 2017).

   ii. The half-life of iNO is extremely short, about 5 seconds. Once NO crosses the vascular endothelium, it is rapidly bound by hemoglobin-forming methemoglobin. The quantity of methemoglobin depends on iNO concentration and concurrent nitrate-based drug therapy. If the methemoglobin level is excessive, a reduction in iNO or other nitro-based vasodilators is warranted. Ultimately

NO metabolites are excreted primarily by the kidneys as nitrates and nitrites. Methemoglobin levels should be noted on routine blood gas analysis.

   iii. NO should not be abruptly discontinued if used for more than a short time because rebound effects can occur. To wean NO, titrate down in several steps, pausing several hours before reducing further; monitor for hypoxemia.

2. *Surfactant Replacement Therapy*

   a. *Description.* Surfactant is produced by type II alveolar epithelial cells in the lung. Surfactant is composed mainly of lipids with only 5% to 10% proteins. Surfactant function includes preventing lung collapse during exhalation, lessening the WOB (VO_2), optimizing surface area for gas exchange and ventilation–perfusion matching, optimizing lung compliance, protecting the lung epithelium and facilitating clearance of foreign material, preventing capillary leakage of fluid into alveoli, and defending against microorganisms.

   b. *Indications.* Exogenous surfactant administration is most commonly used for prophylaxis or treatment of preterm infants with RDS. Surfactant may be redosed in the first 48 hours of presentation. Surfactant is not used in pediatric acute respiratory distress syndrome (PARDS) and only used in neonates (Schnapf & Kirle, 2010)

   c. *Nursing considerations* (Schnapf & Kirle, 2010)

   i. Prophylactic surfactant is administered after a period of stabilization in the first 15 minutes of life.

   ii. Surfactant should only be administered by intratracheal instillation using specialized techniques.

   iii. The patient should be sedated and paralyzed to avoid a cough reflex during endotracheal administration of surfactant.

   iv. Although repositioning the infant has been recommended, it is not necessary to move the infant into different positions during instillation as exogenous surfactant has remarkable spreading properties.

   v. Side effects include the following: cyanosis, bradycardia, reflux of surfactant into the ETT, and airway obstruction. Therapy can rapidly affect oxygenation and lung compliance. Rales and moist breath sounds may occur transiently.

vi. Do not suction airways for 1 hour after dosing unless substantial obstruction occurs.

3. *Sildenafil* (Lexicomp Online, 2016)

a. *Description.* Sildenafil inhibits phosphodiesterase type 5 (PDE-5) in smooth muscle of pulmonary vasculature where PDE-5 is responsible for the degradation of cyclic guanosine monophosphate (cGMP). Increased cGMP concentration results in pulmonary vasculature relaxation; vasodilation in the pulmonary bed and the systemic circulation (to a lesser degree) may occur.

b. *Indications.* PH

c. *Nursing considerations*

i. Typically administered orally although IV formulations exist.

ii. Patients should avoid grapefruit juice as it may increase serum levels/toxicity of sildenafil.

iii. Nursing should monitor heart rate, blood pressure, and oxygen saturation.

iv. Should also monitor for a prolonged erection in males as this can lead to a permanent disability.

H. Bronchodilators and Anti-Inflammatory Agents

1. Direct bronchodilation can be achieved through anticholinergic blockade, direct smooth muscle relaxants, or beta-adrenergic stimulation.

2. *Beta-Agonist Medications* (Lexicomp Online, 2017)

a. *Description.* Dilation of the airways can be achieved through the administration of beta-agonist agents, specifically the beta2 receptors, found in the smooth muscle of the airways.

b. *Indications* include the relief of acute bronchospasm and management of asthma exacerbations.

c. *Nursing considerations*

i. Adverse side effects are dose related: tachycardia, tremors, headache, nausea, and sleep disturbances. Nurses should monitor serum potassium levels, oxygen saturation, heart rate, PFTs, respiratory rate, use of accessory muscles during respiration, suprasternal retractions, and/or arterial or CBGs (if the patient's condition warrants) (Lexicomp Online, 2017).

3. *Anti-Inflammatory Agents* (Lexicomp, Online 2017)

a. *Description.* Conditions, such as asthma, acute respiratory distress syndrome (ARDS), and postextubation stridor, are mediated by an inflammatory process triggered by environmental or endogenous stimuli. The host inflammatory mechanisms normally provide protection, but in specific settings the process appears to cause injury. Anti-inflammatories will not provide immediate treatment for bronchospasm; effects are noted 24 to 36 hours after administration of high-dose steroids.

b. *Indications.* A component of some daily preventative medications for asthma may include inhaled steroids. High-dose enteral or IV steroids are used for acute exacerbations. Steroid treatments are commonly used for croup-like illnesses and postextubation stridor. Corticosteroids (glucocorticoids) are synthetic preparations of the endogenous hormones. They exert general anti-inflammatory effects, such as the suppression of hypersensitivity, immune responses, and metabolic effects, with an influence on lipid, protein, and carbohydrate metabolism and sodium retention.

i. Dexamethasone is often prescribed to treat upper airway edema and asthma exacerbations.

ii. Methylprednisolone and prednisone are therapies for management and rescue in asthma exacerbations.

c. *Nursing considerations.* Glucocorticoids interact with many other drugs; therefore, taking the patient's medication history is essential before administering these drugs.

i. Many adverse reactions occur in patients receiving steroids, including sodium and water retention, hyperglycemia, hypokalemia, hypertension, and CNS changes ranging from dysphoria to mood disorders.

ii. Patients receiving long-term therapy are at risk for osteoporosis, ulcers, hyperlipidemia, and increased susceptibility to infection with symptoms that may be suppressed by the steroids.

d. *Nonsteroidal agents.* Nonsteroidal anti-inflammatory agents (NSAIDs) have not proven useful in the treatment of pulmonary disorders. In particular, a subset of patients with reactive airway disease (RAD) may exhibit asthma symptoms from the use of aspirin. In addition, aspirin should not be used in pediatric patients under the age of 18 years because of its clear association with Reye syndrome.

e. *Leukotriene inhibitors.* These agents block or inhibit the synthesis of cysteinyl leukotriene (c-leukotriene), a mediator that causes bronchoconstriction, mucus secretion, increased vascular permeability, and eosinophil migration to the airways. The release of c-leukotriene from mast cells, eosinophils, and basophils appears not to be blocked by steroids. Because of the prolonged duration of onset, they are not intended for treatment of an acute episode of asthma.

f. *Anticholinergic agents.* Ipratropium and tiotropium may be used to treat bronchospasm with asthma and as a bronchodilating agent in BPD and neonatal RDS. They block the action of acetylcholine at parasympathetic sites in bronchial smooth muscle causing bronchodilation; local application to nasal mucosa inhibits serous and seromucous gland secretions.

AIRWAY-CLEARANCE THERAPIES

Airway clearance may be impaired in patients with disorders that are associated with abnormal cough mechanics (muscle weakness), altered mucus rheology (CF), altered mucociliary clearance (primary ciliary dyskinesia), or structural defects (bronchiectasis). A variety of interventions is used to enhance airway clearance with the goal of improving lung mechanics and gas exchange, and preventing atelectasis and infection. Airway-clearance therapies (ACTs) are indicated for individuals whose function of the mucociliary escalator and/or cough mechanics are altered and whose ability to mobilize and expectorate airways secretions is compromised. Early diagnosis and implementation of ACT, coupled with medical management of infections and airway inflammation, can reduce morbidity and mortality associated with chronic pulmonary and neurorespiratory disease (Table 2.10; Lester & Flume, 2009; McCool & Rosen, 2006; Strickland, 2015; Strickland et al., 2013).

TABLE 2.10   Types of Airway-Clearance Therapies

Assisted Techniques	
Chest physiotherapy (percussion, postural drainage, and vibration)	• Physical therapy techniques have been employed alone and in combination to facilitate airway clearance and to render cough more effective. • These maneuvers are established as the standard of care in patients with CF and in selected patients with other pulmonary conditions as a way to enhance the removal of tracheobronchial secretions. • However, chest physiotherapy is time-consuming, may require assistance of a therapist/caregiver, and may be uncomfortable or unpleasant.
Manually assisted cough	• Paradoxical outward motion of the abdomen during cough may occur in individuals with neuromuscular weakness or structural defects of the abdominal wall; this paradoxical motion contributes to cough inefficiency. Reducing this paradox either by manually compressing the lower thorax and abdomen or by binding the abdomen should theoretically improve cough efficiency. • The manually assisted cough maneuver consists of applying pressure with both hands to the upper abdomen following an inspiratory effort and glottic closure. • A disadvantage is that this requires the presence of a caregiver and is often not well tolerated and ineffective in patients with stiff chest walls, osteoporosis, who have undergone abdominal surgery, or who have intraabdominal catheters.
Unassisted Techniques	
FET, also called huff-coughing	• This maneuver consists of one or two forced expirations without closure of the glottis starting at middle to low lung volume, followed by relaxed breathing. • Huff-coughing is as effective as directed cough in moving secretions proximally.
Autogenic drainage	• This technique uses controlled expiratory airflow during tidal breathing to mobilize secretions in the peripheral airways and move them centrally. • Three phases: (1) Unstick the mucus in the smaller airways by breathing at low lung volumes. (2) Collect the mucus from intermediate-sized airways by breathing at low to middle lung volumes. (3) Evacuate the mucus from the central airways by breathing at middle to high lung volumes. The individual then coughs or huffs to expectorate the mucus. • Technique can be performed in a seated position without the assistance of a caregiver. • Most commonly used in CF.

(continued)

TABLE 2.10 Types of Airway-Clearance Therapies *(continued)*

Respiratory muscle strength training	• Strengthening the inspiratory muscles may enhance cough effectiveness by increasing the volume of air inhaled during the inspiratory phase of the cough, whereas strengthening the muscles of exhalation may improve cough effectiveness by increasing intrathoracic pressure during the expiratory phase. • In patients with neuromuscular weakness and impaired cough, expiratory muscle training is recommended to improve peak expiratory pressure, which may have a beneficial effect on cough.
Devices	
PEP	• The administration of PEP from 5 to 20 cm H_2O delivered by facemask is believed to improve mucus clearance by either increasing gas pressure behind secretions through collateral ventilation or by preventing airway collapse during expiration.
Oscillatory devices (flutter, intrapulmonary percussive ventilation, high-frequency chest-wall oscillation)	• High-frequency oscillations can be applied either through the mouth or chest wall causing the airways to vibrate, thereby mobilizing secretions. These devices can be used with the patient seated or supine. • The "flutter" device is a plastic pipe with a mouthpiece at one end and a perforated cover at the other end. Within the device, a high-density stainless steel ball rests in a circular cone and creates a valve. Exhaling through the device creates oscillations in the airway, the frequency of which can be modulated by changing the inclination of the pipe. • The IPV uses small bursts of air at 200 to 300 cycles per minute along with entrained aerosols delivered through a mouthpiece. The putative mechanisms for efficacy include bronchodilation from increased airway pressure, increased airway humidification, and cough stimulation. • The method of high-frequency oscillation applied to the chest wall has been referred to as either high-frequency chest compression or high-frequency chest-wall oscillation. These devices are designed to oscillate gas in the airway.
Mechanical insufflation–exsufflation	• Modalities directed at increasing the volume inhaled during the inspiratory phase of cough also increase cough effectiveness. The inability of patients with respiratory muscle weakness to achieve high lung volumes contributes to cough ineffectiveness. Cough efficiency can be further enhanced when the initial inspiration is followed by the application of negative pressure to the airway opening for a period of 1–3 sec. Peak cough flows can be increased.
Electrical stimulation of the expiratory muscles	• Electrical stimulation of the abdominal muscles can also increase expiratory pressures and has the advantage of not requiring the presence of a caregiver. Coughs produced by electrical stimulation are associated with expiratory flows equal to the manually assisted coughs.

CF, cystic fibrosis; FET, forced expiratory technique; IPV, intrapulmonary percussive ventilator; PEP, positive expiratory pressure.

CONGENITAL ANOMALIES OF THE PULMONARY SYSTEM

Congenital Diaphragmatic Hernia

A. Definition

Congenital diaphragmatic hernia (CDH) occurs in anywhere from one in 2,000 to one in 5,000 live births. It is characterized by the incomplete formation of the fetal diaphragm and usually occurs on the left side. Anomalies associated with this condition include neural tube defects, cardiac defects, and midline anomalies (Abel, Bush, Chitty, Harcourt, & Nicholson, 2012; Grover et al., 2015).

B. Pathophysiology

1. This defect allows herniation of the abdominal contents into the thoracic cavity affecting fetal lung development. It compresses the lung on the affected side but also shifts the mediastinum to the opposite side and compresses the contralateral lung, resulting in various degrees of bilateral pulmonary hypoplasia (Abel et al., 2012).

2. The diaphragm forms during the eighth to 10th week of fetal life and separates the abdominal and thoracic cavities.

C. Clinical Presentation

1. The diagnosis of CDH is usually made antenatally. From birth, infants may present with a variety of signs and symptoms. Typically, the abdomen is scaphoid, the chest funnel shaped, and the trachea and mediastinum deviated to the contralateral side. The infant may be entirely well or suffer from problems ranging from choking episodes, to apneic episodes, to acute respiratory failure (Abel et al., 2012).

2. The infant may have tachypnea and marked retractions.

3. Breath sounds are decreased or absent on the affected side and the heart sounds are shifted to the unaffected side.

D. Patient Care Management

1. The management of CDH is no longer a surgical emergency. The initial management is to stabilize the baby and optimize respiratory function. Delayed surgical repair has become generally more accepted (Abel et al., 2012).

2. Operative repair may be by thoracotomy or by subcostal or transverse abdominal approaches. The laparoscopic repair has been described. The principle of repair is reduction of herniated viscera, identification and excision of any hernia sac, and repair of the defect (Abel et al., 2012).

3. More aggressive support includes the use of ECMO. Infants who are symptomatic within the first 6 hours of life have the highest mortality. The distressed newborn has a scaphoid abdomen and diminished or no breath sounds on one side. Infants who are maintained on gentle ventilation methods are less likely to require ECMO (Hansel, 2010).

4. Endotracheal intubation is performed after birth. Umbilical arterial and venous access are immediately established.

5. Chylothorax is a well-recognized complicating factor of CDH repair.

6. Postoperative failure to thrive due to gastroesophageal reflux and oral dysfunction is common (Abel et al., 2012).

7. Nursing care for the infant with CDH focuses on avoiding conditions that increase PVR and is discussed within the context of PH. Conditions that should be prevented include hypoxemia, acidosis, hypothermia, and hypoglycemia.

8. Nursing should minimize noise, excessive light, and invasive procedures.

E. Outcomes

1. The overall prognosis for fetuses with CDH is poor, with the major cause of death being pulmonary hypoplasia and/or its associated abnormalities. The time of diagnosis is related to outcome with those diagnosed early faring the worst. Other poor prognostic indicators include evidence of liver within the chest and cardiac disproportion before 24 weeks gestation. Isolated left-sided hernias, an intra-abdominal stomach, and diagnosis after 24 weeks are favorable prognostic factors (Abel et al., 2012).

2. Survival after repair varies between 39% and 95%.

3. The infant typically has an extensive hospital course.

4. Respiratory Findings

   a. Lung function may be normal or there may be obstructive or restrictive disease.

   b. Bronchial hyperreactivity is described but suggests dysfunction rather than inflammation.

Tracheoesophageal Fistula

A. Definition

Esophageal atresia is a congenital anomaly in which the esophagus is segmented with a blind pouch separating the upper and lower portion. In most instances, there is also a fistula connecting the distal esophagus and trachea. There are several types of tracheoesophageal deformities. The three main types include esophageal atresia with distal tracheoesophageal fistula (TEF), isolated esophageal atresia, and TEF without esophageal atresia (H-type). The most common type is esophageal atresia with distal TEF (Abel et al., 2012; Keckler & Schropp, 2010).

B. Pathophysiology

The esophagus and trachea develop embryologically at the same time. The development of the esophagus and trachea is believed to occur by the proliferation of endodermal cells on the lateral walls of the diverticulum.

These cell masses become ridges of tissue that divide the foregut into two separate channels forming the esophagus and trachea. This process is completed by 36 days after fertilization. During the fourth week of fetal life, interruptions in development may result in abnormalities of the esophagus with and without fistula formation between the two structures (Abel et al., 2012; Keckler & Schropp, 2010).

C. Clinical Presentation

1. Maternal history of polyhydramnios is common.

2. The infant typically presents with regurgitation of saliva. The diagnosis is made by careful placement of a nasogastric (NG) tube into the blind pouch. A simple chest radiograph reveals a curled tube in the proximal esophageal pouch.

3. An infant with an H-type TEF usually presents at 3 to 4 months of age with a history of respiratory distress, pneumonia, and some degree of cyanosis with feedings.

4. Direct bronchoscopic visualization is the diagnostic study of choice (Abel et al., 2012; Keckler & Schropp, 2010).

D. Patient Care Management

1. Preoperative stabilization is essential.

2. After repair, the infant may require ventilatory support. The infant may require neuromuscular blockade and prolonged mechanical ventilation if there is concern that the anastomosis is under tension.

3. Oropharyngeal or nasopharyngeal suctioning is performed with a suction catheter that is marked at the time of surgery to avoid the anastomosis site.

4. An extrapleural chest tube and drain are placed at the time of surgery; an assessment of the color and consistency of the drainage is important. The presence of mucus in the collecting chamber may indicate a leak at the site of anastomosis.

5. Gastric decompression is essential with either an NG or gastrostomy tube. Often, an NG tube will remain in place for an extended period of time to stent the surgical site.

6. Successful transition from NG/gastrostomy tube (G-tube) feedings to oral feedings takes several weeks and may require assessment and support from speech therapy (Abel et al, 2012; Keckler & Schropp, 2010).

E. Outcomes

1. Survival rate is more than 95%.

2. The most significant complication is stricture or recurrent fistula formation.

3. Infants have persistent respiratory symptoms in 50% of cases. Complications range from apnea and bradycardia to aspiration, recurrent pneumonia, and even respiratory arrest.

4. The largest single cause of persistent respiratory disease is gastroesophageal reflux. This is treated both medically and surgically (Abel et al., 2012; Keckler & Schropp, 2010).

Choanal Atresia

A. Definition

Choanal atresia is the most common cause of true nasal obstruction. It occurs in approximately one in 10,000 live births. It can be unilateral or bilateral, isolated or associated with other congenital abnormalities. Unilateral choanal atresia is twice as common as bilateral choanal atresia (Greenough, Murthy, & Milner, 2012; Keckler & Schropp, 2010).

B. Pathophysiology

The exact embryologic malformation causing choanal atresia is unknown; however, certain theories now point to a failure of mesodermal flow to reach preordained positions in the facial process. Any abnormalities in this flow would affect the normal penetration of the nasal pits and the thinning that allows breakthrough at the anterior choana (Greenough et al., 2012; Keckler & Schropp, 2010).

C. Clinical Presentation

1. The clinical presentation may be severe, with immediate respiratory distress that requires intubation or an oral airway.

2. Infants with unilateral choanal atresia may be asymptomatic until the nonaffected nare becomes blocked with secretions. Infants with bilateral choanal atresia classically appear normal when crying and mouth breathing, but respiratory difficulty appears as soon as they try to breathe through the nose.

3. Can be diagnosed on CT, but MRI should also be employed to determine whether there are intracranial connections (Greenough et al., 2012; Keckler & Schropp, 2010).

D. Patient Care Management

1. Nasal causes of obstruction are relieved by an oral airway.

2. Surgical intervention includes opening the bony membrane that is blocking the airway and inserting tubes to maintain the airway; these are sutured in place for at least 4 weeks (Greenough et al., 2012; Keckler & Schropp, 2010).

E. Outcomes

1. The prognosis following reconstruction is excellent and generally without complication; the most significant complication is restenosis of the choanae. This is managed by repeated dilatations of the choanae.

2. Rarely, tracheostomy or long-term intubation may be required when choanal atresia is complicated by reconstructive maneuvers for other craniofacial abnormalities (Greenough et al., 2012; Keckler & Schropp, 2010).

Tracheomalacia

A. Definition

1. An abnormal collapse of the trachea due to localized or generalized weakness of the tracheal wall leading to respiratory obstruction

2. Commonly acquired as a complication of intubation of premature infants

3. Occurs in primary and secondary forms and either form can be congenital

4. *Primary.* An intrinsic abnormality of the tracheal wall

5. *Secondary.* Extrinsic compression of the tracheal wall.

6. *Congenital.* Usually associated with cardiovascular abnormalities, which may include double aortic arch, anomalous innominate artery, and pulmonary artery sling

    a. May also be associated with bronchomalacia and with other tracheal abnormalities such as TEF or laryngeal cleft.

B. Clinical Presentation

1. Clinical manifestations are variable and diagnosis is only reliably made by endoscopy.

2. There is likely to be stridor, which is usually expiratory because the obstruction is predominately intrathoracic.

3. There are usually recurrent episodes of stridor and dyspnea during which the child may become cyanosed and moribund. Such spells may be precipitated by severe crying, coughing, or feeding.

4. Symptoms are usually present in the immediate neonatal period but may deteriorate during the first or second year of life.

C. Patient Care Management

1. The condition is generally self-limiting and, if mild, requires no active treatment.

2. If severe, it is important to carefully monitor and document episodes that may represent airway collapse. Agitation and attempts by the infant to forcefully exhale cause airway collapse and complicate management, sedation and muscle relaxation may be indicated in some patients undergoing mechanical ventilation. Unexplained periods of increased respiratory distress and arterial desaturation are noteworthy, especially in an infant on long-term mechanical ventilation.

3. Family should be taught CPR, especially if the episodes are severe.

4. In more severe cases, active treatment may be considered, including surgery for abnormal vasculature (vascular ring), aortopexy, tracheostomy, CPAP (through facemask, nasal mask, or tracheostomy), segmental resection, internal stents, and/or cartilage grafting.

5. Bronchodilators may worsen tracheomalacia in some infants and children and should be used with caution.

D. Outcomes

Generally, children outgrow the condition by 1 to 2 years of age (Greenough et al., 2012; Keckler & Schropp, 2010).

Tracheal Stenosis

A. Definition

A rare but potentially life-threatening disorder that often leads to severe respiratory insufficiency. In most cases, stenotic lesions are composed of complete tracheal rings of cartilage. The severity of symptoms correlates with the length of affected trachea, the presence of concomitant respiratory conditions, degree of luminal narrowing, and any bronchial involvement.

B. Pathophysiology

1. Tracheal stenosis is characterized by narrowing of the tracheal lumen. The anomaly has three distinct types: generalized hypoplasia (the entire length of the trachea is narrowed), funnel-like stenosis (subglottic tracheal diameter is of normal caliber; however, the trachea narrows more distally), and subsegmental stenosis (a short segment of trachea is narrowed in an hourglass fashion).

2. Tracheal stenosis is often associated with abnormal bronchial branching patterns.

3. Frequently associated with other cardiovascular and extrathoracic anomalies.

C. Clinical Presentation

1. Tracheal stenosis presents clinically with a wide variety of symptoms. The severity of airway symptoms generally corresponds with the degree of airway obstruction.

2. *Minimal Symptoms.* Tracheal stenosis may be diagnosed incidentally or during a workup for biphasic wheeze. Children/adolescents might not be diagnosed until they develop exercise-associated respiratory difficulties.

3. *Symptomatic Neonate.* This group of patients develops respiratory distress within the first few hours of life. Presenting symptoms include stridor, cyanotic spells, and coarse cough. Assisted ventilation is often required.

4. *Symptomatic Infant.* Tracheal stenosis usually presents with respiratory symptoms near the end of the first year of life when physical activity increases or in the face of a respiratory illness. Symptoms of airflow limitation, wheeze, exertional shortness of breath, and increased WOB become apparent.

D. Patient Care Management

1. A subset of infants will outgrow their tracheal stenosis, but surgical intervention is often inevitable for symptomatic patients.

2. Treatment requires a multidisciplinary team.

3. Surgical options include resection and primary anastomosis, rib cartilage tracheoplasty, peridcardial

patch tracheoplasty, and slide tracheoplasty. Slide tracheoplasty is recognized as the procedure of choice.

4. There is no established protocol for postoperative management.

5. Major postoperative complications include anastomotic breakdown with subsequent air leak, tracheal narrowing secondary to excessive granulation tissue formation, or restenosis at the suture line.

E. Outcomes

Any child presenting with the symptom of airway narrowing should undergo evaluation with direct laryngoscopy and bronchoscopy after discharge (Abel et al., 2012; Hofferberth, Watters, Rahbar, & Fynn-Thompson, 2015, 2016; Walsh & Vehse, 2010).

UPPER AIRWAY INFECTIONS

Acute Epiglottitis

A. Definition

1. Acute epiglottitis is a severe life-threatening medical emergency. It is a rapidly progressive infection of the epiglottis and surrounding area (Figure 2.15).

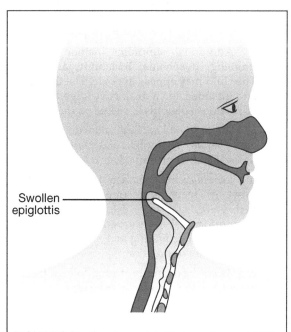

Swollen epiglottis

FIGURE 2.15 Swollen epiglottis in acute epiglottitis.

2. It is a serious obstructive inflammatory process that occurs primarily in children 2 to 5 years old but can occur from infancy to adulthood (Conlon, 2013).

3. The obstruction is supraglottic as opposed to subglottic obstruction of laryngitis.

4. The responsible organism is usually *Haemophilus influenzae* type b (Hib) although other infectious organisms include *Streptococcus pyogenes, Streptococcus pneumoniae,* or *Staphylococcus aureus.*

B. Pathophysiology

Thickened epiglottis and aryepiglottic folds lead to narrowing of the airway and turbulent gas flow. Pulmonary edema may occur from an increased transmural pressure gradient from pulmonary vasoconstriction resulting from alveolar hypoxia as well as the negative pleural pressure generated against the airway obstruction (Conlon, 2013).

C. Clinical Presentation

1. *History* usually reveals acute onset of symptoms, including high fever, sore throat, dyspnea, and rapidly progressing respiratory obstruction. The child may go to bed asymptomatic to awaken later with symptoms. The child usually appears sicker than clinical findings suggest.

2. *Physical Examination*

    a. The child often insists upon sitting upright and leaning forward with the chin thrust out, mouth open, and tongue protruding (tripod position).

    b. Additional symptoms include dysphagia, drooling, dysphonia, irritability, and anxiety. The child may appear hypoxic. The throat is red and inflamed and a distinctive large, cherry-red, edematous epiglottis is visible on throat exam.

    c. Throat should not be examined without emergency airway equipment and high-level personnel available for an immediate difficult intubation.

    d. *Presentation* is characterized by an abrupt onset of fever, sore throat, drooling, muffled voice, and hyperextension of the neck. Respiratory distress is usually mild to moderate. Stridor is a late finding and suggests near-complete airway obstruction.

    e. *Assess* the degree of stridor, color, retractions, air entry, and level of consciousness.

3. *Diagnostic Tests*

    a. If *epiglottitis* is suspected, invasive or anxiety-provoking procedures should be avoided.

Also avoid direct oral cavity examination because depression of the tongue could force the enlarged epiglottis over the laryngeal opening and agitate the patient.

    b. An anterior–posterior (AP) radiograph of the neck may not reveal a swollen epiglottis. A lateral neck radiographic examination, however, is diagnostic and is always indicated in the presence of upper airway lesions.

    c. Obtain blood cultures to identify the organism after airway control is established.

4. *Clinical Course.* Acute infection usually resolves in 24 to 72 hours with antibiotics; most patients have concomitant bacteremia.

5. *Differential Diagnosis.* Distinguish epiglottis from laryngotracheobronchitis by presentation, lateral neck radiographic examination, or direct visualization in the operating room (Table 2.11; Conlon, 2013).

D. Patient Care Management

1. *Prevention.* The Hib vaccine has significantly reduced the incidence of this disease in children and therefore is strongly recommended for infants.

2. *Direct Care.* If epiglottitis is strongly suspected, the patient should be taken directly to the operating room for direct laryngoscopy and subsequent intubation. Before endotracheal intubation or tracheotomy is performed, keep the child comfortable and disturb him or her as little as possible. Allow the patient to maintain a comfortable position. Supplemental oxygen can be administered while the child is sitting in a parent's lap. Ceftriaxone, cefotaxime, or a combination of ampicillin and sulbactam should be given parenterally, pending culture and susceptibility reports. Antibiotics should be continued for 7 to 10 days. The use of corticosteroids for reducing edema may be beneficial during the early treatment phase.

3. *Supportive Care.* This includes admission to the PICU for close monitoring. Use sedation and arm restraints or muscle relaxants to prevent self-extubation, and decrease movement of the ETT in the larynx. Deliver oxygen as necessary. Monitor closely for postobstructive pulmonary edema. Criteria for extubation may include air leak around the artificial airway or direct examination of the epiglottis. Extubation is performed in the PICU or operating room with intubation and emergency tracheostomy equipment available.

TABLE 2.11   Diagnostic Features of Infectious Causes of Stridor

Diagnostic Factors	Acute Laryngotracheobronchitis	Acute Epiglottitis	Acute Bacterial Tracheitis	Acute Spasmodic Laryngitis
Age range	3 mo–3 y	2–6 y	2–4 y	1–3 y
Etiology	Viral	Bacterial	Bacterial	Viral with allergic component
Pathology	Inflammation of subglottic region, trachea, bronchi, bronchioles	Inflammation of epiglottis, aryepiglottic folds, and surrounding tissue	Acute infectious process in the trachea	Signs of inflammation are absent or mild
Onset	Gradual	Acute	Variable	Gradual
Signs and symptoms	Hoarseness Barking cough Stridor	High fever Drooling Dysphagia Dysphonia Distress Inspiratory stridor Sniffing position	High fever Inspiratory stridor Drooling May mimic epiglottitis	Recurrent paroxsymal attacks of laryngeal obstruction that occur chiefly at night
Diagnosis	History and physical examination	History and physical examination Swollen supraglottis on direct visualization	Thick purulent secretions	History and physical examination
Radiographic signs	Subglottic narrowing "steeple sign"	Increased epiglottic shadow on lateral neck x-ray examination	Subglottic irregularity; "steeple sign" may be present	Usually not performed
Treatment	Mist hydration Racemic epinephrine Steroids	Antibiotics Airway management with endotracheal tube	Antibiotics Airway control	Usually managed at home with cool-mist humidity
Course	Obstructive signs decrease over a period of 3–4 d	Improvement 36–48 hr after antibiotics are initiated	Improvement 36–48 hr after antibiotics are initiated May require tracheostomy	Usually a quick recovery within 12–24 hr

Source: Conlon, P. (2013). The child with respiratory dysfunction. In M. Hockenberry & D. Wilson (Eds.), *Wong's essentials of pediatric nursing* (9th ed., pp. 706–761). St. Louis, MO: Elsevier.

4. *Complications.* Intubation has been reported to have fewer complications than tracheostomy. These include self-extubation and obstruction from secretions. Patients who undergo intubation rather than tracheostomy have shorter periods of artificial airway support and hospitalization.

5. *Outcome.* Given appropriate management of the airway during the initial stabilization, there should be no long-term sequelae for this disease (Conlon, 2013).

Acute Laryngotracheobronchitis

A. Definition

1. Acute laryngotracheaobronchitis (LTB) is an inflammatory swelling of the submucosa in the subglottic area. *Croup* is a general medical term that refers to this inflammatory process, which results in stridor, cough, and hoarseness (Conlon, 2013).

2. LTB is the most common croup syndrome.

3. LTB primarily affects children younger than 5 years of age and peaks between 9 and 18 months of age. There is a tendency for LTB to recur in children who have had one episode. LTB can be either viral or bacterial in origin and is usually preceded by an upper respiratory infection. Viral LTB accounts for 85% of reported cases. The parainfluenza viruses (types 1, 2, and 3) account for about 75% of cases; other viruses associated with this disease include influenza A and B, adenovirus, and RSV. Nonviral LTB may result from asthma, angioneurotic edema, foreign-body aspiration, or subglottic stenosis following endotracheal intubation (Conlon, 2013).

B. Pathophysiology

The term *laryngotracheobronchitis* refers to a viral infection of the glottic and subglottic regions. In children, the cricoid cartilage makes up the narrowest segment of the upper airway. Swelling and secretions in this subglottic region increase resistance to airflow, leading to respiratory distress (Figure 2.16).

C. Clinical Presentation

1. *History.* Following an upper respiratory infection, LTB has a gradual onset of symptoms, which include rhinorrhea, coryza, and low-grade fever. Symptoms vary over several days, with stridor worsening at night. Parents may report that the child went to bed and later awoke with a barky, brassy cough.

2. *Physical Examination.* Clinical manifestations are produced by subglottic obstruction. Clinical

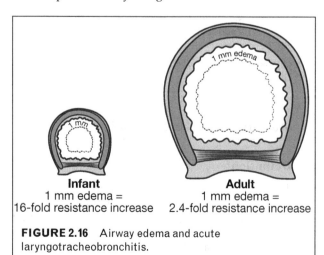

FIGURE 2.16 Airway edema and acute laryngotracheobronchitis.

Infant
1 mm edema =
16-fold resistance increase

Adult
1 mm edema =
2.4-fold resistance increase

signs of respiratory failure are predictive of severity. The onset of LTB is noted by the development of a barking cough and hoarseness. The patient may also demonstrate inspiratory stridor and thin, copious secretions. The degree of nasal flaring, tracheal tugging, and retraction of the chest muscles depends on the degree of airway resistance. The larynx is nontender on palpation. A low (rather than high) fever helps to differentiate LTB from bacterial tracheitis and epiglottitis. Normal alveolar gas exchange and low oxygen saturation are seen only when complete airway obstruction is imminent.

3. *Diagnostic Tests.* An AP chest radiograph demonstrates a funnel-shaped narrowing of the glottis and subglottic airway ("steeple sign"). A lateral radiograph of the neck demonstrates a normal epiglottis. Radiographs should be considered only after airway stabilization.

4. *Clinical Course.* Monitor closely for cyanosis, pallor, weakness, or other signs of hypoxemia. Hypoxemia, hypercarbia, tachycardia, and respiratory acidosis may develop if obstruction is severe.

5. *Differential Diagnosis.* See Table 2.11 for comparison of LTB, epiglottitis, bacterial tracheitis, and acute spasmodic laryngitis.

D. Patient Care Management

1. *Direct Care*

    a. The most important nursing function in the care of children with LTB is continuous, vigilant observation and accurate assessment of respiratory status.

    b. Although rare, intubation may be necessary for increased WOB, pallor, cyanosis, decreased level of consciousness, worsening hypoxemia or hypercarbia, or respiratory distress unresponsive to treatment. Intubation is necessary if respiratory distress is refractory to medical intervention. Development of an air leak can indicate readiness for extubation. The trend away from early intubation of children with LTB emphasizes the importance of nursing observations and the ability to recognize impending respiratory failure.

    c. Racemic epinephrine produces topical mucosal vasoconstriction of the precapillary arterioles, thereby reducing mucosal edema. Indications include moderate-to-severe stridor that does not respond to cool mist. Racemic epinephrine can be very effective; however, rebound swelling may occur after the effects wear off.

d. Oral steroids are often given as a single dose of dexamethasone.

e. Antibiotics are not indicated.

f. A helium–oxygen gas mixture (heliox; 30% oxygen plus 70% helium) may be used for severe croup. The lower density provides less turbulent flow than oxygen alone, and it reduces the WOB by decreasing the resistance to turbulent gas flow through a narrowed airway. It is not recommended as a standard treatment of croup.

2. *Supportive Care*

a. Minimize disturbances and minimize anxiety.

b. Provide cool, humidified oxygen by face mask or through a tube held in front of the patient by the parent. Use humidification and adequate hydration to liquefy secretions. Control fever using antipyretics. Administer IV fluids to ensure adequate hydration. Once epiglottitis and bacterial tracheitis have been ruled out, antibiotic therapy is not needed.

c. Children with mild croup are allowed to drink as long as their respiratory status is stable.

d. Parents are encouraged to try whatever comforting measures work best for the child.

3. *Complications.* Intubation should be performed by a skilled practitioner to limit complications of intubation. ETT size should be 0.5 to 1 mm smaller than that predicted for the patient's age to aid in passing through the narrowed airway and avoid exacerbating subglottic inflammation.

E. Outcomes

Children with mild croup (no stridor at rest) can be managed at home. Parents are taught the signs of respiratory distress and instructed to summon professional help early if needed. Children with labored respirations and stridor or other respiratory symptoms should receive medical attention. Home care includes monitoring for worsening symptoms, continued humidity, adequate hydration, and nourishment (Conlon, 2013; Petrocheilou et al., 2014).

Acute Spasmodic Laryngitis

Acute spasmodic laryngitis is distinct from laryngitis and LTB and is characterized by recurrent paroxysmal attacks of laryngeal obstruction that occur chiefly at night. Signs of inflammation are absent or mild, and it is followed by an uneventful recovery. The child feels well the next day. Some children appear to be predisposed to the condition; allergies or hypersensitivities may be implicated in some cases. Management is the same as for infectious croup (Conlon, 2013).

Bacterial Tracheitis

A. Definition

1. Bacterial tracheitis is an infection of the mucosa of the upper trachea. It is a distinct entity with features of both croup and epiglottitis.

2. It usually occurs in children younger than 3 years and may cause airway obstruction that is severe enough to cause respiratory arrest.

3. It is a rare illness, but is the most common potentially life-threatening upper airway infection in children (Conlon, 2013).

B. Pathophysiology

1. Bacterial tracheitis is thought to be a complication of LTB and although *S. aureus* is the most frequent organism responsible, *Moraxella catarrhalis*, *S. pneumoniae*, and *H. influenzae* have been implicated. Complete airway obstruction may occur as a result of copious, mucopurulent secretions.

2. There is marked subglottic edema with ulceration, erythema, and pseudomembraneous formation on the tracheal surface, and thick mucopurulent tracheal secretions.

3. The epiglottis and arytenoids are usually normal in appearance although epiglottis and bacterial tracheitis may coexist (Balfour-Lynn & Davies, 2012).

C. Clinical Presentation

1. *History.* Patients may present with symptoms resembling LTB or epiglottitis. Patients typically have a prodrome of symptoms consistent with viral upper respiratory tract infection such as rhinorrhea, low-grade fever, cough, sore throat, and hoarse voice.

2. *Physical Examination.* Patients typically become rapidly more symptomatic with respiratory distress, increased WOB, airway compromise, higher fever, and toxic appearance.

3. *Diagnostic Tests*

   a. Bacterial tracheitis should be diagnosed by direct visualization with *bronchoscopy with bronchial alveolar lavage*.

   b. Obtain *blood cultures* to identify the organism after airway control is established.

   c. A lateral neck x-ray shows subglottic swelling.

4. *Clinical Course*

   a. Many patients require intubation and mechanical ventilation for 3 to 7 days.

   b. Frequent tracheal suction is necessary.

   c. The decision to extubate is based on clinical improvement with reduction of fever, decreased airway secretions, and the development of an air leak around the ETT.

D. Patient Care Management

1. Management is focused on the maintenance of a patent airway and treatment of blood pressure instability.

2. Initially IV broad-spectrum antibiotics are administered and refined once cultures and sensitivities are known. Antibiotics are usually given for 10 to 14 days.

3. Corticosteroids may be given before extubation.

4. Patients may require tracheostomy but this occurs much less often than previously reported (Balfour-Lynn & Davies, 2012; Conlon, 2013).

E. Outcomes

The mortality rates for bacterial tracheitis are as high as 18% to 40%. There is also significant morbidity associated with bacterial tracheitis and may include respiratory and cardiopulmonary arrest, respiratory failure, pneumonia, septic shock, toxic shock syndrome, ARDS, and multiple organ dysfunction syndrome.

LOWER AIRWAY INFECTIONS

Bronchitis

A. Definition

Bronchitis is defined as a nonspecific inflammation of the bronchioles and can be classified as acute or chronic.

B. Pathophysiology

1. Acute bronchitis is usually associated with a viral illness, most commonly parainfluenza, RSV, and rhinovirus. Inflammation of the large airways leads to destruction of the ciliated epithelium. A secondary bacterial infection can also develop due to the weakened tissue.

2. Chronic bronchitis symptoms last longer than 2 weeks and are usually a symptom of another condition.

C. Clinical Presentation

1. The initial phase includes upper respiratory symptoms.

2. Includes a dry, brassy cough that may or may not be productive.

3. Coarse breath sounds or rhonchi may be heard on lung exam.

D. Patient Care Management

1. For acute bronchitis, care is primarily supportive, including analgesia, hydration, antivirals, antibiotics, cough suppressants, and bronchodilators.

2. Complications of pneumonia, rhinosinusitis, or otitis can occur in chronically ill or undernourished children.

3. Treatment of chronic bronchitis depends on the underlying cause.

E. Outcomes

Malaise may continue for another week after the cough lessens (Camerda & Goodman, 2011; Conlon, 2013).

Bronchiolitis

A. Definition

Bronchiolitis is an acute inflammatory disease of the lower respiratory tract that results in the obstruction of small airways.

B. Pathophysiology

1. Viral replication in the epithelial cells of the airways results in direct injury of the respiratory epithelium. Abnormal secretions combined with edema of the submucosal layer cause obstruction of the small airways and diffusion impairment. Multiple areas of atelectasis produce ventilation–perfusion mismatching and abnormal gas exchange.

2. The principal abnormality in gas exchange is hypoxemia. Most infants are able to maintain normocarbia despite ventilation–perfusion mismatch by increasing their respiratory rate. Hypercarbia and respiratory failure develop when the infant becomes fatigued and V_E falls.

C. Etiology

1. Bronchiolitis is predominantly caused by RSV, accounting for 60% to 85% of cases (Da Dalt, Bressan, Martinolli, Perilongo, & Baraldi, 2013). Recent data suggest that up to 30% of infants with severe bronchiolitis are coinfected by two or more viruses (Mansbach et al., 2012). Causes after RSV include rhinovirus, parainfluenza, adenovirus, and mycoplasma. RSV and adenovirus can cause long-term complications.

2. Infants who are at risk of severe RSV include children with major chronic pulmonary disease, such as CF, neuromuscular disorders, BPD, prematurity, immunodeficiency, and congenital heart disease. More severe disease is also seen in boys, infants who were not breastfed, and those of lower socioeconomic status.

3. Bronchiolitis most commonly occurs during winter and early spring.

D. Clinical Presentation

1. *History.* Generally, there is a 3- to 7-day history of upper respiratory tract infection with fever and known exposure. Fever is usually present; however, temperatures are generally lower than in bacterial pneumonia.

2. *Physical Examination.* Will demonstrate cough, sneezing, rhinorrhea, and respiratory distress with tachypnea, retractions, wheezing, prolonged expiration, rales, and irritability. Infants may also present with poor feeding, low-grade fever, apnea, and cyanosis. Tachypnea is the most consistent clinical manifestation. Auscultation of the chest may reveal crackles and wheezing throughout the thoracic cavity.

3. *Diagnostic Tests*

   a. Diagnosis and severity of disease are based on history and physical examination.

   b. Radiographic or laboratory studies are not routinely recommended.

   c. Rapid viral antigen tests are available for many common viruses.

4. *Clinical Course.* Viral bronchiolitis generally has a clinical course of 7 to 10 days with peak symptoms at 48 to 72 hours. Severe cases may require mechanical ventilation for apnea, hypoxemia, or respiratory failure.

E. Patient Care Management

1. Most infants with mild signs of respiratory distress can be treated as outpatients with supportive measures.

2. Nasal suctioning to improve airway patency especially before feeding in infants can be beneficial.

3. NG feeding has proved a safe alternative to IV fluid administration in children with bronchiolitis.

4. Apnea may occur and requires mechanical ventilation.

5. Heated, humidified, high-flow oxygen through a nasal cannula may be used in the inpatient management of bronchiolitis. The high flow delivers positive airway pressure to keep the alveoli open and reduce ventilation–perfusion mismatch and small airway microatelectasis.

6. Hypertonic saline 3% should not be used in infants in the emergency room. Using hypertonic saline 3% in the emergency room does not reduce hospital admission rates (Da Dalt et al., 2013). May be used in hospitalized infants and children (Ralston et al., 2014).

7. Bronchodilators have proven ineffective in the treatment of bronchiolitis. A small portion of patients will respond to bronchodilators. If this therapy is used, the practitioner should auscultate before and after treatment for treatment to be effective.

8. Guidelines do not recommend the routine use of systemic corticosteroids, chest physiotherapy, and antibacterial medications. (Ralston et al., 2014).

F. Outcomes

Impaired oxygenation may continue for several weeks after apparent clinical recovery. Recurrent episodes of wheezing can be seen into childhood (Coates, Camerda, & Goodman, 2016; Da Dalt et al., 2013; Mansbach et al., 2012; Ralston, et al., 2014; Teshome, Gattu, & Brown, 2013).

Pneumonia

A. Definition and Etiology

1. Pneumonia is a lower respiratory tract infection that causes inflammation of the lung parenchyma that is typically associated with fever and respiratory symptoms.

2. Worldwide, pneumonia is the single largest cause of death in children under 5 years of age.

3. The most likely etiologic agent depends on the age of the patient, how the organism was acquired (community or nosocomial), and the presence of underlying disease.

    a. In neonates aged 0 to 3 months, maternal flora, such as group B *Streptococcus*, are common causes.

    b. In infants older than 3 months up to 5 years of age, over half of pneumonias are associated with viral respiratory infections.

    c. In school-age children older than 5 years, atypical organisms, such as *Mycoplasma pneumoniae* and *Chlamydophila pneumoniae*, are more common causes.

4. Children fully immunized against Hib and *S. pneumoniae* are less likely to be infected with these pathogens.

5. Compromised host defenses may predispose a patient to pneumonia, including the following:

    a. Bypass of nasal defenses from endotracheal intubation or tracheostomy

    b. Pulmonary aspiration from CNS injury or secondary to gastroesophageal reflux or tracheoesophageal fistula

    c. Abnormal airway secretion or mucociliary clearance from infections, BPD, or CF and in neurologically devastated patients

    d. Underlying chronic disease or poor nutrition

    e. Diseases that alter the immune system

    f. Secondary bacterial infection after influenza

B. Pathophysiology

1. Invading organisms initiate the inflammatory response, which then causes alveolar edema. The edema is a medium for the multiplication of organisms. An inflammatory process of the lungs may involve the interstitial tissue and pleura, leading to lung consolidation, reduced lung compliance, and decreased V_C and total lung capacity.

2. Mode of transmission of the organism is through inspiration of microorganisms, aspiration of oropharyngeal secretions, or systemic circulation. The location of the pneumonia on chest radiograph may help to differentiate the type of pneumonia. The neurologically devastated patient who has poor secretion control is at risk for developing aspiration pneumonia. Generally, *lobar pneumonia* involves one or more lobes of the lung and is observed with bacterial processes. *Bronchopneumonia* involves terminal bronchioles. *Interstitial pneumonia* involves the alveolar walls, producing a hazy, diffuse radiographic pattern characteristic of viral pneumonia.

C. Clinical Presentation

1. *History.* May include mild upper respiratory tract infection or sudden fever, cough, and chest pain. In infants, an upper respiratory tract infection and diminished appetite can lead to the abrupt onset of fever, restlessness, and respiratory distress. Examine for etiologic or precipitating factors.

2. *Physical Examination*

    a. Infants may present with lethargy, poor feeding, or irritability.

    b. Nasal flaring, grunting, retractions, tachypnea, and tachycardia represent respiratory distress. Cyanosis may be present.

    c. Lung exam is a key part of the assessment. Fine crackles, dullness, or diminished breath sounds may be heard. Findings consistent with consolidated lung parenchyma may include dullness to percussion, egophony, bronchophony, or tactile fremitus. Wheezing is more common in viral pneumonia than in bacterial pneumonia.

    d. Abdominal distention may be prominent because of gastric dilation from swallowed air.

    e. The liver may seem enlarged because of downward displacement of the diaphragm secondary to hyperinflation of the lungs.

    f. Signs of dehydration may be seen.

    g. In primary atypical pneumonia, patients may present with repetitive staccato cough with tachypnea, cervical adenopathy, crackles. Wheezing is rarely heard.

3. *Diagnostic Tests*

  a. *Radiographic imaging*

    i. In children with symptoms consistent with community acquired pneumonia, a chest radiograph is not routinely needed to make the diagnosis. A chest radiograph may be indicated in the following situations:

      1) Severe disease, hypoxemia, or significant respiratory distress that requires hospitalizations

      2) Inconclusive clinical findings

      3) To rule out other causes of respiratory distress such as heart disease or foreign body

      4) Failure to improve on adequate antibiotic coverage

      5) To include in workup for young infant with a fever and an unknown source and leukocytosis

    ii. Chest radiograph findings: The chest radiograph confirms the diagnosis of pneumonia and may indicate a complication such as a pleural effusion or empyema. Pneumonia can initially produce a patchy infiltration with fluffy margins. Later, bacterial pneumonia causes more segmental or lobar disease with more homogenous opacification of the involved area of the lung. Aspiration pneumonia usually develops in the portion of the lung that is dependent at the time of aspiration. Bronchopneumonia produces perihilar congestion from inflammation of terminal bronchioles. Pleural effusion may represent empyema, most often associated with bacterial infection.

    iii. Chest x-ray may lag behind clinical symptoms.

  b. *Laboratory testing*

    i. For children who may be hospitalized, a CBC with differential is usually done. Electrolytes to assess for dehydration may also be included.

    ii. Cultures of blood and sputum should be obtained in hospitalized children with severe disease or children not responding to empiric therapy. Sputum or tracheal secretions are of limited value and examined only to note the predominant flora and the presence of neutrophils. A tracheal aspirate from a newly intubated patient may be of some diagnostic value. Reliable reagents for the rapid detection of RSV, parainfluenza, influenza, adenovirus, and many other viruses are available and may be useful.

  c. *Invasive testing*

    i. Quantitative bronchoalveolar lavage (BAL) or protected brush specimen may be indicated to reduce some of the diagnostic confusion that may be created by sputum specimen contamination. However, BAL does not always recover the pathogens that produce pneumonia.

    ii. Lung biopsy may be indicated in the child with severe disease or in the immunosuppressed host. This will provide evaluation of lung tissue and a culture obtained under sterile setting to guide more definitive treatment.

4. *Clinical Course*

  a. The clinical course depends on the patient's age, the cause of pneumonia, and the clinical presentation. On occasion, extrapulmonary manifestations of bacterial pneumonia, such as dehydration and obtundation, result in patient admission to the ICU.

  b. Complications of pneumonia include lung abscess, necrotizing pneumonia, pneumatocele, empyema, pleural effusion, bronchopleural fistula, and pneumothorax.

D. Patient Care Management

1. *Prevention*

  a. Active and up-to-date immunizations against influenza, pertussis, Hib, and *S. pneumoniae*.

  b. Immunocompromised patients should receive scheduled trimethoprim–sulfamethoxazole (Septra) as prophylaxis against *Pneumocystis carinii* pneumonia.

  c. Identify and treat pregnant women with *Chlamydia trachomatis*.

2. *Direct Care*

  a. Patients are monitored for signs of increasing respiratory distress, cardiovascular compromise, and altered mental status.

  b. Oxygen delivery should maintain saturations of greater than 90%. Intubate and provide mechanical ventilation for respiratory failure.

3. *Supportive Care*

  a. If the patient is dehydrated, a fluid bolus of 10 to 20 mL/kg is administered. Hydration maintenance can be achieved with IV fluids. If the course is prolonged, enteral feedings are initiated.

b. Antimicrobials are administered for age group and suspected organism. Duration of antimicrobial therapy in based on patient status, causative organism, and severity. Treatment of nosocomial pneumonia involves the use of antimicrobial agents directed at the identified pathogen or, if it is unknown, at the most likely etiologic agent based on the clinical setting and available diagnostic information.

c. Children who fail to improve after 48 to 72 hours of antibiotic coverage should undergo further investigation.

E. Outcomes

1. Respiratory complications of pneumonia include pleural effusion, empyema, pneumatocele, necrotizing pneumonia, lung abscess, bronchopleural fistula, and pneumothorax (Gereige & Laufer, 2013).

2. Most children will make an uneventful recovery. Children with recurrent pneumonia should be referred for pulmonary evaluation (Bradley et al., 2011, Conlon, 2013; Gereige & Laufer, 2013; Kelly & Sandora, 2016; Newman et al., 2012).

OTHER INFECTIONS OF THE RESPIRATORY TRACT

Pertussis

A. Definition

1. Pertussis, or "whooping cough" is an acute respiratory tract infection caused by *Bordetella pertussis* and may also be caused by *Bordetella parapertussis*.

2. Highly contagious and particularly threatening in young infants.

3. Pertussis can result in encephalopathy, seizures, and pneumonia.

4. Incidence is highest in the spring and summer months.

5. A single attack confers lifetime immunity.

B. Pathophysiology

1. The organism is transmitted by aerosol droplets from infected to susceptible humans. After transmission, adhesion of the bacteria to ciliated cells of the upper and lower respiratory tract establishes colonization, followed by multiplication and spread on the epithelium, local mucosal damage, and finally induction of respiratory symptoms.

2. Invasiveness is extremely rare.

3. The precise mechanisms during infection are unknown.

4. The pathology of pertussis causes inflammation, congestion, and infiltration of the respiratory mucosa with lymphocytes and granulocytes and leads to accumulation of viscous secretions in the lumen of the bronchi, bronchial obstruction, and occasional atelectasis.

C. Clinical Presentation

1. *Catarrhal Stage.* Begins with symptoms of an upper respiratory tract infection, including coryza, sneezing, lacrimation, cough, and low-grade fever. Symptoms continue for 1 to 2 weeks when dry hacking cough becomes more severe.

2. *Paroxysmal Stage.* Coughing is the most prevalent symptom. The cough is most common at night and consists of short, rapid coughs followed by sudden inspiration associated with a high-pitched crowing sound or "whoop." During paroxysms, cheeks become flushed or cyanotic, eyes bulge, and tongue protrudes. Paroxysm may continue until thick mucus plug is dislodged. Vomiting frequently follows an attack. This stage generally lasts 4 to 6 weeks and is followed by a convalescent stage.

3. Infants younger than 6 months may not have the characteristic whoop cough but may have difficulty maintaining adequate oxygenation with the amount of secretions.

D. Patient Care Management

1. Most children can be managed at home with supportive care, but admission to the hospital can occur (severe respiratory symptoms and/or apnea).

2. Preventive care includes encouraging immunization and antibiotic therapy (erythromycin, azithromycin, and clarithromycin).

3. Supportive care includes hospitalization, increased oxygen intake and humidity, adequate fluids, and intensive care management and mechanical ventilation if needed for infants younger than 6 months of age.

4. Complications include pneumonia, apnea (infants <1 year of age), atelectasis, PH (critical pertussis), otitis media, seizures, hemorrhage (scleral, conjunctival, epistaxis, and pulmonary hemorrhage), weight loss and dehydration, hernias, prolapsed rectum, syncope, sleep disturbance, rib fractures, and incontinence.

5. If hospitalized, nursing management should include the following:

   a. Maintain isolation with droplet precautions.

   b. Obtain nasopharyngeal culture for diagnosis.

   c. Encourage oral fluids; offer small amounts frequently.

   d. Ensure adequate oxygenation during paroxysms; position infant on side to decrease chance of aspiration with vomiting.

   e. Provided humidified oxygen; suction as needed to prevent choking on secretions.

   f. Observe for signs of airway obstruction (increased restlessness, apprehension, retractions, cyanosis).

   g. Rarely, infants progress to needing ECMO.

   h. Household contacts should be treated with prophylactic antibiotics. Nursing should encourage compliance.

   i. Nursing should encourage all patients to obtain pertussis vaccination.

   j. Nursing should also encourage healthcare workers, pregnant women, and all contacts with infants (babysitters/grandparents) to receive pertussis boosters.

E. Outcomes

1. Pertussis symptoms usually last for 6 to 10 weeks but may persist for longer.

2. Mortality rates are high in children younger than 6 months of age (Berger et al., 2013; Cherry, 2013; Conlon, 2013; Lopez, Crus, Kowalski, & Raphael, 2014).

TUBERCULOSIS

A. Definition

1. TB is the second leading cause of death from an infectious disease. Ten to 15 million people in the United States are infected with TB.

2. Case rates of TB for all ages are higher in urban, low-income areas among non-White racial and ethnic groups.

3. TB is caused by *Mycobacterium tuberculosis*, an acid-fast bacillus. Children are susceptible to the human (*M. tuberculosis*) and the bovine (*Mycobacterium bovis*) organisms.

4. The source of TB infection in children is usually an infected member of the household or frequent visitor to the home. The airway is the usual portal of entry for the organism.

B. Pathophysiology

1. Transmission is usually person to person and occurs via inhalation of mucus droplets that become airborne when an infected individual coughs, sneezes, speaks, laughs, or sings. After drying, the droplet nuclei can remain suspended in the air for hours. Only small droplets can reach alveoli. Droplet nuclei also can be produced by aerosol treatments, sputum induction, aerosolization during bronchoscopy, and through manipulation of lesions or processing of tissue or secretions in the hospital or laboratory.

2. After inhaling *M. tuberculosis*, the majority of children do not develop disease but rather develop latent TB infection. These children have a positive TB skin test and clinical or radiographic evidence of TB disease. In a portion of children, infection results in pathologic changes and associated clinical disease.

3. Following infection, all children progress through an asymptomatic incubation period generally lasting 3 to 8 weeks. The subsequent development of clinical disease is determined by the interaction of the host and the organism and is highly age dependent. Younger children (younger than 2 years) are at greatest risk for both the development of disease and severe manifestations of disease. After the age of 10 years, children are more likely to manifest adult-type disease.

C. Clinical Presentation

May be asymptomatic or produce a broad range of symptoms, including fever, malaise, anorexia, weight loss, cough (may or may not be present; progresses slowly over weeks to months), aching pain and chest tightness, and/or hemoptysis. Symptoms occur with progression, including increased respiratory rate, poor expansion of the lung on the affected side, diminished breath sounds and crackles, dullness to percussion, persistent fever, generalized symptoms, pallor, anemia, weakness, and weight loss.

D. Patient Care Management

1. Diagnosis is based on the information derived from physical examination, history, tuberculin skin testing, blood testing, radiographic examinations, and cultures of the organism.

2. The TST is the most important indicator of whether a child has been infected with the tubercle bacillus. A positive reaction indicates that the individual has been infected and has developed sensitivity to the bacillus. The test is usually positive 2 to 10 weeks after initial infection. It does not confirm the presence of active disease.

3. The term *latent tuberculosis infection (LTBI)* is used to indicate infection in a person with a positive TST, no physical findings of disease, and normal chest radiograph findings. Most children are asymptomatic when a positive skin test is found and most of them do not go on to develop the disease.

4. The terms *TB disease* or *clinically active TB* are used with a child who has clinical symptoms or radiographic manifestations caused by the organism.

5. Medical management of LTBI disease in children and adolescents consists of adequate nutrition, pharmacotherapy, prevention of unnecessary exposure to other infections that further compromise the body's defenses, and sometimes surgical procedures.

6. For the child with clinically active TB, the goal is to achieve sterilization of the TB lesion. Anti-TB drugs kill or inhibit multiplication of *M. tuberculosis* organisms, thereby arresting progression of infection and preventing most complications. For treatment of disease, these drugs must always be used in recommended combination and dosage to minimize emergence of drug-resistant strains. Use of nonstandard regimens for any reason should be undertaken only in consultation with an expert in treating TB. Commonly used drugs for treatment of TB include ethambutol, isoniazid, pyrazinamide, and rifampin. Treatment for drug-resistant TB may include amikacin, capreomycin, cycloserine, ethionamide, kanamycin, levofloxacin, para-aminosalicylic acid, and/or streptomycin.

7. The goal of treatment is to achieve killing of replicating organisms in the TB lesion in the shortest possible time. Achievement of this goal minimizes the possibility of resistant organisms. The major problem limiting successful treatment is poor adherence to prescribed treatment regimens. The use of direct observation of therapy (DOT) decreases the rates of relapse, treatment failures, and drug resistance; therefore, DOT is recommended strongly for treatment of all children and adolescents with TB disease in the United States.

8. For TB disease, a 6-month, four-drug regimen consisting of rifampin, isoniazid, pyrazinamide, and ethambutol for the first 2 months and isoniazid and rifampin for the remaining 4 months is recommended for the treatment of pulmonary disease, pulmonary disease with hilar adenopathy, and hilar adenopathy disease of infants, children, and adolescents when a multidrug-resistant strain is not suspected. In the 6-month regimen with four-drug therapy, rifampin, isoniazid, pyrazinamide, and ethambutol are given once a day for at least the first 2 weeks by DOT. An alternative to daily dosing between 2 weeks and 2 months of treatment is to give these drugs twice or three times a week by DOT. After the initial 2-month period, a DOT regimen of isoniazid and rifampin given two or three times per week is acceptable.

9. Surgical procedures may be required to remove the source of infection in tissues that are inaccessible to pharmacotherapy or that are destroyed by disease. Orthopedic procedures may be performed for correction of bone deformities, and bronchoscopy may be done for removal of a tuberculous granulomatous polyp.

10. Children with TB receive their care in ambulatory settings, outpatient departments, schools, and public health settings. Most children are not contagious and require only standard precautions. Children with no cough and negative sputum smears can be hospitalized in a regular patient room. However, airborne precautions and a negative pressure room are required for children who are contagious and hospitalized with active TB disease. Infection control for hospital personnel in contagious cases should include the use of a personally fitted air-purifying N95 or N100 respirator.

E. Outcomes

1. Most children recover from primary TB infection and are unaware of its presence. However, very young children have a higher incidence of disseminated disease.

2. TB is a very serious disease during the first 2 years of life, during adolescence, and in children who are HIV positive. Except in cases of TB meningitis, death seldom occurs. Antibiotic therapy has decreased the death rate and the hematogenous spread from primary lesions (Conlon, 2013; Kimberlin, Brady, Jackson, & Long, 2015; Perez-Velez, 2012; Swaminathan & Rekha, 2010).

PULMONARY DYSFUNCTION CAUSED BY NONINFECTIOUS IRRITANTS

Foreign-Body Aspiration

A. Definition

1. Foreign-body aspiration is an important cause of accidental death in infants and children. Toddlers younger than 3 years of age account for 60% to 80% of foreign-body aspirations. Beginning at age 8 to 10 months, the curious infant has developed thumb–forefinger grasp, enabling placement of objects into the mouth, and has learned to crawl. By 1 to 2 years of age, the toddler is climbing.

2. Severity is determined by the location, type of object aspirated, and extent of obstruction.

3. Dry vegetable matter, such as a seed, nut, or piece of carrot or popcorn that does not dissolve and that may swell when wet, causes a particularly difficult problem. The high fat content of potato chips and peanuts may cause the added risk of lipoid pneumonia. "Fun foods" are the worst offenders in terms of choking. Offending foods in order of frequency of choking are hot dogs, round candies, peanuts or other nuts, grapes, cookies, biscuits, other meats, caramels, carrots, peas, apples, celery, popcorn, sunflower seeds, orange seeds, cherry pits, watermelon seeds, gum, and peanut butter. Other items include burst latex balloons, plastic or glass beads, marbles, pen or marker caps, buttons or disk batteries, and coins (Conlon, 2013).

    a. *Disk-battery ingestion.* Although most button battery ingestions are benign, passing through the gut without a problem, in recent years the number of debilitating or fatal battery ingestions has dramatically increased. These disastrous outcomes occur when batteries get stuck in the esophagus, usually in small children. Large-diameter button batteries, especially 20-mm-diameter lithium coin cells, are implicated in most of these serious cases, but other battery types and smaller button batteries may also get stuck and cause serious problems. Burns and life-threatening complications can occur if batteries aren't removed from the esophagus within 2 hours. Batteries beyond the esophagus rarely cause a problem and can usually be left to pass spontaneously if the patient remains asymptomatic. Serious complications have also been seen when small batteries are placed in the nose or ear—another situation in which urgent removal is critical (National Capital Poison Center, n.d.).

    b. Batteries cause tissue injury through three interacting mechanisms. These mechanisms come into play when a battery is lodged in the gut, ear, nose, or other orifice, rather than free floating and in transit. The mechanisms include generation of an external electrolytic current that hydrolyzes tissue fluids and produces hydroxide at the battery's negative pole, leakage of battery contents, and physical pressure on adjacent tissue. Most severe complications following battery ingestions occur in the esophagus. Batteries must become lodged or impacted for tissue damage to occur. Batteries moving freely in the gut or surrounded by volumes of fluid do not cause focal tissue damage due to the failure of enough hydroxide to accumulate at one location to produce focal damage. The esophagus is especially susceptible to foreign-body retention due to its several anatomic areas of narrowing and weak peristalsis (National Capital Poison Center, n.d.).

    c. Most serious battery ingestions are not witnessed. Consider the possibility of a battery ingestion in every patient with acute airway obstruction; wheezing or other noisy breathing; drooling; vomiting; chest pain or discomfort; abdominal pain; difficulty swallowing; decreased appetite or refusal to eat; or coughing, choking, or gagging with eating or drinking. Suspect a button battery ingestion in every presumed "coin" or other foreign-body ingestion (National Capital Poison Center, n.d.).

    d. X-rays obtained to locate the battery should include the entire neck, esophagus, and abdomen. Batteries located above the range of the x-ray have been missed, as have batteries assumed to be coins or cardiac monitor electrodes. On physical exam, check both ear canals and the nasal cavity to exclude battery insertion. Anticipate complications based on battery position and orientation. Damage will be more severe in tissue adjacent to the negative pole (National Capital Poison Center, n.d.).

    e. Batteries lodged in the esophagus are surgical emergencies and need to be removed immediately. Serious burns can occur in 2 hours. Do not delay removal because a patient has eaten recently. Endoscopic removal is preferred as it allows direct visualization of tissue injury. Patients with esophageal injury should be admitted and observed due to the high risk of local edema developing with worsening symptoms, especially airway compromise when the battery is lodged high in the esophagus. In stable, well-appearing children, a clear liquid diet can be started after an esophagram shows no evidence of perforation.

The esophagram is obtained at least 1 to 2 days after battery removal, earlier (1 day) for cases with mucosal injury only, and later for cases with deeper injury. Diet may be advanced to soft as tolerated, but all children who have had an esophageal battery removed should be limited to soft foods for a full 28 days to avoid mechanical damage to a healing esophagus. In children with more severe injuries, subsequent care and diagnostic intervention are guided by clinical manifestations (National Capital Poison Center, n.d.).

f. Patients with batteries removed from the upper esophagus should be monitored carefully for voice changes, respiratory distress, or stridor. If any of these are present or suggested, the cords should be visualized under direct laryngoscopic view in the awake patient to confirm bilateral vocal cord mobility. Unilateral or bilateral vocal cord paralysis is a common complication of battery ingestion due to damage to the recurrent laryngeal nerve(s). Paralysis may be delayed and not detected for days or weeks (National Capital Poison Center, n.d.).

B. Pathophysiology

1. Foreign-body location may be supraglottic, glottic, subglottic, tracheal, bronchial, or esophageal. The manifestations of aspiration depend on the size of the foreign body, its composition, its location, the degree of blockage, and the duration of obstruction. Except in the rare instance of impending asphyxia due to an impacted laryngeal foreign body, time exists for a careful history, physical examination, and radiologic examination. History is of paramount importance in the diagnosis. Carefully consider the information described by the caretaker for the characteristic history of a choking or gagging episode, followed by a coughing spell. Most inhaled foreign bodies travel distally into the tracheobronchial tree, but laryngeal impaction occasionally occurs and accounts for the highest rate of mortality in the aerodigestive tract. Smaller nonobstructing objects bypass the supraglottis, glottis, and trachea and lodge most commonly in the right mainstem bronchus. Depending on the size, location, and nature of the foreign body, local irritation produces complaints that include cough, inspiratory stridor, hoarseness, wheezing, shortness of breath, and fever, symptoms that mimic the more common diseases of the respiratory tract. Symptoms may occur within hours of the aspiration or weeks later. Some aspirated foreign bodies may go unrecognized for weeks or longer.

2. The absence of symptoms after a witnessed choking episode does not exclude the presence of a retained foreign body. Following the initial episode of paroxysmal coughing, an asymptomatic lag period occurs.

C. Clinical Presentation

1. *History.* The initial episode is frequently associated with choking and coughing. Often symptoms subside, and the child presents at a later time with diverse symptoms, such as coughing, wheezing, recurrent or protracted pneumonia, and fever. The right bronchus is more often the site of the foreign body than the left bronchus, but the airway might be blocked anywhere from the posterior pharynx to the bronchus (Figure 2.17).

2. *Physical Examination.* Examination findings may be normal or reveal nonspecific signs, such as decreased air entry, wheezing, rhonchi, or inspiratory stridor. Patients with laryngeal foreign bodies have stridor, dyspnea, cyanosis, cough, and voice change. Total airway obstruction can occur. Patients with bronchial foreign bodies present with cough, asymmetric breath sounds, wheezing, dyspnea, and fever.

3. *Diagnostic Tests.* After a thorough history and physical examination, plain neck and chest radiographs should be obtained. About 10% of aspirated foreign bodies are radiopaque making the diagnosis easy. However, the majority of foreign bodies are not obvious and changes are seen secondary to obstruction

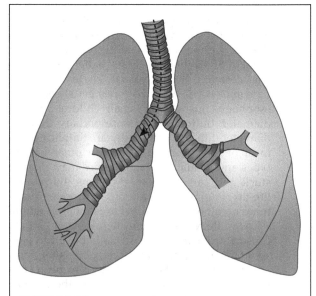

FIGURE 2.17 Anatomy of mainstem bronchus.

of the airway by the object. Anteroposterior and lateral views of the neck and chest may reveal signs of a partially obliterated tracheobronchial air column. The classic radiologic abnormality is unilateral hyperlucency on an expiratory film. Indirect radiologic signs include atelectasis, pneumonia, pneumothorax, and expiratory shift of the mediastinum. Foreign-body aspiration can never be excluded on the basis of chest radiography alone. A final diagnosis is only achieved at the time of bronchoscopic evaluation.

D. Clinical Course

Clinical course depends on the degree of obstruction, location of the foreign body, nature of the object, and availability of equipment or personnel.

1. For life-threatening airway obstruction follow basic life support (BLS) emergency measures for the choking child as outlined in the following section. Emergent bronchoscopy should be performed if these maneuvers are unsuccessful.

2. Before removal of the foreign body, a quiet environment should be provided and vital signs and respiratory distress must be watched carefully. Monitor for changes in the heart rate, respiratory rate, increased retractions, pallor, or cyanosis.

3. Following removal, respiratory effort should continue to be monitored, observing for signs of airway obstruction from edema at the site where the foreign body was removed.

E. Patient Care Management

1. *Prevention*

  a. Caregivers should be instructed to limit the availability of nuts, jewelry, small objects, latex balloons, popcorn, and hot dogs to children younger than 3 years.

2. *Emergency Care*

  a. Follow pediatric advanced life support recommendations. If the child still has adequate air exchange and an effective cough, no attempt should be made to dislodge the foreign body before definitive management with a bronchoscopy. If the child has inadequate air exchange, administer back blows and chest thrusts in infants and abdominal thrusts in children (Conlon, 2013).

3. *Respiratory Care*

  a. Monitor closely for signs of deterioration such as changes in heart rate, respiratory rate, increase in severity of sternal retractions, or increased oxygen requirement.

  b. Immediate removal of the foreign body is the most effective intervention for acute aspiration. Laryngoscopy and/or bronchoscopy may be performed for direct visualization of the airway and removal of the foreign body.

4. *Supportive Care*

  a. Administer oxygen as indicated.

  b. Perform vigorous pulmonary toilet.

  c. Antibiotic therapy should be used if a culture of respiratory secretions shows infection.

F. Outcomes

Pronounced local inflammation or granulation may be seen in the airway with long-standing foreign bodies. If the foreign body is not readily removed, obstruction from edema, erosion with infection, perforation, and hemorrhage may develop. Generally, the outcome is good if appropriate and timely management is provided (American Academy of Pediatrics, 2010; Conlon, 2013; National Capital Poison Center, n.d.; Singh & Parakh, 2014).

Aspiration Pneumonia

A. Definition

1. Aspiration pneumonia occurs when food, secretions, inert materials, volatile compounds, or liquids enter the lungs and cause inflammation and a chemical pneumonitis. Aspiration of fluid or foods is a particular hazard in the child who has difficulty with swallowing or is unable to swallow because of paralysis, weakness, debility, congenital anomalies, or absent cough reflex or in the child who is force-fed especially while crying or breathing rapidly (Conlon, 2013).

2. Altered anatomy of function of the trachea or esophagus may predispose to aspiration of secretions or stomach contents (Table 2.12).

3. Aspiration pneumonia is an important phenomenon in the critically ill patient. When normal airway protective mechanisms are impaired, gastric contents may be aspirated into the airways. This may occur as a result of a decreased level of consciousness or the presence of an ETT, which inhibits the child's ability to occlude the larynx.

B. Pathophysiology

1. Initial parenchymal injury occurs from direct epithelial damage. Indirect damage occurs from the generation of toxic radicals, inflammatory

TABLE 2.12   Causes of Aspiration Pneumonitis

Altered level of consciousness	Drugs, alcohol, anesthesia, seizures, central nervous system disorders
Altered anatomy of trachea or esophagus	Tracheal or esophageal abnormalities, endotracheal tube, tracheostomy
Altered function of swallow or esophageal motility	Loss of normal reflexes, which prevent aspiration of stomach contents; gastroesophageal reflux, especially when associated with neurologic or anatomic impairment
Inhalation injury	Inhalation of toxic substances such as gastric acids or hydrocarbons

cells, and activation of the complement system. Pneumonitis, or inflammation of lung parenchyma, may involve pleura, interstitium, and airways. To be classified as pneumonia, alveolar consolidation must be present.

C. Clinical Presentation

1. *History.* To treat the patient appropriately, it is important to know the nature of the aspirated material. Determine the events surrounding the aspiration episode, such as level of consciousness and feeding history. The severity of the lung injury depends on the pH of the aspirated material (Conlon, 2013).

2. *Physical Examination.* Patients may demonstrate increased cough and fever, acute dyspnea, wheezing, and cyanosis progressing to pulmonary edema. Observe for increased WOB, retractions, and increased respiratory rate. Auscultate for absent breath sounds, crackles, or wheezing in the affected lobes. Aspiration of oral secretions manifests with signs similar to acute bacterial pneumonia. Rarely aspiration causes immediate death from asphyxia; more often, the irritated mucous membrane becomes a site for secondary bacterial infection.

3. *Diagnostic Tests*

   a. *Chest radiographic* changes following aspiration are related to irritation, inflammation, and pneumonia. Aspiration pneumonia characteristically produces patchy opacification in the lung bases and perihilar infiltrations. Radiographs may demonstrate slight hyperventilation to diffuse infiltrates or alveolar densities. Infiltrates are most likely to be observed in the right upper lobe in a patient who was supine at the time of aspiration. Chest radiograph changes may worsen over the first 72 hours and then begin to clear. Radiographic abnormalities may persist for 4 to 6 weeks.

   b. *ABG levels* should be evaluated if hypoxemia and hypercarbia are clinically significant.

   c. *Pulse oximetry* gives a continuous measurement of oxygen saturation.

4. *Clinical Course*

   a. Presentation and management of aspiration pneumonia depend on the nature and quantity of the aspirated material.

   b. Materials with an acidotic pH may produce immediate pulmonary symptoms that worsen over the first 24 hours. Chemical burns increase alveolar capillary membrane permeability with subsequent extravasation of fluid into interstitium and alveoli. Often lung volume decreases, and then ventilation–perfusion mismatch and hypoxia occur. Acidotic fluid produces airway irritation, bronchospasm, peribronchial hemorrhage, and necrosis. Alkalotic materials can also cause devastating airway and lung injury.

   c. Materials with a normal pH can induce hypoxia or pulmonary edema, but generally there is little necrosis.

   d. Irritant gases cause direct injury to the mucosal surface. Epithelial cells become edematous, then necrotic, going through three phases. The acute phase is characterized by pulmonary edema, hypoxemia, and respiratory failure. The delayed phase is characterized by pulmonary edema, airway obstruction, and superinfection. The long-term phase involves reactive airways and interstitial fibrosis.

5. *Differential Diagnosis.* Evaluate for foreign-body aspiration. Generally, cough, dyspnea, and wheezing are seen with foreign-body aspiration (see Foreign-Body Aspiration discussion). Differentiate between acute bacterial or viral pneumonia by history, chest radiograph, secretions, and tracheal aspirate (if available).

D. Patient Care Management

1. *Prevention*

   a. Care of the child with aspiration pneumonia is the same as that described for the child with pneumonia from other causes. However, the major focus of nursing care is on prevention of aspiration. Proper feeding techniques should be carried out, and preventive measures should be used to prevent aspiration of any material that might enter the nasopharynx.

   b. The presence of an NG feeding tube or a history of GERD places the child at risk for aspiration.

   c. Children who are at risk for swallowing difficulties as a result of illness, physical debilitation, anesthesia, or sedation are kept on nothing per os (NPO) status until they can properly swallow fluids effectively.

2. *Direct Care*

   a. NG feedings should be monitored closely. Feeding tubes should be checked before the initiation of bolus feedings; continuous feedings should also be evaluated properly for tube placement.

   b. If gastroesophageal reflux is suspected follow reflux precautions.

   c. Consider the use of transpyloric feedings if an ETT has been placed or if there is a significant risk of reflux or poor gastric emptying.

3. *Supportive Care*

   a. High oxygen concentrations, mechanical ventilation, and high PEEP may be necessary.

   b. Choice of antibiotics depends on the patient's age and the cause of aspiration. Prophylactic antimicrobials have not been proven beneficial and allow overgrowth of resistant organisms. Antibiotic therapy should be reserved for known or suspected secondary infection.

   c. Reflux aspiration can often be treated medically through elevation of the head and torso during sleep; antacids; GI motility-enhancing agents; and small, frequent, thickened feedings.

   d. Optimal medical therapy for reflux.

   e. Surgical management by a Nissen fundoplication can be done if medical management fails. Occasionally, patients continue to aspirate secretions from the mouth and nose and a Nissen will not help in these cases.

E. Outcomes

Prognosis is generally good. Mild restrictive or obstructive defects, such as bronchiectasis (dilation of the bronchi from bronchial wall damage) and reactive airways disease, have been observed.

Acute Pulmonary Embolism

A. Definition

1. Pulmonary embolism (PE) occurs when materials traveling in the bloodstream become impacted in the pulmonary arterial bed. PE may occur after trauma or surgery and may complicate a number of illnesses and treatments.

2. Thromboembolism is the most commonly occurring form of PE and appears when a blood clot travels from a peripheral vessel through the right side of the heart and lodges in the pulmonary arterial bed.

3. Pulmonary thromboembolism may complicate sickle cell anemia, rheumatic fever, and bacterial endocarditis, and may occur with sepsis or severe dehydration.

4. Risk factors in children include presence of a central venous catheter, immobility, heart disease, ventriculoatrial shunt, oral contraceptive use, and trauma.

5. PE is infrequently diagnosed in children although clinicians should always have a high index of suspicion, especially when treating a child with the acute onset of respiratory distress or cardiovascular shock.

B. Pathophysiology

The degree of cardiopulmonary disturbance observed in PE depends on two elements: the previous functional status of the heart and lungs and the severity of the pulmonary venous occlusion. A major pathophysiologic consequence of an acute PE is increased alveolar dead space. This increase in alveolar dead space occurs because lung units continue to be ventilated, but have diminished or absent perfusion. Pulmonary infarction is an uncommon sequela of PE owing to the fact that the lung has three sources of oxygen: pulmonary arteries, the airways, and the bronchial arteries.

C. Clinical Presentation

1. Hypoxemia is common in acute PE.

2. The child with a PE is dyspneic, tachypneic, and may complain of acute chest pain.

3. Breath sounds may be clear or there may be scattered crackles.

4. Radiographic findings are nonspecific and may include atelectasis, localized infiltrates, or a pleural effusion.

5. Fever is also often present without other signs of infection.

6. Supportive radiographic tests include a pulmonary angiogram, V/Q scan, and/or helical CT scan (can be performed quickly in critically ill patients). PFTs may give abnormal results, but they are again nonspecific.

D. Patient Care Management

1. Treatment consists of oxygen, hemodynamic support, anticoagulation, and thrombolytic therapy and goes beyond attempts to lyse the thrombus.

2. In patients with acute respiratory failure, endotracheal intubation and mechanical ventilation are instituted to ensure adequate tissue oxygenation and carbon dioxide removal. High PEEP may be necessary to achieve oxygenation; however, this main impair venous return.

3. Once the diagnosis is established, heparin and/or low-molecular-weight heparin therapy is initiated to prevent further thrombus. Dosing is adjusted according to the activated partial thromboplastic time (aPTT). Approximately 24 to 48 hours after heparin therapy is initiated, warfarin is begun so that there is an overlap of at least 5 days. Fibrinolytic agents may also be used. Catheter-based interventions are potentially lifesaving in selected patients with massive PE. Surgical embolectomy may be an effective strategy for patients with a massive PE with contraindications that preclude use of thrombolysis.

4. Nursing priorities include maintaining supplemental oxygen and ventilatory support if it becomes necessary, evaluating the child's cardiopulmonary status, and assessing the effects of therapy.

5. Pulse oximetry monitoring helps ensure adequate oxygenation. The adequacy of ventilation can be determined by evaluating the child's respiratory rate and effort and periodically monitoring ABGs. In addition, cardiovascular assessment, including heart rate, blood pressure, strength of peripheral pulses, warmth of extremities, and adequacy of urine output, helps determine the need for inotropic support or volume expansion.

6. Because hemorrhage is the major complication of heparin administration, it is especially important to monitor coagulation studies and signs of bleeding.

7. Invasive procedures should be avoided or minimized.

E. Outcomes

Outcomes vary substantially depending on patient characteristics (Dijk, Curtin, Lord, & Fitzgerald, 2012; Jaff et al., 2011; Khaleghi, Richardson, Hall, Streeter, & Carpenter, 2014; Michaels et al., 2009; Motti Eini et al., 2013; Patocka & Nemeth, 2012).

Pulmonary Edema

A. Definition and Pathophysiology

1. The movement of fluid into the alveoli and interstitium of the lungs caused by extravasation of fluid from the pulmonary vasculature.

2. There are two main types of pulmonary edema: cardiogenic and noncardiogenic.

3. Cardiogenic pulmonary edema is caused by an increase in pulmonary capillary pressure resulting from an increase in pulmonary venous pressure. It can be caused by excessive IV fluid administration, left ventricular failure, heart valve disorder (aortic regurgitation, aortic stenosis, mitral regurgitation), myocardial ischemia, myocarditis, sepsis, acute tachydysrhythmia, or coronary arteriosclerosis.

4. Noncardiogenic pulmonary edema is caused by various conditions that result in increased pulmonary capillary permeability.

    a. Subtypes include permeability pulmonary edema (caused by PARDS), high-altitude pulmonary edema (caused by rapid ascension to heights greater than 12,000 feet), or neurogenic pulmonary edema (after CNS insult such as seizures, head injury, or cerebral edema).

    b. Some less common forms of pulmonary edema include reperfusion pulmonary edema (after the removal of thromboemboli from the lung or lung transplant), reexpansion pulmonary edema (caused by rapid reexpansion of a collapsed lung), or pulmonary edema that results from opiate overdose (methadone or heroin), salicylate toxicity (chronic), aspiration (foreign body), inhalation injuries, near-drowning, pulmonary embolis, viral infections, or pulmonary veno-occlusive disease.

c. Other causes include aspiration, traumatic injury, organ dysfunction caused by sepsis, multiorgan failure, alcoholism or substance abuse, pregnancy, chronic renal impairment, malnutrition, hypertension, or a blood transfusion.

B. Clinical Presentation

Symptoms include extreme shortness of breath, cyanosis, tachypnea, diminished breath sounds, anxiety, agitation, confusion, diaphoresis, orthopnea, respiratory crackles, expiratory wheezing (in young infants), heart murmur, S3 gallop, cool peripheries, jugular venous distention, nocturnal dyspnea, cough, pink frothy sputum (if severe), tachycardia, hypertension, and hypotension (if caused by left ventricular dysfunction).

C. Patient Care Management

1. Management depends on the cause but can include oxygen therapy, PEEP via CPAP, and intubation with ventilator support if respiratory failure occurs. If edema is severe, PEEP should not be interrupted to suction.

2. If ventricular failure is the cause, medications, such as diuretics, digoxin, positive inotropes, and vasodilators, may be started and the child may be placed on a sodium and fluid restriction. Morphine may be prescribed to relieve dyspnea.

3. The primary goal of management is to determine the cause and treat the underlying condition.

4. In frank pulmonary edema, suctioning of secretions does not help and may cause harm due to disconnection of ventilator circuit and loss of PEEP.

5. Pulse oximetry is monitored and vital signs are observed closely for any deterioration.

6. The nurse should note changes in oxygen saturation, end-tidal CO_2, and ABG values.

7. An ongoing assessment of the child's cardiopulmonary status is needed.

8. Oxygen, medications, and treatments are administered as prescribed.

9. The nurse should closely monitor intake and output, electrolytes, and comfort.

10. The child should be monitored for restlessness, anxiety, and air hunger.

11. Children should be given the opportunity to express and discuss fears and anxieties.

D. Outcomes

Outcomes vary depending on the primary cause of pulmonary edema (Conlon, 2013; Matthay, 2014).

Pediatric Acute Respiratory Distress Syndrome

A. Definition

1. ARDS in children is different from ARDS in adults. In the absence of identification of these differences, however, children have been characterized as having acute lung injury (ALI) and ARDS based on the adult definitions originating in 1994. Seventeen years later, a second consensus conference was convened with the intent of improving the feasibility, reliability, and validity of ALI/ARDS definitions. This was again conducted without specific consideration of children (Table 2.13; Pediatric Acute Lung Injury Consensus Conference Group, 2015).

2. These concerns prompted the organization of the Pediatric Acute Lung Injury Consensus Conference. A panel of experts met over the course of 2 years to develop a taxonomy to define PARDS and to make recommendations regarding treatment and research priorities.

B. Pathophysiology

1. There may be a difference in the progression and outcome from ARDS in children as compared with adults. Future studies are required to examine whether there are differences in the progression and/ or outcome of ARDS between adults and children or between children of different ages.

2. Biomarker and genetic studies may provide insight into the pathophysiology of PARDS in children.

C. Ventilatory Management

1. There are no outcome data on the influence of mode during conventional mechanical ventilation.

2. In any mechanically ventilated pediatric patient, the Pediatric Acute Lung Injury Consensus Conference Group recommends controlled ventilation to use tidal volumes in or below the range of physiologic

TABLE 2.13   Definition of PARDS

Age	Exclusion of patients with perinatal-related lung disease (prematurity-related lung disease, perinatal lung injury, or other congenital abnormalities)
Timing	Symptoms of hypoxemia and radiographic changes must occur within 7 d of known clinical insult
Edema	Respiratory failure is not fully explained by cardiac failure or fluid overload
Chest imaging	Imaging findings of new infiltrate consistent with acute pulmonary parenchymal disease are necessary to diagnose PARDS

Oxygenation	Noninvasive mechanical ventilation
	    PARDS (no severity stratification)
	    Full-face-mask bilevel ventilation or CPAP >5 cm H_2O
	    PF ratio <300
	    SF ratio <264
	Invasive mechanical ventilation
	    Mild 4 < OI < 8; 5 < OSI < 7.5
	    Moderate 8 < OI < 16; 7.5 < OSI < 12.3
	    Severe OI > 16; OSI > 12.3

Special populations	
Cyanotic heart disease	Standard criteria should be used for age, timing, origin of edema, and chest imaging with an acute deterioration in oxygenation not explained by underlying cardiac disease.
Chronic lung disease	Standard criteria should be used for age, timing, and origin of edema with chest imaging consistent with new infiltrate and acute deterioration in oxygenation from baseline, which meet previous oxygenation criteria.
Left ventricular dysfunction	Standard criteria should be used for age, timing, and origin of edema with chest imaging changes consistent with new infiltrate and acute deterioration in oxygenation, which meet previous criteria not explained by left ventricular dysfunction.

CPAP, continuous positive airway pressure; OI, oxygenation index; OSI, oxygen saturation index; PaO_2/FiO_2 ratio is the ratio of arterial oxygen partial pressure to fractional inspired oxygen (PF ratio); PARDS, pediatric acute respiratory distress syndrome; PF, partial pressure of arterial oxygen (PaO_2) fraction of inspired oxygen (FiO_2); SF, (SpO_2) fraction of inspired oxygen (FiO_2).

Source: Modified from Pediatric Acute Lung Injury Consensus Conference Group. (2015). Pediatric acute respiratory distress syndrome: Consensus recommendations from the pediatric acute lung injury consensus conference. *Pediatric Critical Care Medicine, 16*(5), 428–439. doi:10.1097/PCC.0000000000000350

tidal volumes for age/body weight (i.e., 5–8 mL/kg predicted body weight) according to lung pathology and respiratory system compliance.

3. The Pediatric Acute Lung Injury Consensus Conference Group recommends using patient-specific tidal volumes according to disease severity. Tidal volumes should be 3 to 6 mL/kg predicted body weight for patients with poor respiratory system compliance and closer to the physiologic range (5–8 mL/kg ideal body weight) for patients with better preserved respiratory system compliance.

4. In the absence of transpulmonary pressure measurements, an inspiratory plateau pressure limit of 28 cm H_2O is recommended, allowing for slightly higher plateau pressures (29–32 cm H_2O) for patients with increased chest wall elastance (i.e., reduced chest wall compliance).

5. *PEEP/Lung Recruitment.* PEEP levels of greater than 15 cm H_2O may be needed for PARDS.

a. Markers of oxygen delivery, respiratory system compliance, and hemodynamics should be closely monitored as PEEP is increased.

b. PEEP should be slowly increased and decreased.

6. *High-Frequency Ventilation.* May be considered as an alternative ventilatory mode in hypoxic respiratory failure in patients with moderate to severe PARDS.

7. High-frequency jet ventilation (HFJV) and high-frequency percussive ventilation (HFPV) are not recommended for routine ventilatory management. HFPV may be considered in patients with PARDS and secretion-induced lung collapse that cannot be resolved with clinical care.

8. Liquid ventilation is not recommended.

9. Cuffed ETTs are recommended to maintain PEEP.

10. *Gas Exchange.* Oxygenation and ventilation goals are titrated based on the perceived risks of the toxicity of the ventilator support required. For mild PARDS with a PEEP less than 10 cm H_2O, oxygen saturation generally should be maintained at 92% to 97%. After optimizing PEEP, lower oxygen saturation levels (88%–92%) should be considered with a PEEP of at least 10 cm H_2O.

   a. When oxygen saturation is less than 92% monitoring of central venous saturation and markers of oxygen delivery is recommended.

   b. Permissive hypercapnia may be considered for moderate to severe PARDS.

   c. A pH of 7.15 to 7.20 with lung protective strategies is recommended. Exceptions to permissive hypercapnia should include intracranial hypertension, severe PH, select congenital heart disease lesions, hemodynamic instability, and significant ventricular dysfunction.

   d. Bicarbonate supplementation is not routinely recommended.

D. Noninvasive Support

1. Noninvasive positive-pressure ventilation (NPPV) is considered early in disease management of children at risk for PARDS to improve gas exchange, decrease WOB, and potentially avoid complications of invasive ventilation.

2. Intubation should be considered in patients receiving NPPV who do not show clinical improvement or have signs and symptoms of worsening disease.

3. Children should be monitored for skin breakdown, gastric distention, barotrauma, and conjunctivitis.

4. Heated humidification should be used.

5. Sedation should be used with caution.

6. NPPV is not recommended for children with severe disease.

E. Extracorporeal Support

1. ECMO should be considered to support children with PARDS where the cause of respiratory failure is believed to be reversible or the child is likely to be suitable for consideration for lung transplantation.

2. Careful consideration of quality of life should be considered.

F. Pulmonary-Specific Patient Care Management and Monitoring

1. Treatment involves supportive measures to maintain adequate oxygenation and pulmonary perfusion, treatment of infection or the precipitating cause, and maintenance of adequate cardiac output.

2. iNO is not recommended for routine use (may be considered in patients with PH or severe right ventricular dysfunction).

3. Surfactant therapy is not recommended.

4. Prone positioning is not routinely recommended. It may be considered in severe cases of PARDS.

5. At a minimum, nurses should monitor respiratory frequency, heart rate/rhythm, pulse oximetry, and noninvasive blood pressure. Specific alarms should be available when the monitored variables fall outside predefined ranges.

6. Nurses must continuously evaluate the patient's response to ventilator assistance, including observation of chest excursion and patient comfort and auscultation of lung fields, to assess the adequacy of aeration and the length of inspiratory and expiratory times.

7. Chest imaging is necessary for the diagnosis of PARDS and to detect complications. Imaging frequency is patient dependent.

8. Hemodynamic monitoring is recommended during PARDS in particular to guide volume expansion.

9. Maintaining a clear airway is essential to the patient with PARDS. Suctioning must be performed with caution to minimize the risk of derecruitment.

Routine instillation of isotonic saline is not recommended prior to suctioning. However, it may be indicated in children with thick tenacious secretions.

10. Chest physiotherapy is not recommended as a standard of care.

11. Corticosteroids are not recommended for routine use in PARDS.

12. Pediatric patients with PARDS should receive minimal yet targeted sedation to facilitate their tolerance to mechanical ventilation and to optimize oxygen delivery, VO$_2$, and WOB.

13. Nurses should assess pain with valid and reliable pain and sedation scales to monitor, target, and titrate sedation and facilitate communication. Sedation should be managed by a goal-directed protocol with daily sedation goals established by the team. An individualized sedation weaning plan is developed by the team and managed by the bedside nurse.

14. A neuromuscular blockade (NMB) may be considered if sedation alone is inadequate to achieve mechanical ventilation. When used, NMB should be monitored and titrated to the goal effect. Monitoring may include effective ventilation, clinical movement, and train-of-four response. If full chemical paralysis is used, the team should consider a daily NMB holiday to allow periodic assessment of the NMB and sedation.

15. Enteral nutrition is preferred over parenteral nutrition when tolerated. Enteral nutrition monitoring, advancement, and maintenance should be managed with a goal-directed protocol that is collaboratively managed by the interprofessional team.

16. Patients should receive total fluids to maintain adequate intravascular volume, end-organ perfusion, and optimal delivery of oxygen. Fluid balance should be monitored and titrated to maintain adequate intravascular volume while aiming to prevent positive fluid balance.

17. Blood transfusion should be considered in children with a hemoglobin concentration less than 7.0 g/dL.

18. Psychological and developmental support of the patient and family are important.

G. Morbidity and Long-Term Outcomes

1. Patients should have routine screening for pulmonary function abnormalities within the first year after discharge, including a minimum of respiratory symptom questionnaires and pulse oximetry.

2. Children who are developmentally able should perform spirometry within the first year following hospital discharge.

3. Patients should be referred to a pediatric pulmonologist for further assessment if deficits in pulmonary function are identified.

4. Physical, neurocognitive, emotional, family, and social function should be evaluated within 3 months of hospital discharge for children with moderate to severe PARDS. In younger children, this should be performed before the start of school.

SMOKE-INHALATION INJURY

A. Definition

1. A number of noxious substances that may be inhaled are toxic to humans. They are primarily products of incomplete combustion and cause more deaths from fires than flame injuries. The severity of the injury depends on the nature of the substances generated by the material burned, whether the victim is confined in a closed space, and the duration of the contact with the smoke.

2. Three distinct syndromes of pulmonary complications occur in children with inhalation injury:

   a. Early carbon monoxide poisoning, airway obstruction, and pulmonary edema

   b. ARDS occurring within 24 to 48 hours or later in some cases

   c. Late complications of bronchopneumonia and pulmonary emboli

B. Pathophysiology

1. Heat injury involves thermal injury to the upper airway. Air has low specific heat; therefore, the injury goes no further than the upper airway. Reflex closure of the glottis prevents injury to the lower airway.

2. Chemical injury involves gases that may be generated during the combustion of materials such as clothing, furniture, and floor coverings. When in smoke, acids, alkalis, and their precursors can produce chemical burns. These substances can be carried deep into the respiratory tract.

   a. Synthetic materials are especially toxic producing gases such as oxides of sulfur and nitrogen, acetaldehyde, formaldehyde, hydrocyanic acid, and chlorine. Heated plastics are the source of extremely toxic vapors, including chlorine and hydrochloric acid from polyvinylchloride, and hydrocarbons, aldehydes, ketones, and acids from polyethylene. Irritant gases, such as nitrous oxide and carbon dioxide, combine with water in the lungs to form corrosive acids; aldehydes cause denaturation of proteins, cellular damage, and edema of pulmonary tissues.

b. Chemical burns to the airways are similar to burns on the skin except they are relatively painless because the tracheobronchial tree is relatively insensitive to pain.

c. Inhalation of small amounts of noxious irritants produces alveolar and bronchiolar damage that can lead to obstructive bronchiolitis. Severe exposure causes further injury, including alveolar capillary damage with hemorrhage, necrotizing bronchiolitis, inhibited secretion of surfactant, and formation of hyaline membranes.

3. Systemic injury occurs from gases that are nontoxic to the airways (carbon monoxide and hydrogen cyanide). However, these gases cause injury and death by interfering with or inhibiting cellular respiration. Carbon monoxide is responsible for more than half of all fatal inhalation poisonings.

C. Clinical Presentation

1. Respiratory distress may occur early in the course of smoke inhalation as a result of hypoxia, or patients who are breathing well on admission may suddenly develop respiratory distress. Intubation equipment should be readily available.

2. During the first 24 to 48 hours following injury, pulmonary edema is associated with the toxicity of inhaled gases and fluid resuscitation. After 48 hours, the effects of atelectasis and pneumonia become evident as a clinical picture similar to ARDS develops.

D. Patient Care Management

1. Vital signs and assessments are performed frequently.

2. Pulmonary status is carefully observed and maintained.

3. Pulmonary care may be facilitated by bronchodilators, inhaled corticosteroids, humidification, chest percussion, and postural drainage.

4. Bronchoscopy may be required to clear heavy secretions.

5. Fluid requirements are greater than for those children suffering surface burns alone. Accurate measurement of intake and output is essential.

6. Hyperbaric oxygen therapy may be indicated for the child with carbon monoxide poisoning.

7. Further, HFPV has been shown to improve oxygenation and ventilation at lower peak inspiratory pressure and with minimal effects on hemodynamics. An additional benefit is its ability to enhance the recruitment and mobilization of secretions from the lung periphery to the central airways, thus potentially resolving atelectasis and preventing pneumonia. It shows promising results in inhalation injury.

E. Outcomes

Long-term sequelae of inhalation injury include bronchiolitis obliterans, bronchiectasis, tracheal stenosis (associated with prolonged intubation), or tracheostomy (Conlon, 2013; Toon, Maybauer, Greenwood, Maybauer, & Fraser, 2010; Walker et al., 2015).

Environmental Tobacco Smoke Exposure

A. Parental or family smoking is an important cause of morbidity in children. Children exposed to passive or environmental tobacco smoke have an increased number of respiratory illnesses, respiratory symptoms, and reduced performance on PFTs. Ear infections are also increased in children who have smoking parents. Indoor exposure to tobacco smoke has been linked to asthma in children. Maternal cigarette smoking is associated with increased respiratory symptoms and illnesses in children; decreased fetal growth; increased deliveries of low-birthweight, preterm, and stillborn infants; and a greater incidence of sudden infant death syndrome (SIDS). Antenatal maternal smoking has emerged as a significant risk factor for SIDS. The risk for diagnosis of early-onset asthma in the first 3 years of life is associated with in utero exposure to maternal smoking. Exposure to tobacco smoke during childhood may also contribute to chronic lung disease in the adult (Conlon, 2013).

B. Nurses must provide information about the hazards of environmental smoke exposure in all their interactions with children and their family members. Nurses have an important role in providing parents with affordable smoking-cessation-education resources. In addition, nurses also have a role in educating adolescents about avoiding tobacco products (Conlon, 2013).

LONG-TERM RESPIRATORY DYSFUNCTION

Asthma, Chronic/Acute

A. Definition

1. *Asthma* is defined as a chronic inflammatory disorder of the airways characterized by recurring symptoms, airway obstruction, and bronchial hyperresponsiveness. In susceptible children, inflammation causes recurrent episodes of wheezing, breathlessness, chest tightness, and cough, especially at night or in the early morning. The airflow limitation or obstruction is reversible either spontaneously or with treatment. Inflammation causes an increase in bronchial hyperresponsiveness to a variety of stimuli.

2. Asthma is classified into four categories based on symptom indicators of disease severity. The categories are intermittent, mild persistent, moderate persistent, and severe persistent. These categories provide a stepwise approach to the pharmacologic management, environmental control, and educational interventions for each category.

3. Asthma prevalence, morbidity, and mortality are increasing in the United States. These increases may result from worsening air pollution, poor access to medical care, and underdiagnosis or undertreatment.

4. Asthma is the most common chronic disease of childhood, the primary cause of school absences, and the third leading cause of hospitalizations in children younger than the age of 15 years (Conlon, 2013).

B. Pathophysiology

1. Airflow limitation in asthma is recurrent and caused by a variety of changes in the airway, including the following:

   a. *Bronchoconstriction*. In asthma, the dominant physiological event leading to clinical symptoms is airway narrowing and a subsequent interference with airflow. In acute exacerbations of asthma, bronchial smooth muscle contraction (bronchoconstriction) occurs quickly to narrow the airways in response to exposure to a variety of stimuli, including allergens or irritants.

   b. *Airway edema*. As the disease becomes more persistent and inflammation more progressive, other factors further limits airflow. These include edema, inflammation, mucus hypersecretion and the formation of inspissated mucus plugs, as well as structural changes, including hypertrophy and hyperplasia of the airway smooth muscle.

   c. *Airway hyperresponsiveness*. Airway hyperresponsiveness—an exaggerated bronchoconstrictor response to a wide variety of stimuli—is a major, but not necessarily unique, feature of asthma. The mechanisms influencing airway hyperresponsiveness are multiple and include inflammation, dysfunctional neuroregulation, and structural changes; inflammation appears to be a major factor in determining the degree of airway hyperresponsiveness.

   d. *Airway remodeling*. In some persons who have asthma, airflow limitation may be only partially reversible. Permanent structural changes can occur in the airway; these are associated with a progressive loss of lung function that is not prevented by or fully reversible by current therapy. Airway remodeling involves an activation of many of the structural cells, with consequent permanent changes in the airway that increase airflow obstruction and airway responsiveness and render the patient less responsive to therapy. These structural changes can include thickening of the sub-basement membrane, subepithelial fibrosis, airway smooth muscle hypertrophy and hyperplasia, blood vessel proliferation and dilation, and mucous gland hyperplasia and hypersecretion.

2. Inflammation has a central role in the pathophysiology of asthma. Airway inflammation involves an interaction of many cell types and multiple mediators with the airways that eventually results in the characteristic pathophysiological features of the disease: bronchial inflammation and airflow limitation that result in recurrent episodes of cough, wheeze, and shortness of breath. The processes by which these interactive events occur and lead to clinical asthma are still under investigation.

   a. *Inflammatory cells*, including lymphocytes, mast cells, eosinophils, neutrophils, dendritic cells, macrophages, resident cells of the airways, and epithelial cells, all play a role in inflammation.

   b. *Inflammatory mediators*. Chemokines, cytokines, cysteinyl-leukotrienes, and NO contribute to inflammation.

   c. *Immunoglobulin E*. Immunoglobulin E (IgE) is the antibody responsible for activation of allergic reactions and is important to the pathogenesis of allergic diseases and the development and persistence of inflammation. IgE attaches to cell surfaces via a specific high-affinity receptor. The mast cell has large numbers of IgE receptors; these, when activated by interaction with antigen, release a wide variety of mediators to initiate acute bronchospasm and also to release proinflammatory cytokines to perpetuate underlying airway inflammation. Other cells, basophils, dendritic cells, and lymphocytes also have high-affinity IgE receptors.

C. Clinical Presentation

1. *Cough.* Cough may be hacking, paroxysmal, irritative, and nonproductive. Cough becomes rattling and productive of frothy, clear, gelatinous sputum.

2. *Respiratory-Related Signs.* Shortness of breath; prolonged expiratory phase; audible wheeze; malar flush/red ears; lips may become deep, dark red; may progress to cyanosis of nail beds or circumoral cyanosis; restlessness, apprehension, and prominent sweating increase as the attack progresses; older children may prefer to sit upright with shoulders in a hunched-over position, hands on the bed or chair and arms braced (tripod position) and to speak in short, panting, or broken phrases.

3. *Chest.* Hyperresonance on percussion; coarse, loud breath sounds; wheezes throughout the lung fields; prolonged expiration, crackles, and generalized inspiratory and expiratory wheezing; increasingly high pitched.

4. *With Repeated Episodes.* Barrel chest develops with elevated shoulders, accessory muscles are used for respiration, facial appearance changes (flattened malar bones, dark circles beneath the eyes, narrow nose, and prominent upper teeth).

5. Symptoms occur or worsen in the presence of exercise, viral infection, animals with fur or hair, house-dust mites, mold, smoke (tobacco, wood), pollen, changes in weather, with strong emotional expression, airborne chemicals or dusts, and menstrual cycles.

6. *Differential Diagnostic Possibilities for Asthma*

   a. Upper airway diseases occur, including allergic rhinitis and sinusitis.

   b. Obstructions involving large airways occur, including foreign body in trachea or bronchus, vocal cord dysfunction, vascular rings or laryngeal webs, laryngotracheomalacia, tracheal stenosis, or bronchostenosis, enlarged lymph nodes or tumor.

   c. Obstructions involving small airways occur, including viral bronchiolitis or obliterative bronchiolitis, CF, BPD, heart disease.

   d. *Other:* Recurrent cough not due to asthma, aspiration from swallowing-mechanism dysfunction or gastroesophageal reflux, cough secondary to drugs (angiotensin-converting enzyme [ACE] inhibitors).

D. Diagnostic Evaluation

1. The diagnosis is determined primarily on the basis of clinical manifestations, history, physical examination, and, to a lesser extent, laboratory tests.

2. *PFT.* Provides an objective method of evaluating the presence and degree of lung disease, as well as the response to therapy. Spirometry can generally be performed reliably on children by the age of 5 or 6 years. Spirometry testing should be performed at the time of initial assessment of asthma, after treatment is initiated and symptoms have stabilized, and at least every 1 to 2 years to assess the maintenance of airway function. In most cases, PFT should not be performed during an acute exacerbation as spirometry can exacerbate symptoms.

3. *Allergy Testing.* Skin-prick testing and serological testing for allergen-specific IgE may be used to identify environmental allergens that trigger asthma. It is recommended that all patients with year-round asthma symptoms be tested for allergens.

4. *Additional Laboratory Testing.* A CBC with differential may show a slight elevation in the WBC count during acute asthma, but elevations to more than $12,000/mm^3$ or an increased percentage of band cells may indicate a respiratory infection. The presence of eosinophilia of greater than $500/mm^3$ may suggest an allergic or inflammatory disorder.

5. *Imaging.* Frontal and lateral radiographs may show infiltrates and hyperexpansion of the airways with the anteroposterior diameter on physical examination indicating an increased diameter. Radiography may assist in ruling out a respiratory tract infection.

E. Therapeutic Management

1. *Allergen Control.* Nonpharmacologic therapy is aimed at the prevention and reduction of exposure to airborne allergens and irritants.

2. *Drug Therapy.* Pharmacologic therapy is used to prevent and control asthma symptoms, reduce the frequency and severity of asthma exacerbations, and reverse airflow obstruction.

a. Long-term-control medications are used to achieve and maintain control of inflammation.

b. Quick-relief medications treat symptoms and exacerbations.

c. *Corticosteroids.* Anti-inflammatory drugs are used as first-line drugs to treat reversible airflow obstruction, control symptoms, and reduce bronchial hyperresponsiveness in chronic asthma. These medications may be administered parenterally, orally, or by inhalation.

> i. Oral medications are metabolized slowly with an onset of action up to 3 hours after administration and peak effectiveness occurring within 6 to 12 hours. Oral systemic steroids may be given for short periods of time to gain prompt control of inadequately controlled persistent asthma or to manage severe persistent asthma.
>
> ii. Corticosteroids should be given at the lowest effective dose.
>
> iii. Side effects may include cough, dysphonia, and thrush.

d. *Beta-adrenergic agonists.* These are used for the treatment of acute exacerbations and for the prevention of exercise-induced bronchospasm (EIB). These drugs bind with the beta receptors on the smooth muscle of the airways, allowing smooth muscle to relax. Other effects of the drug help stabilize mast cells to prevent the release of mediators.

e. *Long-acting beta agonists.* These medications are added to anti-inflammatory therapy for long-term prevention of symptoms. These medications are never administered alone for asthma.

f. *Theophylline.* This is a methylxanthine drug used to relieve symptoms and prevent attacks. Only rarely used, it may be considered in the emergency department (ED)/hospital when the child is not responding to maximum therapy.

g. *Leukotriene inhibitor.* Leukotriene modifiers block inflammatory and bronchospasm effects. These are used for long-term control.

h. *Anticholinergics.* May also be used for relief of acute bronchospasm. When used in combination with beta agonists, may be helpful in acute severe asthma.

i. *Monoclonal antibodies.* Omalizumab (Xolair) blocks the binding of IgE to mast cells. Blocking this interaction eventually inhibits the inflammation that is associated with asthma.

j. *Antibiotics.* May be used for patients exhibiting clear signs of a bacterial infection but are otherwise not indicated.

k. *Magnesium sulfate.* May be used in emergency situations. It is a physiologic calcium antagonist and has a direct effect on calcium uptake in smooth muscle, causing relaxation.

3. *Exercise.* EIB is an acute, reversible, usually self-terminating airway obstruction that develops during or after vigorous activity, reaches its peak 5 to 10 minutes after stopping the activity, and usually stops in another 20 to 30 minutes. Patients with EIB have cough, shortness of breath, chest pain or tightness, wheezing, and endurance problems during exercise, but an exercise challenge in a laboratory is necessary to make the diagnosis.

a. Exercise is advantageous for children with asthma and most children can participate in all sports/activities with minimal difficulties provided their asthma is under good control. Appropriate pretreatment with a short-acting beta agonist usually permits full participation in strenuous exertion.

4. *Breathing Exercises.* Breathing exercises help produce physical and mental relaxation, improve posture, strengthen respiratory muscles, and develop more efficient patterns of breathing. These exercises are not recommended during acute, uncomplicated exacerbations of asthma.

5. *Hyposensitization.* Hyposensitization is recommended for asthma patients when there is evidence of a relationship between asthma symptoms and unavoidable exposure to an allergen to which the patient is sensitive, when symptoms occur all year or at least during a major portion of the year, and when symptom control is difficult with drug therapy because multiple medications are required, the patient is not responsive to available drugs, or the patient refuses to take the medications.

F. Nursing Care Management of Acute Exacerbations

1. *Acute Asthma Care/Critical Care Management*

a. Status asthmaticus does not respond to routine therapy and necessitates hospitalization. Children whose asthma has caused even one episode of respiratory failure may be more likely to have repeated episodes of respiratory failure and catastrophic complications.

i. The child in status asthmaticus is usually pale and restless, has severe wheezing, and is sometimes cyanotic. Respiratory rate and heart rate are elevated, and a pulsus parodoxus of more than 15 mmHg may be detected. Vomiting and abdominal pain and distention are common, as is dehydration.

ii. As airway obstruction increases during an acute attack, ABGs change through a characteristic series of stages. Arterial oxygen tension (PaO_2) is decreased because of a reduced V/Q ratio caused by the simultaneous occurrence of air trapping and atelectasis.

iii. Initially the hypoxemia stimulates the respiratory drive and the $PaCO_2$ decreases with a normal or slightly elevated pH. Eventually, as muscle fatigue develops and compensatory mechanisms fail, the $PaCO_2$ begins to rise, producing respiratory acidosis. Respiratory rate and breath sounds decrease, and extreme restlessness is followed by stupor and unconsciousness. With progression, the $PaCO_2$ increases even more, pH falls with a superimposed metabolic acidosis, and PaO_2 becomes markedly reduced.

b. Treatment is directed at ensuring oxygenation and adequate V_A while reversing the primary airway abnormalities: bronchospasm, mucosal edema, and overproduction of secretions.

c. Oxygen should be administered.

d. Generally, initial management begins with administration of continuous beta agonists. Often anticholinergic agents are considered.

e. Parenteral corticosteroids are started immediately. Enteral corticosteroids are just as effective; however, the child may not be able to tolerate them. Do not delay steroid administration due to lack of IV access.

f. Heliox therapy may be considered.

g. IV magnesium sulfate is also administered early in the course (not proven but may be adjunctive therapy).

h. Most patients respond well to therapy. However, a small minority will show signs of worsening ventilation, whether from worsening airflow obstruction, worsening respiratory muscle fatigue, or a combination of the two.

i. Signs of impending respiratory failure include declining mental clarity, worsening

fatigue, and progressive hypercapnia. Exactly when to intubate is based on clinical judgement. Clinicians should be aware that hypotension commonly accompanies the initiation of positive-pressure ventilation (PPV) and close attention should be paid to maintaining or replacing intravascular volume.

j. Permissive hypercapnia or controlled hypoventilation is the recommended ventilator strategy to provide adequate oxygenation and ventilation while minimizing high airway pressures and barotrauma. It involves administration of as high an FiO_2 as necessary to maintain adequate arterial oxygenation, acceptance of hypercapnia, and treatment of respiratory acidosis. Adjustments are made to the V_T, ventilator rate, and I:E ratio to minimize airway pressures. Bronchodilators are continued.

k. Nurses must continuously monitor patients in status asthmaticus. Frequent evaluations are necessary to assess the efficacy of medications.

l. Respiratory assessments include respiratory rate and effort as well as the quality of air movement on auscultation.

m. The child's level of consciousness is frequently assessed because a decreased mental status may signal impending respiratory failure.

n. Caring for the child with asthma after endotracheal intubation presents additional challenges. Routine maneuvers to maintain airway patency may irritate airway receptors and trigger bronchospasm and hypoxia. Heavy sedation and in some patients neuromuscular blockade may be required.

o. The risk of developing a pneumothorax is great in mechanically ventilated patients with asthma. Pneumothorax should be suspected if there is a sudden clinical deterioration with hypoxemia, acidosis, hypotension, or unilateral absence of breath sounds. If ventilation is not effective, ECMO may be considered.

2. *Long-Term Asthma Care*

a. Once over status asthmaticus, nursing care may begin with review of the health history of the child, the home/school/play environment, and parent/child attitudes about the condition.

b. Nurses should provide asthma education.

c. They should obtain information on how asthma affects the child's everyday activities and self-concept, the child's and family's adherence to the prescribed therapy, and their personal treatment goals. Every effort is made to build a partnership between the child/family and healthcare team. In general, the child and family's satisfaction with asthma control and with the quality of care should be assessed.

d. The nurse should also assess the child and family's perception of the severity of disease and their level of social support.

e. One of the major emphases of nursing care is outpatient management by the family. Parents/children are taught how to prevent exacerbations, to recognize and respond to symptoms of bronchospasm, to maintain health and prevent complications, and to promote normal activities.

3. *Support Child or Adolescent and Family.* The nurse can provide support in a number of ways. Children/families need education on their condition and reassurance from the healthcare team that they can learn to control and cope with their asthma and live a normal life.

G. Complications

Catastrophic complications include hypoxic brain injury and death. Other complications include secondary bacterial infection, pneumothorax, and sudden airway closure from severe bronchospasm causing respiratory arrest.

H. Prognosis/Outcome

Some children's asthma symptoms may improve at puberty, but up to two thirds of children with asthma continue to have symptoms through adulthood. The prognosis for control or disappearance of symptoms varies in children from those who have rare and infrequent attacks to those who are constantly having wheezing or are subject to status asthmaticus. In general, when symptoms are severe and numerous, when symptoms have been present for a long time, and when there is a family history of allergy, there is a greater likelihood of a poor prognosis. Risk factors that may predict the persistence of symptoms into adulthood (from infancy) include atopy, male gender, exposure to environmental tobacco, and maternal history of asthma. Many children who outgrow their exacerbations continue to have airway hyperresponsiveness and cough as adults.

I. Risk factors for asthma deaths include early onset, frequent attacks, difficult-to-manage disease, adolescence, history of respiratory failure, psychologic

problems, dependency on or misuse of asthma drugs, presence of physical stigmata, and abnormal PFT results (Conlon, 2013; National Heart, Lung, and Blood Institute & National Asthma Education and Prevention Program, 2007).

Cystic Fibrosis

A. Definition

CF is an autosomal recessive disorder of the cystic fibrosis transmembrane regulation gene (CFTR). Mutation of the CFTR causes defective epithelial ion transport leading to dehydrated, viscous secretions. Abnormal secretions obstruct tubular structures in the upper and lower airways, vas deferens, gut, liver, and pancreas.

B. Etiology and Incidence

1. CF is caused by two disease-causing mutations in CFTR. CFTR is the principal chloride channel of epithelial cells and controls ion transport. This defective channel leads to imbalances in electrolytes and fluids at the cell surface leading to abnormal secretions and inflammatory responses.

2. In the Unites States, CF is the most common fatal genetic disease affecting the Caucasian population. The incidence of CF is approximately one in 3,000 to 4,000 births in non-Hispanic Caucasian births and considerable less in other ethnic groups (Cystic Fibrosis Foundation, 2016; Farrell et al., 2017).

C. Clinical Presentation

1. Due to widespread CF newborn screening, at least 64% of infants are diagnosed in the first year of life (Farrell et al., 2017).

2. Newborns with CF may present with meconium ileus.

3. Failure to thrive; recurrent or chronic pulmonary infections; large, bulky, foul-smelling stools; and salty-tasting skin are clinically suspicious for CF.

4. Physical exam findings may include wheezing or crackles on lung exam, nasal polyps, digital clubbing, or rectal prolapse.

D. Diagnostic Studies

1. Pilocarpine iontophoresis sweat test is the gold standard for diagnosis of CF.

2. Genetic analysis of CFTR is also available.

3. Since 2010, newborn screening for CF is performed in all 50 states.

E. Patient Care Management

Treatment regimens for infants and children with CF are complicated and individualized. Patient care is managed by a multidisciplinary team at a CF-accredited center. Regimens typically include nutritional support that may or may not include pancreatic enzyme replacement, ACT, and inhaled antibiotics.

F. Outcomes

Life expectancy for people with CF has continued to increase with advances in treatments and therapies. Respiratory disease is the main source of morbidity and mortality. Some patients will have progressive respiratory failure and need lung transplantation (Borowitz et al., 2009; Cystic Fibrosis Foundation, 2016; Farrell et al., 2017; Lahiri et al., 2016).

Bronchiectasis

A. Definition

Bronchiectasis is an abnormal and permanent dilatation of the bronchi. Chronic inflammation, destruction of ciliated epithelial cells, and accumulation of secretions leads to airflow obstruction and recurrent infections.

B. Pathophysiology

1. CF is the most common cause of significant bronchiectasis. Other conditions that predispose children include impaired immune dysfunction, ciliary dyskinesia, foreign-body aspiration, aspiration of gastric contents, infection, or clinical syndromes or congenital tracheobronchomegaly. There are three main mechanisms that lead to bronchiectasis:

    a. Obstruction

    b. Chronic inflammation

    c. Congenital forms related to abnormal cartilage formation

C. Clinical Presentation

1. Patient complains of cough and purulent sputum production.

2. Physical exam findings may include crackles or wheezing on lung exam. Digital clubbing can also

be seen. Dyspnea and hypoxemia are seen in severe cases. Obstructive, restrictive, or mixed patterns on pulmonary function studies can be seen, depending on the severity of disease. Growth failure and malnutrition can also be seen.

3. Bronchiectasis is best defined by high-resolution CT, which proved to be the most sensitive and specific noninvasive method of diagnosis.

D. Patient Care Management

1. The goal of treatment is to prevent further progression of lung damage and decline in lung function. This requires treatment of the underlying cause.

2. Treatment may include chest physiotherapy, antibiotics, and bronchodilators.

3. Surgical intervention may be considered for select patients.

E. Outcomes

Prognosis for children with bronchiectasis has improved with earlier diagnosis and more effective treatments and therapies (Bonavita & Naidich, 2012; Chalmers et al., 2014; Feldman, 2011; Redding, 2009).

Obstructive Sleep-Disordered Breathing

A. Definition

1. Obstructive sleep apnea syndrome (OSAS) is defined as a disorder of breathing during sleep with prolonged partial upper airway obstruction or a complete obstruction that disrupts normal respiration during sleep and normal sleep patterns.

2. Common symptoms include nightly snoring, interrupted or disturbed sleep patterns, enuresis, and daytime neurobehavioral problems.

3. Children with OSAS usually do not exhibit daytime sleepiness as do adults with the exception of obese children.

4. If untreated, obstructive sleep-disordered breathing may result in complications such as growth failure, cor pulmonale, PH, poor learning, behavioral problems, attention deficit hyperactivity disorder, and death.

B. Pathophysiology

1. The pathophysiology of OSAS remains poorly understood. OSAS occurs when the upper airway collapses during inspiration. Such collapse is a dynamic process that involves interaction between sleep state, pressure-flow airway mechanics, and respiratory drive.

2. When resistance to inspiratory flow increases or when activation of the pharyngeal dilator muscle decreases, negative inspiratory pressure may collapse the airway.

3. Although childhood OSAS is associated with adenotonsillar hypertrophy, it is not caused by large tonsils and adenoids alone.

4. OSAS is the combined result of structural and neuromuscular variables within the upper airway.

C. Clinical Presentation

1. Nighttime signs and symptoms include snoring, paradoxical chest and abdomen motion, retractions, witnessed apnea, snorting episodes, difficulty breathing, cyanosis, sweating, and disturbed sleep.

2. Daytime symptoms can include mouth breathing, difficulty waking, moodiness, nasal obstruction, daytime sleepiness, hyperactivity, and cognitive problems.

3. With severe cases, OSAS is associated with cor pulmonale, failure to thrive, developmental delay, PH, and even death.

D. Patient Care Management

1. OSAS is diagnosed by polysomnography (PSG). PSG is indicated when the clinical assessment suggests the diagnosis of OSAS in children.

2. A common treatment for sleep-disordered breathing in children is adenotonsillectomy, provided there is evidence of adenotonsillar hypertrophy. PSG is indicated following adenotonsillectomy to assess for residual OSAS in children with preoperative evidence for moderate to severe OSAS, obesity, craniofacial anomoalies that obstruct the upper airway, and neurologic disorder.

3. Children with OSAS are at risk for respiratory compromise postoperatively as a result of upper airway edema, increased secretions, respiratory depression secondary to analgesic and anesthetic agents, and postobstructive pulmonary edema. Patients may require cardiorespiratory monitoring for 24 hours postoperatively to ensure their stability.

4. CPAP and BiPAP may be helpful in older children with sleep-disordered breathing whose condition persists after surgical intervention.

5. CPAP/BiPAP is a long-term therapy with frequent assessments to evaluate the required amount of pressure and the overall effectiveness of the intervention.

6. Tracheostomy may be required for children with craniofacial syndromes in which there is partial or complete upper airway obstruction.

7. Nursing care of the child with sleep-disordered breathing involves early detection by observation of the infant's or child's sleep patterns and active participation in the diagnostic polysomnography.

8. Counseling families of children with sleep-disordered breathing may involve counseling for dietary modifications, exercise programs, weight management, use of CPAP/BiPAP equipment, and direct postoperative care after surgical intervention of tonsillectomy or adenoidectomy.

9. Nursing can help the child and family cope with the chronic illness diagnosis if intervention, such as CPAP or BiPAP, is required.

E. Outcomes

One of the major drives to treat any medical condition is the prevention of morbidity and mortality. The consequences of untreated OSAS in children can be serious. Sleep-disordered breathing can lead to substantial morbidities affecting the CNS, the cardiovascular and metabolic systems, and somatic growth, ultimately leading to a reduced quality of life (Aurora et al., 2011; Conlon, 2013; Ehsan & Ishman, 2016; Tan, Gozal, & Kheirandish-Gozal, 2013).

PULMONARY HEMORRHAGE

A. Definition and Etiology

1. Bleeding in the lower respiratory tract in children is rare but can be life-threatening. Hemoptysis, the expectoration of blood, is an acute manifestation and gives a rough measure of the amount of pulmonary hemorrhage. *Pulmonary hemosiderosis* is a term to describe persistent or recurrent bleeding.

2. Causes of pulmonary hemorrhage include bronchitis and bronchiectasis (especially in CF), acute or chronic infection, pneumonia or abscess, TB, or chest trauma. Cardiovascular causes include increased pulmonary venous pressure, arteriovenous (AV) malformation, and pulmonary emboli. Autoimmune disorders and rare immune-related vascular disease as a cause of pulmonary hemorrhage is generally limited to older children. Aspiration of maternal blood can be a cause in the neonate.

3. Acute idiopathic pulmonary hemorrhage of infancy is described as an episode of pulmonary hemorrhage in a previously healthy infant who is younger than 1 year of age and no other cause for bleeding can be found.

B. Pathophysiology

1. The pathophysiology of pulmonary hemorrhage depends on the etiology. The hemorrhage can be focal, resulting from infection, trauma, or foreign bodies— or diffuse caused by abnormalities of alveolar capillaries. The diagnosis of pulmonary hemorrhage is generally achieved by finding evidence of blood or hemosiderin in the lung. Within 48 to 72 hours of an episode of bleeding, alveolar macrophages convert the iron from erythrocytes into hemosiderin.

2. Prior suggestions of an association between acute idiopathic pulmonary hemorrhage of infancy and toxic mold exposure have not been supported on subsequent review.

C. Clinical Presentation

1. *History.* The severity of patient presentation can vary greatly. This may or not include respiratory distress or hemoptysis. Older children or young adults may report a warm or "bubbling" sensation in the chest wall.

2. *Physical Examination*

    a. Rapid and large-volume blood loss manifests as symptoms of cyanosis, respiratory distress, and shock. The infant or child may vomit large quantities of swallowed blood.

    b. Respiratory distress and hypoxia can be severe, requiring immediate endotracheal intubation and ventilation.

    c. Chronic, subclinical blood loss may manifest as anemia, fatigue, dyspnea, or altered activity tolerance.

D. Diagnostic Tests

1. Acute hemorrhage is usually accompanied by a drop in hematocrit, an increase in reticulocyte count, and a stool positive for occult blood.

2. Diagnosis is most readily confirmed with detection of hemosiderin-laden macrophages in sputum or gastric aspirate using Prussian blue staining. If the patient is unable to expectorate sputum from lower airways, sputum induction or a flexible bronchoscopy with BAL may be needed to obtain the sample.

3. Chest radiograph should be performed and may indicate the site and extent of the bleeding. Normal radiograph does not rule out pulmonary hemorrhage.

4. Culturing of BAL samples for bacteria, viruses, and fungi helps to exclude infectious processes.

E. Clinical Course

The clinical course depends on the etiology of the hemorrhage and the extent of bleeding.

F. Patient Care Management

1. *Direct Care.* Plasmapheresis has been used successfully during acute massive hemorrhage in Goodpasture syndrome and possibly other autoimmune diseases as well.

2. *Supportive Care.* Infants and children are admitted to ICUs for close monitoring of respiratory and hemodynamic status. Degree of anemia is followed closely. Rapid blood transfusions may be warranted. PPV may be used to reduce hemorrhage. With diffuse hemorrhage, corticosteroid and immunosuppressive agents may be beneficial.

3. Complications include severe respiratory failure, anemia, and end-organ failure from hypoxia.

G. Outcomes

Resolution of Pulmonary Hemorrhage. Prognosis of patient depends on underlying disease process (Agarwal et al., 2005; Dine & Werner, 2008; Godfrey, 2004; Nevin, 2016).

PULMONARY HYPERTENSION

A. Definition and Etiology

1. PH is a rare disease in newborns, infants, and children that is associated with significant morbidity and mortality. In the majority of pediatric patients, PH is idiopathic or associated with congenital heart disease and rarely is associated with other conditions such as connective tissue or thromboembolic disease (Jaff, et al., 2011).

2. PH is defined as "a resting mean pulmonary artery pressure greater than or equal to 25 mmHg" (Hoeper et al., 2013, D43). Classification of pediatric PH is challenging due to the many diseases associated with PH across the life span.

3. The World Health Organization (WHO)/World Symposium and Panama classifications have been applied to children with PH; however, controversies persist regarding the relative utility of each system.

B. Pathophysiology

1. *Vasoconstriction*. In young children, the pathobiology suggests failure of the neonatal vasculature to relax, in addition to a striking reduction in arterial number/surface area. However, with time, the changes become fixed with a vasodilator-unresponsive component, which appears to be temporally related to the development of thickened vascular media and adventitia with dramatic increases in the deposition of structural matrix proteins, such as collagen and elastin, in the pulmonary artery wall. In older children, intimal hyperplasia and occlusive changes as well as the plexiform lesion are found in the pulmonary arterioles.

2. With increasing age, intimal fibrosis and plexiform lesions are seen more frequently.

3. Endothelial dysfunction appears to be a key factor in mediating the structural changes that occur in the pulmonary vasculature. The integrity of the pulmonary vascular endothelium is critical for maintaining vascular tone, homeostasis, leukocyte trafficking, transduction of luminal signals to abluminal vascular tissues, production of growth factors and cell signals with autocrine and paracrine effects, and barrier function (Budhiraja, Tuder, & Hassoun, 2004, p. 159).

4. The vascular endothelium is recognized as an important source of locally active mediators that contribute to the control of vasomotor tone and structural remodeling, and appears to play a crucial role in the pathogenesis of PH. These may include increased thromboxane, endothelin, and serotonin, and decreased prostacycline and NO as well as vascular endothelial growth factor and xanthine oxidoreductase.

5. The endothelial cell dysfunction seen leads to the release of vasoproliferative substances in addition to vasoconstrictive agents that ultimately result in progression of pulmonary vascular remodeling and progressive vascular obstruction and obliteration.

C. Classification of PH

During the Fifth World Symposium held in 2013 in Nice, France, the consensus was to maintain the previous clinical classification of PH (Table 2.14). Some modifications and updates were proposed according to new data published in the preceding years. It was also decided in agreement with the Task Force on Pediatric PH to add some specific items related to pediatric PH in order to have a comprehensive classification common for adults and children (Simonneau et al., 2013).

D. Clinical Presentation

1. *History*

   a. The presenting symptoms in children with PH are highly variable.

TABLE 2.14 Updated Classification of Pulmonary Hypertension

1.	PAH
1.1	Idiopathic PAH
1.2	Heritable PAH
1.2.1	BMPR2
1.2.2	ALK-1, ENG, SMAD9, CAV1, KCNK3
1.2.3	Unknown
1.3	Drug and toxin induced
1.4	Associated with:
1.4.1	Connective tissue disease
1.4.2	HIV infection
1.4.3	Portal hypertension
1.4.4	Congenital heart diseases
1.4.5	Schistosomiasis
1'	Pulmonary veno-occlusive disease and/or pulmonary capillary hemangiomatosis
1"	PPHN

(continued)

TABLE 2.14 Updated Classification of Pulmonary Hypertension *(continued)*

2.	Pulmonary hypertension due to left heart disease
2.1	Left ventricular systolic dysfunction
2.2	Left ventricular diastolic dysfunction
2.3	Valvular disease
2.4	Congenital/acquired left heart inflow/outflow tract obstruction and congenital cardiomyopathies
3.	Pulmonary hypertension due to lung diseases and/or hypoxia
3.1	Chronic obstructive pulmonary disease
3.2	Interstitial lung disease
3.3	Other pulmonary diseases with mixed restrictive and obstructive pattern
3.4	Sleep-disordered breathing
3.5	Alveolar hypoventilation disorders
3.6	Chronic exposure to high altitude
3.7	Developmental lung diseases
4.	CTEPH
5.	Pulmonary hypertension with unclear multifactorial mechanisms
5.1	Hematologic disorders: chronic hemolytic anemia, myeloproliferative disorders, splenectomy
5.2	Systemic disorders: sarcoidosis, pulmonary histiocytosis, lymphangioleiomatosis
5.3	Metabolic disorders: glycogen storage disease, Gaucher disease, thyroid disorders
5.4	Other: Tumoral obstruction, fibrosing mediastinitis, chronic renal failure, segmental PH

CTEPH, chronic thromboembolic pulmonary hypertension; PAH, pulmonary arterial hypertension; PH, pulmonary hypertension; PPHN, persistent pulmonary hypertension of the newborn.

Source: Simonneau, G., Gatzoulis, M., Adatia, I., Celermajer, D., Denton, C., Ghofrani, A., . . . Souza, R. (2013). Updated clinical classification of pulmonary hypertension. *Journal of the American College of Cardiology, 62*(25), D34–D41.

b. Infants with PH often present with signs of low cardiac output (tachypnea, tachycardia, poor appetite, failure to thrive, lethargy, diaphoresis, and irritability).

c. Infants and older children may develop cyanosis with exertion due to right-to-left shunting through a patent foramen ovale (PFO) or congenital heart disease (CHD).

d. Children without adequate shunting may present with syncope due to the inability to achieve an adequate cardiac output with exertion.

e. After early childhood, children present with symptoms similar to those of adults.

f. In older children, the most common symptoms are exertional dyspnea and chest pain.

2. *Physical Examination*

a. Murmurs with a prominent S_2 are often heard. Point of maximal impulse (PMI) may be displaced to the subxiphoid area.

b. Jugular venous distention may be present.

c. Hepatomegaly may be present.

d. Ascites and peripheral edema may occur in severe cases.

e. Clubbing and cyanosis may be present in children with underlying lung disease.

f. Varying degrees of dyspnea occur on exertion.

3. *Diagnostic Evaluation* (Hoeper, et al., 2013; Kaestner, et al., 2016)

a. The evaluation and care of pediatric PH patients should be provided or comanaged by specialty PH centers. Routine visits should be performed at a minimum of every 3 to 6 months with more frequent visits with advanced disease or after initiation or changes in therapy.

b. Echocardiography is the noninvasive test of choice for initial screening for PH. It is useful for identifying potential causes of PH, evaluating RV function, and assessing related comorbidities.

c. ECG is used to assess for rhythm disturbances.

d. *Cardiac catheterization.* The goals for cardiac catheterization in children with PH are to confirm the diagnosis and assess the severity of the disease, to assess the response to pulmonary vasodilators before starting therapy, to evaluate the response to or the need for changes in therapy, to exclude other potentially treatable diagnoses, to assess operability as part of the assessment of patients with systemic to pulmonary artery shunts, and to assist in the determination of suitability for heart or heart–lung transplantation.

e. *Other imaging studies*

i. Chest x-ray is often normal.

ii. CT may yield valuable information on disease pathogenesis.

iii. V/Q scan is commonly used to assess ventilation–perfusion mismatch owing to airway or vascular obstruction and has been useful in determining the presence of PE, determining asymmetrical blood supply after surgical repair of obstructed pulmonary arteries, and assessing abnormal chest radiograph findings.

iv. MRI remains the gold standard for assessing the RV.

f. *Physiological assessments*

i. Six-minute-walk test monitors changes in longitudinal follow-up.

ii. Cardiopulmonary exercise testing is frequently used to evaluate and follow up patients with PH. Useful for monitoring maximal O_2 consumption, CO_2 elimination, maximal cardiac output, and anaerobic threshold.

g. *Biomarkers*

i. B-type natriuretic peptide (BNP) and NT-proBNP are released from the atria and ventricles in response to volume overload and stretch. BNP levels are inversely proportional to prognosis in PH.

h. *Sleep study.* Recommended in the following situations: diagnostic evaluation of patients with PH at risk for sleep-disordered breathing and indicated in the evaluation of patients with poor responsiveness to PH-directed therapies.

i. Genetic testing. May be considered for patients with idiopathic PH and hereditary PH.

E. Patient Care Management

1. *General Measures*

a. Annual influenza vaccination as well as pneumococcal vaccination are recommended unless there are contraindications.

b. Administer antipyretics for temperature elevations greater than 38° C (101° F) to minimize the consequences of increased metabolic demands.

c. Aggressive therapy is needed for pulmonary hypertensive crises occurring with episodes of pneumonia or during upper respiratory tract infection.

d. Decongestants with pseudophedrine should be avoided because they exacerbate PH.

e. Diet and/or medical therapy should be used to prevent constipation as Valsalva maneuvers transiently decrease venous return to the right side of the heart and may precipitate syncopal episodes.

f. Therapy of acute PH in the ICU (Galiè et al., 2013)

i. Oxygen is indicated in children with ventilation–perfusion mismatch based on arterial saturations of less than 95%. Oxygen works as a potent pulmonary vasodilator and a weak systemic vasoconstrictor.

ii. Sodium bicarbonate may be used in PH crisis as acidosis elevates PVR and impairs the effect of inotropic and vasopressor drugs.

iii. Sedation. Anxiety and agitation increase PVR and VO_2 and should be avoided.

iv. Anesthesia, intubation, and insertion of invasive lines are among the most crucial steps in the management of a child with PH with imminent deterioration.

v. Mechanical ventilation is indicated in severe PH with profound cyanosis, respiratory or metabolic acidosis not responding to initial therapy, respiratory failure, or in cardiopulmonary arrest.

vi. Fluid management. RV in patients with significant PH is preload dependent. Volume loss is poorly tolerated and in an acute PH crisis, volume challenge may be useful but hemodynamic monitoring is mandatory.

vii. Medication management

1) Anticoagulation. Recommended for most patients.

2) Calcium channel blockade. Inhibit calcium influx through the slow channel into cardiac and smooth muscle cells. Their usefulness for select patients with PH is based on the ability to cause pulmonary vasodilation. Acute vasodilator testing during right heart cardiac catheterization is a critical part of the initial assessment of patients with PH to determine appropriate treatment course. Chronic calcium channel blockade is

efficacious for patients who demonstrate an acute response to vasodilator testing.

3) Prostaglandins. These have been shown to improve hemodynamics, quality of life, and exercise capacity. Treatment often requires a continuous IV/subcutaneous delivery system.

4) Prostacyclin analogs. These medications produce vasodilation and decrease platelet adherence to the endothelium. They also disaggregate platelets that have already clumped, increase red blood cell flexibility, decrease blood viscosity, and inhibit platelet aggregation.

5) Endothelin receptor antagonists. These are promising drugs for the treatment of PH. These medications improve exercise capacity, quality of life, and cardiopulmonary dynamics. These medications block the vasoconstrictive effects of endothelin receptors.

6) NO. This is an inhaled vasodilator that exerts selective effects on the pulmonary circulation.

7) Phosphodiesterase inhibitors. These medications promote pulmonary vasodilation.

8) Elastase inhibitors. Statins have been shown to exert numerous effects on vascular wall function.

9) Cardiac glycosides, diuretics, antiarrhythmic therapy, inotropic agents, and nitrates may be used.

- Children with right-sided heart failure may benefit from digitalis in addition to diuretic therapy.

- Although malignant arrhythmias are rare in PH, treatment is appropriate for documented cases.

- Inotropic support may be used during PH crisis.

- Nitrates have been used to treat chest pain in children.

viii. Nonpharmacologic therapy includes intra-arterial communication (may be lifesaving in selected patients), Potts shunt (aortopulmonary shunt), ECMO (a bridge to recovery or to transplant), ventricular assistive devices (VADs), and transplantation.

F. Prognosis and Outcomes

PH remains a significant source of morbidity and mortality in many childhood diseases. PH remains distinct from adult disease. Long-term outcomes remain poor. Pediatric PH has been understudied and little is understood about the natural history, fundamental mechanisms, and treatment of childhood PH. The American Heart Association and American Thoracic Society Joint Guidelines for Pediatric PH (Abman et al., 2015) provides recommendations for the diagnosis and treatment of PH in children that highlights key gaps in our knowledge and will serve as a source of ideas for promoting new research (Abman et al., 2015; Galiè et al., 2013; Hoeper et al., 2013; Hopper, Abman, & Ivy, 2016; Kaestner et al., 2016; Simonneau et al., 2013).

THORACIC TRAUMA

A. Definition and Etiology

1. Thoracic trauma is frequently associated with head and abdominal trauma; the mortality rate is higher in this instance. The mortality rate from thoracic trauma is reported to be 26% and can be as high as 33% when penetrating injuries are involved. Thoracic trauma is frequently associated with head, abdominal, and spine trauma, making the mortality rate higher (Bruzoni & Krummel, 2012).

2. In the pediatric age group, because of chest-wall resiliency, physiologic aberrations can occur with trauma that does not fracture or penetrate.

3. The interruption of satisfactory respiration and circulation secondary to chest injury is frequently complicated by blood loss and hypotension and all three factors must be quickly reversed for survival.

4. Restoration of the normal cardiopulmonary function fundamentally depends on a clean airway, intact chest and diaphragm, and unrestricted heart–lung dynamics.

B. Pathophysiology

1. *Rib Fractures.* These are unusual in children because of the extreme flexibility of the osseous and cartilaginous framework of the thorax. Crush and direct-blow injuries are the usual etiologic factors.

a. In addition, manual compression of the lateral chest wall, rickets, tumors, and osteogenesis imperfecta have been associated with fracture.

b. Multiple fractures of the middle ribs can be seen in cases of battered child syndrome.

c. Violence to the chest wall may produce pulmonary and cardiac lacerations and contusions, various pneumothoraces, and hemothorax. Critical respiratory distress may also follow multiple anterior rib fractures (leading to a flail chest).

d. The clinical picture includes local pain that is aggravated by motion. Tenderness is elicited by pressure applied directly over the fracture or on the same rib. The fracture site may be ecchymotic and edematous.

e. The clinical manifestations may range from these minimal findings to the severest form of ventilatory distress with a flail chest and lung injury.

f. Treatment requires control of pain in order to permit unrestricted respiration. Displacement requires no therapy. Thoracentesis and chest tube insertion should be done promptly for hemothorax and pneumothorax. Shock should be managed by appropriate replacement therapy and oxygen.

2. *Traumatic Pneumothorax* (Figures 2.18 and 2.19). Traumatic, simple, tension, and open pneumothorax are rare in infants and children, in whom a very mobile mediastinum would compound the cardiorespiratory distress usually encountered in such injuries. The injuries are formidable and require specific maneuvers to reverse a malignant change of events.

a. The creation of a tension pneumothorax in which intrapleural pressure is at or exceeds atmospheric pressure requires a valvular mechanism through which the amount of air entering the pleural space exceeds the amount escaping it. The positive intrapleural pressure is dissipated by a mediastinal shift, which compresses the opposite lung in the presence of an ipsilateral pulmonary collapse and angulates the great vessels entering and leaving the heart. Intrapleural tension can be increased by traumatic hemothorax, and respiratory exchange and cardiac output are critically diminished.

b. The etiologic possibilities, in addition to chest wall and lung trauma, include rupture of the esophagus, pulmonary cyst, emphysematous lobe, and postoperative bronchial fistula.

c. Clinical findings may include external evidence of a wound, tachypnea, dyspnea, cyanosis with hyperresonance, absence or transmission of breath sounds, and dislocation of the trachea and apical cardiac impulse. The hemithoraces may be asymmetric, the involved side being the larger.

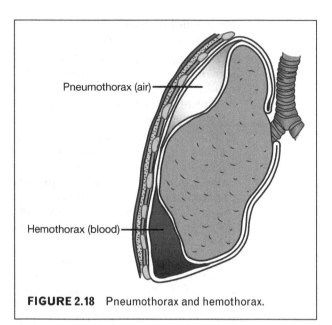

FIGURE 2.18 Pneumothorax and hemothorax.

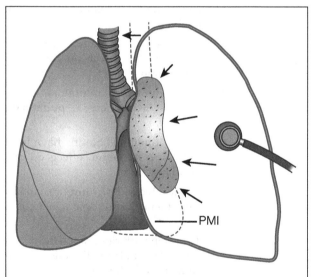

FIGURE 2.19 Tension pneumothorax.

PMI, point of maximal impulse.

d. Chest tube insertion is indicated for a tension or simple pneumothorax.

e. Prompt relief and pulmonary expansion can be anticipated if the source of the intrapleural air has been controlled.

f. An open sucking pneumonthorax in which atmospheric air has direct entrance and exit from a relatively free pleural space is also an urgent thoracic emergency. The access is almost invariably accomplished through a large traumatic hole in the chest wall.

i. The emergency management of this critical situation is prompt occlusion of the chest-wall defect by bulky sterile dressings and measures to prevent conversion of this open pneumothorax into a tension pneumothorax. Simultaneous pleural decompression by closed intercostal tube drainage is essential. After systemic stabilization, more formal surgical debridement, reconstruction, and closure can be done in the operating room.

ii. Subcutaneous emphysema usually results from injury to the pulmonary ventilator system.

3. *Hemothorax* (Figure 2.18). Blood in the pleural cavity is the most common sequelae of thoracic trauma regardless of type. The source of the bleeding is either systemic (high pressure) from the chest wall or pulmonary (low pressure). Hemorrhage from pulmonary vessels is usually self-limiting unless major tributaries have been transected.

a. Intrapleural blood eventually clots and becomes organized fibrous tissue.

b. The immediate findings are those of blood loss compounded by respiratory distress and perhaps hemoptysis. The trachea and apical pulse impulse are dislocated, the percussion note is flat, and the breath sounds are indistinct. The actual diagnosis is confirmed by thoracentesis after adequate radiographic studies if time allows.

c. Chest tube insertion evacuates the blood.

4. *Tracheobronchial Trauma.* Rupture of the trachea or bronchus in infants and children is usually preceded by a severe compression injury of the chest or a sharp blow to the anterior part of the neck. This discontinuity of a major airway is characterized by intrathoracic tension phenomena; later, stricture at the site of rupture leads to a loss of lung function by sepsis and atelectasis.

a. Rapidly progressive interstitial emphysema, pneumomediastinum, tension pneumothorax, and hemoptysis are fairly specific.

b. Bronchoscopic demonstration of the rupture is always necessary.

c. The initial management of bronchial rupture is concerned with the maintenance of a patent airway and decompression of the pleura and mediastinum by one or more intercostal tubes connected to closed drainage. Confirmatory endoscopy and bronchoplasty are followed by little or no loss of pulmonary functions distal to the narrowed segment.

5. *Posttraumatic Atelectasis.* With pulmonary contusion from any source, production of tracheobronchial secretions is stimulated but elimination is impeded by airway obstruction, pain, and depression of cough.

a. The clinical findings are dyspnea and cyanosis, an incessant unproductive cough with wheezing and audible rattling, and gross rhonchi and rales.

b. Adjunctive therapies may be considered in instances of chest trauma by frequent position changes, insistence on coughing, small amounts of depressant drugs (using the smallest dose possible), oxygen, humidification, antibiotics, diuretics, IV colloid, and minimal hydration.

6. *Cardiac Trauma.* This should be suspected after penetration of any part of the chest, lower part of the neck, or upper part of the abdomen. The possibility of heart injury also exists in the presence of blunt trauma to the anterior or left hemithorax with laceration by fractured sternum or ribs, or severe compression between the sternum and vertebral column. Blood loss with perforation varies between exsanguination, either internal or external, and minimal bleeding with or without acute cardiac tamponade. Nonpenetrating trauma can produce various degrees of myocardial contusions ranging from a small area of edema to a ruptured chamber.

7. *Traumatic Rupture of the Thoracic Aorta.* Many injuries of this type are associated with life-threatening injuries in other organs such as the abdomen and head.

8. *Injuries to the Esophagus.* Perforation of the esophagus in the neonatal age group can occur in the delivery room from extreme positive-pressure resuscitation or aspiration with a stiff catheter. In later infancy and childhood, rupture can follow ingestion of lye or a solid foreign body, esophagoscopy, or dilation. Spontaneous rupture proximal to an esophageal web has been described.

a. Hyperthermia, hypotension, and chest and neck pain mirror the mediastinitis. Pneumomediastinum, tension pneumothorax, subcutaneous emphysema, and hematemesis may be encountered.

b. A tension pneumothorax must quickly undergo decompression followed by prompt closure of the esophageal defect, mediastinal drainage, and dosing of antibiotics.

9. *Traumatic Blunt Rupture of the Diaphragm.* Blunt-trauma rupture of the diaphragm may occur with severe trauma. It is more common on the left than on the right. Significant cardiorespiratory abnormalities may occur in the early stages. If the rupture is not initially diagnosed, intestinal obstruction may be the leading symptom at the time of late diagnosis.

10. *Thoracoabdominal Injuries.* In infants and children, combined injury to the thorax and abdomen, including diaphragm rupture, is usually preceded by a violent traffic accident or other form of sudden, jolting impact.

    a. The clinical signs of upper abdominal tenderness, rigidity, and rebound tenderness almost uniformly accompany lower chest trauma and are explained by the abdominal distribution of intercostal nerves.

    b. Diaphragm rupture can occur with minimal soft tissue injury.

    c. The preliminary management of combined thoracoabdominal injuries must provide an adequate airway and circulation, gastric decompression, and evaluation and control of other injuries.

C. Clinical Presentation

1. *History.* It is important to learn the details of the mechanism of injury to pinpoint possible sites of injury.

2. *Physical Examination*

    a. Children with significant intrathoracic injuries may not have suggestive external evidence of these injuries. The primary survey during trauma resuscitation includes a rapid thoracoabdominal examination, including rapid assessment of airway and breathing. The absence of breath sounds implies the presence of a pneumothorax or hemothorax. However, because of the hyperresonance of the infant's thoracic cavity, breath sounds may be transmitted to the contralateral side. Observe for chest-wall ecchymosis, bruising, abrasions, sensation of crepitus, point tenderness over a rib, or a displaced trachea.

    b. Tension pneumothorax causes severe respiratory distress, distended neck veins, contralateral tracheal deviation, and poor systemic perfusion. There may be hyperresonance to percussion, decreased chest expansion, and diminished breath sounds on the side of the injury.

    c. Hemothorax manifests with signs similar to those of tension pneumothorax. Tachycardia and hypotension may result from decreased venous return to the heart.

    d. In tracheobronchial injury, small tears may present with subcutaneous emphysema, dyspnea, sternal tenderness, and hemoptysis. Complete transection presents with severe respiratory distress and failure.

    e. Rib fractures may cause palpable crepitus, rib deformity, and asymmetric chest-wall movement. Pain leads to splinting of the thorax with impaired ventilation.

    f. Aortic and great vessel injuries should be suspected if the patient develops midscapular back pain, unexplained hypotension, upper extremity hypertension, bilateral femoral pulse deficits, large initial chest tube output, sternal fracture, or widened mediastinum demonstrated by radiographic examination of the chest.

3. *Diagnostic Tests*

    a. Radiographic evaluation of the chest is standard in thoracic trauma cases (Table 2.15).

TABLE 2.15 Radiographic Evaluation of the Chest on Trauma

Hemothorax	Fluid assumes a dependent position Complete opacification of the hemothorax with accumulation of pleural fluid The trachea and mediastinum may be shifted away A lateral decubitus view may help confirm the presence of free pleural fluid
Pneumothorax	Presents with unilateral hyperlucency
Tension pneumothorax	Underlying lung will collapse Trachea and mediastinum will be shifted away from the side of the pneumothorax
Rib fractures	Rib and thoracic spine fractures are evaluated Excludes other chest and upper abdominal injuries
Cardiac tamponade, aortic, and great vessel injuries	High mediastinal-width to chest-width ratio Blurring of the aortic knob Tracheal deviation Widened peritracheal stripes Increased heart size with tamponade

b. ABG monitoring is used to evaluate for hypoxia, hypercarbia, and respiratory acidosis.

c. CT scan may be a useful adjunct in the evaluation and management of blunt chest trauma.

d. Bronchoscopy is used to confirm the diagnosis of rupture of the trachea or bronchus.

e. Angiography is the diagnostic test of choice if large vessel injury is suspected.

f. ECG can be used to evaluate for ischemic changes, premature atrial or ventricular contractions, and other arrhythmias that occur with myocardial contusion.

D. Patient Care Management

1. *Direct Care.* Care involves assessment and establishment of an airway, checking breathing and circulation, and correction of life-threatening injuries.

2. *Supportive Care.* Continue with chest tube evacuation of air or blood as long as necessary. Provide rigorous pulmonary toilet to prevent atelectasis (postural drainage, cough). If the patient is receiving mechanical ventilation, provide frequent suctioning and monitor peak inspiratory pressures. Use antibiotics only for a confirmed infection. Provide oxygen as necessary.

E. Outcomes

Most pediatric trauma-related mortality occurs before admission to the hospital, whether in the field or in the emergency department. Initial stabilization of the pediatric trauma victim includes rapid cardiopulmonary assessment, basic airway maneuvers, vascular access skills, and cardiopulmonary stabilization (Bruzoni & Krummel, 2012; Guidry & McGahren, 2012; Miller, 2006; Rodgers & McGahren; 2010; Tovar, 2008).

RESPIRATORY EMERGENCY

Respiratory Failure

A. Definition and Etiology

1. Effective pulmonary gas exchange requires clear airways, normal lungs and chest wall, and adequate pulmonary circulation.

2. Respiratory insufficiency is applied to two situations: (a) Where there is increased WOB but gas exchange is near normal and (b) when normal blood-gas tensions cannot be maintained and hypoxemia and acidosis develop secondary to carbon monoxide retention.

3. *Respiratory failure* is defined as the inability of the respiratory apparatus to maintain adequate oxygenation of the blood with or without carbon dioxide retention.

a. This process involves pulmonary dysfunction that generally results in impaired alveolar gas exchange, which can lead to hypoxemia or hypercapnia.

b. Respiratory failure is the most common cause of cardiopulmonary arrest in children.

c. Respiratory arrest is the complete cessation of breathing.

d. Apnea is the cessation of breathing for more than 20 seconds or for a shorter period when associated with hypoxemia or bradycardia.

i. Apnea can be central, in which respiratory efforts are absent; obstructive, in which respiratory efforts are present; and mixed in which both central and obstructive components are present.

4. Respiratory dysfunction may have an abrupt or insidious onset.

5. Respiratory failure can occur as an emergency situation or may be preceded by gradual and progressive deterioration of respiratory function.

B. Pathophysiology

1. Most clinical manifestations are nonspecific and are affected by variations among individual patients and differences in the severity and duration of inadequate gas exchange.

2. *Cardinal Signs.* The cardinal signs are restlessness, tachypnea, tachycardia, and diaphoresis. It should also be noted that in a patient who has been tachypneic, a decrease in respiratory rate may indicate impending failure.

3. *Early Signs.* Mood changes, headache, altered depth and pattern of respirations, hypertension, exertional dyspnea, anorexia, increased cardiac output and renal output, CNS symptoms, flaring nares, chest-wall retractions, expiratory grunt, wheezing, or prolonged expiration are all signs.

4. *More Severe Hypoxia.* Severe hypoxia is associated with hypotension/hypertension, altered vision, somnolence, stupor, coma, dyspnea, depressed respirations, bradycardia, and cyanosis.

C. Diagnostic Evaluation

Diagnosis is determined by the combined application of three sources of information:
- Presence or history of a condition that might predispose the patient to respiratory failure
- Observation of respiratory failure
- Measurement of ABGs, including pH

D. Patient Care Management

1. If respiratory arrest occurs, the primary objectives are to recognize the situation and immediately initiate resuscitative measures such as airway positioning, administration of oxygen, CPR, suctioning, and intubation.

2. Interventions, such as administering supplemental oxygen, positioning, stimulating, suctioning, and early intubation, may avert an arrest.

3. The principles of management are to maintain ventilation and maximize oxygen delivery, correct hypoxemia and hypercapnia, treat the underlying cause, minimize extrapulmonary organ failure, apply specific and nonspecific therapy to control oxygen demands, and anticipate complications.

4. Family support is aimed at keeping the family informed of the child's status and helping them cope with a near-death experience or an actual death.

Cardiopulmonary Resuscitation

A. Definition and Etiology

Cardiac arrest in children is less often of cardiac origin than from prolonged hypoxemia secondary to inadequate oxygenation, ventilation, and circulation. Some causes of cardiac arrest include injuries, suffocation, smoke inhalation, or infection. Respiratory arrest is associated with a better survival rate than cardiac arrest (Conlon, 2013).

B. Resuscitation Procedure

1. In 2010, the American Heart Association (AHA) implemented some changes in CPR guidelines. These guidelines were updated in 2015 and 2017 and are presented here.

  a. Rescuers should continue to initiate CPR with CAB (compressions, airway, and breathing) sequence instead of A-B-C (airway, breathing, and compressions). This CAB sequence reduces the amount of time to wait to initiate chest compressions.

  b. For simplicity in CPR training, in the absence of sufficient pediatric evidence, it is reasonable to use the adult BLS recommended chest compression rate of 100/min to 120/min for infants and children. It is reasonable that for pediatric patients (birth to the onset of puberty) rescuers provide chest compressions that depress the chest at least one third the anterior–posterior diameter of the chest. This equates to approximately 1.5 inches (4 cm) in infants to 2 inches (5 cm) in children. Once children have reached puberty, the recommended adult compression depth of at least 5 cm, but no more than 6 cm, is used for the adolescent of average adult size.

  c. Conventional CPR, using chest compressions with rescue breaths, should be provided for infants and children in cardiac arrest (Atkins et al., 2018).

2. If rescuers are unwilling or unable to deliver breaths, compression-only CPR for infants and children may administered (Atkins et al., 2015, 2018; Conlon, 2013).

3. *Pulse Check*

  a. The patient should be reassessed for a pulse every 2 minutes of CPR and should not be assessed for longer than 10 seconds.

  b. The carotid or femoral pulse may be used in a child. In an infant the brachial pulse is preferred.

4. *Chest Compression*

  a. *External chest compression* consists of serial, rhythmic compressions of the chest to maintain circulation to the vital organs until the child achieves spontaneous vital signs or advance life support can be provided.

  b. *Infants.* Placement of the fingers for compression is at a point on the lower sternum just below the intersection of the sternum and an imaginary line drawn between the nipples. Rescuers should use two fingers on the sternum. When two rescuers are present, the two-thumb encircling hands technique may be used.

  c. *Lone-rescuer CPR.* 30 compressions to two breaths.

  d. *Two-rescuer CPR.* 15 compressions to two breaths.

  e. *Child 1 to 8 years.* Compressions are applied to the lower half of the sternum. Rescuer should use the heel of one or two hands.

5. *Open the Airway.* For effective CPR the victim is placed on the back on a firm, flat surface. To open the airway, the head is positioned with a head tilt–chin lift maneuver (healthcare providers may use a jaw thrust). One hand should be placed on the victim's forehead while applying firm, backward pressure with the palm to tilt back the head. The fingers of the free hand are placed under the bony portion of the lower jaw near the chin to lift and bring the chin forward.

6. *Give Breaths*

  a. *Infants.* Bag valve mask (BVM) or operator's mouth covers the infant's nose and mouth.

  b. *Children.* Children are ventilated through the mouth while the nostrils are firmly pinched for airtight contact.

  c. A gentle rise of the chest is a sufficient indicator of adequate inflation and indicates that the airway is clear.

7. *Medications*

  Medications are used to:

  a. Correct hypoxemia

  b. Increase perfusion pressure during chest compressions

  c. Stimulate spontaneous or more forceful myocardial contraction

  d. Accelerate cardiac rate

  e. Correct metabolic acidosis

  f. Suppress ventricular ectopy (Atkins et al., 2015; Conlon, 2013)

Airway Obstruction

A. Attempts at clearing the airway should be considered for children in whom aspiration of a foreign body is witnessed or strongly suspected and in unconscious, nonbreathing children whose airways remain obstructed despite usual maneuvers to open them.

B. In a conscious choking child, attempt to relieve the obstruction only if the child is unable to make any sounds, the cough becomes ineffective, and/or there is increasing respiratory difficulty with stridor.

C. Infants

1. A combination of back blows (over the spine between the shoulder blades) and chest thrusts (on the sternum, the same location as for chest compressions) is recommended to relieve the foreign-body obstruction.

2. A choking infant is placed face down over the rescuer's arm with the head lower than the trunk and supported. For additional support, the rescuer should support the arm firmly against the thigh. Up to five quick sharp back blows are delivered (less force than with an adult). After the delivery of back blows, the rescuer turns the infant and places him/her supine on the rescuer's thigh and up to five quick downward chest thrusts are applied in rapid succession.

3. Back blows and chest thrusts are continued until the object is removed or the infant becomes unconscious. At that time CPR should be initiated.

D. Children

1. A series of subdiaphragmatic abdominal thrusts (Heimlick maneuver) is recommended for children older than 1 year of age. The maneuver creates an artificial cough that forces air and the foreign body out of the airway. The procedure is carried out with the child in a standing, sitting, or lying position.

2. The thrusts are delivered to the upper abdomen with a fisted hand at a point just below the rib cage. Up to five thrusts are repeated in rapid succession until the foreign body is expelled.

3. The child may vomit after relief of the obstruction and should be positioned to prevent aspiration (Conlon, 2013).

BPD (CHRONIC LUNG DISEASE OF PREMATURITY)

A. Definition

1. BPD is also known as *neonatal chronic lung disease* or *chronic lung disease of prematurity*.

2. In 1967, Northway first described BPD as persistent chronic respiratory symptoms, need for supplemental oxygen, and abnormal finding on chest radiograph. Advances in care of premature infants have changed the presentation of BPD. With the use of surfactant, antenatal glucocorticoid therapies and less aggressive mechanical ventilation and management of these neonates, survival has increased. The overall incidence of BPD has not changed despite the management strategies.

3. The "old" BPD was characterized by airway injury, inflammation, and parenchymal fibrosis, typically following mechanical ventilation and oxygen therapy for acute respiratory distress.

4. The "new" BPD is now more commonly seen in infants born at earlier gestational ages and characterized by disruption of normal lung development.

5. The definition of BPD is continuously evolving and varies among institutions.

6. Criteria from the National Institute of Child Health and Human Development (NICHHD) are based on timed assessments of infants according to their gestational age (Ehrenkranz et al., 2005).

    a. Infants less than 32 weeks gestational age are assessed at 36 weeks or when discharged home, whichever comes first.

    b. Infants greater than 32 weeks gestational age are assessed between 29 and 55 days of age or when discharge home, whichever comes first.

7. These infants require supplemental oxygen for at least 28 postnatal days and have abnormal chest radiographs at 36 weeks correct age. Based on the extent of support needed, these infants are classified as having mild, moderate, or severe BPD (Ehrenkranz et al., 2005).

    a. *Mild.* Breathing on room air

    b. *Moderate.* Require oxygen at less than 30%

    c. *Severe.* Require oxygen at greater than 30% and/or PPV

B. Etiology

Even with advances in perinatal and neonatal care over the past few decades, BPD continues to be a common complication of prematurity. Reported incidence of BPD varies throughout centers due to differences in neonatal risk factors, care practices, and definitions used. For infants with gestational ages of 22 to 28 weeks, the incidence of BPD is around 40% (Stoll et al, 2010). BPD results in significant morbidity and mortality, especially in very-low-weight and extremely low-weight infants. Ninety-seven percent of cases are seen in infants with birth weight less than 1,250 g (Bowen & Maxwell, 2014). BPD in infants greater than 32 weeks gestation is now rare and more extreme preterm newborns (24–26 weeks gestation) are surviving.

C. Pathophysiology

1. BPD is the response of the lung to acute injury at critical periods of lung growth that is multifactorial and not entirely understood. There are several risk factors that are associated with BPD, including prematurity, mechanical lung overdistention or volutrauma, oxygen toxicity, pulmonary or systemic infections, pulmonary vascular damage and edema, and deficiency or dysfunction of lung surfactant.

2. ALI, inflammatory responses, cytokines activation

    a. *Airway damage.* Metaplasia and smooth muscle hypertrophy lead an increase in mucus production, which leads to airway obstruction and atelectasis.

    b. Pulmonary vascular disease with increased permeability and smooth muscle hypertrophy lead to pulmonary edema and PH.

    c. Interstitial damage due to alteration in growth factors leads to impaired development of alveoli and capillaries.

D. Clinical Presentation

1. Signs and symptoms of BPD include tachypnea, retractions, failure to thrive, increase in ventilatory requirements or inability to wean, hypoxia, hypercapnia, respiratory acidosis, crackling, wheezing, and bronchospasm.

2. Some premature infants have no or very mild initial respiratory distress but go on to become chronically oxygen dependent.

3. Increased intrathoracic pressure may cause the syndrome of inappropriate antidiuretic hormone (SIADH), causing fluid and sodium retention.

4. Chronic hypoxemia may lead to cor pulmonale.

5. Abnormalities of the airway, aspiration, lobar hyperinflation, atelectasis, and copious endotracheal secretions are common.

6. PH may evolve to right ventricular failure, tachycardia, hepatomegaly, periorbital edema, and a prominent S_2 or a gallop rhythm.

7. Pulmonary exacerbation of BPD is usually triggered by a viral infection.

E. Invasive and Noninvasive Diagnostic Tests

1. *Chest Radiographs*

    a. Bilateral changes occur with fine granular opacification consistent with atelectasis or edema.

    b. Large airway collapse may also be seen.

2. CT scans can show multifocal areas of hyper-aeration, as well as linear and triangular subpleural opacities.

3. Serial pulmonary function testing may assist in assessing treatment modalities for BPD. Changes in PFTs correlate with radiographic findings.

4. Tracheomalacia, bronchomalcia, or both can be seen with bronchoscopy.

5. ABGs are not diagnostic of BPD but are used to assess for acidosis, hypercarbia, and hypoxia.

6. Echocardiograms are used to evaluate for PH.

7. Cardiac catheterization is not routinely performed.

8. Using pulse oximeters or transcutaneous oxygen monitoring is a reliable and noninvasive way to monitor arterial oxygenation. Pulse oximeters are easy to use and can monitor oxygen levels during feedings, crying, and sleeping.

F. Patient Care Management

1. *Oxygen Therapy*

a. Supplemental oxygen is used to avoid intermittent or prolonged periods of hypoxemia that can lead to impaired lung growth, cardiovascular and pulmonary vascular complications, and poor growth.

b. The goal of oxygen therapy is to maintain the oxygen level to adequately perfuse tissues and prevent PH and cor pulmonale, which can develop as a result of chronic hypoxemia, and also to reduce supplemental oxygen as quickly as possible to prevent oxygen toxicity.

c. Typically, oxygen saturations should be targeted between 90% and 95% and need to take into account gestational age. For very premature infants, saturations greater than 95% should be minimized to avoid oxygen toxicity. In the presence of congenital heart disease or PH, target saturations are based on specific patient needs.

d. If an infant's oxygen requirement increases, consider GERD, aspiration, congenital heart disease, or a new pneumonia.

e. Assessment of the infant's breathing room air should include noting growth patterns; if the patient stops growing, oxygen therapy may be reinstituted.

2. *Mechanical Ventilation*

a. Early use of CPAP may prevent or attenuate the need for invasive mechanical ventilation.

b. Weaning from ventilation may be prolonged in some infants and should be done slowly (see "Mechanical Ventilation" section).

c. Tracheostomy or home ventilation may be required in some patients with severe BPD.

3. *Growth and Nutrition*

a. Adequate nutrition is essential for normal growth and maturation of the lung. Ensure adequate protein and energy intake in the first few weeks after birth. Increased calorie and protein intake is required to meet the needs of the infants due to increased metabolic needs and rapid growth requirements.

b. Increased WOB necessitates a higher basal caloric requirement and increased VO_2. Calories should not be withheld because of the possibility of fluid overload. If necessary, diuretics can be adjusted.

c. VO_2 ideally is measured with a metabolic cart to provide accurate caloric requirement calculations. Otherwise, taking daily weights on the same scale and under the same conditions provides an estimation of basal metabolic requirements.

d. The enteral route is preferred for feedings. Because fluids are often restricted, infant formulas can be modified to increase caloric content, but the high osmotic load of high-calorie formula may cause intolerance in some infants. Complicating factors in providing adequate nutrition include the following:

  i. Gastroesophageal reflux

  ii. Constipation due to high-calorie formula and insufficient fluid intake

  iii. Poor suck and swallow or oral aversion

  iv. Risk for developing necrotizing enterocolitis due to decreased mesenteric flow

  v. Trace element and vitamin deficiencies

e. Speech therapy is essential for preventing and treating oral aversion.

4. *Fluid Management*

a. Infants with BPD poorly tolerate excess or even normal amounts of fluid. These infants have a tendency to accumulate these extra fluids in their lungs. This can lead to decline in lung function, hypoxemia, hypercapnia, and longer time on the ventilator.

b. In infants who are fluid restricted, it is critical to maintain total energy and macronutrient provision. This can be achieved using fortifiers to increase caloric density (Poindexter & Martin, 2015).

5. *Pharmacologic Interventions*

  a. *Bronchodilators*

    i. Bronchodilators can worsen lung function in infants with airway malacia as it can exacerbate wheezing.

    ii. Bronchodilators can reduce airway resistance but this is short lived and they can cause cardiovascular side effects such as tachycardia and hypertension.

    iii. Bronchodilators are more commonly used during acute exacerbations of airway obstruction.

  b. *Corticosteroids*

    i. Overall, the use of steroids in the BPD population is controversial and evolving.

    ii. Typically, use of systemic glucocorticoid therapy is limited to:

      1) Infants with severe BPD who require substantial persistent ventilatory and oxygen support

      2) Acute respiratory exacerbation

    iii. There is controversy about the use of inhaled corticosteroids in BPD. Overall, inhaled glucocorticoids may provide some short-term pulmonary benefit while avoiding the adverse effects of systemic administration. However, whether postnatal administration of inhaled glucocorticoids (such as budesonide) prevents BPD without increasing undesirable outcomes, including mortality, requires further study.

  c. *Methylxanthines*

    i. Medications, such as aminophylline (although rarely used) and caffeine, have shown to reduce airway resistance and potential other benefits such as respiratory stimulation and respiratory muscle contractility.

  d. *Diuretics*

    i. Diuretic therapy, including furosemide, hydrochlorothiazide, and spironolactone, is used to mobilized fluid and improve lung compliance.

    ii. Infants on chronic diuretic therapy should be monitored for electrolyte imbalance, ototoxicity, and metabolic alkalosis.

6. *Monitor for Infection*

  a. Monitor closely for signs and symptoms of infections.

  b. If quantity or quality of secretions changes, a tracheal secretion sample is collected for culture and Gram stain to evaluate for infection. If pneumonia is suspected, a CBC, blood culture, and chest radiograph are obtained.

7. *Prevention*

  a. Prevention of viral illnesses is essential for infants and children with BPD.

  b. Stay up to date on regular vaccines.

  c. Ensure proper hand hygiene is used by all caregivers.

  d. RSV prophylaxis with palivizumab should be considered based on the guidelines from the American Academy of Pediatrics.

    i. For premature infants (<32 weeks gestation) and those who have an oxygen requirement for at least the first 28 days after birth, palivizumab prophylaxis should be given for the RSV season during the first year of life.

    ii. During their second year of life, palivizumab prophylaxis should be considered if the child with BPD has required medical support within 6 months prior to the start of RSV season.

G. Complications and Long-Term Outcome

1. Long-term outcomes in this population have improved over time and mortality rate for BPD is low. When death does occur, common causes include respiratory failure, infection, or intractable PH and cor pulmonale.

2. During early childhood, readmission is common for respiratory distress associated with lower respiratory infections. RSV infections can be life-threatening.

3. Survivors of prematurity have high rates of abnormal PFT (obstruction with response to bronchodilator therapy) at school age when compared to peers without BPD. They also have been found to have significantly more respiratory symptoms and asthma treatments compared with controls.

4. BPD poses a significant risk for neurodevelopmental compromise. Postnatal infection and/or sepsis, periventricular leukomalacia, severe intraventricular hemorrhage, hearing impairment, and severe retinopathy of prematurity (ROP) are all important confounding variables that can greatly affect an infant's neurodevelopmental outcome (Groothuis & Makari, 2012). Assessment and referral to early-intervention programs for developmental delays and movement disorders are strongly recommended.

5. For infants with ROP, close follow up with ophthalmology should continue until mature retinal exam.

6. Ongoing follow-up care should involve a multidisciplinary care team, including the pediatrician, pulmonologist, speech therapist, nutritionist, and developmental specialists (Bowen & Maxwell, 2014; Darlow & Morley, 2015; Doyle & Anderson, 2009; Ehrenkranz et al., 2005; Groothuis & Makari, 2012; Islam, Keller, Aschner, Hartert, & Moore, 2015; Moore et al., 2012; Murthy et al., 2014; Poindexter et al., 2015; Poindexter & Martin, 2015; Schulzke & Pillow, 2010; Stoll et al., 2010).

PHYSIOLOGIC PRINCIPLES OF MECHANICAL VENTILATION

A. Objectives of Mechanical Ventilation

1. *Improve pulmonary gas exchange.*

2. *Relieve respiratory distress* by relieving upper and lower airway obstruction, reducing VO_2, and relieving respiratory fatigue.

3. *Manage pulmonary mechanics* by normalizing and maintaining the distribution of lung volume and providing pulmonary toilet.

4. *Provide airway protection* in patients with decreased level of consciousness or with neuromuscular disorders.

5. *Provide general support* for hemodynamically unstable patients.

6. *Prevent further lung injury.*

B. Physiologic Principles

1. *Pulmonary Function* (Table 2.16).

TABLE 2.16 Pulmonary Function

RR	=	Infant: 30–40 bpm Child: 20–30 bpm
Inspiratory time	=	Infant: 0.4–0.6 sec Child: 0.6–1 sec
Inspiratory flow	=	Infant: 2–3 L/min Child: 8–15 L/min
V_T	=	$\dfrac{\text{Inspiratory time} \times \text{Flow rate}}{RR}$
V_E	=	$V_T \times RR$
V_{DS}	=	2 mL/kg (40%–50% of V_T)
V_A	=	$(V_T - V_{DS}) \times RR$
FRC	=	30 mL/kg
V_C	=	Infant: 33–40 mL/kg Child: 40–50 mL/kg
TLC	=	Infant: 63 mL/kg Child: 70–75 mL/kg

$$\text{Compliance } (C_L) = \Delta\text{Volume}/\Delta\text{Pressure}$$
$$\text{or}$$
$$C_L = \frac{V_T}{\text{Plateau pressure}}$$

FRC, functional residual capacity; RR, respiratory rate; TLC, total lung capacity; V_A, alveolar ventilation; V_C, vital capacity; V_{DS}, physiologic dead space; V_E, minute ventilation; V_T, tidal volume.

a. V_T. Equals volume of air inspired with each inspiratory effort. The normal V_T in a spontaneously breathing patient is 4 to 7 mL/kg. The calculated V_T is the product of inspiratory time and flow rate: $V_T = T_I \times$ Flow.

b. V_E. Equals total volume of gas inspired over a period of 1 minute; V_E is the product of respiratory rate and V_T: $V_E = RR \times V_T$.

c. V_A. Equals the volume of air available for gas exchange in the alveoli that accounts for the presence of dead space: $V_A = (V_T - V_D) \times RR$.

d. *Dead-space ventilation* (V_D). Equals the volume of gas occupying airway lumina that does not participate in gas exchange. Normally, V_D is approximately 2 mL/kg. Therefore, it comprises approximately one third of the V_T.

e. *FRC.* Equals the volume of gas in the lungs at end-expiration that maintains alveolar distention: FRC ~30 mL/kg.

f. V_C. Equals the volume of gas measured after a forced (maximal) expiration following maximal inspiration: $V_C = 40 - 50$ mL/kg.

2. *Relationship of pressure (P), flow (F), and resistance (R) is expressed by the equation: $P = F \times R$*

a. *Pressure.* The driving pressure to transfer flow to the alveoli is directly proportional to flow and resistance; that is, if either flow or resistance increases, pressure will increase.

b. *Resistance.* Resistance is a force that impedes the flow of gas. It is inversely proportional to the diameter of the airway. Factors that increase resistance should be minimized, such as appropriate size and length of the ETT and ventilator circuit, treatment of airway edema, and secretions.

c. *Inspiratory flow.* Appropriate flow rates through an oxygen delivery system or ventilator must provide adequate V_E under a variety of clinical conditions.

3. *Compliance*

a. *Compliance* is the relationship between volume and pressure within a closed space. A change in either volume or pressure will alter compliance.

a. For example, a patient with severe parenchymal lung disease will have decreased compliance ("stiff lung") requiring a greater amount of inspiratory pressure to maintain the same V_T.

b. *Total lung compliance* is the summation of chest-wall compliance and lung compliance (see Figure 2.4).

c. *Lung compliance* is determined by the elasticity of lung tissue and the presence of surfactant in alveoli (which prevents alveolar collapse).

d. *Chest-wall compliance* is determined by the contour of the thoracic cage, the structural integrity of the thorax and external impedance, such as a distended abdomen.

C. Physiologic Interface Between a Ventilator and a Child

1. *MAP.* MAP is the average airway pressure measured at the proximal airway, from one inspiration to the beginning of the next. MAP directly affects the PaO_2. It is determined by V_T, peak inspiratory pressure (PIP), flow rate, respiratory rate, and end-expiratory pressure.

2. V_T. Small absolute V_Ts are observed in infants and small children, necessitating a ventilator that is capable of regulating V_T to as low as 20 mL (for full-term infants). Infants and small children are not capable of increasing V_T spontaneously because of the structural contour of their chest wall and increased compliance. With respiratory distress, the child will instead increase respiratory rate.

3. *Respiratory Rate (RR).* The RR observed in children is faster to compensate for the inability to increase V_T and also because of increased metabolic rate. Shorter inspiratory times are observed in children. The spontaneous inspiratory time is determined by lung compliance, airway resistance, and flow rate. A "stiff" lung or narrowed airway may necessitate a longer inspiratory time on the ventilator.

4. *Peak Inspiratory Pressure.* The principal determinants of PIP include lung compliance, inspiratory time, airway resistance, and V_T. Minimizing PIP is a lung-protective strategy to avoid volutrauma. Normal PIPs in spontaneously breathing newborns are 10 to 12 mmHg; in older infants and small children, they are approximately 12 to 15 mmHg. Adolescents and adults are characteristically 20 mmHg or less.

5. *Inspiratory Flow.* Flow patterns and flow rate are more variable from breath to breath in infants and young children. Constant flow is more typical of an adolescent or adult. Appropriate flow rates through an oxygen delivery system or a ventilator must be ensured to provide adequate V_E under a variety of clinical conditions. In addition, flow patterns can be manipulated on most ventilators to optimize V_A and to provide flexibility for the patient. An example is a "decelerating flow" pattern in which a large proportion of the flow is delivered on the initiation of a breath, with the remainder of the flow delivered more slowly, to enhance distribution of oxygen to alveolar units.

6. *PEEP*. PEEP is a mechanism provided at end-expiration to maintain FRC (Figure 2.20). Some conditions are characterized by decreased FRC (restrictive diseases) in which PEEP is a primary therapeutic intervention to prevent alveolar collapse at end-expiration.

7. *Synchronization*. The smooth interaction between the ventilator and the patient is an important goal. Spontaneous breathing should be maintained and supported whenever feasible. Selection of a ventilation strategy appropriate to the child's physiologic needs and individual comfort should allow good synchronization.

D. Positive-Pressure Ventilation

1. *Positive-Pressure Ventilators*. PPV creates a positive pressure at the proximal airway that exceeds

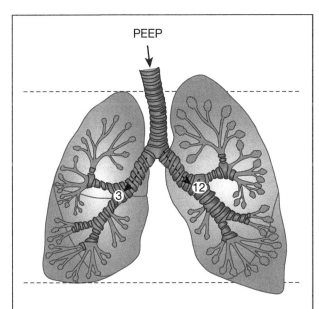

FIGURE 2.20 Effect of PEEP on FRC. In restrictive disease without PEEP, there is increased negative intrapleural pressure at FRC. Alveolar pressures are equal (note the left side of illustration). With the addition of 12 cm H_2O PEEP, pressure is increased. Alveolar distention is maintained at end expiration. Patients with ARDS typically develop patchy atelectasis requiring higher PEEP to maintain FRC.

ARDS, acute respiratory disease syndrome; FRC, functional residual capacity; PEEP, positive end-expiratory pressure.

Note: The numbers show the effect of 3 cm PEEP and 12 cm PEEP.

alveolar pressure, forcing gas flow to the lungs. The *mode* of ventilation is used as a broad term to describe several phases of PPV. One method for understanding PPV is illustrated in Figure 2.21. The three principal mechanisms are mode, control, and phase variables.

2. *Mode*. A strict definition of *mode* describes the type of breath (mandatory or spontaneous) that the ventilator allows to the patient as well as how much support the ventilator will give each spontaneous breath. Following is a sampling of possible modes available on a wide variety of current ventilators on the market. Although some names of modes may be proprietary in nature, they are included for clinician awareness due to their frequent use in the pediatric critical care setting.

a. *Controlled mandatory ventilation (CMV)*. The ventilator controls every breath with preset parameters. The patient cannot initiate spontaneous breaths.

b. *Assist/control ventilation (A/C)*. The ventilator breaths are regulated as in CMV; however, if the patient initiates a breath, the ventilator will complete the effort with the preset mechanisms. The patient does not exert much work except for the initial effort.

c. *Intermittent mandatory ventilation (IMV)*. A preset respiratory rate with other preset limits is delivered to the patient. The patient can breathe spontaneously from the circuit, but the ventilator does not interface with these efforts. If the patient should be midway into a spontaneous breath, when the machine timing initiates a breath, the patient will receive a larger, more uncomfortable breath.

d. *Synchronized intermittent mandatory ventilation (SIMV)*. The ventilator has a preset IMV rate and settings. The patient can breathe spontaneously from the circuit. If the patient initiates a breath within the timing window before the next ventilator-timed breath, the ventilator will synchronize its timing with the patient and likewise support the patient.

e. *Pressure support ventilation (PSV)*. PSV allows the patient to breathe spontaneously, providing pressure/flow support with each effort. The pressure support is predetermined by the clinician. When spontaneous effort is sensed, gas flow is delivered until the airway pressure reaches the preset limit. The higher the pressure, the greater the support for the patient (decreased respiratory work). The patient can continue inspiration with a variable flow rate and variable

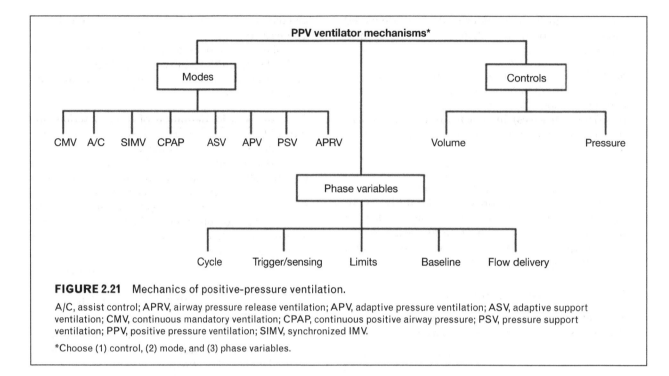

FIGURE 2.21 Mechanics of positive-pressure ventilation.

A/C, assist control; APRV, airway pressure release ventilation; APV, adaptive pressure ventilation; ASV, adaptive support ventilation; CMV, continuous mandatory ventilation; CPAP, continuous positive airway pressure; PSV, pressure support ventilation; PPV, positive pressure ventilation; SIMV, synchronized IMV.

*Choose (1) control, (2) mode, and (3) phase variables.

inspiratory time, whereas the preset airway pressure is sustained. PSV can be used alone or with SIMV facilitating "muscle conditioning."

f. *Adaptive support ventilation (ASV).* ASV is similar to *mandatory minute ventilation (MMV)*, in which the minute ventilation is preset based on patient's ideal weight. ASV allows the patient to breathe spontaneously but with a backup RR if the patient becomes apneic. The ventilator compares both the patient's V_T and RR to its internal targets and adjusts either or both to achieve the preset V_E with the lowest possible PIP. MMV, on some ventilators, utilizes a preset IMV rate rather than a backup rate, and the V_T may be determined by the clinician.

g. *Adaptive pressure ventilation (APV).* APV is a 0-pressure-regulated, volume-controlled type in which a target V_T is preset, as are the IMV rate, inspiratory time, and PEEP. In APV, the ventilator monitors lung compliance and airway resistance and continuously adjusts the PIP to deliver the V_T at the lowest possible pressure (thus a variable PIP). Some ventilators do not automatically adjust PIP; instead, it is established by the clinician.

h. *Continuous positive airway pressure.* CPAP is a mode in which the patient is breathing spontaneously with preset end-expiratory pressure. There is no backup IMV rate in this mode; PSV can be added for support of patient-initiated breaths.

i. *Airway pressure release ventilation (APRV).* APRV is a mode of ventilation that provides a form of pressure control in which the inspiratory time, frequency, PEEP, and PIP are preset, with V_T and V_E variable. It allows spontaneous patient inhalation and exhalation at a preset high CPAP (T-high) for a preset time (e.g., 3 seconds). Periodically, the CPAP/PEEP is released for 1 to 2 seconds to allow greater exhalation and therefore CO_2 removal (T-low).

j. *Neurally adjusted ventilatory assist (NAVA).* NAVA is an increasingly popular form of ventilation in infants and children that encourages patient comfort, control, and support. A noninvasive catheter (Edi catheter) featuring electrodes is introduced into the esophagus and allows for visual monitoring of the electrical activity of the diaphragm (Edi) and serves as a trigger for spontaneous inspiration. The Edi also allows for optimal ventilatory support as NAVA will proportionately assist the patient according to the diaphragm's activity (Edi). The patient remains in control of his or her respiratory pattern as well as V_T.

3. *Controls.* The control variable regulates inspiration.

a. *Pressure control.* The PIP is regulated throughout the inspiratory cycle. It may be set above the patient's PIP to ensure that patient does not exceed the desired PIP, or it may be set to *limit* the patient's PIP at a lower level (Figure 2.22). The V_T volume is determined by the difference

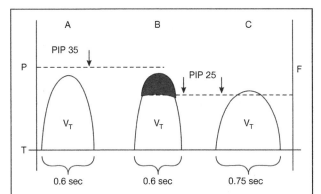

FIGURE 2.22 The relationship among V_T, PIP, flow, and T_I. (A) V_T is a function of flow and T_I and is represented by the area under the curve. If F and T_I are kept constant, pressure limiting a breath will result in decreased V_T (B is shown in black). (C) In order to maintain a constant V_T when a pressure limit is set, either the T_I must be increased or the flow rate must be increased.

PIP, peak inspiratory pressure; T_I, inspiratory time; V_T, tidal volume.

between the PIP and PEEP, or delta P (ΔP). A target V_T is established first by setting the desired PEEP, then setting the PIP at a level that allows the desired V_T. This is a lung-protective strategy to minimize high-peak pressures while ensuring an adequate V_T. It is commonly used in patients with decreased C_L (stiff lungs). The disadvantage is that, as compliance changes, V_T will be altered. With improving compliance at the same PIP, V_T will increase with the risk of volutrauma.

b. *Volume control.* The V_T is assured throughout inspiration, with variable PIP. A preset inspiratory time and flow rate, plus IMV, PEEP, and PSV, are clinician determined; the flow rate, or I time, is variable, regulated by the patient's lung compliance. PIP is variable according to lung compliance. The disadvantage of this control is that a high PIP may be generated, either acutely (because of airway resistance) or more insidiously, as lung compliance diminishes, with a potential for barotrauma. A high-PIP alarm is set, usually 5 to 10 mmHg higher than the patient's PIP.

4. *Phase Variables.* These variables are the mechanisms that can be selected to match individual patient needs to achieve an optimal ventilation strategy and synchronization.

a. *Cycle.* The cycling mechanism determines the end of inspiration. The choices are volume-, time-, or flow-cycled ventilation. Currently,

pressure-cycled ventilation is rarely used. If a patient is in time-cycled ventilation, inspiration will last only as long as the preset T_I. T_I is one factor of V_T (the other being flow rate). Therefore, the time-cycled mode is a type of volume-controlled ventilation.

b. *Trigger and sensing mechanism.* The trigger is the mechanism that *initiates* inspiration. The trigger may be a preset IMV rate or patient-initiated breath, which is detected by either a flow or pressure sensor. The sensing mechanisms allow the patient to trigger the ventilator. *Pressure sensors* are activated when the patient generates a preset level of negative pressure in the circuit as the patient initiates inspiration. *Flow sensors* are activated when the patient initiates inspiration, displacing a preset level of flow from the circuit. *Placement* of these sensors and their *sensitivity* are important with the goal of minimizing the WOB. Ideally, a sensor is positioned at the proximal airway and the flow is accessible at the proximal airway rather than from the ventilator port. A flow sensor generally requires less patient effort than a pressure sensor, and therefore it is preferable for most infants and children.

c. *Flow delivery.* The rate of flow during inspiration determines distribution of gas in the lungs. The availability of flow determines the ease with which the patient can access flow. The pattern of flow delivery—fast, gradual, or slow—will influence patient comfort and synchronization as well as distribution of gas flow in the lungs.

 i. Continuous circuit flow provides immediate access to flow with minimal patient effort; demand flow requires the patient to inspire the volume of air within the entire inspiratory limb of the circuit before the gas is actually delivered to the patient. The latter imposes a greater WOB and is less desirable for infants and small pediatric patients.

 ii. Fast flow delivery in the initial portion of inspiration is often useful for patients who have noncompliant lung disease or a mixed state in which there is both overdistention and collapse. This flow pattern is described as decelerating flow.

d. *Limits.* Mechanisms that regulate inspiration to provide safety mechanisms. High pressure, time, and flow limits are set, depending on the selected strategies for individual ventilation.

e. *Baseline variables.* Variables that regulate the expiratory phase. PEEP is used to maintain FRC.

In children with tracheomalacia, PEEP also appears to "stent" open the airways, which may have a natural tendency to collapse at end expiration.

E. Selection of Ventilation Variables

1. The choice of mechanisms is guided by the respiratory compliance of the patient, the ability to breathe spontaneously, and predicted clinical course of the underlying disease. Clinical assessment of the patient after choosing a mode is important as sometimes patients do not respond in the expected manner to ventilator settings and need to try different modes.

2. Preservation of spontaneous breathing efforts should be maintained whenever possible. The ventilator should have the capability of both allowing spontaneous breathing and providing supported breaths in synchrony with the patient's effort.

F. Alternative Ventilation Strategies

1. *Inverse-Ratio Ventilation*

a. *Conventional modes* of ventilation use inspiratory:expiratory (I:E) time ratios of typically 1:2 to 1:4. With inverse-ratio ventilation (IRV), the ratio is reversed. The I:E is greater than 1:1 and often 2:1 or more. Lengthening the inspiratory time allows more time for distribution of gas throughout the lungs. The usual sequence of changes that evolves to IRV is a gradual lengthening of the inspiratory time to a point when inspiration is greater than expiration. Lengthening the inspiratory time can cause increased V_T as well as increased PIP, which must be monitored. The $PaCO_2$ may eventually rise with the shorter exhalation time, but permissive hypercapnia is frequently tolerated.

b. *IRV* is employed when the usual strategies for enhancing oxygenation have failed. IRV is thought to allow MAP and V_T to be maintained at relatively lower levels without increasing PEEP, provided air trapping does not occur. Patients almost always require sedation and paralysis when receiving ventilation in this mode (Table 2.17)

2. *High-Frequency Ventilation*

a. Historically, high-frequency ventilation (HFV) has been used to provide an alternative to patients for whom conventional ventilation is failing. In more recent years, HFV has been used

TABLE 2.17 Expected Ventilator Requirements Associated With Pathophysiologic Conditions

Conditions	Patient Requirements
Infectious disease (e.g., epiglotitis)	Normal V_T/PIP Normal FiO_2
Facial abnormalities/tracheomalacia	Spontaneous breathing, requires little ventilation unless sedated

Surfactant deficiency
  RDS
  ARDS
Pneumonitis
Fibrosis
Pulmonary edema
Excessive PEEP
	Ensure adequate V_T and normal FRC
	Monitor exhaled V_T and MAP
	Guard against overdistention (too much V_T)
	May require patient paralysis or heavy sedation
	Severe disease or complications (e.g., air leak syndrome): faster rates, lower V_T, permissive hypercarbia

Spinal muscular atrophy
Guillian–Barré syndrome
Spinal cord injury
CNS alterations
  Sedation
  Altered consciousness
  Central apnea
	Normal V_T, low to normal PIPs
	Normal PaO_2/low FiO_2
	Spontaneous breathing with support is preferable when possible
	Monitor exhaled V_T on PSV breaths

ARDS, acute respiratory distress syndrome; CNS, central nervous system; FiO_2, fractional inspired oxygen; FRC, functional residual capacity; MAP, mean airway pressure; PaO_2, arterial oxygen partial pressure; PEEP, positive end-expiratory pressure; PIP, peak inspiratory pressure; PSV, pressure support ventilation; RDS, respiratory distress syndrome.

earlier in the course of illness for specific reasons, including ventilation of low-birth-weight infants, prevention of barotrauma with severe restrictive lung disease, treatment for bronchopleural fistulas, airway disruptions, and severe pulmonary interstitial edema with markedly reduced CL. With HFV, the shearing effect of repetitive opening and closing of alveoli, from PIP to PEEP (ΔP), is minimized compared with conventional ventilation. The two most commonly used are high-frequency oscillation ventilation (HFOV) and HFJV.

   i. *HFOV*. This ventilator uses a piston pump to drive a volume of gas into the lungs at a frequency of 60 to 3,600 per minute (1–60 Hz). Exhalation is active (generated by the piston motion), unlike other high-frequency ventilators. Not only does this facilitate CO_2 removal, but it diminishes the potential for volume stacking (inadvertent PEEP/MAP). The delivered V_T is less than or equal to the anatomic deadspace (V_D).

   ii. A *conventional ETT* is used with this ventilator, making the transition from a conventional ventilator to an HFOV somewhat easier than with other high-frequency ventilators.

   iii. *Adequate lung inflation* at the start of this ventilatory technique is essential to avoid extensive microatelectasis. The MAP is initially set approximately 3 to 5 mmHg higher than the patient's MAP on the conventional ventilator. After stabilization, the MAP can then be weaned.

   iv. *Four mechanisms* of HFOV are MAP, power amplitude (ΔP), the frequency in hertz (Hz), and T_I.

    1) MAP determines lung expansion and FRC and is the principal mechanism for regulating oxygenation. An estimation of adequate lung volume can be made from a chest radiograph, in which the lung fields should be expanded to 8 to 10 ribs. Greater expansion than this may overly distend the lung, increasing resistance to gas delivery. Lower MAPs may cause microatelectasis to develop.

    2) The power amplitude (ΔP) regulates the "tidal volume." This mechanism determines the amplitude (or change in position) of the piston. Increasing amplitude will increase V_T to a point at which the V_T actually begins to diminish secondary to inadequate inspiratory time.

With experience, a "gestalt" impression of chest "bounce" provides a quick estimate of appropriate ΔP, which may range from 30 to 80.

    3) Frequency measured in hertz is similar to the IMV rate on a conventional ventilator, but it also directly influences V_T. The "optimal" hertz set point is that which facilitates CO_2 removal (in conjunction with ΔP). Delivered V_T will *decrease* at a threshold (individual) level. An increasing CO_2 can indicate that either the hertz is too high or the ΔP is too low.

    4) Inspiratory time: If inspiratory and expiratory time constants are equal, then the inspiratory time theoretically would be set at 50% (I:E = 1:1). However, the time constants are rarely equal, and an inspiratory time of 50% will cause air trapping with this form of ventilation. Conventionally, a 33% inspiratory time is used.

   v. Determining initial HFOV settings

    1) MAP should be determined first, generally set three to five times higher than the MAP on the patient's conventional ventilator.

    2) Amplitude selection, estimated from the ΔP of the conventional ventilator, is a safe place to start. If CO_2 retention occurs, the amplitude can be increased, assuming MAP is optimized. The goal is to look for a "plateau" with ABGs to determine the optimal MAP and optimal amplitude.

    3) Frequency. Neonates generally require 10 to 15 Hz; infants, 8 to 10 Hz; young preschool age children, 6 to 8 Hz; and older children, 4 to 6 Hz. It is prudent to start on the lower end of the range to avoid air trapping (volume stacking).

    4) Inspiratory time. Manufacturer recommendations suggest a 33% inspiratory time (66% expiratory time), altering only if all other maneuvers to improve ventilation fail. Volume stacking can occur with shorter expiratory times, which might be first noted with an MAP measurement that is drifting higher than the setting.

   vi. HFJV. HFJV is a technique of ventilation that delivers a burst of gas from a high-pressure source at supraphysiologic frequencies, with a rate of 60 to 600 pulses per minute. The burst is delivered through a port of a specialized ETT, providing a V_T that is approximately equal to V_D (± 2 mL/kg). Exhalation is *passive* around the jet cannula into the continuous-flow circuit of the tandem ventilator. *HFJV* is used in tandem with a conventional ventilator to provide gas flow for entrainment. The V_T is both the burst of gas and the gas entrained from a tandem conventional ventilator at a set peak airway pressure. Disadvantages of HFJV are air trapping causing hypercarbia and overdistention and concern for reintubation in an emergency with the specialized ETT.

vii. *Inspiratory driving pressure* provides the primary mechanism for regulating V_T delivery. The driving pressure range is 0 to 50 PSI.

viii. A *valve device* on the expiratory limb of the circuit provides PEEP.

ix. *Respiratory rate* is regulated by a valve that creates timed flow interruption. The rate is adjusted to between 60 and 150 breaths per minute.

x. *Inspiratory time* is set as a percentage of the total respiratory cycle, from 10% to 50%. Inspiratory times greater than 40% generally will not allow adequate expiratory time.

3. *Extra Corporeal Membrane Oxygenation*

   a. *ECMO* uses a cardiopulmonary bypass machine, which provides an alternative method for gas exchange or cardiovascular support in patients for whom conventional therapy has failed.

   b. *Candidates for ECMO.* Patients for whom ventilation strategies are failing or who are in severe cardiac failure refractory to standard therapy are candidates for ECMO. ECMO therapy is applied only to patients with potentially resolvable single-organ failure and potential for good neurologic outcome. Criteria for respiratory patients vary among hospitals but may include the following:

      i. Oxygenation index greater than 40 with maximal conventional therapy, which predicts 77% mortality

      ii. Alveolar-arterial gradient ($A\text{-}aDO_2$) greater than 580 mmHg with PIPs above 40, together defining a 81% mortality rate in children

      iii. Static compliance less than 0.5 mL/cm H_2O/kg

   c. *Contraindications for ECMO* include the following:

      i. Irreversible conditions

      ii. Previous head bleeds in neonates

      iii. Pulmonary hemorrhage

      iv. Contraindication to heparinization

   d. *Application.* The success with ECMO in neonates for respiratory failure has been well established. For reasons that remain unclear, ECMO support for respiratory failure has not been as successful in pediatric patients as in neonates.

   e. *Cardiac bypass.* Cannulation of a major artery and vein is used for both cardiac and pulmonary failure; the blood is diverted from the vein (usually the subclavian or femoral), through the membrane oxygenator, and back to the artery (often the carotid artery in an infant).

   f. *Pulmonary bypass.* Two major veins are cannulated to divert blood to the oxygenator and returned to the right atrium. This requires good cardiac function to maintain normal cardiac output. Veno–veno bypass is preferred, when possible, to avoid arterial vascular injury or compromise.

   g. See Chapter 3 for more information.

4. *Negative Pressure Ventilation*

   a. *Negative pressure ventilators* are used for patients with either neuromuscular disease or central apnea. The patient must have a patent airway, and the structural qualities of the lung must be normal. Negative pressure ventilation (NPV) generates lung expansion with a ventilator that uses negative pressure, rather than positive pressure, using a device that surrounds the chest. The operating mechanism mimics a spontaneously breathing patient.

   b. *Devices.* The historical model is an "iron lung" tank ventilator, used in the mid-20th century for polio patients. More recent devices include the "shell" device, called a *cuirasse*, which surrounds only the thorax like a clam shell. The difficulty is in obtaining a tight seal, requiring some precision in sizing. Another device, called a *raincoat*, is aptly named and functions in the same manner as the shell.

   c. *Principle of operation.* With the thorax enclosed in a shell or tank, negative pressure is created inside the shell, creating a "vacuum" pressure. The thoracic cage expands outward with this vacuum effect, thus increasing lung volume (and therefore decreasing alveolar pressure). A pressure gradient now exists between the mouth (atmospheric pressure) and the lung (subatmospheric pressure), causing air to fill the lungs. The ventilator is preset to release the negative pressure (an IMV rate), allowing the natural recoil of the lungs to allow exhalation.

d. *Limitations.* The seal of the tank or shell must be very tight. Dilation of the great vessels is exaggerated, diminishing cardiac output. NPV is cumbersome if the child requires 24-hour-a-day ventilation.

e. *Nursing care issues.* Children who need 24-hour-a-day NPV may be at risk for aspiration. Gastric jejunal tubes are indicated for enteral feedings. Hypothermia may also occur because of convective cooling from air being pulled through the collar. Skin integrity may be compromised. Finally, anxiety and claustrophobia may occur.

f. NPV is a method that can avoid a tracheostomy and perhaps is best suited for patients who do not require full-time ventilation, such as those with night apnea (Ondine's curse).

5. *Noninvasive Positive-Pressure Ventilation*

a. *NPPV* provides positive-pressure support through a nasal mask or nasal prongs without the use of an ETT, which is more invasive. A simple positive-pressure ventilator is used to deliver CPAP or BiPAP.

b. *Indications for NPPV.* Patients with acute respiratory failure may avoid intubation with early use of NPPV. Airway reflexes should be intact. NPPV may also facilitate earlier extubation in some patients as a bridge from intubation to spontaneous breathing. Patients with neuromuscular syndromes and apnea syndromes are also potential candidates for NPPV. All patients should have a normal respiratory drive.

c. *Principle of operation.* NPPV is a pressure-controlled mode with continuous flow. For simple CPAP or expiratory positive airway pressure (EPAP), a baseline expiratory pressure is set as on a conventional ventilator. The patient breathes spontaneously, with the expiratory pressure maintaining FRC. BiPAP provides both inspiratory positive airway pressure (IPAP) and EPAP. The patient can breathe spontaneously; when the BiPAP ventilator senses patient effort, it delivers flow to achieve the higher pressure until patient demand ceases. A backup IMV rate can be set as well.

d. *Clinical considerations.* Patients must have normal airway secretions and adequate cough and gag reflexes and must demonstrate a sustained effort to breathe spontaneously. Complications include unrecognized ventilatory insufficiency, pressure injury to the skin, aspiration, and gastric distention. Gastric feedings are determined individually; infants and smaller children may be safer with jejunal feedings than with gastric feedings, although more recent research has found no difference in rates of aspiration between NG and jejunal feedings.

INTUBATION

A. Objectives

1. Establish airway patency.

2. Provide a conduit for positive-pressure mechanical ventilation.

B. Interfaces

1. Noninvasive ventilation can be provided with a BVM, full-face mask, or nasal mask.

2. Invasive ventilation can be provided with a supraglottic airway device, nasal or orally placed ETT, or tracheostomy.

C. Equipment

1. ETT

a. ETT size can be estimated with the following formula: ETT size (millimeters) = (16 + age in years)/4.

b. Children younger than 8 years old can usually be intubated with an uncuffed ETT as their narrow subglottis provides a good seal.

2. Supraglottic airway device

3. Stylet

4. Laryngoscope with appropriate size blade and functioning light

5. Resuscitation bag and mask

6. High-flow oxygen source

7. Suction

D. Monitoring

1. Pulse oximeter

2. Cardiorespiratory monitor

3. End-tidal CO_2

E. Procedure

1. Clear airway of secretions or obstructive materials.

2. Place child's head in the "sniffing" position. This allows best visualization of the glottis.

3. Preoxygenate with 100% oxygen.

4. Sedation and amnesiacs should be given. Sometimes a muscle relaxant is also given.

5. BVM after medications are administered to support ventilation.

6. Place the laryngoscope into the vallecula and visualize the vocal cords.

7. Pass the ETT through the vocal cords.

8. If unsuccessful, resume BVM ventilation before another attempt.

9. If successful, verify position by auscultation (verify equal bilateral breath sounds), end-tidal CO_2, chest x-ray or bronchoscope visualization (if available).

10. Secure the airway in place.

F. Difficult Airway

1. *Cannot Mask Ventilate*

    a. Improper head or airway positioning

       i. Optimize chin lift/jaw thrust.

       ii. Insert a shoulder roll.

       iii. Add cricoid pressure.

       iv. Use a two-person BVM technique.

       v. Ensure equipment is working properly.

       vi. Consider increasing sedation.

    b. Upper airway obstruction

       i. Insert oropharyngeal airway.

    c. Laryngospasm

       i. Provide adequate anesthesia.

    d. Gastric distention

       i. Pass orogastric (OG)/NG tube.

    e. Consider a supraglottic airway device

2. *Cannot Intubate*

    a. Continue to optimize oxygenation with 100% FiO_2.

    b. Optimize head position.

    c. Have rescue medications and personnel available if child decompensates.

    d. Call for assistance from airway specialist.

       i. Bronchoscopic intubation

       ii. Rigid bronchoscopy with jet ventilation

       iii. Surgical tracheostomy

       iv. If no airway specialist available, consider surgical cricothyroidotomy

          1) Surgical cricothyroidotomy has serious complications and should only be performed by properly trained individuals in life-threating situations.

PATIENT CARE MANAGEMENT AND MONITORING OF THE CHILD ON MECHANICAL VENTILATION

A. Patient Care Management

1. *Airway Management.* The goal is to maintain position and patency of the ETT. Retaping of the ETT should always be done with immediate availability of a skilled clinician who can reintubate the patient if necessary. A bag-mask circuit and suction should always be maintained at the bedside. If erosion of the lip, gumline, or tongue occurs, frequent repositioning of the tube is necessary. Some devices are available that can secure the tube in a midline position without pressure on any surface.

2. *Suctioning* the ETT should be performed per hospital standards and when there is evidence of increased airway secretions. Lightly sedated patients may indicate this by coughing. Increased PIP may be noted, and auscultation of the lungs may reveal upper airway rhonchi.

    a. Always preoxygenate the patient before suctioning.

    b. The suction catheter should be an appropriate size to allow ease of insertion. Insertion distance should be known and documented to avoid suctioning below the tip of the ETT.

c. Sterile technique is important to avoid contamination and possible ventilator-associated pneumonia (VAP). In-line suction catheters work well for most patients, particularly those patients with high MAPs, to avoid excessive volume loss (derecruitment).

d. Routine instillation of normal saline should not be necessary if the humidification is adequate. Tenacious secretions, however, occasionally require instillation (0.5–2 mL); after administration, allow several ventilator breaths to disperse the fluid or provide bag-valve assistance. Chronically tenacious secretions may also respond to deoxyribonuclease (DNAse), an agent commonly used to break up sticky secretions with patients who have CF.

3. *Assessment* of the child receiving mechanical ventilation:

a. *General observations.* Observe the comfort of the child, the synchrony between patient and ventilator, chest excursion, color and perfusion, and level of consciousness. It should be noted that a patient on HFOV will not be able to be assessed for ventilator synchrony or chest excursion. Clinicians will rather assess for the presence of adequate "chest wiggle," ranging from the clavicles to the mid-thigh bilaterally.

b. *Auscultation.* Note the symmetry of breath sounds; recall that the thin chest walls of infants transmit breath sounds to the opposite side. Evaluate the quality of breath sounds, noting adventitious sounds, wheezing, or diminished aeration. Absent or severely diminished aeration over one entire lung is an urgent finding, reflecting either a pneumothorax, lung collapse, bronchial obstruction, malpositioned ETT, or a consolidation (e.g., pneumonia, atelectasis). Observe chest excursion and expansion (appropriate to the size of the child); observe from the foot of the bed to best appreciate asymmetry in chest expansion.

c. *Note the WOB.* VO_2 is greatly increased with increased WOB.

d. *Insertion distance of the ETT* should be verified and documented at frequent intervals.

e. *Note the volume and quality of secretions.* VAP is a leading cause of nosocomial infection; a change in the quality of the secretions, especially in the presence of a fever, should prompt further investigation.

f. *Evaluate* for the presence of an air leak around the ETT; ideally, an air leak will be present at a PIP of 25 mmHg or less.

g. *Palpation.* Note the presence of crepitus, inspiratory crackles, or bony abnormalities. Note any points of tenderness.

B. Monitoring of the Child During Mechanical Ventilation

1. *Arterial Blood Gases*

a. The conventional approach to verifying adequate oxygenation and ventilation is by periodic sampling of arterial blood with the goal of achieving normal blood gas values. However, capillary blood gas (CBG), a much less invasive sampling procedure, provides reliable measurements of pH and $PaCO_2$, which can be used for correlating, trending, and management decisions.

b. *Permissive hypercarbia* is a strategy for guiding ventilator manipulations that allows hypercarbia to exist with normal oxygenation, pH greater than 7.25, $PaCO_2$ of 45 to 80 mmHg, and no evidence of cerebral dysfunction. The benefit of permissive hypercarbia is that it facilitates lower V_T ventilation, thereby minimizing the incidence of ALI.

2. *Pulse Oximetry.* As a noninvasive monitoring tool, pulse oximetry should be used continuously. The oximetry probe should be routinely changed in order to avoid burns.

3. E_TCO_2 *Monitors.* E_TCO_2 monitors are useful for infants and children for trending, weaning, and monitoring hyperventilation therapy. They are also essential for quick recognition of ETT dislodgement.

4. *Transcutaneous CO_2 Monitoring* (see earlier discussion)

5. *Alarms.* Ensure activation of ECG monitoring alarms. Appropriate ventilator alarms should be used according to the modes selected.

6. *Serial Chest Radiographs.* Radiographs are important to verify ETT position and to evaluate pulmonary processes. The decision for x-ray examinations should be determined by the individual needs of each patient.

7. *Monitoring of Neuromuscular Blockade.* "Twitch monitoring" or train-of-four monitoring with a cutaneous nerve stimulator may be used for patients who receive a neuromuscular blocker to assess the level of paralysis. It is performed every 6 to 8 hours to ensure that the minimum amount of medication is used. Alternatively, one can discontinue the paralytic agent every 12 to 24 hours to assess for return of neurological function ("drug holiday"). The incidence of myopathy in patients who have been paralyzed, particularly those who are concurrently receiving steroids, is significant and should be considered on a daily basis.

8. *Monitoring Ventilator Parameters*

a. Monitor V_T continuously in pressure-controlled modes; deviations of greater than 10% should be reported to the therapist for remediation.

b. Monitor PIPs if in a volume-controlled mode; increasing PIP may indicate airway secretions or worsening lung compliance. Uncontrolled PIPs put the patient at risk for barotraumas.

c. Monitor *PEEP* and observe for the presence of "auto-PEEP," which occurs with breath stacking or patient-ventilator asynchrony.

d. Monitor patient efforts to breathe. How much pressure support does the patient require? Is the chest excursion adequate with the pressure support? Is the patient able to access flow to initiate a breath (sensitivity)? If in a spontaneous mode are the patient's V_T and RR adequate to meet V_E requirements?

e. Ventilator graphics can provide a visual assessment of the patient's pulmonary dynamics and patient–ventilator interface. Overdistention, auto-PEEP, change in CL, and airway obstruction can be observed on these waveforms (Figure 2.23).

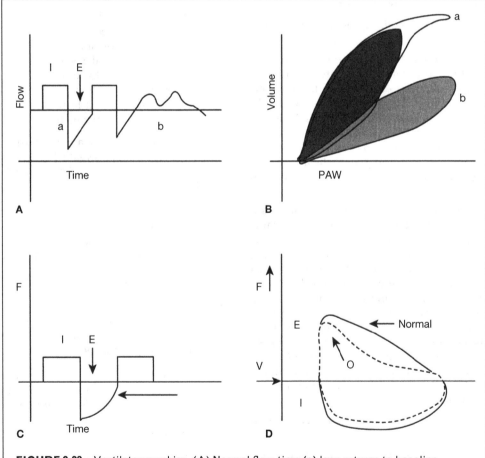

FIGURE 2.23 Ventilator graphics. (A) Normal flow-time (a) loop returns to baseline with normal contour; (b) patient dysynchrony. (B) Volume–pressure loop (gray); (a) overdistention; (b) decreased compliance. (C) Flow-time loop with auto-PEEP/airway trapping; inspiration begins before expiration curve returns to baseline. (D) Flow-volume loop with normal contour and obstruction (dotted line).

E, expiration; I, inspiration; PAW, pulmonary airway pressure; PEEP, positive end expiratory pressure.

C. Supportive Care of the Child on Mechanical Ventilation

1. *Equipment Function*

   a. The nurse should be knowledgeable about the mode of ventilation, the ventilator control, and phase variables selected.

   b. Alarm activation and both temperature and humidity of the ventilator should be noted. The temperature should ideally be that of standard body temperature (37° C).

2. *Fluids and Electrolytes*

   a. Fluid retention may occur because of underlying disease or SIADH secondary to PPV.

   b. Calculation of input and output of fluid is essential for all patients. Fluid restriction may be used in some settings, but urine output should still be maintained at greater than 1 mL/kg per hour and hemodynamic stability ensured.

   c. Daily weights are valuable in evaluating fluid therapy and should be performed in all patients. Bed scales facilitate this task.

   d. Metabolic alterations affect electrolytes and pH. Permissive hypercarbia causes bicarbonate retention and chloride excretion.

3. *Nutrition*

   a. Early nutrition should be initiated for all patients. Enteral feedings are preferred and can be administered via NG or nasojejunal tube, even in the presence of hypoactive bowel sounds.

   b. Formal nutrition screening should be done early and serially. Indirect calorimetry is the optimal assessment tool, when available, but is usually unnecessary.

   c. Restriction of carbohydrates to less than 30% of metabolic needs may be necessary for patients with ventilatory insufficiency. Excess carbohydrate loads produce excess CO_2 (respiratory quotient [RQ] $\geq$1), thus increasing ventilatory work to remove the CO_2. In some cases this is the cause for difficulty in weaning from a ventilator.

4. *Skin Care*

   a. Patient repositioning is done as often as tolerated at a minimum of every 2 hours. When feasible, the prone position offers significant benefit for lung aeration as well by improving ventilation–perfusion matching, although early results of a multicenter trial do not demonstrate a difference in outcomes. Use dermal protection on pressure points. High-risk patients, especially those who do not tolerate turning, may require pressure reduction or relief from specialized mattresses. Careful inspection of all pressure points should be documented at least every 8 hours.

5. *Mobilization of Pulmonary Secretions*

   a. Adequate humidification should be ensured, with proper temperature regulation. Low temperatures may cause secretions to become thick and sticky. High and low temperatures may affect the patient's core body temperature.

   b. Assess the patient for airway secretions and suction as indicated. Maintain sterile technique for suctioning. Use of chest physiotherapy either by manual technique or by the vibrating vest technique may be beneficial.

6. *Sedation and Pain Management*

   a. Sedation is frequently needed for optimal ventilator management and for patient comfort. However, noninvasive measures should always be offered first, including the presence of parents, a favorite blanket or toy, ear plugs to block out noise (especially with high-frequency ventilators), and darkening the room.

   b. Assess the patient's need for pain medication: The presence of an ETT, suctioning, and ventilator breaths is uncomfortable at the least and often painful.

   c. Conventional pharmacologic therapy usually includes a benzodiazepine or a narcotic. The choice in medications is determined individually. Many centers are using dexmedetomidine and a narcotic to reduce delirium.

   d. Children who are paralyzed, pharmacologically or otherwise, must have both sedation and pain medication. Monitor for increased pupil size, tachycardia, or increased blood pressure to determine the adequacy of sedation and pain management.

7. *Psychological Needs of the Child and Family*

   a. Communication barriers and sometimes a diminished level of consciousness alter the child's expressive language and family relationships. Strategies for minimizing barriers include picture boards for preschoolers, picture or alphabet boards for school-age children, or predetermined hand signals. A dry-erase board is appreciated by children old enough to write messages.

   b. Provide sedation as needed for comfort, but also provide environmental relief through family presence, family voices on tape, or stories or music on cassettes.

c. Establish a night–day routine for the patient as early as possible. Include the family in this plan and, optimally, post the plan on the patient's door or at the bedside.

d. Balance the needs for patient safety with developmental needs. Restraints are usually necessary but can be removed when there is supervision.

D. Strategies for Weaning From Ventilation

1. *Indications for Readiness.* Many strategies have been proposed, but currently there is no one documented method for ensuring a successful weaning-to-extubation process. The following criteria are goals to achieve before extubation is actually considered:

a. Hemodynamic stability

b. SaO_2 greater than 90% with an FiO_2 of 0.4 or less (oxygen saturation may depend upon cardiac history/status)

c. PEEP of 5 cm H_2O or lower

d. Adequacy of respiratory muscles to sustain spontaneous ventilation ($V_T \geq 5$ mL/kg)

e. $PaCO_2$ in a range acceptable for the patient

f. Presence of an adequate gag and cough reflex

g. Adequate level of consciousness

h. Adequate respiratory effort, with an NIF greater than −20 to −25 cm H_2O on serial measurements

i. Pain control is adequate without excessive sedation

j. Patient has ability to control his or her own secretions

2. *Possible Weaning Approach.* There is no one accepted method for weaning trials and there is no evidence to support the use of one technique over another:

a. *Before weaning,* parameters to be monitored for each patient should be clearly identified. They may include SaO_2, $PaCO_2$, respiratory rate, V_T, and general effort and color. All patients should have ECG monitoring and pulse oximetry during this process. There are numerous weaning strategies available.

b. The more commonly employed techniques include *spontaneous trials* with SIMV or PSV to maintain baseline FRC.

i. Trials of spontaneous breathing without PSV support may be used to verify readiness to extubate or as a method of improving muscle endurance. To assess for readiness to extubate, many suggest a 1- to 2-hour trial to observe WOB, V_T, and aeration. Spontaneous trials may be also used for "muscle conditioning" in which planned trials of a stated duration, several times a day, are performed, noting patient tolerance during each. With each successive trial, the time is gradually increased while observing effort, exhaled V_T, and when applicable, ABGs. Clinicians may consider allowing for a period of rest (i.e., 6 to 8 hours; nighttime may be optimal) for a full recovery.

ii. PSV + spontaneous trials provide enough support to overcome the resistance of the ETT; PSV is weaned, by 1 to 2 cm H_2O every 4 to 8 hours, as tolerated (although this is highly variable), observing trends in exhaled V_T and respiratory rate as support is withdrawn. PSV spontaneous trials can be approached similarly to that with SIMV (when IMV rate is weaned to zero). Again, careful observation of the patient, including spontaneous V_T, WOB, and adequacy of aeration is required. Depending on ETT size, the reccommended *minimum* level of PSV is as follows:

ETT Size	PSV
3.0–3.5	10
4.0–4.5	8
>5.0	6

1) Be aware that, with reduction in PSV, fatigue or atelectasis may not be apparent for 3 to 6 hours or more.

2) SIMV with PSV weaning: Weaning from this mode can be accomplished either by first weaning the PSV to the recommended minimum and then weaning the IMV rate or vice versa. The rate of IMV changes and subsequent weaning of PSV should be guided by an individualized plan and assessment criteria. The temptation to accelerate the weaning process in patients who have been

intubated for more than a few days may result in atelectasis or a collapsed lung, thereby delaying the entire process.

E. Complications of Mechanical Ventilation

1. *Causes of acute deterioration* in an intubated child can be evaluated using the mnemonic DOPE: dislodgement, obstruction, pneumothorax (or other air leaks), equipment failure.

2. *Complications From Longer Term Ventilation*

   a. *Oxygen toxicity.* Patients receiving greater than 50% FiO_2 for prolonged periods of time may develop parenchymal changes from oxygen exposure. Oxygen should be treated as a medication with strict adherence to prescription guidelines. Continuous monitoring of O_2 is strongly recommended. The lowest acceptable SpO_2 measurement for the child should be clearly established while FiO_2 is maintained at the lowest possible level.

   b. *ALI.* Alveolar overdistention is responsible for the development of pulmonary injury. Cyclic opening and closing of lung units with large volumes cause injury by "shearing" forces. Exhaled V_T volumes should be continuously monitored and documented every 1 to 2 hours. Parameters for "acceptable" exhaled volumes should be established for each patient. If the patient is not pressure limited, PIP should be noted; if PIP increases, it is indicative of airway secretions or changes in lung compliance.

   c. *Barotrauma* has been reported in patients who are receiving mechanical ventilation. High PIPs or distending pressures or sudden changes in either may cause alveolar rupture. Continuous observation of lung volumes and pressures is required to minimize the occurrence of this complication (Pediatric Acute Lung Injury Consensus Conference Group, 2015).

   d. *Atelectasis* occurs from nonuniform distribution of V_T, inadequate V_T, and adsorption atelectasis. Patient positioning may affect the site of atelectasis. Patient repositioning (including head elevation) should be done every 1 to 2 hours. The prone position is useful for lower lobe aeration and should be used when feasible.

   e. *Pneumonia.* VAP is recognized as a significant cause of morbidity in the PICU:

      i. ETT becomes quickly colonized with bacteria, most commonly gram-negative organisms, thus providing entry to the lungs.

      ii. Aspiration is a constant risk. The presence of an ETT does not guarantee protection for patients. An NG tube is usually recommended for drainage. Current research questions the practice of the routine use of gastric acid neutralization by such agents as histamine-2 blockers. It is thought that alkaline gastric secretions impose a greater risk for nosocomial pneumonia than acidic.

      iii. The head of the bed should be elevated 30 degrees in all ventilated patients if not contraindicated.

      iv. The CBC with differential and temperature surveillance may be evaluated while the ETT is in place. When a *new* ETT is placed in a patient with a pneumonic process, tracheal aspirate specimens for Gram stain and culture can be useful. However, the specimens should be interpreted in conjunction with clinical factors, types of organisms, and evidence of inflammatory cell infiltration.

      v. Decreased cardiac output caused by compression of the great vessels secondary to elevated intrathoracic pressures (especially high levels of PEEP) is a potential problem. This can be remediated with adequate volume (preload) expansion.

      vi. A central vascular line for monitoring central venous pressure (CVP) or pulmonary pressures may be used in hemodynamically unstable patients.

      vii. SIADH may occur because of stimulation of thoracic receptors, causing third spacing or fluid retention. Hourly urine output measurements and serial serum sodium and protein measurements allow early detection.

      viii. *Complications from intubation* include postextubation edema, tracheal ulcerations, vocal cord injury, granulomas or polyp formation, sinusitis, and airway obstruction resulting from a plugged ETT or bronchospasm.

      ix. Helium and oxygen admixture (Heliox) is an intervention used for airway disease that has had notable success in children. Helium is a lighter atom than oxygen and therefore the transfer of helium provides more laminar flow; it acts as a carrier of oxygen lower into the respiratory tract.

      x. All newly extubated children should be positioned upright with humidified air or oxygen. No sedative agents should be administered. Be cautious with deep tracheal suctioning because it might stimulate laryngospasm.

xi. Pharmacologic management of the patient receiving mechanical ventilation is usually required; if the patient has been on narcotic or benzodiazepine therapy for longer than 5 to 7 days, withdrawal symptoms may occur with abrupt discontinuation.

THE CHILD DEPENDENT ON TECHNOLOGY: PATIENT CARE MANAGEMENT, INCLUDING EMERGENCY CARE

A. Definition

1. Due to dramatic and rapidly developing advances in both medicine and technology, children with once unmanageable diagnoses, such as congenital anomalies, extreme prematurity, or severe critical illness, are now able to live much longer, fuller, and more productive lives than any time in history. Although many definitions exist for the technology-dependent child, the standard definition refers to children who need "both a medical device to compensate for the loss of a vital bodily function and substantial and ongoing nursing care to avert death or further disability" (Mesman, Kuo, Carrol, & Ward, 2013, p. 451). Although such a definition encompasses children dependent upon various forms of technology, such as IV nutrition or dialysis, for the purpose of this text, we limit our scope of reference to those of the pediatric population who require a tracheostomy tube, suction and monitoring devices, and/or mechanical ventilation.

2. Although they may not fit the strictest interpretation of the definition given earlier, it is important to briefly highlight other forms of supportive therapies and technologies for children with chronic pulmonary needs. Noninvasive mechanical ventilation is frequently used for children with sleep disorders as well as various possible airway anomalies. CPAP as well as BiPAP can be administered via numerous appliances such as nasal pillows, partial-face masks, or full-face masks. Special attention must be given to periodically assessing the child for proper interface fit, compliance of use, and efficacy. Some noninvasive ventilators allow for "on-demand" ventilation such as Sip and Puff ventilation, allowing a child to take a breath on demand via a triggering device (often a dental straw) where they will then receive a preset positive-pressure breath. Such a method is often beneficial for neuromuscular patients with weakening respiratory muscles; the periodic positive-pressure offsets the WOB allowing the patient to maintain activities of daily living (ADL).

B. Prevalence and Etiology

The prevalence of this population is quite marginalized in comparison to the pediatric population at large, with an estimated 5,000 tracheostomy procedures taking place annually in the United States (Peterson-Carmichael & Cheifetz, 2012). The origins of these tracheostomy placements primarily stem from chronic lung issues (requiring long-term mechanical ventilation) or for management of upper airway obstructions. Table 2.18 outlines these and other potential causal factors.

C. Collaborative Care

1. *Interdisciplinary Team Members.* Children who are dependent on technology to sustain their basic life functions require complex and intricately coordinated care, spanning multiple specialties and healthcare disciplines. Patient-centered care may be provided through a comanaged medical home for each child. Such cohesive collaboration among a diverse team of providers is rapidly becoming the standard of care in order to best meet the needs of this population. A typical team consists of partnerships between a generalist provider (such as a pediatrician) and a combination of subspecialists determined by the child's diagnoses, for example a pediatric pulmonologist, otolaryngologist, neurologist, and gastroenterologist. Due to the great burden that is placed upon family caregivers and parents of the technology-dependent

TABLE 2.18 Causal Factors for Tracheostomy

Etiology	Incidence (%)
Airway management	63
Chronic respiratory disease	23
Central hypoventilation	9
Neuromuscular weakness	6

Source: Peterson-Carmichael, S., and Cheifetz, I. (2012). The chronically critically ill patient: Pediatric considerations. *Respiratory Care, 57*(6), 993–1003. doi:10.4187/respcare.01738

child, further services are often provided by interdisciplinary team members such as a nurse case manager, a respiratory therapist, a social worker, a speech and language pathologist (SLP), a physical therapist, an occupational therapist, and a dietician/nutritionist. In addition to this, family caregivers are frequently supported by a team of healthcare practitioners, including home care nursing services (via nursing agency or private duty), home medical equipment (HME) provider-supplied respiratory therapists, and service technicians.

2. *Care Settings.* Care coordination for those who are technology dependent not only encompasses who is caring for the child, but where care is being provided. Care for the child with a tracheostomy and/or ventilator most universally takes place according to a bilevel model. First, as an inpatient, tracheostomies and other forms of technology are introduced in the acute care hospital. This discharging facility frequently becomes part of the medical home and will be part of the continuum of care in the future when acute care is required during episodes of severe illness or complication. Second, care is transitioned to the home with competently trained family caregivers (typically prepared by the discharging facility and HME provider) and home care nursing services. Care in this alternate setting is in almost every instance more cost-effective, in addition to the other benefits it provides such as increased quality of life for the child and his or her caregivers along with a decreased risk of infection. This model stands in stark contrast to the adult population for whom the majority of out-of-hospital care is provided in the subacute setting such as in the long-term acute care (LTAC) facility or a skilled nursing facility (SNF). Although a few such facilities do exist nationwide for the technology-dependent child, they are the exception rather than the rule.

D. Special Situations

1. *Emergency Care.* Caregivers, both professional and family/lay, must be thoroughly prepared and skilled in the various emergent scenarios that can present themselves specific to the child with a tracheostomy and/or long-term mechanical ventilator. Many of these issues arise from complications with the tracheostomy tube itself. For instance, the child may unintentionally become decannulated, meaning the tracheostomy tube is dislodged from the stomal opening. Clinicians must be diligent

to replace the tracheostomy tube as soon as possible, particularly for those patients who are ventilator dependent. Further problems can arise if difficulty is encountered when replacing the tube into the stoma. If severe obstruction or complications are present, it may become impossible to reintroduce the tube into the trachea. Under such circumstances the patient may require manual ventilation, if so, the stoma must be covered with gauze and tape to provide traditional bag-mask ventilation via the mouth. Bag-mask-to-stoma ventilation can also be utilized in circumstances in which severe upper airway obstruction is present, preventing proper ventilation via the previous method.

2. A second emergent scenario that frequently arises is that of tracheal tube obstruction. Most often, this is a result of mucus plugging secondary to poor humidification and/or bronchial hygiene or increased secretions or bleeding. In such situations, caregivers are trained to first attempt tracheal suctioning in an effort to clear a partially obstructed tube. When this fails to provide adequate resolution, the obstructed tracheostomy tube must be removed and replaced with a new tube. Attention is then given to identifying the underlying cause of the plug and implementing appropriate interventions to prevent future occurrences.

3. A third emergent scenario—respiratory arrest—may ultimately arise when either of the situations are not adequately addressed or resolved. As in all emergencies, perform resuscitation breathing for the patient, giving attention to proper and corrective airway management. The tube may need to be suctioned or immediately exchanged for a new tube. As previously mentioned, bag-mask ventilation with a covered stoma or bag-mask-stoma procedures may be essential for successful resuscitation. If not appropriately corrected, full CPR efforts may become necessary.

4. *Hospital Readmission.* Any trauma, insult, or similar emergency to those described previously may necessitate a hospital readmission for further diagnostics, treatment, and recovery. Hospital clinicians must make every effort to maintain the continuum of care provided in the home while optimizing and reevaluating all aspects of patient care. In an effort to provide a smooth transition, many institutions continue to use the patient's home ventilator during hospitalization. This prevents possible errors in ventilator management

and settings along with providing optimum comfort for the child.

E. Monitoring the Child Dependent on Technology

1. *Importance of Monitoring.* The most recent clinical practice guidelines of the American Thoracic Society for chronic, pediatric home ventilation recommend monitoring the technology-dependent child, particularly when the child is unobserved or asleep (Sterni et al., 2016). Although there is the potential for sleep disturbance and alarm fatigue for the caregiver (due to nuisance alarming), the benefits far outweigh the possible disadvantages.

2. *Standard Equipment.* The most widely recommended and used monitor for the mechanical ventilator-dependent child is a continuous pulse oximeter (may either be recorded or nonrecorded). Particularly in the infantile population, hypoxemia is most likely to be one of the earliest indicators of circumstances leading to inadequate ventilation, including airway obstruction or equipment malfunction. Cardiopulmonary monitoring via an apnea monitor may also be utilized; however, it is recommended to a lesser degree in the literature due to its limited scope of benefit; it is used mainly for children with central apneas or bradycardic events (Sterni et al., 2016). In addition, great attention must be given to the optimization and maintenance of adequate alarms on the mechanical ventilator. Most of the commonly used portable ventilators on the market offer various combinations of high-pressure alarms (indicating possible obstructions) or low-pressure and/or minute-volume alarms (indicating possible air leak or circuit disconnection). It is imperative that a monitoring device is used outside of the mechanical ventilator alarms as studies have shown that these alarms are not always sensitive to all dangerous situations (such as decannulation of a patient with a particularly small-diameter tracheostomy tube).

3. *Preparation and Intervention.* It is imperative for all trained caregivers to remain prepared at all points to intervene when an emergency or crisis presents itself. An essential component of preparation requires the proper supplies and equipment to be present with the child *at all times*. Table 2.19 includes the minimum necessary emergency equipment that must be immediately available to the technologically dependent child.

F. Supportive Care of the Child Dependent on Technology

Weight Management and Monitoring. Children who have a tracheostomy and/or long-term mechanical ventilator must be continually evaluated for proper development and growth. The correlation between weight gain and length gain must be considered in this evaluation as linear growth is highly reflective of lung growth. If proper respiratory support is not being offered, the required calories necessary for the increased WOB will be consumed regardless, creating a deficit leading to either a lack of appropriate weight gain or actual weight loss. Weight gain in technology-dependent children can be devastating and can be precipitated by a feeding regimen that

TABLE 2.19 Tracheostomy Emergency Supplies and Equipment

Portable suction machine (preferably battery operated)
Suction catheters
Manual resuscitator bag (with appropriately sized mask)
Same-sized tracheostomy tube
Next-size-smaller tracheostomy tube (often referred to as a *downsize*)
Extra tracheostomy ties
Water-soluble lubricant (for tracheostomy tube insertion)
Normal saline vials
Scissors
Medical tape

does not account for limited activity. In addition to this, attention should also be offered to the proper overall development of the child. These rehabilitative concerns, such as the ADL, mobility, and communication skills, are continually assessed and addressed by the comprehensive therapy teams, including physical, occupational, and speech therapists. A plethora of assistive devices exist to meet needs across the spectrum of disabilities. Of particular note to the tracheostomy population is the ability to restore speech (vocalized communication) via the Passy Muir speaking valve (or other similar device). Initial and ongoing assessment, both inpatient and outpatient, is crucial to the continued success of this intervention.

G. Liberation From Technology

Transitioning away from the use of the mechanical ventilator is the first step in liberation from technological dependence. As long as clinical stability has been present for a determined length of time by the provider team, caregivers may initiate the weaning process, ranging from a reduction in prescribed mechanical ventilator settings, such as the amount of pressure support or PEEP offered to actual time spent off of the ventilator, frequently referred to as a *sprint* or *trial*. During this time off of the ventilator, the child may be supplemented with heated and humidified medical air via a trach collar mask in order to facilitate proper bronchial hygiene and secretion management. As tolerated, this time free from technological support is lengthened and increased in a stepwise, methodical fashion until respiratory support may no longer be required at all. At such a point, it is possible for the tracheostomy tube to be temporarily occluded via a removable cap, restoring the upper airway and offering a demonstration of how the child may tolerate complete removal of the tracheostomy tube. Finally, prior to decannulation, many providers complete additional testing, such as an overnight sleep study (nocturnal polysomnogram), a 12-hour recorded pulse oximetry study and flexible bronchoscopy, to discern whether the underlying pathologies are adequately resolved.

H. Complications

1. Over time, the impact of the child dependent upon technology becomes great, both for the patient's family as well as the community at large. One of the greatest and most readily documented consequences of this dependence is felt by the child and his or her family. Numerous studies cite fatigue and burnout for the family caregiver as having one of the greatest impacts, the effects reach multiple domains such as emotional health, social functioning, and family relationships (Duma, 2012). From a more global perspective, advances in technology have also created new needs and financial barriers that must be collectively overcome by families, providers, and communities.

2. Clinically speaking, various complications beyond those emergencies noted previously may arise. For instance, scar tissue (granulomas/fibromas) may be found both within the trachea as well as around the stomal site, possibly leading to bloody secretions, difficulty in placing the tracheostomy tube, and ventilatory obstruction. Furthermore, frequent topical infection around the stoma or within the trachea can develop, even leading to hospital readmission.

LUNG TRANSPLANTATION

A. Definition and Etiology

1. Lung transplant is a therapeutic option for children and infants with untreatable or end-stage diseases of the lungs or of the pulmonary vascular system. Lung transplantation for pediatric patients can prolong life and also improve quality of life. Since 1986, almost 2,000 pediatric lung transplants have been reported to the Heart-Lung Transplant Registry (Benden et al., 2014). Children have undergone heart–lung, single-lung, bilateral-lung, and living donor bilobar transplantation. Bilateral lung transplantation is performed for nearly all children because of concerns over the growth potential of the transplanted lungs.

2. CF is the most common indication for pediatric lung transplant. Other less common indications include idiopathic pulmonary fibrosis, surfactant protein deficiencies, childhood interstitial lung disease, congenital heart disease, and retransplantation. See Table 2.20 for additional indications for lung transplantation.

B. Pathophysiology

1. Recipients of lung transplant have end-stage parenchymal or vascular lung disease with significant impact on ADL and quality of life.

2. Candidates with primary PH frequently have poor right ventricular function with increased CVP, hepatomegaly, jugular distention, periorbital edema, and pulmonary effusion.

TABLE 2.20 Indications for Lung Transplantation

CF
Idiopathic pulmonary arterial hypertension
Retransplantation related to chronic rejection
Congenital heart disease, often with Eisenmenger's syndrome
Idiopathic pulmonary fibrosis
Obliterative bronchiolitis, not retransplant
Retransplant, not obliterative bronchiolitis
Desquamative interstitial pneumonitis
Pulmonary vascular disease
Eisenmenger's syndrome
Pulmonary fibrosis, other
Surfactant protein B deficiency
Chronic obstructive pulmonary disease/emphysema
Bronchopulmonary dysplasia
Bronchiectasis

CF, cystic fibrosis.

Source: Benden, C., Goldfarb, S. B., Edwards, L. B., Kucheryavaya, A. Y., Christie, J. D., Dipchand, A. I., . . . Stehlik, J. (2014). The registry of the International Society for Heart and Lung Transplantation: Seventeenth official pediatric lung and heart–lung transplantation report—2014; focus theme: Retransplantation. *Journal of Heart and Lung Transplantation, 33*(10), 1025–1033. doi:10.1016/j.healun.2014.08.005

3. Candidates with congenital heart disease, Eisenmenger's syndrome, or pulmonary AV malformation may demonstrate profound cyanosis, clubbing, polycythemia, and hypoxemia exceeding the child's normal values.

4. Candidates with surfactant dysfunction have refractory respiratory failure and progressive PH.

C. Candidate Evaluation

1. Candidates selected for single-lung transplantation require normal heart function or reversible right ventricular dysfunction and absence of pulmonary infection.

2. Candidates for double-lung transplantation require normal heart function or reversible right ventricular dysfunction but may have some infectious processes present. Both heart and lungs must be transplanted in children with a complex, nonrepairable cardiac defect or inadequate cardiac function in addition to end-stage pulmonary disease. Previous thoracotomy or sternotomy is not an absolute contraindication to transplantation.

3. Patients with CF are difficult to evaluate for transplant because the course of decline can be unpredictable. In addition to the severity of the disease, rate of change in lung function, frequency of exacerbations, nutritional status, comorbidities, and colonization or infection with certain bacteria should also be taken into consideration. An FEV_1 below 30% or rapid decline in FEV_1 may indicate the need to refer for lung transplant (Lynch, Sayah, Belperio, & Weigt, 2015).

4. Invasive and noninvasive diagnostic studies for transplant evaluation may include the following:

a. Laboratory tests including blood chemistry and hematology studies, viral serology for HIV, hepatitis B and C, CMV, Epstein–Barr virus (EBV), varicella, toxoplasma, and antibodies to childhood immunizations

b. Chest radiograph

c. CT scan of neck and chest

d. ECG

e. Cardiac echo

f. Bone density scan

g. Complete PFTs

h. Exercise study with pulse oximetry such as a 6-minute walk

i. Quantitative V/Q scan

5. Absolute contraindications include systemic disease affecting other organ systems.

a. Active infection with HIV, hepatitis B or C, TB

b. Malignancy

c. Renal, liver, or left ventricular failure

d. Irreversible or progressive CNS or neuromuscular disease

6. Other considerations regardless of diagnosis, all lung transplant candidates should possess the following (Faro et al., 2007).

a. A clear diagnosis or adequately delineated trajectory of illness despite optimal medical therapy that puts the individual child at risk of dying without a lung transplant.

b. An adequate array of family support personnel.

c. Adequate access to transplant services and medications after transplantation.

d. Adequate evidence of willingness and ability on the part of patient and parent to adhere to the rigorous therapy, daily monitoring, and reevaluation schedule after transplant.

D. Donor Evaluation

1. Donor availability remains a major limitation to the applicability of transplantation for end-stage lung disease.

2. *Donor Criteria*

a. Ideally younger than 55 years old.

b. ABO blood type compatibility.

c. Clear chest radiograph.

d. Arterial oxygen tension should be more than 300 mmHg on an inspired oxygen fraction

of 1.0 with an appropriate V_T and 5 cm H_2O PEEP.

e. Gram stain and sputum cultures free of bacteria, fungus, and significant number of WBCs.

f. No aspiration or sepsis.

g. Within a reasonable size range of the recipient. Height is used as the most accurate correlate to lung size. Height that falls within 15% to 20% of the recipient height is probably suitable.

h. A history of limited cigarette smoking is probably acceptable if other parameters of the evaluation fall within the guidelines.

i. Absence of pulmonary contusions, chest tubes, tracheostomies.

j. Mild pulmonary contusions and subsegmental atelectasis would not necessarily exclude a donor as long as these criteria are met.

k. Flexible bronchoscopy should be performed to examine the airways for erythema suggestive of aspiration of gastric contents. In addition, this provides an opportunity to assess the nature and quantity of pulmonary secretions. The presence of purulent secretions that do not clear well with suctioning should exclude the donor even if the chest radiograph is clear and the oxygenation is adequate.

3. *Relative Contraindications.* Donors are excluded in the presence of positive HIV serology, active hepatitis, history of asthma, TB, or other significant pulmonary disease.

E. Patient Care Management

1. *Ventilatory Support and Weaning.* In the majority of patients, standard ventilation and weaning techniques are sufficient. Typically weaning can occur quickly during the first few hours to days after transplant. In patients transplanted for PH, weaning may take longer.

2. *Provide and Monitor Immunosuppression.* Protocols differ from one center to another but most use a triple-drug immunosuppression approach. Drug regimens generally include cyclosporine or tacrolimus in combination with azathioprine or mycophenolate mofetil and prednisone.

3. *Monitor and Treat Rejection*

a. Surveillance bronchoscopies are performed on a schedule basis to assess graft acceptance. Acute rejection is treated with high-dose steroids. Persistent or recurrent rejection may be treated with lympholytic therapy or the daily immunosuppressive regimen may be modified.

4. *Infection and Infection Prophylaxis*

a. Donors and potential candidates are screened by serologic testing of hepatitis A, B, C, and D viruses, herpes virus, EBV, HIV, toxoplasma, and CMV.

b. Infections after lung transplant are common due to immunosuppression, transmission from donor, and presence of hospital-acquired infections.

c. Children are monitored, and cultures are obtained to screen for signs of infection, including fever or temperature instability, increasing quantity or a change in the nature of the pulmonary secretions, increasing respiratory distress, worsening ABGs, leukocytosis or leukopenia, and radiographic changes.

d. Routine postoperative care includes thorough pulmonary toilet using strict aseptic technique.

e. Serologic follow-up is performed on patients who have negative results at the time of transplant. Skin testing for TB and energy are routine.

f. Sputum cultures are obtained on a routine basis from patients with CF to guide prophylaxis.

g. During the perioperative period, antibiotic coverage is planned to cover bacterial sensitivities from the donor culture and adjusted if necessary based on surveillance cultures.

5. *Monitor Systemic Perfusion Parameters.* Strict monitoring of input and output in the postoperative period is critical to avoid pulmonary edema.

6. *Monitor Nutritional Status.* Monitor intake, output, and weight and calculate caloric requirements. Nutritional consults should be sought for patients with previous malnourishment (e.g., patients with CF). Provide an enteral or parenteral diet as ordered. Monitor the child's wound healing.

7. *Pain Management.* Pain control is essential after lung transplantation. Undertreated pain can result in poor respiratory effort and the subsequent development of pneumonia and atelectasis. Pain control is also crucial to facilitate weaning for mechanical ventilation and promote appropriate breathing (Cason et al., 2015).

8. *Physical Rehabilitation.* Exercise training can help in optimizing functional capacity and fitness pre-transplant and improve outcomes and quality of life posttransplant (Wickerson et al., 2016).

F. Complications of Lung Transplantation

1. There are predictable timelines for complications following lung transplantation.

a. *Immediate posttransplant phase.* First month after transplantation

i. Typically, flexible bronchoscopies are performed within 24 to 48 hours post-transplant to obtain lower airway cultures and assess the integrity of the airway anastomosis.

ii. Complications related to surgery, rejection, or infection can be seen in this phase.

b. *Early phase.* One to 6 months after transplantation

i. Complications in this phase include infection due to opportunistic and viral pathogens and medication side effects.

c. *Late phase.* Greater than 6 months after transplantation

i. Bronchiolitis obliterans and malignancies are commonly seen in this phase.

ii. Posttransplant lymphoproliferative disease (PTLD) is the most common malignancy in children and occurs more in solid-organ transplant and in patients with CF. This incidence for PTLD increases at 5-year posttransplant (Table 2.21).

G. Survival and Mortality

1. Overall survival in pediatric lung transplantation is similar to the expected survival in adults.

2. The 1- and 5-year actuarial survival for children undergoing lung transplantation is approximately 82% and 52%, respectively (Benden et al., 2014). Most deaths after pediatric lung transplantation occur shortly after transplantation.

3. More than 80% of lung transplant patients report no activity limitations up to 5 years posttransplant (Benden et al., 2014).

4. Infections, graft failure, surgical complications, and bronchiolitis obliterans are the common causes of death in pediatric lung transplant (Benden et al., 2014; Camargo et al., 2014; Cason et al., 2015; Faro et al., 2007; Hayes, Benden, Sweet, & Conrad, 2015; Kirkby & Hayes, 2014; Kotloff & Thabut, 2011; Lynch et al., 2015; Weill et al., 2015; Wickerson et al., 2016).

TABLE 2.21   Complications of Lung Transplantation

Postoperative period
  Ischemia of the anastomosis site
  Bleeding
  Infection
  Systemic hypertension
  Phrenic nerve paresis

First 3 months
  Hypertension
  Rejection
  Infection

First year
  Viral infection
  Rejection
  Hypertension

After first year
  Viral infection
  Rejection
  PTLD

PTLD, posttransplant lymphoproliferative disease.

CASE STUDIES WITH QUESTIONS, ANSWERS, AND RATIONALES

Case Study 2.1

A 2-year-old female is admitted to the PICU with right middle lobe (RML) and right lower lobe (RLL) pneumonia. The patient and her family were initially on vacation in Florida when she developed a cough and intermittent fevers lasting for 7 days. Upon returning home, the patient was taken to the emergency room. She had an overall normal exam with a chest x-ray showing complete consolidation and atelectasis of the RML and RLL. She was prescribed azithromycin for 5 days and an albuterol inhaler. She followed up in her primary care provider's office 1 day later with a continued cough and response to albuterol and she was sent home with 5 days of oral steroids. She returned to the primary care provider 3 days later with continued cough and the decision was to continue the prescribed course. She was seen in the emergency department 10 days later with fever. Physical exam findings included oxygen saturation of 97% and decreased breath sounds. Repeat chest x-ray showed RML and RLL consolidation with a right pleural effusion (similar to earlier finding). At this point, she was admitted for further workup to include IV antibiotics, chest CT, and/or bronchoscopy.

1. What piece of history would be the most important for the team to elicit from the family?
    A. Travel to Florida
    B. Observation of any choking or gagging episodes
    C. When the symptoms first started
    D. Older siblings

2. What would you be most concerned about for this child?
    A. Foreign-body aspiration
    B. Immune dysfunction
    C. CF
    D. Asthma

A chest CT was performed and showed dense areas of opacification, ground glass opacities, and tree-in-bud pulmonary opacities within the right middle and lower lobes consistent with pneumonia and areas of atelectasis. Mild irregularity and narrowing of the bronchus intermedius. Apparent bronchiectatic changes within the right middle and lower lobes. Right hilar and right paratracheal lymphadenopathy.

3. Can a chest x-ray/chest CT be considered a definitive diagnostic test for a foreign body?
    A. Yes
    B. No

Bronchoscopy was performed as the patient failed further management with IV antibiotics. Flexible bronchoscopy showed normal upper airway anatomy, normal tracheal anatomy, normal mucosa, and copious amounts of thick yellow white secretions in the bronchus intermedius, RML, and RLL. A foreign body identified as a cylindrical cap was identified in the distal portion of the bronchus intermedius, completely occluding it.

4. What supportive care measures should be performed by the hospital care team?
    A. Administer oxygen
    B. Perform vigorous pulmonary toilet
    C. Continue antibiotic therapy
    D. All of the above

5. How should the bronchiectasis be managed?
    A. Chest physiotherapy
    B. Hypertonic saline
    C. Antibiotic therapy
    D. All of the above

Case Study 2.2

Patient is a 4-year-old female admitted to the PICU with sanguineous mucus plugging her tracheostomy. Patient has a history of prematurity of 24 5/7 weeks; chronic, steroid-dependent interstitial lung disease; history of ARDS related to adenovirus pneumonia; and asthma. She is ventilator dependent. Patient has a known fibroma around her tracheostomy site. Patient has suffered from rhinorrhea the last several days but has been afebrile.

Since she started with nasal symptoms, her mom has noticed increased bloody secretions through the tracheostomy with suctioning. The morning of admission, the patient's mother awoke to a pulse oximeter alarm with an oxygen saturation in the low 80s. Emergency medical services were called and the patient presented to the PICU.

1. What should the caregiver at home perform first?
   A. Suction the tracheal tube
   B. Change the tracheal tube
   C. Perform bag-valve-mask ventilation
   D. Call 911

2. What standard equipment should the family have at home when caring for a child dependent on technology?
   A. Pulse oximeter
   B. Apnea monitor
   C. Car seat
   D. Shower chair

3. What would you be most concerned about for the cause of the bleeding?
   A. Known granuloma
   B. Recent infection
   C. Pulmonary hemorrhage
   D. Both A and B

The patient was discharged home approximately 5 days after admission as no further episodes of bleeding occurred during the hospitalization. A bronchoscopy was performed that showed no further evidence of bleeding. The patient presented back to the PICU approximately 10 days after discharge again after coughing up bloody secretions through the tracheostomy. She required multiple tracheostomy changes at home and complained of difficulty breathing. Her caregivers at home called emergency medical services and patient presented to the hospital. The patient had a bedside bronchoscopy performed showing irritated tracheal mucosa with a film of exudates with areas of recent bleeding, but no active bleeding. A new tracheostomy was inserted without difficulty.

4. The patient should have a tracheal culture performed before administration of antibiotics for presumed tracheitis?
   A. True
   B. False

5. The child dependent on technology requires complex, coordinated care with a primary care provider, subspecialists (pulmonology, otolaryngology, neurology, gastroenterology), nursing, respiratory therapy, social work, dietary services, speech/language pathology, physical therapy/occupational therapy, and home care services (nursing and medical equipment providers).
   A. True
   B. False

Answers and Rationales

Case Study 2.1

1. **B.** The characteristic history of a choking or gagging episode, followed by a coughing spell given by the caregivers should be carefully considered.

2. **A.** Toddlers younger than 3 years of age account for 60% to 80% of foreign-body aspirations.

3. **B.** Foreign-body aspiration can never be excluded on the basis of chest radiography alone. A final diagnosis is only achieved at the time of bronchoscopic evaluation.

4. **D.** All options are supportive care measures for the patient.

5. **D.** *Bronchiectasis* is defined as irreversible dilation of the bronchial tree. Typically, the segmental and subsegmental bronchi become irregularly shaped and dilated leading to a loss of the typical funnel configuration that allows smooth central flow of secretions. In addition, ciliary activity in the area of the dilation is inadequate and further contributes to the difficulty in mobilizing secretions. Medical management depends on the severity of the disease. Chest physiotherapy, hypertonic saline, and antibiotic therapy are warranted.

A leading cause of accidental death in the toddler is foreign-body aspiration. The degree of respiratory sequelae depends on the nature of the material aspirated. Mobile infants and toddlers are at particularly high risk by virtue of their tendency to place objects in their mouths. The preferred location for objects small enough to be ingested is the right middle lobe bronchi, which has the most direct and straight connection to the trachea.

Case Study 2.2

1. **A.** Caregivers, both professional and family/lay, must be thoroughly prepared and skilled in the various emergent scenarios that can present themselves, specific to the child with a tracheostomy and/or long-term mechanical ventilator. Many of these issues arise from complications with the tracheostomy tube itself.

An emergent scenario that frequently arises is that of tracheal tube obstruction. Most often, this is a result of mucus plugging secondary to poor humidification and/or bronchial hygiene or increased secretions or bleeding. In such situations, caregivers are trained to first attempt tracheal suctioning in an effort to clear a partially obstructed tube. When this fails to provide adequate resolution, the obstructed tracheostomy tube is to be removed and replaced with a new tube. Attention is then given to identifying the underlying cause of the plug and implementing appropriate interventions to prevent future occurrences.

2. **A.** The most recent clinical practice guidelines of the American Thoracic Society for chronic, pediatric home ventilation recommend monitoring the technology-dependent child, particularly when the child is unobserved or asleep. The most widely recommended and used monitor for the mechanical ventilator-dependent child is a continuous pulse oximeter (may either be recorded or nonrecorded). Particularly in the infantile population, hypoxemia is most likely to be one of the earliest indicators of circumstances leading to inadequate ventilation, including airway obstruction or equipment malfunction.

3. **D.** Both the known granuloma and infection may contribute to bleeding in our patient.

4. **A.** A tracheal culture should be performed first to guide appropriate antibiotic therapy.

5. **A.** Children who are dependent upon technology to sustain their basic life functions require complex and intricately coordinated care, spanning multiple specialties and healthcare disciplines. Patient-centered care may be provided through a comanaged medical home for each child. Such cohesive collaboration among a diverse team of providers is rapidly becoming the standard of care in order to best meet the needs of this population.

REFERENCES

Abel, R., Bush, A., Chitty, L., Harcourt, J., & Nicholson, A. (2012). Congenital lung disease. In R. Wilmott, T. Boat, A. Bush, V. Chernick, R. Deterding, & F. Ratjen (Eds.), *Kending's disorders of the respiratory tract in children* (8th ed., pp. 317–357). Philadelphia, PA: Elsevier.

Abman, S. H., Hansmann, G., Archer, S., Ivy, D., Adatia, I., Chung, W. K., . . . Wessel, D. (2015). Pediatric pulmonary hypertension: Guidelines from the American Heart Association and American Thoracic Society. *Circulation, 132,* 2037–2099. doi:10.1161/CIR.0000000000000329.

Agarwal, H., Taylor, M., Grzeszczak, M., Lovvorn, H., Hunley, T., Jabs, K., & Shankar, V. (2005). Extra corporeal membrane oxygenation and plasmapheresis for pulmonary hemorrhage in microscopic polyangiitis. *Pediatric Nephrology, 20*(4), 526–528. doi:10.1007/s00467-004-1724-5

American Academy of Pediatrics. (2010). Policy statement—prevention of choking among children. *Pediatrics, 125*(3), 601. doi:10.1542/peds.2009-2862

Atkins, D., Berger, S., Duff, J., Gonzales, J., Hunt, E., Joyner, B., . . . Schexnayder, S. (2015). Part 11: Pediatric basic life support and cardiopulmonary resuscitation and emergency cardiovascular care. *Circulation, 132*(Suppl. 2), S519–S525. doi:10.1161/CIR.0000000000000265

Atkins, D., de Caen, A. R., Berger, S., Samson, R. A., Schexnayder, S. M., Joyner, B. L., . . . Meaney, P. A. (2018). 2017 American Heart Association focused update on pediatric basic life support and cardiopulmonary resuscitation quality. *Circulation, 137,* e1–e6. doi:10.1161/CIR.0000000000000540

Aurora, R., Zak, R., Karippot, A., Lamm, C., Morgenthaler, T., Auerbach, S., . . . Ramar, K. (2011). Practice parameters for the respiratory indications for polysomnography in children. *Sleep, 34*(3), 379–388. Retrieved from https://aasm.org/resources/practiceparameters/pppolysomnographychildren.pdf

Balfour-Lynn, I. M., & Davies, J. C. (2012). Acute infections that produce upper airway obstruction. In R. Wilmott, T. Boat, A. Bush, V. Chernick, R. Deterding, & F. Ratjen. (Eds.), *Kending's disorders of the respiratory tract in children* (8th ed., pp. 424–436). Philadelphia, PA: Elsevier.

Benden, C., Goldfarb, S. B., Edwards, L. B., Kucheryavaya, A. Y., Christie, J. D., Dipchand, A. I., . . . Stehlik, J. (2014). The registry of the International Society for Heart and Lung Transplantation: Seventeenth official pediatric lung and heart–lung transplantation report—2014; focus theme: Retransplantation. *Journal of Heart and Lung Transplantation, 33*(10), 1025–1033. doi:10.1016/j.healun.2014.08.005

Berger, J., Carcillo, J., Shanley, T., Wessel, D., Clark, A., Holubkov, R., . . . Nicholson, C. E. (2013). Critical pertussis illness in children, a multicenter prospective cohort study. *Pediatric Critical Care Medicine, 14*(4), 356–365. doi:10.1097/PCC.0b013e31828a70fe

Bonavita, J., & Naidich, D. P. (2012). Imaging of bronchiectasis. *Clinics in Chest Medicine, 33*(2), 233–248. doi:10.1016/j.ccm.2012.02.007

Borowitz, D., Robinson, K., Rosenfeld, M., Davis, S., Sabadosa, K., Spear, S., . . . Accurso, F. (2009). Cystic fibrosis foundation evidence-based guidelines for management of infants with cystic fibrosis. *Journal of Pediatrics, 155*(6 Suppl.), S73–S93. doi:10.1016/j.jpeds.2009.09.001

Bowen, P., & Maxwell, N. (2014). Management of bronchopulmonary dysplasia. *Paediatrics and Child Health, 24*(1), 27–31. doi:10.1016/j.paed.2013.06.007

Bradley, J., Byington, C., Shah, S., Alverson, B., Carter, E., Harrison, C., . . . Swanson, J. T. (2011). Executive summary: The management of community-acquired pneumonia in infants and children older than 3 months of age: Clinical practice guidelines by the Pediatric Infectious Diseases Society and the Infectious Diseases Society of America. *Clinical Infectious Disease, 53*(7), 617–630. doi:10.1093/cid/cir625

Bruzoni, M., & Krummel, T. (2012). Disorders of the respiratory tract caused by trauma. In R. Wilmott, T. Boat, A. Bush, V. Chernick, R. Deterding, & F. Ratjen (Eds.), *Kending's disorders of the respiratory tract in children* (8th ed., pp. 1036–1045). Philadelphia, PA: Elsevier.

Budhiraja, R., Tuder, R. M., & Hassoun, P. M. (2004). Endothelial dysfunction in pulmonary hypertension. *Circulation, 109,* 159–165. doi:10.1161/01.CIR.0000102381.57477.50

Camargo, P., Pato, E., Campos, S., Afonso, J., Carraro, R., Costa, A., . . . Pêgo-Fernandes P. M. (2014). Pediatric lung transplantation: 10 years of experience. *Clinics, 69*(Suppl. 1), 51–54. doi:10.6061/clinics/2014(Sup01)10

Camerda, L. E., & Goodman, D. M. (2016). Wheezing, bronchiolitis, and bronchitis: Bronchitis. In R. Kliegman, B. Stanton, J. St. Geme, & N. Schor (Eds.), *Nelson's textbook of pediatrics* (20th ed., pp. 2044–2050). St. Louis, MO: Elsevier.

Cason, M., Naik, A., Grimm, J. C., Hanna, D. Faraone, L., Brookman, J. C., . . . Hanna, M. N. (2015). The efficacy and safety of epidural-based analgesia in a case series of patients undergoing lung transplantation. *Journal of Cardiothoracic and Vascular Anesthesia, 29*(1), 126–132. doi:10.1053/j.jvca.2014.07.023

Chalmers, J., Goeminne, P., Aliberti, S., McDonnell, M., Lonni, S., Davidson, J., . . . Hill, A. (2014). The bronchiectasis severity index: An international derivation and validation study. *American Journal of Respiratory and Critical Care Medicine, 189*(5), 576–585. doi:10.1164/rccm.201309-1575OC

Cherry, J. (2013). Pertussis: Challenges today and for the future. *PLOS Pathogens, 9*(7), e1003418. doi:10.1371/journal.ppat.1003418

Conlon, P. (2013). The child with respiratory dysfunction. In M. Hockenberry & D. Wilson (Eds.), *Wong's essentials of pediatric nursing* (9th ed., pp. 706–761). St. Louis, MO: Elsevier.

Coates, B., Camerda, L. E., & Goodman, D. M. (2016). Wheezing, bronchiolitis, and bronchitis. In R. Kliegman, B. Stanton, J. St. Geme, & N. Schor (Eds.), *Nelson's textbook of pediatrics* (20th ed., pp. 2044–2050). St. Louis, MO: Elsevier.

Cystic Fibrosis Foundation. (2016). *Cystic Fibrosis Foundation Patient Registry annual data report 2015.* Bethesda, MD: Author. Retrieved from https://www.cff.org/Our-Research/CF-Patient-Registry/2015-Patient-Registry-Annual-Data-Report.pdf

Da Dalt, L., Bressan, S., Martinolli, F., Perilongo, G., & Baraldi, E. (2013). Proceedings and selected abstracts of the 4th international conference on clinical neonatology treatment of bronchiolitis: State of the art. *Early Human Development, 89* (Suppl. 1), S31–S36. doi:10.1016/S0378-3782(13)70011-2

Darlow, B. A., & Morley, C. J. (2015). Oxygen saturation targeting and bronchopulmonary dysplasia. *Clinics in Perinatology, 42*(4), 807–823. doi:10.1016/j.clp.2015.08.008

de Caen, A., Berg, M., Chameides, L., Gooden, C., Hickey, R., Scott, H., . . . Samson, R. (2015). Part 12: Pediatric advance life support: 2015 American Heart Association guidelines update for cardiopulmonary resuscitation and emergency cardiovascular care. *Circulation, 132*(Suppl. 2), S526–S542. doi:10.1161/CIR.0000000000000266

Dijk, F., Curtin, J., Lord, D., & Fitzgerald, D. (2012). Pulmonary embolism in children. *Paediatric Respiratory Reviews, 13*(2), 112–122. doi:10.1016/j.prrv.2011.09.002

Dine, A. P., & Werner, S. L. (2008). Pediatric hemoptysis with pulmonary hemorrhage and respiratory failure: A case report. *American Journal of Emergency Medicine, 26*(5), 639.e3–639.e4. doi:10.1016/j.ajem.2007.10.035

Doyle, L., & Anderson, P. (2009). Long-term outcomes of bronchopulmonary dysplasia. *Seminars in Fetal and Neonatal Medicine, 14*, 391–395. doi:10.1016/j.siny.2009.08.004

Dreyfus, L., Javouhey, E., Denis, A., Touzet, S. & Bordet, F. (2017). Implementation and evaluation of a paediatric nurse-driven sedation protocol in a paediatric intensive care unit. *Annals of Intensive Care, 7*(1), 36. doi: doi:10.1186/s13613-017-0256-7

Duma, H. (2012). Rehabilitation considerations for children dependent on long-term mechanical ventilation. *International Scholarly Research Network ISRN Rehabilitation, 2012.* doi:10.5402/2012/756103

Ehrenkranz, R., Walsh, M., Vorh, B., Jobe, A., Wright, L., Fanaroff, A., . . . Poole, K. (2005). Validation of the National Institutes of Health Consensus definition of bronchopulmonary dysplasia. *Pediatrics, 116*(6), 1353–1360. doi:10.1542/peds.2005-0249

Ehsan, Z., & Ishman, S. (2016). Pediatric obstructive sleep apnea. *Otolaryngologic Clinics of North America, 49*(6), 1449–1464. doi:10.1542/peds.2005-0249

Farrell, P., White, T., Ren, C., Hempstead, S., Accurso, F., Derichs, N., . . . Sosnay, P. (2017). Diagnosis of cystic fibrosis: Consensus guidelines from the Cystic Fibrosis Foundation. *Journal of Pediatrics, 181*(Suppl.), S4–S15.e1. doi:10.1016/j.jpeds.2016.09.064

Faro, A., Mallory, G. B., Visner, G. A., Elidemir, O., Mogayzel, P. J., Danziger-Isakov, L., . . . Waltz, D. (2007). American Society of Transplantation executive summary on pediatric lung transplantation. *American Journal of Transplantation, 7*(2), 285–292. doi:10.1111/j.1600-6143.2006.01612.x

Feldman, C. (2011). Bronchiectasis: New approaches to diagnosis and management. *Clinics in Chest Medicine, 32*(3), 535–546. doi:10.1016/j.ccm.2011.05.002

Fouzas, S., Prifitis, K. N., & Anthracopoulos, M. B. (2011). Pulse oximetry in pediatric practice. *Pediatrics, 128*(4), 740–752. doi:10.1542/peds.2011-0271

Galiè, N., Corris, P., Frost, A., Girgis, R., Granton, J., Jing, Z., . . . Keogh, A. (2013). Updated treatment algorithm of pulmonary arterial hypertension. *Journal of the American College of Cardiology, 62*(Suppl. 25), D60–D72. doi:10.1016/j.jacc.2013.10.031

Gentile, M. A., Heuer, A. J., & Kallet, R. H. (2017). Analysis and monitoring of gas exchange. In R. Kacmarek, J. Stoller, A. Heuer, R. Chatburn, & R. Kallet (Eds.). *Egan's fundamentals of respiratory care* (11th ed., pp. 369–399). St. Louis, MO: Elsevier.

Gereige, R., & Laufer, P. M. (2013). Pneumonia. *Pediatrics in Review, 34*(10), 438–456. doi:10.1542/pir.34-10-438

Godfrey, S. (2004). Pulmonary hemorrhage/hemoptysis in children. *Pediatric Pulmonary, 37*(6), 476–484. doi:10.1002/ppul.20020

Greenough, A., Murthy, V., & Milner, A. (2012). Respiratory disorders in the newborn. In R. Wilmott, T. Boat, A. Bush, V. Chernick, R. Deterding, & F. Ratjen. (Eds.), *Kending's disorders of the respiratory tract in children* (8th ed., pp. 358–385). Philadelphia, PA: Elsevier.

Groothuis, J., & Makari, D. (2012). Definition and outpatient management of the very low-birth-weight infant with bronchopulmonary dysplasia. *Advances in Therapy, 29*(4), 297–311. doi:10.1007/s12325-012-0015-y

Grover, R., Murthy, K., Brozanski, B., Gien, J., Rintoul, N., Keene, S., . . . Children's Hospitals Neonatal Consortium. (2015). Short-term outcomes and medical and surgical interventions in infants with congenital diaphragmatic hernia. *American Journal of Perinatology, 32*(11), 1038–1044. doi:10.1055/s-0035-1548729

Guidry, C., & McGahren, E. (2012). Pediatric chest I: Developmental and physiologic conditions for the surgeon. *Surgery Clinics of North America, 92*, 615–643. doi:10.1016/j.suc.2012.03.013

Hayes, D., Benden, C., Sweet, S., & Conrad, C. (2015). Current state of pediatric lung transplantation. *Lung, 193,* 629–637. doi:10.1007/s00408-015-9765-z

Hoeper, M., Bogaard, H., Condliffe, R., Frantz, R., Khanna, D., Kurzyna, M., . . . Badesch, D. (2013). Definitions and diagnosis of pulmonary hypertension. *Journal of the American College of Cardiology, 62*(25), D42–D50. doi:10.1016/j.jacc.2013.10.032

Hofferberth, S., Watters, K., Rahbar, R., & Fynn-Thompson, F. (2015). Management of congenital tracheal stenosis. *Pediatrics, 136*(3), e660–e669. doi:10.1542/peds.2014-3931

Hofferberth, S., Watters, K., Rahbar, R., & Fynn-Thompson, F. (2016). Evolution of surgical approaches in the management of congenital tracheal stenosis: Single-center experience. *World Journal for Pediatric and Congenital Heart Surgery, 7*(1), 16–24. doi:10.1177/2150135115606627

Hopper, R., Abman, S., & Ivy, D. (2016). Persistent challenges in pediatric pulmonary hypertension. *Chest, 150*(1), 226–236. doi:10.1016/j.chest.2016.01.007

Islam, J., Keller, R., Aschner, J., Hartert, T., & Moore, P. (2015). Understanding the short- and long-term respiratory outcomes of prematurity and bronchopulmonary dysplasia. *American Journal of Respiratory and Critical Care Medicine, 192*(2), 134–156. doi:10.1164/rccm.201412-2142PP

Jaff, M. R., McMurtry, M. S., Archer, S. L., Cushman, M., Goldenberg, N., Goldhaber, S., . . . Zierler B.K. (2011). Management of massive and submassive pulmonary embolism, iliofemoral deep vein thrombosis, and chronic thromboembolic pulmonary hypertension: A scientific statement from the American Heart Association. *Circulation, 123,* 1788–1830. doi:10.1161/CIR.0b013e318214914f

Kaestner, M., Schranz, D., Warnecke, G., Apitz, C., Hansmann, G., & Miera, O. (2016). Pulmonary hypertension in the intensive care unit. Expert consensus statement on the diagnosis and treatment of paediatric pulmonary hypertension. The European Paediatric Pulmonary Vascular Disease Network, endorsed by ISHLT and DGPK. *Heart, 102,* ii57–ii66. doi:10.1136/heartjnl-2015-307774

Keckler, S., & Schropp, K. (2010). Surgical disorders in childhood that affect respiratory care. In B. Walsh, M. Czervinske, & R. DiBlasi (Eds.), *Perinatal and pediatric respiratory care* (3rd ed., pp. 482–497). St. Louis, MO: Saunders.

Kelly, M., & Sandora, T. (2016). Community acquired pneumonia. In R. Kliegman, B. Stanton, B., J. St. Geme, & N. Schor (Eds.), *Nelson's textbook of pediatrics* (20th ed., pp. 2088–2094). St. Louis, MO: Elsevier.

Khaleghi, T., Richardson, T., Hall, M., Streeter, S., & Carpenter, S. (2014). Increasing rates of pulmonary embolism: A retrospective analysis of pediatric tertiary care hospitals. *Blood, 124*(21), 204. Retrieved from http://www.bloodjournal.org/content/124/21/204

Kimberlin, D. W., Brady, M. T., Jackson, M. A., & Long, S. S. (Eds.). (2015). *Red book: 2015 report of the Committee on Infectious Diseases* (30th ed.). Elk Grove Village, IL: American Academy of Pediatrics.

Kirkby, S., & Hayes, D., Jr. (2014). Pediatric lung transplantation: Indications and outcomes. *Journal of Thoracic Disease, 6*(8), 1024–1031. doi:10.3978/j.issn.2072-1439.2014.04.27

Kost, S., & Roy, A. (2010). Procedural sedation and analgesia in the pediatric emergency department: A review of sedative pharmacology. *Clinical Pediatric Emergency Medicine, 11*(4), 233–243. doi:10.1016/j.cpem.2010.08.002

Kotloff, R. M., & Thabut, G. (2011). Lung transplantation. *American Journal of Respiratory and Critical Care Medicine, 184*(2), 159–171. doi:10.1164/rccm.201101-0134CI

Lahiri, T., Hempstead, S. E., Brady, C., Cannon, C. L., Clark, K., Condren, M. E., . . . Davis, S. D. (2016). Clinical practice guidelines from the Cystic Fibrosis Foundation for preschoolers with cystic fibrosis. *Pediatrics, 137*(4). doi:10.1542/peds.2015-1784

Lanken, P., Terry, P., DeLisser, H., Fahy, B., Hansen-Flaschen, J., Heffner, J., . . . Yankaskas, J. (2008). An official American Thoracic Society clinical policy statement: Palliative care for patients with respiratory diseases and critical illnesses. *American Journal of Respiratory and Critical Care Medicine, 177*(8), 912–927. doi:10.1164/rccm.200605-587ST

Lester, M., & Flume, P. (2009). Airway-clearance therapy guidelines and implementations. *Respiratory Care, 54*(6), 733–750. Retrieved from https://pdfs.semanticscholar.org/d81c/e8c9ffbb7e8228ecd5279440ec27d97f5e48.pdf

Lexicomp Online. (2016). Pediatric & neonatal Lexi-Drugs. Retrieved from http://webstore.lexi.com/Pediatric-Lexi-Drugs

Lopez, M., Cruz, A., Kowalkowski, M., & Raphael, J. (2014). Trends in hospitalizations and resource utilization for pediatric pertussis. *Hospital Pediatrics, 4*(5), 269–275. doi:10.1542/hpeds.2013-0093

Lynch, J., Sayah, D., Belperio, J., & Weigt, S. (2015). Lung transplantation for cystic fibrosis: Results, indications, complications, and controversies. *Seminars in Respiratory and Critical Care Medicine, 36*(2), 299–320. doi:10.1055/s-0035-1547347

Mansbach, J., Piedra, P., Teach, S., Sullivan, A., Forgey, T., Clark, S., . . . Camargo, C. A. (2012). Prospective multicenter study of viral etiology and hospital length of stay in children with severe bronchiolitis. *Archives of Pediatric and Adolescent Medicine, 166*(8), 700–706. doi:10.1001/archpediatrics.2011.1669

Matthay, M. (2014). Resolution of pulmonary edema. Thirty years of progress. *American Journal of Respiratory and Critical Care Medicine, 189*(11), 1301–1308. doi:10.1164/rccm.201403-0535OE

McCool, F., & Rosen, M. (2006). Nonpharmacologic airway clearance therapies: ACCP evidence-based clinical practice guidelines. *Chest, 129*(1 Suppl.), 250S–259S. doi:10.1378/chest.129.1_suppl.250S

Mehta, H., Kashyap, R., & Trivedi, S. (2014). Correlation of end tidal and arterial carbon dioxide levels in critically ill neonates and children. *Indian Journal of Critical Care Medicine, 18*(6), 348–353. doi:10.4103/0972-5229.133874

Mesman, G., Kuo, D., Carroll, J., & Ward, W. (2013). The impact of technology dependence on children and their families. *Journal of Pediatric Healthcare, 27*(6), 451–459. doi:10.1016/j.pedhc.2012.05.003

Michaels, L., Beckman, M., Thornburg, C., Marquez, K., Kulkarni, R., Pipe, S., . . . Manco-Johnson, M. (2009). The CDC Hemostasis and Thrombosis Centers (HTC) pilot sites: Data from the pediatric registry. *Blood, 114*(22), 2990. Retrieved from http://bloodjournal.org/content/114/22/2990

Miller, L. (2006). Chest wall, lung, and pleural space trauma. *Radiologic Clinics of North America, 44*(2), 213–224. doi:10.1016/j.rcl.2005.10.006

Moore, T., Hennessy, E. M., Myles, J., Johnson, S. J., Draper, E. S., Costeloe, K. L., & Marlow, N. (2012). Neurological and developmental outcome in extremely preterm children born in England in 1995 and 2006: The EPICure studies. *BMJ, 345,* e7961. doi:10.1136/bmj.e7961

Motti Eini, Z., Houri, S., Cohen, I., Sion, R., Tamir, A., Sasson, L., & Mandelberg, A. (2013). Massive pulmonary emboli in children does fiber-optic-guided embolectomy have a role? Review of the literature and report of two cases. *Chest, 143*(2), 544–549. doi:10.1378/chest.11-2759

Murthy, K., Dykes, F., Padula, M., Pallotto, E., Reber, K., Durand, D., . . . Evans, J. (2014). The Children's Hospitals neonatal database: An overview of patient complexity, outcomes and variation in care. *Journal of Perinatology, 34,* 582–586. doi:10.1038/jp.2014.26

National Capital Poison Center. (n.d.). Mechanism of battery-induced injury. Retrieved from http://www.poison.org/battery/mechanism-of-injury

National Heart, Lung, and Blood Institute, & National Asthma Education and Prevention Program. (2007). *Expert panel report 3: Guidelines for the diagnosis and management of asthma.* Bethesda, MD: U.S. Department of Health and Human Services National Institutes of Health. Retrieved from https://www.nhlbi.nih.gov/files/docs/guidelines/asthgdln.pdf

Neunhoeffer, F., Kumpf, M., Renk, H., Hanelt, M., Berneck, Bosk, A., . . . Hofbeck, M. (2015). Nurse-driven pediatric analgesia and sedation protocol reduces withdrawal symptoms in critically ill medical pediatric patients. *Pediatric Anesthesia, 25*(8), 786–794. doi:10.1111/pan.12649

Nevin, M. A. (2016). Pulmonary hemorrhage and hemoptysis. In R. Kliegman, B. Stanton, J. St. Geme, J., & N. Schor (Eds.), *Nelson's textbook of pediatrics* (20th ed., pp. 2123–2128). St. Louis, MO: Elsevier.

Newman, R., Hedican, E., Herigon, J., Williams, D., Williams, A., & Newland, J. (2012). Impact of a guideline on management of children hospitalized with community-acquired pneumonia. *Pediatrics, 129*(3), e597–e604. doi:10.1542/peds.2011-1533

Patocka, C., & Nemeth, J. (2012). Pulmonary embolism in pediatrics. *Journal of Emergency Medicine, 42*(1), 105–116. doi:10.1016/j.jemermed.2011.03.006

Pediatric Acute Lung Injury Consensus Conference Group. (2015). Pediatric acute respiratory distress syndrome: Consensus recommendations from the Pediatric Acute Lung Injury Consensus Conference. *Pediatric Critical Care Medicine, 16*(5), 428–439. doi:10.1097/PCC.0000000000000350

Perez-Velez, C. (2012). Pediatric tuberculosis: New guidelines and recommendations. *Current Opinion in Pediatrics, 24,* 319–328. doi:10.1097/MOP.0b013e32835357c3

Peterson-Carmichael, S., & Cheifetz, I. (2012). The chronically critically ill patient: Pediatric considerations. *Respiratory Care, 57*(6), 993–1003. doi: doi:10.4187/respcare.01738

Petrocheilou, A., Tanou, K., Kalampouka, E., Malakasioti, G., Giannios, C., & Kaditis, A. (2014). Viral croup: Diagnosis and a treatment algorithm. *Pediatric Pulmonology, 49,* 421–429. doi:10.1002/ppul.22993

Poindexter, B., Feng, R., Schmidt, B., Aschner, J., Ballard, R., Hamvas, A., . . . Jobe, A. (2015). Comparisons and limitations of current definitions of bronchopulmonary dysplasia for the Prematurity and Respiratory Outcomes Program. *Annals of the American Thoracic Society, 12*(12), 1822–1830. doi:10.1513/AnnalsATS.201504-218OC

Poindexter, B., & Martin, C. (2015). Impact of nutrition on bronchopulmonary dysplasia. *Clinics in Perinatology, 42*(4), 797–806. doi:10.1016/j.clp.2015.08.007

Ralston, S. L., Lieberthal, A. S., Meissner, H. C., Alverson, B. K., Baley, J. E., Gadomski, A. M., . . . Hernandez-Cancio, S. (2014). Clinical practice guideline: The diagnosis, management, and prevention of bronchiolitis. *Pediatrics, 134*(5), 1474–1502. doi:10.1542/peds.2014-2742

Redding, G. J. (2009). Bronchiectasis in children. *Pediatric Clinics of North America, 56*(1), 157–171. doi:10.1016/j.pcl.2008.10.014

Rodgers, B., & McGahren, E. (2010). Thoracic trauma in children. In B. Walsh, M. Czervinske, & R. DiBlasi (Eds.), *Perinatal and pediatric respiratory care* (3rd ed., pp. 674–691). St. Louis, MO: Saunders.

Schnapf, B., & Kirley, S. (2010). Fetal lung development. In B. Walsh, M. Czervinske, & R. DiBlasi (Eds.), *Perinatal and pediatric respiratory care* (3rd ed, pp. 1–11). St. Louis, MO: Saunders.

Schulzke, S. M., & Pillow, J. J. (2010). The management of evolving bronchopulmonary dysplasia. *Paediatric Respiratory Reviews, 11*(3), 143–148. doi:10.1016/j.prrv.2009.12.005

Simonneau, G., Gatzoulis, M., Adatia, I., Celermajer, D., Denton, C., Ghofrani, A., . . . Souza, R. (2013). Updated clinical classification of pulmonary hypertension. *Journal of the American College of Cardiology, 62*(25 Suppl.), D34–D41. doi:10.1016/j.jacc.2013.10.029

Singh, H., & Parakh, A. (2014). Tracheobronchial foreign body aspiration in children. *Clinical Pediatrics, 53*(5), 415–419. doi:10.1177/0009922813506259

Spahn, J., & Szefler, S. (2008). Pharmacology of the lung and drug therapy. In L. Taussig (Ed.), *Pediatric respiratory medicine* (2nd ed., pp. 219–233). St. Louis, MO: Mosby.

Sterni, L., Collaco, J., Baker, C., Carroll, J., Sharma, G., Brozek, J., . . . Halbower, A. C. (2016). An official American Thoracic Society clinical practice guideline: Pediatric chronic home invasive ventilation. *American Journal of Respiratory and Critical Care Medicine, 193*(8), e16–e35. doi:10.1164/rccm.201602-0276ST

Stoll, B. J., Hansen, N. I., Bell, E. F., Shankaran, S., Laptook, A. R., Walsh, M. C., . . . Higgins, R. D. (2010). Neonatal outcomes of extremely preterm infants from the NICHD Neonatal Research Network. *Pediatrics, 126*(3), 443–456. doi:10.1542/peds.2009-2959

Strickland, S. (2015). Year in review 2014: Airway clearance. *Respiratory Care, 60*(4), 603–605. doi:10.4187/respcare.04095

Strickland, S., Rubin, B., Drescher, G., Haas, C., O'Malley, C. A., Volsko, T. A., . . . Hess, D. R. (2013). AARC clinical practice guideline: Effectiveness of nonpharmacologic airway clearance therapies in hospitalized patients. *Respiratory Care, 58*(12), 2187–2193. doi:10.4187/respcare.02925

Swaminathan, S., & Rekha, B. (2010). Pediatric tuberculosis: Global overview and challenges. *Clinical Infectious Diseases, 50*(Suppl. 3), S184–S194. doi:10.1086/651490

Tan, H., Gozal, D., & Kheirandish-Gozal, L. (2013). Obstructive sleep apnea in children: A critical update. *Nature and Science of Sleep, 5,* 109–123. doi:10.2147/NSS.S51907

Teshome, G., Gattu, R., & Brown, R. (2013). Acute bronchiolitis. *Pediatric Clinics of North America, 60*(5), 1019–1034. doi:10.1016/j.pcl.2013.06.005

Toon, M., Maybauer, M., Greenwood, J., Maybauer, D., & Fraser, J. (2010). Management of acute smoke inhalation injury. *Critical Care and Resuscitation, 12*(1), 53–61. Retrieved from https://www.cicm.org.au/CICM_Media/CICMSite/CICM-Website/Resources/Publications/CCR%20Journal/

Previous%20Editions/March%202010/11_2010_Mar_Rev-Management-of-acute.pdf

Tovar, J. (2008). The lung and pediatric trauma. *Seminars in Pediatric Surgery, 17*(1), 53–59. doi:10.1053/j.sempedsurg.2007.10.008

Walker, P., Buehner, M., Wood, L., Boyer, N., Driscoll, I., Lundy, J., . . . Chung, K. (2015), Diagnosis and management of inhalation injury: An updated review. *Critical Care, 19*, 351. doi:10.1186/s13054-015-1077-4

Walsh, B., & Vehse, N. (2010). Pediatric airway disorders and parenchymal lung diseases. In B. Walsh, M. Czervinske, & R. DiBlasi (Eds.), *Perinatal and pediatric respiratory care* (3rd ed., pp. 554–581). St. Louis, MO: Saunders.

Weill, D., Benden, C., Corris, P. A., Dark, J. H., Davis, R. D., Keshavjee, S., . . . Glanville, A. (2015). A consensus document for the selection of lung transplant candidates: 2014—An update from the Pulmonary Transplantation Council of the International Society for Heart and Lung Transplantation. *Journal of Heart and Lung Transplantation, 34*(1), 1–15. doi:10.1016/j.healun.2014.06.014

Weiner, D., Halfaer, M., & Allen, J. (2008). Respiratory effects of anesthesia and sedation. In L. Taussig (Ed.), *Pediatric respiratory medicine* (2nd ed., pp. 347–357). St. Louis, MO: Mosby.

West, J. (2012). *Respiratory physiology the essentials* (9th ed.). Baltimore, MD: Lippincott Williams & Wilkins.

Wickerson, L., Rozenberg, D., Janaudis-Ferreira, T., Deliva, R., Lo, V., Beauchamp, G., . . . Mathur, S. (2016). Physical rehabilitation for lung transplant candidates and recipients: An evidence-informed clinical approach. *World Journal of Transplant, 6*(3), 517–531. doi:10.5500/wjt.v6.i3.517

3 CARDIOVASCULAR SYSTEM

Louise Callow and Alissa Scheffer

DEVELOPMENTAL ANATOMY AND PHYSIOLOGY

A. Embryologic Development of the Heart

1. *Formation of the Heart Tube.* Days 15 to 23 (Table 3.1)

2. *Formation of the Heart Loop.* Days 23 to 28 (Figure 3.1)

    a. Structure of the cardiac wall in the fully developed heart

        i. The pericardium

        ii. The epicardium

        iii. The myocardium

        iv. The endocardium

        v. Papillary muscles and chordae tendineae

3. *Formation of Embryonic Ventricles.* Days 22 to 35 (Figure 3.2)

4. *Formation of Cardiac Septa.* Days 27 to 45

    a. Chambers of the fully developed heart

        i. The atria

        ii. The ventricles

5. *Division of the Truncus Arteriosus (TA).* Days 32 to 33

6. *Formation of Cardiac Valves.* Days 34 to 36

    a. Cardiac valves in the fully developed heart (Figure 3.3)

        i. Atrioventricular (AV) valves

        ii. Semilunar valves

7. *Formation of the Great Veins.* Weeks 4 to 7

B. Genetic Signals to Embryonic Development

1. As more is learned about the human genome, gene control of cardiac embryonic events continues to unfold and is constantly changing, with much more yet to be learned. Genetic control of heart development includes a cascade of signaling molecules that trigger myocardial transcription factors. The transcription factors cause cardiac-specific proteins to be formed. These proteins regulate the growth of muscle types and looping effector genes, resulting in the formation of the normal heart (Pierpont et al., 2007).

2. *Key signaling molecules* include bone morphogenic proteins (BMPs) and fibroblast growth factors (FGFs). BMPs control cell division, cell death, cell migration, and differentiation. FGF signals proteins that cause angiogenesis (blood vessel formation).

3. *Key transcription factors* include the following:

    a. NKX2-5 transcription factor, which is cardiac specific, is expressed throughout the heart from the earliest stages and controls differentiation from embryo to cardioblast.

    b. Endothelin 1 and other factors, which differentiate cardioblasts into Purkinje-type cells.

    c. Myocyte-enhancing transcription factor 2 (MEF2) and GATA transcription factors, which cause the cardioblasts to form into the heart tube.

4. *Cardiac-specific proteins* that result from transcription factor production control the development of the cardiac chambers.

    a. Ventricular differentiation is controlled by the MEF2C and Irx4 genes.

    b. Formation of the valves is controlled by Smad-6 and NF-ATC transcription factors, calcineurin, and transforming growth factor β (TGF-β).

    c. Ventricular differences (right from left) are controlled by d-Hand for the right and NKX2-5 stimulation of e-Hand for the left ventricle (LV).

    d. Ufd1 activates d-Hand and Neuropilin 1 activates migration of neural crest cells to form the conotruncus, aorta, and aortic arch.

    e. PAX 3 gene signals growth of the aortic outflow tract; Forkhead transcription factor Mfh 1 signals growth of the transverse arch. Gridlock gene signals growth in the area of the coarctation, and FAP2b signals development of the area of the ductus arteriosus.

TABLE 3.1 Embryological Development

Developmental Event	Gestation	Embryogenesis
Formation of the heart tube	Days 15–23	Endothelial tubes fuse to the endocardial tube, and the heart begins to beat from a focus in the sinus venosus.
Formation of the heart loop	Days 23–28	The initial straight tube now loops. Looping determines the sidedness of the heart and the correct relationship of the heart segments to each other.
Formation of embryonic ventricles	Days 23–35	The region of the tube proximal to the fold becomes the embryonic ventricle.
Formation of cardiac septa	Days 27–45	The medial walls of the expanding ventricles fuse, forming the major portion of the ventricular septum; an extension of the endocardial cushions and the truncal conus create the membranous septum. Atrial septation and connection of the common pulmonary vein to the left atrium are closely related during atrial septation.
Division of the truncus arteriosus	Days 32–33	Outflow tracts divide by fusion of the conotruncal cushions and spiraling follows the course of cushion development.
Formation of the cardiac valves	Days 34–36	The mitral valve and tricuspid valve form from endocardial cushions, and the tricuspid valve also forms from the conus septum. The semilunar valves form at the interface of truncal cushions and aorticopulmonary septum.
Formation of the great veins	Weeks 4–7	Three primitive systems, the vitelline, the umbilical, and the cardinal venous systems, form the venous pattern through the process of vasculogenesis.

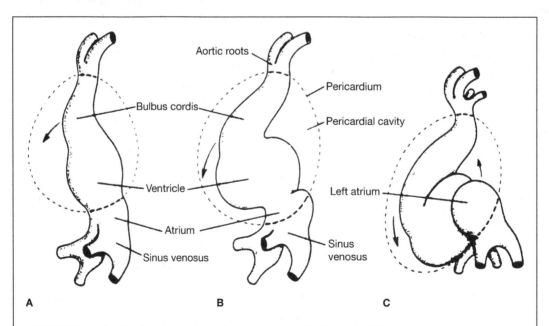

FIGURE 3.1   Cardiac looping to the right as seen from the left side. (A) At 8 somites, (B) at 11 somites, and (C) at 16 somites. Dashed line indicates the parietal pericardium. The atrium gradually assumes an intrapericardial position.

Source: Reprinted with permission from Adams, F. H., Emmanoulides, G. C., & Riemenschneider, T. A. (2016). *Moss' heart disease in infants, children, and adolescents* (9th ed.). Philadelphia, PA: Elsevier.

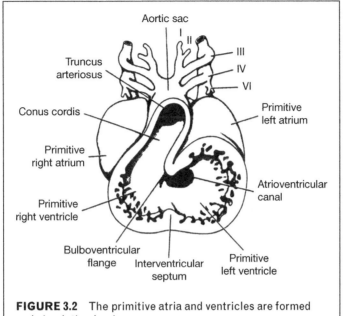

FIGURE 3.2 The primitive atria and ventricles are formed and circulation begins.

Source: Reprinted with permission from Adams, F. H., Emmanoulides, G. C., & Riemenschneider, T. A. (2016). *Moss' heart disease in infants, children, and adolescents* (9th ed.). Philadelphia, PA: Elsevier.

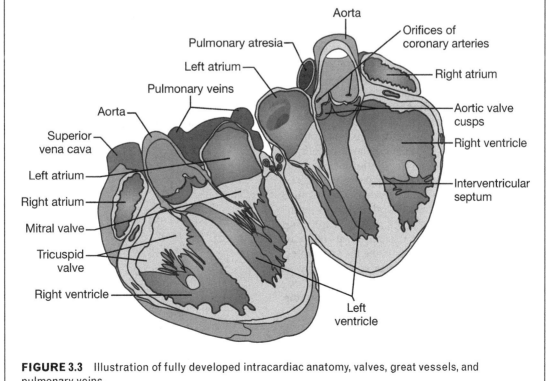

FIGURE 3.3 Illustration of fully developed intracardiac anatomy, valves, great vessels, and pulmonary veins.

C. Systemic Vasculature in the Fully Developed Heart

1. *Systemic vessels* supply tissues with oxygen and nutrients and remove metabolic wastes. The diameter of the vessels (especially the arterioles) and viscosity of the blood create systemic vascular resistance (SVR). Tissue perfusion is controlled via local chemical reactions and nerves that dilate or constrict blood vessels.

2. *Major Components of the Systemic Vasculature*

a. An artery is a high-pressure circuit composed of strong, compliant, elastic-walled vessels carrying blood from the heart to the capillary beds. Elastic fibers within the arterial wall enable the wall to stretch during systole and recoil during diastole.

b. Arterioles are the major vessels controlling SVR and arterial pressure. Arterioles are controlled by the autonomic nervous system and by autoregulation. They contain smooth muscle innervated by sympathetic α-adrenergic nerve fibers. Stimulation causes constriction of the vessels; decreased adrenergic discharge dilates the vessels controlling blood distribution to various capillary beds. Arterioles may give rise to metarterioles (precapillaries) or give rise directly to capillaries, where flow is regulated through constriction or dilation.

c. The capillary system allows the exchange of oxygen and carbon dioxide and solutes between blood and tissues and permits fluid volume transfer between plasma and the interstitium. Capillary filtration is related to hydrostatic and osmotic pressures across membranes. Increased hydrostatic pressure leads to movement of fluid from vessel to interstitium via osmosis. Greater capillary osmotic pressure leads to fluid movement from interstitium into vessels. Capillaries lack smooth muscle. Diameter changes are passive because of precapillary and postcapillary resistance. Because of their narrow lumens, capillaries can withstand high internal pressures without rupturing. Laplace's law states that the tension in the wall of the vessel necessary to balance the distending pressure is lessened as the radius of the blood vessel decreases. Diffusion is the most important process in moving substrates and wastes between the blood and tissues via the capillary system.

d. The venous system stores approximately 65% of the total volume of blood in the circulatory system. Venules receive blood from capillaries and serve as collecting channels and capacitance (storage) vessels. Veins are capacitance vessels that conduct blood to the heart within a low-pressure system surrounded by skeletal muscles. When muscles contract, they compress veins, moving blood toward the heart. Valves in veins prevent retrograde blood flow. Under normal conditions, the venous pump keeps the venous pressure in the lower extremities at 25 mmHg or less. Gravity has profound effects on the erect, mobile individual. Pressure can rise to 90 mmHg in the lower extremities, which results in swelling and a decrease in blood volume because of leakage of fluid from the circulatory system into the interstitium.

3. *Coronary Vasculature in the Fully Developed Heart* (Figure 3.4)

a. Arteries branch off the base of the aorta, supplying blood to the conduction system and myocardium.

b. The right coronary artery (RCA) supplies the sinoatrial (SA) node (55% of hearts), the AV node (90% of hearts), the right atrium (RA), right ventricle (RV) muscles, and the inferoposterior wall of the LV. Eighty percent of the time, a branch of the RCA called the *posterior descending artery* is the terminal portion of the RCA, resulting in a right dominant coronary system. Located in the posterior interventricular groove, it supplies the RV, LV, and the posterior part of the interventricular septum. The RCA gives off a posterior lateral branch that descends from the lateral side of the heart to the apex. It supplies the anteroposterior surface of the RV.

c. The left coronary artery (LCA) branches into the left anterior descending artery (LAD), which supplies the anterior part of the interventricular septum, the anterior wall of the LV, the right bundle branch (RBB), and the anterosuperior division of the left bundle branch (LBB).

d. The circumflex artery, also branching off from the LCA (into major branches of the circumflex artery and one or more obtuse marginal branches, supplies the AV node (10% of hearts), the SA node (45% of hearts), and the posterior surface of the LV via the obtuse marginal branches.

e. Veins return desaturated blood to the heart. They consist of the great cardiac veins, the small cardiac veins (both drain into the coronary sinus, which drains into the RA), and the thebesian vessels (which drain blood into the RA through the atrial wall; Hazinski, 2013).

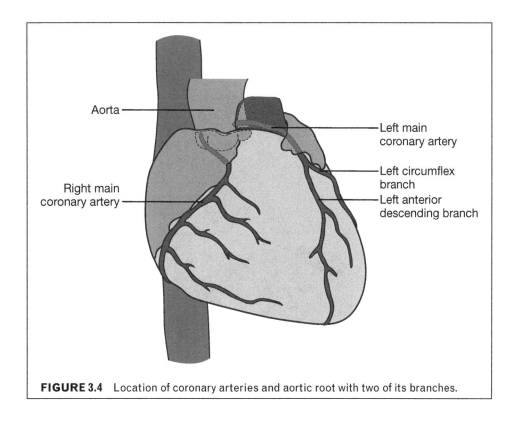

FIGURE 3.4 Location of coronary arteries and aortic root with two of its branches.

D. Embryonic, Neonatal, and Pediatric Cardiovascular Physiology

1. *Fetal Circulation* (Figure 3.5)

   a. Gas exchange occurs in the placenta.

   b. Umbilical venous blood (the most highly saturated) returns via the umbilical vein from the placenta and accounts for 42% of fetal cardiac output (CO). From the umbilical vein, about half the fetal blood flows through the ductus venosus to the inferior vena cava (IVC) and the other half enters the hepatic portal system.

   c. There is a preferential flow of more highly saturated blood through the foramen ovale into the left atrium (LA) and LV to the ascending aorta and to the brain and myocardium.

   d. The superior vena cava (SVC) flow is directed to the tricuspid valve and the RV, along with coronary sinus blood. Blood flows from the RV to the pulmonary trunk, and about 8% of RV output perfuses the pulmonary artery (PA). The rest of the RV output flows through the ductus arteriosus to the aorta. Parallel circulation

exists in the fetus: the RV pressure equals the LV pressure.

   e. Vascular pressure reflects streaming with RA pressure greater than the LA pressure, PA pressure greater than the aortic pressure, and the umbilical vein pressure higher than that of the IVC.

   f. The fetal myocardium is less compliant because of the lower ratio of contractile to noncontractile fibers (30% in fetus; 60% in adult).

2. *Transitional Circulation*

   a. Interruption of the umbilical cord creates increased SVR and decreased IVC return to the heart. The primary change in circulation after birth is a shift from gas exchange in the placenta to gas exchange in the lungs.

   b. Peripheral vascular resistance (PVR) rapidly decreases in the first 12 to 24 hours of life, and pulmonary blood flow increases. The reduction to normal PVR occurs slowly over 14 to 21 days. This process may be delayed in preterm infants.

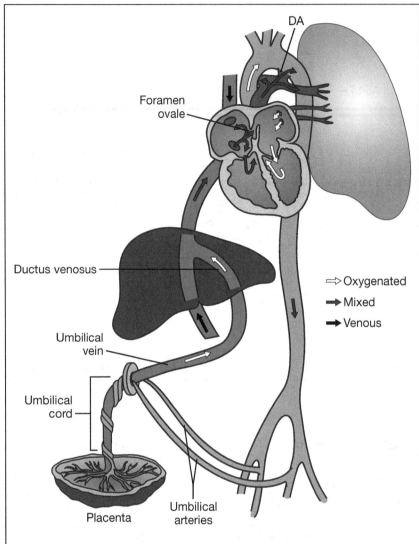

FIGURE 3.5 Fetal circulation with oxygenated placental blood entering umbilical veins, shunting through the ductus venosus, and entering the right side of the heart. Mixed venous blood shunts through the foramen ovale and ductus arteriosus, eventually returning to the aorta and placenta via the umbilical artery.

DA, ductus arteriosus.

c. The ductus arteriosus constricts primarily in response to increased arterial PO_2 and is influenced by the loss of placental prostaglandin. The ductus arteriosus in the mature infant is functionally closed 12 to 24 hours after birth, but closure can be reversed with prostaglandin E1 (PGE1). Anatomic closure from fibrosis usually occurs within 2 weeks. The RV ejects all blood into the pulmonary circulation when the ductus arteriosus closes and the PVR decreases. The foramen ovale closes as a result of increased LA pressure from increased pulmonary venous blood return. The ductus venosus closes soon after birth.

d. Rapid loss of the low resistance placental circuit increases the SVR and LV pressure, and LV and RV outputs equalize.

3. *Neonatal and Pediatric Circulation* (Figure 3.6)

   a. The neonatal myocardium functions at near maximum CO. There is a relatively fixed stroke volume (SV) in the first weeks of life. The larger ratio of noncontractile to contractile muscle fibers disappears after about 1 week.

   b. The neonatal myocardium responds to stress by a combination of hyperplasia and hypertrophy. Increased heart rate (HR) produces little change in CO because of a high resting HR in the neonate and newborn. However, because the neonatal myocardium operates high on its CO curve and SV is limited, the CO can be increased by increasing HR more than by increasing contractility. Increased afterload will result in a drop in CO. The neonatal myocardium is extremely sensitive to increases in afterload.

4. *Peripheral Blood Vessel Physiology*

   a. The local mechanism for tissues to control their own blood flow is known as *autoregulation*. Two major hypotheses exist:

      i. Myogenic response hypothesis. As pressure rises, vessels stretch, stimulating the contraction of smooth muscles (feedback mechanism). As pressure decreases, smooth muscles relax.

      ii. Metabolic hypothesis. Because of the normal metabolic activity of the tissues, carbon dioxide, potassium, lactate, prostaglandins, and phosphates accumulate and cause vasodilation, which increases the blood flow to the area of activity to flush these waste products away.

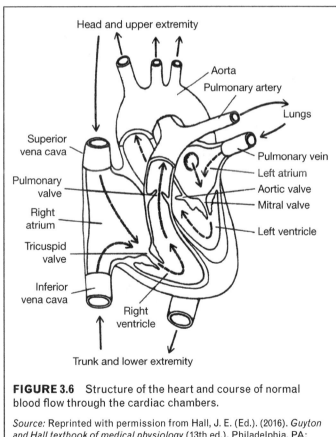

FIGURE 3.6 Structure of the heart and course of normal blood flow through the cardiac chambers.

Source: Reprinted with permission from Hall, J. E. (Ed.). (2016). *Guyton and Hall textbook of medical physiology* (13th ed.). Philadelphia, PA: Elsevier.

b. There is a delicate balance between the two mechanisms involved in the myogenic response: Myogenic response → vasoconstriction → decrease in blood supply → local increase in metabolites → vasodilation → wastes removed.

c. Autonomic regulation of vessels

  i. Sympathetic nervous system fibers secrete norepinephrine at nerve endings, producing vasoconstriction. In arterioles, this mechanism helps regulate blood flow and arterial pressure. In veins, this mechanism helps to vary the amount of blood stored. Venoconstriction causes an increase in venous return to the heart.

  ii. Parasympathetic nervous system fibers secrete acetylcholine at nerve endings (cholinergic effect), producing vasodilation (Figures 3.7 and 3.8).

d. Stretch receptors. Baroreceptors (pressoreceptors)

  i. Receptor sites are located in the aortic arch, carotid sinus, venae cavae, pulmonary arteries, and atria. Sensitive to arterial pressures, the receptor sites are activated by elevated blood pressure (BP) or increased blood volume, resulting in stretching of the arterial walls. The impulse is transmitted from the aortic arch and the carotid sinus to the medulla. Sympathetic action is inhibited and the vagal reflex dominates, resulting in decreased HR and contractility, dilation of the systemic vasculature, and normalized BP.

  ii. In response to decreased BP, the vagal tone decreases and the sympathetic system becomes dominant, resulting in increased HR and contractility and arterial and venous constriction and BP elevation to near normal.

e. The vasomotor center in the medulla (also called *cardioaccelerator center* or *cardiac center*) consists of the vasoconstrictor and vasodepressor areas.

  i. Stimulation of the vasoconstrictor area causes increased HR, SV, and CO and, ultimately, increased arterial BP. Venoconstriction, which decreases stores of blood in the venous system, increases venous return and increases SV.

  ii. Inhibition of the vasoconstrictor area stimulates the vasodepressor area, which causes vasodilation. An increase in storage of blood in the venous capacitance system occurs, thereby decreasing SV, CO, and arterial BP.

  iii. The vasomotor center works with stretch receptors and chemoreceptors located in the carotid sinus and aortic arch. A rise in BP stimulates the carotid sinus, which inhibits the vasoconstrictor area. This induces vasodilation via stimulation of the vasodepressor area. A fall in oxygen saturation, a rise in carbon dioxide, or a fall in pH stimulates chemoreceptors, which then stimulate the vasoconstrictor center and cause a rise in arterial BP (Hazinski, 2013).

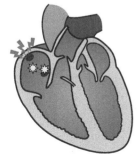

Sympathetic system activates cardiac β₁ adrenergic receptors

Cardiac Excitatory Effects

↑ rate of SA node pacing
↑ rate of conduction
↑ force of contraction
↑ irritibility of foci

FIGURE 3.7 The sympathetic system activates cardiac β₁ adrenergic receptors.

SA, sinoatrial.

Parasympathetic system activates cholinergic receptors

Vagus nerve

Cardiac Inhibitory Effects

↓ rate of SA node pacing
↓ rate of conduction
↓ force of contraction
↓ irritibility of atrial and junctional foci

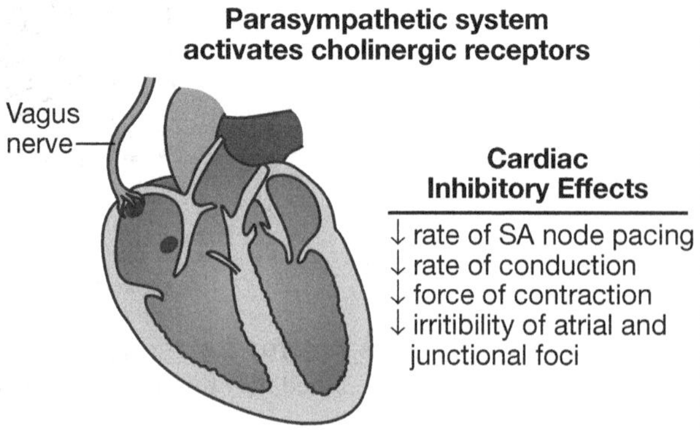

FIGURE 3.8 The parasympathetic system activates cholinergic receptors.

SA, sinoatrial.

E. Neurohormonal Control of the Fully Developed Heart

1. *Autonomic Nervous System*

   a. Sympathetic stimulation initiates the release of norepinephrine. Stimulation of α-adrenergic fiber results in arteriolar vasoconstriction. Stimulation of β-adrenergic (β_1) fiber increases SA node discharge, thereby increasing the HR (positive chronotropy); increasing the force of myocardial contraction (positive inotropy); and accelerating AV conduction time (positive dromotropism).

   b. Parasympathetic stimulation initiates the release of acetylcholine, which stimulates the action of the right vagus nerve (affecting the SA node) and the left vagus nerve (affecting AV nodal conduction tissue). The rate of SA node discharge is decreased and slows the HR (negative chronotropy). It may slow conduction through AV tissue (negative dromotropism).

2. *Natriuretic peptides* are produced by the atria, ventricles, and brain and act as regulators of extravascular fluid volume and BP through control of sodium and water by countering the effects of the renin–angiotensin–aldosterone system.

   a. Atrial natriuretic peptide (ANP) is produced by the atria in response to atrial-wall tension from increased intravascular volume. Levels in the blood vary significantly with changes in position, exercise, and pacing. ANP reduces sympathetic tone, increases venous capacitance, and shifts intravascular fluid to the extravascular space by increased vascular endothelial permeability. A natural diuresis reduces the extravascular volume by directly affecting the renin–angiotensin–aldosterone receptors in the kidney. ANP reduces peripheral vascular resistance and lowers BP. It lowers the activation of vagal blockers, thus suppressing the reflex tachycardia and vasoconstriction that goes with reduced preload (Colucci & Chen, 2017).

   b. Brain natriuretic peptide (BNP) is produced by the ventricles in response to ventricular wall tension and volume expansion. Its effects are similar to those of ANP, producing natriuresis, diuresis, and vasodilation and counteracting the effects of the renin–angiotensin–aldosterone system. BNP also appears to prevent myocardial fibrosis, vascular smooth muscle cell proliferation, and thrombosis. BNP levels in blood are more stable than ANP levels. Both ANP and BNP levels rise rapidly after birth in response to increased LV volume and pressure during transition to extrauterine life. Then levels drop to normal within 2 weeks of life. Gender-related differences are noted after puberty (greater in females). Elevations in BNP are seen in volume overload and ventricular dilation.

   c. C-type natriuretic peptide is produced mostly by the central nervous system (CNS), kidneys, and vascular endothelial cells.

3. *Chemoreceptors* are located in the carotid and aortic bodies and are sensitive to changes in PO_2, PCO_2, and pH. They affect HR and respiratory rate via stimulation of the vasomotor center in the medulla.

4. *Stretch receptors* respond to pressure and volume changes. Stretch receptors located in the atria, large veins, and PA produce the Bainbridge reflex. An increase in venous return stretches the receptors. Afferent nerve impulses transmit to the vasomotor center in the medulla. The medulla increases efferent impulses, increasing HR and CO, and enabling the heart to pump out all the blood returned to it.

5. *During the respiratory reflex* inspiration decreases intrathoracic pressure, increasing venous return to the heart. Inspiration stimulates stretch receptors in the lungs and thorax. Impulses from the stretch receptors inhibit the vasomotor center in the medulla. This inhibition decreases vagal tone, causing an increase in the HR, which allows the heart to pump out the extra blood. This reflex results in "sinus arrhythmia," which may occur in a normal heart.

F. Variables That Affect CO

1. *Cardiac Output* $= SV \times HR$. The cardiac index can be used in children because of the potential variation in CO by body size. Cardiac index is equal to CO divided by body surface area (BSA). CO is the amount of blood being pumped by the heart to the tissues and is measured in liters per minute.

2. *SV* is the amount of ventricular volume pumped during systole. SV is affected by preload, afterload, and contractility. The ejection fraction (the volume ejected vs. volume remaining in the ventricle at the end of systole) is calculated by dividing the SV by the end-diastolic volume and is expressed as a percentage.

3. *Preload* is the resting force in the myocardium, which is determined by the volume in the ventricles at the end of diastole (left ventricular end-diastolic volume [LVEDV] reflected by left ventricular end-diastolic pressure (LVEDP). Preload can be related to such variables as the volume of blood returned from veins, stretch, and fiber length. An increase in

preload stretches myocardial muscle fibers, causing more forceful subsequent ventricular contractions, increasing SV and CO. An increase in preload is accomplished by increasing the blood volume returning to the ventricles (Figure 3.9). The Frank–Starling law states that there is a direct relationship between the volume of blood in the heart at the end of diastole and the force of contraction during the next systole. The preload or ventricular filling pressure reflects the initial sarcomere length, which influences the development of myocardial force. Muscle fibers may reach a point of stretch beyond which contraction is no longer enhanced and SV decreases. Increased preload may be related to mitral insufficiency, aortic insufficiency, ventricular septal defect (VSD), atrial septal defect (ASD), patent ductus arteriosus (PDA), fluid overload, and vasoconstrictors.

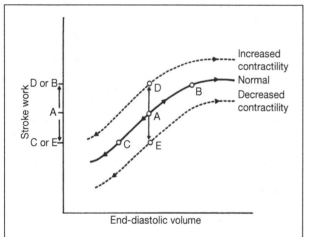

FIGURE 3.9 The work of the heart varies with changing end-diastolic volume according to the Frank–Starling relationship. The work of the heart can also be varied by changes in contractility. The solid curve (CAB) describes normal myocardial contractility, and point A represents the basal state. Changes in cardiac work that result from alterations in venous return shift the work of the heart along this normal curve. Cardiac work can be increased from A to B by enhanced venous return and decreased from A to C by a reduction in venous return. The work of the heart can also be changed by modifications in myocardial contractility. A positive inotropic agent can increase cardiac work from A to D, even with constant end-diastolic volume. Cardiac work can be decreased from A to E by a negative inotropic agent without change in end-diastolic volume.

Source: Reprinted with permission from Katz, A. M. (2011). *Physiology of the heart* (5th ed.). Philadelphia, PA: Lippincott Williams & Wilkins.

Decreased preload may be related to mitral stenosis (MS), hypovolemia, and vasodilators (Hall, 2016).

4. *Afterload* is the initial resistance that must be overcome by the ventricles to open the semilunar valves and propel blood into the systemic and pulmonary circulatory systems (Hall, 2016).

   a. Afterload is clinically measured as SVR and peripheral vascular resistance (PVR).

   b. SVR = mean arterial pressure (MAP) – central venous pressure (CVP)/systemic blood flow.

   c. Systemic blood flow is a value measured in resistance units. The resistance units times 80 converts resistance units into dynes per second per square centimeter.

   d. Normal SVR = 900 – 1,400 dynes/sec/cm^2

   e. Factors that increase afterload include fixed anatomic obstructions, peripheral arterial vasoconstriction, systemic hypertension, pulmonary hypertension, polycythemia, and vasoconstrictors. Excessive afterload increases LV or RV stroke work, increases myocardial oxygen demand/consumption, and may result in LV or RV failure.

   f. Factors that decrease ventricular afterload include vasodilators and sepsis. This will decrease RV or LV stroke work, potentially decrease myocardial oxygen demand/consumption and thereby improve LV or RV function.

5. *Contractility* is the strength and efficiency of contraction (force generated). Positive inotropic drugs, sympathetic stimulation, and hypercalcemia can act to increase the contractile state of the myocardium. Factors that can decrease contractility of the myocardium include negative inotropic drugs, hypoxia, hypercapnia, intrinsic depression attributable in part to long-standing congestive heart failure (CHF), parasympathetic stimulation, metabolic acidosis, hypocalcemia, hypoglycemia, hypomagnesemia, hyponatremia, hyperkalemia, the condition of the myocardium, and intrinsic myocardial disease (Hall, 2016).

6. *HR and rhythm* can alter CO with excessively high or low HRs. Tachycardia will decrease filling time of the ventricle-limiting CO and coronary perfusion. Bradycardia effects CO through the decreased ability to meet oxygen delivery due to reduced supply from lower HRs (Figure 3.10). Some arrhythmias, primarily heart block, and junctional rhythms decrease synchrony between atrial and ventricular contraction altering adequate emptying and/or filling of the atria or ventricle and can affect CO (Hall, 2016; Hazinski, 2013).

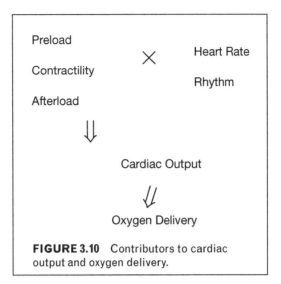

Preload

Contractility

Afterload

× Heart Rate

Rhythm

⇓

Cardiac Output

⇓

Oxygen Delivery

FIGURE 3.10 Contributors to cardiac output and oxygen delivery.

G. Arterial Pressure

Factors that can affect arterial *BP* include CO, HR, SVR, arterial elasticity, blood volume, blood viscosity, age, BSA, exercise, and anxiety.

1. Pulse pressure is a function of SV and arterial capacitance. This difference between systolic and diastolic BP is expressed in millimeters of mercury ($P_s - P_d$).

2. MAP is the average pressure in the aorta based on the volume of blood in the arterial system and the elastic properties of the arterial walls. It is calculated by MAP = systolic BP + (2 × diastolic BP)/3.

3. Regulation of arterial pressure is also under the control of the renin–angiotensin–aldosterone system and involves renin, a protease secreted by the kidney that converts angiotensin I to angiotensin II. Release of renin from the kidney is stimulated by stretch receptors in juxtaglomerular cells that are sensitive to changes in BP. Decreased BP, a rise in sympathetic output, or a fall in sodium concentration results in increased renin secretion. Increased BP results in decreased renin secretion. Angiotensin II is the most potent vasoconstrictor known, producing arteriolar constriction and an increase in systolic and diastolic pressures.

4. Other mechanisms include capillary fluid shift mechanisms, local control mechanisms, and the renal-fluid volume process. With a rise in arterial pressure, the kidneys excrete more fluid, causing a reduction in extracellular fluid and blood volume; this reduces circulating blood volume and potentially CO, leading to normalization of arterial pressure. With a fall in arterial pressure, the kidneys retain fluid, causing increased intravascular volume and, it is hoped, increased CO, which may result in normalization of arterial pressure.

ANATOMY OF THE CARDIAC CONDUCTION SYSTEM

A. SA Node (Figure 3.11)

The SA node is the pacemaker of the heart because it possesses the fastest rate of automaticity (spontaneous generation of impulses).

B. Internodal Atrial Pathways

Internodal atrial pathways, which consist of the anterior tract (Bachmann's), middle tract (Wenckebach's), and posterior tract (Thorel's), conduct impulses from the SA node through the RA to the AV node.

C. Bachmann's Bundle

Bachmann's bundle conducts impulses from the SA node to the LA.

D. AV Node

The AV node (AV junction) delays impulse transmission between atria and ventricles, allowing time for ventricular filling following atrial contraction and before ventricular systole. The AV node controls the number of

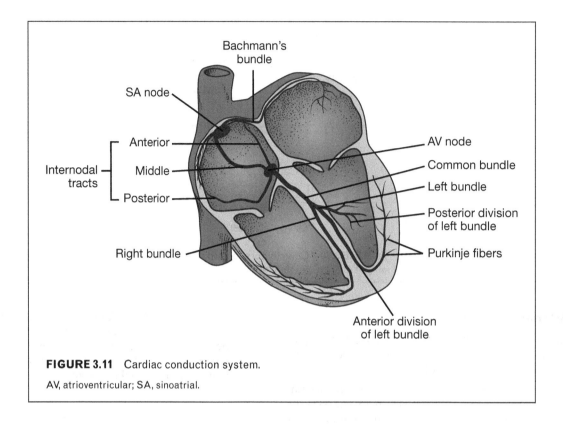

FIGURE 3.11   Cardiac conduction system.

AV, atrioventricular; SA, sinoatrial.

impulses (if the atrial rate becomes excessive) reaching the ventricles, thereby having some control over HR.

E. Bundle of His

The bundle of His is composed of thick fibers arising from the AV node that travel over the crest of the ventricular septum on its right side to the bundle-branch system.

F. Bundle-Branch System

The bundle-branch system is composed of pathways that arise from the bundle of His. The RBB is a direct continuation of the bundle of His that transmits impulses down the right side of the interventricular septum toward the RV myocardium. The bundle divides into three parts (anterior, lateral, and posterior), dividing further to become parts of the Purkinje system. The LBB separates into the left posterior fascicle (which transmits impulses over the posterior and inferior endocardial surfaces of the LV) and the left anterior fascicle (which transmits impulses to the anterior and superior endocardial surfaces of the LV).

G. Purkinje System

The Purkinje system arises from the distal portion of the bundle branches and transmits impulses into the subendocardial layers of both ventricles. It provides for depolarization (from endocardium to epicardium) followed by ventricular contraction and ejection of blood from the ventricles.

ELECTROPHYSIOLOGY

A. Properties of the Myocardial Conduction System

   1. *Automaticity* is the ability to generate impulses spontaneously. The cardiac muscle is the only muscle in the body with this property.

   2. *Rhythmicity* is the regularity of impulse generation. These impulses should follow the normal conduction system previously outlined.

   3. *Conductivity* is the ability to transmit impulses. This is assuming the conduction system of the heart remains intact and is not blocked or altered by medication, trauma, hypoxia, or congenital disease processes.

4. *Excitability* is the ability to respond to stimulation. This includes both the parasympathetic and sympathetic nervous system simulation.

B. Excitation–Contractile Process of Cardiac Muscle

1. The sodium and unbound calcium ion concentrations are greater outside the cell, and the potassium ion concentration is greater inside the cell. The resting membrane potential (RMP) for myocardial muscle fibers is –80 to –90 mV.

2. Depolarization can result from chemical, electrical, or mechanical stimulation. The stimulus reduces the RMP to a less negative value (depolarization). The threshold potential is the voltage level, where an action potential (AP) is produced. For all cardiac tissue except the SA and AV nodes, the threshold potential is –60 to –70 mV. For the SA and AV nodes, the threshold potential is –30 to –40 mV. Reaching the threshold causes changes in the membrane. The permeability of the cell membrane is altered, opening specialized channels in the membrane, which permits the passage of sodium and calcium ions into the cell. The AP is the graphic representation of this change (Figure 3.12).

3. The AP produced during depolarization is transmitted to the interior of the cell via T tubules, which transmit the AP to all myofibrils. Calcium is stored in the lateral sacs of the sarcoplasmic reticulum and is released during the AP. Calcium enters the interior of the cell, causing an interaction between actin and myosin filaments through a complex interaction with enzymes. Actin filaments move progressively inward on myosin filaments as successive electrochemical interactions take place (interdigitation). The result is shortening of sarcomeres and then of muscle fibers and thus myocardial contraction. Relaxation of muscle fibers occurs when free calcium is pumped back into the sarcoplasmic reticulum.

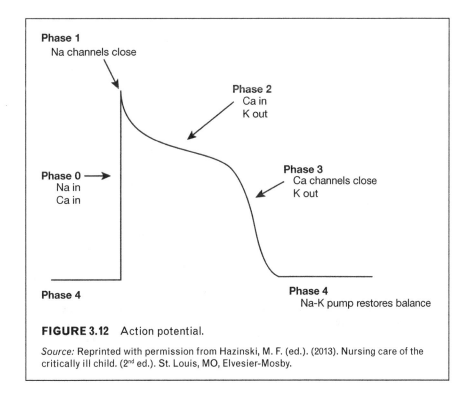

FIGURE 3.12 Action potential.

Source: Reprinted with permission from Hazinski, M. F. (ed.). (2013). Nursing care of the critically ill child. (2nd ed.). St. Louis, MO, Elvesier-Mosby.

4. *The "gate" theory* proposes fast channels of the membrane specific for sodium may be controlled by the following:

    a. The activation gate opens the fast channels as the RMP becomes less negative, allowing a rapid influx of sodium into the cell, which causes depolarization (phase 0 of the AP).

    b. The deactivation gate closes the channels impeding the influx of sodium into the cell. Closure of the gates is complete by phase 1.

5. *A return to the RMP* results from an inward current of calcium and potassium ions that diffuse out of the cell.

    a. Phase 2, the plateau phase, occurs as calcium flows in and potassium flows out.

    b. Phase 3, the rapid depolarization phase, occurs as the calcium channels close and potassium rapidly moves out of the cell.

    c. Phase 4, the resting phase, of the sodium–potassium pump regulates the concentration of cations in the cell. This pump, found in the cell membrane, actively pumps excess sodium out of the cell and pumps in the potassium.

        i. Unlike other cells of the heart that require another stimulus to depolarize them once they have been repolarized, the SA and AV nodes spontaneously depolarize (generate impulses) in phase 4. This spontaneous depolarization is due to the steady influx of sodium and the efflux of potassium ions, raising the nodal tissues back to the threshold potential and initiating an AP. This phenomenon is known as *automaticity*.

C. Refractoriness of Heart Muscle

1. *Absolute refractory period* encompasses phases 0, 1, 2, and part of 3 of the APs. During this period of time, the cell cannot respond to another stimulus and produce an AP.

2. *Relative refractory period* (the latter part of phase 3) is a period when a strong stimulus can cause depolarization.

3. *Supernormal period* occurs at the end of phase 3. During this time, a very weak stimulus that would not normally elicit an AP can evoke a response and cause depolarization.

4. The *vulnerable period* is the point at the very beginning of the relative refractory period. A stimulus at this time (which corresponds to the peak of the T wave on the ECG) can result in myocardial electrical chaos. The R-on-T phenomenon occurs when a premature QRS complex interrupts the previous beat's T wave, which may result in ventricular tachycardia (VT) or ventricular fibrillation (VF).

D. Physiologic Response to Depolarization and Repolarization

1. Electrical depolarization of the atria is represented by the P wave on the ECG. Following atrial depolarization, the pressure in the atria rises higher than the diastolic pressure in the ventricles, forcing blood from the atria into the resting ventricles.

2. Electrical depolarization of the ventricles occurs, producing the QRS complex on the ECG. Isometric or isovolumetric contraction is the first phase of ventricular contraction (systole). Ventricular pressure rises while ventricular volume remains stable because the semilunar valves have not yet opened. The increased pressure in the ventricles closes the AV valves. As ventricular pressure exceeds great vessel pressure, the semilunar valves open. Blood from the ventricles is rapidly ejected into the great vessels. As the outflow of blood from the ventricles decreases, the pressure in the ventricles also decreases, falling below the pressure in the great vessels. This causes a backflow of blood from the great vessels to the ventricles, which closes the semilunar valves. The dicrotic notch on the arterial pressure tracing represents closure of the aortic valve.

3. Repolarization of the ventricles occurs during mechanical systole and produces the T wave on the ECG. Atrial repolarization is not seen on the ECG as it occurs during ventricular depolarization.

4. Isometric or isovolumetric relaxation occurs when ventricular pressure falls rapidly following semilunar valve closure. Intraventricular volume remains static before the AV valves open. A "v" wave is produced on the atrial pressure curve during isometric relaxation related to blood flow into the atria from the pulmonic and systemic circuits. As ventricular pressure remains lower than atrial pressure, the AV valves open to initiate the rapid-filling phase (Figure 3.13).

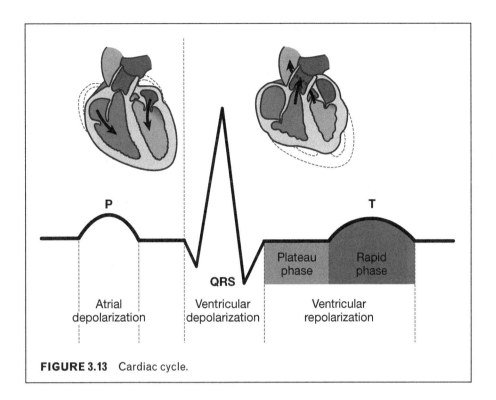

FIGURE 3.13 Cardiac cycle.

CARDIOVASCULAR ASSESSMENT

A. History

1. *Gestational and Birth History* (Fillipps & Bucciarelli, 2015)

a. Maternal and paternal congenital heart disease (CHD) history, family heart disease history, acquired and CHD history are important to screen for specific genetic and familial transmission of specific congenital or acquired cardiac disease.

b. Maternal health history, serologies, exposures and infections, medications (prescribed and illicit), gestational diseases, and alcohol exposure outline potential environmental factors known to cause congenital cardiac disease. They may also guide maternal and infant care during and immediately after delivery. Gaining knowledge of these exposures and appropriate treatment regimens is essential to providing care for the neonate with heart disease and potential need for early operative intervention.

c. Birth history, Apgar scores, screening saturations, birth weight, and gestational age guide care surrounding potential birth trauma with end-organ complications and additional risks associated with cardiopulmonary bypass (CPB) that influence decision making regarding interventions if needed.

d. If the infant had a fetal diagnosis of CHD, a conformational postnatal echocardiogram (echo) and electrocardiogram will be performed shortly after delivery. Assessment for further intervention to prevent compromise to the newborn's cardiovascular stability can be performed at the time of delivery.

2. *General History* (Bates, 2017)

a. The *chief complaint* is the patient's or parents' description of why they are seeking evaluation.

b. History of present illness will determine the onset, description, course, and duration of the specific symptom complex. Evaluate exacerbations and remissions of signs and symptoms, including the following:

i. Feeding pattern. Note the duration, frequency, associated distress, volume taken, if stopping to rest or breathe during eating, and caloric supplementation required (poor feeding/weight gain is the earliest sign of CHF).

ii. Fatigue. Note whether the child tires while feeding or playing.

iii. Edema. Assess for presence of orbital and sacral edema.

iv. Diaphoresis. Note the location, degree, and precipitating factors.

v. Dyspnea, tachypnea. Note whether these occur with or without activity.

vi. Color. Obtain information if available regarding the oxygen saturation with or without activity; skin color, and saturation in each extremity (differential cyanosis). Acrocyanosis may be present in distal portions of the extremities, around the mouth and nail beds and can be a normal variant in newborns that increases when crying. Cyanosis is always abnormal. Mottling or pallor can be a sign of poor CO.

vii. Squatting. This occurs in children with cyanotic lesions (specifically, tetralogy of Fallot) or when repairs are delayed or the defect is undiagnosed (generally children without previous medical care).

viii. Growth. Graph against normal limits for height (>2 years)/length (<2 years), weight, and head circumference. With CHF, weight will fall below normal limits before height does. Head circumference is preserved until CHF is long-standing.

ix. Frequency of infections. Particularly note respiratory illnesses but include any past history of sepsis or bacteremia and strep throat.

x. Syncope. Is there an associated prodrome, is there associated dizziness, is there a particular time of occurrence or stimulating factor?

xi. Capillary refill is normally 3 to 4 seconds and may be prolonged due to cardiovascular compromise.

xii. Clubbing of the nailbeds indicates long-standing arterial desaturation.

xiii. Palpitations. Are they with or without chest pain, are they felt in the neck or throat, do they start rapidly, or are they gradual in onset?

c. Past history and family history include all previous illnesses, injuries, and family history of similar disease (i.e., history of CHD and early onset coronary artery disease).

i. Obtain prenatal and perinatal history, including in vitro fertilization, prenatal care, and fetal diagnosis.

ii. Family history should include evaluation of inheritance risk of single gene chromosomal disorders or multifactorial syndromes associated with CHD (Tables 3.2–3.4). Determination of a family history of sudden or unexplained death at a young age is important information in that it may represent a potentially inherited cardiac disease.

iii. Explore environmental exposures, include drug teratogens, external radiation exposure, smoking, maternal systemic diseases, and infectious exposure of the fetus (Table 3.5).

iv. There is a slightly higher risk (2.5%–16%) of CHD if one parent or sibling has CHD, especially the mother.

d. Psychosocial history includes the use of nonprescription drugs or alcohol during pregnancy or taken by the child, daily living patterns, relationships with significant others, recreational habits, educational level of the child and parents, and developmental level of the child. Potential exposure of the child to abuse in the home or by a caregiver should be explored.

e. The medication history should include all medications prescribed or obtained over the counter, including herbal remedies, dosages, and reason for use.

B. Physical Examination

1. *Inspection*

a. Assess the general appearance.

i. Note size for age (height, weight, and head circumference graphed against normal limits), activity level, level of consciousness, and physical characteristics of chromosomal defects (genetic phenotypes, i.e., Down syndrome).

b. Assess the skin and mucous membranes.

i. Note pallor, cyanosis, or mottling. Skin color is influenced by vasoconstriction/vasodilation. Cyanosis is evident if saturation is less than 85%, which is equivalent

TABLE 3.2   Single-Gene Defects Associated With Congenital Heart Disease

Name/Locus	Gene Defect	Phenotype	CV Effect
Marfan's—15q21	Defect for fibrillin, alters growth factor β-binding sites, 80 mutations found	Skeletal: Tall stature, arachnodactyly, scoliosis Ocular: Retinal detachments Neonatal: valves	Progressive dilation of AO root with catastrophic aortic dissection, AI, MVP
Holt-Oram—12q24	Mutation of transcription factor TBX5	Malformed thumb, hypoplasia of thenar eminence, radial aplasia	80% ASD; also VSD, AVC; conduction abnormalities
Familial ASD—5q34	Mutation of transcription factor NKX2-5		ASD and conduction abnormalities; also TOF, DORV, Ebstein's, muscular VSD
Char Syndrome—6q12-21	Defect of transcription factor AP-2b, role in neural crest differentiation	Facial: Short philtrum, duck-bill lips, ptosis, low-set ears Skeletal: Abnormal fifth digit	PDA
Duchenne's MD—Xp21	Mutation of dystrophin gene	Skeletal and smooth muscle weakness	Dilated cardiomyopathy
Barth Syndrome—Xq28		Immunologic: Cyclic neutropenia Renal: Organic aciduria Somatic: Skeletal myopathy, growth failure	Dilated cardiomyopathy
Alagille's—20p12	Mutation of JAG1, codes for cell surface receptor, results in arteriohepatic dysplasia	Hepatic: Liver dysfunction, decreased number of bile ducts Other: Eye, skeletal, kidney	67% diffuse peripheral PA stenosis, hypoplasia of pulmonary vascular tree TOF, PA, coarctation, ASD, PDA, VSD
Noonan's—12q24.1	Mutation of PTPN11 gene, encodes nonreceptor protein tyrosine phosphatase SHP2	Skeletal: Short stature, shield chest, webbed neck, peripheral edema Face: Hypertelorism, downward slant eye, rotated ears low-set posteriorly Head: Deafness, delays, 25% cognitive impairment Hematologic: Factor XI deficiency, platelet dysfunction, Von Willebrand's disease	80% heart disease; 40% valvar PS not responsive to balloon dilation; 15% partial AVC; 10% hypertrophic cardiomyopathy; 9% coarctation; also ASD, PDA, mitral valve defects, TOF
Wolff–Parkinson–White—7q34-36	Mutation of γ-2 regulatory subunit of AMP-activated protein kinase (PRKAG2)		Short PR interval, prolonged QRS, slurred upstroke of R wave (delta wave) Prone to SVT

AI, aortic insufficiency; AMP, adenosine monophosphate; AO, aorta; ASD, atrial septal defect; AVC, atrioventricular canal defect; CV, cardiovascular; DORV, double-outlet right ventricle; MD, muscular dystrophy; MR, mitral regurgitation; MVP, mitral valve prolapse; PA, pulmonary atresia; PDA, patent ductus arteriosus; PS, pulmonary stenosis; SVT, supraventricular tachycardia; TOF, tetralogy of Fallot; VSD, ventricular septal defect.

Source: Retrieved from https://onlinelibrary.wiley.com/doi/epdf/10.1111/chd.12317

TABLE 3.3 Chromosomal Defects Associated With Congenital Heart Disease

Name/Locus	Gene Defect	Phenotype	CV Effect
Williams—7q11.23	Monosomy of allele for elastin gene	Face: Elfin faces, stellate pattern to iris Behavior: "Cocktail party personality" Mental: Developmental delay with language skills preserved	Supravalvar AS Supravalvar PS Renal artery stenosis
Down-21	Trisomy of 21	Face: Flattened profile, epicanthal folds, upslanting palpebral fissures, excess nuchal skin, simian crease Mental: Cognitive impairment, hypotonia GI: Duodenal atresia, Hirschsprung's, imperforate anus 15% hypothyroidism	40% heart disease 45% AVC 35% VSD 8% ASD 5% TOF with or without AVC
Patau-13	Trisomy 13	Head: Microcephaly, sloping forehead, cleft lip and palate Seizures, cerebral malformations Overlapping fingers with postaxial polydactyly Severe cognitive impairment	80% heart disease VSD, ASD, PDA, PS coarctation, dextrocardia
Edwards-18	Trisomy 18	Head: Microcephaly, prominent occiput, narrow forehead, cleft lip and palate, low-set ears IUGR, single umbilical artery Extremities: Clenched hands with overlapping digits, rocker bottom feet	90% heart disease VSD, ASD, PDA, PS, TOF, bicuspid AO valve, TGA, coarct, polyvalvar thickening
Turner's—45X		Skeletal: Short stature, broad chest with widely spaced nipples, peripheral edema Excess nuchal skin, ovarian dysgenesis Mental: Normal intelligence	23% heart disease 50% bicuspid AO valve 33% coarctation also AS, PAPVR, VSD, ASD 25% multiple cardiac anomalies
DiGeorge/ velocardiofacial (CATCH-22)—22q11	Contiguous gene syndrome with 25 genes in deleted region	Face: Cleft palate, high-arching palate Neck: Aplasia/hypoplasia of parathyroids, thymus Learning disabilities, renal anomalies, growth delay, psychiatric disorders	75% conotruncal defects 25%–30% truncus arteriosus 25%–40% IAA 20% TOF 25% R aortic arch
Cat eye syndrome—22p	Tetrasomy of 22p	Facial: Coloboma of iris, down-staring palpebral fissures, periauricular tags/pits	TAPVR LSVC

AO, aorta; AS, aortic stenosis; ASD, atrial septal defect; AVC, atrioventricular canal defect; coarct, coarctation of the aorta; CV, cardiovascular; GI, gastrointestinal; IAA, interrupted aortic arch; IUGR, intrauterine growth restriction; LSVC, left superior vena cava; PAPVR, partial anomalous pulmonary venous return; PDA, patent ductus arteriosus; PS, pulmonary stenosis; R, right; TAPVR, total anomalous pulmonary venous return; TGA, transposition of the great arteries; TOF, tetralogy of Fallot; VSD, ventricular septal defect.

TABLE 3.4   Multifactorial Inheritance Syndromes Associated With Congenital Heart Disease

Name/Locus	Gene Defect	Phenotype	CV
Heterotaxy syndrome	Mutation of Xq26.2 Mutation of ZIC3 gene	Situs ambiguous Asplenia-polysplenia syndrome Lung lobation altered Malrotation	Dextrocardia Other, usually complex heart defects
Jervell-Lange-Nielsen—Romano-Ward	Mutation of K$^+$ ion channel gene Six mutations 11p15.5 defect in encoding K$^+$ ion channel for phase 3 repolarization 7q35 defect in encoding Ca activated K$^+$ channel 3p21 Na channel defect 4q25? Calcium–calmodulin kinase defect	Congenital deafness from ion flow deficit in stria	Prolonged QT, syncope, sudden death Prolonged QT, syncope, sudden death
Familial hypertrophic	Defect of sarcomeric proteins at 1q3, 19p12.2q13.2, 11p11, 7q3, 3p21, 12q23, 15q14, 14q1		Asymmetric left ventricular hypertrophy with acute obstruction or ventricular arrhythmias

CV, cardiovascular.

TABLE 3.5   Fetal Environmental and Systemic Exposures Associated With Cardiac Anomalies

Exposure	Cardiac Anomaly
Thalidomide	Truncus, TOF, VSD, PDA
Fetal alcohol	VSD, ASD, TOF
Amphetamines	VSD, PDA, ASD, TGV
Trimethadione	VSD, TOF
Anticonvulsants	PS, AS, coarct, PDA, TGV, TOF, HLHS
Sex hormones	VSD, TGV, TOF
Lithium	Ebstein's anomaly, tricuspid atresia, ASD
Retinoic acid	TOF, TGV, DORV, truncus, VSD
Rubella	PDA, PS, AS, coarct, VSD, ASD
Mumps	Endocardial fibroelastosis
Coxsackie	Myocarditis
HIV	Dilated cardiomyopathy
CMV	Myocarditis, fetal heart block
Parvovirus B19	Myocarditis, nonimmune hydrops fetalis with high output heart failure

(continued)

TABLE 3.5 Fetal Environmental and Systemic Exposures Associated With Cardiac Anomalies *(continued)*

Exposure	Cardiac Anomaly
Diabetes	TGV, VSD, hypertrophic cardiomyopathy
Lupus erythematosus	Congenital complete heart block
Phenylketonuria	TOF, VSD, ASD
Thyroid dysfunction	SVT, cardiomyopathy
Friedreich's ataxia	CHB, PVCs, cardiomyopathy

AS, aortic stenosis; ASD, atrial septal defect; CHB, complete heart block; CMV, cytomegalovirus; coarct, coarctation of the aorta; DORV, double-outlet right ventricle; HLHS, hypoplastic left heart syndrome; PDA, patent ductus arteriosus; PS, pulmonary stenosis; PVC, premature ventricular contraction; SVT, supraventricular tachycardia; TA, truncus arteriosus; TGV, transposition of the great vessels; TOF, tetralogy of Fallot; VSD, ventricular septal defect.

to 5 g of reduced hemoglobin per 100 mL of blood. The degree of visible cyanosis is dependent on total hemoglobin and its saturation. Respiratory cyanosis decreases with crying (improved respiratory effort) and oxygen. In cardiac disease, cyanosis increases with crying (increased resistance to pulmonary blood flow and shunting) and remains unchanged with oxygen administration. *Acrocyanosis* (cyanosis of the extremities) is normal in the newborn with vasomotor instability. Note the distribution of cyanosis over the body. *Peripheral* cyanosis (extremities, perioral [around the mouth]) may represent hypothermia or decreased flow, whereas central cyanosis (mucous membranes) indicates reduced hemoglobin saturation. *Chronic* cyanosis stimulates erythropoiesis and polycythemia, which cause increased blood viscosity and an increased risk of spontaneous cerebrovascular accidents, brain abscess, thrombocytopenia with short platelet survival, reduced platelet aggregation with hemorrhagic abnormalities (which may cause operative bleeding), and vascular sheer stress producing increased PVR, even in the face of decreased pulmonary blood flow.

ii. Note edema, which is more common in the periorbital and sacral areas of infants.

iii. Note the patient's temperature. Skin temperature is influenced by the environment and by CO and assists in describing the level of decreased perfusion (i.e., cold to knee, cold to midthigh).

iv. Note the presence of diaphoresis at rest and/or with crying/exercise/feeding.

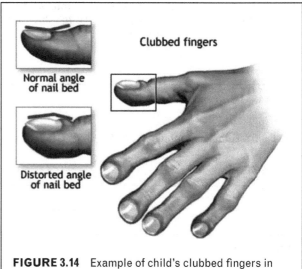

FIGURE 3.14 Example of child's clubbed fingers in contrast to normal fingers.

c. Observe the extremities

i. Note clubbing of nail beds indicated by a flattened angle of the nail base to 180 or more degrees (normal is about 160 degrees). Clubbing develops after decreased oxygen saturation persists longer than 6 months (Figure 3.14).

ii. Compare both sides for equal growth, particularly length, in children requiring multiple catheterization procedures or with a history of arterial occlusions from monitoring lines.

iii. Note the color of the nailbeds, palms, and soles of feet.

d. Observe the chest and precordium for visible pulsations.

i. An active precordium with heaves or thrusts over the precordium is noted in volume overload such as left-to-right shunts or aortic or mitral insufficiency.

ii. Note the shape, contour, and symmetry of the chest, Harrison's groove in older children, and the visible point of maximal intensity of cardiac impulse (point of maximal impulse [PMI]).

e. Observe the neck for jugular venous distention.

2. *Palpation*

a. Precordium

i. Note the PMI, normally found at the fifth left intercostal space (LICS), medial to the midclavicular line after 7 years or at the fourth LICS before 7 years. Lateral displacement of the PMI away from the left sternal border (LSB) indicates elevated diaphragm or left ventricular hypertrophy (LVH). Medial displacement toward the sternum indicates right ventricular hypertrophy (RVH) or an abnormally small LV.

ii. Seven areas should be palpated (Figure 3.15), including the supraclavicular, aortic, pulmonary, tricuspid, mitral, epigastric, and ectopic areas.

iii. Thrills. Use the ball portion of the palm of the hand to palpate for thrills (feels like a vibration or a cat purring).

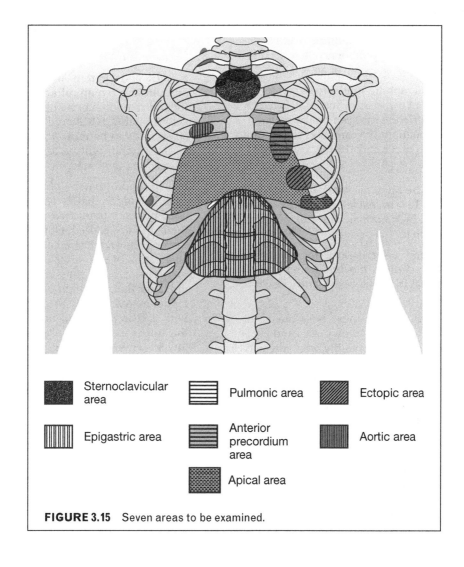

Sternoclavicular area

Pulmonic area

Ectopic area

Epigastric area

Anterior precordium area

Aortic area

Apical area

FIGURE 3.15 Seven areas to be examined.

1) In the aortic area, thrills indicate aortic stenosis (AS).

2) In the pulmonic area with radiation to the left side of the neck, thrills indicate pulmonic stenosis.

3) In the apical area during systole, thrill indicates mitral regurgitation (MR) and during diastole, MS.

4) If felt in the suprasternal notch area, thrill may indicate AS, pulmonic stenosis, or a PDA.

5) If felt in the intercostal spaces (ICSs), thrill may indicate coarctation of the aorta with collateral circulation.

6) If felt in the mid to lower LSB, a VSD may be indicated.

iv. Lifts are pulsations noted under the palm of the hand. Pulsation in the pulmonic area indicates MS or hypertension. Lifts in the tricuspid area may indicate a VSD, elevated RV pressure, pulmonary stenosis (PS), pulmonary hypertension, or an ASD.

v. Friction rubs are similar to the sensation of rubbing two pieces of material together. Pericardial friction rubs can be heard continuously throughout the cardiac cycle. Pleural friction rubs occur only during respiration.

b. Peripheral pulses

i. These are rated on a scale of 0 to 4, with 0 = absent; 1+ = palpable but thready, easily obliterated; 2+ = normal; 3+ = full; 4+ = full and bounding.

ii. Common arterial sites for palpation include the carotid, brachial, radial, femoral, popliteal, dorsalis pedis, and posterior tibialis.

iii. Obtain simultaneous assessments of upper and lower extremity pulses and evaluate their strength, equality, and intensity as an indication of coarctation of the aorta. In the presence of a coarctation without a widely patent PDA, the lower extremity pulses are weak and the upper extremity pulses are strong and full.

iv. Strong, bounding pulses are found in a PDA, aortic regurgitation, AV fistulas, and TA. Waterhammer pulses may be found with aortic insufficiency or a PDA secondary to low diastolic pressure. Delayed, weak pulses are found in cardiac tamponade, AS,

MS, CHF, shock, and hypoplastic left heart syndrome (HLHS). Pulsus alternans (alternating pulse waves, every other beat weaker than the preceding beat) indicates a weak heart muscle, as seen in severe hypertension or LV failure.

c. Capillary filling time is evaluated by compressing the extremity with moderate pressure and noting the time required for the blanched area to reperfuse. Normal capillary filling time is less than 3 seconds with the extremity at the level of the heart.

d. The liver is palpated starting in the lower abdomen and pressing upward at the right costal margin until the liver edge is palpated. The liver edge of an infant is normally 3 cm below the costal margin. The liver edge of a 1-year-old is at 2 cm below the margin; the liver edge of a 4- to 5-year-old child is at 1 cm below. By adolescence, the edge is either not palpable or is at the costal margin (Duderstadt, 2014).

3. *Auscultation*

a. HR and rhythm are assessed together by auscultating the apical area. Asses the regularity and rate for expected limitations for age and activity status. HR should be counted for at least 60 seconds to be most accurate. The regularity of the rhythm will be assessed over the same 60-second time frame.

b. To appropriately obtain an accurate BP, a cuff bladder that is at least two thirds the circumference and two thirds the length of the extremity is used. Obtain four extremity BP readings during the initial assessment to rule out coarctation of the aorta. Thigh pressure is equal to upper extremity pressure until a child is 1 year old; after that, the thigh pressure may be higher. Upper extremity pressures are higher in patients with a coarctation and no ductus arteriosus. If the upper extremity pulses are lower than the lower extremity pulses, a reverse coarctation may be present. This can be seen with ductal stents that obstruct antegrade aortic flow.

c. Note the pulse pressure. Low diastolic pressure increases the pulse pressure and may indicate a PDA, a large systemic to PA shunt, PA to aorta collaterals, or aortic regurgitation. Decreased pulse pressure may indicate AS, vasoconstriction, low CO, or cardiac tamponade. A narrowed pulse pressure with both low systolic and higher diastolic BP may indicate cardiac tamponade.

d. Pulsus paradoxus is an exaggeration of the normal physiologic response to inspiration. Usually on inspiration there is a fall of less than 10 mmHg in arterial systolic pressure. In pulsus paradoxus, the drop exceeds 10 mmHg during normal inspiratory effort. It can also be found in pericardial effusion, hypovolemia, pericardial tamponade, significant asthma, shock, or hypovolemia.

e. Heart sounds (Figure 3.16)

i. S_1 represents closure of the mitral and tricuspid valves and the beginning of systole. The mitral component of S_1 is loudest at the apex. The tricuspid component of S_1 is loudest at the fifth ICS to the left of the sternum. S_1 is louder than S_2 at the apex. S_1 is increased in intensity from MS, anemia, fever, exercise, and hyperthyroidism. S_1 is decreased in intensity from first-degree AV block, MR, shock, cardiomyopathy, hypothyroidism, and left bundle-branch block (LBBB). A split S_1 denotes separation of mitral and tricuspid sounds and is normally heard in the tricuspid area. If audible at the anterior axillary line, it is more likely an aortic ejection click (Park, 2016).

ii. S_2 represents closure of the aortic and pulmonic valves at the beginning of diastole. The aortic component of S_2 is loudest at the second right intercostal space (RICS). The pulmonic component of S_2 is loudest at the second LICS. S_2 is heard best in the aortic and pulmonic areas. Increased intensity may be normal or may indicate hypertension or coarctation. Decreased intensity (best heard in the aortic area) indicates AS. Decreased intensity (best heard in the pulmonic area)

indicates pulmonic stenosis or tricuspid atresia. A split S_2 (best heard in the pulmonic area during inspiration) is physiologically related to the increased venous return to the RV, thus delaying closure of the pulmonary valve, and may be normal. A fixed split of S_2 represents delayed closure of the pulmonic valve from increased pulmonary blood flow through the RV as in ASD and total anomalous pulmonary venous return (TAPVR). A widely split S_2 may occur with delayed activation of the RV from right bundle-branch block (RBBB), LV pacing, or ectopic beats. A single S_2 may be heard in tetralogy of Fallot, pulmonary atresia or stenosis, and transposition of the great vessels (TGV; Park, 2016).

f. Extra heart sounds (Park, 2016)

i. S_3 is caused by the rapid entry of blood into the ventricles. S_3 is best heard at the apex with the bell and may be a normal finding in children. S_3 sounds like "Ken-tuc-ky." A loud S_3, or ventricular gallop, is a pathologic finding caused by resistance to ventricular filling related to increased volume load or decreased compliance. It occurs in MR, CHF, tricuspid insufficiency, left-to-right shunts, and anemia. It is likely the result of tensing of the chordae tendinae with rapid filling of the ventricle (Figure 3.16).

ii. S_4 is produced by atrial contraction, is best heard at the apex, and is almost never a normal finding in children. It is a dull, low-pitched heart sound occurring late in diastole from contraction of the atria as they force the final bolus of blood into stiff ventricles prior to ventricular systole. It sounds like "Ten-nes-see." It can indicate AS, pulmonic stenosis, hypertension, heart failure (HF), and anemia.

iii. Clicks occur in mid- to late systole and are loudest over the mitral or tricuspid auscultation region. They are the result of systolic prolapse of the mitral or tricuspid valve accompanied by valve regurgitation. They can also be noted in the pulmonary or aortic region due to stenosis from a bicuspid valve.

iv. Snaps occur during diastole shortly after the S_2. They are the result of opening of the mitral or tricuspid valves. The more severe the stenosis, the shorter the interval between aortic closure and the opening snap.

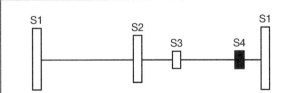

FIGURE 3.16 Diagram showing the relative relationship of the heart sounds. Filled bar shows an abnormal heart sound.

Source: Reprinted with permission from Park, M. K. (2016). *Park's The Pediatric Cardiology Handbook* (5th ed.). Philadelphia, PA: Saunders-Elsevier.

g. Murmurs are heard because of turbulent flow through an abnormal opening or obstructed area. The following are evaluated (Park, 2016):

i. Timing of systolic murmurs

1) Systolic ejection murmurs are heard between S_1 and S_2 (early, mid, or late). The intensity increases and then decreases known as *crescendo–descendo*. Holosystolic murmurs that are blowing and higher pitched and are heard throughout systole without change in intensity correlate with valve regurgitation and VSDs, and are the result of ventricular pressure exceeding atrial pressure at the onset of systole with immediate flow back across the regurgitant valve or the result of LV pressure exceeding RV pressure prior to the opening of the aortic valve in VSD. Generally, the smaller the VSD, the louder the murmur because of the increased turbulence. Midsystolic ejection murmurs begin after S_1 in mid- to late systole and may be accompanied by a midsystolic ejection click. They are usually crescendo—decrescendo (Figure 3.17).

ii. Intensity of systolic murmurs is based on a scale:

1) Grade I. Barely audible (not heard in all positions)

2) Grade II. Just easily audible (not heard in all positions)

3) Grade III. Heard well in all positions

4) Grade IV. Heard well, a palpable thrill

5) Grade V. Louder, can be heard with stethoscope partly off chest

6) Grade VI. Heard with stethoscope off chest

iii. Timing of diastolic murmurs

1) Early decrescendo murmurs are high pitched and blowing and are often the result of regurgitant flow through a valve.

2) Mid- to late "rumbling" diastolic murmurs result from turbulent flow across a stenotic valve. They occur less commonly from increased flow across the mitral or tricuspid valve. This murmur becomes louder at the end of diastole, when atrial contraction accelerates flow across the stenotic valve (Figure 3.18).

iv. Intensity of diastolic murmurs is based on a 4-point scale:

1) Grade I. Barely audible

2) Grade II. Faint but immediately audible

3) Grade III. Easily heard

4) Grade IV. Very loud

v. Continuous murmurs are heard throughout the cardiac cycle without an audible break between systole and diastole. They are the result of blood flow from an area of high pressure to low pressure, most often caused by a PDA or systemic to pulmonary shunt (Figure 3.18).

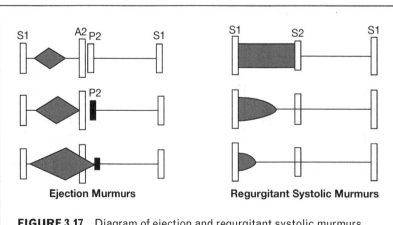

Ejection Murmurs   **Regurgitant Systolic Murmurs**

FIGURE 3.17 Diagram of ejection and regurgitant systolic murmurs.

Source: Reprinted with permission from Park, M. K. (2016). *Park's The Pediatric Cardiology Handbook* (5th ed.). Philadelphia, PA: Saunders-Elsevier.

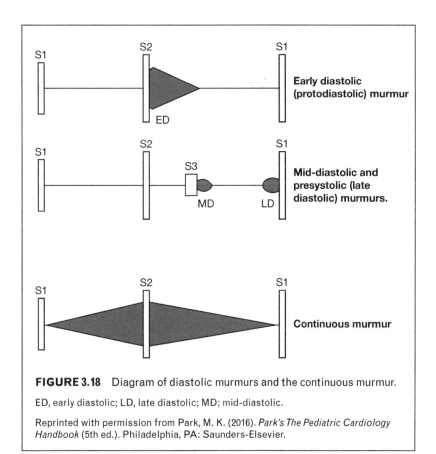

FIGURE 3.18 Diagram of diastolic murmurs and the continuous murmur.

ED, early diastolic; LD, late diastolic; MD; mid-diastolic.

Reprinted with permission from Park, M. K. (2016). *Park's The Pediatric Cardiology Handbook* (5th ed.). Philadelphia, PA: Saunders-Elsevier.

vi. To-and-fro murmurs are distinguishable from continuous murmurs in that they do not go past S_2. They have a discrete systolic and diastolic component. They are commonly noted in patients with RV–PA valved conduits or Sano shunts.

vii. Location of heart murmurs

1) Apical area (with some extension up to the pulmonic area): Murmurs of mitral insufficiency or stenosis, subaortic stenosis, aortic insufficiency, aortic ejection click of AS, and click or late systolic murmur of mitral valve prolapse

2) Tricuspid area (with some extension up to the pulmonic area): Murmurs of tricuspid insufficiency or stenosis, pulmonary insufficiency, VSD, and aortic insufficiency

3) Aortic area. Murmurs of AS or insufficiency

4) Pulmonic area. Murmurs of PS or insufficiency, ASD, pulmonary ejection click, and PDA

5) Note areas of the murmur's radiation specifically to other areas of chest, axilla, or back

viii. Pitch and quality of the murmur

1) High-pitched murmurs are heard with the diaphragm of the stethoscope and low-pitched murmurs are heard with the bell of the stethoscope.

2) The quality of a murmur is described as blowing, rumbling, harsh, or musical (Duderstadt, 2014).

C. Noninvasive Diagnostic Studies

1. *Laboratory studies* to be ordered may include electrolytes with renal function, hepatic function tests and total and direct bilirubin, complete blood count (CBC), lipid profile, calcium (total and ionized), magnesium, BNP levels, troponin levels, lactate levels, and a clotting profile (prothrombin time [PT], partial thromboplastin time [PTT], activated clotting time [ACT], bleeding time, and platelet count.

2. *Pulse oximetry* uses changes in infrared light to evaluate the level of saturated hemoglobin, providing an indirect measurement of oxygen saturation (normal 96%–100%). Pulse oximetry can be used to evaluate or trend cyanosis or to assess tolerance of procedures (suctioning, sedation). Pulse oximetry is performed routinely prior to discharge in all newborns to assess for potential cardiac disease (Mahle, Newburger, et al., 2014).

3. *Chest Radiograph.* This evaluates heart size by estimation of the cardiothoracic ratio, which is determined by cardiac width compared with the thoracic width of the chest (Herring, 2012). The normal cardiothoracic ratio is 50% or less. A large thymus in infants may be mistaken for cardiomegaly. Cardiac borders are evaluated on an anterioposterior film (Figure 3.19). The right border indicates the RA. The left lower border indicates the LV; the LA blends into the ventricular shadow unless it is significantly enlarged. The first convexity above the apex is the PA. The second convexity above the apex is the aortic arch. Specific defects can be identified from abnormal borders. A boot-shaped heart can indicate tetralogy of Fallot related to RV hypertrophy with apex upturned. A convex shoulder of the aorta is seen in transposition of the great arteries (looks like an egg with a narrow superior mediastinum). Increased pulmonary vascularity is indicated by arteries that appear enlarged and extend into the lateral third of the lung field as seen in ASD, VSD, PDA, TAPVR, truncus, transposition, and AV canal (Figure 3.20). Decreased pulmonary vascularity is noted when the hilum appears small, lung fields are empty and devoid of vessels, and the x-ray image appears dark/black. This may be

noted in tetralogy of Fallot, tricuspid atresia, Ebstein anomaly, severe pulmonary hypertension, and transposition with PS (Figure 3.21).

a. Lung fields/lung health are assessed by looking for atelectasis, effusion, pneumothorax, pneumonia, and volume loss/expansion. The diaphragm location and margin of diaphragm should be sharp.

b. Diaphragms should be located at symmetrical positions on each side of the chest. Elevation

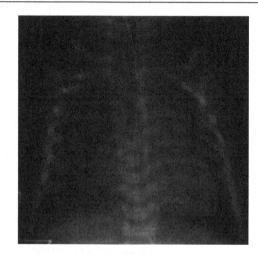

FIGURE 3.20 Chest x-ray with evidence of increased pulmonary vascularity.

Courtesy of Children's National Medical Center.

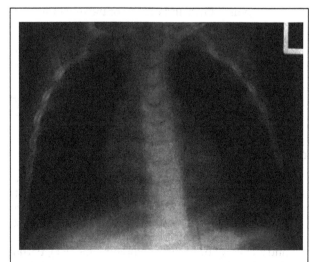

FIGURE 3.19 Heart borders as seen on anterioposterior chest x-ray.

Courtesy of Children's National Medical Center.

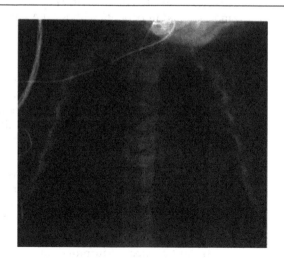

FIGURE 3.21 Chest x-ray with evidence of decreased pulmonary vascularity.

Courtesy of Children's National Medical Center.

of the diaphragm on one side suggests paralysis of diaphragm or subpulmonic effusion.

c. Assessment of any invasive monitoring lines or tubes should be performed on every x-ray obtained when these are present. Endotracheal tube (ETT), nasogastric or transpyloric tube, chest tubes, intracardiac lines, pacemaker leads (temporary or permanent), stents, coils, artificial valves, ventricular assistive device (VAD) and extracorporeal membrane oxygenation (ECMO) cannulas, central venous line (CVL), umbilical artery catheter (UAC), and umbilical venous catheter (UVC) should be evaluated. A comparison to location on the previous x-ray should be performed.

d. Abnormal bony structures may be associated with syndromes or from injury during delivery and should be noted and recorded.

4. *Electrocardiogram.* ECG provides a noninvasive examination of HR, rhythm, conduction abnormalities,

and provides clues to diagnosis of certain cardiomyopathies, congenital heart defects, and hypertension. It can detect electrolyte imbalances, including hypocalcemia (prolong ST segment), hyperkalemia (shortens ST segment), hypokalemia (flat T waves, PR interval is prolonged), and hyperkalemia (tall, peaked T waves; Park & Guntheroth, 2006).

a. Horizontal lines are a measurement of time. Each small block equals 0.04 second, and each larger dark block equals 0.2 second, with use of standard paper speed of 25 mm/sec.

b. Vertical lines represent a measurement of voltage with each small block equal to 0.1 mV or 1 mm and each larger block equal to 0.5 mV or 5 mm (if gain of ECG is set to standard of 1 mV = 10 mm).

5. *ECG Waves and Intervals* (Figure 3.22)

a. The P wave represents atrial depolarization. It is measured from the beginning of the P wave

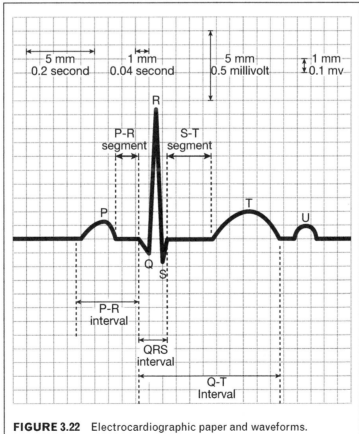

FIGURE 3.22 Electrocardiographic paper and waveforms.

to the end of the wave, when it returns to the baseline. Usually, it is less than 0.08 second. The normal amplitude is less than 2.5 mm (3 mm in the neonate), and it is usually gently rounded with all waves having the same appearance. Right atrial enlargement is noted by tall, peaked P waves greater than 2.5 mm. Left atrial enlargement (LAE) demonstrates a wide, notched P wave.

b. The PR interval represents atrial depolarization and conduction through the AV node. It is measured from the beginning of the P wave to the beginning of the QRS complex. The normal PR interval is 0.12 to 0.20 second (shorter in younger children with faster HRs). A prolonged PR interval is an indication of first-degree heart block (Table 3.6).

c. The QRS interval represents ventricular depolarization. It is measured from the beginning of the QRS to the end of the QRS. Normal duration is 0.06 to 0.10 second. Prolonged QRS duration may indicate interventricular conduction delay. Although commonly called the *QRS complex*, the first initial downward deflection is labeled Q, the first upward deflection is labeled R, the first downward deflection after the R wave is labeled S, and any other deflections are labeled with an accent to indicate "prime," such as rSR'. The size of the wave is indicated by a capital or small letter; waves over 5 mm are in capitals.

d. The T wave represents ventricular repolarization and should be in the same direction as the QRS complex. The T wave may change

configuration with hypokalemia (flattened) or hyperkalemia (peaked).

e. The ST segment represents ventricular repolarization. It is measured from the end of the QRS to the beginning of the T wave. The ST segment should not vary more than 1 mm from the baseline. Elevations may indicate ischemia and inflammation. Depression may indicate strain or ischemia.

f. The QT interval represents summation of depolarization and repolarization and varies with the HR. It is measured from the beginning of the QRS to the end of the T wave. The QT interval must be corrected for HR. The normal is less than 0.45 second.

g. The 12-lead ECG in children should include a recording of V_3r or V_4r, or both. These leads are placed on the right side of the chest in the same positions that the V_3 and V_4 leads are placed on the left side of the chest. The purpose of the V_3r and V_4r leads is to provide an opportunity for analysis of the strong right-sided forces in young children.

6. *ECG Analysis*

a. The rate is calculated by counting specific wave patterns during a determined time, such as 6 seconds. An alternative method (used if the rate is regular with no respiratory rate [RR] variation) is to estimate the rate by noting the position of one wave on a dark line and then noting the next time the wave falls on a dark line. It is essential to remember the six consecutive numbers: 300, 150, 100, 75, 60, and 50. If it

TABLE 3.6 Maximal PR Intervals

Age	HR (bpm) <71	HR (bpm) 71–90	HR (bpm) 91–110	HR (bpm) 111–130	HR (bpm) 131–150	HR (bpm) 151
1 mo	0.11	0.11	0.11	0.11		
1–9 mo	0.14	0.13	0.12	0.11		
10–24 mo	0.14		0.10			
3–5 y	0.16	0.16	0.13			
6–13 y	0.18		0.16	0.16		

HR, heart rate.

Source: From Engorn, B., & Flerlage, J. (2015). *The Harriet Lane handbook* (12th ed.). Philadelphia, PA: Elsevier, Saunders.

is one large block, the rate is 300 per minute; two large blocks equal 150 per minute; and so on. The rate can also be determined in regular rhythm by dividing 1,500 by the number of small blocks between complexes. The number of QRS complexes in a 6-second strip is multiplied by 10 (60 seconds) to determine the HR. This is accurate when the rhythm is regular and there is no R-to-R variability. The rate should be determined for both the atrial rhythm (the P wave) and the ventricular rhythm (QRS rate). The HR should always be appropriate for age and situation (Park, 2010).

b. The rhythm is considered regular if the RR interval and PP interval have a variation of less than three small blocks. Note whether the rhythm is regularly irregular.

c. The P-wave to QRS ratio should be a consistent 1:1. P waves should be upright in leads I, II, and AVF, which represents normal sinus rhythm (NSR) and if not, an arrhythmia should be suspected. Evaluate size of P wave for indications of right atrial enlargement (P wave >2.5 mm in V1) or LAE (P wave >2 mm in lead II and V1 or notched P wave; Figure 3.23).

d. The PR interval should be normal for age and HR.

e. The QRS interval should be less than or equal to 0.10 second and have a normal configuration. Evaluate for right or LVH. Axis of QRS

assists with diagnosis of specific congenital heart defects, ventricular hypertrophy. Assess for bundle-branch block (BBB), which may be present in repaired or unrepaired CHD. A significantly prolonged QT interval may be an indication for internal cardioverter defibrillator (ICD) placement due to risk of VT.

f. The corrected QT interval (QTc) adjusts the QT interval for heart rate and is used in pediatrics. The QTc and ST segment are evaluated. If abnormal, further evaluation for conduction delays and channelopathies may be indicated.

7. *Holter Monitoring.* Holter monitoring provides a 24-hour record of ECG activity. It is used to document arrhythmias and/or conduction disorders at rest and at stress as well as the frequency of their occurrence. Patients and parents use a diary to record patient activity as well as symptoms to allow correlation of symptoms with cardiac events captured on the monitor. This monitor typically records continuously for 48 hours but can be used for longer periods of time if necessary (Moss & Adams, 2016).

a. Data that can be obtained from a Holter monitor include basic heart rhythm and range of HR, the number of premature beats, the frequency and type of arrhythmia, ST segment changes, precipitating and/or terminating events for a cardiac arrhythmia, and correlation of activity with ST segment changes in the event of chest pain.

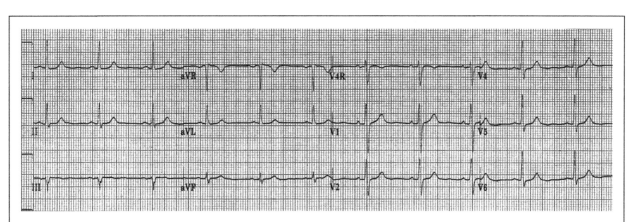

FIGURE 3.23 Morphology of QRS complex.

b. Indications for Holter placement include a determination of whether symptoms, such as syncope, chest pain, and palpitations, are arrhythmia based; to screen patients at high risk for sudden cardiac death (SCD); to evaluate pacemaker function; to assess the effect of sleep/exercise on arrhythmia; to evaluate efficacy of medical management of arrhythmia; and to follow progression of disease states known to develop VT or other potentially lethal arrhythmia.

c. It is the preferred test in patients with frequent (daily or near daily) symptoms, syncope, palpitations, atrial fibrillation, at risk of SCD.

d. The advantages of this test are its noninvasive nature and provision of rhythm detail over an extended period of time and with multiple activity levels. Therefore, brief and nonsustained arrhythmia events can be captured. The Holter is cost-effective, can be used on an outpatient basis, and does not require the patient to push a button when rhythm irregularly is felt. The patient or family mail the device back to the cardiology department unless used on an inpatient basis. These monitors can be placed for a variety of reasons, including symptoms of chest pain, palpitations, and syncope or for assessment and monitoring of the heart rhythm. Monitoring of the cardiac rhythm can be done to monitor sleep and exercise HRs, to monitor pacemaker function or for routine screening for the patient with CHD, those patients at increased risk of SCD, and/or to determine the effect or response to antiarrhythmic therapy.

e. Limitations to its use include noncompliance of the patient either in not wearing the device or in using the event diary. There is a possibility of infrequent arrhythmia events not being captured during the Holter monitoring period.

8. *Exercise Stress Testing.* Stress testing is used to evaluate ECG and simultaneous clinical response to specific stimuli (Balady & Morise, 2015). Exercise stress testing is used to evaluate myocardial oxygen supply and demand; evaluate or provoke arrhythmias; evaluate BP response to exercise; assess aerobic power and "functional" status (or level of conditioning); provide information for the need for further diagnostic testing; evaluate adequacy of current medical therapy; and evaluate chest pain, palpitations, or syncope.

a. A cycle or treadmill with ECG, BP, oxygen consumption, and CO trend recordings is used. VO_2 measurements may or may not be included because of the equipment required, technical

capabilities, and the ability of the child to wear or tolerate the equipment. The Bruce protocol tests the level of exercise tolerance/symptoms by increasing the speed and incline of the treadmill every 3 minutes until failure or symptoms occur. The patient is continuously monitored for ECG and HR/rhythm. The best predictor of exercise capacity in children is the endurance time, or the length of time of the exercise test.

b. Normal response to dynamic exercise would show an HR, CO, and VO_2 increase. Systolic BP increases with the intensity of the workload, but diastolic BP may remain unchanged. Mean BP rises mildly. SV increases with work, particularly from rest to moderate effort. Inappropriate increases in CO are seen in patients with cardiomyopathy, left ventricular outflow tract obstruction, coronary artery disease, or with the onset of ventricular or atrial arrhythmias. Excessive response in BP can be seen in patients who have undergone coarctation of the aorta repair, those with hypertension, those with inappropriate dilation of the vascular bed in response to stress with the potential to develop hypertension, and patients with aortic regurgitation. Failure of the BP to increase with progressive increases in exercise is interpreted as an inadequate ability to increase CO. Increased arrhythmia with exercise highlights the need for more thorough arrhythmia evaluation. ST segment changes are abnormal under all conditions. Sustained ST depression of 2 mm or more at 60 to 80 seconds warrants further investigation.

c. Contraindications to testing include acute illnesses, such as myocarditis, pericarditis, endocarditis, asthma, thrombophlebitis/pulmonary embolus or infarction, myocardial infarction (MI), serious noncardiac disease, severe symptomatic AS, and febrile illness or chronic illnesses such as CHF and thyroid, renal, and hepatic dysfunction (relative contraindication depending on patient condition). Serious arrhythmia is an absolute contraindication for stress exercise testing. Special care is required in AS, cardiomegaly, hypoxemia, anemia, uncontrolled arrhythmias/tachycardia/bradycardia/heart block, severe systemic or pulmonary hypertension, hypertrophic cardiomyopathy (HCM), moderate valvar disease or psychiatric disorders that preclude the ability to follow instructions. Exercise testing should immediately be terminated for decreased BP despite an increased exercise workload, angina, dizziness or near syncope, signs of decreased perfusion, serious ventricular arrhythmias (VT, premature ventricular contraction [PVCs]), and patient request. Relative reasons for termination include ST depression greater than 3 mm, chest pain, fatigue, shortness of breath, wheezing, leg cramps, and less serious arrhythmia (supraventricular tachycardia [SVT], sinus tachycardia).

d. Complications of exercise stress testing include arrhythmias (SVT, VT PVCs), hypotension, and syncope.

9. *Autonomic Testing*. This is used to evaluate vasomotor syncope.

a. Following placement of intravenous (IV) lines, the patient is placed in specific positions (flat, then 60–80 degrees) before and after drug administration (i.e., isoproterenol, propranolol). The patient's HR, rhythm, and BP as well as symptoms as described by the patient are monitored for appropriate response to the medications and changes in patient angle. Complications include arrhythmias (asystole, bradycardia), hypotension, and cardiovascular collapse. This test is also known as a *tilt table test*.

10. *Echocardiography*. Echocardiography is utilized to visualize cardiac structures, evaluate diastolic and systolic cardiac function, determine valve gradients, predict right ventricular and PA pressures, diagnose congenital heart defects, and identify thrombus and/or possible endocarditis (Solomon & Gillia, 2015). Echo uses sound waves to represent a multidimensional image of the heart from which one can measure the density of tissue and the elastic properties of the heart (Figure 3.24).

a. The M-mode echo gives a graph of lines for each surface seen by the probe with space between surfaces. It allows the most accurate measurement of the dimensions of structures.

b. Two-dimensional transthoracic echo provides a cost-effective, easy-to-obtain, and accurate one-dimensional view of cardiac structures, veins, arteries, and systolic and diastolic function and is used to identify congenital abnormalities. It is not the best tool for images of posterior cardiac structures. The orientation varies with locations of the probe.

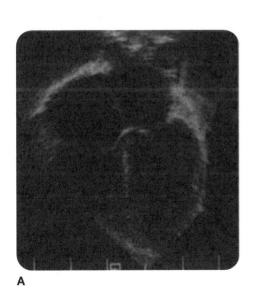

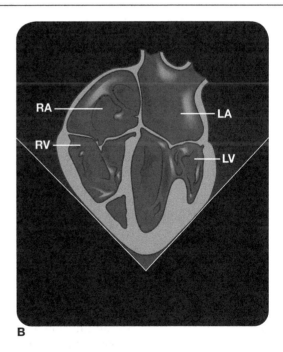

A   B

FIGURE 3.24 Echocardiographic image (A) and diagram (B) of apical four-chamber view of cardiac structures.

LA, left atrium; LV, left ventricle; RA, right atrium; RV, right ventricle.

Source: (A) Reprinted with permission from Snider, A. R., & Serwer, G. A. (2001). *Echocardiography in pediatric heart disease.* St. Louis, MO: Mosby.

i. If the ultrasound (US) is aligned and there is adequate tricuspid regurgitation (TR), estimates of right ventricular pressure and PA pressure can be obtained. Gradients across valves, VSDs, pulmonary arteries, or aorta and surgical shunts can be obtained. Residual postoperative defects can be identified.

ii. Using bubble studies, definition of residual shunts or baffles leaks can be made with the ability to then direct care.

iii. Echocardiographic guidance of procedures, such as drainage of pericardial or pleural effusions, placement of invasive monitoring lines such as Swan–Ganz catheters, balloon atrial septostomy, and closure of intracardiac shunts with device placement, is another use for transthoracic echo.

iv. It can assess the function of diaphragms, presence of vegetation or thrombus in the heart, tumors, and effusions.

v. The parasternal view reveals left-sided structures, including the LA, mitral valve, LV, and aortic valve.

vi. The apical view shows all four chambers of the heart (most similar to drawings of the heart).

vii. The subcostal view demonstrates the right ventricular outflow tract (RVOT), the RA, and the RV.

viii. The suprasternal view shows the aortic arch.

c. Three-dimensional echo provides more detailed views of specific structures, allowing measurement of borders and clearer definition of structural anatomy and measurement of atrial and ventricular volumes, particularly if configuration is not usual.

d. Doppler echo measures the velocity of blood flow and is useful to assess the pressure gradient across a valve.

e. Transesophageal echo (TEE) is used to look at cardiac structures when transthoracic echo is not feasible or adequate, such as in an adult or obese patient or in the operating room when assessing adequacy of surgical repair. It is often used to define atrial thrombus prior to cardioversion, assess for vegetations, assess the adequacy of surgical repair during the intraoperative period, and assess for weaning off CPB. It requires placing the echo probe orally into the esophagus. In the nonoperative patient, sedation may be necessary to prevent gagging. Assessment of aortic dissection is also best performed by TEE. Airway or oropharyngeal anomalies preclude placement of the TEE probe. Compression of the tracheobronchial tree is possible from the TEE probe and monitoring of ventilatory status is necessary in any patient undergoing TEE.

f. Contrast echo uses the forceful injection of dextrose and water, saline, or blood into a peripheral or central vein to produce microcavitation, which appears as a cloud of "bubbles" inside cardiac structures visualized by echo. Contrast echo is used to detect intracardiac right-to-left shunts, identify flow patterns, and validate structures.

g. Three-dimensional echo is used to assess a three-dimensional view of cardiac morphology, valve structure, size, and location of septal defects, and abnormalities of the ventricular myocardium, especially in noncompaction LV and endocardial fibroelastosis. This type of echo can be used to reconstruct cardiac anatomy for use in planning surgical interventions.

h. Fetal echo can assess for the presence of CHD in the fetus as early as 12 weeks gestation. In most institutions it is a routine screening tool for any parent with a history of CHD or history of children with CHD. It can be used to assess cardiac anatomy for structural abnormalities as well as fetal arrhythmia and effects of arrhythmia on the myocardium. It will assess for the effects of maternal disease on the fetal heart, including diabetes mellitus and connective tissue disease such as lupus. If the fetus has known or suspected chromosomal abnormalities, fetal echo can define cardiac effects. It is used to identify and quantitate fetal hydrops, diaphragmatic hernia, associated cardiac defects, and omphalocele. It can determine polyhydramnios or oligohydramnios. In mothers with known drug exposure, such as alcohol, lithium, amphetamines, antiseizure medications, and nonprescription drugs, assessment of cardiac effects in function or structure can be noted prenatally.

11. *Computerized Tomography (CT)*. CT is an important tool used to accurately evaluate CHD and is particularly helpful in delineating extracardiac anatomy and vasculature (Figure 3.25; Lim, 2015). It can be used in conjunction with echo and cardiac catheterization. It is used frequently when extracardiac anatomy is not well defined with echo or catheterization. It can be used postoperatively to evaluate potential postoperative extracardiac complications, specifically abscess/infection and pulmonary emboli.

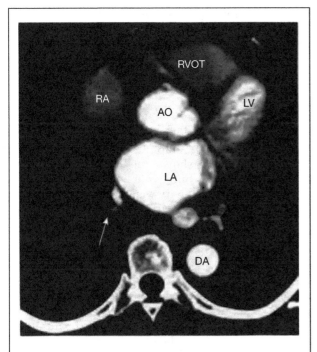

FIGURE 3.25 High cardiac level imaging on CT.

AO, aorta; DA, ductus arteriosus; LA, left atrium; LV, left ventricle; RA, right atrium; RVOT, right ventricular outflow tract.

Source: Reprinted with permission from Herring, W. (2012). *Learning radiology* (2nd ed.). Philadelphia, PA: Elsevier.

a. Advantages of CT/CT angiography (CTA) include improved definition of extracardiac anatomy and vasculature. Three-dimensional reconstruction of images allows for improved understanding of anatomy and is used to guide future planned interventions.

b. Disadvantages include the amount of radiation exposure encountered by the patient. It may require intubation/sedation/general anesthesia depending on the length of the scan and or use of angiography.

12. *MRI/MR Angiography (MRA).* MRA is helpful in characterizing morphologic abnormalities and their physiologic effects. It provides the ability to evaluate the morphology of the heart chambers, mural thrombi, coronary arteries, and detail the extracardiac vasculature (pulmonary arteries and arch; Lim, 2015).

a. The advantages of MRA are that it can provide access to heart chamber function and anatomy (Figure 3.26) as well as great vessel anatomy in greater detail than echo or catheterization. It also does not expose the patient to radiation as with CT scanning.

b. MRI/MRA testing is a disadvantage in patients who require intubation and general anesthesia, particularly infants and children who can't lay still or follow instructions for breath holding. Cardiac MRA (cMRA) most often will require

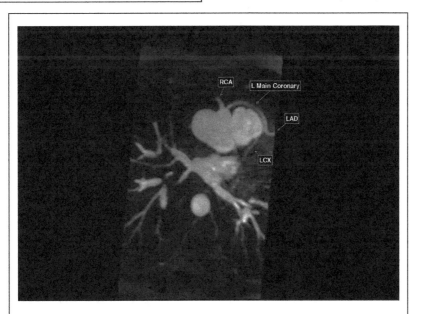

FIGURE 3.26 Cardiac MRI.

L, left; LAD, left anterior descending artery; LCX, left circumflex artery; RCA, right coronary artery.

Courtesy of Michigan Medicine, University of Michigan, CS Mott Children's Hospital, Congenital Heart Center.

a sedated and/or intubated and anesthetized patient. Specific intracardiac devices can interfere with quality of the study due to artifact. Certain devices, such as a permanent pacemaker, prohibit the use of MRI/MRA. Most stents, sternal wires, vessel closure devices, and septal defect closure devices are MRI/MRA compatible.

13. *Nuclear Medicine Testing*

a. Lung perfusion studies utilize radioisotopes injected into a vein in the upper extremity to measure quantitative blood flow to each lung. A lung perfusion study is a minimally invasive imaging study and potentially can be performed at the bedside if necessary (Udelson, Diliszian, & Bobow, 2015).

b. Cardiac perfusion studies utilize a radioactive tracer injected through a peripheral IV. A cardiac perfusion study is a noninvasive imaging study that is done without radiation exposure. The scan measures blood flow to the heart muscle at rest and also can be used during exercise to assess coronary blood flow and to identify areas of underperfusion, hypokinesis, or akinesis of the myocardium (Udelson et al., 2015).

c. A multigated acquisition (MUGA) scan evaluates ventricular function of the left and right heart using a radioactive isotope to examine motion abnormalities of the heart wall. It is also a noninvasive nuclear medicine test without radiation exposure (Udelson et al., 2015).

14. *Cardiac Catheterization*

a. Diagnostic therapies

i. Angiography. The right ventriculogram shows the RV size and structure, RV outflow tract, TR, PA anatomy, and pulmonary venous return to the left side of the heart. The left ventriculogram shows the LV size, function, structure, and outflow tract, and left-to-right shunting patterns. The aortogram shows the aortic arch structure, aortic regurgitation, and coronary anatomy. Selective coronary angiography demonstrates coronary blood supply. Cardiac catheterization is a means to measure the pressures and saturations in cardiac chambers and great vessels. Cardiac catheterization reveals variations from normal values (Figure 3.27).

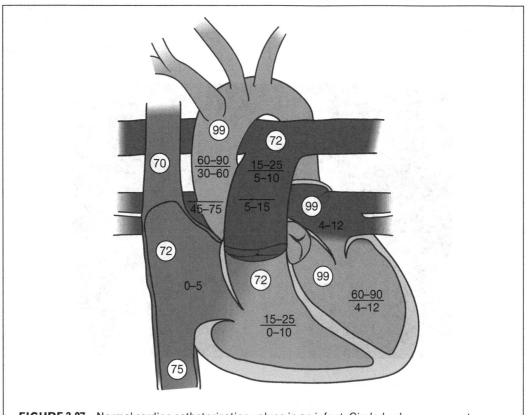

FIGURE 3.27 Normal cardiac catheterization values in an infant. Circled valves represent expected saturations; numbers without circles represent pressures.

ii. In situations of obstruction or mixing lesions, values will reflect the alterations in blood flow. Cardiac catheterization is a means to measure the pressures and saturations in cardiac chambers and great vessels and determine variations from normal values.

iii. CO is measured by the Fick or thermodilution method (Davidson, Kinley, & Bhatt, 2015).

1) $CO = SV \times HR$

2) $CI = CO/BSA$ in m²; normal is 2.5 to 4 L/min/m²

iv. Pulmonary flow (Qp) is $VO_2/(Cpv\text{-}Cpa)$

v. Systemic flow (Qs) is $VO_2/(Cao\text{-}Cmv)$

(Note: Cpv-Cpa is oxygen content pulmonary vein-oxygen content of pulmonary artery. Cao-Cmv is oxygen content aorta-oxygen content of mixed venous; $Qp = VO_2/PV$ saturation-PA saturation; $Qs = VO_2/aortic$ saturation-mixed venous saturation)

vi. PVR is the mean PA pressure (PAP) − mean left atrial pressure (LAP)/Qp. The normal value in children is 1–3 Wood units/m². PVR is higher in the neonate and begins to fall to the normal range by 6 to 8 weeks of age.

vii. SVR is the mean aortic pressure − mean right atrial pressure (RAP)/Qs. The normal SVR for children is about 20 units/m² and for infants about 10 units/m² (Table 3.7).

viii. Cardiac catheterization can be used for cardiac biopsy for identification of rejection in a transplanted heart, biopsy for diagnosis of infectious etiology or continued inflammatory response in myocarditis, and to assess for cellular disease such as mitochondrial disease.

b. Interventional therapies

i. Balloon dilation of cardiac valves, including the pulmonary, aortic, mitral, and tricuspid, is used to relieve stenosis of the valve. Balloon dilation of vessels has been used with peripheral systemic arteries, native aorta or recoarctation of the aorta, the PA and its branches, and the pulmonary veins.

ii. Placement of occluding coils will embolize an abnormal arterial supply or will occlude a PDA.

iii. Interventational catheter can be used for placement of vascular stents in the RVOT, a valved conduit or coarcation can be performed.

iv. ASD closure devices, VSD closure devices, and PDA occluders can be placed during an interventional catheter.

v. Other treatments include balloon atrial or blade atrial septostomy, placement of an intracardiac left atrial drain, foreign-body removal endomyocardial biopsy for diagnosis of sarcoidosis, myocarditis, and rejection in the heart transplant patient.

c. Complications of catheterization include arrhythmias from catheter manipulation; air embolization; allergic reaction to contrast; myocardial

TABLE 3.7 Hemodynamic Values Obtained From Pulmonary Artery Catheter

Measurement	Calculation	Normal Values
Cardiac index	$\dfrac{CO}{BSA}$	3–4.2 L/min/m²
Stroke volume	$\dfrac{CO}{HR} \times 1000$	1 mL/kg/contraction
Systemic vascular resistance index	$\dfrac{MAP-CVP}{CI} \times 80$	700–1,600 dynes/sec/cm/m²
Peripheral vascular resistance index	$\dfrac{MPAP-PCWP}{CI} \times 80$	20–130 dynes/L/m²

BSA, body surface area; CI, cardiac index; CO, cardiac output; MAP, mean arterial pressure; MPAP, mean pulmonary artery pressure; PCWP, pulmonary capillary wedge pressure.

infarction; arterial and venous thrombosis (and emboli); perforation of the heart, valves, or vessels; shock; acidosis; hypotension (from HF, stress in a critically ill child); blood loss; infection; and death.

Electrophysiologic studies are used to evaluate the location and characteristics of abnormal rhythms and the medical therapies to treat them (Kugler, 2016; Moss & Adams, 2015). Pretesting includes an echo, ECG, and CBC. The child may also require an exercise stress test, Holter monitoring, and signal-averaged ECG. The patient is on nothing-by-mouth (NPO) status 4 to 6 hours before the procedure depending on the type of sedation and anesthesia planned. Premedication with a sedative, analgesic, or amnestic agent is required. Anesthesia and intubation may be used if an extended period of sedation is anticipated. A large sheath is placed for threading of catheters to identify the location of abnormal electrical tissue of the heart. Multiple catheters can be placed in various locations inside the heart. Common locations include the high RA, coronary sinus, bundle of His, RV, and LV. Pacing through these catheters evaluates conduction intervals as well as stimulates extrasystoles to determine sources of arrhythmias (Said & Kugler, 2016).

  a. Stimulation of specific abnormal rhythms (such as SVT, VT) may be used to test antiarrhythmic medications. Radiofrequency ablation or cyroablation can be used to eliminate abnormal conduction pathways or areas that generate ectopic beats. Ablation cures roughly 90% of SVT, but there may be recurrences. It can improve the arrhythmia by decreasing the incidence of arrhythmia and improving medication control of other arrhythmias with medication.

  b. Complications (in addition to those related to cardiac catheterization) include uncontrollable arrhythmias, which may result in cardiac arrest and death, varying degrees of conduction disorders, and a higher risk of intracardiac clotting when multiple catheters are placed in the LV or LA or the length of the study is prolonged.

CARDIOVASCULAR MONITORING

A. HR and Rhythm

  1. Continuous ECG monitoring is useful for rapid identification and response to rhythm changes. Continual monitoring is required in known arrhythmias and anomalies that predispose to acute arrhythmia, during the cardiac surgery postoperative period, initiation of antiarrhythmic medications, and drug overdoses. Modified chest lead (MCL)-1 or limb leads (such as leads I, II, III, AVR, AVF) are often used for monitoring.

  a. Lead placement (Figure 3.28)

      i. Ground lead. Right shoulder midclavicular line

      ii. Negative lead. Left shoulder midclavicular line

      iii. Positive lead. Fourth ICS, right sternal border

  b. MCL-1 allows detection of arrhythmias, BBB, and differentiation of aberrancy. MCL-1 typical pattern is negative, similar to V_1.

  2. Monitoring rules assess the impact of rhythm on the patient through assessment of perfusion and BP to determine whether the arrhythmia affects CO.

  a. The hierarchy providing the most accurate information is to begin with the 12-lead ECG with all leads recorded simultaneously with standardized amplitude size, then recording on monitor paper, followed by evaluation of the monitor screen.

  b. Consider the progression and pattern of arrhythmias, the impact of surgery on the conduction system, ST segment changes, and the usual rhythms that occur with the use of specific drugs.

B. Hemodynamic Measurements

  1. *Arterial pressure monitoring* is indicated in situations for which a continuous BP reading is desirable, frequent blood sampling is required, and/or vasoactive medications are in use.

  a. Insertion can be obtained by percutaneous placement or by using the surgical cut-down technique. The radial site is frequently used. The dorsalis pedis; posterior tibialis; femoral, temporal, and axillary arteries are alternative sites. The Allen test is used to assess ulnar patency or perfusion prior to insertion in the radial site. The Allen test consists of occluding both the radial and ulnar arteries until the patient's fingers and palm blanch and then releasing only the ulnar artery supply to determine whether the alternative blood supply to the hand is adequate if the catheter or clot occludes the radial artery.

  b. Monitoring equipment required includes nondistensible tubing, heparinized infusion fluid, and a transducer. The phlebostatic axis corresponds to the RA (Figure 3.29).

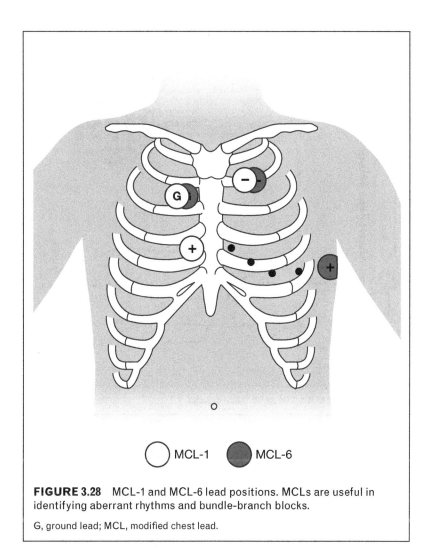

FIGURE 3.28 MCL-1 and MCL-6 lead positions. MCLs are useful in identifying aberrant rhythms and bundle-branch blocks.

G, ground lead; MCL, modified chest lead.

c. A normal waveform (Figure 3.30) has a clear dicrotic notch. When the arterial catheter is unstable in the vessel it will present a fling waveform with an exaggerated systolic peak. A dampened waveform can be related to occlusion by a clot, absorption by air bubble, a kink in the catheter or monitoring tubing, nonpulsatile flow (as seen with ECMO), or a loose connection. Absence of a waveform can be related to a displaced or clotted line, nonperfusing rhythm, equipment malfunction, or arterial spasm.

d. Complications include hemorrhage, ischemia, hematoma, arterial spasm, infection, arterial thrombosis, and inaccurate readings.

2. *CVP monitoring* is indicated for assessment of blood volume (preload) and RV function. In the absence of pulmonary vascular disease, MS, or elevated PVR, the CVP may be an indirect measurement of left heart filling. The venous catheter may be used for infusion of large-volume, hypertonic solutions, vasoactive agents, and caustic electrolyte supplementations.

a. Insertion sites used include the internal jugular, external jugular, femoral and subclavian veins, and transthoracic placement into the RA.

b. Monitoring equipment includes nondistensible tubing, infusion fluid, transducer, and ECG monitor during placement. Choices involved in the selection of the catheter include nonthrombogenic material, the number of lumens, the size of the catheter in relation to blood vessels, and the length of the catheter.

c. Normal waveform components (Figure 3.31) include the a wave, which reflects mechanical atrial systole; x descent, which reflects the decrease in RA volume during relaxation; c wave,

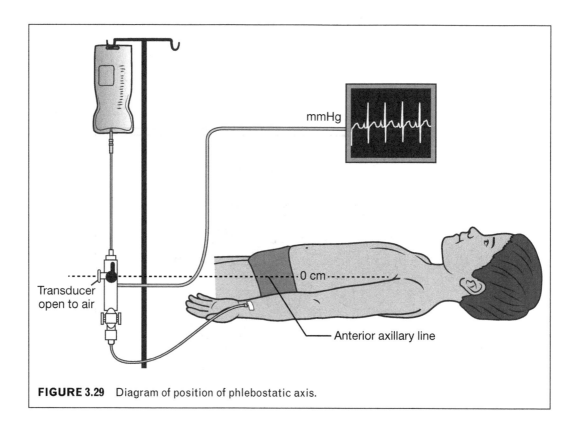

FIGURE 3.29   Diagram of position of phlebostatic axis.

which reflects the increase in RA pressure from closure of the tricuspid valve; v wave, which reflects mechanical atrial diastole; and y descent, which reflects emptying of the RA into the RV. CVP waveforms can change with arrhythmia.

d. Abnormally high readings occur as a result of RV, LV, or biventricular dysfunction, TR, tricuspid stenosis, pulmonary hypertension, hypervolemia, and cardiac tamponade. Abnormally high false readings can occur due to catheter obstruction or kinking.

e. Abnormally low values occur in the presence of hypovolemia regardless of etiology and in states of hyperactive/hyperdynamic ventricular contractility.

f. Complications of placement and use include arrhythmias, pneumothorax, infection, air embolism or thromboembolism, hemorrhage, vessel perforation or thrombosis, poor venous return, and inaccurate readings.

3. *PA and pulmonary artery wedge pressure (PAWP) monitoring* are indicated for use in the diagnosis of cardiopulmonary failure, management of shock, evaluation of abnormal PVR, treatment of patients with known pulmonary arterial hypertension (PAH) at risk of pulmonary hypertensive crisis, and

measurement of CO. The PA catheter may also provide an indirect measure of left heart function and volume status.

a. Insertion can be achieved through a percutaneous technique, cut-down technique, or transthoracic insertion at the time of cardiothoracic surgery. The PA can be accessed through the femoral, internal jugular, or subclavian veins. The catheter is advanced through the right heart structures into the PA with continuous ECG monitoring and monitoring of the waveform on the catheter as it passes through the right heart.

b. Monitoring equipment requirements are the same as for CVP, with two pressure lines for the CVP and PA ports. Cardiac emergency drugs should be available because of the risk of ventricular arrhythmias from the catheter tip touching the RV wall during passage of the catheter. A defibrillator should be available because of the risk of ventricular arrhythmias deteriorating into a rhythm that requires cardioversion or defibrillation. Blood should be available in case of perforation during insertion.

c. Normal waveform (Figure 3.32) components include the a wave, which reflects LA systole; the

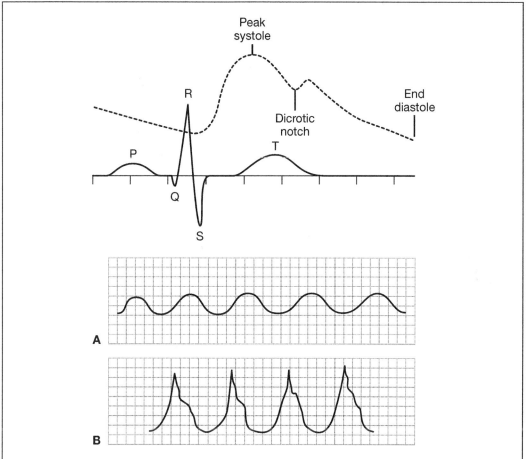

FIGURE 3.30 Diagram of arterial waveform (dotted line) in relation to cardiac cycle by electrocardiography. (A) Dampened waveform; (B) waveform affected by "fling."

Source: Reprinted with permission from Hazinski, M.F. (ed.). (2013). Nursing care of the critically ill child. (2nd ed.). St. Louis, MO, Elsevier-Mosby.

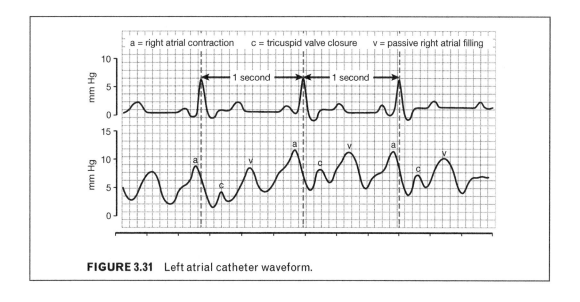

FIGURE 3.31 Left atrial catheter waveform.

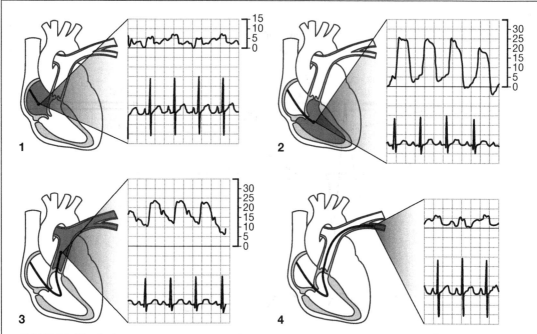

FIGURE 3.32 Catheter positions and waveforms for monitoring the pulmonary artery. (1) Catheter in right atrium (RA) with RA pressure tracing measuring A wave, V wave, and mean pressure. (2) Catheter in right ventricle (RV) with right ventricular pressure tracing measuring systolic and end diastolic right ventricular pressure. (3) Catheter in the pulmonary atresia (PA) with PA tracing measuring PA systolic and diastolic pressure. (4) Catheter in the pulmonary capillary with wedge tracing measuring PAWP.

PAWP, pulmonary artery wedge pressure.

x descent, which reflects decreased LA volume; the c wave, which reflects closure of the mitral valve; the v wave, which reflects LA filling (diastole); and the y descent, which reflects opening of the mitral valve.

d. Pressure readings:

i. RA pressure is the same as the CVP. RV pressure is normally 20 to 30 mmHg/0 to 5 mmHg, with a mean pressure of 2 to 6 mmHg. High pressure is related to pulmonary hypertension and elevated PVR, PS or other RVOT obstruction, VSD with left-to-right shunting, RV failure, constrictive pericarditis, cardiac tamponade, and chronic LV failure.

ii. The PA pressure is normally 20 to 30 mmHg/6 to 10 mmHg, with a mean of less than 12 mmHg. High PA pressure results from increased PVR, resulting from vascular disease, pulmonary parenchymal disease, MS, LV failure, or pulmonary vascular changes from increased pulmonary blood flow.

iii. Pulmonary capillary wedge pressure (PCWP) is usually 4 to 12 mmHg. High pressure is related to LV failure, MS, MR, cardiac tamponade, hypervolemia, or constrictive pericarditis. Low pressure is related to hypovolemia or vasodilation. PA diastolic pressure readings may be used to avoid risks associated with balloon inflation.

iv. Thermodilution CO can be obtained if there is no intracardiac shunt. Injection of cold saline into the RA will flow past the thermistor PA catheter and provide a measurement of CO.

e. Complications include arrhythmias, pulmonary infarction, PA rupture, pulmonary embolism, balloon rupture, knotting of the catheter, hemorrhage, injury to the tricuspid or pulmonary valve, and infection.

4. *LA monitoring* is indicated for direct measurement of LA filling pressure to measure LVEDP, or for indirect measure of LV compliance (Flori, Johnson, Hanley, & Fineman, 2000). The left atrial catheter is inserted in the operating room through the left atrial appendage into the LA for direct pressure measurement of LA pressure. Monitoring equipment may include air filter, nondistensible tubing, transducer, and infusion to maintain line patency only.

a. Careful assessment for bleeding with removal of the line is necessary. Assessment of coagulation studies and platelet counts should be performed prior to line removal if concerns exist regarding clotting in the patient. If the patient is systemically anticoagulated at the time of line removal, the coagulation values should be normalized prior to removal.

b. Complications include arrhythmia, perforation, hemorrhage and tamponade at removal, entrapment in a prosthetic mitral valve, inaccurate readings, and systemic air or clot thrombosis.

C. Hemodynamic Calculations

1. *CO is measured by* the area under the curve for change in blood temperature (thermodilution technique; Dominico & Herrera, 2015).

a. The Fick equation for CO measurement uses oxygen consumption and the arteriovenous oxygen content difference to calculate CO. This equation can calculate Qp and Qs separately. $CO (L/min) = VO_2/(AOsat–MVsat) \times Hgb \times 1.36 \times 10$.

b. *CI = CO/BSA*; enter height and weight to calculate BSA; normal: 2.5 to 4 L/min/m².

c. *PVR* is calculated using the mean PA pressure – PAWP (or LA pressure)/CI × 80; normal: 37 to 250 dynes/s/cm² or 0.5 to 3 Wood units.

d. *SVR* is calculated using the MAP – CVP/CI × 80; normal: 900 to 1,400 dynes/sec/cm² or 11 to 17.5 Wood units.

e. *Qp:Qs* is the ratio of pulmonary to systemic blood flow. $Qp/Qs = AO_{sat} – MV_{sat}/PV_{sat} – PA_{sat}$. The pulmonary venous saturation can be assumed to be 95% to 99% if there is no lung disease. Normal: Qp:Qs is 1:1.

f. With intracardiac right-to-left shunt (i.e., tetralogy of Fallot) pulmonary blood flow will be less and the Qp:Qs will be less than 1:1.

g. With an intracardiac left-to-right shunt (i.e., VSD) the pulmonary blood flow will be increased and the Qp:QS will be greater than 1:1.

h. In single-ventricle patients, the pulmonary arterial saturation and arterial saturation are equal.

2. *Oxygen consumption (VO₂)* is the rate that oxygen is removed from the blood for tissue perfusion.

a. $VO_2(mL)2/min) = CO(L/min) \times (CaO_2(mL/dL) \times 10$.

3. *Oxygen delivery (DO₂)* is the amount of oxygen delivered to the cells each minute (L/min).

a. Oxygen delivery (DO_2) = arterial blood oxygen content × CO or $DO_2 (mL/min) – [(PaO_2 \times 0.003) + (Hgb \times 1.34 \times SaO_2)] \times CO$.

b. Oxygen delivery can be compromised by severe decrease in O_2-carrying capacity (anemia, hypoxia), low arterial hemoglobin O_2 saturation, low CO.

4. *Arterial–venous oxygen delivery difference (a–vO2 difference)* is an indication of how much oxygen is removed from the blood at the capillary level. $A–VDO_2 = CaO_2–CvO_2$.

a. With low DO_2, oxygen extraction is increased to maintain normal VO_2. If increased extraction is insufficient to maintain VO_2, then CO will increase.

b. If both increased extraction and increased CO are insufficient to increase VO_2, then DO_2 will fall below critical DO_2 levels and a shift to anaerobic metabolism will occur.

c. Low a-vDO2 may be result in increased extraction (i.e. sepsis) or decreased delivery (low CO syndrome [LCOS])

5. *CaO₂ is the arterial oxygen content* and is calculated by $(Hbg \times SaO_2 \times 1.36) + (0.003 \times PaO_2)$.

6. *CmvO₂* is the mixed venous oxygen content $(Hgb \times 1.36 \times SvO_2)$.

7. *SvO₂* is classically measured from the PA. In CHD with intracardiac mixing lesions, the SVC is the preferred sampling site.

a. Normal SvO_2 is 70% to 75% with normal systemic oxygen saturations.

8. *Alveolar-arterial gradient (A-a gradient)* is the difference between alveolar oxygen concentration and arterial oxygen concentration.

a. Normal value is 5 to 10 mmHg in infants and increases with age (for each decade increase by 1). Age in years/4 + 4.

b. Not useful in patients with intracardiac shunts.

c. Assists in determining source of hypoxemia: Extrapulmonary course of hypoxemia includes low cardiac output or shock. Intrapulmonary source of hypoxemia includes pneumonia or ARDS.

d. Aa gradient = $[150 - 5/4(PCO_2)] - PaO_2$.

e. A normal A-a gradient in a patient with hypoxia indicates hypoventilation (i.e., neuromuscular disorder, CNS disease, high altitude).

f. In contrast, a high A-a gradient suggests a diffusion problem or ventilation–perfusion (V–Q) mismatch (i.e., pneumonia, CHF, ARDS, pulmonary embolus, atelectasis, pneumothorax; see Chapter 2).

9. *Coronary perfusion pressure (CPP)* is especially important in congenital lesions with severe left ventricular outward tract obstruction (LVOTO), coronary stenosis, or systemic to pulmonary shunts.

a. Coronary perfusion pressure (mmHg) = arterial diastolic BP – LVEDP.

b. Low CPP results in decreased perfusion of cardiac muscle, and can lead to endocardial and/or myocardial ischemia.

D. SvO$_2$ Monitoring

1. *Indications* include the assessment of oxygen supply—demand balance, monitoring of tissue oxygenation, management of shock states, and evaluation of parallel circulation in patients with a single ventricle.

2. *Oxygen content (CaO$_2$)* is determined by PaO$_2$, SaO$_2$, and hemoglobin. Oxygen delivery (DaO$_2$) is determined by CaO$_2$, CO, and tissue demand. Hemodynamic monitoring can help estimate CO, and blood gas analysis can provide CaO$_2$. Oxygen consumption (VO$_2$) indirectly reflects tissue demand: $CaO_2 - PvO_2 = VO_2$.

3. *One monitoring mechanism* used for SvO$_2$ monitoring is a PA catheter with a fiber-optic tip, which uses light to reflect off blood saturation (the same concept as pulse oximetry). It is floated into place like a PA line, or it is directly placed through the chest wall during surgery. The traditional PA line is used for intermittent analysis of PvO$_2$. Other tools include SVC lines, such as FloTrac, for continuous SVO$_2$ measurement.

4. *Interpretation of SvO$_2$ values* is influenced by the hemoglobin level. Anemia, cyanide toxicity, and increased hemoglobin affinity impair tissue extraction of oxygen and affect SvO$_2$ accuracy. CO, PaO$_2$, SaO$_2$, and VO$_2$ also influence values. If other factors are stable, SvO$_2$ can be used to estimate changes in CO and physiologic states of increased oxygen demand.

a. Normal SvO$_2$ ranges from 60% to 80%. Low SvO$_2$ can indicate low CO or increased demand (that the body cannot meet) such as fever, infection, shivering, burns, or stresses such as endotracheal suctioning. High SvO$_2$ can indicate low metabolic rate from anesthesia, use of paralytics, β-blockade, hypothermia, or high-output cardiac failure from sepsis (in which maldistribution of blood flow allows peripheral shunting in capillary beds and a defect in cellular oxygen utilization). Right-to-left intracardiac shunting can raise SvO$_2$ (Jesurum, 2001).

b. Continuous monitoring can be used to assess the patient's tolerance of procedures that increase VO$_2$ or to assess response to therapy directed at increasing CO.

E. Noninvasive Monitoring

1. *Noninvasive infrared spectroscopy (NIRS)* is used to determine regional venous oxyhemoglobin saturation via continuous monitoring with sensor pads. Placement in the lumbar area assesses renal tissue oxygenation (Durandy, Rubatti, & Couturier, 2010). Abdominal wall placement assesses splanchnic tissue oxygenation. Forehead placement assesses cerebral tissue oxygenation. Factors that may affect measurement are increased superficial tissue, body wall edema, or elevated bilirubin.

2. *A pulse contour cardiac output monitor (PiCCO)* is used to determine CO via two methods: (a) transpulmonary thermodilution-derived measurements and (b) pulse contour analysis of arterial waveform. It requires arterial and central venous catheter placement.

3. *PediaSat™* monitors oxygen delivery and consumption via continuous ScvO$_2$ monitoring with a central venous catheter.

4. *Capnography (ETCO$_2$)* monitors exhaled carbon dioxide via continuous monitoring with a sensor placed in line with the ETT or with a special nasal cannula with a sensor in extubated patients. It displays graphical data of end-tidal carbon dioxide and can replace arterial or venous blood gas measurement for the effectiveness of ventilation. Transcutaneous CO$_2$ monitoring using a probe to monitor CO$_2$ is another noninvasive method of monitoring the adequacy of ventilation and gas exchange.

5. *Cerebral perfusion pressure (CPP)* determines the adequacy of cerebral blood flow by measuring the difference between MAP and CVP (MAP–CVP/RA = CPP). This measurement requires continuous arterial and venous pressure monitoring. It is vital in patients with high CVP, marginal MAP, and/or cyanosis as low CPP can be a prelude to hypoxic–ischemic injury of the brain. In lesions with elevations in CVP due to single-ventricle physiology or RV dysfunction with elevation in right ventricular end-diastolic pressure (RVEDP) and RAP and low CO, the CPP should be monitored to be assured of adequate brain perfusion.

PEDIATRIC CARDIOVASCULAR PHARMACOLOGY

A. Vasoactive and Inotropic Agents

1. *Vasoactive and inotropic agents* work through α- and β-adrenergic receptors on cells. The α_1 receptors cause blood vessels to vasoconstrict. β_1 receptors innervate cardiac muscle and increase AV conduction, HR, and contractility. β_2 receptors innervate vascular smooth muscle in the lungs, and stimulation results in bronchodilation. β_2 receptors also cause arterial vasodilation. In addition, phosphodiesterase inhibitors improve contractility through the cyclic adenosine monophosphate (cAMP) system without any interaction of the α and β receptors. All patients receiving vasoactive infusions should have continuous ECG monitoring and careful monitoring of peripheral IV sites if agents are not infused centrally. Continuous assessment of hemodynamic parameters and tissue perfusion is key to assessing effectiveness of dose/therapy.

2. *Catecholamines*

  a. Dobutamine (Dobutrex)

    i. Action. Increases *contractility*, coronary blood flow, and HR by acting on β_1-adrenergic receptors of the heart. It may cause mild vasodilation by lowering CVP. It has mild α_1 affects.

    ii. Uses. To improve CO by increasing contractility of the heart without increasing vasoconstriction and afterload.

    iii. Side effects. The side effects are ventricular and atrial tachycardia, hypertension or hypotension, ventricular ectopy, headache, palpitations, and chest pain.

    iv. Pharmacokinetics. Onset of action is 1 to 10 minutes and the duration is 2 to 3 minutes. It is metabolized in the tissue and liver. It is excreted in the urine.

    v. Interactions. If used in patients with monoamine oxidase inhibitors (MAOIs), it may result in severe and prolonged hypertension. It is incompatible with alkaline solutions or those containing $NaHCO_3$.

    vi. Nursing implications. Observe for initial decrease in diastolic BP. Use with caution in a patient who is hypovolemic as dobutamine may result in significant hypotension. Observe closely for ventricular ectopy or atrial tachycardia/arrhythmia. Monitor CVP and PAP (if catheter in place) as both may decrease at start of infusion.

    vii. Dose. The dose is 5 to 20 mcg/kg/min (Taketomo, 2016).

  b. Dopamine (Intropin)

    i. Action. Dopamine acts on α-adrenergic receptors to constrict blood vessels and thus increase CO at high doses (>15 mcg/kg/min); also it causes selective vasodilation of renal and mesenteric vessels at low doses (<5 mcg/kg/min); dose-specific response.

    ii. Uses. Dopamine is used to increase CO, BP, and urine flow and as an adjunct in the treatment of shock or hypotension. In low dosages it is used to promote renal perfusion.

    iii. Side effects. Dopamine may cause arrhythmias, tachycardia, hypertension, slough of extravasation, decreased renal perfusion (high doses), and increased PVR.

    iv. Pharmacokinetics. Its onset of action is 5 minutes, it has a duration of less than 10 minutes; it is metabolized in the liver and excreted in urine as metabolites.

    v. Interactions. May cause hypertensive crisis when combined with an MAOI; is incompatible with alkaline solutions and $NaHCO_3$.

    vi. Nursing implications. With initiation of therapy, watch for tachycardia/tachyarrhythmias.

    vii. Usual dosage (Taketomo, 2016)

      1) Low dose. Administer 1 to 50 mcg/kg per minute for increased renal blood flow and urine output.

      2) Intermediate dosage. Administer 5 to 15 mcg/kg/min for increased renal blood flow, HR, cardiac contractility, CO, and BP.

3) High dose. Administer more than 15 mcg/kg/min, which begins to provide α-adrenergic effects with vasoconstriction and increased BP.

4) In the neonate, infant, and child the range is 1 to 20 mcg/kg/min to a maximum dose of 50 mcg/kg/min.

5) In the adolescent and the adult, the range is 1 mcg/kg/min up to 50 mcg/kg/min.

6) If dosages greater than 20 mcg/kg/min are required, consider changing to a more direct-acting vasopressor.

c. Epinephrine

i. Action. Catecholamine stimulates α-, β_1-, and β_2-drenergic receptors, resulting in the relaxation of smooth muscle of the bronchial tree, cardiac stimulation with increased myocardial oxygen consumption, and dilation of the skeletal muscle vasculature. At low doses (0.01–0.02 mcg/kg/min), epinephrine can cause vasodilation via β_2 receptors. Higher doses can cause vasoconstriction of vascular and skeletal smooth muscle. Effects of bronchodilation are mediated through stimulation of the α and β receptors.

ii. Uses. Epinephrine is used to treat bronchospasms, bronchial asthma, anaphylactic reactions, cardiac arrest, transient AV block, hypotension, and severe low CO.

iii. Side effects. May cause hypertension with resultant cerebral hemorrhage and stroke, chest pain, myocardial ischemia, palpitations, SVT, tachyarrhythmia/tachycardia, dyspnea, hyperglycemia, vasoconstriction, and ventricular ectopy. It may also cause renal insufficiency from vasoconstriction, nausea and vomiting, and skin necrosis if the infusion infiltrates into the subcutaneous tissue.

iv. Pharmacokinetics. The onset of action when administered via IV is 1 minute with a half-life of 2 minutes. It is metabolized in the liver and excreted in the kidney.

v. Interactions. Hypertensive crisis may result in a patient who is taking an MAOI. It may enhance the vasopressor effect of direct acting α and β agonists. It may enhance the arrhythmogenic effect of general anesthetics. SSRIs may increase the hypertensive effect of epinephrine.

vi. Nursing implications. Observe for tachyarrhythmias with initiation and progression of therapy. Observe closely for significant hypertension and follow changes in neurologic status. Follow glucose levels for sustained hyperglycemia. Assess for signs of decreased renal and limb perfusion from excessive vasoconstriction. If using epinephrine for bronchodilation, observe closely for rebound bronchospasm. Follow the patient's respiratory status closely for the development of pulmonary edema or dyspnea if not on a ventilator. If the patient is hypovolemic, correct this prior to the initiation of an epinephrine infusion.

vii. Dose. Administer 0.02 to 1 mcg/kg/min of a continuous infusion, titrating to patient effect and tolerance (Taketomo, 2016).

d. Isoproterenol (Isuprel) α_1 and β_2 agonist

i. Action. Catecholamine increases levels of cAMP, causing smooth muscle relaxation, bronchodilation, and pulmonary vasodilation, as well as increases in HR and contractility.

ii. Uses. Epinephrine is used to treat bronchospasm, heart block, bradyarrhythmias, shock, and reactive airway disease.

iii. Side effects. Tachyarrhythmias, ischemic ECG changes, hyperglycemia, palpitations, chest pain or angina, decreased diastolic BP, and increased myocardial oxygen consumption are the major and most important side effects of this medication.

iv. Pharmacokinetics. The half-life of epinephrine is 2.5 to 5 minutes. It is metabolized in the liver, lungs, and gastrointestinal tract.

v. Interactions. It may enhance the hypertensive and tachycardiac effect of sympathomimetics. It may decrease serum theophylline derivatives. The concomitant use of inhalation anesthetics may enhance the arrhythmogenic effect of isoproterenol.

vi. Nursing implications. Observe for the presence of tachycardia and tachyarrhythmias or ventricular arrhythmias. Observe for ECG changes indicating myocardial ischemia or complaints of chest pain and angina. Observe for a decrease in the diastolic BP and signs of worsening CHF as the myocardial oxygen demand and consumption increase faster than the supply. Flushing, headache, and dizziness may make the patient uncomfortable.

vii. Dose. Administer 0.05 to 2 mcg/kg/min (Taketomo, 2016).

e. Norepinephrine bitartrate (Levophed)

i. Action. Catecholamine, which affects both α- and β-adrenergic receptors in cardiovascular tissue, causes constriction of blood vessels, increased contractility of the heart, and increased coronary blood flow. The α effects are greater than the β effects.

ii. Uses. Epinephrine is used to treat hypotension and shock following adequate fluid resuscitation.

iii. Side effects. Causes tachyarrhythmias, tissue slough with extravasation, increased right and left ventricular afterload, increased myocardial oxygen demand, VT in patients with associated hypoxemia and hypocarbia, anxiety, and dsypnea.

iv. Pharmacokinetics. Onset is within 1 to 2 minutes; duration is short, generally 1 to 2 minutes; crosses the placenta excreted in the urine.

v. Interactions. Causes hypertensive crisis with MAOI; ineffective in alkaline solutions or those with $NaHCO_3$.

vi. Nursing implications. Evaluate ventricular function, kidney perfusion, and bowel perfusion due to an acute increase in afterload. Observe peripheral perfusion for decreased perfusion from vasoconstriction. Carefully assess infusion sites to avoid extravasation. Follow BP or MAP, HR, and intravascular volume status.

vii. Dose. In infants and children the initial dose is 0.05 to 0.1 mcg/kg/min; maximum dose is 2 mcg/kg/min. In adults the initial dose is 8 to 12 mcg/min titrated to the desired response. The usual adult maintenance range is 2 to 4 mcg/min (Taketomo, 2014).

f. Vasopressin

i. Action. An endogenous hormone that stimulates a family of arginine vasopressin (AVP) receptors, oxytocin receptors, and purinergic receptors that act to mediate systemic vasoconstriction and reabsorption of water in the renal tubules. It can cause smooth muscle contraction in the gastrointestinal tract by stimulating muscular V_1 receptors and release of procatin and ACTH via AVPR1b receptors.

ii. Uses. Vasopressin is used to increase blood flow to the heart and brain during severe hypotension for patients with diabetes insipidus; as an adjunct in the treatment of acute and massive gastrointestinal hemorrhage; for the treatment of persistent pulmonary hypertension in neonates, cadaveric organ donation; and the treatment of pulseless cardiac arrest and VF or tachycardia.

iii. Side effects. Hypertension, bradycardia, water intoxication, hyponatremia, abdominal cramps, mesenteric ischemia, decreased platelet count, increased serum bilirubin, renal insufficiency, bronchoconstriction, venous thrombus, and increased myocardial oxygen demand are the major side effects of norepinephrine.

iv. Pharmacokinetics. The potential exists for the drug or its metabolites to be excreted in breast milk. The onset of action is in less than 1 minute, with a peak effect in 15 minutes. The half-life is 10 minutes. It is not absorbed by the gastrointestinal tract and is destroyed by trypsin in the gastrointestinal tract. It is metabolized in the liver and kidney and excreted in the urine.

v. Interactions. There is a decreased effect when used with lithium, epinephrine, and heparin. Use with caution in patients with renal disease and those with a history of a seizure disorder, cardiovascular disease, and vascular disease.

vi. Nursing implications. Intense vasoconstriction may decrease renal, bowel, and peripheral perfusion. Assess closely for evidence of decreased peripheral perfusion and urine output. Assess for abdominal distension and bloody stools. Follow serum electrolytes closely, specifically serum sodium.

vii. Dose. Administer 0.0003 to 0.002 units/kg/min via continuous infusion for severe hypotension (Taketomo, 2014).

g. Phenylephrine hydrochloride (Neo-Synephrine)

i. Action. This is a potent, direct-acting α_1-adrenergic stimulator with virtually no β-adrenergic activity. It elevates systolic and diastolic BP via systemic arteriolar vasoconstriction, and increases the SVR greater than it affects the PVR. The increase in the SVR results in dose-dependent increases in systolic and diastolic BP and reductions in HR and CO.

    ii.   Uses. It is used for hypercyanotic spells as seen in tetralogy of Fallot, SVT, and severe hypotension.

    iii.   Side effects. It can cause hypertension; reflex bradycardia; and decreased CO, especially in patients with poor ventricular function. It can cause an excessive increase in the SVR and vasoconstriction with resultant ischemia to vital end organs. Extravasation may potentially result in tissue ischemia and necrosis.

    iv.   Pharmacokinetics. Its onset is immediate, with a half-life of 5 minutes, and a duration of 15 to 20 minutes. It is metabolized by liver and excreted in the kidney.

    v.   Interactions. It potentiates the actions of MAOIs.

    vi.   Nursing implications. This medication can produce intense vasoconstriction; therefore, observe for adequate perfusion to vital end organs, especially the kidney, bowel, and the periphery. Monitor the BP carefully for hypertension. Monitor the HR and rhythm as tachycardia and ventricular arrhythmias may result.

    vii.   Dose. Neonates, infants, children, and adolescents: IV bolus, 5 to 20 mcg/kg/dose; IV infusion, 0.1 to 0.5 mcg/kg/min titrated to desired effect as an initial dose. Increase to 2 mcg/kg/min for shock or intraoperative hypotension. For patients with infundibular spasms as seen in hypercyanotic spells, the dose can be increased up to 5 mcg/kg/min (Taketomo, 2016).

h.   Digoxin (Lanoxin): Cardiac glycoside

    i.   Action. Digoxin inhibits the sodium–potassium ATPase pump in myocardial cells and increases intracellular sodium, which increases calcium influx and increases contractility. For SVT, it acts by suppressing the AV node conduction and increases the effective refractory period and decreases conduction velocity.

    ii.   Uses. It is used for the treatment of mild to moderate HF, to decrease the ventricular response rate in fast atrial arrhythmias, and to treat fetal tachycardia in the absence of hydrops.

    iii.   Side effects. Atrial or ventricular arrhythmias can result, all degrees of AV block may occur, as can prolongation of the PR interval without arrhythmia, laryngeal edema, and facial edema. Toxicity is manifested by arrhythmia and bradycardia, blurred vision or yellow halo, nausea, vomiting, and anorexia.

    iv.   Pharmokinetics. For oral dosing, the onset of action is 1 to 2 hours with a peak effect between 2 and 8 hours. In IV dosing the onset of action is 5 to 60 minutes and the peak effect is 1 to 6 hours. It is metabolized in the stomach and gastrointestinal tract and excreted by the kidney. The half-life of digoxin is determined by the age of the patient. In a preterm infant the half-life is 61 to 170 hours; in the infant it is 8 to 25 hours; in the child it is 18 to 36 hours; and in the adolescent and adult it is 36 to 48 hours.

    v.   Interactions. Multiple medication interactions occur with the use of digoxin therapy. In particular, interactions with other antiarrhythmic medications may potentiate the side effects of either medication.

    vi.   Nursing implications. Assess HR prior to dose administration to assure HR greater than 60 beats per minute (bpm) and assess for lower HRs that may indicate AV block or bradycardia related to digoxin toxicity. Dose adjustment is required in renal impairment and is also required with concomitant use of other antiarrhythmics (e.g., amiodarone, flecainide, or procainamide). Follow the PR interval for prolongation (note any pacemaker). Assess the potassium level, watching for hypokalemia, the calcium level for hypercalcemia, and the magnesium level for hypomagnesium. Evaluate the therapeutic response of digoxin administration by noting improvements in CHF symptoms. Teach the family the signs of digoxin toxicity such as poor feeding or appetite, nausea, vomiting, and visual changes. Digoxin immune Fab (Digibind) is the antidote to digoxin and can be used in an acute and symptomatic digoxin toxicity.

    vii.   Dose. The total digitalizing dose (TDD) and maintenance dose vary with age and whether dosing is done via IV or PO. The TDD is administered over 24 hours in increments of ½, ¼, and ¼ dosing. In patients younger than 10 years of age, the dosing is BID and in those older than 10 years of age it may be daily, depending on cardiologist preference and patient compliance (Taketomo, 2014).

3. *Phosphodiesterase Inhibitors*

   a. Milrinone

      i. Action. It improves cardiac contractility and CO and decreases PVR and SVR without increasing myocardial oxygen demand or HR by inhibiting phosphodiesterase cAMP in the cardiac and smooth vascular muscle. This medication has a positive inotropic and vasodilatory profile with little or no chronotropic activity.

      ii. Uses. Ventricular failure and LCOS, CHF, and pulmonary hypertension are the main indications for use of milrinone.

      iii. Side effects. Hypotension, atrial and ventricular ectopy can be seen. On occasion, headache and angina are reported.

      iv. Pharmacokinetics. The peak action is seen within 2 minutes, with a duration of 2 hours, and a half-life of 1.7 to 2.7 hours. It is 80% to 85% eliminated unchanged in urine.

      v. Interactions. Incompatible with furosemide and procainamide when using with a continuous infusion of lasix. There is an increased risk of hypotension in patients receiving other medications that reduce the SVR such as angiotensin-converting enzyme (ACE) inhibitors.

      vi. Nursing implications. Assess for improvement in cardiac function and decreased signs of LCOS or CHF. Assess for decrease in SVR by noting increased perfusion to peripheries and urine output. Observe for onset of new arrhythmias, either atrial or ventricular. May require the administration of volume at the onset of therapy to maintain preload in the face of vasodilation.

      vii. Dose. Load 50 mcg/kg over 10 minutes, then infuse 0.3 to 0.75 mcg/kg/min to desired effect (Taketomo, 2014).

B. Antiarrhythmic Agents

1. *Antiarrhythmic medications* act to prevent, inhibit, and/or alleviate abnormal heart rhythms caused by irregular electrical activity of the heart. The mechanism of action is classified according to the effect on cardiac AP (Brugada et al., 2013).

2. *Class I* agents act by depressing the fast inward sodium current across the cell membrane, thus slowing the conduction and lengthening the refractory period.

   a. Lidocaine

      i. Action. Lidocaine increases the electrical stimulation threshold of the ventricles, which stabilizes the cardiac membrane.

      ii. Uses. Lidocaine is used for VT and digoxin toxicity.

      iii. Side effects. May cause hypotension, bradycardia, heart block, respiratory depression, seizures, and cardiovascular collapse.

      iv. Pharmacokinetics. Onset of action is in 2 minutes with a duration of action of 20 minutes. It is metabolized in the liver, excreted in the urine, and crosses the placenta.

      v. Nursing implications. Requires ECG monitoring with measurement of PR and QRS duration. Observe closely for ectopy or arrhythmias.

      vi. Dose. Administer 1 mg/kg/dose in the bolus form or 20 to 50 mcg/kg/min if a continuous infusion (Taketomo, 2016).

   b. Procainamide (Pronestyl)

      i. Action. It is a direct membrane depressant that decreases the conduction velocity, prolongs refractoriness, decreases automaticity, and reduces repolarization abnormalities. Depresses the excitability of the cardiac muscle and slows impulse conduction in the atrium, bundle of His, and both ventricles.

      ii. Uses. Used to treat PVCs, atrial fibrillation, junctional ectopic tachycardia (JET), SVT, and VT.

      iii. Side effects. May cause heart block, VT, hypotension and possible cardiovascular collapse, cardiac arrest, and bone marrow suppression. It is a negative inotropic agent.

      iv. Pharmacokinetics. Monitor levels of drug and its metabolites: procainamide (PROC) and metabolite N-acetylprocainamide (NAPA) levels. Both are antiarrhythmics. Therapeutic levels of PROC or NAPA are 4 to 8 mcg/mL and toxic levels are greater than 16 mcg/mL. Toxic side effects can occur at levels between 8 and 10 mcg/mL or higher. A combined drug level of less than 30 mcg/mL is considered therapeutic. Any level greater than 30 mcg/mL is considered toxic. The half-life is 2.5 to 4.7 hours for PROC and 6 to 8 hours for NAPA. The half-life of the medication is prolonged in renal impairment. It is excreted in the kidney.

v. Interactions. This medication should be used extremely cautiously in patients with lupus, torsades de pointe, heart block, or who are on phosphodiesterase type 5 inhibitors.

vi. Nursing implications. Monitor ECG for new or worsening arrhythmias, follow the PR and QRS duration, observe for PVCs, and close BP monitoring for hypotension. Follow the white blood cell count and platelet count at least daily for the initial 3 to 5 days of therapy and report any complaints of aches, sore throat, or new fever due to the concern for marrow suppression with this medication.

vii. Dose. In pediatrics, the loading dose is 3 to 6 mg/kg/dose over 5 to 10 minutes, which may be repeated every 5 to 10 minutes up to a maximum of 15 mcg/kg/dose. The maintenance infusion is 20 to 80 mcg/kg/min as continuous infusion; with a maximum dose of 2 g over 24 hours. These doses should be decreased in liver or renal dysfunction. The loading dose should be reduced in patients with CHF (Taketomo, 2016).

c. Propafenone (Rythmol)

i. Action. It slows conduction in the cardiac tissue by altering transport of ions across the cell membranes. It causes a slight prolongation of the AV nodal refractory period and decreases the rate of rise of the AP without affecting its duration. It decreases spontaneous automaticity by stabilizing myocardial membranes.

ii. Uses. It is used for ventricular arrhythmias, paroxysmal atrial tachycardias (flutter and fibrillation), and paroxysmal atrial tachycardia.

iii. Side effects. May cause complete heart block (CHB), blurred vision, dizziness, headache, chest pain, palpitations, taste alterations, constipation, decreased cardiac conduction, and anorexia.

iv. Pharmacokinetics. Peak action, 3 to 4 hours; half-life, 5 to 8 hours; protein bound, metabolized in liver, excreted in urine as metabolites, crosses placenta, and excreted in breast milk.

v. Interactions. Increases levels of digoxin and warfarin. Toxicity can be induced in combination with amiodarone.

Phenobarbital decreases levels. This medication should not be combined with quinidine, fluoxetine, dofetilide, or tipranavir.

vi. Nursing implications. Monitor ECG, QRS duration, observe for prolongation of QRS or the development of second- or third-degree heart block; monitor for digoxin toxicity.

vii. Dose. In pediatrics, the IV loading dose is 0.1 to 0.2 mg/kg. The maintenance IV dose is 4 to 8 mcg/kg/min in a continuous infusion. The oral dose is 3 mg/kg every 8 hours; no elixir formulation is available (Taketomo, 2016).

3. *Class II* agents are competitive β-adrenergic blockers that reduce sympathetic excitation of the heart.

a. Propranolol (Inderal)

i. Action. This is a nonselective β-blocker of both cardiac and bronchial adrenoreceptors with resultant reductions in HR, myocardial irritability, and force of contraction. It depresses the automaticity of the sinus node and ectopic pacemaker of the heart and decreases the AV and intraventricular conduction velocity. The hypotensive effect is associated with decreased CO, suppressed renin activity, as well as β-blockade. It therefore can exhibit negative inotropic, chronotropic, and dromotropic activity.

ii. Uses. It is used for the management of cardiac arrhythmias, myocardial infarction, tachyarrhythmias, HCM, and hypertension. It can also be used to treat migraines.

iii. Side effects. May cause laryngospasm, bone marrow suppression, bradycardia, hypotension, bronchospasm.

iv. Pharmacokinetics. Onset for IV propranolol is 2 to 5 minutes and the peak is 15 minutes. The duration is 3 to 6 hours when given via IV. It is metabolized in the liver, is excreted primarily in the urine, and crosses the placenta, blood–brain barrier, and is excreted in breast milk.

v. Interactions. Do not use in patients with greater than second-degree AV block or significant sinus bradycardia. Care should be taken when used in patients with pulmonary hypertension, hypoglycemia, hyperthyroidism, Wolff–Parkinson–White syndrome (WPW), and reactive airway disease.

vi. Nursing implications. Monitor ECG and BP for bradycardia and hypotension. Follow serum glucose at the onset of treatment and for 24 hours following increased doses. Assess for sleep disturbance or nightmares and in older male patients assess for erectile dysfunction. Observe closely for manifestations of respiratory compromise, primarily wheezing, or exacerbations of reactive airway disease.

vii. Dose. In pediatrics, the dose for the treatment of arrhythmias via IV is 10 to 20 mcg/kg/dose over 10 minutes with a maximum dose of 1 mg in infants and 3 mg in children. Oral dosing is 1 to 4 mg/kg/d in four divided doses. For the treatment of hypertension in children, the oral dosing is 1 mg/kg/d in two divided doses (1–5 mg/kg/d). In the neonate, treatment for hypertension orally is 0.25 mg/kg every 6 to 8 hours (maximum dose is 5 mg/kg/d) or 0.01 mg/kg via low IV push over 10 minutes every 6 to 8 hours (maximum 0.15 mg/kg every 6–9 hours; Taketomo, 2016).

b. Atenolol (Tenormin)

i. Action. It is a synthetic, β_1-selective (cardioselective) adrenoreceptor blocking agent. It has negative chronotropic properties and decreases the myocardial oxygen demand.

ii. Uses. Atenolol is used for hypertension, tachyarrhythmias.

iii. Side effects. May cause sinus bradycardia, hypotension, bronchospasm, shortness of breath, edema, nausea or loss of appetite, and depression.

iv. Pharmacokinetics. Peak levels for oral administration are achieved 2 to 4 hours after ingestion. The half-life is 6 to 8 hours and the duration is 24 hours. IV administration results in a peak onset of 5 minutes with a half-life of 7 hours. Fifty percent of the oral dose is absorbed from the gastrointestinal tract and excreted by the kidney and the remainder is excreted in the feces. There is no hepatic metabolism.

v. Interactions. Anticholinergics, such as atropine, can increase the drug absorption and nonsteroidal anti-inflammatory drugs (NSAIDs) may decrease drug activity. It may cause hypoglycemia. Caution should be used if given to a patient on calcium channel blockers.

vi. Nursing implications. Monitor HR and rhythm, observing for bradycardia or increase in degree of AV block. Assess breath sounds for wheezing and increased work of breathing. Follow BP for hypotension and glucose levels, especially at the initiation of therapy for hypoglycemia.

vii. Dose. Oral dosing in pediatrics starts at 0.05 to 1 mg/kg/d either once daily or BID. The usual dosage range is 0.5 to 1.5 mg/kg/d. The maximum dosage is 2 g/kg/d not to exceed 1 mg a day (Taketomo, 2016).

c. Esmolol hydrochloride (Brevibloc)

i. Action. It is a short-acting β-adrenergic receptor blocker.

ii. Uses. Used for SVT and hypertension.

iii. Side effects. Hypotension is the most common and most serious side effect. It can also cause infusion site reactions in peripheral IVs.

iv. Pharmacokinetics. Onset of action is within 5 minutes, with a peak effect at 10 to 20 minutes and a half-life of 10 minutes. It is excreted in the kidney.

v. Interactions. Use with digoxin will increase digoxin blood levels by 10% to 20% and potential to cause bradycardic and hypotensive actions of esmolol. It can prolong the action of anticholinesterases. It can increase the risk of MAOI withdrawal rebound hypertension. In patients with depressed myocardial function, the use of esmolol and cardiodepressant calcium channel antagonists can lead to cardiac arrest.

vi. Nursing implications. Monitor ECG and BP to observe for hypotension and bradycardia.

vii. Dose. In pediatrics, an optional IV loading dose of 500 mcg/kg/min followed immediately by an infusion of 50 to 300 mcg/kg/min (Taketomo, 2016).

d. Sotalol (Betapace; Classes II and III)

i. Action. Slows HR and decreases AV node conduction by blocking β-adrenergic activity and increasing AV node refractory time by affecting K^+ channels.

ii. Uses. Used to treat ventricular arrhythmias and difficult-to-control atrial arrhythmias.

iii. Side effects. Causes torsade de pointes, polymorphic VT, bradycardia, dyspnea, fatigue, dizziness.

iv. Pharmacokinetics. Peak action, 2 to 3 hours; half-life, 8 to 12 hours; absorption affected by food, especially milk products; crosses placenta; excreted in breast milk.

v. Interactions. Sotalol antagonizes β agonists.

vi. Nursing implications. Monitor ECG, particularly as therapy is initiated; measure QT interval; assess for bronchospasm; and prepare to treat torsade de pointes with magnesium.

vii. Dose. Dosing for infants, children, and adolescents is 2 mg/kg/d divided every 8 hours with incremental increases by 10 mg/kg/d every 3 days to maximum of 10 mg/kg/d. All doses should be adjusted in renal impairment (Taketomo, 2016).

4. *Class III* agents act on the potassium channels on the cell membrane in phases 2 and 3 of the AP, resulting in uniform lengthening of the AP duration.

   a. Amiodarone hydrochloride (Cordarone)

i. Action. Inhibits both α- and β-adrenergic stimulation, affects sodium–potassium and calcium channels, prolongs the AP and refractory period in myocardial tissue, and decreases AV conduction and sinus node function.

ii. Uses. Used to treat supraventricular and ventricular arrhythmias, JET, atrial fibrillation, or flutter.

iii. Side effects. May cause hepatic toxicity, pulmonary toxicity, fatal gasping syndrome, hypothyroidism or hyperthyroidism, corneal microdeposits, ocular neuritis or neuropathy, bradycardia and hypotension, and photosensitivity with blue skin pigmentation with exposure to sunlight.

iv. Pharmacokinetics. With oral dosing the onset of action is 2 days to 3 weeks, the half-life is 3 to 10 days and is shorter in children than adults, and the duration of effect may last 2 weeks to months. With IV dosing, the onset is within hours and, following completion of an infusion, the effects may last 2 to 3 days up to 1 to 3 weeks. It is metabolized in the liver and stored in fatty tissues. It is excreted in the urine and feces.

v. Interactions. It interacts with any class I antiarrhythmics that prolong the PR interval. It should be used with caution and dosage adjustment of any drug that is metabolized by cytochrome P450 (CYP) enzymes as amiodarone will prolong their effect. Use with warfarin is not contraindicated. Close follow-up of international normalized ratio (INR) should be maintained as elevations with and without bleeding can occur.

vi. Nursing implications. Monitoring ECG with measurement of PR and QRS durations is important as this drug may be prorhythmic. Monitor the BP if using IV infusion for hypotension. With anticipated long-term use, monitor for side effects, the most important which are pulmonary, hepatic, thyroid, and ocular changes. Patients should use sunblock, clothing, and dark glasses as this drug causes intense photosensitivity. Dietary changes, especially the avoidance of grapefruit juice/grapefruit, are also important. Thyroid levels and pulmonary function tests should be monitored with amiodarone therapy.

vii. Dose. For neonates, infants, children, and adolescents, the IV loading dose for tachyarrhythmia is 5 mg/kg (maximum dose is 300 mg) over 60 min. This is followed by an infusion of 5 to 15 mcg/kg/min. The loading dose can be repeated up to two times to a maximum loading dose of 15 mg/kg. The oral loading dose is 10–15 mg/kg/d in one to two divided doses per day for 4 to 14 days and then reduced to 5 mg/kg/d once daily for several weeks and, if no further arrhythmia, decrease dose to 2.5 mg/kg/d to decrease risk of side effects. The oral loading dose is 10 to 20 mg/kg/d in two divided doses for 7 to 10 days, then is reduced to 5 to 10 mg/kg/d daily for no longer than 7 to 12 months if possible. In pediatric advanced life support (PALS), dosing is 5 mg/kg via IV or intraosseous (IO) rapid bolus. This may be repeated twice for a total bolus of 15 mg/kg (Taketomo, 2016).

5. *Class IV* agents selectively depress myocardial slow calcium channels in the SA and AV nodes.

   a. Verapamil (Isoptin)

i. Action. Inhibits calcium ion influx across the cell membrane, producing a slowing of automaticity and conduction of the SA and AV node. It also increases myocardial oxygen delivery in patients with vasospastic angina and relaxes the coronary vascular smooth muscle, causing coronary vasodilation.

ii. Uses. Verapamil is used to treat PSVT, atrial fibrillation, hypertension.

iii. Side effects. May cause CHF, bradycardia, hypotension, asystole, and variable degrees of AV block. It should be avoided for treatment of SVT in infants due to apnea, bradycardia, hypotension, and cardiac arrest.

iv. Pharmacokinetics. For IV use, the onset of action is 1 to 3 minutes with a peak effect in 3 to 5 minutes, the half-life is 2 to 5 hours, and the duration is 10 to 20 minutes. For oral dosing, the peak effect is 1 to 2 hours, the duration is 6 to 8 hours, and the half-life is 2.8 to 7.4 hours. It is metabolized by liver and excreted in urine and feces.

v. Nursing implications. Monitor ECG for bradycardia or advancing AV block and assess for hypotension. Follow periodic liver function tests. Decrease the dose in renal or liver impairment Calcium chloride should be administered for vascular collapse and acute hypotension.

vi. Dose. In infants, the usual IV dose is 0.75 to 2 mg/kg/dose and may be repeated after at least 30 minutes. For children and adolescents up to 15 years of age, the usual IV dose is 2 to 5 mg/dose up to a maximum dose of 5 mg/dose. For adolescents older than 16 years, the initial dose based on PALS guidelines is 0.1 to 0.3 mg/kg/dose up to a maximum dose of 10. For children and adolescents, the oral dosing is 2 to 8 mg/kg/d divided into three doses, with a maximum daily dose of 480 mg/d (Taketomo, 2016).

b. Diltiazem (Cardizem)

i. Action. Calcium channel blockers inhibit slow channel influx in myocardial and arterial smooth muscle, resulting in decreased AP excitation.

ii. Uses. Used to treat hypertension, PSVT, atrial flutter, or atrial fibrillation.

iii. Side effects. May cause bradycardia, heart block, headache, hypotension, and syncope.

iv. Pharmacokinetics. Via oral administration, peak occurs in 2 to 3 hours; sustained release, 6 to 12 hours; half-life, 4 to 8 hours; IV peak, 5 minutes; half-life, 2 hours. It is metabolized in the liver, is passed into breast milk, and is excreted by the kidney.

v. Interactions. Potentiates the action of digoxin. Use cautiously in patients with renal and liver dysfunction. Do not use in patients with HCM or in patients with LV dysfunction as it is a negative inotrope.

vi. Nursing implications. Monitor ECG for bradycardia or increasing AV block. Monitor for hypotension and syncope. Administer oral doses before meals and bedtime.

vii. Dose. There are no IV dose recommendations for pediatric use. For oral use in pediatrics, the initial dose is 1.5 to 2 mg/kg/d in three to four divided doses to a maximum of 3.5 mg/kg/d. For adult IV dosing a load of 0.25 mg/kg/dose bolus over 2 minutes (may be repeated at 0.35 mg/kg per dose after 15 minutes) with an infusion of 0.1 to 0.2 mg/kg/hr can be used for up to 24 hours (Taketomo, 2016).

6. *Miscellaneous Antiarrhythmic Medications*

a. Adenosine (Adenocard)

i. Action. Slows conduction time through the AV node, interrupting the reentry pathways through the AV node and restores NSR. It also causes coronary artery dilation and increases blood flow in normal coronary arteries.

ii. Uses. Adenosine is used to convert supraventricular tachycardia (SVT), to produce AV block to unmask atrial flutter, and to differentiate junction ectopic tachycardia from SVT.

iii. Side effects. Side effects are minimal due to the rapidity of action; can see a period of sinus arrest on administration, short-term conduction blocks or hypotension, and a brief period of chest pain with bolus administration.

iv. Pharmacokinetics. It has a rapid onset of action, generally within 10 seconds but its duration is very brief. The half-life is less than 10 seconds. It is metabolized by vascular endothelial cells and erythrocytes and is rapidly metabolized intracellularly.

v. Interactions. Caffeine, caffeine-containing products, and theophylline will diminish the effect of adenosine. Digoxin may enhance the adverse effects of adenosine. Use with caution if the patient is on carbamazepine.

vi. Nursing implications. Give the medication via IV push as rapidly as possible, followed by a rapid IV flush. Be prepared for a short potential period of bradycardia or sinus arrest before resuming HR. Documentation of the rhythm, response to therapy, and the BP should be provided. When possible, having a temporary pacemaker available in the case of sustained bradycardia or heart block is advisable. Be prepared with analgesic if needed as the IV bolus can cause chest pain.

vii. Dose. The initial IV dose is 100 mcg/kg and this is increased by 100 mcg/kg/dose and repeated at 2 minutes if the rhythm does not covert. The dose is then increased to 300 mcg/kg/dose after another 2 minutes and repeated every 2 minutes until conversion of the arrhythmia or use of another therapy is indicated. A maximum single dose is 12 mg (Taketomo, 2016).

b. Atropine

i. Action. Atropine is an anticholinergic agent that blocks acetylcholine at parasympathetic receptor sites, thus blocking vagal stimulation of the heart.

ii. Uses. It is used to treat sinus bradycardia in addition to correcting other potential causative factors. May be given prior to intubation if concerned about excessive bradycardia during the procedure. May be used to inhibit salivation and secretions. It should not be relied upon for reversal of bradycardia associated with various degrees of heart block. Use with caution in patients with hepatic, renal, or thyroid impairment.

iii. Side effects. Atropine may cause asystole, tachycardia, multiple forms of arrhythmias, laryngospasm, hypotension, and urinary retention.

iv. Pharmacokinetics. Peak occurs within 2 to 4 minutes, half-life is 2 to 3 hours; atropine is excreted by the kidneys, crosses the placenta, is excreted in breast milk; a minimal dosage is required to prevent reflex bradycardia.

v. Interactions. Atropine is incompatible with most drugs. Should not be used in patients with asthma.

vi. Nursing implications. Document the response of HR to dose of medication. Monitor the ECG for new or progressive arrhythmia. Monitor the patient's level of consciousness if possible.

vii. Dose. Atropine is not part of the neonatal resuscitation algorithm. For neonatal dosing, administer 0.02 mg/kg/dose via IV, this may be repeated once in 3 to 5 minutes. There is no minimum dose, but do not exceed 0.02 mg/kg/dose. Pediatric dosing is 0.02 mg/kg/dose, which can be repeated in 3 to 5 minutes or use a maximum single dose of 0.5 mg. The maximum total dose is 1 mg. For adolescents, the maximum single dose is 1 mg and the maximum total dose is 2 mg (Taketomo, 2016).

C. Antihypertensive Agents

1. *IV Agents*

a. Nitroglycerin

i. Action. Nitroglycerin produces a vasodilator effect on the peripheral veins and arteries, with more prominent effect on the veins. It reduces cardiac oxygen demand by decreasing preload. It dilates the coronary arteries and improves collateral flow to ischemic regions of the myocardium.

ii. Uses. Nitroglycerin is used to decrease preload (venous dilator at 1–2 mcg/kg/min) and afterload (arterial vasodilator with decreased SVR at 3 to 5 mcg/kg per minute); it is a selective coronary vasodilator. May be used to treat cardiogenic shock and CHF.

iii. Side effects. May cause hypotension with circulatory collapse, bradycardia, increased intracranial pressure (ICP), headache, flushing, nausea; may potentiate methemoglobinemia in patients also receiving inhaled nitric oxide (iNO). May potentiate hypotension in patients receiving other antihypotensive medications. Contraindicated in patients with HCM.

iv. Pharmacokinetics. For neonate, pediatric, or adolescent patients, the onset of action is immediate as is its peak effect. The duration of the IV medication is 3 to 5 minutes and the half-life is 1 to 4 minutes. It is metabolized in the liver and excreted in the urine.

v. Interactions. Patients with severe anemia should be carefully monitored for increased methemoglobinemia with mitroglycerin is used. Patients on hemodialysis should avoid the use of mitroglycerin due to the potential for severe hypotension. Patients with increased ICP or hemorrhage should not be placed on mitroglycerin as this medication may further increase the ICP. Patients with restrictive cardiomyopathy (RCM) or pericarditis who are dependent on venous return for support of CO should not be placed on nitroglycerin. There are multiple drug interactions with nitroglycerin; however, in general, this medication should not be used in patients who are on systemic or pulmonary vasodilator medications or antihypertensive therapies.

vi. Nursing implications. Nitroglycerin is absorbed into soft PVC bags and tubes, therefore, non-PVC bags and tubing must be used for administration. Volume expansion should be available due to the potential for relative hypovolemia. Follow the BP and observe for hypotension. Note therapeutic effect.

vii. Dose. For neonatal IV dosing, the initial dose is 0.25 to 0.5 mcg/kg/min and can be titrated every 1 minute to the usual dose of 1 to 3 mcg/kg/min and a maximum dose of 5 mcg/kg/min. In the pediatric population, the initial dose remains the same with an increase of 1 mcg/kg/min every 15 to 20 minutes to the usual dose of 1 to 5 mcg/kg/min and a maximum dose of 10 mcg/kg/min. For adolescents, the dose initially is 5 to 10 mcg/min and is titrated every 3 to 5 minutes to a maximum dose of 200 mcg/min (Taketomo, 2016).

b. Nitroprusside (Nipride)

i. Action. Nitroprusside directly relaxes arteriolar and venous smooth muscle causing peripheral vasodilation and decreased peripheral resistance. It increases CO by decreasing preload.

ii. Uses. Nitroprusside is used to treat pulmonary or systemic hypertension and afterload reduction.

iii. Side effects. May cause hypotension and relative hypovolemia with cardiovascular collapse, bradycardia or tachycardia, decreased platelet aggregation, and cyanide toxicity.

iv. Pharmacokinetics. Onset of action is less than 2 minutes, the duration is 1 to 10 minutes, and the half-life is 2 minutes. The thiocyanate elimination is approximately 3 days. It is metabolized by combining with hemoglobin to form cyanide and cyanmethemoglobin. It is excreted in the urine. The excretion of the medication will be prolonged in renal dysfunction.

v. Interactions. It may cause methemoglobinemia and should be suspected if a patient develops signs of impaired oxygen delivery despite adequate CO and arterial PO_2. Cyanide toxicity can occur in patients on infusions with renal and/or hepatic dysfunction.

vi. Nursing implications. Protect infusion from light. It should be mixed only in dextrose solutions. Monitor the patient's cyanide and thiocyanate levels at least daily and more often if there is renal dysfunction. Monitor carefully for hypotension. Monitor CVP for preload manipulation and have volume available should there be a fall in preload. Monitor blood gases closely for acidosis, which is the earliest sign of cyanide toxicity.

vii. Dose. For the neonate, the initial IV dosing is 0.5 mcg/kg/min, titrating to effect with a maximum infusion rate of 10 mcg/kg/min. In the pediatric population, the initial dosing is 0.3 to 0.5 mcg/kg/min, titrating up every 5 minutes for desired effect with the usual dose of 3 to 4 mcg/kg/min and a maximum dose of 10 mcg/kg/min. For the adolescent and young adult, the initial dosing is 0.5 to 4 mcg/kg/min; maximum dose, 10 mcg/kg per minute (Taketomo, 2016).

c. Labetalol

i. Action. Blocks α-, $β_1$-, and $β_2$-adrenergic receptor sites.

ii. Uses. Labetalol treats hypertension.

iii. Side effects. May cause hypotension, edema, bradycardia, CHF, bronchospasm, and hypoglycemia. It may mask the symptoms of hyperthyroidism.

iv. Pharmacokinetics. The onset of action orally is 20 minutes to 2 hours, the peak effect is 2 to 4 hours, the half-life is 6 to 8 hours, and the duration is 8 to 12 hours. The IV onset is within 5 minutes, the peak is 5 to 15 minutes, the duration is 16 to 18 hours, and the half-life is approximately 5.5 hours. Labetalol is metabolized in the liver and is excreted in the urine.

v. Interactions. Use with caution in patients with asthma, bradycardia, pulmonary edema, cardiogenic shock.

vi. Nursing implications. Monitor BP, HR, and ECG for hypotension and bradycardia. Follow serum glucose levels for hypoglycemia.

vii. Dose. In pediatrics, the initial oral dose is 1 to 3 mg/kg/d in two divided doses to a maximum daily dose of 10 to 12 mg/kg/d. For IV dosing the initial dose is 0.2 to 1 mg/kg/dose to a maximum dose of 40 mg. IV dosing should be reserved for hypertensive crises. Dosing should be adjusted in renal or hepatic impairment (Taketomo, 2016).

d. Enalaprilat

i. Action. Enalaprilat is an ACE inhibitor. It prevents conversion of angiotensin I to angiotensin II, a potent vasoconstrictor, and this results in lower levels of angiotensin II, which causes an increase in plasma renin activity and a reduction in aldosterone secretion.

ii. Uses. Treats hypertension, afterload reduction, and HF when oral medications cannot be used.

iii. Side effects. May cause hypotension, nausea, diarrhea, headache, dizziness, hyperkalemia, hypoglycemia, angioedema, neutropenia, deterioration of renal function, and cough.

iv. Pharmacokinetics. The onset of action is less than 15 minutes, the peak effect is 1 to 4 hours, the duration is 6 hours, and the half-life is 6 to 12 hours depending on age. It is excreted unchanged primarily in the urine, with a small amount in the feces.

v. Interactions. Use carefully in patients with AS as a decline in systemic BP may reduce the coronary filling pressure. Use with caution in patients with HCM as there may be an increase in outflow obstruction with decreased afterload.

vi. Nursing implications. Monitor BP for hypotension, monitor renal function, and use with caution in patients with renal dysfunction. Monitor serum glucose and potassium levels and the white blood cell (WBC) count. Assess for angioedema and anaphylactoid reactions.

vii. Dose. For the neonate dosing is 5 to 10 mcg/kg/dose IV every 8 to 24 hours as determined by clinical response. For infants and children, the dose is 5 to 10 mcg/kg/dose every 8 to 24 hours to desired effect and to a maximum dose of 1.25 mg/dose. For adolescents, the dose is 0.625 to 1.25 mg/dose every 6 hours to a maximum of 5 mg/dose every 6 hours. All doses must be adjusted in patients with renal impairment (Taketomo, 2016).

e. Phentolamine

i. Action. It competitively blocks α-adrenergic receptors (nonselective) to produce brief antagonism of circulating epinephrine and norepinephrine to reduce hypertension caused by alpha effects of these catecholamines. It can minimize tissue injury due to extravasation of these and other sympathomimetic vasoconstrictors. It has a positive inotropic and chronotropic effect on the heart.

ii. Uses. Phentolamine is used to treat hypertensive episode, pre- or intraoperative treatment and prophylaxis, and pheochromocytoma. Causes extravasation with tissue injury of sympathomimetic vasoconstrictors.

iii. Side effects. May cause hypotension, postoperative pain, nasal congestion

iv. Pharmacokinetics. Bioavailability is 100% when taken submucosally.

v. Interactions. It may potentiate hypotension when combined with other agents that lower BP.

vi. Nursing implications. Monitor BP for hypotension, monitor for bradycardia, orthostasis, and the site of extravasation for skin color and perfusion.

vii. Dose. For the pediatric population, the dose is 0.05 to 0.1 mg/kg/dose. No dosage adjustment is needed in hepatic or renal impairment (Taketomo, 2016).

f. Fenoldopam

i. Action. This is a selective postsynaptic dopamine agonist (D_1-receptors) that exerts hypotensive effects by decreasing peripheral vasculature resistance with increased renal blood flow, diuresis, and natriuresis (Reuter-Rice & Bolick, 2014).

ii. Uses. This is a postsynaptic dopamine agonist that exerts its antihypertensive effect by decreasing the peripheral vascular resistance. Subsequently it increases renal blood flow resulting in diuresis and natriuresis. It has minimal adrenergic effects.

iii. Side effects. May cause tachycardia or bradycardia, T-wave inversion, hypotension, hypokalemia, elevation in blood urea nitrogen (BUN) and creatinine and liver transaminases.

iv. Pharmacokinetics. The onset of action is 5 minutes with a peak effect within 15 minutes and a duration of 1 hour. The half-life is 3 to 5 minutes. It is metabolized in the liver and excreted in the urine, with a small amount in the feces.

v. Interactions. It may potentiate hypotension when combined with other agents that lower BP.

vi. Nursing implications. Monitor for hypotension and tachycardia. Assess renal function for increased BUN and creatinine and hepatic function tests for elevated transaminases. Monitor serum potassium levels for hypokalemia. Monitor ECG for T-wave inversion.

vii. Dose. The initial dose in pediatrics is 0.2 mcg/kg/min and may be increased every 20 to 30 minutes to 0.3 to 0.5 mcg/kg/min with a maximum dose of 0.8 mcg/kg/min. There are no guidelines for dose adjustment with renal or hepatic impairment (Taketomo, 2016).

g. Clonidine

i. Action. Central α-adrenergic agonist. It stimulates α$_2$-adrenoceptors in the brain stem, activating an inhibitory neuron and resulting in reduced sympathetic outflow from the CNS. This produces a decrease in peripheral resistance, renal vascular resistance, HR, and BP.

ii. Uses. Clonidine treats hypertension.

iii. Side effects. May cause bradycardia and AV block, prolonged QT interval, agitation, depression, drowsiness, nightmares, delirium, dry mouth, dry eyes, and dizziness.

iv. Pharmacokinetics. Clonidine may be administered orally or transdermally. When taken orally, the peak effect is in 1 to 3 hours, the half-life is 6 to 7 hours. It is metabolized in the liver and excreted in the kidney.

v. Interactions. It may potentiate hypotension when combined with other agents that lower BP. It may potentiate the SA and AV nodal blocking properties of some medications.

vi. Nursing implications. Monitor HR for bradycardia and BP for hypotension. Monitor ECG for prolonged QT interval. Assess for changes in level of consciousness, sleep disturbance, and/or agitation. Encourage a sleep protocol to prevent delirium when possible. The medication should be tapered over 2 to 4 days to prevent rebound hypertension.

vii. Dose. In pediatrics, the initial dose is 5 to 10 mcg/kg/d in divided doses every 8 to 12 hours and increased gradually as needed, with a usual dosage range of 5 to 25 mcg/kg/d in divided doses every 6 hours and a maximum dose of 0.9 mg/d. Dosage adjustment in renal impairment is recommended (Taketomo, 2016).

h. Hydralazine (Apresoline)

i. Action. Decreases BP through direct vasodilation of arterioles with little to no effect on the veins and decreased systemic resistance.

ii. Uses. Essential hypertension when oral dosing of medications is not an option. Main use is IV treatment of severe essential hypertension/hypertensive crisis when urgent decrease in BP is required.

iii. Side effects. May cause shock, tachycardia, bone marrow suppression, hypotension, and lupus-like syndrome.

iv. Pharmacokinetics. The onset of action via IV administration is 10 to 80 minutes, the peak effect is in 1 to 2 hours, the half-life is 3 to 7 hours, and the duration is up to 12 hours. It is metabolized in the liver and excreted in the kidney.

v. Interactions. It may potentiate hypotension when combined with other agents that lower BP. Use is contraindicated in patients with rheumatic mitral valve diseases. May increase PA pressure in these patients.

vi. Nursing implications. Monitor closely for hypotension, especially with IV forms of the medication. Administer slow IV push and have volume expanders available. The oral form of this medication should be administered with food.

vii. Dose. In neonates, the IV initial dose is 0.1 to 0.5 mg/kg/dose every 6 to 8 hours to a maximum dose of 2 mg/kg/dose. For oral neonatal dosing, administer 0.025 to 1 mg/kg/dose every 6 to 8 hours to a maximum daily dose of 7 mg/kg/d. In the infant, the IV dosing is 0.1 to 0.5 mg/kg/dose every 6 to 8 hours, with a maximum dose of 2 mg/kg/dose. The child and adolescent IV dose is 0.15 to 0.2 mg/kg/dose every 4 to 6 hours to a maximum daily dose of 20 mg/dose. The oral dosing is the same for infants, children, and adolescents at 0.75 to 3 mg/kg/d every 6 to 12 hours, with a maximum daily dose of 7 mg/kg/d. The dose should be adjusted in renal impairment (Taketomo, 2016).

2. *Oral Agents*

a. Captopril (Capoten)

i. Action. Captopril is an ACE inhibitor, renin–angiotensin antagonist, which selectively suppresses the renin–angiotensin–aldosterone system and reduces aldosterone secretion, resulting in arterial and venous dilation.

ii. Uses. Treats hypertension, afterload reduction, and HF.

iii. Side effects. May cause acute reversible renal failure, neutropenia, bronchospasm, hypotension, cough, rash, neutropenia, thrombocytopenia, hyperkalemia, hyponatremia, and increased serum creatinine.

iv. Pharmacokinetics. The onset of action is within 15 minutes, with a peak effect in 1 to 1.5 hours, a duration of 2 to 6 hours, and a half-life of 3.3 hours in infants; 1.5 hours in children; and 1.7 hours in adolescents. It is metabolized by the liver, it crosses the placenta and is excreted in breast milk. It is excreted in the urine, 50% as unchanged drug.

v. Interactions. Causes increased hypotension with diuretics, adrenergic blockers, and other medications that have hypotensive effects. Use with potassium-sparing diuretics may cause hyperkalemia. Use with AS may decrease coronary artery perfusion pressure and result in ischemic changes. Use with caution in patients with renal insufficiency.

vi. Nursing implications. Follow CBC for a decreased WBC or platelet count. Monitor the BP prior to and an hour after doses initially to assure tolerance and lack of hypotension. Monitor HR and ECG for changes of hyperkalemia. Follow serum electrolytes and renal function, especially with drug initiation and dosage increase.

vii. Dose. The dosing in neonates is 0.05 to 0.1 mg/kg/dose every 8 to 24 hours; can titrate up to 0.5 mg/kg/dose. For the infant and child, dosing begins at 0.15 to 0.3 mg/kg per dose every 8 hours to a maximum dose of 6 mg/kg/d divided every 8 hours. In children and adolescents, the initial dose is 0.3 to 0.5 mg/kg/dose every 8 hours, titrating as needed to a maximum dose of 6 mg/kg/d in three divided doses (Taketomo, 2016).

b. Enalapril maleate (Vasotec)

i. Action. Vasotec is an ACE inhibitor, renin–angiotensin antagonist, which selectively suppresses the renin–angiotensin–aldosterone system and reduces aldosterone secretion, resulting in arterial and venous dilation.

ii. Uses. Is used to treat hypertension, afterload reduction, and HF.

iii. Side effects. May cause hypotension, headache, dizziness, renal insufficiency, hyperkalemia, skin rash, cough.

iv. Pharmacokinetics. The onset of action is 1 hour, the peak effect is in 4 to 6 hours, the duration is 12 to 24 hours, and the half-life is 10 hours in the neonate; 2.7 hours in the infant and child; and 2 hours in the adolescent. It is metabolized in the liver, it is excreted in breast milk and in urine and feces.

v. Interactions. Causes increased hypotension with diuretics, adrenergic blockers, and other medications that have hypotensive effects. Use with potassium-sparing diuretics may cause hyperkalemia. Use with AS may decrease coronary artery perfusion pressure and result in ischemic changes. Use with caution in patients with renal insufficiency.

vi. Nursing implications. Monitor BP before and after doses for hypotension and therapeutic effect. Have volume expansion available for hypotension. Follow potassium levels for hypokalemia and BUN and creatinine for renal function. Assess for the rare occurrence of angioedema or anaphylactoid reactions. Follow the WBC count for neutropenia.

vii. Dose. Neonatal dosing is 0.04 to 0.1 mg/kg/d every 24 hours; for infants, children, and adolescents, the initial dose is 0.08 mg/kg/dose once daily to a maximum of 5 mg/d and adjusted according to BP. On occasion in children older than 7 years of age and adolescents, the dose has been increased to 7.5 to 10 mg/d and tolerated. Doses should be adjusted in renal impairment (Taketomo, 2016).

c. Nifedipine (Procardia)

i. Action. It inhibits calcium influx across the cell membrane during cardiac depolarization and dilates peripheral arteries and reduces peripheral vascular resistance, lowering the arterial BP. It increases myocardial oxygen delivery in patients with vasospastic angina.

ii. Uses. Nifedipine is used for systemic or pulmonary hypertension and high-altitude pulmonary edema.

iii. Side effects. May cause CHF, myocardial ischemia, hypotension, disturbed sleep, dizziness, blurred vision, cough, and joint stiffness.

iv. Pharmacokinetics. The onset of action is 20 minutes, with a peak effect of 30 minutes to 6 hours and a half-life of 2.5 hours in adults; there is no data for pediatrics. It is metabolized in the liver and is excreted in the urine and feces.

v. Interactions. Cimetidine, ciprofloxacin, and erythromycin will increase the effects of nifedipine. Quinidine levels are decreased with concomitant administration. Use with caution in patients with HCM. Use of calcium channel blockers in HF has been shown to have no effect or worsen outcomes in adults and it may only be used in patients when other medications are not tolerated.

vi. Nursing implications. Monitor BP for hypotension. It is difficult to administer in young children because it is available only as a sublingual capsule that might require aspiration to obtain the appropriate dose.

vii. Dose. In children and adolescents using the extended release form of the medication, the initial dose is 0.25 to 0.5 mg/kg/d once daily or in two divided doses per day. Titrate to dose effect with a maximum dose of 3 mg/kg/d 10 mg/dose (Taketomo, 2016).

D. Anticoagulation and Antiplatelet Agents

1. *Anticoagulation With IV Medications*

   a. Heparin

      i. Action. Potentiates the action of antithrombin III and thereby inactivates thrombin (as well as activated coagulation factors IX, X, XI, XII, and plasmin) and prevents the conversion of fibrinogen to fibrin; heparin also stimulates release of lipoprotein lipase (lipoprotein lipase hydrolyzes triglycerides to glycerol and free fatty acids; Giglia et al., 2013; Rummell, 2013).

      ii. Uses. Heparin is used to treat systemic anticoagulation, thromboprophylaxis (severe ventricular dysfunction, mechanical prosthetic valve, synthetic shunt, mechanical circulatory support), and to maintain central-line patency.

      iii. Side effects. Thrombocytopenia, heparin-induced thrombocytopenia (HIT), hemorrhage.

      iv. Pharmacokinetics. Heparin potentiates antithrombin III and inactivates thrombin. It prevents fibrinogen from converting to fibrin. It also stimulates the release of lipoprotein lipase. It has a rapid onset of action, in 20 to 30 minutes following IV initiation. The half-life elimination is dependent on age. In the preterm infant, the half-life is shorter, approximately 35 to 41 minutes. In the infant and older child, the half-life is a mean of 1.5 hours. The half-life of a bolus is 30 to 60 minutes. It is excreted rapidly through nonrenal mechanisms and does not require adjustment with renal impairment.

      v. Interactions. Heparin interacts with many medications, specifically medications that have antiplatelet properties. Use with caution in preterm infants; it causes bleeding and thrombocytopenia.

      vi. Nursing implications. Monitor platelets, hemoglobin, hematocrit, signs of bleeding; fecal occult blood test; activated PTT (aPTT; or antifactor Xa activity levels) or ACT. Use with caution—many concentrations are available. Monitor PTT 4 to 6 hours after initiation of continuous infusion and with each titration.

      vii. Dose. IV bolus is 50 to 75 units/kg/dose. Continuous IV infusion: 10 to 20 units/kg/hr (continuous infusions are titrated to achieve therapeutic PTT; Taketomo, 2016).

   b. Argatroban

      i. Action. Highly selective thrombin inhibitor.

      ii. Uses. Used for anticoagulation effect in patients with HIT.

      iii. Side effects. May cause bleeding.

      iv. Pharmacokinetics. This has a direct and highly selective thrombin inhibitor. It reversely binds to the active thrombin site of free and clot-associated thrombin. It will inhibit fibrin formation; activation of coagulation factors V, VIII, XIII; activation of protein C; and platelet aggregation. It is hepatically metabolized. The onset of action is immediate with a time to peak steady state of 1 to 3 hours. The half-life is 39 to 51 minutes and in hepatic impairment is 181 minutes.

      v. Interactions. Argatroban may elevate PT/INR levels in the absence of warfarin, may require monitoring with chromogenic factor X assay.

      vi. Nursing implications. Monitor platelets, hemoglobin, hematocrit, aPTT, signs and symptoms of bleeding.

      vii. Dose. The initial continuous infusion dose is 0.75 mcg/kg/min. Continuous infusions are titrated to achieve therapeutic aPTT (Taketomo, 2016).

2. *Anticoagulation With Subcutaneous Agents*

   a. Enoxaparin

      i. Action. Inhibits thrombosis by inactivating factor Xa (FXa).

      ii. Uses. Used for prophylaxis and treatment of thrombus.

      iii. Side effects. May cause bleeding.

      iv. Pharmacokinetics. Enoxaparin is metabolized in the liver and excreted in the urine. Clearance of the drug is decreased by 30% in patients with CrCl less than 30 mL/

min. The peak effect occurs in 3 to 5 hours and the half-life of the drug is 4.5 to 7 hours.

v. Interactions. Use with caution with NSAID due to increased bleeding risk.

vi. Nursing implications. Monitor CBC with platelets, stool occult blood tests, serum creatinine and potassium; antifactor Xa activity. Dosing adjustments may be needed with changes in renal function. Anti-Xa levels should be drawn 4 to 6 hours after administration, often after 2 to 4 doses to assess therapeutic level.

vii. Dose. In infants 1 to younger than 2 months: Prophylaxis: Administer a 0.75 mg/kg/dose every 12 hours; treatment: administer 1.5 mg/kg/dose every 12 hours. In infants 2 months or older and children younger than 18 years: Prophylaxis: Administer 0.5 mg/kg/dose every 12 hours; treatment: administer 1 mg/kg/dose every 12 hours (Taketomo, 2016).

b. Fondaparinux

i. Action. Selectively binds to antithrombin III (ATIII); neutralizes factor Xa, which disrupts the blood coagulation cascade and inhibits thrombin formation and thrombus development.

ii. Uses. Used for prophylaxis and treatment of deep vein thrombosis (DVT), pulmonary embolism.

iii. Side effects. May cause bleeding, thrombocytopenia, injection site irritation, fever.

iv. Pharmacokinetics. Peak concentration is 3 hours after SQ administration, elimination is prolonged with renal impairment.

v. Interactions. Not recommended if weight is less than 50 kg or in patients with renal impairment or thrombocytopenia.

vi. Nursing implications. Safety and efficacy in pediatric patients have not been established. Do not give intramuscularly (IM). Not recommended in patients with a platelet count less than 100,000.

vii. Dose. Administer 2.5 to 10 mg SQ daily (Taketomo, 2016).

3. *Anticoagulation With Oral Agents*

a. Warfarin

i. Action. Reduces functional vitamin K, which impairs vitamin K-dependent coagulation factors II, VII, IX, and X.

ii. Uses. Prophylaxis and treatment of venous thrombosis, pulmonary embolism, and thromboembolic disorders; prevention and treatment of thromboembolic complications in patients with prosthetic heart valves.

iii. Side effects. May cause hemorrhage, hemoptysis, and bruising.

iv. Pharmacokinetics. This is a vitamin K antagonist. Hepatic synthesis of coagulation factors II, VII, IX, X, and proteins C and S will require the presence of vitamin K. Warfarin competitively inhibits vitamin K complex and depletes functional vitamin K reserves and thus reduces synthesis of these active clotting factors. It does not need to be adjusted in renal impairment. It is metabolized in the liver. The onset of action is 24 to 72 hours, with a peak effect in 5 to 7 days. The duration of effect is 2 to 5 days. The half-life is 20 to 60 hours and is highly variable. The time to a peak level is 4 hours following an oral dose. Younger children generally require higher doses to achieve desired effects. Onset: 24 to 72 hours.

v. Interactions. The diet should be well controlled with avoidance of foods or supplements rich in vitamin K. Alcohol binge drinking can increase the INR by decreasing the metabolism of warfarin. Chronic alcohol use increases warfarin metabolism and decreases the INR. Warfarin causes multiple drug interactions.

vi. Nursing implications. Monitor the parameter: PT/INR.

vii. Dose. Administer 0.1 to 0.2 mg/kg (initial loading dose). Titrate dose to achieve therapeutic INR (Murray et al., 2015; Taketomo, 2016).

b. Apixaban

i. Action. Apixaban is a selective active site inhibitor of free and clot-bound FXa, resulting in decreased thrombin generation and thrombus formation.

ii. Uses. Used for prophylaxis and treatment of DVT or pulmonary embolism.

iii. Side effects. May cause bleeding.

iv. Pharmacokinetics. Absorption affected by food intake.

v. Interactions. Multiple drug interactions, including antifungal medications (ketoconazole), NSAIDs, antiplatelet agents, and some antiepilepsy medications (phenytoin, carbamazepine).

vi. Nursing implications. Safety and efficacy for pediatric dosing is not established; no specific monitoring has been determined.

vii. Dose. Administer 2.5 to 10 mg orally twice daily (Taketomo, 2016).

c. Rivaroxaban

i. Action. Selectively inhibits factor Xa without the need of a cofactor (i.e., antithrombin III) for activity.

ii. Uses. Used to treat acute coronary syndrome, atrial fibrillation, treatment and prophylaxis of DVT, and pulmonary embolism.

iii. Side effects. May cause bleeding.

iv. Pharmacokinetics. Hepatic metabolism, is eliminated by kidneys, food increases bioavailability.

v. Interactions. Has multiple drug interactions, including antifungal medications (ketoconazole), NSAIDs, antiplatelet agents, and some antiepilepsy medications (phenytoin, carbamazepine).

vi. Nursing implications. Safety and effectiveness in pediatric patients have not been established. No therapeutic lab monitoring has been established.

vii. Dose. Administer 5 to 30 mg/d once or twice daily (Taketomo, 2016).

4. *Anticoagulation With Antiplatelet Agents*

a. Aspirin

i. Action. Inhibits platelet aggregation by inhibiting cyclooxygenase-1 and 2 (COX-1 and 2) enzymes.

ii. Uses. Treats Kawasaki disease; thrombus prophylaxis (shunts, single ventricle anatomy, bioprosthetic valves, ventricular dysfunction, coronary stenosis, or injury).

iii. Side effects. May cause bleeding, GI upset.

iv. Pharmacokinetics. Is metabolized primarily by the liver.

v. Interactions. Certain foods may increase salicylate accumulation.

vi. Nursing implications. Monitor serum salicylate concentration. Avoid use with liver impairment due to increased risk for bleeding.

vii. Dose. Administer 1 to 5 mg/kg/d. Higher doses of 80 to 100 mg/kg/d divided into four doses daily may be used in Kawasaki disease (Taketomo, 2016).

b. Clopidogrel

i. Action. Decreases platelet aggregation by blocking the P2Y12 component of adenosine diphosphate (ADP) receptors on the platelet surface (Li & Newburger, 2010).

ii. Uses. Is used to reduce atherothrombotic events.

iii. Side effects. May cause bleeding.

iv. Pharmacokinetics. It does not need to be adjusted with renal or hepatic impairment. It is metabolized in the liver. The duration of action is 5 days after the medication is discontinued. Absorption is rapid. The half-life is 6 hours and the time to peak effect is 45 minutes.

v. Interactions. Interacts with grapefruit juice.

vi. Nursing implications. Monitor mean inhibition of platelet aggregation.

vii. Dose. In infants younger than 24 months: Administer 0.2 mg/kg/dose once daily; in children older than 2 years: administer 1 mg/kg once daily (Taketomo, 2016).

c. *Dipyridamole*

i. Action. Inhibits platelet aggregation and may cause vasodilation by inhibiting the activity of adenosine deaminase and phosphodiesterase.

ii. Uses. Prevents thrombosis.

iii. Side effects. May cause abdominal distress, hepatic insufficiency.

iv. Pharmacokinetics. Absorption is slow and variable.

v. Interactions. Caffeine and more than 200 drugs are known to interact with dipyridamole.

vi. Nursing implications. Avoid administration distal to the stomach.

vii. Dose. Oral: Administer 3 to 6 mg/kg/d in three divided doses (Taketomo, 2016).

E. Pulmonary Hypertension Agents

1. *Prostanoids*

a. Epoprostenol, treprostinil, iloprost

i. Action. Stimulates vasodilation of pulmonary and systemic arterial vascular beds.

ii. Uses. Treats pulmonary hypertension.

iii. Side effects. May cause flushing, hypotension, bradycardia.

iv. Pharmacokinetics. Hepatic metabolism, renal excretion, half-life is greater than 6 minutes.

v. Interactions. Use with caution with medications that cause hypotension.

vi. Nursing implications. IV medication should have a designated line. Avoid abrupt discontinuation of medication.

vii. Dose. Epoprostenol. Administer 2 to 80 nanograms/kg/min. Treprostinil: Safety and effectiveness are not established in pediatric patients. Iloprost: Initial dose used in a study, 7.5 mcg/d INHALED if 10 kg or less; 12.5 mcg/d if 10 to 20 kg; 17.5 mcg/d if 20 to 30 kg; 22.5 mcg/d if 30 to 40 kg; 30 mcg/d if 40 kg or greater; administer in divided doses six times/d; adjust dose and frequency (up to nine times/d) based on patient tolerance and clinical condition (Taketomo, 2016).

2. *Endothelin-1 Receptor Antagonists*

   a. Bosentan, ambrisentan, macitentan

   i. Action. An endothelian receptor antagonist that blocks endothelin receptors on endothelium and vascular smooth muscle (stimulation of these receptors is associated with vasoconstriction).

   ii. Uses. Used to treat pulmonary hypertension.

   iii. Side effects. May cause flushing, hypotension, headache, hepatic dysfunction.

   iv. Pharmacokinetics. May be taken with food. This medication requires biotransformation to an active metabolite. The active metabolite irreversibly blocks the P2Y12 component of ADP receptors on the platelet surface, which prevents activation of the receptor complex and reduces platelet aggregations. Platelets blocked by clopidogrel are affected for the remainder of their lifespan (7–10 days).

   v. Interactions. Causes multiple drug interactions.

   vi. Nursing implications. Monitor liver aminotransferases and hemoglobin; is a teratogen.

   vii. Bosentan dose (weight-based dosing). Children 2 years or older, administer

initial 0.75 to 1 mg/kg/dose twice daily for 4 weeks (maximum dose: 62.5 mg) then increase to maintenance dose of 2 mg/kg/dose twice daily (maximum dose: ≤40 kg: 62.5 mg; maximum dose: >40 kg: 125 mg); adolescents less than 40 kg, initial and maintenance dose of 62.5 mg twice daily; adolescents greater than or equal to 40 kg, initial: administer 62.5 mg twice daily for 4 weeks, increase to maintenance dose of 125 mg twice daily. Ambrisentan dose: The safety and effectiveness of ambrisentan has not been established in pediatric patients. Macitentan dose: The safety and efficacy of macitentan has not been established in pediatric patients (Taketomo, 2016).

3. *Phosphodiesterase Type 5 (PDE-5) Inhibitor*

   a. Sildenafil, tadalafil

   i. Action. Inhibits PDE-5 in smooth muscle of pulmonary vessels, which results in pulmonary vasculature relaxation.

   ii. Uses. Treats pulmonary hypertension.

   iii. Side effects. May cause flushing, headache, GI distress.

   iv. Pharmacokinetics. Hepatic metabolism, is excreted primarily in stool, absorption is slowed by high-fat meal.

   v. Interactions. Do not combine with grapefruit juice; interacts with multiple medications.

   vi. Nursing implications. Higher doses are associated with increased mortality. Monitor BP, O_2 saturation.

   vii. Sildenafil dose. Initial dose is 0.3 mg/kg/dose every 8 hours, increase gradually to a goal of 3 mg/kg/d (maximum dose: 10 mg PO TID; Taketomo, 2016).

4. *Nitric Oxide Therapy*

   a. Inhaled nitric oxide

   i. Action. Inhaled pulmonary vasodilator, increases intracellular cyclic guanosine monophosphate (GMP), which leads to vasodilation of vessels.

   ii. Uses. Treats hypoxic respiratory failure associated with pulmonary hypertension.

   iii. Side effects. May cause hypotension, methemo-globinemia.

   iv. Pharmacokinetics. Systemic absorption occurs after inhalation, binds with hemoglobin and oxyhemoglobin. Excreted in urine.

v. Interactions. Use caution with medications that cause hypotension.

vi. Nursing implications. Use with caution in patients with left-sided obstructive lesions, may follow methemoglobin levels while on iNO. Rebound pulmonary hypertension may occur with discontinuation. Must wean, do not abruptly discontinue.

vii. Dose. Administer 1 to 20 ppm, higher dosage amounts are sometimes used to achieve effect (Abman et al., 2015; Taketomo, 2016).

F. Diuretic Agents

1. *Loop Diuretic Agents*

   a. Furosemide (Lasix)

      i. Action. Inhibits reabsorption of sodium and chloride in the ascending loop of Henle and distal renal tubule; increases excretion of water, sodium, chloride, magnesium, and calcium.

      ii. Uses. Treats fluid overload, pulmonary edema, HF, hypertension, hyperkalemia.

      iii. Side effects. May cause hypokalemia, hyponatremia, ototoxicity, metabolic alkalosis, dehydration.

      iv. Pharmacokinetics. Eliminated by the kidneys; oral and IV doses do not have the same bioavailability.

      v. Interactions. Lasix has multiple drug interactions.

      vi. Nursing implications. Monitor electrolytes, I/O, BP.

      vii. Dose. Oral—Administer 0.5 to 2 mg/kg/dose four times daily.

      viii. IV—Administer 0.5 to 2 mg/kg/dose four times. Infusion: Administer 0.05 to 0.5 mg/kg/hr; max dose (adult): 80 mg/dose (Taketomo, 2016).

   b. Ethacrynic acid (Edecrin)

      i. Action. Inhibits reabsorption of sodium and chloride in the ascending loop of Henle and distal renal tubule, increases excretion of water, sodium, chloride, magnesium, and calcium.

      ii. Uses. CHF and pulmonary edema.

      iii. Side effects. May cause ototoxicity.

      iv. Pharmacokinetics. Onset of action is within 30 minutes.

      v. Interactions. Has multiple drug interactions.

      vi. Nursing implications. Monitor serum electrolytes, BP, renal function, hearing.

      vii. Dose. Oral; 1 mg/kg/dose daily. IV: Administer 1 mg/kg/dose; repeat doses are not routinely recommended (Taketomo, 2016).

   c. Butemadine (Bumex)

      i. Action. Inhibits reabsorption of sodium and chloride in the ascending loop of Henle and distal renal tubule; increases excretion of water, sodium, chloride, magnesium, and calcium.

      ii. Uses. Treats fluid overload, pulmonary edema, HF, hypertension.

      iii. Side effects. May cause hypokalemia, hyponatremia, ototoxicity, metabolic alkalosis, dehydration.

      iv. Pharmacokinetics. Partial metabolism occurs in the liver. Time to peak serum concentration is 0.5 to 2 hours.

      v. Interactions. Do not take with antihypertensives.

      vi. Nursing implications. Monitor electrolytes, I/O.

      vii. Dose. Oral: Administer 0.01 to 0.1 mg/kg/dose twice daily. IV: Administer 0.01 to 0.1 mg/kg/dose four times daily (maximum dose: 10 mg/day); may be given as a continuous infusion (Taketomo, 2016).

2. *Thiazide Diuretic Agents*

   a. Chlorothiazide

      i. Action. Inhibits sodium and chloride reabsorption in the distal tubules causing increased excretion of sodium, chloride, and water, resulting in diuresis. Loss of potassium, hydrogen ions, magnesium, phosphate, and bicarbonate also occurs.

      ii. Uses. Treats HF and edema.

      iii. Side effects. May cause hypokalemia, hypercalcemia, hypochloremic alkalosis, nephritis.

iv. Pharmacokinetics. Onset occurs within 15 minutes of IV doses and within 2 hours of oral dose.

v. Interactions. May interfere with tests for parathyroid function.

vi. Nursing implications. Often used synergistically with loop diuretics, typically administered prior to loop diuretic. Monitor electrolytes, renal function, I/O, BP.

vii. Dose. Oral: Administer 10 to 30 mg/kg/d divided four times daily. IV: Administer 2 to 20 mg/kg/d divided four times daily (Taketomo, 2016).

3. *Potassium Sparing Diuretic Agents*

a. Spironolactone

i. Action. Spironolactone is an aldosterone antagonist, which promotes water excretion.

ii. Uses. Antihypertensive and potassium sparing; this is not a strong diuretic; it is also used in HF.

iii. Side effects. May cause hyperkalemia.

iv. Pharmacokinetics. Is metabolized in the liver. Peak serum concentration occurs in 1 to 3 hours.

v. Interactions. Do not combine with ACE-I.

vi. Nursing implications. Monitor electrolytes (K, Na). Monitor renal function. Use with caution if patient is on an ACE-I or other medications that increase serum potassium.

vii. Dose. Oral: Administer 1 to 3 mg/kg daily or twice daily (Taketomo, 2016).

b. Eplerenone

i. Action. Inhibits the binding of aldosterone, thereby promoting water excretion.

ii. Uses. Treats HF, hypertension.

iii. Side effects. May cause gynecomastia, hyperkalemia.

iv. Pharmacokinetics. May be taken with food.

v. Interactions. Use cautiously with ACE-I and aldosterone receptor blockers (ARBs).

vi. Nursing implications. Not approved for use in children.

vii. Dose. Oral: Administer 25 to 50 mg daily (Taketomo, 2016).

G. Miscellaneous

1. *Carvedilol (Coreg)*

a. Action. α_1- and β-adrenergic blocking agent that reduces BP with peripheral vasodilation.

b. Uses. Used to treat CHF.

c. Side effects. May cause dizziness, bronchospasm, bradycardia.

d. Pharmacokinetics. Peak effect occurs in 7 to 14 days; half-life is 8 hours; protein bound, metabolized in liver.

e. Interactions. Rifampin decreases drug levels; cimetidine increases levels; carvedilol may increase digoxin levels or mask tachycardia from hypoglycemia caused by insulin.

f. Nursing implications. Monitor liver function; monitor for effectiveness as seen by signs and symptoms of CHF.

g. Dose. Approved for use in adults. Administer 3.125 mg orally every 12 hours, up to 25 mg every 12 hours (Taketomo, 2016).

2. PGE_1 *(Alprostadil, Prostin)*

a. Action. Vasodilation occurs with relaxation of smooth muscles.

b. Uses. Used to maintain the patency of ductus arteriosus in infants with ductal-dependent CHD; is a pulmonary vasodilator.

c. Side effects. Apnea occurs in 10% of patients; fever, flushing, hypotension may occur.

d. Pharmacokinetics. Onset is in 15 minutes to 3 hours; half-life, 5 to 10 minutes; metabolized in lungs and excreted through kidneys.

e. Interactions. Potentiates effects of warfarin.

f. Nursing implications. Evaluate effectiveness by increased blood oxygenation, increased pH and decreasing lactate, increased BP, return of pulses, and distal perfusion (depending on the type of congenital heart lesion); monitor ECG, RR, BP, temperature. Monitor for apnea and seizures.

g. Dose. Administer 0.03 to 0.1 mcg/kg/min of infusion; may start at higher doses and titrate down once ductus is fully open (Taketomo, 2016).

CARDIOVASCULAR RESUSCITATION

A. Cardiopulmonary Failure

1. Assess pulmonary and cardiovascular function and assess for signs of impending cardiac arrest. Respiratory decompensation is the primary reason for cardiac arrest in the pediatric population. Children with CHD have a higher likelihood of primary cardiac arrest.

2. Respiratory failure is related to inadequate exchange of gases, either carbon dioxide or oxygen, due to a primary pulmonary process or intrinsic lung disease. Inadequate respiratory work, either tachypnea or bradypnea, will also cause respiratory compromise and potential decompensation (see Chapter 2 for an in-depth discussion of respiratory failure).

3. Initial assessment of respiratory failure includes level of consciousness, work of breathing or audibly abnormal sounds heard without auscultation, and skin discoloration, such as mottling, pallor, and cyanosis. Types of respiratory distress include upper airway obstruction, lower airway obstruction, lung tissue disease, and disordered control of breathing (American Heart Association [AHA], 2015).

   a. The first and most important intervention is to assess whether the patient is in a life-threatening situation and exhibiting absent or agonal respirations, respiratory distress, or cyanosis. Assess the rate, effort, chest expansion and air movement, lung and airway sounds, and oxygen saturation by pulse oximetry. Pulse oximetry, however, does not provide information about effectiveness of ventilation. Transcutaneous or end tidal CO_2 monitoring, if available, aids in the assessment of effective ventilation.

   b. There may be tachypnea, apnea (central, obstructive, or mixed), or bradypnea. Periodic breathing is an irregular pattern with pauses of up to 10 to 15 seconds. Tachypnea is usually the first symptom of increased work of breathing resulting from airway obstruction, pulmonary parenchymal disease, or a chest-wall disorder. In the presence of nonpulmonary disease, tachypnea without distress usually results in a normal pH. Bradypnea results from fatigue, hypothermia, and CNS depression. Minute ventilation may be low.

   c. Respiratory effort may show increased work of breathing as recognized by retractions (subcostal, substernal, or intercostal), nasal flaring, head bobbing, and seesaw breathing (AHA, 2015).

    i. Stridor is related to upper airway obstruction from the supraglottic space to the lower trachea. Associated symptoms include tachypnea, increased inspiratory respiratory effort, a change in the voice/cry, or the presence of a barking cough.

    ii. Prolonged expiration and wheezing are usually related to lower airway obstruction and can be due to bronchial or bronchiolar obstruction caused by bronchiolitis or reactive airway disease. Associated symptoms include tachypnea, increased respiratory effort, and cough.

    iii. Grunting is due to premature glottic closure with chest-wall contraction during early expiration. Infants grunt to increase airway pressure (auto PEEP) to preserve or increase functional residual capacity (FRC). Grunting is usually a sign of pulmonary disease and can be caused by pulmonary edema, pneumonia, atelectasis, and adult respiratory distress syndrome.

    iv. Rales are representative of lung tissue or interstitial disease from infection or pulmonary edema.

    v. Disordered control of breathing produces signs of inadequate or irregular respiratory rate, effort, or both. Central apnea may be present. Causes are generally related to neurologic disorders.

   d. Air entry is evaluated by chest expansion and auscultation of breath sounds.

    i. Asymmetry of chest movement during inspiration or decreased expansion can result from airway obstruction, atelectasis, pneumothorax, hemothorax, pleural effusions, mucus plug, or foreign-body aspiration. It can also result from patient fatigue in situations of prolonged increased respiratory work.

    ii. Breath sounds should be equal bilaterally, auscultated to the base in both lung fields. Evaluate both intensity and pitch over all lung fields. Change in pitch may suggest atelectasis, pneumothorax, or effusion.

   e. Cyanosis is an inconsistent and unreliable sign of distress. It may occur early in polycythemic infants or late in anemic children.

4. *Assessment of circulation* includes HR and rhythm, peripheral and central pulses, capillary refill time, skin color and temperature, and BP. Symptoms of circulatory failure include tachycardia, diminished pulses, slow capillary refill, cool or cold extremities, diminished level of consciousness or response to pain, and low BP (AHA, 2015).

a. Tachycardia may be present as a compensatory mechanism as the heart attempts to compensate for poor oxygen delivery. Bradycardia is a final common pathway for cardiopulmonary failure. Arrhythmia may be a cause of or result of circulatory or pulmonary failure.

b. Perfusion can be assessed with capillary filling time (normal <2 seconds), temperature of extremities, and palpation of peripheral (radial, dorsalis pedis, posterior tibial) and central (femoral, brachial, carotid, axillary) pulses. Diminished circulation is present before hypotension.

c. Hypotension results when compensation can no longer be maintained and the patient is then considered to be in uncompensated shock.

d. Alterations in color can be a result of poor perfusion or inadequate hemoglobin concentrations. Cyanosis is not noted until at least 5 g/dL of hemoglobin are desaturated. Central cyanosis can be the result of lower ambient oxygen concentration, alveolar hypoventilation, diffusion defect, ventilation/perfusion imbalance, or intracardiac shunt.

B. Pediatric Advanced Cardiac Life Support Protocols

1. *Initiation of PALS protocols* in the pediatric population should occur as soon as the child is noted to be without response to stimulus or has an HR less than 60. Key to an organized and effective resuscitation, roles should be identified immediately upon beginning cardiopulmonary resuscitation (CPR). All providers involved in the effort should have an identified role, specifically, the person identified to function in the role of the team leader (AHA, 2015; Atkins et al., 2018).

2. *Airway and Ventilation*

a. The goal is to anticipate and recognize problems of impending cardiopulmonary failure and to provide oxygen when these signs and symptoms present. Identification of the exact etiology of the child's respiratory decompensation can be determined following oxygen administration.

b. If the cause is identified, it should be immediately treated. Maintaining a patent airway is vital (Figure 3.34). Noninvasive respiratory support may be helpful early, but if distress progresses to respiratory failure, intubation is necessary. Oropharyngeal airways may be useful for airway patency in the unconscious child but may stimulate

vomiting in a conscious child. Nasopharyngeal airways are better tolerated by conscious patients. Measurement for an oral airway is from the tip of the nose to the tragus of the ear.

c. A bag-valve-mask device with an airtight seal and oxygen reservoir is held in place with a one-hand head tilt–chin-lift maneuver using the E-C technique. This provides the highest oxygen concentration without intubation. Hyperextension of the neck should be avoided to prevent airway obstruction.

d. Endotracheal intubation is necessary during resuscitation and for most postresuscitation care. Cuffed ETTs can be utilized in all ages with 3.0 or greater airways. Correct ETT placement may be evaluated by symmetric chest movement, equal breath sounds, end-tidal CO_2, stable oxygen saturation and HR on the bedside monitor, $ETCO_2$ detection, and chest x-ray. Other assessments, which may or may not indicate proper tube placement, include the absence of breath sounds over the stomach, condensation in the ETT during expiration, and skin color.

3. *Circulatory Support*

a. Upon identification of impending or present cardiac arrest, chest compressions are initiated. If the HR is less than 60 bpm in infants or the child has signs of poor perfusion (unable to produce a palpable pulse and BP) compressions are indicated. High-quality CPR is the foundation for basic and advanced cardiac life support and management of cardiac arrest.

b. Sudden cardiac arrest in children is not common and is usually related to a cardiomyopathy, anomalous coronary artery, long QT syndrome or other channelopathies, myocarditis, drug intoxications, or commotio cordis. To increase a successful resuscitation effort, assess for and intervene when there are reversible conditions such as hypovolemia, hypoxia, acidosis, hypoglycemia, hypo- or hyperkalemia, hypothermia (5 Hs), tension pneumothorax, tamponade, toxins, coronary, or pulmonary thrombosis (4 Ts). Prompt recognition and treatment of an arrhythmia may prevent cardiac arrest. Depending on the arrhythmia and the degree of cardiovascular decompensation, medication (i.e., adenosine) can be used prior to direct current (DC) cardioversion for conversion of the arrhythmia. If using synchronized cardioversion for SVT/VT, the dosage recommendation is 0.5 to 1 J/kg, increasing to 2 J/kg for subsequent attempts (AHA, 2015; Atkins et al., 2018).

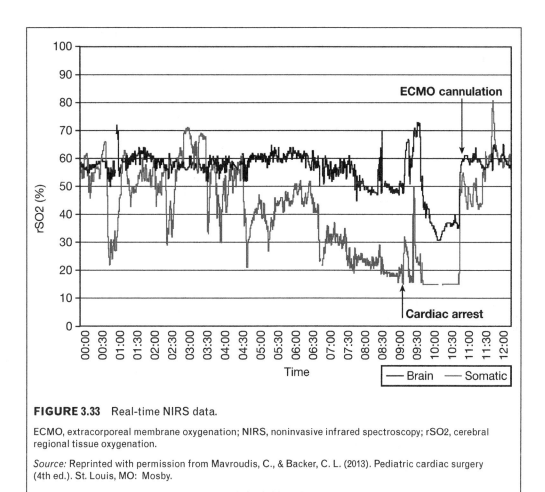

FIGURE 3.33 Real-time NIRS data.

ECMO, extracorporeal membrane oxygenation; NIRS, noninvasive infrared spectroscopy; rSO2, cerebral regional tissue oxygenation.

Source: Reprinted with permission from Mavroudis, C., & Backer, C. L. (2013). Pediatric cardiac surgery (4th ed.). St. Louis, MO: Mosby.

c. Resuscitation begins with compressions (cardiac), then assessing airway, then breathing. The compression rate is at least 100 to 120 per minute for all ages, for children younger than 12 years of age the ratio is 30 compressions to two breaths for one- and two-person CPR. For adults and children older than 12 years of age, the ratio is 30:2 for one- or two-person CPR (Neumar et al., 2015). The depth of compressions is 5 to 6 cm for adults/children older than 12, one third the anterior–posterior diameter of the chest or approximately 5 cm for children age 1 to 12 years, and 4 cm for infants younger 1 year. One hand is used to deliver compressions in children 1 to 8 years of age, and two hands are used for children and adolescents older than 8 years of age. For infants, hands can encircle the chest with two thumbs doing compressions (preferred if possible) or two fingers placed in the same location as in encircling hand technique. To allow for adequate filling of the heart, complete recoil of the chest following compression is important (Atkins et al., 2018).

d. Breathing should be performed at a ratio of one breath every 6 to 8 seconds, or 8 to 10 breaths/min. For rescue breathing only, the ratio is one breath every 3 to 5 seconds. Each breath should take no greater than 1 second assuring effective chest rise without overinflation. Overinflation from rescue breathing will result in gastric distension and possible aspiration.

e. Automatic electrical defibrillation (AED) is used for resuscitation in the nonhospital setting. Current AEDs can detect pediatric shockable and nonshockable rhythms and are now often equipped with pediatric pads and cables that adjust energy doses. An AED can now be used for all children younger than 8 years of age or less than 25 kg. All children older than 8 years of age or greater than 25 kg should have the standard adult AED pad–cable system. Children weighing less than 25 kg but between 1 and 8 years of age should have the AED with attenuated dose or use the adult system if the attenuated system is not available. Infants younger than 1 year of age should only use AED with dose attenuator or manual defibrillation. In extreme circumstances in which no pediatric pads or attenuator are available, an adult AED can be used in infants (AHA, 2015).

f. Electrical defibrillation is required when VF or pulseless VT is present. Ideally, pads should be of a size to be in complete contact with the chest but not touching each other. Front-to-back positioning may be helpful. The AHA recommends a starting dose of 2 J/kg of body weight. This can be doubled to 4 J/kg and repeated (twice) if it is ineffective. If the child is still unresponsive, epinephrine or antiarrhythmics (amiodarone or lidocaine) or both and correction of acidosis should be tried to convert fine fibrillation to coarse fibrillation. For children greater than 10 kg (roughly >1 year of age) large adult pads/paddles should be used. In children younger than 1 year of age or less than 10 kg, the small infant pads/paddles should be used (AHA, 2015).

g. Rhythm check/pulse check should be performed every 2 minutes, for no longer than 5 to 10 seconds. It is vital not to stop effective compressions for any prolonged period of time to optimize the resuscitative effort.

4. *Vascular access* should be obtained as soon as possible. Priorities for vascular access are peripheral, central venous, IO and, if unable to obtain vascular access, endotracheal medications can be administered.

a. IO vascular access (Figure 3.35) is an effective, safe, and temporary mechanism for medication and fluid administration into the vascular space during resuscitation. Access is successful if the needle is placed in the bone marrow, as evidenced by lack of resistance after the needle passes through the bony cortex; the needle stands upright without support; bone marrow can be aspirated; and there is free flow of infusions. Location of IO placement can include distal tibia, anterior superior iliac spine, distal radius, distal ulna, or the sternum.

b. Central venous vascular access is essential, permitting infusion of larger volumes of fluid and more direct infusion of medications. Recommended sites include the femoral, internal jugular, or subclavian veins.

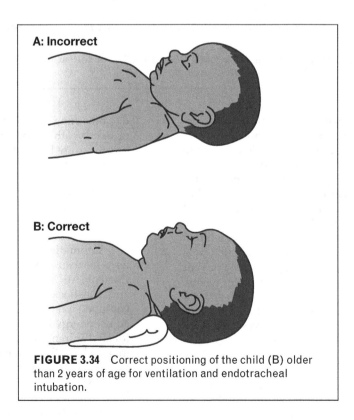

FIGURE 3.34 Correct positioning of the child (B) older than 2 years of age for ventilation and endotracheal intubation.

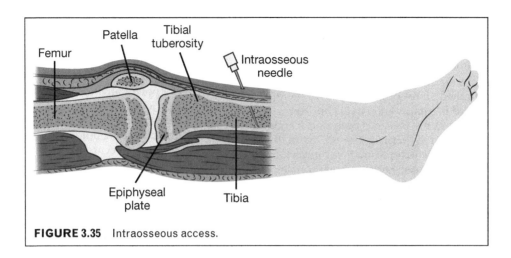

FIGURE 3.35 Intraosseous access.

c. Until vascular access is achieved or in the event that no access can be obtained, lipid–soluble medications may be given via the ETT. These medications include lidocaine, epinephrine, atropine, naloxone, and vasopressin. The drug levels and therapeutic effects achieved are unpredictable. The optimal dose is unknown but the recommended ETT dose is greater than IV/IO. Medications should be diluted in up to 5 mL of saline before instillation and injected deeply into the tracheobronchial tree, followed by five manual ventilations.

d. Arterial vascular access (Figure 3.36) permits direct BP measurement and a method for blood sampling for oxygen, acid–base, and electrolyte analysis. The radial, femoral, posterior tibialis, and dorsalis pedis arteries can be cannulated. The Allen test should be performed to ensure the adequacy of collateral circulation before cannulation of the radial artery.

5. *Pharmacologic Support*

a. Oxygen should be given in all arrest situations, for all hypoxemic patients, or for patients with signs of respiratory distress. Delivery should be in the highest concentration possible. Oxygen should not be withheld even if the measured arterial oxygen tension is high because tissue delivery may be severely compromised. One potential exception is the child with shunt-dependent circulation from specific congenital heart defects in which high oxygen concentrations may further inhibit systemic circulation.

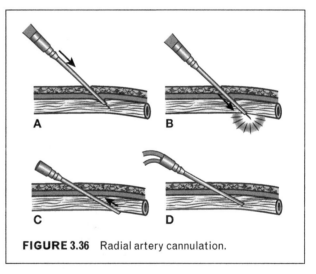

FIGURE 3.36 Radial artery cannulation.

b. Isotonic crystalloid is utilized to expand circulating blood volume in shock and is vital in preventing the progression of shock or cardiac arrest. Consider fluid resuscitation in all forms of shock. If fluid resuscitation is required, PALS guidelines recommend 20 mL/kg as the initial infusion volume.

c. Epinephrine is used for hemodynamic instability, bradyarrhythmias, and inotropic support. It may be helpful in converting fine fibrillation to coarse fibrillation following unsuccessful electrical defibrillation. Epinephrine doses should be repeated every 3 to 5 minutes during resuscitation. Vasopressin at a dose of 40 units may be given to replace the first or second dose of epinephrine. Dopamine or norepineph-rine may be used as adjuncts for hypotension. Vasopressin is effective for increasing SVR and BP without effect on HR or rhythm. Other medications to be considered include glucose because limited stores of glycogen may be rap-idly depleted in infants and small children; cal-cium chloride in the presence of hypocalcemia, hyperkalemia, or hypermagnesemia or in the presence of suspected or known calcium chan-nel blocker overdose. Sodium bicarbonate is indicated for severe metabolic acidosis, hyper-kalemia, hypermagnesemia, tricyclic antide-pressant poisoning, or sodium channel–blocker poisoning (AHA, 2015).

d. Arrhythmia therapy recommended in the PALS algorithms includes antiarrhythmic medi-cations such as atropine, adenosine, amiodarone, procainamide, and lidocaine (see "Pediatric Cardiovascular Pharmacology" section). Defibrillation, synchronized cardioversion, vagal maneuvers, and transcutaneous pacing may be used for specific patient circumstances (see sec-tion "Arrhythmias" and "Myocardial Conduction System Defects").

6. *Neonatal Resuscitation* (AHA, 2015)

a. The neonate should be protected against excessive heat loss. A method to maintain the neonate's body temperature during resuscita-tion should be available.

b. The neonate's neck should be only slightly extended and the head should be maintained in the sniffing position (see B. in Figure 3.34). Ensure a patent airway by suctioning first the mouth and then the nares. Respiratory effort and rate should be evaluated immediately. Stimulation to increase respiratory effort should not be done more than twice before further methods of respi-ratory support (intubation) are used. Indications for assisted ventilation include apnea, HR less than 100 bpm, and persistent central cyanosis in maximal oxygen environment unless known cyanotic CHD is present.

c. Bradycardia (HR <100 bpm) requires ini-tiation of resuscitation protocols and oxygen/ventilatory support. Chest compressions should be initiated for an HR of less than 60 bpm or 60 to 80 bpm but not increasing with adequate ventilation. Compressions can be accomplished using both thumbs side by side on the sternum or two fingers placed one fingerbreadth below the nipple line.

C. ECPR/ECLS

1. *ECPR* (extracorporeal cardiopulmonary resusci-tation; CPR with ECM cannulation) is beneficial if cardiac arrest occurs in infants or children from a reversible or potentially reversible cause. Indications include a patient following surgery for CHD with a long CPB or aortic cross-clamp time that results in ventricular dysfunction, with ventricular stun from inadequate myocardial protection intraopera-tively, or who has residual lesions that are unable to be confirmed in the operating room. Patients with newly diagnosed cardiomyopathy presenting in cardiogenic shock generally have a good likelihood of regaining function to either be discharged or be managed medically regardless of requiring a trans-plant later in life. Patients with hypothermia, drug toxicity sepsis, and respiratory infections can often be resuscitated with ECPR until the infection has cleared or other etiology has been treated and suf-ficient cardiac function for ECMO withdrawal has returned (AHA, 2015).

2. ECPR requires that high-quality CPR and PALS are provided and there is no anticipated nonrevers-ible end-organ failure. It is vital that the time for cannulation and initiation of ECMO is within 30 to 90 minutes from the beginning of high-quality PALS (Figure 3.33). Time frames longer than this are associated with significant end-organ damage, particularly hypoxic–ischemic brain injury and acute renal failure.

D. Postresuscitation Care

1. Once return of spontaneous circulation (ROSC; Figure 3.37) has been established, continue to assess and support the cardiovascular, respiratory, and neurologic systems. The goal is to avoid early and late morbidity and mortality caused by hemody-namic instability and respiratory complications or multiorgan failure and brain injury. During this time, investigation of underlying causes for the arrest or respiratory compromise are undertaken (Hazinski, 2013).

2. Monitoring of the patient should include HR and rhythm, BP and pulse pressure, and SpO_2. If not placed during resuscitation, placement of central access with multiple venous access ports should be secured for ongoing administration of medications and volume replacement. CVP read-ings can guide volume replacement therapy and can be used for SVO_2 and electrolyte monitoring. Echo assessment of function or possible cardiac

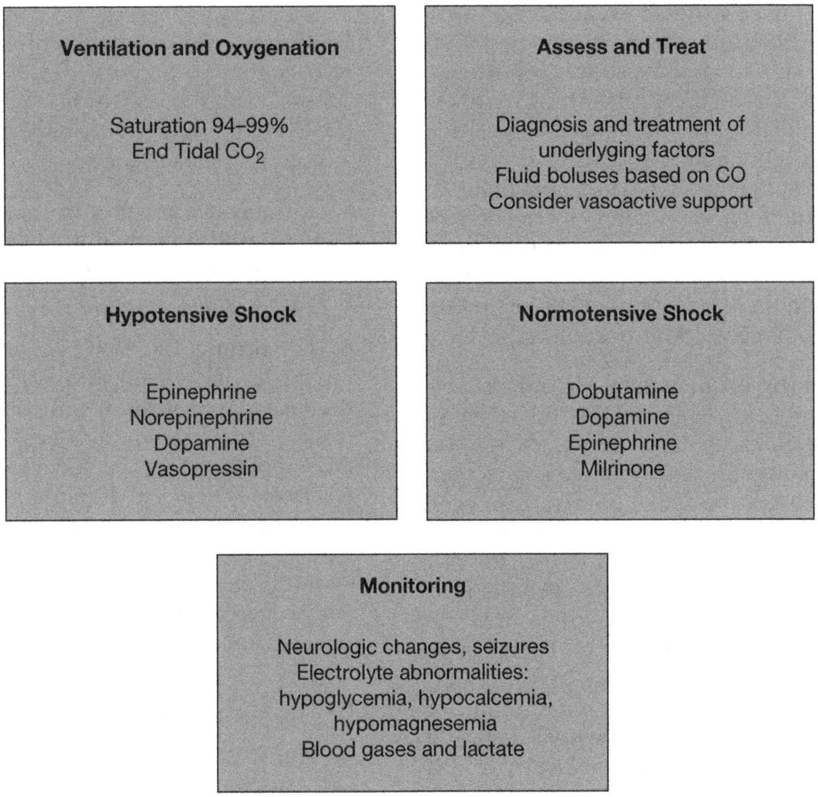

FIGURE 3.37   Management of shock following resuscitation.

anomalies that may have caused the decompensation, $ETCO_2$ for ventilatory adequacy, and NIRS monitoring for regional perfusion are obtained. Serial blood gas measurements, including lactate, electrolyte assessment, hemoglobin and hematocrit assessment, renal function, and troponin/BNP measurements assist with determination of responses to therapy and guide further intervention. Monitor exposure and environment, including the child's core temperature. A Foley catheter with a temperature monitor should be inserted to monitor temperature and urine output as an indirect indication of CO.

3. *Maintain Airway Patency and Administrator Humidified Oxygen.* Delivery of oxygen is titrated by arterial blood gas or pulse oximetry measurement. Maintain effective breathing and continuously evaluate ventilation. The goal for

oxygen saturation is 94% to 99%. If there is concern for adequate ventilation remember DOPE (*D*isplacement of the tube, *O*bstruction of the tube, *P*neumothorax, *E*quipment failure). Placement of an NG tube for gastric decompression can also improve ventilation.

4. Assessment and maintenance of adequate *BP* and perfusion, treatment of arrhythmias, diagnostic tests, and SVO_2 monitoring will optimize recovery. Assess peripheral circulation while adding continuous ECG monitoring, BP recording, and evaluation of end-organ perfusion and level of consciousness. Hypotension should be aggressively treated with medications or preload manipulation. Tissue oxygenation should be maximized, including transfusion of blood products as indicated by patient status. Myocardial contractility should be supported through lusitrophy and vasoactive agents.

Calcium levels should be monitored and calcium replaced if low. Preload should be addressed with volume replacement guided by perfusion and CVP. Afterload (SVR) should be reduced to support ventricular function. This is altered primarily by phosphodiesterase inhibitors or mechanical ventilation for LV afterload reduction. HR can be supported with chronotropic agents and correction of inadequate oxygenation or ventilation. Correction of arrhythmia with medications or mild hypothermia may be needed. Transcutaneous or transvenous pacing may be required for control of HR or rhythm not controlled with medications or cooling.

5. Serial neurologic examinations should be performed frequently to evaluate for intracranial hypertension, seizures, or focal findings. Sedation and pain management are key to decreasing oxygen demand/consumption and to optimizing oxygen delivery. The smallest effective doses should be used. Neuromuscular blockade may reduce the risk of tube dislodgement and decrease oxygen demand in situations for which ventilation pressures are high, there is patient–ventilatory asynchrony, or to protect a difficult airway. Avoidance of hyperthermia and induced hypothermia for a minimum of 12 to 24 hours has been shown to be neurologically protective in adults. Consider CT, cranial US, or MRI if there is concern regarding the child's neurologic status and potential for intraventricular hemorrhage (IVH) or brain edema. Long-term EEG monitoring will assist with early diagnosis and guide treatment of subclinical seizures in the paralyzed or heavily sedated patient. The key is to support CO and oxygen delivery to optimize neurologic function. Permissive mild hypertension may be needed. Ventilation should maintain normal CO_2, hyperventilation can be initiated if signs of cerebral edema are present. Observe for and treat seizures aggressively. Toxicology screening will guide therapeutic treatment if a substance is found. Ensure electrolyte balance, primarily glucose, calcium, and magnesium.

6. The gastrointestinal system is supported by avoiding distension with placement of an nasogastric tube. If an ileus results, ensure appropriate electrolyte replacement. Ensure adequate gastrointestinal function prior to enteral feeding and consider total parenteral nutrition (TPN) until adequate bowel perfusion has returned, lactate levels remain normal, and vasoactive support is stable and/or decreasing. Follow hepatic function tests, ammonia, amylase, and lipase to ensure there has been no ischemic injury to the liver.

7. Assess the hematologic system and replace red cells and platelets as indicated. Assess for evidence of thrombocytopenia related to the cardiac arrest or underlying disease state if one is present. Assess WBC counts for indications of infection as a result of resuscitation or as potential etiology for the arrest. Assess coagulation studies for evidence of DIC related to the underlying etiology of the arrest or as a result of the resuscitation.

8. Infection is treated with broad spectrum antibiotics until culture results are obtained. Measure inflammatory markers inclusive of CRP, sedimentation rate, and procalcitonin.

9. Renal function must be assessed closely by following urine output and BUN/creatinine. Avoid the use of nephrotoxic medications and adjust dosing of all medications based on creatinine and GFR. Follow drug levels when possible. Follow electrolytes, weight, and intake and output closely. Maintain preload, contractility, and reduce afterload to ensure optimal oxygen delivery and CO. Careful titration of vasoactive medications prevents decreased blood flow to the splanchnic and renal vascular beds.

E. Parental Presence

1. Notify parents as soon as possible once the need for resuscitation has been identified. Parents should be provided with staff support during the resuscitation process whether present at the bedside, in a separate waiting area, or on the phone (AHA, 2015).

2. Family members may express the desire to be present during resuscitation. Presence during resuscitation may assist families in adjusting to death with less anxiety and depression and more constructive grief behavior related to witnessing all efforts made to resuscitate their child.

3. Parents or family members may ask not to be present during the final moments of their child's life. Although healthcare providers should offer the opportunity for the family to be present, respect for the decision to remain separate from their child is needed (Jabre et al., 2013).

4. Surveys of healthcare providers have found that family members are not disruptive and help staff to view the child in more humane terms when present during resuscitation (Curley et al., 2012).

5. Survivors of resuscitation express satisfaction that family members were present (Curley et al., 2012).

6. Development of a hospital protocol is suggested to establish how to support family members during resuscitation. A facilitator helps to prepare the family for what they will see and remains with the family to answer questions and provide comfort. Routine grief protocols, such as bathing, hand prints and foot-prints, hair clippings, or other interventions may be helpful for families in the initial hours following the death of their child (Curley et al., 2012).

MECHANICAL CARDIAC SUPPORT

A. Indications–Contraindications for MCS

1. *ECMO*

a. The patient demonstrating severe and non-refractory postcardiotomy LCOS in the operating room or who is unable to be weaned from CPB may benefit from the use of ECMO support to provide time for myocardial recovery. LCOS immediately postoperatively as evidenced by hypotension, elevated lactate or plateau without decline, and refractory response to preload and contractility manipulation are indications for early ECMO support. Early initiation postoperatively assists in minimizing or avoiding end-organ damage and complications (Duncan, 2013; Mesher & McMullan, 2014).

b. Patients with CHD with persistent low CO despite adequate surgical repair documented by echo or cardiac catheterization are candidates for ECMO support.

c. ECMO support may be required for patients with cardiomyopathies unresponsive to medical management as supportive therapy while waiting for transplant. Some patients may have clinical improvement and are weaned from support but need to avoid complications of end-organ function in order to remain active transplant candidates (Thiagarajan, 2016).

d. Systemic illness, particularly respiratory infections with the inability to provide adequate ventilation without excessively high pressures and risk of barotrauma, will benefit from ECMO support. Failure of high-frequency ventilation to maintain adequate gas exchange but with anticipated recovery of pulmonary function can also be well supported with ECMO.

e. Post resuscitation (E-CPR/ECLS).

f. ECMO may be used as a bridge to transplant or other form of MCS.

g. In general, venoarterial (VA) ECMO provides both MCS and gas exchange. ECMO functions as support for patients with severe respiratory failure or severe cardiac failure or both. ECMO is indicated for patients needing short-term MCS, those too small for ventricular assist devices (VAD), or those who have other contraindications for support with a VAD (Mesher & McMullan, 2014).

2. *Ventricular Assist Device*

a. Support of ventricular failure while awaiting cardiac transplant can be achieved using a VAD. It will allow for improved nutritional and physiological condition of the patient entering the transplant operation. The duration of VAD therapy is anticipated to be longer than that achieved with ECMO support (O'Connor & Rossano, 2014).

b. VAD therapy may be destination therapy for HF in patients not meeting criteria for heart transplant (O'Connor & Rossano, 2014).

c. VAD may be indicated for a perceived longer time period of support in patients while awaiting recovery of ventricular function. Subsequent weaning from MCS can be attempted with a VAD. VAD support protects end-organ function and maintains the patient's ability for exercise and nutritional competence (O'Connor & Rossano, 2014).

3. *Contraindications to MCS*

a. Evidence of nonreversible end-organ function is a contraindication for either ECMO or VAD placement. This includes neurologic injury, which is life limiting.

b. Active systemic infection, whether viral, bacterial, or fungal, is a relative contraindication to MCS until the infection has been treated and blood cultures are negative for 48 hours, generally.

c. Relative contraindications include HCM in which the VAD may impede ventricular filling and preload to the device. Severe aortic regurgitation will prohibit decompression and emptying of the ventricle and prohibit adequate support with either ECMO or VAD.

d. Single-ventricle physiology is not a contraindication for ECMO with the exception of the aforementioned issues and is not an absolute contraindication to VAD support. There is increasing experience with successful use of a VAD in single-ventricle patients; however, the lack of a pulmonary ventricle may compromise preload and VAD effectiveness. Mortality with single-ventricle VAD's may be higher as compared to patients with a two-ventricle circulation. Pulmonary venous blood will continuously flow into the systemic ventricle and therefore a pulsatile VAD may not be able to completely remove the entire volume of the heart. Pulsatile VADs may cause pulmonary diastolic flow reversal, resulting in pulmonary venous congestion (Adachi, Burki, Zafar, & Morales, 2015).

e. Part of the decision for VAD or ECMO support and/or the viability of VAD support is determination of the need for LVAD only or biventricular support and the ability to implant a biVAD in the patient (Figure 3.38).

B. Management of ECMO

1. *Initiation of ECMO*

a. Maintain adequate preload and have volume readily available. Generally, the patient will require volume replacement with packed red blood cells to maintain adequate preload to the failing ventricle and due to blood loss during ECMO cannulation (Table 3.8; Butt, Heard, & Peek, 2013).

b. Modulate the SVR to optimize ECMO flow.

i. Consider the use of afterload-reducing agents such as milrinone and nitroprusside.

ii. Provide adequate analgesia and sedation, avoid elevations in temperature or excessive cooling, and monitor for seizures.

2. *Respiratory Support on ECMO*

a. Gas exchange occurs through the oxygenator of the ECMO circuit. Ventilator settings are used to maintain lung volume and expansion, prevent atelectasis and the potential for infection in collapsed alveoli, and optimize respiratory mechanics for eventual weaning from MCS.

b. Respiratory support should provide adequate pulmonary venous saturation for myocardial and coronary oxygenation and to avoid systemic desaturation due to pulmonary venous desaturation and V–Q mismatch. Expansion of the lungs to FRC minimizes increases in PVR, which add afterload to the RV or single ventricle when attempting to wean from ECMO support (Figure 3.39).

3. *Neurologic Assessment and Sedation While on ECMO*

a. Utilize analgesia and sedation as appropriate but avoid routine pharmacological paralysis if possible to optimize assessment of neurologic status.

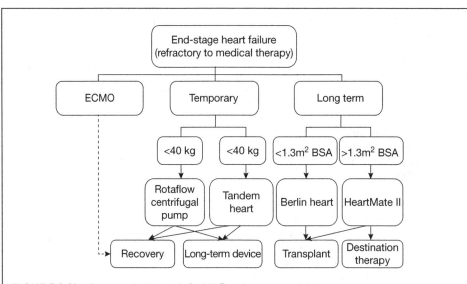

FIGURE 3.38 Proposed algorithm for VAD selection in children.

BSA, body surface area; ECMO, extracorporeal membrane oxygenation; VAD, ventricular assist device.

Source: Reprinted with permission from O'Connor, M. J., & Rossano, J. W. (2014). Ventricular assist devices in children. *Current Opinion in Cardiology, 29,* 113–121. doi:10.1097/HCO.0000000000000030

TABLE 3.8 Extracorporeal Membrane Oxygenation

	VA	VV
Description	Blood drains into the ECMO circuit from the venous circulation and returns to the arterial circulation	Blood drains into the ECMO circuit from the venous circulation and returns to the venous circulation
Indication	Cardiorespiratory failure	Isolated respiratory failure (ARDS, infectious, etc.)
Initiation	Consider after conventional medical therapy has been optimized and there is continued deterioration in cardiorespiratory status with evidence of inadequate tissue oxygenation and/or end-organ dysfunction ECPR	Consider if • oxygenation index >35 • alveolar–arterial oxygen difference >605 • PaO_2 < 35–60
Cannulation sites	Right IJ/right carotid artery Open chest RA/aorta Femoral vein/femoral artery • May require retrograde perfusion catheter May also consider need for LA vent if LA hypertension or LV not fully decompressed	Double lumen cannula • Right IJ • Right femoral vein
Gas exchange	To improve oxygenation: • Increase flow • Increase native CO • Increase membrane FiO_2 To improve CO_2 exchange: • Increase sweep gas	To improve oxygenation: • Increase flow • Increase native CO • Increase membrane FiO_2 To improve CO_2 exchange: • Increase sweep gas
Cardiac output	ECMO Flow (mL/kg/min) • Neonates: 100–150 • Kids/adults: 75–100 • Shunted SV: 160–200, or may consider placement of surgical clip on the shunt Pulsatility dependent on preload and native heart contractility	Relies on native function Preload, contractility, and afterload Vasoactive infusions Oxygen potent inotrope

ARDS, acute respiratory distress syndrome; CO, cardiac output; ECMO, extracorporeal membrane oxygenation; eCPR, extracorporeal cardiopulmonary resuscitation; IJ, internal jugular; LA, left atrium; LV, left ventricle; RA, right atrium; SV, stroke volume; VA, venoarterial; VV, veno-venous.

b. Consider EEG for any suspicion of seizures, especially if using neuromuscular blockade. Placement of continuous EEG monitoring diagnoses subclinical seizures and allows evaluation and treatment of evolving or present neurologic complications. Serial cranial US is recommended to assess for IVH. Emergent CT scans can be done for further evaluation or for early and continued assessment in patients too old for surveillance cranial US.

C. Weaning ECMO

1. Once the patient has achieved evidence of ventricular ejection by arterial waveform and echo demonstrates return of ventricular function with reduction of ECMO flow, attempts to completely wean from bypass can be attempted (Duncan, 2013).

2. Optimization of hemodynamic function with vasoactive support prior to weaning is initiated with particular attention to regulation of adequate BP for perfusion, but avoiding hypertension and increased afterload. Volume should be available to support preload. HR and rhythm are supported as necessary by medication or pacemaker. Normal rhythm and rate improve CO, decrease myocardial oxygen demand, and ensure adequate filling and emptying of the ventricle.

3. Evaluation of lung fields with (CXR) prior to the weaning procedure determines the need for

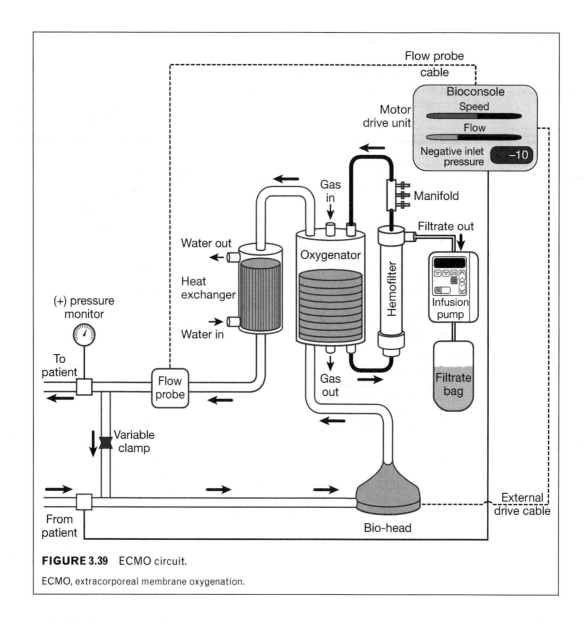

FIGURE 3.39 ECMO circuit.

ECMO, extracorporeal membrane oxygenation.

pulmonary recruitment, increased ventilator settings at the time of weaning, and the need for increased diuresis or drainage of effusions. Ventilation at FRC optimizes PVR and ventricular afterload as well as preload. Ventilator settings are set to promote FRC at the lowest mean airway pressure (MAP) possible. If significant elevations in ventilator pressures or FiO$_2$ are needed to maintain ventilation, reassess pulmonary status and patient readiness for ECMO weaning.

4. Consider cardiac catheterization in postoperative cardiac patients on ECMO who have an anatomic

repair that cannot be adequately assessed through bedside echo. Cardiac catheterization should also be considered for those patients requiring support not demonstrating cardiac recovery beyond 48 to 72 hours postoperatively. Early identification and repair of residual defects can prevent unnecessary time on ECMO and associated exposure to the inherent risks of bypass.

5. Continuous monitoring of vital signs and hemodynamic status throughout ECMO weaning guides real-time interventions and ensures the patient is tolerating withdrawal of MCS. It is necessary to monitor parameters, including NIRS; arterial blood gases and lactate; SVO_2 and A–V O_2 difference; electrolytes, particularly potassium, calcium, and glucose; and urine output.

6. *Decannulation* occurs once the patient has been off ECMO for a period of time to allow assessment of the patient's ability to maintain CO and end-organ function. Decannulation involves removal of the ECMO cannulas after a period of patient stability off ECMO support. If cannulated through the carotid or jugular vessels, repair of the vessel often accompanies decannulation to optimize cerebral blood flow in the future. If cannulated through the chest for postcardiotomy ECMO, decannulation may be performed at bedside or in the operating room. In this latter circumstance, sternal closure may be delayed to allow for adjustment to the new hemodynamics that occur off ECMO support (Duncan, 2013).

D. Nursing Care of Patients Receiving ECMO Support

1. Cannula insertion site care involves placement of a semipermeable transparent or gauze dressing to the site, per institutional guidelines. Monitor the site for signs and symptoms of infection (erythema, drainage, swelling), pressure-related injury (erythema, ulceration, breakdown), bleeding, and loose or dislodged sutures (Nieves et al., 2013).

2. Repositioning should occur every 2 hours as tolerated. Cannula placement may restrict position changes. Use caution to avoid cannula dislodgement or kinking when moving the patient or providing daily care. Maintain the proper body alignment. Use caution with prone positioning and ensure adequate sedation, line, and cannula stabilization while moving into and out of the prone position to maintain adequate ECMO flow and cannula dislodgement. Monitor skin integrity, utilize pressure relief devices, and implement institution-specific pressure ulcer prevention guidelines. The patient's bed may need to be elevated to maintain adequate ECMO flow.

3. Neurological assessment and monitoring should be performed at least hourly. Monitor responsiveness, pupil reactivity, and presence of abnormal movement or posturing. Avoid hyperthermia. Employ NIRS monitoring, cranial US or continuous EEG monitoring per institutional guidelines.

4. Management of sedation and analgesia is paramount to ensure security of the cannulas. Adequate sedation and analgesia minimize oxygen consumption. Optimal sedation/analgesia is aided by routine use of developmentally appropriate sedation/analgesia tools. Some patients may require neuromuscular blockade. Also, some patients may require higher doses of medication to achieve goal sedation levels due to tolerance and/or absorption of some of the medications by the ECMO circuit. Titrate benzodiazepine and/or opioid analgesia infusions to goal sedation level. Patients may require neuromuscular blockade. May require higher doses to achieve goal sedation levels as tolerance may develop and the circuit absorbs some of the drug.

5. Management of bleeding should be anticipated secondary to use of anticoagulation for ECMO, especially in the acute postoperative patient. Frequently reassess hemostasis. Laboratory studies may include ACT, platelet count, fibrinogen level, aPTT, and PT. Replace coagulation factors and blood transfusions per institutional guidelines to maintain adequate blood volume and appropriate hemostasis. Monitor for blood loss and bleeding. Removal of catheters, venipuncture/ heel sticks, and IM injections should be deferred while patient is anticoagulated. Use caution with ETT suctioning to avoid mucosal bleeding. When ETT suction is required, use a soft catheter and low suction level.

6. Infection assessment and monitoring are imperative due to the invasive cannulation sites coupled with invasive monitoring lines and immune compromise from critical illness. Strict aseptic technique should be adhered to with cannula placement or care. Body temperature is regulated by ECMO circuit and due to thermoregulation inherent in the ECMO circuit, patients may not mount a fever in response to infection or other potential triggers. Surveillance blood, urine, and respiratory cultures and routine monitoring of inflammatory markers are performed per institutional guidelines, generally, every 48 hours. Institutional guidelines to prevent ventilator-associated pneumonia (VAP) should be implemented, including elevation of head of bed as tolerated and oral hygiene prophylaxis.

7. Respiratory assessment and monitoring is maintained to prevent secondary pulmonary processes that may prohibit future weaning from ECMO support. Mechanical ventilation support is often

minimized with settings to maintain lung volume and minimize atelectasis. Monitor for bilateral aeration with hourly assessments. Routine ETT suctioning at a shallow depth, with caution to avoid trauma to the carina, ensures mucus clearance and prevents ETT obstruction. Some patients may benefit from lung recruitment maneuvers, including periods of added PEEP and proning. The ventilator settings are adjusted when weaning ECMO support. Emergency ventilator settings should be easily visible and accessible to all caregivers in the event of abrupt circuit failure.

8. Nutrition/electrolyte optimization promotes recovery, cardiac function, and pulmonary status. Parenteral nutrition may be given until the patient is stable on ECMO support. Anticipate initiation of enteral feeds when hemodynamically possible without the risk of bowel complications. Administration of gastrointestinal prophylaxis with H_2 blockers or a proton-pump inhibitor is indicated to prevent gastric ulcer associated with stress and anticoagulation. Monitor the patient's fluid status closely, including urine output and edema. Stress response to ECMO and potential inadequate circulatory support lead to decreased urine output and increased body edema. If diuretic therapy does not maintain an adequate fluid balance or if there has been acute kidney injury, the patient may also require hemofiltration while on ECMO. Routine assessment and correction of fluid and electrolyte imbalance is imperative to optimize organ function.

9. Multidisciplinary collaboration best promotes the safety of the child while on ECMO. Clear and direct communication with an ECMO specialist, collaboration with the multidisciplinary team, and prompt reporting of any clinical changes to providers are optimal for patient safety and reduce complications.

10. Complications of ECMO include bleeding from anticoagulation, fresh surgical incisions, and cardiac surgery; neurologic complications (ischemic/embolic stroke, IVH); respiratory complications (lack of lung expansion on rest ventilator settings); acute renal insufficiency or failure; and liver dysfunction. Patients with chest cannulation have an increased risk of mediastinal infection compared with those who are cannulated in the neck or groin. Patients cannulated in the neck can have compromised perfusion of the cerebral vessels and those cannulated in the groin can have compromised perfusion in the lower extremity. Also, those with neck and groin cannulation usually require vessel repair following decannulation. To prevent lower extremity ischemia, reperfusion catheters may be inserted.

E. Ventricular Assist Devices

1. The types of VADs in use are categorized as either pulsatile or nonpulsatile (Adachi et al., 2015). Pulsatile devices (Berlin heart, Thoratec) have a paracorporeal chamber with a fixed SV and an inner membrane controlled by a pneumatic drive system (Almond, 2013). Suction from the drive system fills the device in diastole and positive pressure during systole ejects the blood into the systemic circulation (Figure 3.40). Nonpulsatile VADs, also known as *continuous flow VADs*, include the HeartMate II, DeBakey, and Impella (Steffen et al., 2016).

    a. VADs come in varying sizes and are small enough for circulatory support in infants and small children.

    b. The incidence of ischemic stroke is higher than in adult patients, and these patients require complex and aggressive anticoagulation treatment.

2. Continuous flow, nonpulsatile systems are implanted intracorporeally and contain an axial-flow impeller pump that provides a continuous forward flow of blood. These pumps have an external power source. In early use, these devices have been shown to have a lower complication rate and overall improved outcome to transplantation as compared to pulsatile systems in the pediatric population.

3. Neurologic evaluation on the VAD is consistent with the evaluation on ECMO. It is hoped that these patients will rehabilitate sufficiently to extubate and remain ambulatory. Changes in neurologic function may be easier to assess in this population as compared to ECMO patients because generally, VAD patients are more alert, interactive, and mobile.

4. Weaning from VAD support is indicated once full pulsatile flow is noted by echo, arterial waveform, or BP measurement when the VAD flow is decreased. Echo performed while the flow is reduced can be used to determine function, response to preload manipulation, and response to vasoactive administration. If CO and DO_2 can be maintained without VAD support, decannulation can be performed, usually in the operating room.

5. Goals of care and management of patients with VADs include the following (Kirklin, 2015):

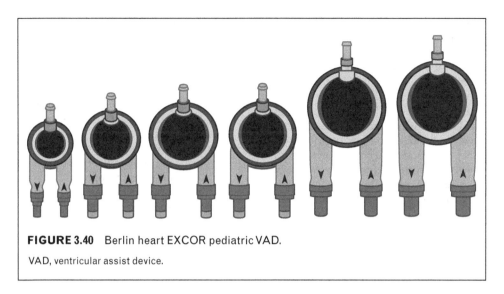

FIGURE 3.40 Berlin heart EXCOR pediatric VAD.

VAD, ventricular assist device.

a. Wound and device exit-site care are needed to promote healing, stabilize the cannulas, and prevent infection. Aseptic technique should be utilized per the VAD manufacturer's recommendations. The type of antiseptic varies per manufacturer as some substances may be harmful to the components of a particular VAD. Routine monitoring of the site for signs and symptoms of infection (erythema, drainage, swelling), pressure-related injury (erythema, ulceration, breakdown), and bleeding is necessary. Monitor skin integrity, utilize pressure-relief devices, and implement institution-specific pressure ulcer prevention guidelines as indicated.

b. Safety for the patient is maintained by securing the device to the child to prevent accidental dislodgement. Utilize an abdominal binder or a manufacturer-provided binder to provide support and offer stabilization to VAD cannula(s). Use caution to avoid inadvertent dislodgement of cannulas during care or activities, including physical and occupational therapies. Review the manufacturer's emergency procedures for loss of power, VAD failure, tubing disconnection, and inadvertent cannula removal as these procedures vary among devices. Review the location of backup devices, power consoles, batteries, and power packs.

c. Hemodynamic assessment and monitoring are important as all patients on VADs are dependent on preload for filling of the VAD and therefore for CO. Monitor CVPs closely in order to maintain an adequate intravascular volume status. Correct hypertension and cannula obstruction as the VAD's output is compromised in the presence of high SVR. Monitor and treat arrhythmias and hypotension in order to maximize VAD function and cardiac support. Monitor for symptoms of cardiac tamponade in case internal cannula erosion or dislodgement occur. Monitor the capillary refill time and quality of the peripheral pulses (in patients with pulsatile devices) as a way to monitor adequate systemic perfusion. Peripheral pulses may be absent or difficult to assess in patients with continuous devices. Monitor oxygen delivery with serial serum lactate and mixed venous saturation sampling.

d. Neurological assessment and monitoring of patient responsiveness, pupil reactivity, presence of abnormal movement or posturing are extremely important for both hemorrhagic stroke due to anticoagulation and embolic stroke caused by cannulas. Risk of seizures, hemorrhage, and stroke associated with VADs can be devastating and result in removal from the transplant list or death.

e. Management of sedation and analgesia ensures appropriate assessment and treatment of pain and the safety of the cannula placement. Routine assessment with developmentally appropriate tools is also important for ongoing rehabilitation for patients who may need to remain hospitalized while on a VAD or while awaiting recovery or transplant.

f. Management of bleeding and anticoagulation is paramount to avoid stroke, hemorrhage, and device malfunction from emboli or clot. Replacement of coagulation factors and blood transfusions per institutional guidelines may be needed to maintain adequate blood volume and appropriate hemostasis. The manufacturer generally provides anticoagulation recommendations; however, the patients' care providers often tailor anticoagulation to account for individual patient needs. Thrombus formation within the device is a risk. Monitor the device frequently with inspection of tubing, connections, valves, and VAD chambers for the presence of fibrin or thrombus.

g. Monitor for local or systemic infection by watching for fever, laboratory changes reflecting infectious or inflammatory process, erythema, drainage, or swelling at the cannula insertion site. This can potentially prevent systemic infection and allow earlier initiation of treatment. Acute and active infections are a contraindication to performing orthotopic heart transplantation, and may necessitate a change in transplant-list status for patients awaiting heart transplantation.

h. Respiratory clearance exercises, such as incentive spirometry or bubble blowing, optimize pulmonary function and prevent infection. Early mobilization is key to overall recovery and to improve respiratory status. Mechanical ventilation in the initial postoperative course is generally indicated. When stable, the goal is to extubate the patient and promote mobility. Patients may require medication (sildenafil, iNO) to treat pulmonary hypertension or right-sided HF in order to promote optimal VAD function and cardiac recovery.

i. Nutrition and electrolyte assessment, monitoring, and delivery will promote adequate caloric intake and protein balance to maintain an anabolic state, prevent infection, promote wound healing, and foster rehabilitation of the child's physical status. Parenteral nutrition may be given until the patient is stable enough for enteral nutrition from a physiologic state or is taking adequate calories enterally. It is important to initiate enteral feeds when possible and monitor fluid status closely. Monitor closely for decreased urine output and increased body edema as this may signal inadequate VAD support of CO. The goal is for assessment and correction of fluid and electrolyte imbalances.

6. Complications include stroke, IVH, seizures, or encephalopathy. Hematologic complications are generally related to the need for anticoagulation and include bleeding and hemorrhage. Gastrointestinal complications can arise from poor bowel perfusion and resultant ischemia, from disruption of the peritoneum as part of the VAD implantation particularly with paracorporeal pulsatile VAD. Immunologic issues primarily involve formation of antihuman leukocyte antigen (HLA) antibodies due to the immunologic response to the VAD tubing or to the CPB circuit when undergoing VAD placement and to the blood products that may be required during placement or in routine postoperative care. This response may limit donor acceptability for transplant. The degree of immunologic reaction is specific to the type of device chosen.

HEART FAILURE IN CHILDREN

A. Definition

CHF, also referred to as HF, is a condition in which the heart is unable to provide adequate CO or regional blood flow to meet the circulatory and metabolic requirements of the body. HF may result from disorders of the pericardium, myocardium, endocardium, heart valves, or great vessels. It can result from congenital and/or acquired forms of heart disease. These include structural abnormalities that place a pressure or volume load on the heart muscle or intrinsic myocardial dysfunction as seen in pediatric cardiomyopathies. As there is increased understanding of the clinical and pathophysiologic syndrome, HF is now classified as right and/or left HF and systolic and/or diastolic HF with associated circulatory and neurohormonal abnormalities. HF can present in fetal life as well as in infants and older children/adolescents.

B. Pathophysiology

1. HF is a constellation of signs and symptoms, composed of both structural and functional abnormalities. The signs and symptoms expressed are primarily a result of increased filling pressures and metabolic and neurohormonal activation (Kirk et al., 2014).

a. Structural heart disease includes obstruction to ventricular inflow or outflow and valve insufficiency. Single ventricle lesions result in ventricular volume overload. Cardiomyopathies result in systolic (reduced contractility) and diastolic (failure of adequate ventricular relaxation and inadequate filling) HF. Hemodynamics, symptoms, outcomes, and treatments vary based on the diagnosis of right heart or left heart disease or a combination and whether it is systolic, diastolic, or combined HF.

 i. Systolic right HF is the inability of the right heart to provide adequate pulmonary blood flow. Increased right heart preload and signs/symptoms of systemic venous congestion result. This can be related to structural abnormalities (valvar stenosis/atresia), increased RV afterload from increased PAP/PVR, IPAH, or from volume overload from a left-to-right intracardiac shunt.

 ii. Systolic left HF is the inability of the left heart to provide adequate systemic blood flow and oxygen delivery. This results in increased left heart preload and/or increased left heart afterload, resulting in signs and symptoms of pulmonary congestion and low CO. It can be related to structural abnormalities (valvar/LVOTO obstruction), increased SVR, or volume and pressure overload from single-ventricle lesions or systemic to pulmonary shunts. It can also be a result of pediatric cardiomyopathy whether primary or secondary in etiology.

 iii. Diastolic right HF is the result of inadequate filling of the right heart during diastole due to ventricular restriction or noncompliance. This results in decreased CO to the pulmonary circuit and decreased return to the LA, compromising left-sided CO. In addition, ventricular noncompliance increases end-diastolic pressures and hence right atrial pressure, causing symptoms of venous congestion. Right-sided diastolic failure can be caused by pediatric cardiomyopathies, long-standing left-to-right shunting lesions, and right-sided obstructive CHD.

 iv. Diastolic left HF is the result of inadequate filling of the left heart during diastole due to ventricular restriction or noncompliance. This results in decreased CO to the systemic circulation and symptoms of CHF. In addition, ventricular noncompliance increased the LVEDP and hence left atrial pressure, causing symptoms of pulmonary congestion. Left-sided diastolic failure can be the result of pediatric cardiomyopathies, left-sided obstructive lesions, prolonged pressure and volume overload from systemic to pulmonary shunts, and congenital endocardial fibroelastosis.

2. Mechanisms of cardiac reserve support a balance of oxygen delivery to demand and consumption. They include increased HR and SV, increased oxygen extraction at the cellular level, redistribution of blood flow to vital organs, cardiac dilation from volume overload, anaerobic metabolism, and cardiac hypertrophy (Figure 3.41; Hall, 2016).

3. Systemic compensatory response as triggered by inadequate oxygen delivery to the body includes the following (Hall, 2016):

a. The renin–angiotensin–aldosterone system is activated with resultant salt and water retention to augment preload. The physiologic result is an increase in contractility from stretching of the muscle tissue, but will eventually result in pulmonary and systemic congestion with edema.

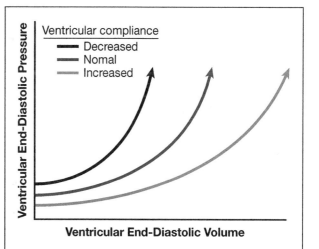

FIGURE 3.41 Ventricular compliance illustrated by ventricular end-diastolic pressure curve.

b. Activation of the sympathetic nervous system results in vasoconstriction to maintain BP for adequate perfusion. This increases afterload to the failing ventricle and increases myocardial oxygen demand and consumption.

c. Sympathetic stimulation also increases HR to provide increased oxygen delivery but reflexively increases myocardial oxygen demand and consumption. Chronic stimulation leads to desensitization.

d. Release of cAMP results in calcium uptake to increase myocardial contractility, overloading the system that pumps calcium out of the cell during diastole, which results in decreased diastolic relaxation. Calcium elevations result in transient electrical depolarizations, predisposing the patient to arrhythmias.

e. Hypertrophy of the cardiac muscle is a normal response to pressure or volume in an attempt to increase the number of myocardial cells sharing the workload of providing CO. Eventually, the hypertrophy exceeds the coronary artery's ability to deliver oxygen to the hypertrophied muscle, with a result in energy and oxygen starvation at the capillary level, including myocyte necrosis. Necrosis leads to fibroblast and collagen deposition within the thinned dilated heart.

f. Desensitization of β-adrenergic receptors decreases energy use and the functioning number of receptor molecules (downregulation), which decreases myocardial contractility.

C. Etiology of Left HF

1. *Obstruction* of forward flow can result from defects such as mitral or AS/atresia or coarctation of the aorta.

2. *Volume overload* can be due to shunting (i.e., VSD, atrioventricular septal defect [AVSD]) or systemic to pulmonary shunts.

3. *Muscular underdevelopment* may occur, such as in HLHS or other single-ventricle variants. Endocardial fibroelastosis may result from inadequate coronary perfusion of the endocardium during fetal life. Secondary cardiomyopathies will result in muscle disease and HF with disease progression.

4. *Decreased myocardial contractility* may result from ischemia, inflammation, or fibrosis. Specific metabolic and neurohormonal disease states or acute electrolyte imbalances will decrease contractility. Congenital anomalies of the coronary arteries can result in systolic HF from decreased coronary perfusion.

5. *Arrhythmias* can cause a failure of the cardiac chambers to fill or empty adequately or failure to contract (e.g., tachyarrhythmias, atrial, or ventricular) normally to provide maximized CO. Severe symptomatic bradycardia will decrease oxygen delivery by decreasing the volume of oxygen delivery pumped to the systemic circulation.

6. *Systemic hypertension and increased afterload* to the LV will trigger cell hypertrophy and eventual HF.

7. *Cardiomyopathies*, primary or secondary, will most often result in progressive systolic and/or diastolic HF (Kirk et al., 2014).

D. Etiology of Right HF

1. *Obstruction* of forward flow can result from defects such as tricuspid, PS, or PA stenosis. The RVOT may be obstructed by infundibular stenosis as seen in tetralogy of Fallot or excessive muscle bundles as in a double-chamber RV.

2. *Volume overload* can be due to left-to-right shunting (i.e., VSD).

3. *Muscular underdevelopment* may occur, such as in pulmonary atresia or a single RV.

4. *Decreased contractility* may result from ischemia, inflammation, or fibrosis. Cardiomyopathy and specific neurohormonal and metabolic diseases may result in decreased RV function. Certain congenital heart defects, such as pulmonary atresia with intact ventricular septum, include coronary abnormalities that effect systolic function.

5. *Arrhythmias* cause an inability of the ventricle to empty and/or fill the ventricle completely and result in inadequate oxygen delivery. Patients with atrial dilation (valvar regurgitation) or Fontan palliation have atrial stretch, which predisposes them to atrial arrhythmias, most notable are atrial flutter/ fibrillation. In addition, RV dilation, specifically in tetralogy of Fallot with pulmonary regurgitation, increases the risk of ventricular arrhythmia. Any patient with previous atrial surgery (Senning/ Mustard operation, Fontan palliation) or ventriculomy (a requirement for placement of an RV-PA conduit for repair or from previous placement of a transannular patch) has scar tissue that places him or her at an increased risk of reentry tachycardias, both atrial and ventricular. Specific cardiomyopathies also are characterized by arrythmia and sudden decrease in CO.

6. *Idiopathic or acquired PA hypertension/pulmonary vascular obstructive disease (PVOD)* or elevations in the PVR will increase RV afterload and eventually result in RV failure.

E. Clinical Signs and Symptoms

1. *Sympathetic stimulation* results in increased HR, arrhythmias, peripheral vasoconstriction with decreased peripheral pulses, mottled and cool skin, and diaphoresis (Hall, 2016).

2. *The renin–angiotensin–aldosterone mechanism* promotes sodium and water retention and results in oliguria, peripheral edema, ascites, jugular vein distension (JVD), and weight gain from fluid retention.

3. *Systemic venous engorgement/right HF* is characterized by increased liver and/or spleen size (hepatosplenomegaly), jugular venous distention, peripheral or periorbital edema, ascites, pleural effusion, or a combination of these signs.

4. *Pulmonary venous engorgement/left HF* results in tachypnea, rales, and wheezing that does not clear until the HF is treated, increased respiratory effort, retractions, nasal flaring, pulmonary edema, and a gray/cyanotic color.

5. *Systemic symptoms* include some or all of the following: irritability, fatigue or lethargy, exercise intolerance, poor appetite with abdominal pain or prolonged feeding with diaphoresis/tachypnea and fatigue, change in responsiveness, poor weight gain, a gallop heard on auscultation, diaphoresis, oliguria, pallor, peripheral cyanosis, and decreased capillary refill. Pulsus alternans or pulsus paradoxus can be seen as compensated HF evolves into decompensated HF.

6. *Redistribution of blood flow* occurs secondary to the vasoconstricting and vasodilating effects of neurohormonal agents such as norepinephrine, renin–angiotensin–aldosterone, vasopressin, ANP, BNP, dopamine, and paracrine agents. Although protective for the heart and brain, redistributed blood flow may result in impairment of other organ systems. Long-term redistribution of blood flow may result in decreased gut perfusion, in

paralytic ileus, or necrotizing enterocolitis (NEC), and an inability to tolerate enteral feedings. Decreased hepatic perfusion results in decreased metabolic function and clotting abnormalities, reduced skin or peripheral perfusion may result in necrotic changes, skeletal muscle may atrophy, and decreased glomerular filtration rate can result in acute kidney injury.

F. Diagnostic Studies

1. The history is often a clue to the etiology of HF. Poor growth from birth, a family history of CHD or cardiomyopathy, and maternal illnesses, specifically connective tissue disorders, provide valuable information in diagnosis. Previous health issues, particularly exposure to environmental toxins, chemotherapy, or chest radiation therapy are important clues to potential etiologies. Physical examination is consistent with the preceding clinical presentation. Neurologic alterations may occur related to hypoxia, as a response to elevations in CVP causing decreased brain perfusion. Symptoms include confusion, irritability, a change in level of consciousness, somnolence, agitation, and irritability. Due to decreased CO and sluggish blood flow, patients with HF have an increased risk for thrombus formation and embolic stroke.

2. Chest x-ray is useful for recognition of cardiomegaly, increased pulmonary vascular markings and edema, pleural effusion, and chest deformities (Figure 3.42).

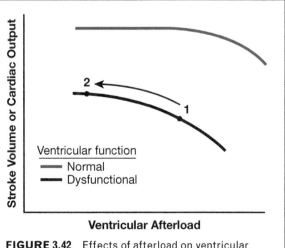

FIGURE 3.42 Effects of afterload on ventricular function.

3. ECG findings can reveal associated conduction disorders or arrhythmias that assist with the diagnosis of specific structural abnormalities or myopathies.

4. Echo establishes the presence or absence of structural defects, including abnormalities of the coronary arteries. It identifies the presence of pericardial effusions, cardiomyopathy, chamber hypertrophy, and chamber volume overload. Measurements of systolic and diastolic dysfunction can be obtained for further evaluation by the cardiologist.

5. PA catheter placement can provide measurements of CO/index, filling pressures, and an estimation of LVEDPs and left-sided preload to guide medical management and response to interventions.

6. Cardiac catheterization is used to evaluate structural defects, quantify CO, perform a myocardial biopsy, and to make additional determinations about potential causes of HF. Right heart cardiac catheterization can also provide information regarding PVR and vascular reactivity, if evaluated.

7. SVO_2 measurements provide information about changes in CO and tissue (myocardial) oxygen delivery (balance of consumption and demand). Improvements in SVO_2 measurement can be used to guide interventions. A normal SVO_2 is 65% to 75% in a patient without cyanotic heart disease. In patients with cyanotic heart disease, interpretation of the SVO_2 is dependent on the systemic arterial saturation.

8. Laboratory studies show dilutional changes in serum sodium and hemoglobin, anemia (including relative anemia in cyanotic CHD), hypocalcemia, hypoglycemia, medication levels (specifically antiarrhythmic medications), and abnormal results suggesting end-organ dysfunction. These include liver and renal function tests and coagulation profiles. Acute elevations in WBC and platelets, related to an inflammatory response, are seen in acute decompensated HF. Anemia can be seen in both systolic and diastolic HF. Serum lactate and base deficit measurement may indicate the level of oxygen delivery deficit. Brain natriuretic peptide (BNP) levels can assist with the diagnosis of symptomatic HF or cardiomyopathy (systolic or diastolic). BNP trends also assist with prognostication of cardiomyopathy and decompensated HF, follow the progression/response to therapy, and can be helpful in differentiating the etiology of shortness of breath in the emergency department.

BNP levels tend to be higher in children with HF associated with left heart dysfunction and volume overload and can be used to differentiate all New York Heart Association (NYHA) classes. BNP levels greater than 16.5 pg/mL and NT-pro BNP 514 pg/mL have a high sensitivity for screening a patient with subclinical HF. If HF has been long-standing, it is possible the BNP level may be normal due to burn out of the response to ventricular dilation. Inflammatory markers are being investigated in pediatrics, as increased C-reactive protein (CRP) in adults has been associated with the degree of systolic HF and vascular disease. Inflammatory reactions are known to be significant in the remodeling process seen in pediatric HF (Chow et al., 2017; Libby, Gerszten, & Ricker, 2015).

9. Cardiac MRI (cMRI)/MRA can be used to assess tissue characteristics, ventricular mass index, and ischemia. cMRI/MRA may better define the coronary and great vessel anatomy as compared to echo, and does not require radiation as compared to CT. Use of cMRI/MRA may be limited by the often necessary need for heavy sedation or intubation. In general, cMRI/MRA is used only in patients for whom echo cannot provide the detail necessary for diagnosis.

G. Goals and Patient Management

1. *General Management of Compensated HF*

   a. The goal of therapy is to reduce symptoms, preserve long-term ventricular function, and prolong survival through antagonism of the neurohormonal compensatory mechanisms.

   b. Improve CO and oxygen delivery balanced to demand/consumption.

   i. Provide supportive therapy to increase oxygen supply (supplemental oxygen, semi-Fowler position, bronchodilators) or decrease oxygen demand (normothermia, reduce activity, keep infant/child in a restful state, support enteral feedings or parental supplementation, increased caloric intake, and mechanical ventilation).

   ii. Support SV through adequate preload and avoidance of tachycardia to promote better filling and emptying of the heart. Treatment of arrhythmias is key to promoting adequate time for atrial and ventricular filling and emptying, especially with myocardial dysfunction. Prevention of anemia and transfusions for nonhemodiluted anemia increases oxygen delivery and improves CO as noted by improvement in MVO_2. Treatment of symptomatic anemia may be at higher relative hemoglobin levels in patients with cyanotic heart disease.

iii. Cardiac resynchronization therapy (CRT) has been shown to be most beneficial for patients with an EF of less than 35%, complete LBBB, a prolonged QRS interval for age, and those who meet the criteria for NYHA Class II to IV. CRT therapy can also be considered for left ventricular dysfunction from cardiomyopathy, CHD or congenital/long-standing heart block treated with the use of a VVI or DDD pacemaker mode requires non-physiologic depolarization due to RV lead placement. CRT eliminates this and can allow normal depolarization and improve ventricular function (Curtis et al., 2013).

iv. Reduction of afterload can be done through the use of ACE inhibitors or ARBs. Maintain normothermia to avoid vasoconstriction from hypothermia, pain, or agitation. RV afterload can also be treated with the use of iNO and eventual conversion to PDE-5 inhibitors such as sildenafil or tadalafil.

v. ICDs are indicated for survivors of SCD or those with a high risk of ventricular arrhythmia and sudden death. This can include patients with HCM, Brugada syndrome, Long QT syndrome, and some other channelopathies. Patients with marked LV dysfunction, ARVM (arrhythmogenic right ventricular myopathy), unexplained syncope, or a family history of SCD may also be considered for ICD implantation (Rossano, Cabrera, & Shaddy, 2016).

vi. Improve contractility and ventricular remodeling with ACE inhibitors or ARBs and digoxin.

vii. Preload manipulation and fluid status management should be optimized to promote optimal ventricular filling and CO and prevent volume overload.

1) Assessment of edema, weight, and breath sounds is performed frequently. Fluid and sodium restrictions may be indicated, specifically in older patients. Electrolyte levels for sodium and potassium levels related to volume overload and diuretic management are followed closely and replacements given to support myocardial and cellular function.

2) Preload manipulation should achieve adequate ventricular filling while avoiding overdilation and volume overload.

3) Diuretic management will treat volume overload, effusions, ascites, and pulmonary edema. Careful assessment of serum electrolytes and the effect of diuretics on renal function is essential.

2. *Prevent complications* related to thromboembolic events in patients with severely decreased systolic function, with evidence of thrombus on imaging study, or with previous thromboembolic event. Certain pediatric cardiomyopathies, particularly RCM and left ventricular noncompaction cardiomyopathy (LVNC), predispose patients to mural and ventricular thrombi. Use of enoxaparin or warfarin in addition to or in place of aspirin therapy may be indicated.

3. Management of compensated, preserved ejection fraction HF (HFpEF)

a. Defined as an LVEF of greater than or equal to 40%

b. Pharmacologic therapy (Rossano, Cabrera, Jefferies, et al., 2016):

i. ACE inhibitors assist with remodeling and are recommended for use with both symptomatic or asymptomatic HF. Use in single ventricle HF may be considered.

ii. Angiotensin II receptor blocking agents (ARBS) include aldosterone inhibitors to augment natriuresis.

iii. Digoxin is not recommended for children with asymptomatic HF as there is no improved survival data to support its use. Recent data in the interstage population for HLHS has shown increased survival to stage 2 palliation and digoxin is recommended in this population (Brown et al., 2016).

iv. β-Blockers may be cardioprotective in some cardiomyopathies, but detrimental in others. Careful diagnosis and use are essential. β-Blockers also can be harmful in pressure overloaded ventricles, as often seen in CHD, repaired or palliated (Kirk et al., 2014).

v. Diuretics include loop diuretics, thiazides, and metolazone. Nesiritide may be considered to promote diuresis refractory to other IV or oral diuretic regimens.

4. Management of compensated, reduced ejection fraction HF (HFrEF)

a. Defined in general as HF with an LVEF of less than or equal to 40% (Kirk et al., 2014).

b. Pharmacologic therapy (Rossano, Cabrera, Jefferies, et al., 2016):

i. Diuretics are used for management of preload.

ii. Management of hypertension with an ACE inhibitor or ARB is recommended.

iii. Medical therapy for HFrEF is limited in modality and efficacy.

c. Nutritional competency with caloric supplementation via a nasogastric or gastrostomy tube as needed is vital. The use of parenteral nutrition in patients unable to tolerate enteral feeding should be considered.

5. *Management of Decompensated HF*

a. Presentation

i. These patients may present with tachycardia-mediated decompensation. Laboratory studies show respiratory acidosis, elevated lactate, hyponatremia, and hypochloremia (likely dilutional or in response to chronic diuretic treatment), elevated serum creatinine, and elevation of the BNP indicating ventricular dilation and volume overload.

ii. Symptoms of marked respiratory distress with low CO and compromised perfusion are generally present and progress.

iii. Echocardiographic evidence of decreased systolic and/or diastolic function is present. Increased AV valve regurgitation as a result of ventricular dilation may also be seen.

iv. Chest x-ray may show effusions and/or pulmonary edema.

b. *Treatment* is aimed at optimizing the DO_2 through decreasing oxygen demand and consumption (Jefferies, Hoffman, & Nelson, 2010).

i. Mechanical ventilation may be required.

1) Positive-pressure ventilation decreases systemic venous return and preload to the RA. This will, in turn, reduce volume overload to the right heart. As long as adequate preload for CO is maintained, this reduction in systemic venous pressure can assist with diuresis and control of edema symptoms. Positive-pressure ventilation also increases the afterload to the RV and therefore should be used cautiously in patients with decompensated right HF or single-ventricle physiology. It will decrease afterload to the LV and can be beneficial for the failing LV.

2) Negative-pressure ventilation will increase systemic venous return and right atrial pressure, thereby augmenting preload and subsequent right heart CO and left heart preload.

3) Mechanical ventilation to achieve FRC is the key to optimizing CO regardless of whether the patient has right or left HF or HFpEF, HFrEF, or combined HF.

ii. HR and rhythm should be optimized.

1) Avoidance of tachycardia to promote adequate filling and emptying of the ventricle and coronary perfusion is key.

2) Antiarrhythmic medications (amiodarone, procainamide) should be used cautiously to achieve NSR and avoid further alterations in preload and SV and hence decreased systolic function.

3) Antiarrhythmic therapies are also important to provide AV synchrony and achieve and/or maintain NSR. The loss of the atrial kick reduces CO by as much as 15% and is significant in patients with decompensated HF.

iii. Afterload reduction is key to promote CO and end-organ function. Right heart and left heart afterload reduction should be considered separately, especially in patients with CHD (Rossano, Cabrera, Jefferies, Naim, & Humlicek, 2016).

1) Phosphodiesterase inhibitors decrease afterload and prevent or reduce hypertension. They may assist with decreasing pulmonary pressures and right heart afterload reduction.

2) Pulmonary vasodilators, such as iNO, may be indicated for right heart or single-ventricle pulmonary hypertension.

3) Nesiritide has positive lusitropic properties and promotes natriuresis and may be a beneficial vasodilator in acute decompensated HF.

iv. Preload

1) Optimization of preload to support ventricular filling and CO is important.

2) Avoidance of volume overload with distension of the ventricle and decreased CO is managed with diuretics. Careful and ongoing assessment of fluid status, BP, and renal function is essential.

v. Contractility to improve systolic function of right and/or left ventricular function is necessary to provide adequate CO and end-organ perfusion (Rossano, Cabrera, Jefferies, et al. 2016).

1) Discontinuation of β-blockers may be indicated in some patients; however, the addition of β-blockers, such as carvedilol, may be beneficial for long-term chronic HF.

2) Treatment of hypotension is often required. Vasoactive agents are chosen by the clinical assessment of DO2 and the physiologic response. Medications include phosphodiesterase inhibitors, dopamine, dobutamine, epinephrine, vasopressin, and calcium chloride infusions. Levosimendan is a promising new agent for the treatment of decreased contractility in systolic decompensated HF. It increases both inotropy and vasodilation but is a calcium sensitizer.

3) For HF related to correctable congenital defects, surgery is indicated when optimal medical management has failed.

4) Mechanical cardiac support is not a cure but may provide a bridge to recovery or transplantation while protecting end-organ function and optimizing the patient's overall nutritional and physical condition. It may also be indicated as destination therapy in patients with recalcitrant HF.

c. End-organ support is vital to recovery. In patients who will eventually require cardiac surgery or orthotopic heart transplant (OHT) for treatment of their HF, end-organ function will be a factor in determining whether the patient is a candidate for these procedures.

d. Nutritional competency is as vital as it is in compensated HF (Costello, Gellatly, Daniel, Justo, & Weir, 2014).

6. *Patient and family education* should include teaching about diet, medications, and signs and symptoms of CHF.

SHOCK

A. Definition

1. *Shock* is a complex syndrome of decreased tissue perfusion resulting in an inadequate supply of oxygen and nutrients to body cells. It is most often characterized by inadequate peripheral and end-organ perfusion. There can be normal, increased, or decreased systolic BP. Low CO is most often present in the pediatric patient in a shock state.

B. Etiology and Pathophysiology

1. Shock can be a result of inadequate blood volume or oxygen-carrying capacity, inappropriate distribution of blood volume and flow, impaired cardiac contractility, or obstructed blood flow (Hazinski, 2013).

2. When oxygen demand increases or delivery decreases the tissues extract an increased amount of oxygen. The deficit will progress until the body switches to anaerobic metabolism, which occurs when the demand exceeds delivery. Adequate oxygen delivery is dependent on cardiac output, which is the product of heart rate (rate and rhythm) times stroke volume (preload, afterload, contractility).

3. *Compensated shock* is identified by a normal systolic BP with clinical evidence of inadequate tissue perfusion. The body utilizes several compensatory mechanisms to maintain adequate oxygen delivery (Pomerantz & Roback, 2016).

a. *Tachycardia.* This is especially relevant for newborns and infants because they function at the upper limits of SV routinely, and HR is the only means to modulate SV. As tachycardia increases, the ventricular filling and emptying time shortens, compromising SV and CO.

b. *Increase in SVR and vasoconstriction.* This increases afterload to the ventricle. If SVR increases, even with a fall in CO, BP and oxygen delivery *can be maintained. If SVR falls and CO is decreased,* oxygen delivery decreases, and BP will fall.

c. There is an increase in the contractility of the heart muscle, resulting in increased strength of cardiac contraction.

d. There is an increase in the venous smooth muscle tone, which increases venous return to the heart and augments preload.

4. *Decompensated shock* is identified when physiologic attempts to maintain systolic BP, tissue perfusion, and oxygen delivery fail (Pomerantz & Roback, 2016).

a. Altered level of consciousness due to decreased brain perfusion is an early symptom.

b. Hypotension is a late sign. It may occur early in shock types associated with decreased SVR, most notably, septic shock.

c. Assess for progression of all symptoms: a further increase in HR, decrease in perfusion and urine output, and prolongation in capillary refill time.

5. *Hypovolemic shock* (inadequate blood volume or oxygen-carrying capacity): Decreased intravascular volume causes decreased venous return, decreased ventricular filling, decreased SV, and decreased CO with decreased blood flow to tissues. Oxygen delivery is compromised to a significant extent, resulting in anaerobic metabolism. Causes include blood loss related to trauma, surgery, gastrointestinal tract bleeding, and intracranial hemorrhage; plasma loss from capillary fluid shifts in sepsis, thermal injury, burns, or nephrotic syndrome; and water loss from vomiting and diarrhea, diuretic administration, diabetes insipidus, or inadequate fluid intake. In hypovolemic shock, preload is decreased, afterload is increased, and contractility is normal or increased. The patient typically presents with tachycardia and tachypnea without distress; adequate systolic BP; narrow pulse pressure; weak or absent peripheral pulses; normal or weak central pulses; delayed capillary refill; cool to cold, pale, mottled diaphoretic skin; dusky/pale extremities; changes in level of consciousness; or oliguria (Pomerantz & Roback, 2016).

6. *Cardiogenic shock* is inadequate perfusion due to myocardial dysfunction. Common causes are CHD, myocarditis, cardiomyopathy, arrhythmias, sepsis, poisoning or drug toxicity, and myocardial injury. This is characterized by extreme tachycardia, high SVR, decreased CO from reduction in SV. Pulmonary congestion leads to pulmonary edema and respiratory compromise. Systemic congestion leads to effusions, ascites, and peripheral edema. Preload is variable, afterload is increased, and contractility is decreased. Decreased coronary perfusion and myocardial ischemia leads to further ventricular dysfunction. Symptoms besides tachycardia include increased work of breathing progressing to respiratory distress and grunting, hepatomegaly, JVD, cyanosis is associated with cyanotic CHD, normal or low BP with a narrow pulse pressure, weak or absent peripheral pulses, normal followed by weak central pulses, delayed capillary refill with cool extremities, cold/pale/mottled/diaphoretic skin, decreased level of consciousness, and oliguria (Pomerantz & Roback, 2016).

7. *Distributive shock* occurs with inappropriate distribution of blood volume with inadequate organ and tissue perfusion. The most common forms are septic shock, anaphylactic shock, and neurogenic shock (head injury, spinal injury). In septic shock, abnormal distribution of blood volume occurs because of decreased SVR and shunting of blood past capillary beds. In anaphylactic shock, venodilation, arterial vasodilation, and increased capillary permeability combine with pulmonary vasoconstriction to reduce

CO. In neurogenic shock, there is a generalized loss of vascular tone leading to severe vasodilation and hypotension. The sympathetic nervous system fails to increase HR, causing CO and oxygen delivery to fall. In the initial stages of distributive shock, SVR may decrease and there is increased blood flow to the skin, also called *warm-dry shock*. High CO with low SVR is a key difference between anaphylactic shock and hypovolemic shock, where CO is low and SVR is high. In distributive shock, preload is normal or decreased, contractility is normal or decreased, and afterload is variable. In classical cases, there is low SVR causing a widened pulse pressure and early hypotension, increased blood flow to some peripheral tissue beds, inadequate perfusion to splanchnic (gut and kidneys) vascular bed. The patient will demonstrate tachypnea without increased work of breathing, tachycardia, bounding peripheral pulses, brisk or delayed capillary refill, warm-flushed skin (warm shock) peripherally, or pale, mottled skin with vasoconstriction (cold shock); hypotension with widened pulse pressure (warm shock); or hypotension with a narrow pulse pressure (cold shock) OR normotension, oliguria, and changes in the level of consciousness (Pomerantz & Roback, 2016).

a. Septic shock is the most common form of distributive shock. It is caused by infectious organisms or their endotoxins stimulating the immune system and triggering activation of inflammatory mediators. Patients may have hyperthermia or hypothermia, elevated or decreased WBC with left shift in differential, metabolic acidosis, and elevated lactate (Weiss & Pomerantz, 2017).

b. Anaphylactic shock is an acute, multiorgan allergic response caused by a severe reaction to a drug, vaccine, food, toxin, plant, venom, or other antigen. This results in the release of immunoglobulin E (IgE), histamine, serotonin, bradykinin, and prostaglandins in response to an anaphylactic reaction. These inflammatory mediators cause vasodilation and capillary leak. It is characterized by venodilation, arterial vasodilation, increased capillary permeability, and pulmonary vasoconstriction. An acute increase in right ventricular afterload may reduce pulmonary blood flow and preload to the LV, with resultant decrease in CO. Acute-phase symptoms occur 5 to 10 minutes after exposure. Presentation commonly includes anxiety or agitation, nausea and vomiting, hives, angioedema, respiratory distress with stridor or wheezing, hypotension, tachycardia.

c. Neurogenic shock is a sudden loss of sympathetic nervous system signal to the smooth muscle in the vessel walls and results in uncontrolled vasodilation. In neurogenic shock, preload and afterload are decreased and contractility is normal. It is characterized by hypotension with a wide pulse pressure and a normal to slow HR.

8. *Obstructive shock* occurs when CO is impaired by a physical obstruction of blood flow. Causes include cardiac tamponade, tension pneumothorax, ductal-dependent congenital heart lesions, and massive pulmonary embolism. The obstruction results in low CO, inadequate tissue perfusion, and an increase in SVR. May initially appear as hypovolemic shock but close examination will demonstrate pulmonary and/or systemic venous congestion. Preload is variable, afterload is increased, and contractility is normal (Pomerantz & Roback, 2016).

C. Clinical Signs and Symptoms

1. *Compensated phase* occurs in response to a deficiency in oxygen delivery, resulting in anaerobic metabolism, and lactic acid production. Vasoconstriction results in cool, pale, or mottled skin with delayed capillary filling time, diminished peripheral pulses, and narrow

pulse pressure. Diaphoresis results in clammy, moist skin. Urine output decreases. Poor skin turgor, dry mucous membranes, and sunken fontanelles are noted if dehydration is present. HR and contractility increase with a rise in CVP and PAWP in cardiogenic shock and a drop in CVP and PAWP in hypovolemic shock. Peripheral vascular resistance and SVR are elevated and cardiac index decreases. Increased rate and depth of breathing result in respiratory alkalosis. Decreased level of consciousness is indicated by atypical response to parents, restlessness, confusion, and lethargy. Pupils may dilate. Infants may demonstrate a weak cry and poor suck (Hazinski, 2013).

  a. Compensatory mechanisms. See Figure 3.43 for compensatory mechanisms for the lack of oxygen delivery and metabolism to tissues.

2. *Uncompensated phase* of shock, in which compensatory mechanisms fail, leads to multisystem organ failure. The cascade of physiologic changes may include the loss of autoregulation in the microcirculation from increases in capillary permeability, leading to third spacing, and decreased venous return. Low CVP, BP, and PCWP occur. Coronary

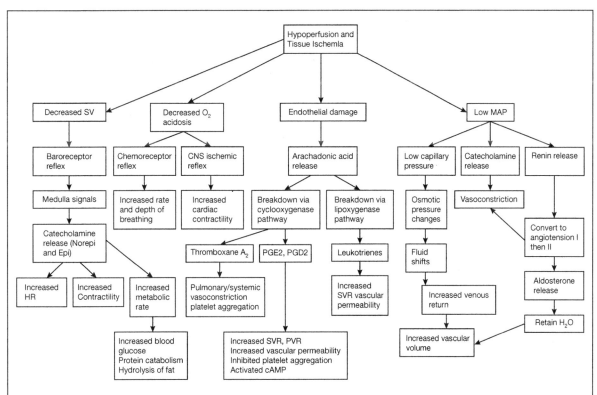

FIGURE 3.43 Compensatory mechanism in response to shock.

cAMP, cyclic adenosine monophasphate; CNS, central nervous system; epi, epinephrine; HR, heart rate; MAP, mean arterial pressure; norepi, norepinephrine; PGD2, prostaglandin D2; PGE2, prostaglandin E2; PVR, peripheral vascular resistance; SV, stroke volume; SVR, systemic vascular resistance.

perfusion suffers, resulting in ischemic changes on the ECG. Mental status deteriorates, and acute renal failure occurs. Gastrointestinal tract ischemia promotes translocation of gram-negative bacteria across damaged mucosa into the circulation, resulting in bowel edema, ulceration, and sepsis. Liver ischemia results in elevated bilirubin and liver enzymes, as well as jaundice and abnormal clotting/coagulopathy. Alveolar ischemia causes decreased surfactant production, leading to alveolar collapse, atelectasis, and decreased compliance. Ischemia to the distal extremities occurs, with necrosis and ulceration of toes and fingers. Irreversible changes may occur during the uncompensated phase of shock (Hazinski, 2013).

3. *Refractory Phase.* This is the last phase of shock, during which irreversible injury continues. Bradycardia and profound hypotension occur with no response to potent vasopressors, leading to organ failure and ultimately death.

D. Diagnostic Evaluation

1. *Chest radiographic* examination demonstrates cardiomegaly and pulmonary congestion.

2. *Echo* evaluates the presence of structural disease, systolic function, valvular structure, systolic time intervals, and ejection fraction, specifically noting hypokinetic areas of the myocardium.

3. *Laboratory studies* include arterial blood gases to determine hypoxia, respiratory or metabolic acidosis, and lactate levels. Electrolytes diagnose hyponatremia, hyperkalemia, hypoglycemia, and hypocalcemia. Obtain CBC with differential to assess for anemia, leukocytosis, and infectious response. Obtain coagulation studies if concern for hemorrhagic shock. Renal and hepatic function studies determine organ function.

4. *PA catheterization*, if anatomically possible, is occasionally performed to measure pressures and CO and evaluate intracardiac shunting. It allows continuous mixed venous O_2 saturation monitoring.

5. SVO_2*, A–VO$_2$ difference* determines the degree of low CO state and oxygen extraction (Gallet et al., 2012).

6. *ECG* can assess for sinus tachycardia versus arrhythmia. Blood, urine, or respiratory cultures, CRP, procalcitonin, and erythrocyte sedimentation rate (ESR) identify potential infectious origin of shock.

E. Goals and Patient Management

1. *Correct the Primary Cause of Shock*

   a. Hypovolemia. Volume replacement is initiated to reverse volume losses.

   b. Distributive. Vasoactive medications are used to increase the SVR and decrease the dilation of the blood vessels. Volume replacement is provided until the vascular bed has an adequate volume status. Steroids are given to treat septic shock that results in adrenal insufficiency and refractory hypotension.

   c. Cardiogenic. Improve oxygenation and blood flow through reduction of metabolic demand and afterload, optimization of preload, increase of myocardial relaxation, and respiratory support.

   d. Obstructive. Quickly identify etiology and treat with chest tube, pneumothorax aspiration, and initiation of PGE$_1$ for ductal patency. For pulmonary embolism, consider administration of anticoagulation and fibrinolytic agents, if severe cardiovascular compromise.

2. *Evaluate cardiovascular function* via an arterial line for continuous BP monitoring, monitor CVP to assess preload, use a PA catheter to assess therapy, monitor SVO_2, and perform perfusion assessment, which includes assessment of BP, skin color, temperature, capillary refill, urine output, and perfusion to organs.

3. Support cardiovascular function and decrease oxygen demand (Bronicki, Taylor, & Baden, 2016).

   a. Optimize preload with fluid resuscitation (20 mL/kg boluses) until responsive. Choose crystalloid versus colloid based on underlying disease process, nature of fluid losses, and patient's baseline hemodynamics. Rate and volume replacement are related to degree of shock and ability of ventricle to handle rapid fluid administration.

   b. Optimize contractility with inotropic agents, vasodilators, cardiac rest, and mechanical support, when necessary (see "Mechanical Cardiac Support" section).

   c. IV access is obtained with large-bore catheters in major vessels. In shock, an IO line can be used to infuse large volumes, blood, and drugs in children when IV access cannot be obtained in a timely manner.

4. *Support End-Organ Function.* Mechanical ventilation provides cardiopulmonary support. Renal support may include diuretics, continuous renal replacement therapy (CRRT), plasmapheresis, or hemodialysis. Prevent any further injury through an assessment of organ systems affected by the redistribution of blood flow.

5. *Provide adequate nutrition* through enteral or parenteral nutrition.

6. *Correct electrolyte abnormalities*, primarily hypoglycemia, hypocalcemia, hyperkalemia, metabolic acidosis.

F. Complications

1. Complications of shock include renal failure, hepatic failure, sepsis, disseminated intravascular coagulation (DIC), or death.

ARRHYTHMIAS AND MYOCARDIAL CONDUCTION SYSTEM DEFECTS

A. Definition

1. *NSR* refers to the initiation of the electrical impulse in the SA node with propagation through the AV node and bundle of His to the Purkinje fibers. It allows contraction of the atrium with a delay at the AV node and then contraction of the ventricle with expulsion of CO to the pulmonary and systemic circulation (refer to "Electrophysiology" section).

2. *An arrhythmia* is an abnormality in the rate, regularity, or site of origin of a cardiac impulse. A disturbance in the conduction of that impulse prevents the normal sequence of activation of the atria and ventricles.

B. Pathophysiology

1. A *reentry mechanism* is the cause of most atrial and ventricular tachyarrhythmias. Excitation impulses are able to travel via two routes; in the reentry circuit, the impulse travels down one pathway and returns up a second pathway. These are two discrete pathways with enough delay on one of the pathways to allow time for a refractory period and recovery. With reentry, the tachycardia will be regular with an abrupt onset and cessation.

    a. *Orthodromic* describes the pathway traveling down the AV node to the ventricles and returning retrograde up the accessory tissue (occurs in 90% of the cases).

    b. *Antidromic* describes the pathway traveling down accessory tissue and returning retrograde up through the AV node (occurs in 10% of cases).

2. *Abnormal automaticity* is a derangement of the AP of cardiac cells, allowing them to reach their threshold voltage prematurely. This usually occurs from injured or abnormal cardiac cells. With abnormal automaticity, there is variation in the HR influenced by sympathetic tone with a gradual increase and decrease of tachycardia. There is an atypical response to antiarrhythmic medications.

3. Triggered activity represents small oscillations in the cell membrane voltage during repolarization, causing the cell to reach the threshold potential.

C. Etiology

1. Factors that may precipitate arrhythmias include the following:

    a. Cellular milieu. Hypoxia, hypotension, electrolyte, or metabolic abnormalities may trigger an arrhythmia or conduction system abnormality.

    b. Disease states. CHD, pulmonary hypertension, CNS diseases, sepsis, myocarditis, acute rheumatic fever, or endocrine or metabolic disease can trigger arrhythmias or result in conduction system defects.

    c. Cardiac procedures, such as cardiac catheterization, can trigger arrhythmias due to catheter placement triggering an arrhythmia due to interference with the conduction tissue.

    d. Cardiac surgery can result in damage to the conduction system from mechanical manipulation, medication or anesthetics, cannulation from CPB, trauma from sutures, resection of ventricular septum for VSD enlargement, and disruption from outflow tract muscle resection. Transient conduction system injury can result from edema caused by surgical trauma, inflammation, ischemia from coronary insufficiency, sutures near the conduction pathway, hemodynamic changes and LCOS, electrolyte shifts, and medication interactions.

    e. Congenital conduction abnormalities include congenital complete heart block, reentry arrhythmias such as WPN syndrome, and channelopathies such as prolonged QT syndrome.

D. Supraventricular Arrhythmias (Figure 3.44)

1. *Sinus arrhythmia* is a normal and common physiologic variation of NSR.

    a. Etiology is related to respiratory variations with the HR increasing with inspiration and decreasing with expiration. It may be marked in children with airway obstruction, asthma, increased ICP, and following atrial surgery.

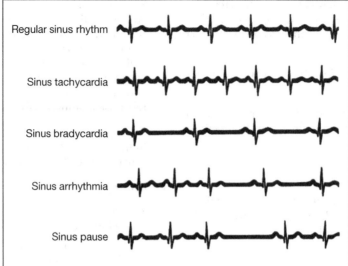

FIGURE 3.44 Normal and abnormal rhythms originating in the sinoatrial node. All rhythms have a P wave in front of each QRS complex with a regular PR interval.

Source: Reprinted with permission from Park, M. K., & Guntheroth, W. G. (2006). *How to read pediatric ECGs* (4th ed.). Philadelphia, PA: Elsevier.

This is a normal phenomenon in the fetus and in most children at all ages.

b. No clinical signs or symptoms are seen, and the child has a benign, irregular pulse.

c. ECG findings include an irregular rhythm; P-P and R-R intervals vary by more than 0.12 second with beat-to-beat variability, upright P waves, one P wave for each QRS complex, and a normal PR interval and QRS configuration.

d. Intervention is not necessary.

2. *Sinus Tachycardia*

a. Etiology is related to increased sympathetic tone, pain, fear, anxiety, anemia, exercise, fever, infection, hypoxemia, hypovolemia, shock, CHF, and pulmonary edema.

b. History, signs, and symptoms. The patient's history may reveal the underlying cause such as presence of infection. The child will have a rapid, regular pulse and may also have palpitations and/or dyspnea. He or she may have decreased perfusion and BP due to CHF, hypovolemia, or shock. The symptoms may only be related to the etiology.

c. ECG findings include regular rhythm, an increased HR, a P:QRS ratio of 1:1, normal PR interval and QRS configuration, and origin of the rhythm in the SA node. Neonates may have

a sinus tachycardia as high as 220 to 250 bpm, overlapping with rates of SVT.

d. Interventions include treating the underlying cause. Digoxin is not effective unless the tachycardia is related to CHF.

3. *SA node conduction disorders, including pause, block, or arrest*, result in a pause in the HR followed by NSR.

a. Etiology of pause, arrest, or block can be related to hypoxemia, digoxin toxicity, hyperkalemia, increased vagal tone, or cardiac surgery. In addition, MI, ischemia, atropine, aspirin toxicity, or infection (myocarditis, rheumatic fever) can be the contributing factors.

b. History, signs, and symptoms. The patient is usually unaware of the arrhythmia or may complain of skipped beats. The palpated pulse has a prolonged pause. CHF and decreased CO may develop if the pauses are frequent. Syncope or near syncope will occur if the pauses are prolonged.

c. ECG findings include a varying or irregular HR, a prolonged pause between QRS complexes, the absence of one or more expected P waves, absent QRS complex unless junctional or ventricular escape beat occurs, and a normal QRS duration. In SA pause, the pause is less than twice the underlying sinus interval. In SA block, the pause is an exact multiple of the underlying sinus interval; the SA node fires but the impulse is not conducted. In SA arrest, the pause is greater than twice the underlying sinus interval.

d. Intervention includes treatment of the underlying cause, atropine for frequent episodes, or a pacemaker for symptomatic episodes.

4. *Sinus bradycardia* causes an HR that is low for the patient's age and clinical state, but the rhythm is normal.

a. Etiology. The most common cause is hypoxia but causes also include surgical disruption of the SA node, use of digoxin or β-blockers, increased vagal tone, increased ICP, hypothermia, hypothyroidism, anorexia, and other medication side effects (i.e., dexmedetomidine).

b. History, signs, and symptoms. There is a slow, regular pulse. In infants, CHF may occur because of the inadequacy of the rate and resultant decreased CO.

c. ECG findings include a P wave before every QRS complex, regular P-P and R-R intervals, a normal QRS configuration, a normal PR interval, and upright P waves.

d. Interventions include oxygen, bag-mask ventilation to assist breathing if needed, and epinephrine or atropine for symptomatic bradycardia. To determine the exact degree of bradycardia when the patient is asleep and awake, 24-hour ECG monitoring is obtained. A stress ECG is performed if the patient is older than 5 years of age and can follow directions to determine the degree of SA node dysfunction. Transesophageal pacing can test automaticity and sinus node recovery time. Invasive study of the SA node should include the AV node function. If the conduction system is intact, permanent atrial demand pacing can be used to protect against prolonged and symptomatic bradycardia with effects on ventricular function.

5. *Sick sinus syndrome* (SSS, bradycardia–tachycardia syndrome) occurs when the HR varies from rates in excess of 180 bpm to severe bradycardia with long sinus pauses. Arrhythmias may include profound sinus bradycardia, SA exit block, sinus arrest with junctional escape, paroxysmal atrial tachycardia, slow or fast ectopic atrial or nodal rhythm, atrial flutter, or atrial fibrillation.

a. Etiology. Causes include disease or ischemia of the SA node from extensive atrial surgery (i.e., Fontan). It may be of idiopathic origin. SSS may occur following cannulation for CPB; hypertrophy of an otherwise anatomically normal heart; fibrosis of areas of the SA node, AV node, or injury to the sinus node artery.

b. History, signs, and symptoms. Patients may experience syncope, seizures, lethargy, poor feeding, seizures, dizziness, exercise intolerance, palpitations, chest pain, or sudden death.

c. ECG findings include an irregular rhythm, variable rate, and P waves that vary in amplitude and morphology.

d. Intervention for symptomatic SSS includes a pacemaker for the bradycardic component. Antiarrhythmics are used for the tachycardic component, generally after pacemaker insertion.

6. *Supraventricular Tachycardia*

a. Etiology. Most often, SVT is due to a reentry mechanism. Patients with SVT can have episodes due to increased automaticity from hypoxemia, electrolyte imbalance, acid–base abnormalities, myocardial disease, digoxin toxicity, and CHD. Most episodes involve reentry occurring from accessory AV conduction tissue or dual AV node pathways (i.e., AV node reentry tachycardia).

b. History, signs, and symptoms. Ongoing SVT often precipitates symptoms of shock and CHF, but older children rarely present in HF or shock. They report palpitations that may be felt in the throat, malaise, and a racing heart. SVT can be well tolerated in most patients, but prolonged excessive HRs can eventually result in CHF.

c. ECG findings include P:QRS ratio of 1:1; a ventricular rate usually greater than 220 bpm in infants and greater than 150 bpm in children; regular P-P and R-R intervals; abrupt onset and termination of tachycardia; normal QRS configuration; and P waves that may be absent, inverted, or superimposed (Figure 3.45).

d. Other findings. Patients with recurrent SVT or ongoing SVT can show evidence of myocardial dysfunction. Electrophysiology studies may reveal an automatic ectopic focus located in the atria or bundle of His, a concealed AV unidirectional retrograde accessory pathway, or a permanent form of reciprocating junctional tachycardia.

e. Interventions include treatment based on the HR, the mechanism of tachycardia, the degree of myocardial dysfunction, and symptoms.

i. For acute SVT, vagal maneuvers are used initially to terminate the arrhythmia.

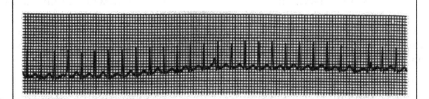

FIGURE 3.45 Electrocardiographic tracing of supraventricular tachycardia with normal QRS complex and regular R-R intervals.

Source: Reprinted with permission from Park, M. K., & Guntheroth, W. G. (2006). *How to read pediatric ECGs* (4th ed.). Philadelphia, PA: Elsevier.

If these are not successful, pharmacologic therapy with adenosine for acute termination of the episode is then utilized. Chronic therapy with propranolol is started if the SVT is recurrent, prolonged, or hemodynamically important. On rare occasions, verapamil can be used in children older than 1 year of age. DC cardioversion or overdrive pacing if pacemaker wires are present is used in hemodynamically compromised patients.

ii. In patients with recurrent or prolonged episodes of SVT, the mechanism of SVT is defined by electrophysiologic study. Following this study, the safety of digoxin use can be determined. Treatment of SVT can be divided into stable and unstable SVT.

iii. Options for therapy include the following:

1) Diving reflex or other vagal maneuvers can be used to terminate hemodynamically stable SVT.

2) Pharmacologic treatments may be useful for breakthrough tachycardia or episodes that present with evidence of hemodynamic intolerance. These medications include adenosine, propranolol, and verapamil. Antiarrhythmic therapy with sotalol, amiodarone, propaferone, and flecainide are reserved for more recalitrant SVT. Digoxin is used occasionally dependent on the type of SVT defined at electrophysiology study. If digoxin is used with amiodarone, the dose should be decreased by 50%.

3) Synchronized cardioversion is used for patients with hemodynamically significant SVT.

4) Overdrive pacing using temporary pacing wires placed after cardiac surgery, transesophageal pacing in intubated patients, or in patients with a permanent pacemaker can be used to convert SVT and maintain NSR with suppression AAI pacing.

5) Radiofrequency or cryoablation may be performed in patients of adequate size (age and weight) for catheter placement if the SVT is not responsive to medical treatment, the child develops severe side effects of the medication, there are medication compliance issues, or the child's lifestyle does not allow effective medication regimens.

7. *Wolff–Parkinson–White Syndrome*

a. Etiology involves the presence of a congenital accessory connection evident on resting ECG that conducts electrical activity faster than the AV node. WPW may be an isolated disease or it may be associated with CHD (especially Ebstein anomaly), Pompe disease, and cardiac myopathies. SVT caused by WPW pathways may occur at any age secondary to the reentry pathways.

b. History, signs, and symptoms. Frequent tachycardia occurs in infancy with decreased episodes in early childhood followed by resumption of symptoms at puberty. Symptoms may include palpitations, lethargy, decreased activity tolerance, or, more rarely, syncope, seizures, and sudden death.

c. ECG findings in WPW may be diagnosed by surface ECG. ECG features include regular rhythm, episodes of SVT, a short PR interval, a wide QRS complex, and the presence of a delta wave (slurred upstroke of the QRS complex appearance).

d. Interventions include medical treatment of frequent episodes of SVT or syncope with propranolol or amiodarone, radiofrequency ablation of an accessory pathway (especially if not responsive to medical therapy), and avoidance of digoxin in children older than 6 to 12 months of age. Vagal maneuvers or DC cardioversion are used for breakthrough tachycardia or in the situation of hemodynamically significant SVT. The biggest issue in patients with WPW is assessing for the risk of SCD. This can only be done when patients are old enough to undergo a treadmill stress test to monitor for the maintenance or resolution of preexcitation on ECG during exercise. Patients with SVT can be treated with propranolol or other antiarrhythmics. Older patients can undergo an electrophysiology study and ablation. Amiodarone is not a preferred medication given its long list of side effects.

8. Junctional Tachycardia

a. Pathophysiology involves an accelerated HR originating in the AV node, the loss of AV synchrony, and decreased CO resulting from the loss of the atrial kick or AV synchrony. This is especially harmful if CO is already compromised by heart disease or cardiac surgery. This type of arrhythmia is common in postoperative cardiac surgery patients and is frequently seen following repair of tetralogy of Fallot and AVSDs.

b. ECG findings show a variable HR ranging from 120 to 200 bpm, a normal and regular QRS complex, and an inverted P wave that may or may not follow the QRS complex. If sustained, the child may require an electrophysiologic study to determine the exact origin of the tachycardia. After cardiac surgery, many patients' arrhythmia resolves within 48 to 72 hours (Figure 3.46).

c. Treatment may not be necessary if the HR is within normal limits and the CO is adequate. Intervention may be required, especially in severely compromised patients. Cooling to a temperature of 35°C, sedation and analgesia to remove endogenous catecholamine responses, inotropic support of CO with careful attention to the tachycardic side effects of vasoactive agents, overdrive pacing when able to capture the HR, chemical paralysis, and medications, such as amiodarone or procainamide, may be used. Dexmetomadate is now commonly used after cardiac surgery and slows the HR as an additional effect.

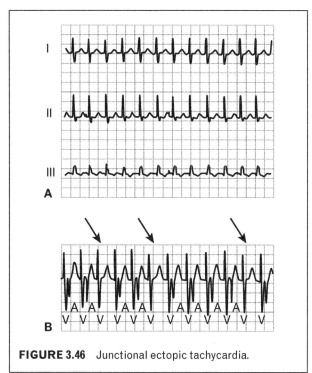

FIGURE 3.46 Junctional ectopic tachycardia.

9. *Atrial Flutter*

a. Pathophysiology and etiology of atrial flutter are related to a dilated, stretched atrial wall resulting from CHD or acquired heart disease, atrial surgery in neonates, hypoxemia, valvular disease, digoxin toxicity, increased sympathetic tone, or infection.

b. History, signs, and symptoms. Clinical signs and symptoms of HF develop if atrial flutter is not treated quickly, depending on the ventricular rate. If the patient is conducting the flutter at higher rates, there is a greater likelihood of hemodynamic instability. Children may have palpitations, angina, dyspnea, or decreased CO. Symptoms are more pronounced if there is underlying cardiac disease, especially if there is associated ventricular dysfunction at baseline.

c. ECG findings include a rapid atrial rate with characteristic sawtooth P waves, a normal QRS configuration, an atrial rate that is usually 300 bpm and regular (but may go as high as 400–450 bpm), a ventricular response rate from 1:1 conduction to various degrees of AV block, and an unidentifiable PR interval. Slower ventricular rates occur if varying degrees of block result in 2:1 or 3:1 flutter conduction (defined as one ventricular contraction in response to every second or third atrial contraction, respectively; Figure 3.47).

d. Intervention in unstable symptomatic children is direct cardioversion. Rapid overdrive atrial pacing may be useful through transesophageal, temporary epicardial wires, if present, or transvenous pacing wires. Medications are given to slow conduction through the AV node, which will decrease the ventricular response rate. Medications are given to increase AV block and decrease the ventricular response rate. These medications include digoxin, propranolol, and verapamil. Medications to help prevent recurrence include sotalol, flecainide, propaferone, and amiodarone. Surgical procedures can be used to improve hemodynamics and relieve atrial stretch or for implantation of an ICD with antitachycardia pacing capability. Electrophysiology study and catheter ablation of the flutter foci may be successful, but the recurrence rate is high.

10. *Atrial Fibrillation*

a. Etiology is related to increased sympathetic tone, hypoxemia, valvular disease, structural heart disease with dilated atria, atrial surgery, digoxin toxicity, or hyperthyroidism. It is not a common arrhythmia in children.

b. History, signs, and symptoms. The patient's history will often include previous cardiac disease or surgery. Clinical signs and symptoms depend on the ventricular response rate. Children may have palpitations, angina, dyspnea, decreased CO, CHF, ischemia, atrial emboli, and an irregular pulse.

c. ECG findings include a wavy baseline with absent or irregular P waves and an "irregularly irregular" ventricular rhythm. With a rapid and irregular atrial rate and no discernible P waves, the atrial rate is not able to be calculated. An irregular and slower ventricular rate is noted; the PR interval is not measurable; and the QRS configuration is normal (Figure 3.48).

d. Interventions can include medications or procedures. Medications can be given to slow the HR, including digoxin and propranolol. They can also be given to convert and maintain NSR (antiarrhythmic medications). Patients can also have cardioversion to return to NSR but it is important to determine the length of time the arrhythmia has been present and confirm that there are no intracardiac thombi as a result of the arrhythmia. Patients with recurrent atrial fibrillation may also undergo atrial fibrillation ablation.

E. Ventricular Arrhythmias

1. *Ventricular arrhythmias* are rare in otherwise normal hearts, occurring in only 10% of pediatric cardiac arrests. They are associated with surgical correction of CHD and can occur in newly transplanted hearts. They are also found in myocarditis, cardiomyopathies, idiopathic hypertrophic subaortic stenosis (IHSS), cardiac tumors, metabolic disturbances, drug toxicity, RV hypertrophy, channelopathies, and QT prolongation. PVCs may be found in utero and in normal children. SCD following the repair of CHD or SCD without known heart disease is most likely due to ventricular arrhythmias (Figure 3.49).

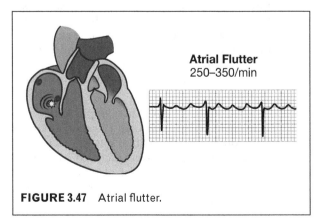

FIGURE 3.47 Atrial flutter.

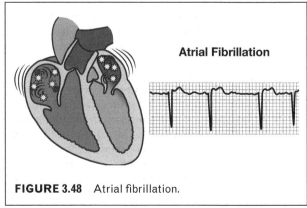

FIGURE 3.48 Atrial fibrillation.

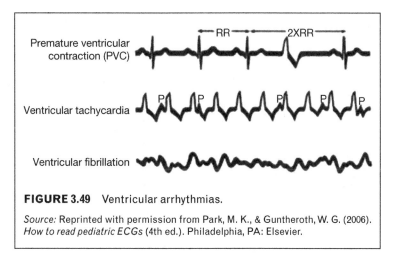

FIGURE 3.49 Ventricular arrhythmias.

Source: Reprinted with permission from Park, M. K., & Guntheroth, W. G. (2006). *How to read pediatric ECGs* (4th ed.). Philadelphia, PA: Elsevier.

2. *Ventricular Tachycardia*

   a. Etiology is related to both reentry and enhanced automaticity resulting from intramyocardial tumor, metabolic disturbances, cardiomyopathy, drug ingestion, drug toxicity, long QT syndrome or other channelopathies, damage to the His–Purkinje system or myocardium (MI, myocarditis, surgery), hypoxemia, acidosis, or hypokalemia. VT is defined as three or more consecutive PVCs. This arrhythmia is uncommon in children who have not undergone intracardiac surgery. In children after cardiac surgery, as many as 18% have nonsustained runs of VT. Torsade de pointes may occur from triggered electrical activity.

   b. History, signs, and symptoms. Patients may experience palpitations, dyspnea, dizziness, anxiety, diaphoresis, angina, decreased level of consciousness, syncope, or decreased BP. VT may be asymptomatic in short bursts, but CO may decrease rapidly with prolonged bursts or short bursts in compromised patients. This rhythm may deteriorate to VF.

   c. ECG findings include a wide, bizarre, abnormal QRS configuration; an HR usually greater than 100 bpm; P waves that are not related to the QRS complex; no discernible PR interval; and a sustained or nonsustained tachycardia. Diagnosis is confirmed by ECG monitor, surface 12-lead ECG, or intracardiac electrophysiology.

   d. Intervention for asymptomatic VT in children with normal hearts may not be warranted in rare situations. The majority of the time, even in asymptomatic patients, treatment is preferred due to the risk of SCD. Medical treatment for VT associated with abnormal myocardial function includes lidocaine, propranolol, procainamide, sotalol, or amiodarone. If present, tumors may be excised. Radiofrequency ablation is used if reentry VT is demonstrated on electrophysiology study. Cardioversion is indicated for acute events of perfusing VT, and defibrillation is used for life-threatening events of nonperfusing VT.

3. *Ventricular Fibrillation*

   a. Etiology includes insults to the His–Purkinje system or myocardium, hypoxemia, electrolyte imbalance, hyperkalemia, electrical shock, drugs, prolonged VT, or long QT syndrome or other channelopathies.

   b. History, signs, and symptoms. Clinical signs and symptoms include loss of consciousness; lack of pulse, respiration, or BP; possible seizure; cyanosis; and clinical death.

   c. ECG findings include a repetitive series of chaotic ventricular waves varying in size and amplitude; complete absence of characteristic P wave, QRS complexes, and T waves; and no measurable HR.

   d. Interventions include cardiopulmonary resuscitation (CPR) plus defibrillation. VF that is not responsive to three successive defibrillation attempts should be treated with medications. The PALS algorithm includes drug–CPR–shock (repeat). See section "Pediatric Advance Cardiac Life Support Protocols."

4. *Long QT Syndrome*

   a. Etiology. Inherited cardiac ion channel disorder associated with either sodium or potassium channels.

b. History, signs, and symptoms. These patients will exhibit one or more of the following: episodes of syncope or aborted SCD, a family history of aborted or SCD, a hearing deficit in 11p15.5 gene disorder, seizures, and palpitations with emotional or physical stress.

c. ECG findings include a prolonged QT interval with a corrected QT interval (QTc) greater than 0.46; an abnormal T-wave configuration (notched, biphasic) with ventricular arrythmias, including R on T VF and VT. In some circumstances, the ECG will have normal QT intervals and therefore close monitoring for prolonged QT intervals on ECG may be more difficult to detect and requires even more diligence. Genetic testing is important to differentiate the type of long QT syndrome.

d. Interventions include medical therapy with β-blocker medications, placement of an internal cardioverter defibrillator, and check of electrolyte balance. Despite therapy, there is a continued risk of sudden death (Kaiser et al., 2015).

F. AV Node Conduction Disorders (Figure 3.50)

1. *First-Degree AV Block*

    a. Etiology. Delay in transmission of intraatrial impulse associated with rheumatic fever, CHD, injury to the AV node, certain cardiac drugs, increased vagal tone, cardiac surgery,

hypoxemia, and ischemia of the conduction system.

    b. History, signs, and symptoms. Usually there are no clinical signs and symptoms. The patient or family will not describe any abnormalities in activity or appetite.

    c. ECG findings include a regular rhythm, a P wave for every QRS complex, a regular P-P and R-R intervals, and a prolonged PR interval for age and HR.

    d. Intervention centers around monitoring because first-degree AV block may progress to second- or third-degree AV block. Treatment is needed only if the cause is drug toxicity.

2. *Second-Degree AV Block*

    a. *Wenckebach (Mobitz type I)*

       i. Etiology includes impaired conduction through the AV node and can be found occasionally in normal hearts or after insults to the AV node, such as inferior MI, hypoxemia, increased vagal tone, and digoxin toxicity.

       ii. History, signs, and symptoms. There usually are no signs or symptoms. If the HR decreases dramatically, CO may decrease. Usually this type of second-degree heart block does not progress.

       iii. ECG findings include a regular P-P interval, an irregular R-R interval, more P

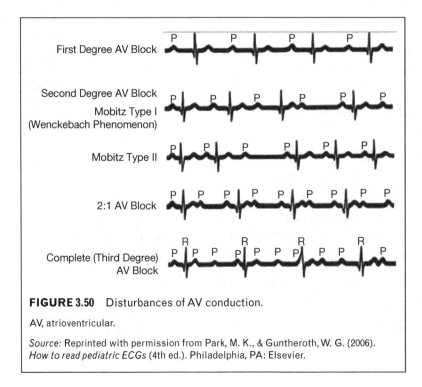

FIGURE 3.50 Disturbances of AV conduction.

AV, atrioventricular.

Source: Reprinted with permission from Park, M. K., & Guntheroth, W. G. (2006). *How to read pediatric ECGs* (4th ed.). Philadelphia, PA: Elsevier.

waves than QRS complexes, and a PR interval that progressively increases until a QRS complex is dropped and then the P:QRS relationship resumes.

    iv. Interventions include treatment of the underlying cause and observation.

  b. *Mobitz type II second-degree heart block*

    i. Etiology. This type of second-degree heart block is more serious and is due to a conduction block in the distal AV conduction system near the bundle of His. It is often related to ischemic changes, insults to the AV node, MI, hypoxemia, cardiac drugs, ischemic disease of the conduction system, CHD, and cardiomyopathy.

    ii. History, signs, and symptoms. A slower HR may diminish CO. Heart block at the level of the bundle of His may progress suddenly and rapidly to CHB with significantly lower HRs and signs and symptoms of CHF or syncope.

    iii. ECG findings include a regular P-P interval, a slower ventricular response, a normal atrial rate, P waves that are upright and normal, a fixed PR interval in the conducted beats, more P waves than QRS complexes, and possibly, an abnormal QRS complex.

    iv. Interventions include treatment of the underlying cause, close monitoring, and consideration for pacemaker placement in symptomatic children.

3. *Complete AV Block (CHB)*

  a. Etiology. This type of heart block occurs within the AV node, junction, or bundle branches and may be congenital or can occur in otherwise structurally normal hearts. Congenital CHB may be diagnosed antenatally and is associated with maternal connective tissue disorders or antinuclear antibodies. Acquired CHB is relatively uncommon in infants and children. It can occur with myopathies, infectious diseases, fibrotic degeneration of the conduction system, CHD, diabetes, collagen disorders or rheumatic fever, surgical interruption of the bundle of His or both bundle branches, and tumors.

  b. History, signs, and symptoms. Symptoms include syncope with lower HRs, decreased exercise tolerance, associated ventricular ectopy, slow HR, decreased CO, and SCD—whether aborted or nonaborted. There is usually normal growth and development, but infants may exhibit signs of CHF if the HR is less than

45 bpm during the first year of life. An evaluation for structural disease should be included in all patients presenting with heart block.

  c. ECG findings include a regular rhythm, an atrial rate greater than the ventricular rate, regular R-R and P-P intervals, and a variable PR interval. The QRS interval will reflect the source of an escape rhythm; for example, a narrow QRS indicates an atrial or junctional origin, whereas a wide QRS may indicate a ventricular origin or a higher origin with aberrant conduction through the ventricles.

  d. Interventions include evaluation of patients with CHB with an ECG, chest radiographic examination, physical examination, echo, Holter monitor, an exercise test every year beginning at the age of 4 to 5 years of age. Permanent cardiac pacing is indicated when syncope or heart failure is present, the heart block is below the bundle of His, the infant has a ventricular rate of less than 55 bpm with frequent or complex ventricular arrhythmias, or the patient has moderate to severe exercise intolerance.

4. *Bundle Branch Block*

  a. Etiology is related to damage to the bundle branch from fibrotic scarring or ischemia. BBB is common following some forms of surgical repair for congenital heart defects such as VSD or tetralogy of Fallot. It can also occur secondary to medications (intraventricular conduction delay), or endocarditis or other infectious processes.

  b. History, signs, and symptoms. Usually there are no clinical signs and symptoms. If all three bundles are blocked—these include the left anterior fascicle, left posterior fascicle, and the RBB—the child will develop CHB and potential asystole.

  c. ECG findings include a QRS width greater than 0.12 seconds or association with other arrhythmias. Diagnosis of RBBB or LBBB is determined with a 12-lead ECG. To evaluate a BBB from a monitor rhythm strip, find a rabbit ear configuration (like the letter "M") in V_1 and a broad, wide S wave in V_6 in RBBB; find a broad, wide S wave in V_1; and a tiny R wave with big "S" wave in V_6.

  d. Interventions include 24-hour ECG monitoring for patients with bifascicular block to assess the development of progressive and denser heart block. Patients are treated with pacemaker implantation if they have BBB with associated heart block or/and those who meet criteria for CRT.

PACEMAKERS AND INTERNAL CARDIOVERTER DEFIBRILLATORS

A. Indications for Cardiac Pacemakers

Pacemakers are used to deliver an electrical impulse (stimulus) to the heart to initiate depolarization and stimulate cardiac contraction. The most common indications for pacemaker placement in the pediatric population are surgically induced heart block, congenital complete heart block, SSS and other symptomatic bradyarrhythmias, long QT syndrome, and neurocardiogenic syncope. Resynchronization therapy can provide a reduction in outflow gradient in symptomatic hypertrophic cardiomyopathy. Conversion to biventricular pacing is used in patients with LV dysfunction to attempt to mimic a more natural conduction impulse and improve LV function.

B. Components of a Pacemaker System

1. The *pulse generator* consists of a battery and is the programmable circuitry of the pacemaker.

2. *Lead wires* conduct impulses from the pulse generator to the heart. An electrode in contact with the heart delivers the impulse. Most leads are bipolar, meaning they contain active and ground leads or positive and negative leads. Unipolar leads use the pacemaker generator itself as the ground pole. Pacemaker wires can be temporary or permanent.

3. *A cable* is used to connect temporary epicardial wires to an external pulse generator.

C. Temporary Cardiac Pacemakers

1. *Transvenous catheters* are placed through the femoral or upper extremity veins with an electrode tip positioned in the RA or RV using bipolar electrodes. This approach may be used for congenital CHB or heart block from myocarditis or infection.

2. *Epicardial wires* are placed directly on the RA or RV or both at the time of open heart surgery. By convention, atrial wires exit to the right chest, ventricular wires exit to the left chest. From the externalized portion of the wire, a contact pin is secured to a cable that connects to the pulse generator. Wires allow both pacing and the ability to have a direct electrogram from the atrial (or ventricular) chambers. Temporary epicardial pacing is indicated for the early postop cardiac surgery patient in heart block or with atrial arrhythmias or sinus bradycardia.

3. An *esophageal pacing probe* passed via the esophagus paces by an impulse traversing the tissue between the electrode and the RA. The probe can pace or record an atrial electrogram. This type of pacing may be used in a patient without temporary epicardial atrial leads that may require atrial pacing or an atrial kick from DDD pacing. Patients generally require heavy sedation to tolerate this type of pacing.

4. *Transthoracic pacing* is accomplished via electrode pads delivering a stimulus through the chest wall. One pad is placed on the anterior chest, and one is placed on the child's back (avoiding the scapula). Noninvasive pacing is not reliable and requires direct electrical impulses to travel through the chest wall, which is painful. Sedation is recommended. Transthoracic pacing may be used during resuscitation, until transvenous pacing can be established or as support during anesthesia induction for other pacer placement.

D. Permanent Cardiac Pacemakers

1. *Transvenous (endocardial) pacing* catheters can be threaded through the subclavian or jugular vein to the RA or RV or both. Transvenous systems are generally used in children who weigh more than 12 kg. Younger or smaller patients require epicardial lead placement as vessel size prohibits transvenous placement. Relative contraindications to transvenous pacing include a lack of venous access to the ventricle (i.e., s/p Fontan), intracardiac right-to-left shunting, elevated PVR, or right ventricular dysfunction or fibrosis (Figure 3.51).

2. *Epicardial leads* are placed through a thoracotomy or sternotomy incision on the epicardial surface of the heart using corkscrew coil, fishhook, or suture electrodes. Epicardial leads may be difficult to place in the presence of scar tissue from repeated operations and resultant adhesions. Epicardial leads are more prone to lead fractures than tranvenous leads.

3. *Generators* are placed in the anterior chest wall or abdominal wall.

E. Pacemaker Functions

1. Nomenclature was defined by the North American Society for Pacing and Electrophysiology (NASPE) and British Pacing and Electrophysiology Group (BPEG) devised a generic code used to communicate pacer functions (Table 3.9; Park, 2016). The first letter describes chamber(s) paced, the second letter describes chamber(s) sensed, and the third letter describes the mode of response to sensing. In permanent pacemakers, additional codes include the fourth letter, which indicates the ability of the pacemaker to respond to programming, and the fifth letter, which indicates the ability of the pacemaker to respond to tachyarrhythmias by burst pacing or shock.

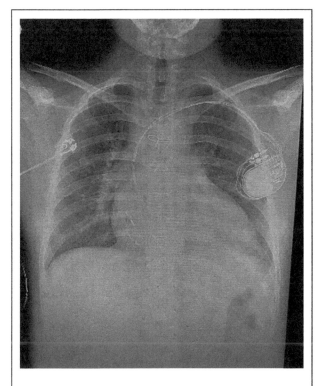

FIGURE 3.51 Standard transvenous lead position in an adolescent.

Courtesy of Michigan Medicine, University of Michigan.

2. Pacemaker capabilities include *pacing* (the ability of the pacemaker to deliver an impulse to the heart), *sensing* (the ability to detect intrinsic cardiac activity), and *capture* (the effectiveness of the pacing stimulus to cause contraction).

3. *Generator Activity Modes (Response to Sensing,* Table 3.10)

    a. Triggered. Will pace in response to sensing no electrical activity (Park, 2016).

    b. Inhibited. Will not pace in response to sensing electrical activity (Park, 2016).

    c. Demand (inhibited and/or triggered) mode. Allows the pacemaker to sense intrinsic cardiac activity and inhibit pacing when it senses intrinsic activity at a rate equal to or above the programmed rate. A pacing stimulus is delivered (triggered) when the intrinsic rate is inadequate. Demand pacing avoids complications caused by competition between the child's intrinsic rate and the pacemaker. AV conduction is required for effective atrial demand pacing. AV conduction is not required for ventricular demand pacing, but AV synchrony is lost. Synchronous AV demand pacing simulates the normal cardiac cycle, but it cannot be used in the presence of atrial arrhythmia (Park, 2016).

    d. Asynchronous or fixed-rate mode. Paces at a continuous set rate without sensing or responding to intrinsic cardiac activity. AV conduction is required for an effective atrial fixed rate pacing mode (Park, 2016).

TABLE 3.9 The NASPE/BPEG Generic (NBG) Pacemaker Code

I	II	III	IV	V
Chamber Paced	Chamber Sensed	Response to Sensing	Rate Modulation	Antitachyarrythmia Function(s)
A = Atrium V = Ventricle O = None D = Dual (A + V)	A = Atrium V = Ventricle O = None D = Dual (A + V)	T = Triggered I = Inhibited O = None D = Dual (T + I)	P = Simple M = Multiprogrammable O = None C = Communicating R = Rate Modulation	P = Pacing S = Shock O = None D = Dual (P + S)

NASPE, North American Society for Pacing and Electrophysiology; BPEG, British Pacing and Electrophysiology Group.

Source: From Mavroudis, C., & Backer, C. L. (2013). *Pediatric cardiac surgery* (4th ed.). St. Louis, MO: Mosby.

TABLE 3.10   Common Pacemaker Modes

Mode	Generator Activity	Indication
AAI—atrial demand	Paces atrium Senses atrium Inhibits pacer if senses atrial activity above set rate	Sinus or high-junctional bradycardias when AV conduction system intact, provides atrial kick
VVI—ventricular demand	Paces ventricle Senses ventricle Inhibits pacer if senses ventricular activity above set rate	Used in emergencies to establish ventricular activity, when AV dissociation present, maintains CO without atrial kick
AOO—atrial asynchronous	Paces atrium Sensing off Triggered to fire at fixed rate	Sinus or high-junctional bradycardias when AV conduction system intact, can trigger atrial arrhythmias, used in emergencies
VOO—ventricular asynchronous	Paces ventricle Sensing off Triggered to fire at fixed rate	Asystole Dangerous as can cause R-on-T with ventricular fibrillation, use DDD or VVI instead
DDD—AV sequential or dual chambered pacing	Paces atrium and ventricle Senses atrium and ventricle Fires only if atrium or ventricle drop below a set rate	Any arrhythmia without AV conduction (blocks) Avoid in atrial fibrillation or flutter as tracks atrial rate Maintains CO with atrial kick

AV, atrioventricular; CO, cardiac output.

e.   Rate-responsive pacing. Pacemaker rate changes in response to changes in patient parameters (Park, 2016).

f.   Pacemakers can monitor and track arrhythmias, including the date, time, and length of duration of the event as well as record an intracardiac electrogram.

4. *Pacemaker Settings*

a.   Mode. See Table 3.10.

b.   Rate. Pacing is activated when the patient's HR is under a preset limit. It is also important to know what the upper HR limit for pacing is to continually assess appropriate pacing.

c.   AV interval. The time between atrial sensing or pacing and ventricular activity (sensing or pacing). Equivalent to the PR interval, it is the time to allow atrial contraction and diastolic filling of ventricle.

d.   The postventricular atrial refractory period is the time when the atrial lead does not sense or respond to intrinsic atrial activity. It is a protective feature to prevent rapid ventricular pacing to atrial ectopy (premature atrial

contractions, atrial flutter, or fibrillation) and to avoid pacing of retrograde P waves.

e.   Capture threshold. The minimum amount of electrical current needed to depolarize the myocardium. It is measured in milliamps (mA). The pacemaker output is usually set at two to three times the capture threshold to allow for a safety margin.

f.   Sensing threshold. The programmed setting for the pacemaker to recognize intrinsic cardiac activity. It is measured in millivolts (mV). Lowering the mV threshold increases pacemaker sensitivity to cardiac impulses, whereas raising the mV decreases the sensitivity.

F. ECG Evidence of Pacemakers (Figure 3.52)

1. *Capture represents* depolarization of the atria or ventricle initiated by the pacemaker impulse. It produces a pacemaker spike displayed on the ECG. An atrial pacing stimulus is followed by a P wave, and a ventricular pacing stimulus is followed by a QRS complex if the respective chambers are captured.

2. *Undersensing* occurs when the pacemaker fails to identify intrinsic depolarization and paces

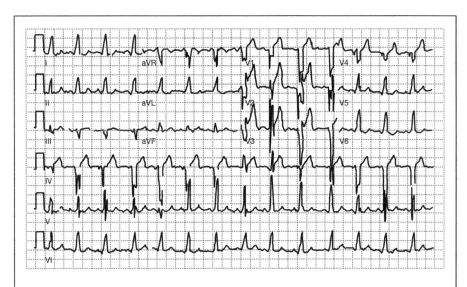

FIGURE 3.52 12-lead ECG with appropriate ventricular sensing and pacing.

Courtesy of Michigan Medicine, University of Michigan, CS Mott Children's Hospital, Congenital Heart Center.

regardless of the chamber activity. This can be caused by lead fracture, high impedance in the lead, a lack of connection to the generator, or a low sensitivity setting.

3. *Oversensing* occurs when the pacemaker detects activity that is not actual cardiac depolarization and inhibits pacing. This can be caused by shivering, chest-wall movement, or ungrounded electrical equipment.

4. *Noncapture* occurs when the pacemaker fires but fails to cause a myocardial depolarization (no P wave or QRS wave). This can be caused by lead fracture or disconnection, low battery, low output settings, or high pacing thresholds from edema or scarring at the lead site (Table 3.11).

G. Complications of Pacemakers

1. *Insertion* can result in local or systemic infection, pneumothorax, myocardial perforation with transvenous placement, arrhythmias, and hematoma or bleeding.

2. *Component problems* are outlined in Table 3.11 and can result in abnormal pacer function.

3. *Bleeding or tamponade* can follow placement of transvenous wires or removal of temporary wires.

4. *Risk of systemic emboli* can occur in children with right-to-left intracardiac shunts with transvenous pacing catheters.

5. *Risk of pulmonary emboli* can occur in children with PA hypertension.

H. Automatic Internal Cardiovertor Defibrillator (AICD or ICD)

1. *Indications for automatic ICD placement* (Kaiser et al., 2015) include SCD survivors, those at risk of ventricular arrhythmias by underlying diagnosis (long QT syndrome, HCM, severely diminished ventricular function), or those with inducible VT on electrophysiology study.

2. *Implantation techniques* include both epicardial patches, which are sutured to the pericardium (usually for children weighing less than 20 kg), or transvenous electrodes.

3. The *ICD generator* can be programmed to sense, pace, overdrive pace, cardiovert, and defibrillate in response to preset recognition criteria for an arrhythmia (rate, QRS duration, number of beats). The device also has an internal memory to allow recording of the rhythm before, during, and after an event.

I. Goals and Patient Management

1. For *temporary pacemakers*, assess the hemodynamic status of the child by his or her vital signs as well as the response to pacing. Evaluate ECG monitoring to determine the underlying rhythm, pacing and sensing thresholds, and appropriate

TABLE 3.11 **Demonstration of Abnormal Pacemaker Function Related to Undersensing, Oversensing, or Noncapture**

	Sample ECG Appearance	Some Possible Clinical Consequences	Some Possible Causes	Corrective Measures
Undersensing Device fails to detect existing cardiac depolarizations, therefore, competes with the native rhythm	These native R waves are not detected ...therefore the pacer emits these unneeded spikes	Competition with a native rhythm Stimulation of dysrhythmias ("R-on-T")	Lead disconnected from pacer or from viable myocardium Sensitivity set too low Lead fracture Low battery	Check connection of lead to pacer Increase sensitivity (turn sensing control to a smaller number) Sensitivity (mV) Reposition or change lead Change battery
Oversensing Device detects noncardiac electrical events and interprets them as cardiac depolarizations, therefore, the device is wrongly inhibited from pacing	Pacing should occur as indicated by the arrows but is inhibited by oversensed noncardiac electrical noise. When the noise ceases pacing resumes.	Pacemaker-dependent patients receive no stimuli from the pacemaker, producing a pause in rhythm and reduction in cardiac output	Electrical potential caused by noncardiac muscle contraction (especially pectorals) is detected and misinterpreted by the device; interference from electrical sources (ungrounded equipment, short circuits) is detected and misinterpreted by the device indicating that sensitivity is set too high	Decrease sensitivity (turn sensing control to a larger number) Sensitivity (mV) Remove all ungrounded electrical equipment or have it evaluated by hospital engineers
Noncapture Device emits stimuli that fail to capture the myocardium	This dual-chamber device paces and captures in the atrium and ventricle from the first two beats. Ventricular capture is then lost; the ventricular pacing spikes are not followed by depolarizations; ventricular escape begins.	Pacemaker-dependent patients receive no stimuli from the pacemaker, producing a pause in rhythm and reduction in cardiac output	Lead disconnected from pacer or from viable myocardium Output set too low in the noncaptured chamber Lead fracture High pacing threshold due to medication or metabolic changes Low battery	Check connection of lead to pacer Increase output in the noncaptured chamber Reposition or change lead Change battery Alter medication regimen; correct metabolic changes

Source: From Witherall, C. L. (1994). Cardiac rhythm control devices. *Critical Care Nursing Clinics of North America, 6,* 95–102.

capture. Ensure normal electrolytes and acid–base balance. Pacemaker wires and equipment should be appropriately grounded to prevent accidental electrocution. Also, properly ground all electrical equipment used by the child, including video and electronic games. Pacemaker dials should be covered to prevent accidental changes in settings. Some pacemakers have locking buttons to prevent an accidental change in programmed settings. Note that some models do not have memory, so that programmed settings are lost if the pacemaker is turned off. A spare battery should be taped to the pacemaker in the event of battery failure, especially in pacemaker-dependent patients. When using a temporary transvenous system, stabilize the extremity associated with the catheter insertion site (avoid leg flexion), and observe the catheter site for signs of infection. Patient and family teaching should include indications for pacing and procedures surrounding placement.

2. For *permanent pacemakers*, assess the hemodynamic status of the child by his or her vital signs as well as the response to pacing. Evaluate ECG monitoring to determine underlying rhythm, pacing and sensing thresholds, and appropriate capture. Teach the patient and family to assess the patient status and to know when they should call for help. Teach the patient and family to report dizziness, syncope, weakness, fatigue, increased symptoms of CHF, redness, swelling, drainage at the incision site(s), palpitations, unresolved or frequent hiccups, fever, decreased feeding, or irritability. Provide the family with information for a medic-alert bracelet and information regarding transmission of transtelephonic pacemaker checks. Stress the importance of always carrying the pacemaker identification card with the patient and physician name, address, and phone number; medications; and the pacemaker type and settings. If the patient moves out of the area, timely referral to a new cardiologist is recommended. Instruct the patient and the family on the appropriate timing to return to normal activity, including school, driving, and exercise (contact sports are to be avoided). Pregnancy generally is well tolerated, depending on any associated disease. Pacemaker generator battery life should be tested regularly via phone transmissions or interrogation, with anticipatory planning for subsequent generator changes (Swerdlow, Wang, & Zypes, 2015).

3. For *ICD* placement, teach the child and family what action to take in the event the ICD deploys a shock. Testing the function of the ICD device should occur in the controlled setting of the electrophysiology laboratory where VT or VF is intentionally induced and terminated to test the device. The ICD function can be checked with a routine device interrogation (Wiley, Demo, Walker, & Shuler, 2016).

4. *Pacemaker interrogation* will be performed at regular intervals as an outpatient, but also following pacemaker insertion, prior to discharge, and any time pacemaker function is questioned. Interrogation may be done to assess ventricular function in different modes and at different HRs during the acute phase of illness. Interrogations can also be done transtelephonically on an outpatient basis (Park, 2016).

   a. Pacemaker interrogation consists of the following:

   i.   Prior to beginning interrogation, the device manufacturer is needed as the programmer for pacemaker interrogation is specific to the device.

   ii.   The interrogation involves placing a device (often called a *wand*) over the generator that communicates to the programmer.

iii.   The battery voltage is checked, which may give insights into the life span of the current generator.

iv.   The pacemaker leads are tested for impedance (300–1,000 Ohms unless high impedance leads are used), sensing (normal atrial sensing is >1 mV; normal ventricular sensing is >5 mV), and threshold testing (ideally atrial threshold will be at or <1 V at 0.4 ms; the ventricular threshold will be at or <1–2 V at 0.4 ms).

v.   The underlying rhythm is documented with acute suspension of pacing or by decreasing the pacemaker rate or threshold until there is a loss of capture and the patient's rhythm is evident. For patients who are pacemaker dependent for HR, care should be exercised in going below rates of 30 and the pacing capability should not be acutely terminated or the risk of asystole is significant.

vi.   The number of mode-switch episodes is documented.

vii.   The sensing threshold is documented.

viii.   The pacing output is set at two times the pacing threshold for pulse voltage and three times for pulse duration.

ix.   The pacemaker will provide a record of high rates.

x.   The pacemaker will provide a history of the percentage of time each chamber is paced and sensed.

xi.   Changes can be made to any function of the pacemaker that best suits the patient's CO and pacemaker needs.

   b. ICD interrogation will be performed at the time of implantation, prior to discharge, any time an ICD shock is delivered, and periodically as an outpatient (Park, 2016).

   i.   The interrogation requires the programmer to be compatible with the ICD device and a device is positioned over the generator as with pacemaker interrogation.

   ii.   The ICD leads are tested, the underlying rhythm is noted, the sensing threshold is documented, the history of high rates is noted, and the number of tachycardia episodes is noted.

   iii.   In addition, the number and appropriateness of ICD shocks can be studied. The time to last full energy charge is noted; normal is less than 15 seconds.

J. Complications

1. Inappropriate sensing, failure to capture, oversensing

2. Inappropriate ICD shock or failure to detect and shock

3. Infection of generator site or endocarditis

4. Lead fracture, generator end-of-life battery failure

5. Pain at generator insertion site

6. Psychological implications of ICD or pacemaker placement

CONGENITAL HEART DISEASE

A. Etiologic Aspects of CHD

1. *Cardiovascular disease* can be familial or acquired. CHD includes all cardiovascular diseases present at birth. CHD occurs in 8% to 10% of every 1,000 live births. CHD may be attributable primarily to genetic factors, with little environmental influence, or attributable to genetic and environmental (multifactorial) interactions (Hazinski, 2013).

2. *Genetic causes* are frequently associated with a syndrome (e.g., Down syndrome). The recurrence risk of the heart lesion in a subsequent birth is related to the recurrence risk of the chromosomal anomaly (Christiansen et al., 2015). A single mutant gene may cause a syndrome, or others may be related to microdeletions and translocations. It may have dominant inheritance (e.g., IHSS, ASD). With dominance, part of the gene is responsible for the trait. Recessive traits must be present in two copies to permit expression. There are autosomal dominant and recessive forms of conduction defects. With Mendelian inheritance, the recurrence risk is high.

3. *Multifactorial inheritance* is responsible for most CHD. Hereditary predisposition to cardiovascular maldevelopment interacts with an environmental trigger at the vulnerable period of cardiogenesis. Generally, the recurrence risk is 1% to 4%. The more common the defect, the more likely it is to recur. Risk increases rapidly with the number of first-degree relatives affected. If two first-degree relatives are affected, the recurrence risk is tripled. If three or more first-degree relatives are affected, the risk is a type C classification with a very high recurrence (Christiansen et al., 2015). Teratogenic exposure in

the mother may contribute to the incidence of CHD, although proof is lacking in some cases. Usually the exposure is of short duration.

4. *Risk to offspring* of the affected parent: Risks are higher for offspring when the affected parent is the mother.

5. There is a 1% incidence of *single-gene hyperlipoproteinemia*. The single most important risk factor is early onset of coronary disease in a first-degree relative younger than 55 years (heredity, 57%–63%). Environmental factors, such as diet, smoking, and exercise, can be manipulated to reduce risk factors.

B. CHD Classifications

1. *Acyanotic cardiac lesions* are those with left-to-right intracardiac shunts (i.e., VSDs). Blood shunts from areas of high to low resistance. The physiology of these defects leads to symptoms of pulmonary overcirculation, which may result in symptoms of CHF (Figure 3.53).

2. *Obstructive cardiac lesions* are characterized by restrictive blood flow in the left heart (systemic circulation) across the stenotic area with hypertensive changes proximal to the obstruction; the physiology of obstructive lesions may include hypoperfusion states distal to the obstruction (Figure 3.54).

3. *Cyanotic cardiac lesions* are those with right-to-left intracardiac shunt with reduced pulmonary blood flow. This is commonly caused by obstruction in the right heart (pulmonary circulation; i.e., tricuspid atresia, TAPVR). This results in intracardiac and/or extracardiac mixing of saturated and desaturated blood and cyanosis. Cyanotic symptoms are related to the degree and number of right-to-left shunts. Cyanosis may also result from anatomically malposed vessels (i.e., TGV; Figure 3.55).

4. *Great vessel lesions* usually occur during looping of the ventricles in embryologic development. The coronary arteries will always be associated with the aorta, regardless of where the aorta arises. The respective circulation may be normal despite anatomic abnormalities or may present with severe cyanosis in the neonatal period (Figure 3.56).

5. *Single-ventricle cardiac lesions* result in ductal-dependent systemic circulation if the hypoplastic ventricle is on the systemic side (aortic outflow) or ductal-dependent pulmonary circulation if the hypoplastic ventricle is on the right side (pulmonary ventricle). Early survival is dependent upon maintaining a PDA, typically requiring a prostaglandin infusion.

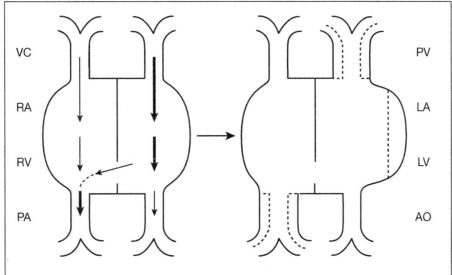

FIGURE 3.53 Diagram of blood flow in ventricular septal defect.

AO, aorta; LA, left atrium; LV, left ventricle; PA, pulmonary artery; PV, pulmonary ventricle; RA, right atrium; RV, right ventricle; VC, vena cava.

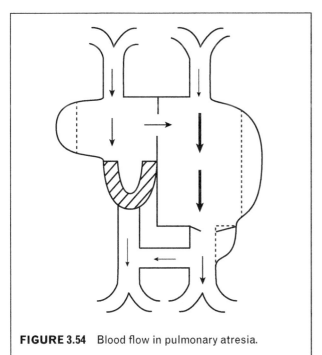

FIGURE 3.54 Blood flow in pulmonary atresia.

C. Acyanotic Cardiac Lesions

1. *Patent Ductus Arteriosus*

   a. Anatomy

   i. Persistence of a normal fetal channel connecting the aorta and PA.

   b. Incidence

   i. In preterm infants the response to the vasoconstrictor stimulus of oxygen is not developed, resulting in persistence of the ductus arteriosus. The incidence of PDA in full-term infants is approximately 4.5% and in preterm infants may be as high as 30% (Mumtaz & Qureshi, 2013). Failure to close in this population is related to a structural defect in the wall of the ductus. Exposure to rubella during the first trimester of pregnancy is associated with PDA.

   c. Pathophysiology

   i. In fetal life, the ductus arteriosus permits flow to be diverted away from the high-resistance pulmonary circulation to the descending aorta and the low-resistance placental circulation.

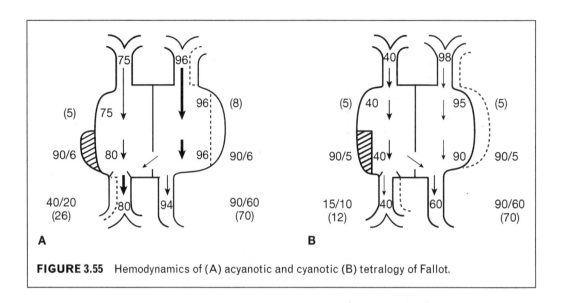

FIGURE 3.55 Hemodynamics of (A) acyanotic and cyanotic (B) tetralogy of Fallot.

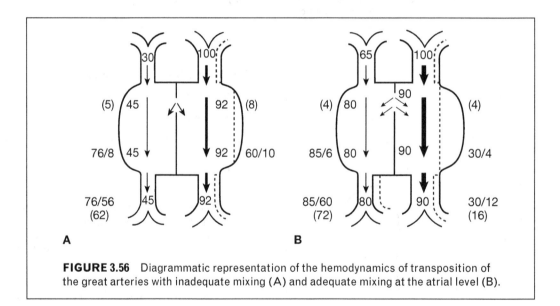

FIGURE 3.56 Diagrammatic representation of the hemodynamics of transposition of the great arteries with inadequate mixing (A) and adequate mixing at the atrial level (B).

ii. Closure of the ductus arteriosus normally occurs from contraction of the medial smooth muscle in the wall of the ductus arteriosus during the first 12 to 24 hours after birth, which is initiated by a rise in the perivascular PO_2 and decrease in endogenous prostaglandin. This produces functional closure; however, the ductus may be reopened at this point in response to a strong stimulus such as acidosis, hypoxemia, or prostaglandins. Anatomic closure occurs between 2

and 3 weeks and is produced by fibrosis of the ductal tissue with permanent sealing of the lumen to produce the ligamentum arteriosum. Following anatomic closure, the ductus cannot be reopened.

iii. In isolated PDA, where the ductus fails to close normally, blood shunts from left to right into the PA and lungs. This occurs as the PVR drops and the pressure in the aorta exceeds that of the PA. Pulmonary blood flow increases, thus increasing venous return to the LA; LA and LV volume overload and CHF ensues. Over time, the increased flow and pressure on the pulmonary circulation changes the pulmonary vasculature, resulting in PA hypertension and increased PVR. Once these changes have progressed from medial hypertrophy and intimal hyperplasia to fibrosis of the pulmonary bed, they are irreversible and result in pulmonary hypertension and reversal of the cardiac shunt. Blood is then shunted right to left, causing cyanosis. This reversal of shunt flow resulting from changes in the pulmonary vascular bed from pressure and volume overload is known as *Eisenmenger syndrome*. Once reversal of shunt flow has occurred, surgical closure of the defect is contraindicated. These children may then be candidates for treatment of pulmonary hypertension (prostacyclin infusion) or heart–lung or lung transplant. In the presence of additional cardiac lesions, the PDA direction can be right-to-left or bidirectional (Mumtaz, Qureshi, Mavroudis, & Backer, 2013a).

iv.   The presence of a large PDA results in a low diastolic pressure. This may adversely affect myocardial function from poor coronary perfusion.

d.   Clinical signs and symptoms

i.   The presentation depends on the size and diameter of the ductus; the degree of shunting, which is based on the length and diameter of the ductus; compensatory mechanisms; and the stage of lung development. Full-term neonates have elevated PVR, and therefore shunting is not so pronounced. Premature infants may have severe low CO and require emergency closure to restore adequate diastolic pressure and perfusion of the myocardium as well as other organs. Small PDAs with small shunts rarely produce symptoms, and growth and development are normal. Moderate and large defects produce symptoms of CHF from the left-to-right shunt and LV volume overload.

ii.   Examination reveals a machine-like continuous murmur auscultated at the left upper sternal border. Poor feeding, irritability, tachycardia, tachypnea, and slow weight gain are often present. The pulse pressure is wide, and peripheral pulses may be strong and collapse suddenly because of low diastolic pressure resulting from ductal shunting of blood into the low-pressure PA. This is referred to as a *water-hammer pulse*.

e.   Diagnostic evaluation

i.   ECG shows prominent LV forces, LA hypertrophy, and possibly RV hypertrophy.

ii.   Chest radiographic examination shows enlargement of the cardiac silhouette with LA and LV enlargement. The MPA segment is prominent. The pulmonary vascular markings are accentuated in moderate to large shunts.

iii.   Echo demonstrates an increased LA diameter. An estimate of the shunt may be made from the LA-to-aorta ratio.

iv.   Cardiac catheterization for diagnosis is rarely performed. If done, it will demonstrate a step-up in oxygen concentration in the PA. The PA pressure and resistance can also be evaluated and may be elevated in large shunts.

f.   Goals and patient medical management

i.   Medical therapy involves control of CHF with medications or closure of the ductus with indomethacin once normal kidney function and an adequate platelet count are ensured.

g.   Goals and surgical patient management

i.   Interventional catheterization can be performed to provide closure with intracardiac device in a small- or moderate-sized ductus. Risk of device closure includes residual shunt, embolization of the coil or device, damage to adjacent structures, and hemolysis.

ii.   Surgical closure involves division or ligation (or both) of the ductus through a left thoracotomy. Postoperative complications are rare but may include damage to the recurrent laryngeal nerve, chylous effusion, bleeding, infection, paralyzed phrenic nerve, ligation of the left PA or descending aorta, or tear in the ductus or aorta.

iii.   Use of video-assisted thoracoscopic surgery is being introduced at some centers. Risks of this procedure, although low, include injury to the recurrent laryngeal nerve, thoracic duct injury with chylous effusion, prolonged exposure to radiation and residual ductus due to inadequate visualization requiring need to convert to thoracotomy.

h.   Complications include bleeding, perforation, inability to ligate ductus, and nerve damage.

2. *Atrial Septal Defect*

    a. Anatomy

        i. Atrial septal defect is a defect in the atrial septum from improper embryologic formation of the septal wall (Figure 3.57).

        ii. Failure of the septum to form in the fetal period results in defects in the atrial septal wall.

    b. Incidence. Occurs in approximately 6% to 10% of live births and is more common in females by a ratio of 2:1 (Backer & Mavroudis, 2013a).

    c. Pathophysiology

        i. The defect is created by failure of the endocardial cushion tissue to seal the septum primum (ostium primum defect), failure of the valve of the fossa ovalis cordis to close (patent foramen ovale [PFO]), or failure of closure of the septal fenestration (ostium secundum defect). Defects allow blood to be shunted from the higher pressure left side of the heart to the lower pressure right side of the heart, resulting in RV volume and pressure overload with RA and RV dilation. Pulmonary vascular changes occur in 10% to 20% of patients with an ASD. By the third to fourth decade of life, atrial arrhythmias, CHF, and paradoxical embolus become problems. Endocarditis is uncommon.

        1) Sinus venosus. High in the septum near the junction of the SVC and RA, or low at the IVC RA junction; may be associated with partial anomalous pulmonary venous return.

        2) Ostium secundum. This is the most common type of ASD and occurs in the region of the fossa ovalis cordis. It may be associated with mitral valve prolapse.

        3) Ostium primum. Low in septum; may involve defects of one or both AV valves.

        4) Unroofed coronary sinus. Coronary sinus blood is diverted to the LA.

        5) Patent foramen ovale. Occurs in central region of the septum, where the fossa ovalis remains open.

    d. Clinical signs and symptoms

        i. Most patients are asymptomatic, but those with large left-to-right shunts may exhibit symptoms of fatigue and dyspnea. Growth retardation is unusual.

        ii. Examination. Auscultation may reveal a systolic ejection murmur at the LSB (pulmonary flow murmur); wide, fixed, split S_2; and a diastolic murmur from large-volume flow across the tricuspid valve.

    e. Diagnostic evaluation

        i. ECG demonstrates RV and RA hypertrophy, right-axis deviation, RBBB, prolonged PR interval, and possibly evidence of junctional rhythm or a SVT.

        ii. Chest radiographic examination may show RVH, RA enlargement, and increased pulmonary vascular markings, but in most cases heart size may be normal.

        iii. Echo confirms the diagnosis in most cases with evidence of RV volume overload, direct visualization of the location and size of defect, and identification of associated defects (most common, anomalous pulmonary veins or PS).

        iv. Cardiac catheterization is rarely indicated. If performed, the catheterization would demonstrate an increase in oxygen saturation in the RA.

    f. Goals and medical patient management. Monitor for spontaneous closure. Refer patients with persistent uncorrected moderate to large defects, left-to-right shunting increases with age resulting in an increased risk of developing heart failure, atrial arrhythmias, and pulmonary hypertension.

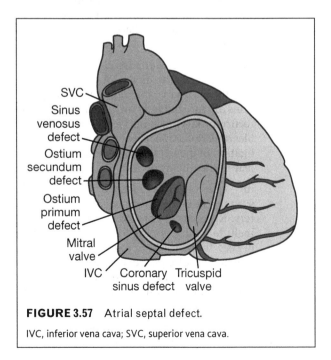

SVC
Sinus venosus defect
Ostium secundum defect
Ostium primum defect
Mitral valve
IVC
Coronary sinus defect
Tricuspid valve

FIGURE 3.57 Atrial septal defect.

IVC, inferior vena cava; SVC, superior vena cava.

g. Goals and surgical patient management

i. Many ASDs close spontaneously (up to 85%), but repair of the defect is low risk and is recommended by school age despite presentation to prevent long-term problems with pulmonary disease and arrhythmia. Adult patients undergoing ASD closure may not benefit from complete resolution of symptoms, specifically arrhythmias, but most likely they will have improved quality of life. Closure of a patent foramen ovale/ASD in an adult presenting with paradoxical embolism is indicated to prevent recurrence and avoid risk of lifelong anticoagulation.

ii. Defects may be closed via a right thoracotomy or through a sternotomy. Current techniques of minimally invasive closure of ASD use a small median sternotomy incision with excellent visualization for the surgeon and improved cosmetic results. Surgical repair requires a short period of cardiopulmonary bypass. The defect may be closed primarily by suturing the tissue edges, or patched with material, like that of the pericardium (Figure 3.58). Generally, these patients are extubated in the operating room or shortly after arriving in the intensive care unit (Winch et al., 2016).

iii. Transcatheter closure of ASD is routinely performed in patients meeting criteria for size, shape, and location of the defect (Figure 3.59). The Amplatzer Septal Occluder (AGA Medical Corp., Golden Valley, MN) device is approved by the Food and Drug Administration for use in small- to

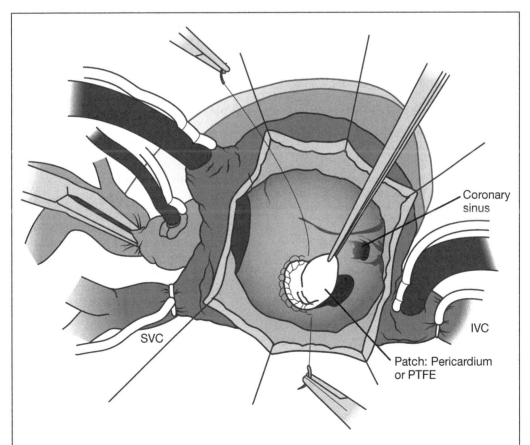

FIGURE 3.58 Closure of an ostium secundum ASD with a patch. Cardioplegia has been delivered and the heart arrested. The right atrium has been opened. The ASD is being closed with a patch—usually of autologous pericardium, although PTFE also can be used.

ASD, atrial septal defect; IVC, inferior vena cava; PTFE, polytetrafluoroethylene; SVC, superior vena cava.

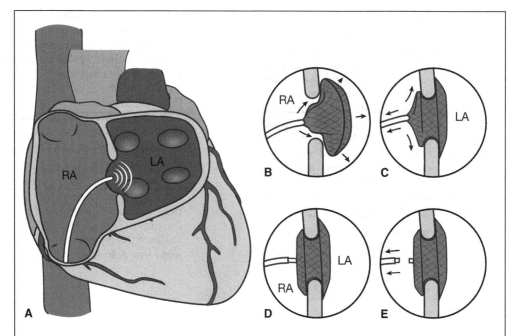

FIGURE 3.59 Implantation of the Amplatzer ASD occluder. (A) The delivery catheter is positioned across the atrial defect. (B) LA disk with self-centering connecting stalk is delivered. (C) The device is withdrawn so that the connecting stalk is within the ASD and the left disk is firm against the atrial septum. (D) RA disk is delivered. (E) Delivery cable is disconnected; the device can no longer be withdrawn back into the atrium.

ASD, atrial septal defect; LA, Left atrium; RA, right atrium.

medium-sized secundum defects. Risks include incomplete closure, embolization of the device, tricuspid valve injury, erosion of tissue, and arrhythmia.

h. *Complications* include atrial arrhythmia, heart block, residual defect, anemia, phrenic nerve injury, air embolus, patch dehiscence, pericardial effusion/postpericardiotomy syndrome, and AV valve regurgitation in ostium primum defects (Heching, Bacha, & Liberman, 2015).

3. *Ventricular Septal Defect*

a. Definition

i. Communication between the RV and LV is created by an opening in the septal wall. Defect results from imperfect embryologic formation of the septal wall.

b. Incidence

i. VSD accounts for 20% of CHD, is the most common CHD excluding bicuspid aortic valve, occurs in isolation in 2/1,000 patients and is slightly more common in girls (Mavorudis, 2013).

c. Pathophysiology

i. Effects of the VSD depend on the size and number of the defects and resistance to flow through the lungs (flow is also affected by the presence of RV outflow tract obstruction). VSDs may present as small defects with normal PVR, moderate defects with variable PVR, or large defects with either mild to moderate or marked elevation of PVR.

d. Classification (Figure 3.60)

i. Perimembranous VSD is the most common type and is located below the crista supraventricularis adjacent to the tricuspid valve. It may be associated with malalignment of the septum.

ii. Infundibular, subpulmonic, subarterial, conal, and supracristal VSDs are positioned in the RV outflow tract under the pulmonary valve.

iii. Inlet VSD is a common defect located under the AV valve posterior and inferior to the membranous septum.

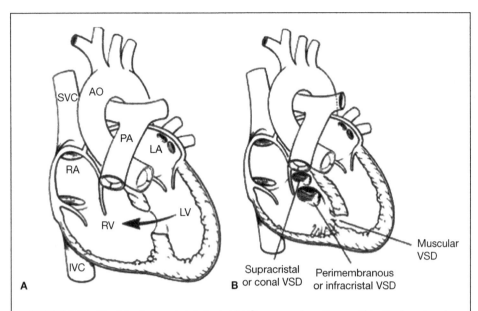

FIGURE 3.60 Ventricular septal defect. (A) Oxygen saturations within the heart and great vessels are depicted. (B) Types of VSDs.

AO, aorta; IVC, inferior vena cava; LA, left atrium; LV, left ventricle; PA, pulmonary artery; RA, right atrium; RV, right ventricle; SVC, superior vena cava; VSD, ventricular septal defect.

Source: Reprinted with permission from Kambam, J. (1994). Atrial septal defect. In J. Kambam (Ed.), *Cardiac anesthesia for infants and children.* St. Louis, MO: Mosby.

iv. Muscular defects are located in the muscular septum. If multiple, they are termed *Swiss cheese* septum.

e. Clinical signs and symptoms

i. Children are usually asymptomatic until 2 to 4 weeks of age, when PVR falls. The drop in PVR allows shunting from the LV to the RV and creates pulmonary overcirculation. Long-term pulmonary overcirculation causes PA hypertension and vascular changes progressing from medial hypertrophy and intimal hyperplasia to fibrosis and Eisenmenger syndrome (rarely before 1 year of age).

ii. Presentation is dependent on the size of the shunt and PVR.

iii. Examination reveals a holosystolic murmur at the LSB, normal S_1, split and increased S_2, possible S_3, thrill at the LSB, active precordium, and a diastolic rumble at the LSB in large defects. The murmur decreases as PVR increases.

f. Diagnostic evaluation

i. Assess the size of the defect, magnitude of hemodynamic overload, and status of pulmonary vasculature.

ii. ECG. Small defects have normal ECG findings. Moderate to large defects have LA enlargement, LVH with or without RVH, left-axis deviation, and BBB.

iii. Chest radiographic examination. Small defects have normal radiographic findings. Moderate to large defects have cardiomegaly, prominent PA segment, and increased pulmonary vascular markings.

iv. Echo confirms the location, size of defect, associated lesions, and LA and LV dilation. Echo also quantifies the degree of RV and PA hypertension.

v. Cardiac catheterization demonstrates an elevated pulmonary-to-systemic flow ratio (Q_p:Q_s), elevated RV and PA pressures, elevated PVR in large defects, and oxygen step-up in the RV and PA.

g. Goals and medical patient management

i. Indications for intervention include CHF, PA hypertension, growth failure, or evidence for LV volume overload. Some defects close spontaneously. Medical management is used for control of CHF (see "Heart Failure in Children" section).

h. Goals and surgical patient management

i. Surgical palliation with a PA band aims at controlling pulmonary blood flow and protecting the pulmonary vascular bed, mainly for large and multiple muscular VSDs in the lower septum, patients with multiple anomalies, and preterm infants. This approach may be indicated as a temporizing measure in cases for which CHF symptoms are significant, yet primary VSD repair is not yet feasible. PA banding via a left thoracotomy decreases the pressure distal to the band to approximately one half the aortic pressure, but it may not restrict flow adequately. Surgery poses the risk of chylothorax, paralyzed hemidiaphragm, and damage to the recurrent laryngeal nerve. Complications include migration of the band, distortion of the vessels, failure to protect the lung vasculature adequately, erosion of the band into the PA, creation of subaortic stenosis from septal hypertrophy, and damage to the pulmonary valve.

ii. Percutaneous device closure is indicated for perimembranous VSDs. Device closure may also be attempted in cases of multiple or difficult-to-reach VSDs, which may require alternative surgical approaches such as ventriculotomy. Device placement avoids ventriculotomy and can be performed in the catheterization laboratory or in the operating room. Disadvantages include peripheral vascular injury from the large venous sheaths, residual shunting, arrhythmia, device migration or embolization, or disruption of papillary muscles.

iii. For large, hemodynamically significant defects, surgical closure is performed at any age to prevent endocarditis and pulmonary veno-occlusive disease (PVOD). Approach is via a sternotomy with use of CPB. Circulatory arrest may be necessary in anatomically difficult lesions or in small patients. Usually defects are closed by a GORE-TEX or Dacron patch as opposed to primarily approximating tissue edges and suturing the defect closed (Silvestry, 2018).

iv. Endocarditis remains a lifelong risk.

i. Complications

i. Systemic hypertension, damage to the aortic valve, heart block, tricuspid insufficiency, residual shunt with low CO, or pulmonary hypertensive crisis are all complications of VSD. Repair before the patient is 2 years of age usually permits normalization of growth and reversal of any related developmental delays (Bronicki & Chang, 2011).

4. *Atrioventricular Septal Defect*

a. Definition

i. A defect that occurs in the atrial and ventricular wall and deficiency of the endocardial cushion tissue, with various degrees of AV valve regurgitation (Backer, & Mavroudis, 2013b; Figure 3.61).

ii. Embryologic deficiency of the endocardial cushion tissue results in ostium primum atrial defect, common AV orifice, inlet VSD, malrotation of the aortic valve, elongation and narrowing of the LV outflow tract, and abnormal attachment of the AV valve to the ventricular septum. AVSD is associated with Down syndrome.

b. Types of AVSD

i. Balanced. Ventricles are equal in size.

ii. Unbalanced. One ventricle is larger; AVSD is classified into forms of single ventricular lesions

iii. Incomplete. There are separate AV valve orifices in addition to the ostium primum defect.

iv. Complete. There is a common AV valve orifice, usually with five leaflets.

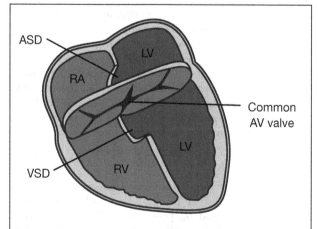

FIGURE 3.61 Anatomy of ASD. Complete AV canal defect. There is a common AV valve with an ostium primum ASD above and a large inlet VSD below.

ASD, atrioventricular septal defect; AV, atrioventricular; LA, left atrium; LV, left ventricle; RA, right atrium; RV, right ventricle; VSD, ventricular septal defect.

c. *Incidence:* Occurs in 4% to 5% of congenital heart defects (Hazinski, 2013).

d. Pathophysiology

i. AVSD is characterized by a large ASD and VSD and a common AV valve. Physiology is similar to ASD and VSD, in which shunting of blood is related to the size of intracardiac septal defects, AV valve competency, PVR, and PA pressure. Usually, left-to-right shunting occurs once PVR decreases, causing pulmonary overcirculation, elevation in PA pressure, and eventual rise in PVR from long-standing pressure and volume overload. A severely regurgitant AV valve leads to early symptoms of CHF and low CO, which may increase PA pressure and PVR and is difficult to treat medically or surgically.

e. Clinical signs and symptoms

i. Symptoms of CHF and pulmonary overcirculation usually occur in early infancy from a large increase in pulmonary blood flow, and are associated with elevated PA pressure and complicated by insufficiency of the common AV valve.

ii. Usually patients with AVSD are small and undernourished (Cooper & Ravishankar, 2013). Oxygen saturation is normal except in the presence of pulmonary vascular disease, which may occur in older children or accelerated disease in an infant. Desaturation can result from ventilation–perfusion (VQ) mismatch from pulmonary changes secondary to a large left-to-right shunt.

iii. Examination: Auscultation reveals a systolic ejection murmur at the LSB, mid-diastolic murmur at the lower LSB and apex from AV valve regurgitation, and a split prominent S_2.

f. Diagnostic evaluation

i. ECG findings are NSR; prolonged PR interval; RA, LA, or bilateral atrial enlargement; BBB, and left-axis or northwest-axis deviation.

ii. Chest radiographic examination shows an enlarged heart, enlarged RA, prominent PA, and increased pulmonary vascular markings.

iii. Echo visualizes the VSD and ASD. Both right- and left-sided components of the common AV valve are displaced into the ventricles and are associated with variable deficiency related to the inflow of the ventricular septum. Echo predicts noninvasive estimates of PA pressure and can quantitate the degree of AV valve regurgitation.

iv. Cardiac catheterization demonstrates an increase in oxygen saturation throughout the right side of the heart; elevated PA pressure and PVR may be present and may or may not be responsive to oxygen.

g. Goals and medical patient management

i. Medical treatment of CHF is usually initiated early. Control of the CHF and optimization of weight gain are goals of medical management. Elective repair is preferred between 3 and 6 months of age (see "Heart Failure in Children" section).

h. Goals and surgical patient management

i. Surgical repair is recommended for any symptomatic infant to prevent early development of pulmonary vascular disease. Surgery involves a sternotomy and CPB. One or two patches are used, depending on the character of the defect and preference of the surgeon (Figure 3.62). The VSD is closed and the AV valve is partially anchored to the patch. The atrial component of the patch is partially sewn in place, the AV valve repair is completed, and the atrial defect is closed.

ii. The post repair competence of the left AV valve (mitral valve) is a significant determinant of optimal long-term outcomes following AVSD repair.

i. Complications

i. Complications include heart block, pulmonary hypertensive crisis (rapid fall in BP and HR with concomitant rise in PAP to systemic or suprasystemic levels treated with hyperventilation; hyperoxygenation; pulmonary vasodilators, including nitric oxide, sedation, and paralysis), residual shunt, and residual AV valve regurgitation or stenosis (Fox, Stream, & Bull, 2014).

ii. Endocarditis remains a lifelong risk.

5. *Double-Outlet Right Ventricle*

a. Definition

i. Origins of both great arteries from a morphologic RV.

ii. Double-outlet right ventricle (DORV) is the result of a failure to achieve conotruncal inversion (rotation) and leftward shift of the

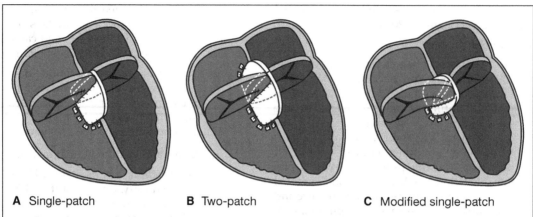

A Single-patch   **B** Two-patch   **C** Modified single-patch

FIGURE 3.62 Schematic three-dimensional reconstruction of the three different surgical techniques: (A) single patch, (B) two patch, and (C) modified single patch.

conal (aortic or pulmonic) segment of both great vessels from the RV.

b. Incidence

   i.   DORV is a rare defect occurring in less than 1% of CHD in a spectrum of transposed complexes (Park, 2016).

c. Pathophysiology

   i.   DORV represents a large continuum of entities, including VSD, TOF, and transposition of the great arteries (Figure 3.63). Both great arteries arise from the RV; usually a VSD is present, and varying degrees of PS may exist. The great arteries may be in normal position, side by side, in dextroposition or levoposition. The VSD may be subaortic, subpulmonic (Taussig–Bing syndrome), or doubly committed (a large VSD related to both semilunar valves).

   ii.   Physiology is based on the degree of PS and the relationship of the VSD to the PA and aorta. Blood enters the right side of the heart normally. RV output flows to the lowest resistance circuit. In the absence of PS, blood flow to the lungs is unrestricted and significant pulmonary overcirculation and PVOD occur. If PS is present, blood may exit more evenly to the PA and aorta (termed *balanced*). The more severe the PA obstruction, the greater the flow to the aorta.

d. Clinical signs and symptoms

   i.   Symptoms of either HF or cyanosis occur along a continuum depending on the anatomic variant of DORV.

   ii.   Subaortic VSD with PS is similar to TOF. Cyanosis, clubbing, exertional dyspnea, polycythemia, RV impulse at LSB, loud systolic ejection murmur, normal S_1, and single S_2.

   iii.   Subpulmonic VSD with or without PS resembles TGV. Cyanosis early, precordial bulge, high-pitched systolic murmur at the upper LSB, and single S_2.

   iv.   Subaortic VSD without PS is similar to a simple VSD. Active precordium, holosystolic murmur at the LSB, and an apical diastolic rumble.

e. Diagnostic evaluation

   i.   ECG shows RVH, right-axis deviation, normal to increased LV forces, first-degree AV conduction delay, and RA enlargement.

   ii.   Chest radiographic examination: With PS, mild cardiomegaly, may have absent main PA segment, and decreased pulmonary vascularity occur. Without PS, cardiomegaly, increased pulmonary vascularity, and prominent main PA segment are seen. With PVOD, "pruning" of the peripheral pulmonary vascular bed occurs (distal lung fields appear dark).

   iii.   Echo displays mitral and semilunar discontinuity, origin of both great vessels from the anterior RV, absence of LV outflow except through the VSD, associated lesions, and accurate position of the VSD.

   iv.   Cardiac catheterization results are variable, depending on anatomy. It is helpful in quantitating PAP and PVR.

f. Goals and medical patient management. Provide symptom management until surgical correction or palliation. Symptoms are variable, dependent on anatomic variance.

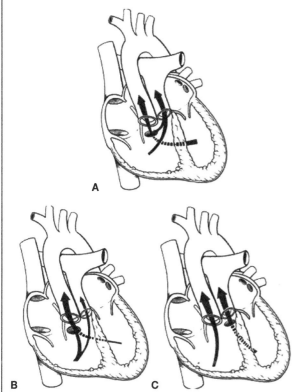

FIGURE 3.63 Three major forms of the double-outlet right ventricle defect are presented. (A) When DORV with subaortic VSD occurs without pulmonary stenosis, the VSD directs left ventricular outflow into the aorta; by doing so, some blood shunts into the pulmonary artery, as shown by the arrows. This defect produces hemodynamics similar to what occurs with a simple VSD. (B) When DORV with subaortic VSD occurs with pulmonary stenosis, the subaortic VSD directs left ventricular outflow into the aorta, as shown by the arrows. If pulmonary stenosis is significant, shunting of right ventricular outflow into the aorta (a right-to-left shunt) will occur. This defect produces hemodynamics similar to tetralogy of Fallot. (C) When DORV with subpulmonic VSD occurs without pulmonary stenosis, the VSD directs left ventricular outflow into the PA and right ventricular outflow to enter the aorta, as shown by the arrows. This action produces hemodynamics similar to the transposition of the great arteries.

DORV, double-outlet right ventricle; PA, pulmonary artery; VSD, ventricular septal defect.

Source: Reprinted with permission from Hazinski, M. F. (Ed.). (2013). *Nursing care of the critically ill child* (3rd ed.). St. Louis, MO: Elsevier-Mosby.

g. Goals and surgical patient management

i. Intracardiac repair involves closing the VSD with separation of flow to great vessels via sternotomy utilizing bypass. The goal is complete anatomic repair. Without PS, early surgery helps to protect the pulmonary vascular bed. Patients may require arterial switch and VSD closure. As an alternative, the anatomy of the VSD and great vessels may best lend itself to intracardiac baffling of the VSD to direct the LV flow into the aorta (Figure 3.64). Neonates may require initial palliation with PA banding for control of CHF while awaiting growth for eventual repair (see sub-section "Ventricular Septal Defect" and the section "Great Vessel Lesions"). Risks associated with VSD closure and arterial switch operation for repair of DORV are the same as each operation (see discussion of VSD and arterial switch operation). Risks associated with intracardiac baffling for repair include residual shunt, low CO/CHF, left ventricular or right ventricular outflow tract obstruction, and heart block, especially if the VSD is enlarged.

ii. In the presence of PS, the VSD is closed to reestablish LV-aortic continuity, and an RV–PA conduit is placed to establish RV to PA continuity (Figure 3.65). This conduit will not grow with the patient and will need to be replaced later in life. If PS is mild, it may require only valvotomy or a transannular patch. For infants with a significant degree of PS, stabilization on prostaglandins followed by palliation with a systemic-to-pulmonary shunt may be necessary, with definitive repair at 6 to 12 months of age.

h. Complications

i. Postoperative complications include arrhythmia, VSD patch dehiscence or residual VSD, aortic obstruction, residual PS, tricuspid insufficiency, and myocardial dysfunction (Bronicki & Chang, 2011).

ii. Endocarditis is a lifelong risk.

6. *Ebstein's Anomaly*

a. Definition

i. Downward displacement of posterior and septal leaflets of the tricuspid valve with an atrialized portion of the RV.

ii. The perforations that result in the formation of the chordae tendineae and papillary muscles fail to develop, resulting in tissue redundancy (Figure 3.66).

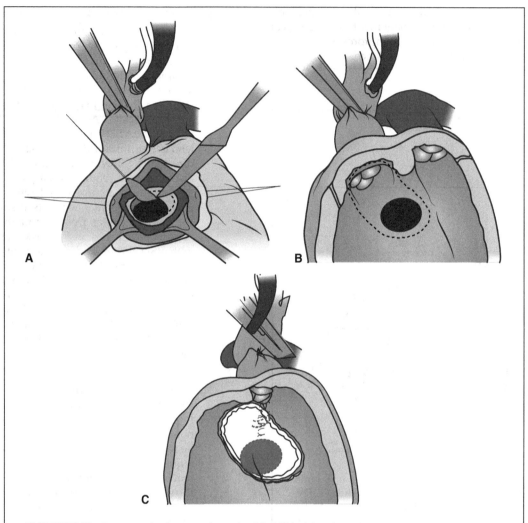

FIGURE 3.64 Intraventricular tunnel repair of DORV with subaortic or doubly committed VSD without pulmonary stenosis. (A) If the VSD is restrictive, it is enlarged by resection of the interventricular septum, indicated by inner dashed line. Outer dashed line indicates the portion of the infundibular septum that may require resection to prevent subaortic stenosis. (B) Enlarging the ventricular septal defect. (C) Creation of a tunnel connecting the VSD to the aorta.

DORV, double-outlet right ventricle; VSD, ventral septal defect.

b. Incidence

   i. Ebstein's anomaly constitutes 0.5% to 1% of CHD cases (Park, 2016).

   ii. Unusually high incidence occurs in infants of mothers who are taking lithium.

c. Pathophysiology

   i. Anatomy of the valve is variable, but there is always redundancy of valve tissue and adherence of medial and posterior leaflets to the RV wall. An atrialized RV (thin-walled upper segment) occurs from downward displacement of the tricuspid valve. The RV function is dependent on the effective size of the remaining ventricular segment. It is common to have associated anomalies, including ASD, PFO, VSD, or WPW.

   ii. Physiology depends on the degree of malformation of the tricuspid valve. Mild

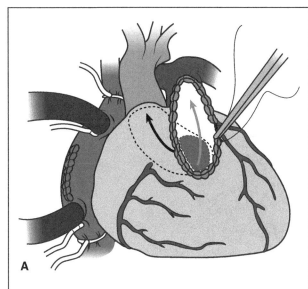

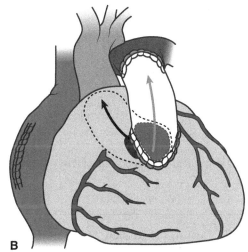

FIGURE 3.65 Reconstruction of the right ventricular outflow tract during repair of DORV with subaortic or doubly committed VSD. (A) Patch enlargement of the right ventricular outflow tract with or without transannular extension into the main PA. (B) The use of a valved, extracardiac conduit to establish continuity between the right ventricle and PA.

DORV, double-outlet right ventricle; PA, pulmonary artery; VSD, ventral septal defect.

anomalies may have normal valve function. With severe malformation, cyanosis can occur from right-to-left shunting through the ASD related to massive TR and elevated RA pressure. Blood enters the RA normally,

but on entering the RV it regurgitates into the RA because of tricuspid insufficiency. In rare circumstances, the tricuspid valve may be stenotic and cause RA dilation resulting from elevated pressure across the stenotic valve.

iii. Tricuspid insufficiency in newborns may improve as neonatal elevation of PVR and hence RV hypertension normally regresses, thus decreasing cyanosis.

d. Clinical signs and symptoms

i. Symptoms vary based on the degree of tricuspid valve deformity. Cyanosis may be noted in the neonate; the cyanosis disappears over the next few weeks and returns by age 5 to 10 years. Severe tricuspid insufficiency in neonates involves low CO, hepatomegaly, and cyanosis. After infancy, dyspnea on exertion and fatigue may occur. Arrhythmias are common (50%). Growth and development are usually normal.

ii. Examination reveals normal cardiac impulse, variable intensity systolic murmur, normal S_1, and possibly a click. If asymptomatic, the S_2 is normal. If symptomatic, the S_2 is diminished or single and an S_3 or S_4 or both may be heard. Hepatomegaly may be present.

e. Diagnostic evaluation

i. ECG findings are always abnormal and show RBBB, a right-axis deviation, right atrial enlargement, and a prolonged PR interval. WPW may occur (in 5%–20% of cases).

ii. Chest radiographic examination in the symptomatic infant demonstrates at least moderate, if not massive, cardiomegaly with decreased pulmonary vascular markings (Figure 3.67). Asymptomatic children have normal to slight enlargement of heart size and normal pulmonary vascular markings with RA enlargement of varying degree.

iii. Echo demonstrates delayed tricuspid valve closure. Valve displacement is present with a sail-like anterior leaflet of the tricuspid valve. Other anatomic findings, specifically, RV size or ASD and eccentric coaptation of the tricuspid valve leaflets, can be defined.

iv. Cardiac catheterization is not necessary to delineate anatomy. But arrhythmias are common, so an electrophysiology

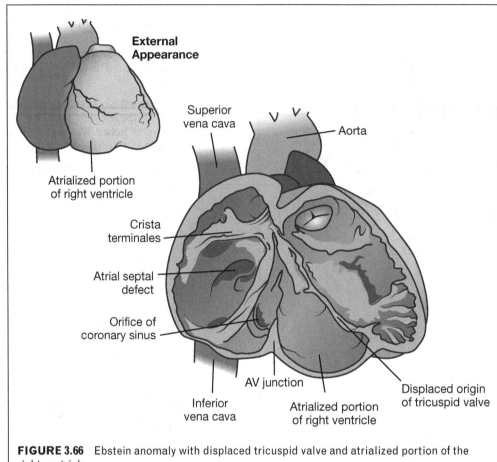

External Appearance

Atrialized portion of right ventricle

Superior vena cava

Aorta

Crista terminales

Atrial septal defect

Orifice of coronary sinus

AV junction

Inferior vena cava

Atrialized portion of right ventricle

Displaced origin of tricuspid valve

FIGURE 3.66 Ebstein anomaly with displaced tricuspid valve and atrialized portion of the right ventricle.

AV, atrioventricular.

study and ablation may be warranted. Cardiac catheterization will also demonstrate the portion of the RV that is functioning as the RA.

f. Goals and medical patient management

i. The goal is to optimize RV output/flow. Improvement in oxygenation by manipulation of PVR with nitric oxide, oxygen, and hyperventilation may be helpful. PGE therapy in the absence of severe RV outflow tract obstruction or tricuspid stenosis can be fatal. For severely symptomatic neonates, prognosis is poor because stabilization of the newborn is difficult.

g. Goals and surgical patient management

i. No surgery may be required if the degree of TR is mild. In moderate or greater TR, tricuspid valvuloplasty with ASD closure or excision of redundant RA wall may be required to relieve cyanosis, preserve RV function, and prevent paradoxical embolus (Figure 3.68). Valvuloplasty is more effective in older patients. Valve rings may be utilized to stabilize a valve repair rather than opting for tricuspid valve replacement. Tricuspid valve replacement is required if valvuloplasty is not effective, usually with plication of the RA.

ii. Tricuspid valve closure to create tricuspid atresia, placement of a systemic-to-pulmonary shunt, and creation of an ASD is utilized in infants with severe Ebstein anomaly. This is done with CPB. These patients will go on to a single-ventricle repair with cavopulmonary shunt and Fontan procedure. Postoperative complications include low CO, RV dysfunction with

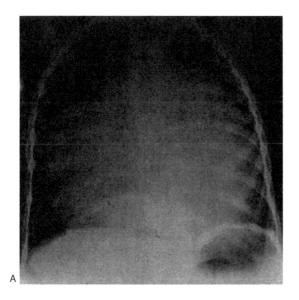 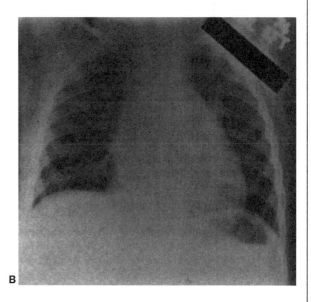

FIGURE 3.67 Chest radiographs of a 2-year-old girl with Ebstein anomaly. (A) Preoperative (cardiothoracic ratio, 0.96). (B) Thirteen days after repair (cardiothoracic ratio, 0.55).

Source: Reprinted with permission from Danielson, G. K., Maloney, J. D., & Devloo, R. A. E. (1979). Surgical repair of Ebstein's anomaly. Mayo Clinic Proceedings, 54, 185.

elevated RV, increased PVR, dysrhythmia, residual TR, and persistent pleural effusions.

iii. Cardiac transplantation for the neonate with severe Ebstein anomaly is another option.

iv. Ablation (radiofrequency or surgical) of WPW may be required.

h. Complications

i. Low CO syndrome, hypotension, arrhythmia (JET, SVT), TR, chylothorax, hypoxemia, stroke, and seizures (Bronicki & Chang, 2011).

ii. Endocarditis is a lifelong risk.

7. *Truncus Arteriosus*

a. Definition

i. A single arterial trunk arises from the base of the heart giving rise to pulmonary, systemic, and coronary circulations.

ii. Conotruncal or truncoarterial separation does not proceed normally. Either a deficiency or an absence of conal (infundibular) septum causes a large VSD.

b. Incidence

i. This accounts for 0.21% to 0.34% of all cases of CHD (Mavroudis, 2013c).

c. Pathophysiology

i. Truncus includes an unrestrictive VSD, a single semilunar valve with possible truncal valve abnormalities, and override of the ventricular septum by the truncal valve. Tricuspid truncal valve occurs in 69% of cases, quadricuspid truncal valve in 22% of cases, and bicuspid truncal valve in 9% of cases. Truncal valve insufficiency is related to thick dysplastic cusps. Truncal valve stenosis is rare (Mavroudis, 2013c).

ii. The type of truncus is differentiated by the existence and location of the main PA and the PA branches (Figure 3.69). Type I has a short main PA segment, which arises from the trunk and then branches into the right and left pulmonary arteries (48%). In type II, the PA arises separately from the trunk but in close proximity to it (29%–48%). In type III, the PA arises separately from the trunk and at some distance from it (6%–10%). In type IV, arteries arising from the descending aorta

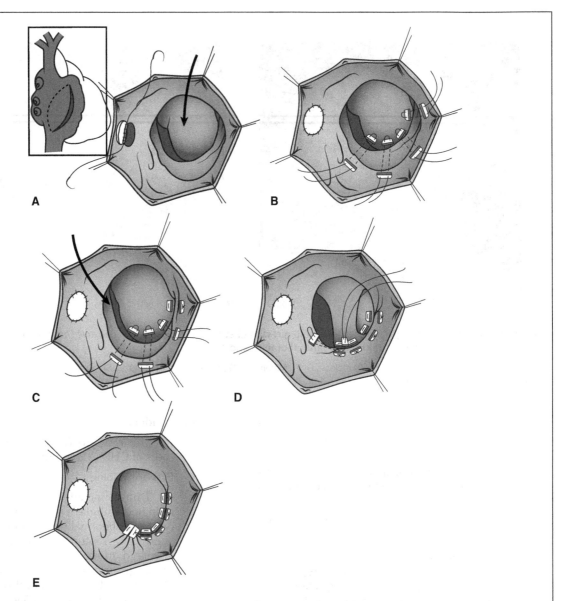

FIGURE 3.68 The surgical repair procedure of an Ebstein anomaly requires several steps. The inset at the left of (A) shows the right atrial appendage to the inferior vena cava; by excising the redundant portion of the right atrium (as shown by the dotted line), the final size of the right atrium becomes normalized. (A) To close the atrial septal defect, the surgeon places a patch over the affected area. The arrow indicates the large anterior leaflet, which displaces the posterior leaflet downward from the annulus. (B) The surgeon utilizes mattress sutures to connect the tricuspid annulus and tricuspid valve. By placing sutures in the atrialized portion of the right ventricle, the atrialized ventricle is plicated; the aneurysmal cavity is eventually obliterated when these sutures are subsequently tied. (C) The clinician ties down the sutures, following a sequential pattern. The arrow shows the hypoplastic, markedly displaced septal leaflet that occurs as a result. (D) Following a posterior annuloplasty, the diameter of the tricuspid annulus is narrowed. The posterior and leftward extent of the annuloplasty are terminated at the coronary sinus to avoid injury to the conduction system; however, additional sutures may be needed to obliterate the posterior aspect of the annuloplasty repair to ensure the valve is completely competent. If corrected adequately, the tricuspid annulus will admit two or more fingers in the adult. (E) After the repair is completed, the anterior leaflet functions as a monocusp valve.

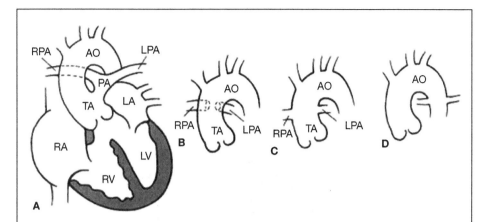

FIGURE 3.69 The anatomic type of persistent TA is determined by the branching patterns of the pulmonary arteries. (A) In type I, the main PA arises from the truncus and then divides into the RPA and LPA branches. (B) In type II, the pulmonary arteries arise from the posterior aspect of the truncus. (C) In type III, the pulmonary arteries arise from the lateral aspects of the truncus. (D) In type IV, or pseudotruncus arteriosus, arteries arising from the descending aorta supply the lungs.

AO, aorta; LA, Left atrium; LPA, left pulmonary artery; LV, left ventricle; PA, pulmonary artery; RA, right atrium; RPA, right pulmonary artery; RV, right ventricle; TA, truncus arteriosus.

Source: Reprinted with permission from Park, M. K. (2016). *Park's The Pediatric Cardiology Handbook* (5th ed.). Philadelphia, PA: Saunders-Elsevier.

supply the lungs (Figure 3.70; Mavroudis, 2013c).

iii. Commonly associated lesions include coarctation and interrupted aortic arch (IAA). Coronary artery anomalies may occur. Extracardiac anomalies occur in about 21% to 30% of children and most often include 22Q11 deletion syndrome, bowel malrotation, and hydroureter. Right aortic arch is more commonly associated with TA than with any other congenital heart defect. Complications of this diagnosis include subendocardial ischemia and PVOD early on from the high pressure and volume of pulmonary flow and progressive truncal valve insufficiency.

iv. Systemic and pulmonary venous blood returns normally and enters the respective ventricle. Ventricular blood mixes through the VSD and exits the heart through the truncus. Blood then flows to the lungs and body, depending on the respective resistance in the systemic and pulmonary circuits. Symptoms appear when the PVR begins to fall, around 2 to 4 weeks of life. In the event of severe truncal valve insufficiency (or more rarely stenosis), low CO and cardiac compromise occur almost from birth.

d. Clinical signs and symptoms

i. History. Symptoms of CHF occur when the PVR drops and pulmonary blood flow increases. In infants with associated DiGeorge syndrome, hypocalcemia and hypomagnesemia are frequently noted.

ii. Examination reveals cyanosis only when PVR is increased; this is a concern for eventual repair. Active precordium, normal S_1, loud ejection click, loud and single S_2, and S_3 heard at the apex are common. In addition, a systolic ejection murmur at the LSB and frequently an apical diastolic murmur can be heard. If truncal valve insufficiency exists, a blowing diastolic high-pitched murmur is heard at the LSB.

e. Diagnostic evaluation

i. ECG shows a normal QRS configuration or minimal right-axis deviation, NSR, biventricular hypertrophy, and LAE.

ii. Chest radiographic examination demonstrates moderate cardiomegaly, increased pulmonary vascular markings, right arch in one third of patients, and dilated truncal root. In the presence of PVOD, enlargement of the PA and a tapering of the distal pulmonary vascular tree occur.

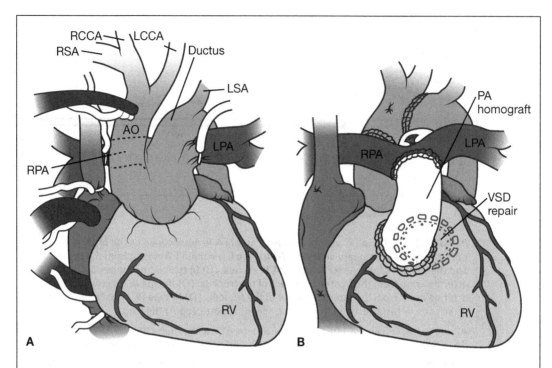

FIGURE 3.70　A patient with truncus arteriosus and interrupted aortic arch can benefit from aortobicaval cardiopulmonary bypass (A), a procedure that is established through bilateral PA constriction (enforced snuggers). In this procedure, the patent ductus arteriosus is utilized to ensure lower extremity flow. (B) To repair the truncus arteriosus with interrupted aortic arch, the surgeon performs a direct aortic reconstruction without using foreign material. Right ventricular-to-PA continuity is ensured through use of the LeCompte maneuver to repair any abnormalities that may exist.

AO, aorta; LCCA, left common carotid artery; LPA, left pulmonary artery; LSA, left subclavian artery; PA, pulmonary artery; RCCA, right common carotid artery; RPA, right pulmonary artery; RSA, right subclavian artery; RV, right ventricle; VSD, ventricular septal defect.

iii.　Echo confirms the diagnosis, and anatomic features are identified. Origin of the pulmonary arteries, VSD location and size, and anatomy of the truncal valve are accomplished. The pressure gradient across the truncal valve and the degree of insufficiency are determined if necessary.

iv.　Cardiac catheterization is not necessary except in complex variants. Right and left ventricular pressures are equal, and there is increased oxygen saturation in the PA. PVR may be elevated, and PA pressure is elevated.

f.　Goals and medical patient management

　i.　Medical management to control CHF is warranted. Irradiated blood should always be used until DiGeorge syndrome can be ruled out.

g.　Goals and surgical patient management

　i.　Repair should not be delayed because PVOD develops rapidly.

　ii.　Surgical repair entails sternotomy and CPB possibly with deep hypothermic circulatory arrest. The VSD is closed to the truncal valve, creating LV-to-truncal valve continuity (Figure 3.71). The PAs are connected to the distal end of the RV conduit; the conduit is then connected to the RV outflow tract, reestablishing RV-to-PA continuity. Truncal valve insufficiency or stenosis is addressed only if severe. Moderate insufficiency or stenoses often improve when the volume load crossing it is decreased after separation of the circulations. In most neonatal repairs, the ASD or PFO is left open to allow bidirectional shunting until RV compliance improves.

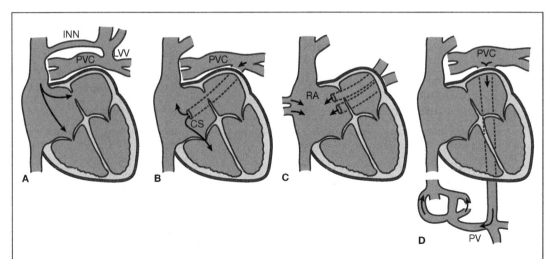

FIGURE 3.71 The four most common anatomic defects in TAPVC. (A) TAPVC drainage to the INN via an LVV. (B) TAPVC from the common PVC to the CS. (C) TAPVC to the RA. (D) Infradiaphragmatic TAPVC from the common pulmonary venous confluence to the PV.

CS, coronary sinus; INN, innominate vein; LVV, left vertical vein; PV, portal vein; PVC, pulmonary venous confluence; RA, right atrium; TAPVC, total anomalous pulmonary venous connection.

h. Complications

i. Complications particular to this operation are conduction disturbances, including heart block, low CO, residual PS or VSD, PA hypertensive crisis, and progressive truncal valve insufficiency (Mahle, Matthews, et al., 2014).

ii. No increased mortality has been found with repair of IAA and TA.

iii. The requirement for truncal valve replacement for severe regurgitation at presentation increases surgical morbidity and mortality. Repair of the valve, even if residual moderate truncal valve stenosis exists, has had improved results (J. Jacobs et al., 2014).

iv. Pulmonary homograft conduits are currently the preferred material for initial establishment of RV to PA continuity because of the ease of use, improved hemostasis, and improved longevity. Failure of a homograft conduit is related to the size of the conduit and the child at implantation, growth of the patient, pulmonary versus aortic homograft, Dacron extension, and extracardiac placement of the valve. Debate continues as to whether the homograft, porcine-valved heterograft, or bovine jugular vein conduit provides the best conduit over time. Branch PA stenosis is not uncommon and requires balloon dilation or patch arterioplasty at reoperation for conduit replacement (J. Jacobs et al., 2014).

v. Endocarditis is a lifelong risk.

8. *TAPVR, Unobstructed*

a. Anatomy. TAPVR occurs when all four pulmonary veins drain anomalously into the right side of the heart. TAPVR is an embryologic error of incorporation of pulmonary veins into the LA (Backer, & Mavroudis, 2013a).

i. TAPVR accounts for 1% of all CHD with a male predominance of infradiaphragmatic veins (Park, 2016).

b. Pathophysiology

i. Pulmonary veins have no connection to the LA. The LA is often small, underdeveloped, and noncompliant. The pulmonary veins may empty in various ways to the RA (Figure 3.71).

ii. Supracardiac pulmonary veins drain to the left SVC or right SVC via the vertical vein, forming a confluence posterior to the LA (50%; Park, 2016).

iii. Intracardiac pulmonary veins drain to the IVC via the vertical vein (frequently obstructed at the level of the diaphragm [20%]; Park, 2016).

iv. Cardiac pulmonary veins drain to the coronary sinus or RA and rarely are obstructed or stenotic (20%; Park, 2016).

v. Mixed pulmonary veins drain via a combination of the preceding variants (10%; Park, 2016).

vi. An ASD is considered part of the complex and is mandatory for survival. One third of cases have other cardiac anomalies such as TOF, TGV, PA, or a single ventricle. The prevalence of TAPVR is increased in patients with asplenia, heterotaxy, and other forms of CHD.

vii. Hemodynamics depends on the distribution of mixed venous blood between the pulmonary and systemic circulation, the size of the ASD, and the degree of obstruction. All venous blood enters the right side of the heart and exits the PA. This creates pulmonary overcirculation and hypertension. For survival, blood must enter the LA via the ASD. If the ASD is small, the LV volume will be low and CO will be severely compromised. If the ASD is large and the LA is compliant, LV volume will be appropriate.

viii. Even if the veins are not obstructed, the increased pulmonary flow creates medial hypertrophy and intimal hyperplasia, ending with PVOD by the third to fourth decade of life when left untreated.

c. Clinical signs and symptoms

i. History. Patients with unobstructed veins present with CHF usually between 2 and 4 weeks of life as PVR decreases and shunting increases.

ii. Examination. With unobstructed veins, there is an increased and split S_2, an S_3, and a systolic ejection murmur at the upper LSB. Although difficult to differentiate from persistent pulmonary hypertension of the newborn during the neonatal period, the diagnosis of obstructed TAPVR must be quickly identified.

d. Diagnostic evaluation

i. Echo confirms the diagnosis and localizes the site of venous drainage. Pulmonary venous obstruction is quantified by Doppler. Associated lesions are defined; RV pressure

and PA hypertension are noted; and PA, RA, and RV volume overload are noted.

e. Goals and medical patient management

i. Medical treatment for CHF is required for patients with unobstructed veins.

f. Goals and surgical patient management

i. Unobstructed veins are repaired early to prevent PVOD. Surgical repair is aimed at returning pulmonary vein flow to the left side of the heart, eliminating obstruction, closing the ASD, and preventing PVOD. Repair is done via sternotomy on CPB using deep hypothermic circulatory arrest. The pulmonary vein confluence is anastomosed to the posterior wall of the LA, or the veins are directed through the ASD by an intraatrial patch, thereby redirecting pulmonary venous return correctly and closing the ASD.

g. Complications

i. Postoperative problems include pulmonary hypertensive crisis, SSS and other atrial arrhythmias, restenosis of the anastomosis, and inability to relieve the stenosis fully (Latus, Delhaas, Schranz, & Apitz, 2015).

ii. Long-term prognosis depends on the presence of diffuse pulmonary vein obstruction, the relief of all existing stenosis, any associated cardiac lesions, and the state of the pulmonary vascular bed. About 10% of these children have a second obstruction usually associated with intracardiac or mixed types of veins. Use of sildenafil for treatment of PA hypertension has proven successful over the long term (Mavourids, 2013).

9. *Anomalous LCA From the PA (ALCAPA)*

a. Definition. An anomalous origin of the LCA occurring when the LCA arises from the PA instead of from the aorta.

b. An anomalous origin of a coronary artery is rare, occurring in 0.25% to 0.5% of patients with congenital cardiac abnormalities (Mavroudis, Doge-Khatami, Backer, & Lorber 2013).

i. The myocardium is perfused by the abnormally arising coronary artery, which has a relatively low perfusion pressure and carries blood with a lower oxygen saturation instead of oxygenated, higher pressure blood from the aorta. This can result in progressive LV ischemia and dilation, which can lead to mitral valve regurgitation.

c. Clinical signs and symptoms. Symptoms are dependent on age and presence of collateral vessels. Most cases present with severe CHF symptoms at a few months of age. Children may be asymptomatic. May develop arrhythmias, angina, or sudden death. Infants may present with irritability, diaphoresis, and poor feeding. Gallop may be present with MR.

d. Diagnostic evaluation. ECG abnormalities/ST segment changes, echo with RCA dilation and retrograde LCA flow, CXR may have cardiomegaly and pulmonary edema.

e. Goals and medical patient management. Stabilize until urgent surgical repair is needed.

f. Goals and surgical patient management. Surgical reimplantation of the LCA into the aorta is needed. MR, if present, rarely requires surgical repair as this should improve as LV function improves.

g. Complications. Low CO, LV dysfunction, arrhythmias, and coronary spasm are the most common complications from repair of the ALCAPA. Death may occur, particularly if there is severe LV dysfunction prior to operation.

D. Obstructive Physiology

1. *Aortic Stenosis*

  a. Valvar

    i. Definition

      1) Malformation of the aortic valve, which causes obstruction to ejection of blood from the LV.

      2) Obstruction occurs at the valve annulus of the LV.

    ii. Incidence

      1) AS occurs more frequently in boys and occurs in about 3% to 6% of congenital heart defects. It may be associated with nonimmunologic hydrops fetalis (Mavroudis, 2013a).

    iii. Pathophysiology

      1) Associated cardiac lesions, such as PDA, VSD, or coarctation, are common. They are not the same. The valve tissue is the tissue the leaflets are made of and the leaflets are the parts of the valve that move. They are essentially the valve.

The tissue comprising the valve leaflets is thick and rigid with diminished commissural separation of varying degrees, but the leaflets themselves are mobile in children.

2) Most often the valve is bicuspid with a single, fused commissure and an eccentrically placed orifice. The valve annulus may be hypoplastic (<4–5 mm). With severe stenosis, the LV develops concentric hypertrophy, decreased LV function, compromised myocardial blood flow, elevated LVEDP, and poststenotic dilation of the ascending aorta.

3) Valvular gradients can give some estimation of the degree of stenosis. This number may be misleading in instances of low CO, in which output across the valve is already diminished and the gradient may be falsely low. Estimations of valvular gradients used to determine severity and to guide interventional decisions are (a) mild: 5 to 49 mmHg, (b) moderate: 50 to 75 mmHg, and (c) severe: greater than 75 mmHg (Park, 2016).

4) Subendocardial or endocardial fibroelastosis may occur in utero if the stenosis is severe and does not regress after repair. Therefore, despite adequate relief of the stenosis, LV function may be permanently compromised.

    iv. Clinical signs and symptoms

      1) Critical AS is a severe form of AS that presents at birth with symptoms of circulatory shock from obstruction to systemic blood flow. Most children with AS are asymptomatic and grow and develop normally. As symptoms occur, they usually involve fatigue, exertional dyspnea, angina pectoris, and syncope with at least moderate AS. Examination reveals LV lift, precordial systolic thrill, systolic aortic ejection murmur or ejection click, S_2 delayed or split S_3, and, on occasion, a diastolic murmur of aortic insufficiency.

    v. Diagnostic evaluation

      1) ECG findings may vary with severity but usually include T-wave inversion, deep S wave in V_1, LV strain, LVH, and ST segment depression.

2) Exercise testing is used to evaluate BP response and ECG changes with exercise. A fall or a lack of rise in systolic BP suggests the presence of severe obstruction.

3) Chest radiographic examination demonstrates normal to minimal enlargement of heart size; rounding of the cardiac apex; LA enlargement if stenosis is severe; pulmonary congestion and enlargement of the PA, RV, and RA; and poststenotic dilation of the ascending aorta.

4) Echo shows diminished systolic valve movement and demonstrates the anatomy of the valve leaflets, an increase in LV wall thickness, transvalvular aortic gradients, end-diastolic dimensions to predict LV peak systolic pressure, and associated cardiac anatomy.

5) Cardiac catheterization is important as a diagnostic tool to establish the site and severity of the stenosis, define associated anomalies, measure CO, and assess valve gradients.

  vi. Goals and medical patient management

1) Congenital AS is a progressive lesion, and most affected children require intervention at least once. The earlier the intervention, the greater the likelihood of further intervention. Intervention is recommended when severe symptoms or LV strain or syncope are present. Stabilization of the neonate with critical AS requires prostaglandin therapy.

  vii. Goals and surgical patient management

1) Interventional catheterization or balloon valvuloplasty is successful in opening the valve in most patients, and the results in neonates are similar to those of surgical valvotomy. Cardiac catheter procedures are difficult in the neonates given the size of catheter required for interventional therapies.

2) Surgical valvuloplasty carries the same risks as balloon procedures; however, stabilization on CPB during the procedure allows time for the ventricle

to rest and to resolve acidosis. It also provides a backup in the presence of malignant ventricular arrhythmias with valve manipulation (Figure 3.72).

3) For stenosis (initial or recurrent) in patients with limited annulus size, enlargement of the entire aortic root is required. The Konno procedure with aortic root replacement involves enlarging the LV outflow tract and aortic annulus and incorporating an aortic valve replacement. This is accomplished through a sternotomy on CPB (Figure 3.73). Risks of this operation include heart block, myocardial failure and low CO, patch dehiscence of the ventricular patch used to enlarge the septum and aortic root, and perivalvular leak.

4) Some patients require valve replacement for progressive stenosis or insufficiency but have an adequate aortic annulus size. A decision regarding the best valve to use for that patient's age, lifestyle, gender, and anatomy is made and the replacement is performed. In most circumstances, these homografts or bioprosthetics require replacement within 5 to 10 years. Prosthetic valves may last 15 to 20 years or longer in older adolescents or adults. In infants and

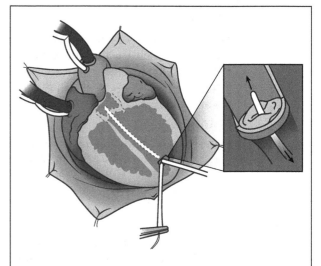

FIGURE 3.72 Operative technique showing antegrade aortic transvalvar dilation with blunt dilators via an apical purse-string suture.

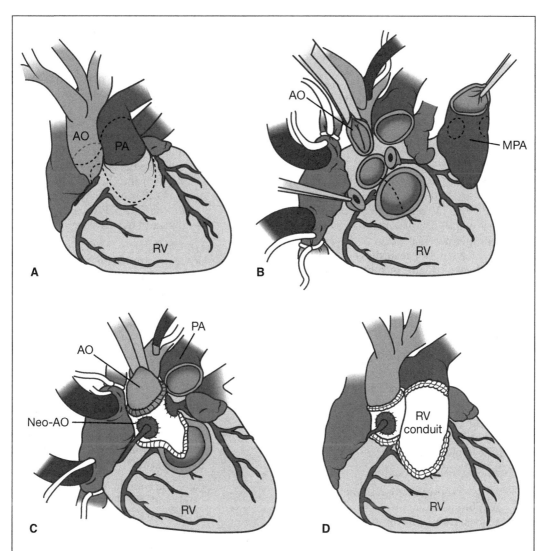

FIGURE 3.73 (A) In preparation for the Ross–Konno procedure, the surgeon will identify the heart's incision and excision boundaries. (B) After cross-clamping the aorta, the surgeon may note antegrade and retrograde cardioplegic arrest during aortic resection, coronary mobilization, and main pulmonary artery harvest; the dotted line indicates the interventricular septal incision. An extra portion of right ventricle is used during the ventriculoseptoplasty in order to harvest the pulmonary autograft. (C) The neoaortic left ventricular outflow reconstruction is completed through placing the pulmonary autograft extension into the interventricular septum and securing in place. (D) The completed Ross–Konno procedure shows the RV conduit securely attached in place following the cardiopulmonary bypass.

AO, aorta; MPA, main pulmonary artery; NEO-AO, neoaortic; RV, right ventricle.

younger children, the valve will likely require replacement within 5 years.

5) In patients with aortic and pulmonary roots of the same or similar size, a Ross procedure can be performed. This operation involves translocating the native pulmonary valve into the aortic root (autograft) and replacing the

pulmonary valve with a homograft. The proposed benefit is that the autograft will grow and be durable in the aortic position, thus not requiring future replacement.

viii. Complications

1) Complications of valvar AS in general include endocarditis, sudden death,

development of valvular insufficiency, and arrhythmias.

2) Risks of Ross or Ross–Konno operation include bleeding, MI from coronary injury during excision of the pulmonary autograft, aortic regurgitation, and low CO.

3) Endocarditis is a lifelong risk.

b. Subaortic stenosis

    i. Definition

1) Subaortic stenosis consists of a membranous diaphragm or fibrous ring encircling the LV outflow tract beneath the base of the aortic valve. Progressive aortic regurgitation may occur and is an indication for surgery regardless of the LVOT gradient or degree of subaortic stenosis.

    ii. Incidence

1) Subaortic stenosis includes 15% to 20% of AS and occurs more often in boys. The incidence is 0.25/1,000 live births (Tchervenkov et al., 2013).

    iii. Pathophysiology. Abnormal blood flow created by membrane can lead to AV insufficiency.

    iv. Clinical signs and symptoms. Exhibited as asymptomatic murmur or increasing exercise intolerance.

    v. Diagnostic evaluation

1) Echo shows dilation of the aortic root. A fibromuscular ring produces thick echoes from a level near the annular attachment of the anterior mitral leaflet.

    vi. Goals and medical patient management: Monitor for increase in gradient, progressive aortic insufficiency, or symptoms associated with LVOTO, such as dyspnea, fatigue, and chest pain.

    vii. Goals and surgical patient management

1) Surgical approach is via median sternotomy using CPB. The obstructing membrane or ring is excised along with resection of LV muscle (myomectomy). Myomectomy has been shown to dramatically reduce recurrence of the stenosis (Figure 3.74).

    viii. Complications

1) Risks specific to this procedure include aortic insufficiency, mitral valve damage, heart block, and creation of a VSD.

2) Endocarditis is a lifelong risk.

c. Supravalvar aortic stenosis (SVAS)

    i. Definition

1) Congenital narrowing of the ascending aorta may be localized or diffuse, hourglass shaped, membranous type, or hypoplastic type. Coronary arteries are subjected to elevated pressure and may be dilated; the lumin may be narrowed by a thick medial layer. The aortic lumen is constricted, and the distal flow is diminished. It is often associated with Williams syndrome (SVAS, PA stenosis, mental retardation, and hypercalcemia in infancy).

    ii. Incidence. LVOT obstructive lesions occur in approximately six in 10,000 live births. Supravalvar AS is the least common form of AS, accounting for 5% to 10% of cases (Tchervenkov et al. 2013).

    iii. Pathophysiology. Significant obstruction can create a hyperdynamic, hypertrophied LV. May have associated coronary artery enlargement and dilatation of the sinuses of Valsalva.

    iv. Clinical signs and symptoms. Loud systolic ejection murmur best heard at the first RICS, accentuated S_2, thrill at the first RICS or suprasternal notch, and higher BP in right arm.

    v. Diagnostic evaluation. *ECG* reveals LVH and RVH if peripheral PA stenosis is present. Chest radiographic examination rarely shows poststenotic dilation. Cardiac catheterization localizes the site of obstruction and degree of hemodynamic alteration. A pressure gradient is found above the aortic valve. Coronary artery problems can be identified, as can the presence and degree of PA involvement (peripheral PS).

    vi. Goals and medical patient management. Mild to moderate AS may be managed conservatively. Monitor for worsening LV hypertrophy.

    vii. Goals and surgical patient management

1) Definitive therapy for SVAS, whether discrete or diffuse, consists of surgical correction of the obstruction. This is done via sternotomy and CPB, an incision is made into the aorta, with a patch placed to enlarge the area (Figure 3.75).

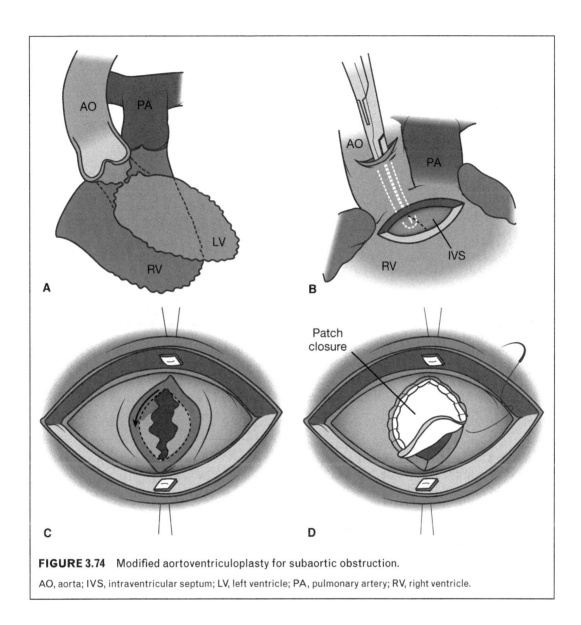

FIGURE 3.74 Modified aortoventriculoplasty for subaortic obstruction.

AO, aorta; IVS, intraventricular septum; LV, left ventricle; PA, pulmonary artery; RV, right ventricle.

viii. Complications may occur if there is diffuse hypoplasia of the aorta or accompanying PA hypoplasia; transfer of the gradients farther down the aorta or to the PA can occur postoperatively resulting in "suicidal RV" and severe low CO. Endocarditis is a lifelong risk.

2. *Coarctation of the Aorta*

   a. Definition. This is a narrowing of the aorta causing elevation of pressure proximally and decreased pressure distally. A local area of intimal thickening and distortion are found, most commonly distal to the contraductal shelf.

   b. Incidence. Coarctation occurs in about 8% to 10% of CHD and is more common in males (Park, 2016).

   c. Pathophysiology. Classification of coarctation is based on the presence or absence of severe isthmus (aortic segment distal to the left subclavian) narrowing and major associated lesions. It is associated frequently with PDA, VSD, AS, aortic insufficiency, bicuspid aortic valve, mitral and tricuspid valve anomalies, and DiGeorge syndrome (usually with interrupted arch). Constriction of the aorta occurs most often at the junction of the ductus and aorta just distal to the left subclavian artery–juxtaductal coarctation.

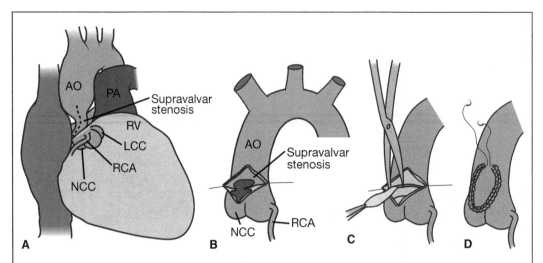

FIGURE 3.75 (A) The dotted line indicates the proposed location for an incision among the aortic cusps to repair a supravalvar aortic stenosis via the one-patch technique. (B) The surgeon will make an incision in the ascending aorta to address its narrowing; to properly address the issue, this incision should extend through the area of supravalvar stenosis into the NCC of the sinus of Valsalva. (C) When resecting the supravalvar fibrous ring, care must be taken to ensure no injury occurs to the orifices of the involved coronary arteries. (D) Upon completion of the procedure, a single patch is augmented to the supravalvar area.

AO, aorta; LCC, left coronary cusp; NCC, noncoronary cusp; PA, pulmonary artery; RCA, right coronary artery; RV, right ventricle.

i. The most severe form of coarctation is the IAA, which is a congenital absence of a portion of the aorta. The types of aortic interruption are based on location. *Type A* is distal to the left subclavian artery (30%); *type B* is distal to the left common carotid artery (43%); and *type C* is between the right and left common carotid arteries (17%; Figure 3.76; Park, 2016). Evaluation of coarctation is an ongoing process because the obstruction can worsen over time, resulting in increased upper extremity hypertension.

ii. Blood exits the LV normally but has varying degrees of difficulty crossing the obstruction. This results in LV hypertension and hypertrophy. In some cases, blood cannot cross the constriction. In this case, the infant is dependent on right-to-left shunting across the ductus to perfuse the distal aorta and body.

iii. As the child grows older, significant aortic collaterals may form to perfuse the aorta distal to the coarctation. Complications of LV failure, long-standing systemic hypertension, stroke, and endocarditis are risks of unrepaired disease.

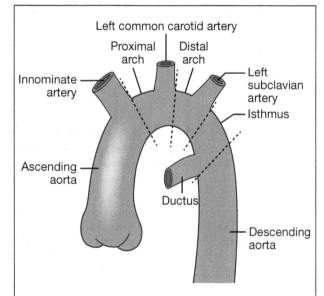

FIGURE 3.76 Depiction of aortic arch in three segments: proximal arch, distal arch, and isthmus. Ductus arteriosus* (* If the ductus remains open, it is referred to as a patent ductus arteriosus [PDA]).

d. Clinical signs and symptoms

i. Patient history and clinical presentation depend on the degree of constriction.

Neonates with severe obstruction present with severe CHF and cardiovascular collapse and require prostaglandin to maintain ductal patency and reestablish systemic flow until surgical correction. Older children rarely have symptoms but may complain of cramps or pain in calves with exercise.

i. Examination of the infant reveals a heaving precordium, equally diminished pulses if the ductus is open, and a nonspecific systolic murmur at the LSB. In the child, examination finds a BP differential between the upper and lower extremities, systemic hypertension, a short systolic ejection murmur at the LSB. A continuous murmur may be present if there are aortic collaterals present.

e. Diagnostic evaluation

i. ECG. RVH and LV strain occur in the infant; increased LV forces and strain occur in the child.

ii. Echo defines anatomy, LV function, and associated lesions.

iii. Chest radiographic examination demonstrates cardiomegaly and possibly increased pulmonary vascular markings in the infant; normal heart size, LV prominence, rib notching, and a prominent descending aorta occur in the child.

iv. Although uncommon, cardiac catheterization can determine associated lesions, anatomy of coarctation, gradient across the coarctation unless there is low CO or a PDA, and descending aortic saturation less than the ascending aortic saturation (from right-to-left shunting at the ductal level). Cardiac catheterization is generally not indicated unless there are complex associated lesions.

f. Goals and medical patient management

i. In the neonate, initial stabilization on prostaglandin and correction of any end-organ failure at diagnostic presentation are required. Short-term stabilization of CHF may be necessary. Medical management is not indicated long term.

g. Goals and surgical patient management

i. Interventions depend on age, degree of constriction, ductal dependency, and associated lesions.

ii. Interventional cardiac catheterization is done primarily for older children or as residual coarctation after repair (Figure 3.77). Risks include aneurysm, recurrent coarctation, difficult vascular access in small infants, and inadequate relief of narrowing. Reduction of collateral vessels following relief of the coarctation by balloon dilation may make operative intervention more hazardous if recoarctation occurs. There is increased risk of paraplegia from low perfusion pressure distal to the aortic cross-clamp during surgery when collateral flow is diminished. CPB may be used to prevent this complication.

iii. Surgical repair is accomplished via thoracotomy with one of the several methods. Subclavian flap angioplasty, end-to-end anastomosis following resection of the coarcted segment (Figure 3.78), patch aortoplasty, and interposition graft are surgical options used. Sternotomy and bypass are used if complete arch reconstruction is required or associated lesions are to be repaired (i.e., VSD, subaortic stenosis). Specific postoperative complications include paradoxical hypertension, mesenteric arteritis (feed slowly, await return of bowel sounds), and paralysis (bypass is used if distal aortic pressure is <40 mmHg).

h. Complications

i. Residual arch obstruction, NEC, recurrent laryngeal nerve injury (Averin, 2012), phrenic nerve injury, hypertension, chylous effusion, and thoracic duct injury are possible complications (Figure 3.79; McElhinnery et al., 2000). Careful attention to enteral feeding protocols is warranted to prevent bowel complications (Owens & Musa, 2009).

ii. Endocarditis is a potential lifelong risk specifically if associated with bicuspid aortic valve.

3. *Interrupted Aortic Arch*

a. Definition. No continuity or complete interruption of the aorta between the ascending and descending aorta. It is classified according to location of the interruption. In type A, the interruption occurs distal to the left subclavian arterial origin; in type B, interruption occurs between the origins of the left common carotid and left

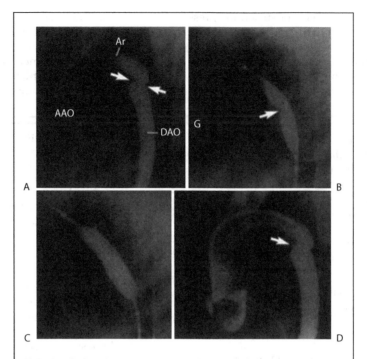

FIGURE 3.77 Balloon angioplasty of recoarctation after surgical repair with subclavian flap. (A) Predilation aortogram demonstrating the narrowed recoarcted segment (arrows). (B) Initial balloon inflation with creation of waist from obstructive shelf. (C) Upon full inflation, the waist is relieved. (D) Postangioplasty aortogram shows successful dilation of recoarcted segment. Note the irregularity of vessel wall in the dilated area (arrow).

AAO, ascending aorta; Ar, aortic arch; DAO, descending aorta; G, guidewire.

Source: Reprinted with permission from Castaneda, A. R., Jonas, R. A., Mayer, J. E., & Hanley F. L. (2006). *Cardiac surgery of the neonate and infant* (2nd ed.). Philadelphia, PA: W. B. Saunders.

subclavian arteries; in type C, interruption occurs proximal to the origin of the left common carotid artery (Figure 3.80).

b. Incidence. Occurs in 1% of all congenital heart defects. Type B is the most common form (>435), followed by type A (approximately 305). Type C is rare (175; Park, 2016).

c. Pathophysiology. Blood flowing in the arteries proximal to the interruption is fully oxygenated, whereas blood flowing distal to the interruption is deoxygenated (via PDA from the PA). Systemic blood flow is dependent on ductal patency. Associated lesions/syndrome: VSD, LVOTO, bicuspid aortic valve, and DiGeorge syndrome.

d. Clinical signs and symptoms. Exhibited as tachypnea, poor perfusion, and poor feeding. Circulatory shock and CHF if ductus arteriosus closes.

e. Diagnostic evaluation. ECG may demonstrate RVH. CXR may demonstrate cardiomegaly and pulmonary overcirculation. Echo to establish specific diagnosis. Genetic microarray to evaluate for DiGeorge syndrome.

f. Goals and medical patient management. Maintain ductal patency with prostaglandin infusion until intervention. Management of circulatory shock, CHF, end-organ damage occur if late diagnosis.

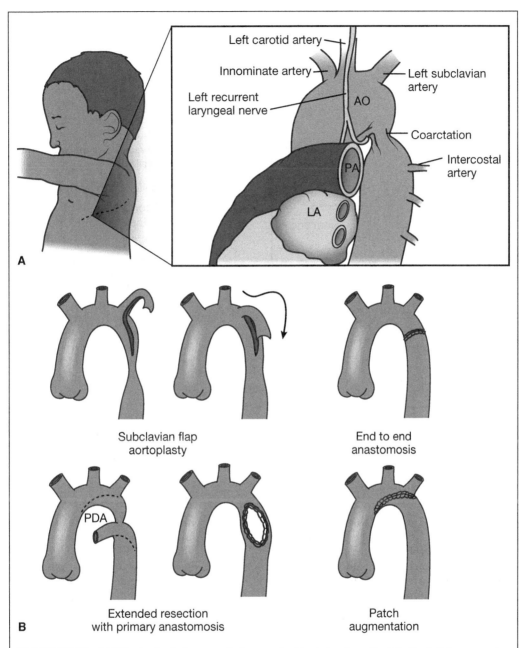

FIGURE 3.78   (A) The typical placement of a surgical incision for a CoA is the left torso, under the armpit, as shown by the dotted line. This provides access to the relevant internal anatomy to correct the coarctation. (B) Four operative procedures are commonly used to repair a CoA: subclavian flap aortoplasty, end-to-end aortic anastomosis, extended resection with primary anastomosis, and patch augmentation.

AO, aorta; CoA, coarctation of the aorta; LA, left atrium; PA, pulmonary artery; PDA, patent ductua arteriosus.

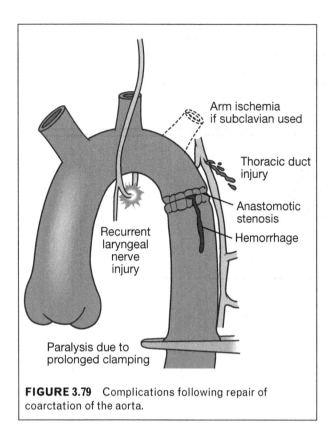

Arm ischemia
if subclavian used

Thoracic duct
injury

Anastomotic
stenosis

Recurrent
laryngeal
nerve
injury

Hemorrhage

Paralysis due to
prolonged clamping

FIGURE 3.79 Complications following repair of coarctation of the aorta.

g. Goals and surgical patient management. Arch reconstruction with CPB with deep hypothermic circulatory arrest, VSD closure, and enlargement of LVOT, if indicated, are necessary (Figure 3.81; Jonas, 2015).

h. Complications. Residual obstruction, anastomotic stenosis, pulmonary hypertension, left ventricular dysfunction, phrenic nerve injury, laryngeal nerve injury, and compression of left bronchus by reconstructed aortic arch (Strychowsky, Rukholm, Gupta, & Reid, 2014).

4. *Mitral Valve Insufficiency*

  a. Anatomy

    i. Mitral valve insufficiency results in failure of the valve leaflets to coapt normally, which allows regurgitation of blood into the LA.

  b. Incidence

    i. Mitral insufficiency is rare.

  c. Pathophysiology

    i. Congenital mitral insufficiency is usually associated with other lesions, such as single-ventricle lesions and AVSD. Isolated insufficiency of the mitral valve may be associated with connective tissue disorders and metabolic diseases. Acquired mitral insufficiency may be associated with CM, Kawasaki syndrome, trauma, and endcarditis. Regurgitation of LV volume into the LA and, depending on the severity of mitral valve incompetence, into the pulmonary veins, causes PA hypertension and elevated PVR over time.

  d. Clinical signs and symptoms

    i. History. Inquire about family history, intrauterine exposures, immunologic or connective tissue disorders, infections.

    ii. Clinical presentation depends on the severity of insufficiency. Examination of patient with mitral regurgitation reveals diffuse apical impulse, active precordium, soft S_1, accentuated S_2, high-frequency blowing or harsh holosystolic murmur at the apex, and a low-frequency apical diastolic murmur. A third heart sound indicates poorly tolerated mitral insufficiency with CHF.

  e. Diagnostic evaluation

    i. ECG shows LA enlargement and LVH.

    ii. Chest radiographic examination shows an enlarged heart with LA and LV enlargement, increased pulmonary vascular markings, and congestion.

    iii. Echo demonstrates an abnormal valve anatomy, increased LA and LV dimensions, normal to increased LV systolic indexes, insufficiency or overlapping of anterior and posterior leaflets, a break in leaflet echo suggesting a cleft, and regurgitant flow into the LA and pulmonary veins if insufficiency is severe.

    iv. Cardiac catheterization reveals elevated PCWP, PA pressure, PVR, LA pressure, LVEDP, LA opacification to a varying degree with LV injection, and a deceptively normal LV ejection fraction because of the ability to eject retrograde to low-pressure atrium.

  f. Goals and medical patient management

    i. Treatment may be medical if the child is not in severe CHF. The child must be watched closely for signs of PA hypertension

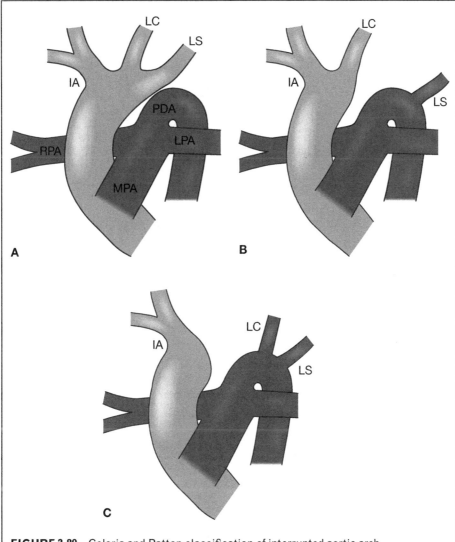

FIGURE 3.80 Celoria and Patton classification of interrupted aortic arch.

IA, innominate artery; LC, left carotid artery; LPA, left pulmonary artery; LS, left subclavian; LSA, left subclavian artery; MPA, man pulmonary artery; PDA, patent ductus arteriosis; RPA, right pulmonary artery.

and the development of PVOD. Afterload reduction and diuretics (see "Pediatric Cardiovascular Pharmacology" section) may be used cautiously.

g. Goals and surgical patient management

i. Surgical intervention is indicated in the presence of severe CHF, ventilator dependency or PA hypertension, and vascular changes. Valvuloplasty may be difficult if there is deficient valve tissue. Prosthetic rings may be used in some cases. Cleft valve or elongated chordae tendineae may

be amenable to repair. Mitral valve replacement is used as a last resort due to operative risks and complexity in infants and children. Relief of mitral insufficiency producing a competent mitral valve may unmask LV dysfunction (Figure 3.82).

h. Complications

i. Endocarditis is a lifelong risk.

ii. Early development of PA hypertension and pulmonary vascular disease occurs.

iii. Pulmonary congestion, pulmonary edema, and pulmonary insufficiency occur.

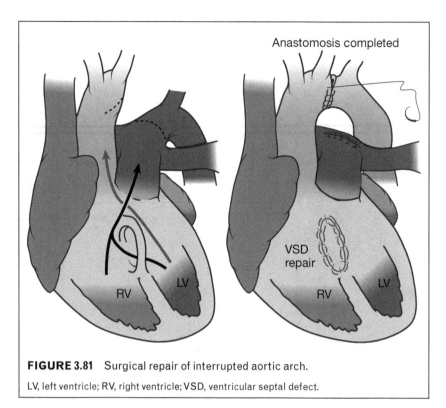

FIGURE 3.81 Surgical repair of interrupted aortic arch.

LV, left ventricle; RV, right ventricle; VSD, ventricular septal defect.

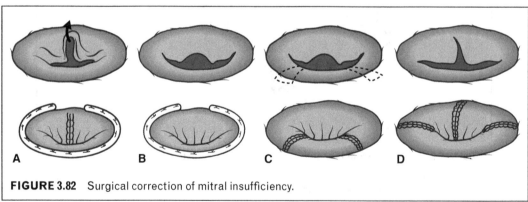

FIGURE 3.82 Surgical correction of mitral insufficiency.

iv. There is an enlargement of the left atrium and predisposition to atrial arrhythmias, primarily atrial flutter/fibrillation.

5. *Mitral Stenosis*

a. Definition

i. Narrowing of the mitral valve orifice restricts blood flow from the LA to the LV.

b. Incidence

i. MS is rare. Congenital MS is usually associated with other lesions when present. Acquired MS may be associated with rheumatic fever, carcinoid causes, systemic lupus erythematosus, rheumatoid arthritis, and some mucopolysaccharidoses.

c. Pathophysiology

i. Congenital MS is a variable expression of developmental abnormality involving the LV. Excessive or abnormal deposition of tissue occurs embryologically.

ii. MS is characterized by the component of the mitral valve that is abnormal. Abnormalities include thick, rolled leaflet margins, abnormal chordae tendineae, papillary muscle hypoplasia, LV endocardial sclerosis, hypoplasia or atresia of the mitral valve, commissure fusion, excessive tissue, parachute mitral valve, or supramitral ring. Left atrial, pulmonary venous, and PCWPs increase relative to resistance to flow across the mitral valve into the LV. Eventually, MS may cause PA hypertension, elevated PVR, and RV dysfunction from PVOD. LV volume load decreases, causing ischemia, fibrosis, and further LV dysfunction and decreased CO (del Nido & Baird, 2012).

d.   Clinical signs and symptoms

   i.   History. Inquire about endocarditis, rheumatic fever, immunologic disorder.

   ii.   Clinical presentation. Timing and type of symptoms of MS are based on the degree of obstruction to LV inflow. The most severe presentation (related to ductal closure with systemic hypoperfusion) is similar to the history of HLHS. A history of frequent pulmonary infections, poor weight gain, irritability, tiring with feeding, diaphoresis, tachypnea, chronic cough, and increased work of breathing are noted.

   iii.   Examination reveals an active RV impulse with PA hypertension, soft S_1, split S_2, possible S_3 or S_4, and a low-frequency mid-diastolic murmur at the apex.

e.   Diagnostic evaluation

   i.   ECG. LA and RA enlargement or RVH suggest PA hypertension and severe MS. Diminished LV forces are noted.

   ii.   Chest radiographic examination demonstrates LA enlargement, prominence of pulmonary vascular markings, and right-sided enlargement.

   iii.   Echo shows decreased mitral valve opening, abnormal posterior leaflet motion, LA enlargement, reduced aortic-wall motion, and diminished LV dimensions. It defines abnormalities of chordae tendineae and papillary muscles and estimates transvalvular gradients, ASD size, and changes in pulmonary vein inflow patterns.

   iv.   Cardiac catheterization reveals mild systemic desaturation and hypoxemia, left-to-right atrial shunt with severe MS, elevation of PA pressure, PVR, PCWP, and LA pressure; a diastolic pressure gradient from the LA pressure to the LVEDP; and a transpulmonary gradient if PVOD has developed.

f.   Goals and medical patient management

   i.   CHF is medically managed, including administration of diuretics +/− digoxin. β-Blockers may be indicated, but should be used cautiously.

g.   Goals and surgical patient management

   i.   Surgical intervention is considered for elevated PAP and PVR. Mitral valve commissurotomy is done via sternotomy and bypass with excision of excess tissue and membranes. Mitral valve replacement is difficult in infants with small annulus size (Figure 3.83). The success of the operation is contingent on mitral valve characteristics and annulus size, LV size, PVR, PA pressure, and age. Older patients have better results if

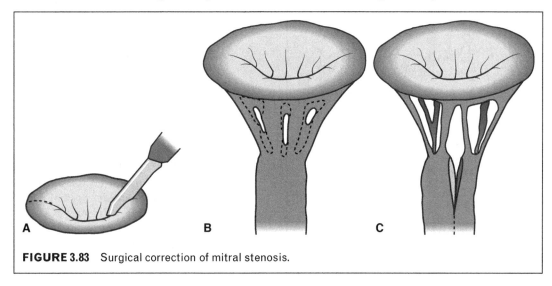

FIGURE 3.83   Surgical correction of mitral stenosis.

no PVOD is present. The mitral valve orifice must be opened to allow adequate LV inflow and pulmonary vein drainage.

   ii.   If mitral valve replacement is performed, systemic anticoagulation is indicated.

 h. Complications

   i.   Endocarditis is a lifelong risk.

   ii.   Early development of PA hypertension and pulmonary vascular disease is a risk due to LA hypertension from mitral stenosis.

   iii.   Pulmonary congestion, pulmonary edema, pulmonary insufficiency may result from LA and PA hypertension as the mitral stenosis worsens.

   iv.   Enlargement of left atrium predisposes the patient to atrial arrhythmias, primarily atrial flutter/fibrillation.

   v.   Immediate postoperative complications can include residual PA hypertension, low CO, arrhythmias, and conduction disturbances.

6. *Pulmonary Stenosis*

 a. Anatomy

   i.   Pulmonary stenosis involves a narrowed pulmonary valve causing obstruction to flow from the RV to the PA, resulting in RVH (Figure 3.84).

   ii.   PS results from an embryologic error in the formation of pulmonary leaflets.

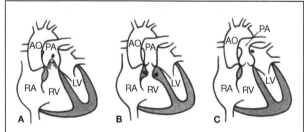

FIGURE 3.84 Anatomic types of PS. (A) Valvular stenosis. (B) Infundibular stenosis. (C) Supravalvular pulmonary stenosis (or stenosis of the main PA). Abnormalities are indicated by arrows.

AO, aorta; LV, left ventricle; PA, pulmonary artery; PS, pulmonary stenosis; RA, right atrium; RV, right ventricle.

Source: Reprinted with permission from Park, M. K. (2016). *Park's The Pediatric Cardiology Handbook* (5th ed.). Philadelphia, PA: Saunders-Elsevier.

 b. Incidence

   i.   It occurs in 8% to 10% of children with CHD (Mavouridis, 2013).

   ii.   Dysplastic pulmonary valve is common in association with Noonan syndrome.

 c. Pathophysiology

   i.   The pulmonary valve is conical or dome shaped and is formed by fusion of valve leaflets. It may be bicuspid (20% of cases). Thickened and immobile leaflets obstruct RV outflow. The endocardium of the infundibulum may be thick and endocardial fibroelastosis may develop. In severe cases, there is tricuspid valve regurgitation and RA dilation. If an ASD or PFO is present, right-to-left shunting can occur, resulting in cyanosis of varying degrees. If PS is severe and significant, right-to-left atrial shunting occurs across the ASD, the RV and pulmonary valve may be hypoplastic. Grading of PS severity is based on transvalvular gradients of (a) mild, 25 to 49 mmHg; (b) moderate, 50 to 75 mmHg; and (c) severe, greater than 75 mmHg (Park, 2016).

 d. Clinical signs and symptoms

   i.   Clinical presentation may vary depending on the degree of PS from an asymptomatic presentation, to mild exertional dyspnea and cyanosis, to severe CHF. Dyspnea and fatigue with exercise are the most common early symptoms and, as stenosis progresses, these symptoms occur even at rest. Growth and development are usually normal. The presence of cyanosis from right-to-left atrial shunting indicates moderate PS.

   ii.   Examination reveals a normal S_1, pulmonary ejection click, and a diastolic ejection murmur (shorter in milder PS, longer in severe PS). The holosystolic murmur of tricuspid insufficiency and soft or absent S_2 are characteristic of severe PS. In the newborn with severe PS, S_2 is almost always single.

 e. Diagnostic evaluation

   i.   ECG is useful to assess the severity of PS. In mild stenosis, normal RV forces are present. Severe RVH and RA enlargement are present in severe stenosis.

   ii.   Chest radiographic examination demonstrates a prominent main PA segment, RVH and downward apex, and cardiomegaly in severe PS only (usually only mild enlargement).

iii. Echo determines function and anatomy of the pulmonary valve and associated lesions, septal and RVH, prominent valve with restricted systolic motion, poststenotic dilation of the PA, and size of the tricuspid valve and RV (small only in severe PS). It is also used to estimate the PVR and valve gradient.

iv. Cardiac catheterization is not required for diagnosis, but it excludes other diagnoses, and may be used to perform interventional therapy. RV pressure is elevated. The valve area and gradient and anatomy are defined. CO is quantified to use in determining the accuracy of the pulmonary valve gradient.

f. Goals and medical patient management

i. Identify neonates requiring emergent intervention for critical PS. Until intervention, maintain ductal patency with PGE_1 in patients with critical PS.

ii. In noncritical PS, conservative management and monitoring is recommended. Intervention is recommended for a pulmonary valve gradient greater than 40 mmHg or RV dysfunction.

g. Goals and surgical patient management

i. Intervention is required for moderate or greater PS. Balloon valvuloplasty is the currently accepted treatment and provides excellent short-term and long-term results. The balloon catheter is inserted across the pulmonary valve and inflated to a size 10% to 20% greater than the annulus (Figure 3.85). Valvuloplasty is not as effective for dysplastic valves and neonates with critical PS, although results in this group are improving. Risks include RV perforation, residual stenosis, and creation of insufficiency.

ii. Surgical valvotomy (Figure 3.86) may be done in cases in which the catheter cannot pass through the pulmonary valve or when associated lesions require surgery. Surgery requires sternotomy and a short period of CPB. Progressive dilators are inserted through the pulmonary valve via incision in the PA to 1 cm greater than the valve annulus. Risks include RV failure, creation of pulmonary insufficiency, and inadequate relief of PS (Karamichalis, Darst, Mitchell, & Clarke, 2013).

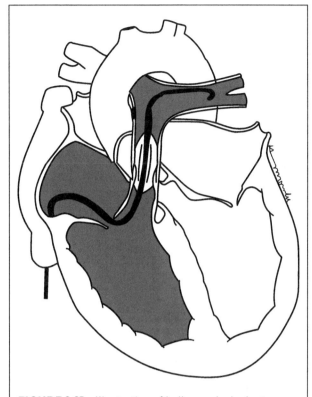

FIGURE 3.85 Illustration of balloon valvuloplasty catheter positioned across the pulmonary valve.

h. Complications

i. Endocarditis is a lifelong risk.

ii. Residual PS may be present immediately after the procedure or may develop over time requiring re-intervention.

iii. Pulmonary insufficiency with dilation of the RV that progresses to RV dysfunction are risks associated with repair of PS.

E. Cyanotic Cardiac Lesions

1. *Tetralogy of Fallot*

   a. Definition

   i. The four classic features are VSD, PS, RV hypertrophy, and overriding aorta.

   ii. Physiology and degree of cyanosis depend on PS of varying degrees. PS is often dynamic and progressive in nature because of the anterior deviation of the infundibular septum, creating subvalvular or infundibular stenosis. Also associated are varying degrees of valvular and supravalvular stenosis (Figure 3.87).

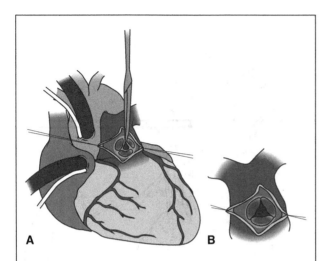

FIGURE 3.86 Technique of pulmonary valvulotomy. (A) Fused leaflet commissures are incised to the PA wall. (B) Completed valvulotomy.

PA, pulmonary artery.

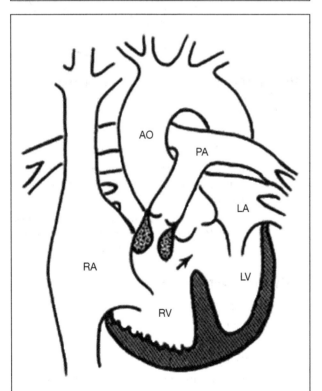

FIGURE 3.87 Anatomy of tetralogy of Fallot with ventral septal defect, pulmonary stenosis, and overriding aorta.

AO, aorta; LA, left atrium; LV, left ventricle; PA, pulmonary artery; RA, right atrium; RV, right ventricle.

Source: Reprinted with permission from Kambam, J. (1994). Atrial septal defect. In J. Kambam (Ed.), *Cardiac anesthesia for infants and children.* St. Louis, MO: Mosby.

iii. Associated anomalies include coronary artery anomalies, AVSD (newborns will present with CHF and cyanosis), absent pulmonary valve (associated with dilated PA and degrees of respiratory compromise from bronchial compression), ASD, or PA (Stewart, Mavroudis, & Backer, 2013).

b. Incidence

i. TOF is the most common form of cyanotic CHD and accounts for as much as 10% of CHD. It is likely related to abnormal septation of the conus. It occurs slightly more often in boys (Mavroudis, 2013a).

c. Genetic syndromes occur in at least 20% of patients PS with TOF. The most common is DiGeorge syndrome (Mavroudis, 2013a).

d. Pathophysiology

i. Blood enters the RV normally. RV outflow obstruction causes shunting across the VSD to the aorta, thereby mixing systemic venous and pulmonary venous return. The severity of the PS determines the severity of the cyanosis. As the aorta handles biventricular CO, it is often dilated.

ii. Classic hypoxic episodes are marked by increasing cyanosis, hyperpnea, and irritability, progressing to unconsciousness, seizures, or cardiac arrest. Episodes occur secondary to a spasm of the infundibulum of the RV outflow tract and/or a drop in the systemic resistance, increasing right-to-left shunting and decreasing pulmonary blood flow. The murmur disappears as no flow passes across the narrowed pulmonary outflow tract. Interventions to break these episodes include sedation, fluid bolus (hematocrit 45%), bicarbonate, oxygen, knee–chest position, and intubation and anesthesia if necessary. Morphine sulfate is the sedation medication of choice during these episodes. IV propranolol (Inderal) or other β-blocker may be used to relax the RV infundibulum and decrease the ventricular response to agitation. Phenylephrine (Neo-Synephrine) IV increases the systolic BP and ideally decreases shunting away from the RV outflow tract. Occurrence of spells may indicate a need for earlier repair.

e. Clinical signs and symptoms

i. Clinical presentation depends on the degree of PS. If stenosis is severe, surgical intervention is indicated. Neonates with severe PS will be ductal dependent. If PS is not severe, symptoms are mild and include dyspnea on exertion, clubbing, squatting, and cyanosis. Hypercyanotic spells may occur in patients with severe PS.

ii. Examination reveals a normal cardiac impulse, normal S_1, single S_2, systolic ejection murmur at the LSB (related to PS), diastolic murmur (with absent pulmonary valve), and a continuous murmur of collaterals or PDA.

f. Diagnostic evaluation

i. ECG shows right axis deviation, RVH, normal conduction, and rarely, ectopy.

ii. Chest radiographic examination demonstrates a boot-shaped heart from absence of the PA segment and upturned cardiac apex from RV hypertrophy, normal or diminished pulmonary vascular markings, and a right aortic arch in 15% to 25% of cases (Mavroudis, 2013a).

iii. Echo is the major diagnostic tool for definition of essential morphology, gradients, and identification of associated lesions (anomalous coronary arteries are often difficult to visualize).

iv. Cardiac catheterization may be necessary to adequately detail the RV outflow tract. It will show equal pressures in the RV and LV. Coronary arteries are often better delineated by cardiac catheterization than by echo.

g. Goals and medical patient management

i. Medical intervention is necessary for hypoxic spells associated with deep cyanosis, hypoxemia, acidosis, or seizures. Maintenance of adequate circulatory volume, and maintenance of a normal hematocrit, sedation, oxygenation, and knee–chest position are utilized to break spells. Inderal may be useful. The presence of hypercyanotic spells is an indication for surgery.

ii. Medical management includes prostaglandins in neonates who are ductal dependent for pulmonary blood flow. Inderal may be useful as interim medical management.

h. Goals and surgical patient management

i. Surgical palliation is provided by a systemic-to-pulmonary shunt (usually a modified Blalock–Taussig shunt with GORE-TEX interposition tube between the subclavian artery and ipsilateral PA) via thoracotomy (Figure 3.88). Too large a shunt causes pulmonary overcirculation, symptoms of CHF, and risk of pulmonary vascular disease. Too small a shunt does not adequately relieve cyanosis. Risks of aortopulmonary shunts include chylothorax, damage to phrenic or recurrent laryngeal nerve, infection, PVOD, and distortion of the PA.

ii. Corrective operation via sternotomy and CPB can be performed at any age. Timing generally depends on severity of right ventricular outflow tract obstruction (RVOTO) symptoms. Repair consists of VSD closure (GORE-TEX patch) directing LV flow to the aorta, relief of RV outflow tract obstruction, and shunt takedown if one was done previously. Infundibular muscle resection or division of muscle bundles with pulmonary valvotomy or transannular GORE-TEX patch results in pulmonary insufficiency (Figure 3.89). In cases of anomalous coronary arteries or small-branch pulmonary arteries, an RV-PA conduit is used (Figure 3.90). Risks of operation include heart block, JET, residual PS, residual RV outflow tract obstruction, VSD, RV dysfunction, pulmonary insufficiency, or damage to the aortic valve. Late reoperation for PS, and/or to place a competent pulmonary valve may be necessary to preserve RV function and exercise tolerance (Kanter, Kogon, Kirshbom, & Carlock, 2010; Redington, 2012).

i. Complications

i. Endocarditis is a lifelong risk.

ii. Late development of arrhythmia, RV dysfunction, pulmonary regurgitation, recurrent PS, RV-PA conduit obstruction or insufficiency, and TR (J. Jacobs et al., 2014) may occur.

2. *Pulmonary Atresia With a VSD (PA/VSD)*

a. Anatomy.

PA/VSD is a form of RVOTO with complete obstruction. Thus, patients are at severe risk of cyanosis. For survival at birth, patients must have either ductal-dependent or collateral-dependent pulmonary blood flow.

b. The incidence of PA/VSD is 1% to 2% of patients with CHD. The incidence is higher in siblings (2.5%–3%) and in children of adults with

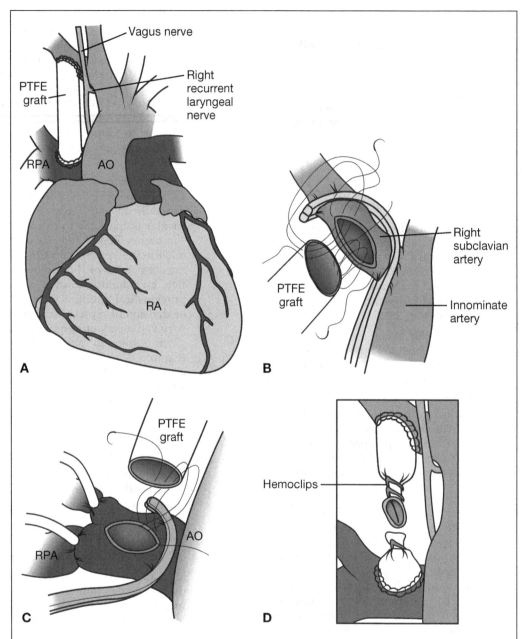

FIGURE 3.88 (A) This modified Blalock–Taussig shunt procedure uses a PTFE graft to increase pulmonary blood flow. (B) Proximal anastomosis can be used to connect the PTFE graft with the right subclavian artery. (C) Distal anastomosis is another method utilized in incorporating a modified Blalock–Taussig shunt procedure with the RPA. (D) This takedown of a modified Blalock–Taussig shunt is performed through use of hemoclips and shunt division.

AO, aorta; PTFE, polytetrafluoroethylene; RA, right atrium; RPA, right pulmonary artery.

TOF (1.2%–8.3%; Mavroudis, Backer, Jacobs, & Anderson, 2013).

c. Pathophysiology

   i. Due to the lack of flow into the native PA, varying degrees of main PA and branch

PA hypoplasia develop. In the most severe forms, there are no true pulmonary arteries and all pulmonary blood flow is supported by the ductus arteriosus or collateral vessels from the aorta, which form small and native pulmonary arteries (Figure 3.91). Collaterals

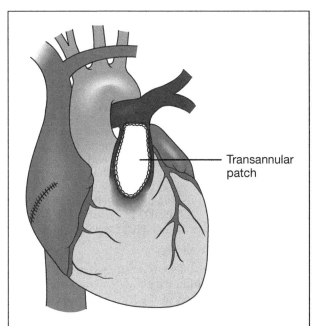

FIGURE 3.89 A transannular patch is often used to enlarge the hypoplastic pulmonary valve annulus and main pulmonary trunk. It is essential to keep the proximal extent of the patch, which extends onto the origin of the left PA, as short as possible for best results.

PA, pulmonary artery.

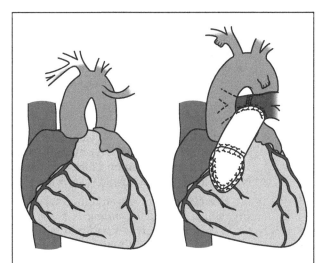

FIGURE 3.90 Technique of repair with insertion of homograft conduit after primary unifocalization in those with absence of both interpericardial pulmonary arteries.

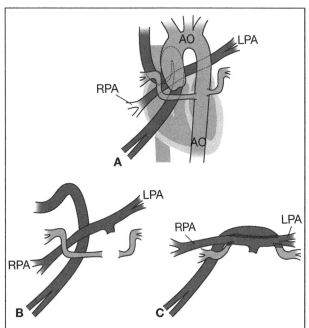

FIGURE 3.91 Diagrams of the anatomy of major AP collateral and true pulmonary arteries and the techniques of unifocalization.

AO, aorta; AP, action potential; LPA, left pulmonary artery; RPA, right pulmonary artery.

are frequently stenotic at either the aortic or pulmonary end and this stenosis is progressive throughout the disease course.

d. Clinical signs and symptoms

i. Many patients present within the first week of life as PDA begins to close and cyanosis is evident. Other patients may not be diagnosed until several months of age because collateral flow masks cyanosis.

ii. Presentation is usually marked by CHF and failure to thrive (FTT) by 3 to 6 months, occasional cyanosis, continuous murmurs of collaterals, and single S_2.

e. Diagnostic evaluation

i. Catheterization is routine at diagnosis to assess the anatomy of the PA, which is extremely variable but frequently is small and nonconfluent.

ii. Chest radiographic examination demonstrates mild to moderate cardiomegaly with no main PA segment and increased pulmonary vascular markings.

iii. ECG reflects RV hypertrophy with right axis deviation, upright and peaked T waves in the right precordial leads and reversal of the R/S ratio. If the RV is hypoplastic, evidence of RV hypertrophy may not be present.

    iv.   Echo findings can be used to accurately determine intracardiac anatomy, presence of patent ductus, and coronary anatomy.

f.   Goals and medical patient management

    i.   Initial management includes evaluation of adequate pulmonary blood flow.

    ii.   If pulmonary blood flow is inadequate, prostaglandin infusion to maintain ductal patency may be utilized. Additional treatment may include administration of volume to increase preload, optimizing oxygen-carrying capacity by increasing hematocrit greater than 40%, using vasoconstrictors to increase SVR thereby driving more flow to the pulmonary system.

g.   Goals and surgical patient management

    i.   Results and long-term outcomes are based on PA architecture and the state of the pulmonary vascular bed at diagnosis.

    ii.   Often the child requires several surgical interventions.

    iii.   Early interventions focus on stabilizing pulmonary blood flow. One surgical approach is PA unifocalization with an RV–PA conduit to promote growth of the proximal and distal PA, which requires CPB. Alternatively, cardiac catheterization for stenting of PDA may be performed.

    iv.   VSD closure with full anatomic repair via median sternotomy and CPB is accomplished only in children who have forward RV output and adequately sized pulmonary arteries, typically evidenced by increasing oxygen saturation, an adequate number of PA segments incorporated into the RVOT, and a predominant left-to-right shunt at catheterization (Reddy & Hanley, 2013).

    v.   A postoperative RV:LV pressure ratio of less than 3:4 to 2:3 is ideal to provide good long-term results. Future operations for conduit replacement resulting from conduit stenosis or regurgitation are expected (Mavroudis, 2013a).

h.   Complications

    i.   Complications of operation include residual VSD, PA stenosis, RV hypertension, aortic regurgitation, and arrhythmia, including CHB. Postoperative cardiac catheterization may be indicated to assess the PA vasculature and the need for balloon or stenting of stenotic vessels.

    ii.   Endocarditis is a lifelong risk.

3.   *Pulmonary Atresia/ Intact Ventricular Septum*

    a.   Definition

        i.   Involves complete obstruction of the RV outflow requiring shunting at the atrial and great-vessel level for survival.

    b.   Incidence

        i.   PA/IVS is an uncommon defect occurring in 4.5 cases/100,000 live births. It represents fewer than 1% of CHDs (Mavroudis, 2013a).

    c.   Pathophysiology

        i.   The defect is characterized by atresia of the pulmonary valve with variable size and function of the RV and tricuspid valve. The RA may be dilated proportional to the degree of tricuspid insufficiency from a lack of RV outflow. An ASD is always present. RV size may be decreased or normal but capable of handling forward CO with relief of obstruction at the pulmonary valve. RV pressure increases relative to the outflow obstruction and can cause tricuspid insufficiency and increased RA pressure. Shunting typically occurs across the ASD into the LA. Flow into the PA and lungs is maintained by a PDA. The LV supports the total CO.

        ii.   Coronary artery anomalies may include fistulous communication between coronary arteries and the RV, which can cause retrograde flow of desaturated blood into the coronary arteries, resulting in ventricular ischemia and even death. Coronary arteries may be stenotic.

    d.   Clinical signs and symptoms

        i.   Clinical presentation is cyanosis evident shortly after birth as the PDA physiologically closes. CHF is uncommon unless the defect is accompanied by tricuspid insufficiency.

        ii.   Examination reveals an S_1, normal intensity, single S_2, and a *continuous murmur of the PDA*. When there is significant tricuspid insufficiency, the child may have a holosystolic murmur.

    e.   Diagnostic evaluation

        i.   ECG shows LV predominance and RA enlargement. ST–T wave changes reflect major underlying coronary anomalies when present.

ii. Chest radiographic examination results are normal in most cases (with decreased pulmonary blood flow). Marked cardiomegaly is present with severe tricuspid insufficiency.

iii. Echo defines an imperforate pulmonary valve, tricuspid valve size and anomalies, and visualization of the ASD and may be able to assess abnormal coronary artery connections.

iv. Cardiac catheterization is indicated for full delineation of all anatomic defects. Low systemic venous saturations, decreased LA saturation from right-to-left shunting, and RV pressure are noted. Coronary artery fistulas and stenosis are visualized.

f. Goals and medical patient management

i. Maintaining ductal patency is mandatory for survival until full diagnostic evaluation and surgical repair are completed.

g. Goals and surgical patient management

i. All operations aim, when possible, at encouraging growth of the tricuspid valve and RV. The surgical approach depends on multiple factors, including predicted RV function and size, the presence of RV-dependent coronary blood flow or coronary artery stenosis, and the size of the tricuspid valve and ASD. The ASD is left open in these infants to provide pressure relief for noncompliant RVs. It is closed only after final palliation in patients with a usable RV with good function. For the diminutive RV, small tricuspid valve inlet, or for patients with RV-dependent coronary blood flow, initial palliation with a systemic-to-pulmonary shunt and progression to a single-ventricle palliation, with a Fontan operation as the final step in the pathway.

ii. For patients with moderate RV hypoplasia and tricuspid valve annulus who may be able to progress to biventricular repair, an RVOT patch and shunt are performed. Repair with ASD closure alone is feasible if the RV/tricuspid valve can handle the entire forward CO. If not, repair with SVC to PA connections and ASD closure may be the best option. In mild RV hypoplasia, the likelihood of a biventricular repair is high. RV to PA continuity is performed initially using a transannular patch or valvotomy (membranous PA).

iii. OHT is a consideration for patients with RV dysfunction and coronary artery stenosis or sinusoids.

h. Complications

i. Early and late mortality of this defect remains high, and consensus has yet to be reached regarding optimal patient management.

ii. Endocarditis remains a lifelong risk.

4. *Tricuspid Atresia (TA)*

a. Anatomy

i. Lack of tricuspid valve formation results in absence of blood flow from RA to RV and poor RV formation in utero. Survival is contingent upon placement of an obligatory right-to-left atrial shunt.

b. Incidence

i. Etiology is agenesis of the tricuspid atresia or failure of trabecular components of the ventricle to develop (single ventricle). TA is an uncommon defect (1%–3% CHD cases; Park, 2016).

c. Pathophysiology

i. Agenesis of the tricuspid valve results in no communication between the RA and RV. TA is associated most often with a small RV, ASD, and an aortopulmonary connection (PDA; Figure 3.92). Physiology and symptoms depend on the degree of PS or PA and the presence or absence and size of the VSD. Because blood cannot exit the RV, it is shunted right to left at the atrial level and systemic desaturation occurs. Blood then flows across the left side of the heart to the RV via the VSD and out to the lungs if there is little or no PS. The result is normal to increased pulmonary blood flow with clinical manifestations of CHF (Mavroudis, 2013a).

ii. With associated PS or PA, there will be little or no flow to the PA. These infants usually have small RVs, are cyanotic early, and are ductal dependent for pulmonary blood flow. With VSD, systemic output may be significantly compromised if the VSD is small or restrictive or becomes so early in life.

iii. In single-ventricle variants of tricuspid atresia, both AV valves empty into one ventricle (known as *double inlet*). Ventricles are differentiated based on trabeculations. These lesions, as with TA, may have normal,

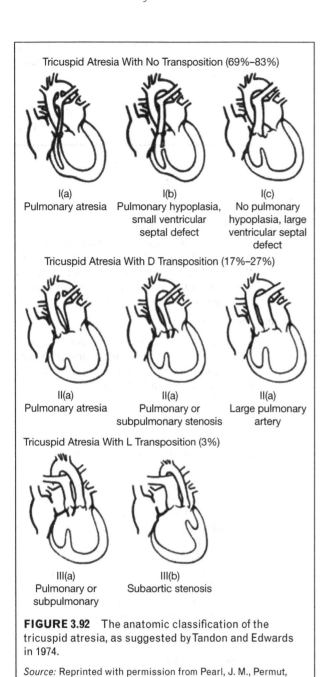

Tricuspid Atresia With No Transposition (69%–83%)

I(a)
Pulmonary atresia

I(b)
Pulmonary hypoplasia, small ventricular septal defect

I(c)
No pulmonary hypoplasia, large ventricular septal defect

Tricuspid Atresia With D Transposition (17%–27%)

II(a)
Pulmonary atresia

II(a)
Pulmonary or subpulmonary stenosis

II(a)
Large pulmonary artery

Tricuspid Atresia With L Transposition (3%)

III(a)
Pulmonary or subpulmonary

III(b)
Subaortic stenosis

FIGURE 3.92 The anatomic classification of the tricuspid atresia, as suggested by Tandon and Edwards in 1974.

Source: Reprinted with permission from Pearl, J. M., Permut, L. C., & Laks, H. (1996). Tricuspid atresia. In A. E. Bauer, et al. (Eds.), Glenn's thoracic and cardiovascular surgery (6th ed.). Stamford, CT: Appleton & Lange.

d. Clinical signs and symptoms

i. Clinical presentation is dependent on the amount of pulmonary blood flow (presence of a VSD, degree of PS or PA). Early cyanosis is common (50%, TA without VSD) and expected (78%, TA without VSD) by 1 month because of the obligatory atrial shunt (Park, 2016). CHF may occur with VSD and no PS. Hypoxic spells occur in 16% to 45% of patients younger than 6 months. Examination reveals a hyperactive apical impulse, clubbing, left precordial prominence, single S_1 and S_2 (most common unless pulmonary blood flow is increased), systolic ejection murmur at the mid to upper LSB from the PS, occasional holosystolic murmur at the LSB if a VSD is present, and a continuous murmur of the PDA or collaterals if PVR is normal.

e. Diagnostic evaluation

i. ECG shows a superior and leftward QRS axis, RA enlargement, absent or diminished RV forces, and increased LV forces.

ii. Echo demonstrates absence of the tricuspid valve and diminished RV size. It also defines associated defects, increased LV dimensions, size of the VSD and ASD, and the relationship of the great vessels.

iii. Chest radiographic examination in tricuspid atresia variants with diminished pulmonary blood flow demonstrates normal to mild cardiomegaly, concave main PA segment, and diminished pulmonary vascular markings. Chest radiographic examination in tricuspid atresia variants with increased pulmonary blood flow demonstrates gross cardiomegaly and increased pulmonary vascular markings.

iv. Cardiac catheterization is not necessary for first-stage palliation, but is indicated to assess adequacy of PVR prior to proceeding to cavopulmonary connection (Glenn, Hemi-Fontan, Fontan). On catheterization, the RV is not entered from the RA, and flow of systemic venous blood from the RA to the LA through the ASD results in decreased saturation of the LA blood. The RA pressure is greater than or equal to the LA pressure. Cardiac catheterization can demonstrate and define the presence of a VSD, collaterals, the relationship of the great vessels, and the degree of PS. If no PS is present and there is a VSD, PA pressure and PVR may be elevated.

increased, or decreased pulmonary blood flow based on the degree of PS. Clinical manifestations, physical examination, diagnostic findings, and interventions depend on the degree of AV valve regurgitation, extracardiac or intracardiac shunting, and pulmonary obstruction.

f. Goals and medical patient management

i. Medical interventions for the infant with tricuspid atresia and PS include initial stabilization with prostaglandin infusion to maintain ductal patency until surgery. Initial treatment for patients with nonrestrictive pulmonary flow involves medical management with the use of CHF medications.

g. Goals and surgical patient management

i. Initial surgical palliation for those with decreased pulmonary blood flow typically involves placement of an aortopulmonary shunt via thoracotomy. Initial palliation in infants with increased pulmonary blood flow may involve ligating the PA and performing an aortopulmonary shunt or PA banding.

ii. In the cohort of TA patients having transposed great vessels and a hypoplastic systemic outflow chamber, a Damus–Kaye–Stansel operation via median sternotomy and CPB may be indicated. This operation is similar to a Norwood operation in that a systemic outflow is created by aortic-to-pulmonary (off the LV) anastomosis, ligation of the PA, and creation of a systemic-to-pulmonary shunt.

iii. Regardless of initial palliation, patients with TA typically undergo staged cardiac reconstruction ending with a Fontan (see the "Diagnostic Evaluation" section). Second-stage palliation is typically either bidirectional Glenn or hemi-Fontan, depending on the venous anatomy and surgeon preference. Fontan operation via lateral tunnel or extracardiac conduit is the final palliation (Figures 3.93 and 3.94).

h. Complications

i. The risk of complications for patients with tricuspid atresia is from cyanosis, stroke, and brain abscess. Patients with CHF from excessive pulmonary blood flow may develop PVOD. All patients are at risk for endocarditis. Atrial arrhythmias are not uncommon. Delayed growth and development may be seen. Complications for patients with tricuspid atresia who undergo the single-ventricle pathway with a Bidirectional Glenn/Hemifontan and the completion Fontan operation can be found in the section on hypoplastic left heart syndrome (HLHS). (Marino, 2013).

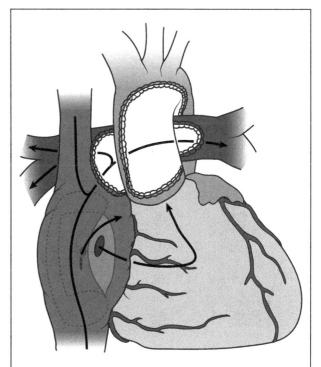

FIGURE 3.93 The completed Fontan procedure showing the systemic venous return from the superior and inferior venae cavae directed to the pulmonary artery.

5. *Total Anomalous Pulmonary Venous Return*

a. Anatomy

i. This defect occurs when all four pulmonary veins drain anomalously via a connection into the right side of the heart instead of the LA.

ii. Variations depend on the drainage site of pulmonary veins.

1) Supracardiac TAPVR. The common pulmonary venous pathway drains into the right SVC through the left vertical vein and the left innominate vein.

2) Intracardiac TAPVR. The common pulmonary venous sinus drains into the coronary sinus or the pulmonary veins enter the RA.

3) Infracardiac TAPVR. A descending vertical vein usually drains the venous confluence, penetrates the diaphragm, and connects with a vessel of the portal system.

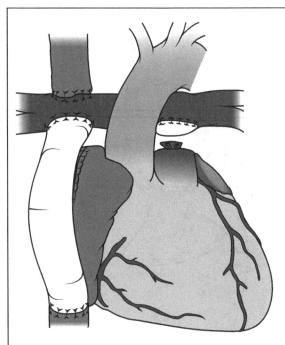

FIGURE 3.94 To create this total cavopulmonary connection, the surgeon combines a right-sided superior cavopulmonary anastomosis with the interposition of a polytetrafluoroethylene graft conduit between the divided inferior vena cava and the underside of the PA confluence. This results in a total extracardiac conduit type of cavopulmonary connection.

PA, pulmonary artery.

Note: Numbers refer to oxygen saturations.

4) Mixed type of TAPVR may also occur. There are two or more sites of anomalous pulmonary venous connections.

b. The incidence of TAPVR ranges from 0.6 to 1.2 per 10,000 live births (Park, 2016)

c. Pathophysiology

i. TAPVR may occur with or without pulmonary venous obstruction (obstructed vs. unobstructed).

ii. If the pulmonary veins are obstructed, blood cannot exit the lungs effectively, creating a critical situation of low CO from LV-volume underloading, severe pulmonary congestion from the obstruction, hypoxemia, and acidosis. Increased pulmonary venous pressure is transmitted to the pulmonary vascular bed, and reflex PA vasoconstriction occurs to prevent pulmonary edema. The result is decreased pulmonary blood flow, RA dilation, RVH, and RV failure (Fox et al., 2014).

iii. Even if the veins are not obstructed, the increased pulmonary flow creates medial hypertrophy and intimal hyperplasia, ending with PVOD by the third to fourth decade of life, if left untreated.

d. Clinical signs and symptoms

i. This is dependent on the degree of pulmonary venous obstruction. Children with obstructed veins have marked respiratory distress, cyanosis, dyspnea, tachycardia, tachypnea, RV heave, a systolic ejection click, increased S_1, a fixed and split S_2, low CO, and acidosis. If the pulmonary venous return is unobstructed, patients may have mild tachypnea, mild arterial desaturation, a widely split S_2, and possibly a pulmonic flow murmur or diastolic rumble.

e. Diagnostic evaluation

i. ECG indicates RA enlargement, RVH, and right axis deviation.

ii. Chest radiographic examination generally demonstrates a small heart with diffuse pulmonary edema if obstructed, or RA and RV dilation and increased pulmonary markings if unobstructed (Figure 3.95).

iii. Echo confirms the diagnosis and localizes the site of venous drainage. Pulmonary venous obstruction is quantified by Doppler. Associated lesions are defined; RV pressure and PA hypertension are noted; and PA, RA, and RV volume overload are noted.

f. Goals and medical patient management

i. In severely obstructed TAPVR, preoperative stabilization with intubation, hyperventilation, hyperoxygenation, and nitric oxide may be needed. ECMO support may be necessary to support CO in the most severe situations until surgical relief of obstruction can be performed.

g. Goals and surgical patient management

i. Repair of obstructed TAPVR is almost always a surgical emergency. Unobstructed veins are repaired early to prevent PVOD. Surgical repair is aimed at returning

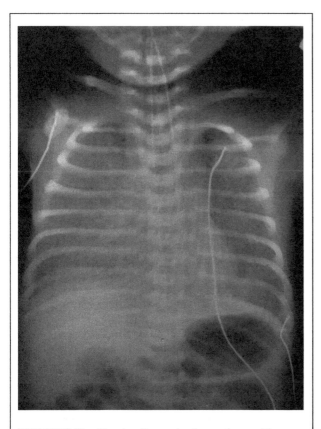

FIGURE 3.95 Chest radiograph of a newborn with obstructed total anomalous venous return below the diaphragm.

Courtesy of Michigan Medicine, University of Michigan.

of volume needed to maintain the BP and thereby decrease extracellular water, edema, and elevated LA/PA pressure (Latus et al., 2015).

h. Complications

i. Postoperative problems include pulmonary hypertensive crisis, SSS and other atrial arrhythmias, restenosis of the pulmonary vein anastomosis, and inability to relieve the stenosis fully.

ii. Long-term prognosis depends on the presence of diffuse pulmonary vein obstruction, the relief of all existing stenosis, any associated cardiac lesions, and the state of the pulmonary vascular bed. About 10% of patients with repaired TAPVR have a second obstruction usually associated with intracardiac or mixed types of veins. Use of sildenafil for treatment of PA hypertension has proven successful over the long term (Ivy et al., 2013).

F. Great Vessel Lesions

1. *D-Transposition of the Great Arteries (D-TGA)*

a. Definition

i. Transposition of the great arteries (TGA) is a ventriculoarterial (VA) discordance in which the morphologic LV gives rise to the PA and the morphologic RV gives rise to the aorta, creating parallel circulations (Figure 3.96). D-looping in utero was incomplete, leaving the aorta and PA malposed (Hermsen & Chen, 2015).

b. Incidence

i. Although the cause is largely unknown, TGA may be due to a left shift in the pulmonary conus. It is more common in boys of normal birth weight and size. TGA is the most common form of cyanotic CHD to present in the newborn period.

ii. TGA accounts for 5% to 7% of CHD (Park, 2016).

c. Pathophysiology

i. "Simple" TGA is associated with ASD, VSD, and PDA 80% of the time. Parallel circulation exists in that the systemic venous blood enters the right side of the heart normally, but exits through the aorta sending deoxygenated blood back to the body

pulmonary vein flow to the left side of the heart, eliminating obstruction, closing the ASD, and preventing PVOD. Repair is done via sternotomy on CPB using deep hypothermic circulatory arrest. The pulmonary vein confluence is anastomosed to the posterior wall of the LA, or the veins are directed through the ASD by an intra-atrial patch, thereby redirecting pulmonary venous return correctly and closing the ASD. In the immediate postsurgical phase, hyperventilation, nitric oxide, and, in some cases, ECMO may be required postoperatively for pulmonary stabilization. LV compliance is poor, and the LA cannot easily dilate. Slow volume infusion prevents further increase and transmission of elevated pressure to the lungs. Use of inotropic agents may decrease the amount

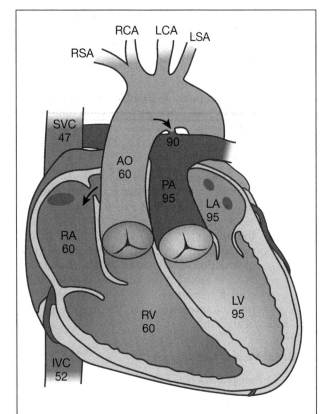

FIGURE 3.96 Transposition of the great arteries. Oxygen saturations in the cardiac chambers and great vessels are depicted with some shunting (mixing) of blood at the atrial level and through a patent ductus arteriosus.

AO, aorta; LA, left atrium; LCA, left carotid artery; LSA, left subclavian artery; LV, left ventricle; PA, pulmonary artery; RA, right atrium; RCA, right carotid artery; RSA, right subclavian artery; RV, right ventricle; SVC, superior vena cava.

Note: Numbers refer to oxygen saturations.

instead of the lungs. Pulmonary venous blood enters the left side of the heart normally, but exits through the PA sending oxygenated blood to the lungs instead of the body. The child requires intracardiac mixing to oxygenated systemic blood to survive. The degree of cyanosis or acidosis depends on the number, location, and size of intracardiac and extracardiac shunts (ASD, VSD, and PDA). Mixing of blood allows systemic saturation of 75% to 90%. LV pressure is maintained at systemic levels for the first 1 to 2 weeks of life. After that, PVR and LV pressure fall. Early

development of PVOD in infants with TGA has been found and is an indication for early repair. PVOD is more common if a VSD is present. PVOD can develop as early as 2 weeks of age and occurs in most patients with unrepaired TGA by 1 year of age (Mavroudis, 2013b).

d. Clinical signs and symptoms

   i. Clinical presentation depends on the degree of shunting. Cyanosis within 24 hours of birth is the most common presentation. If a large VSD is present, the infant may present at 2 weeks of age with CHF.

   ii. Examination reveals cyanosis if there is an intact septum; hepatomegaly, tachycardia, or tachypnea if VSD is present. Patients with severe cyanosis develop clubbing after 6 months. TGA without a VSD reveals a normal S_1, single S_2, continuous murmur of the PDA, and an occasional systolic ejection murmur on auscultation. For TGA with a VSD, auscultation reveals a normal S_1, single S_2, and soft systolic ejection murmur at the LSB.

e. Diagnostic evaluation

   i. ECG shows right-axis deviation, RVH, or biventricular hypertrophy, or findings may be normal for age. In the presence of a VSD, the ECG shows biventricular hypertrophy and a normal QRS axis.

   ii. Chest radiographic examination demonstrates an oval-shaped "egg on a string" silhouette, narrow superior mediastinum, and moderate cardiomegaly that may be normal for age. With a VSD, the chest radiographic examination demonstrates moderate cardiomegaly, a narrow superior mediastinum, and increased pulmonary vascular markings.

   iii. Echo plays a dominant role in diagnosis by establishing major anatomic features and anatomic variants, but it might not define the coronary anatomy.

   iv. Cardiac catheterization may be indicated for balloon atrial septostomy to promote better intra-cardiac mixing prior to complete repair. Findings demonstrate increased saturation with shunting, LV outflow obstruction, and slight increases in atrial pressure. May be indicated to better define coronary anatomy when echo is not sufficient.

f. Goals and medical patient management

i. Medical stabilization with prostaglandin therapy is necessary if atrial communication is not sufficient to provide mixing and oxygenation. Medications to treat CHF may be indicated while awaiting operation if a large VSD is present. Balloon atrial septostomy is indicated if atrial level mixing is restrictive and saturations inadequate. The procedure may be performed at bedside with US guidance or in the catheterization lab.

g. Goals and surgical patient management (Mavroudis, 2013b)

i. Repair via arterial switch (described here) should be performed before the fall of LV pressure and mass regression because the LV will have to handle the systemic pressure load. The LV will become deconditioned over time and then will be unable to handle a normal pressure load.

ii. Timing of repair of transposition with VSD is somewhat elective but operation by 2 weeks of age is preferred to avoid CHF and early development of PVOD. In complex VSD and small patients, a PA band may be used until the infant is older.

iii. Interventional catheterization is used if the ASD is restrictive or surgery is delayed. Balloon septostomy via catheterization tears the atrial septum. Blalock–Hanlon operation or atrial septectomy via sternotomy on bypass is used to excise the atrial septum surgically, to improve mixing and saturation, and to reduce acidosis.

iv. Surgical intervention depends on age at presentation, LV pressures, and associated lesions.

1) Arterial switch operation (Figure 3.97) provides anatomic correction involving transection of both great vessels via median sternotomy using CPB. The pulmonary valve becomes the aortic valve with anastomosis of the distal aorta to the proximal PA and closure of associated shunts. Coronary arteries with a button of PA tissue are transferred to the new aortic root. Criteria for an arterial switch include timing of repair and no fixed PS, which would become AS after the switch. This procedure leaves the LV and mitral valve on the systemic side and avoids a complex intra-atrial baffle, which decreases the risk of significant atrial arrhythmias. Early postoperative problems center on LV dysfunction, low CO, and myocardial ischemia or infarction from kinking or distorting of the coronary arteries during transfer. A common residual defect is the development of supravalvular PS.

2) The Mustard operation or the Senning operation (venous switch) redirects venous inflow via intra-atrial baffling, draining the pulmonary veins via the tricuspid valve to the RV to the aorta and the systemic veins, and draining via the mitral valve to the LV and to the PA. The procedure includes closure of the ASD, VSD, and PDA if present. The RV and tricuspid valves are established as the systemic ventricle and AV valve. Complications include early and late atrial arrhythmias, late RV dysfunction and TR, venous baffle obstruction, and late development of PVOD. This procedure is uncommon. It was utilized before the mid-1980s as the standard surgical treatment for TGA. An arterial switch operation is now the preferred treatment.

v. Late diagnosis of transposition with IVS may require conditioning of the LV. One approach is PA band and placement of a systemic-to-pulmonary shunt. The shunt overloads the LV with volume and pressure to prepare it to accept systemic pressure workloads following an arterial switch operation. The exact length of time from palliation to arterial switch is still not clear, but repair has been done as soon as 2 weeks after palliation measures. Indicators of RV preparation are LV/RV pressure ratio greater than 70%, LV volume/mass normal for age, and LV-wall thickness normal for age.

1) Complex TGA includes TGA with VSD and PS. Palliation with a systemic-to-pulmonary shunt occurs in the neonatal period. Correction is completed in 6 months to 1 year with the Rastelli operation, which reestablishes LV–aortic continuity (Figure 3.98). The VSD is patched to direct LV flow to the aortic valve, and RV–PA continuity is established with an RV–PA conduit. The size of the VSD and

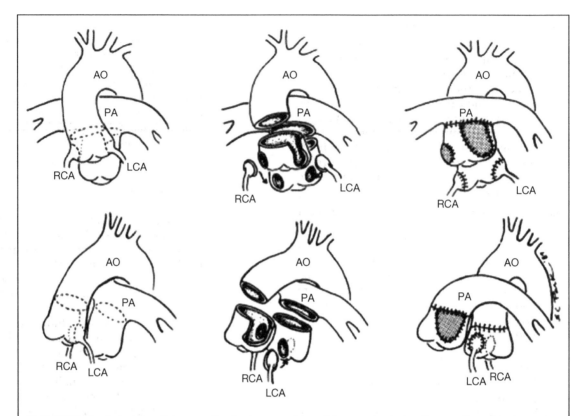

FIGURE 3.97 Arterial switch operation for transposition of the great arteries. Transection of both great vessels followed by anastomosis to the anatomically correct ventricles with coronary transfer.

AO, aorta; LCA, left coronary artery; PA, pulmonary artery ; RCA, right coronary artery.

Source: Reprinted with permission from Kambam, J. (1994). Atrial septal defect. In J. Kambam (Ed.), *Cardiac anesthesia for infants and children*. St. Louis, MO: Mosby.

location to the semilunar valves determine the degree of surgical difficulty. If the VSD is small and enlargement is necessary, the risk of postoperative CHB increases.

h. Complications include endocarditis, risk of cyanosis, CHF, and PVOD. Postoperative complications with the Rastelli operation include arrhythmia, VSD patch dehiscence or residual VSD, aortic obstruction, residual PS, tricuspid insufficiency, and myocardial dysfunction. Endocarditis is a lifelong risk.

2. *L-Transposition of the Great Arteries (L-TGA)*

a. Definition. Levo- or L-looped transposition of the great arteries (L-TGA) is a rare form of CHD characterized by AV and VA discordance.

b. Incidence. This is a rare CHD, occurring in less than 1% of congenital heart lesions (Devaney & Bove, 2013; Mavroudis, 2013b).

c. Pathophysiology. Without additional defects, normal physiologic return of deoxygenated systemic venous blood to the heart and transport of oxygenated pulmonary venous return to the systemic circulation through the discordant ventricles and great arteries is present. Systemic ventricular failure (i.e., systemic HF) is a common late complication in L-TGA patients because the morphological RV is unable to sustain systemic circulation over a life span secondary to an unfavorable tripartite geometric configuration that does not adapt to pressure or volume overload and progressive TR that increases volume overload and contributes to ventricular dysfunction and failure (Figure 3.99).

d. Clinical signs and symptoms. These patients are often asymptomatic unless there are additional cardiac anomalies. Patients with L-TGA are at increased risk for heart block and HF as

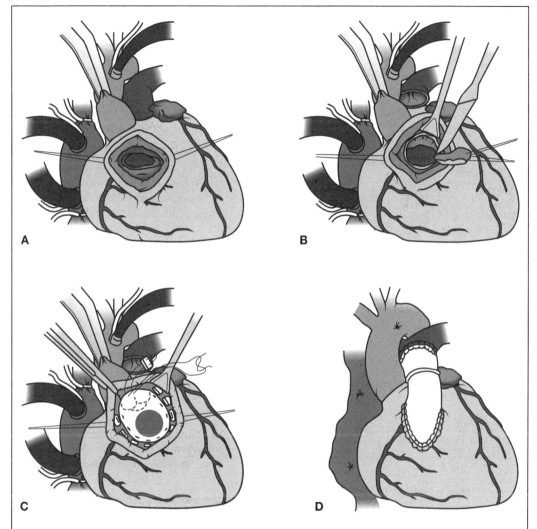

FIGURE 3.98 Stages of the Rastelli operation. (A) In a Rastelli operation, the surgeon performs a right ventricular incision, paying particular attention to not damage the tricuspid valve attachments, ventricular septal defect anatomy, coronary artery distribution, and intended position of the conduit in order to prevent complications. (B) BY performing a comprehensive infundibular resection, the surgeon maximizes left ventricular-to-aortic continuity. (C) Using a large patch, the surgeon closes the ventricular septal defect, which creates a tunnel to the aorta. The surgeon then determines the most appropriate site to open a distal pulmonary atresia in order to ensure distal conduit anastomosis. (D) As shown, following the separation from cardiopulmonary bypass, the valved conduit is securely positioned.

adults due to progressive decline in systemic right ventricular function.

e. Diagnostic evaluation

i. Electrocardiography may show varying degrees of AV block and this is more common than the occasional atrial arrhythmia or WPW. RVH may be present as it is now the systemic pumping chamber. The absence of Q waves in I, V_5, and V_6 or the presence of Q waves in V4r or V_1 is characteristic because of reversed depolarization from LV to RV.

ii. Chest radiography shows a narrow, straight upper mediastinal border due to placement of great vessels. If a VSD is

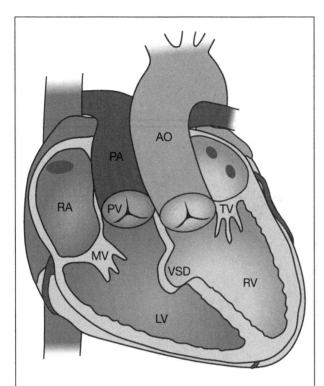

FIGURE 3.99 Congenitally corrected transposition of the great arteries with VSD.

AO, aorta; LV, left ventricle; MV, main ventricle; PA, pulmonary artery; PV, pulmonary ventricle; RA, right atrium; RV, right ventricle; VSD, ventricular septal defect.

present, then increased pulmonary vascular markings and cardiomegaly may be present. If there is AV valve regurgitation, atrial enlargement can be seen.

iii. Echo confirms the diagnosis in the majority of the cases. The AV valves, their relationship to RV or LV, ventricular morphology, and semilunar and great vessel attachments can be well delineated. Associated defects, including arch abnormalities, anatomic location of the VSD, right or left outflow tract obstruction, or AV valve abnormalities, are well seen. The situs of the atria is confirmed.

iv. Cardiac catheterization is rarely necessary but can be used in complex anatomical situations or for hemodynamic data prior to corrective surgery.

f. Goals and medical patient management

i. Requires close monitoring for congenital CHB or development of conduction disorders

as they grow. Placement of a permanent pacemaker may be required to maintain CO and preserve ventricular function. The presence of or development of AV regurgitation and ventricular dysfunction is followed closely either preoperatively or following intervention. Management of HF or treatment with afterload reduction for worsening AV valve regurgitation may be necessary.

g. Goals and surgical patient management

i. Associated lesions determine the timing of surgical intervention and projected readiness of LV if a double switch operation is planned. If the patient has associated PS, placement of an early systemic to pulmonary shunt may be required.

ii. Anatomic repair. Type of surgical repair depends on the presence of a VSD and/or PS: Double Switch—Senning with arterial switch operation—or a Senning Rastelli. May require serial PA banding to train LV (Figure 3.100; Murtuza et al., 2011).

iii. Conventional repair. The focus is on palliative interventions to address associated lesions, such as placement of PA bands for a large VSD or interventions to improve PS or AV valve insufficiency (Devaney & Bove, 2013).

h. Complications. Heart block, atrial arrhythmias, low CO, LV/RV systolic/diastolic dysfunction, and endocarditis remains a lifelong risk.

G. Single Ventricle Physiology

1. *Hypoplastic Left Heart Syndrome*

a. Anatomy

i. CHD characterized by various levels of underdevelopment of left heart structures. The left-sided valves may be small or atretic, the LV cavity nonexistent or hypoplastic, and the ascending aorta miniscule to well formed. In all cases of HLHS, the left-sided heart structures fail to form normally and are not large enough to function as systemic ventricles and valves.

b. Incidence

i. HLHS occurs in 1% of CHD cases or in 0.163/1,000 live births. Research suggests an autosomal-recessive transmission. Recurrence risk in siblings is 0.5%; HLHS is more common in boys, and 10% of infants with HLHS have associated extracardiac malformations (Park, 2016).

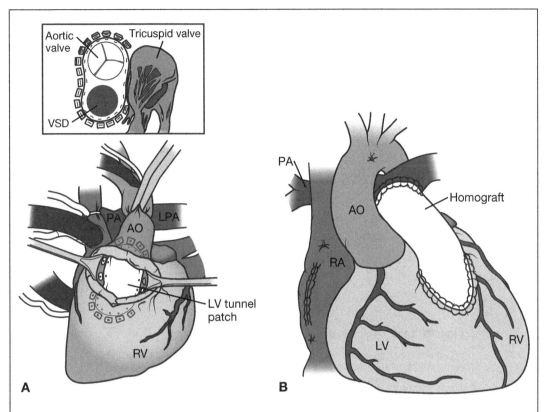

FIGURE 3.100 The Rastelli procedure in anatomic correction of CCTGA.

AO, aorta; CCTGA, congenitally corrected transposition of the great arteries; LPA, left pulmonary artery; LV, left ventricle; PA, pulmonary artery; RA, right atrium; RV, right ventricle.

c. Pathophysiology

i. Right-sided structures, the PA, coronary arteries, and lungs are normal, although the RA, RV, and PA may be dilated. Left-sided structures have variable levels of underdevelopment. Mitral valve atresia or stenosis occurs frequently. Aortic atresia or stenosis (annulus ≤5 mm) occurs. Stenotic valves have a small aortic root with leaflets that are thick, dysplastic, and obstructive. LV hypoplasia occurs in varying degrees (volume <20 mL/m²). There is a non–apex-forming LV (Figure 3.101). The endocardium may be thick or sclerotic. The ascending aorta varies in size but is hypoplastic, usually to the level of the transverse arch (usually 2–3 mm). Coarctation is present in 80% of patients (Feinstein et al., 2012).

ii. Associated lesions are not common with classic HLHS, but may include AVSD, TGV, and univentricular heart. A PDA and ASD are obligatory for survival and are considered part of the complex. On occasion, the ASD is small or restrictive and the newborn presents with obstructed TAPVR, which is associated with increased mortality.

iii. Systemic venous blood returns normally to the RA and flows normally out the right side of the heart. Pulmonary venous blood flows across the ASD to the RA because it cannot exit the left side of the heart if mitral atresia is present. Mixing in the RA desaturates the blood. All blood flows across the tricuspid valve to the RV and to the PA. If mitral or AS is present, a small amount of forward flow out the LV may occur but not enough to support the CO. Blood flows right to left across the PDA to supply systemic blood flow distally and flows proximally to feed the coronary arteries.

d. Clinical signs and symptoms

i. Clinical presentation. Cyanosis is rare at birth; however, as normal involution of the

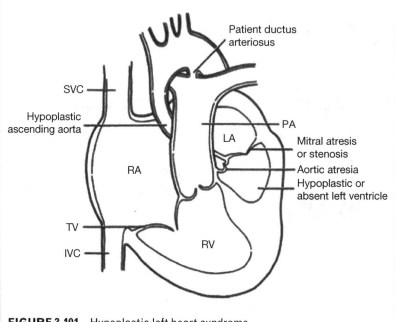

FIGURE 3.101 Hypoplastic left heart syndrome.

IVC, inferior vena cava; LA, left atrium; PA, pulmonary artery; RA, right atrium; RV, right ventricle; SVC, superior vena cava; TV, tricuspid valve.

Source: Reprinted with permission from Callow, L. B. (1992). Current strategies in the nursing care of infants with hypoplastic left-heart syndrome undergoing first-stage palliation with the Norwood operation. *Heart & Lung 20*, 463–470.

PDA occurs, systemic perfusion is compromised. Symptoms of CHF become evident and, if unrecognized, will progress to vascular collapse. Tachypnea, dyspnea, grunting, cool and poorly perfused extremities, lethargy, and pallor or gray color will be noted.

ii. Examination reveals auscultation of crisp, loud heart sounds; a single S_2; a pulmonary ejection click and an S_3; an enlarged liver; a left precordial bulge; a soft systolic ejection murmur; and variable femoral pulses. There may be no gradient with low CO or an open PDA.

e. Diagnostic evaluation

i. ECG demonstrates sinus tachycardia, peaked waves, RA enlargement, RVH, and lack of LV forces and may show ST–T wave changes.

ii. Chest radiographic examination: Levocardia, an enlarged, globular-shaped heart, and variable pulmonary vascular markings (severe pulmonary edema and increased markings if ASD is restrictive) are present.

iii. Echo is a valuable diagnostic tool that defines all anatomic variants of HLHS. Findings include an enlarged RV and PA, mitral valve leaflets are not visualized, the LV cavity is hypoplastic, the LV is nonapex forming, the aortic root is 5 mm or smaller, and hypoplasia of the aortic arch is present. Anatomy and function of the tricuspid valve are evaluated.

iv. Cardiac catheterization is not required initially unless there is an extreme anatomic variant. It will demonstrate an obligatory left-to-right atrial shunt with increased oxygen saturation in the RA, RV, and PA; aortic saturation equal to PA saturation; RV pressures elevated and equal to or in excess of systemic arterial pressure; PCWP and LA and RA pressures equal except in the presence of obstructive ASD, in which PCWP and LA pressure are greater than RA pressure.

f. Goals and medical patient management

i. Ductal patency is maintained while the diagnosis is confirmed and decisions are made for interventions. The typical approach is Norwood procedure with staged reconstruction. Another treatment option is cardiac transplantation, which requires maintenance with prostaglandin therapy until a donor is found. Compassionate care may be offered when there are multiple life-limiting associated noncardiac congenital anomalies or associated cardiac defects that preclude successful staged reconstruction (such as severely obstructed pulmonary veins or ASD) or transplantation. The expectation with compassionate care is death of the newborn will occur within 1 week of birth in 95% of the patients. With the improved outcomes seen with stage reconstruction and the option of transplantation for those who qualify, compassionate care is rarely offered (Feinstein et al., 2012).

ii. Preoperative stabilization. Balance is maintained between systemic and pulmonary blood flow by manipulating SVR and PVR. If the patient is cyanotic with low pulmonary blood flow, interventions include ensuring patency of the ASD and PDA, hyperventilation, hyperoxygenation, and relief of pulmonary congestion (DeMauro, Millar, & Kirpalani, 2014). Pulmonary vasoconstriction and systemic vasodilation are avoided to balance the two circulations, and the hematocrit is maintained at a level between 40 and 55 mL/dL. Conversely, pulmonary overcirculation can occur and result in poor CO (hypotension, acidosis) with good oxygenation (PaO$_2$ usually >45 mmHg). In this case, nitrogen administration with FiO$_2$ less than 21% can help to maintain mild metabolic acidosis (pH 7.35) and pulmonary vasoconstriction to reduce excessive pulmonary blood flow. CO and systemic circulation are maintained with medications to reduce SVR along with optimal circulating volume (Burkhardt, Rücker, & Stiller, 2015). Adequate organ function should be present prior to first surgical intervention (McElhinnery et al., 2000).

g. Goals and surgical patient management

i. First-stage palliative reconstructive surgery with the Norwood operation creates an unobstructed RV outflow tract to prevent ventricular hypertrophy and dysfunction and provide good coronary artery flow (Figure 3.102). Pulmonary blood flow is controlled to prevent PVOD via use of a systemic-to-pulmonary shunt to allow growth of the central main PA. A large ASD (atrial septectomy) is created to allow mixing of venous blood return at the atrial level and promote LA decompression and to avoid elevated PA pressure or PVR. The Norwood operation is aimed at maintaining anatomic and physiologic criteria for an eventual Fontan procedure. The Norwood operation is done via sternotomy with CPB. The aortic arch and RV outflow tract are reconstructed using the proximal PA, aorta, and homograft augmentation. Careful reconstruction of the proximal PA–aortic anastomosis is completed to avoid torsion and obstruction to coronary artery flow. Pulmonary blood flow is created by a systemic-to-pulmonary GORE-TEX shunt (Figure 3.103). Either a modified Blalock–Taussig shunt or an RV-to-PA conduit may be utilized to supply pulmonary blood flow. The Sano operation (RV–PA conduit) is believed to increase diastolic BP by eliminating runoff into the PA from the aorta. This would increase coronary artery perfusion and decrease the risk of ischemia to the ventricle. This is considered especially helpful in small or preterm infants and in those with exceptionally small ascending aortas. Manipulation of systemic and pulmonary resistance has questionable effect on pulmonary blood flow in these circumstances. Long-term concerns with this type of conduit include the long-term effects of a ventriculotomy on a single systemic ventricle and the incidence of sudden occlusion and growth of the central and peripheral PAs (Hornik et al., 2011; Slicker et al., 2013).

ii. Hybrid approach. This is an alternative to stage 1 palliation with the Norwood operation. The hybrid approach for HLHS is a combination of interventional cardiac catheterization (balloon atrial septostomy and placement of a PDA stent) and surgical interventions (placement of PA bands via sternotomy). This approach does not require CPB. This approach may be preferred for infants with HLHS presenting late with end-organ dysfunction, infants with contraindications for CPB, low-birth-weight or premature infants with HLHS, and HLHS patients with significant right ventricular dysfunction or a restrictive or intact atrial septum. These patients will need to be monitored postoperatively for signs of stent or PA band migration, stent stenosis, thrombosis, and systemic perfusion.

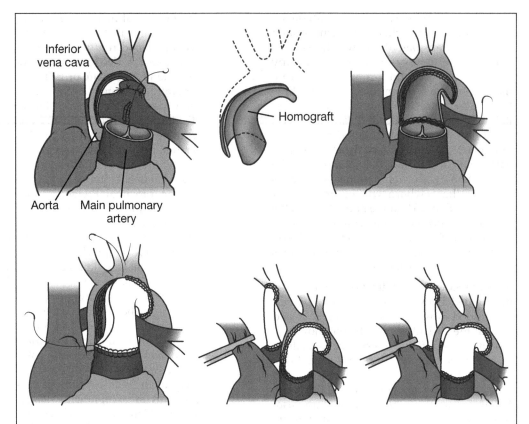

FIGURE 3.102 Surgical reconstruction in hypoplastic left heart syndrome. Using a homograft patch, the aorta is reconstructed and a systemic-to-pulmonary shunt provides pulmonary flow to the now transected pulmonary artery.

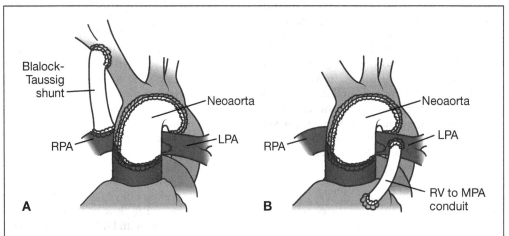

FIGURE 3.103 Stage I Norwood procedure with pulmonary blood flow provided by a modified right Blalock–Taussig shunt.

LPA, left pulmonary artery; MPA, main pulmonary artery; RPA, right pulmonary artery; RV, right ventricle.

1) Mechanical ventilation, anticoagulation, and vasoactive support are often required in the initial postoperative period. These patients will eventually require a comprehensive stage 1 palliation or Norwood procedure. Postoperative complications include an unbalanced flow between systemic and pulmonary circulations and/or severe cardiovascular collapse. The inability to maintain balanced circulation or preoperative obstructed atrial septum may require ECMO for cardiac or pulmonary healing (see section "Mechanical Cardiac Support"). In postoperative Norwood patients, the shunt may be occluded temporarily to permit adequate circulation on ECMO (Tabbutt et al., 2012). Problems with temporary and reversible elevated PVR and severe hypoxemia may be managed by inhalation of nitric oxide. Low CO may respond to reduction of inhaled oxygen to 21% or subatmospheric oxygen reducing pulmonary blood flow and increasing systemic blood flow. Desired oxygen saturations vary between 70% and 80%, depending on the patient's hemodynamic state. Measurement of SvO_2 and calculation of shunt fractions $(Q_p:Q_s)$ can assist in the manipulation of PVR or SVR. Coupling the SvO_2 with serum lactates provides early warning of inadequate CO and the need for treatment of PVR and SVR based on SvO_2 and shunt fractions (Ohye et al., 2012).

iii. Second-stage palliation with bidirectional cavopulmonary shunt or hemi-Fontan is generally performed 3 to 6 months after initial palliation. The purpose of the cavopulmonary shunt is to provide venous blood flow to the lungs and a stable form of oxygenation, remove volume overload from the RV, protect the RV from hypertrophy, and preserve long-term function. It is performed via sternotomy on CPB and may require hypothermic circulatory arrest. If necessary, PA stent or arterioplasty is performed to ensure unobstructed pulmonary blood flow to permit passive flow without excessively high SVC pressures. The pulmonary arteries are repaired as necessary. The SVC is connected end to side with the right or main PA, and flow goes passively from the SVC to the right and left pulmonary arteries by pressure gradient. Full hemodynamic and anatomic catheterization to assess the size and architecture of the pulmonary arteries, PA pressure, pulmonary blood flow, and RV function is commonly performed before cavopulmonary shunt is placed (Figures 3.104 and 3.105).

1) A bulging fontanel; high SVC pressure; irritability; low saturations; and edema of the face, neck, and upper extremities (SVC syndrome) are signs of high venous pressure. PVR is optimized; early heparin use with conversion to aspirin later may prevent thrombus in the low-flow cavopulmonary circuit. Any alteration in PVR will affect pulmonary blood flow because there is no ventricular pump to overcome this added resistance. These patients are prone to pleural effusions. Diuretics are used to reduce volume overload and improve pulmonary mechanics, and ventilatory support techniques are directed at promoting

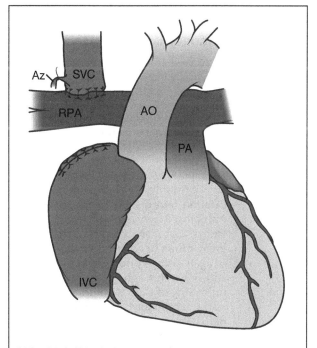

FIGURE 3.104 Bidirectional Glenn.

AO, aorta; Az, azygous vein; IVC, inferior vena cava; PA, pulmonary artery; RPA, right pulmonary artery; SVC, superior vena cava.

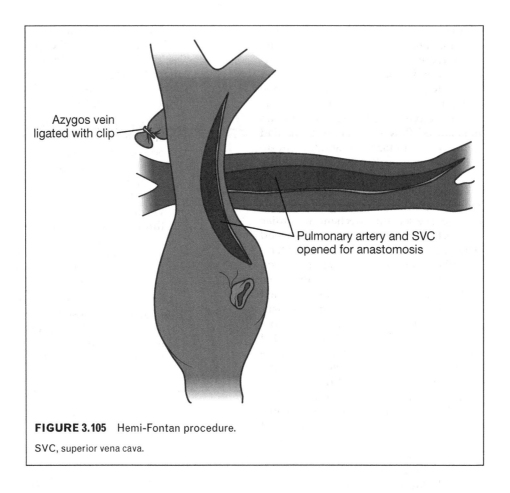

FIGURE 3.105 Hemi-Fontan procedure.

SVC, superior vena cava.

passive pulmonary blood flow. MAP is maintained in a lower range. Early extubation permits physiologic negative pressure ventilation and encourages passive flow to the pulmonary circuit (Mahle, 2016). Spontaneous respiration reduces MAP, also promoting pulmonary flow (DeMauro et al., 2014). Hematocrit should be maintained greater than or equal to 40% to optimize oxygen delivery to tissues. IVC blood still flows through the RV, so complete unloading of the RV volume overload is not accomplished by the second-stage palliation, and mixing of oxygenated and unoxygenated blood occurs with expected saturations of 80% to 85%.

iv. Final-stage physiologic palliation. Fontan procedure is also done for tricuspid atresia and other single-ventricle hearts of diagnostic categories other than HLHS. Recommended age is younger than or equal to 4 years at operation to prevent

ventricular hypertrophy and dysfunction from volume overload and to optimize long-term ventricular function. Full hemodynamic and anatomic catheterization is required before performance of a Fontan procedure to assess for suitability of hemodynamics. Criteria for adequate outcomes include good branch PA architecture without stenosis, normal PA pressure, PVR, and ventricular function. Relative criteria include competent AV valve and NSR. The operation is done via sternotomy on CPB, possibly with circulatory arrest. The lower systemic venous return, IVC, is directed to the PA. A lateral tunnel is sewn inside the RA directing IVC flow to the PA (Figure 3.93). An external IVC-PA conduit (Figure 3.94) is used for systemic or pulmonary venous anatomic aberrations prohibiting previous connections. Often a 3- to 4-mm fenestration is created between the Fontan conduit and the RA to allow a "pop-off" of blood flow to preserve systemic circulation in instances when the pulmonary pressure is transiently elevated. The goal of the Fontan is to achieve passive flow from the systemic veins to the lungs based on the pressure gradient from the SVC or IVC, to the main PA, to the left and right pulmonary arteries, and to the lungs. Relief of any PA stenosis via arterioplasty or stent placement, or both, is indicated to prevent a fixed elevation in PVR. Relief of significant AV valve regurgitation is necessary to prevent elevations in atrial pressure transmitted to the lungs (M. Jacobs, 2013).

h. Complications following Fontan operation

   i. Postoperative care may be complicated by ventricular dysfunction, arrhythmias, elevated PVR, and excessive cyanosis from a baffle leak. Observation of the RA–LA gradient may demonstrate a widening gradient with RA hypertension from increased PVR or a narrow gradient but high LA pressure that may signify LV dysfunction. Ideally, the RA pressure will be less than 15 mmHg, with transpulmonary gradient not greater than 10. Ventilation should be optimized with low MAP, and extubation should occur as early as possible (Miller et al., 2014). Late complications include thromboembolic events, rhythm disturbances, protein-losing enteropathy, aortopulmonary collaterals, pathway obstruction, AV valve regurgitation, and ventricular dysfunction. Neurologic outcomes are encouraging. Resting CO is normal, although at maximal exercise it may be limited. Atrial arrhythmias, primarily SSS and atrial fibrillation or flutter, can occur. Recurrent pleural effusions and hepatic congestion may develop. Long-term ventricular failure requires transplantation. Many Fontan procedures are fenestrated (controlled hole in intra-atrial baffle allowing right-to-left shunting when systemic venous pressures are excessively high). Fenestration in the Fontan procedure is believed to maintain CO and volume load in the ventricle and ease transition to passive flow. The right-to-left shunt and cyanosis continue until the fenestration is closed. If performed, fenestration closure is done weeks to months after the Fontan operation. Initially there is a decrease in CO despite normalization of oxygen saturation in patients with fenestration closure. Improved survival for the Fontan procedure can be related to younger age at operation, refined surgical technique and staging procedures,

and postoperative management. Complex single ventricles, heterotaxy, PA distortion, PAH, or long bypass times during Fontan increase morbidity and mortality (Monagle et al., 2011). Late complications include thromboembolic events, rhythm disturbances, protein-losing enteropathy, development of aortopulmonary collaterals, Fontan pathway obstruction, AV valve regurgitation, and ventricular dysfunction. Neurologic outcomes are encouraging. Resting CO is normal; however, at maximal exercise, it may be limited.

   ii. Endocarditis is a lifelong risk (Fredenburg, Johnson, & Cohen, 2011).

2. *Single Ventricular Variants*

   a. *Definition.* Single ventricular variants are complex cardiac defects that have only one functional ventricle. Examples of right-sided single-ventricle lesions include tricuspid atresia, double inlet LV, and PA. Examples of left-sided single ventricle lesions include HLHS, DORV, heterotaxy variants with PS or atresia.

   b. *Incidence.* Occurrence is rare; appears in five in 100,000 live births (Park, 2016)

   c. *Pathophysiology* is dependent on the constellation of defects. Single-ventricle lesions with increased pulmonary blood flow will be treated as tricuspid atresia with VSD. Patients with single-ventricle variants with decreased pulmonary blood flow will be treated as tricuspid atresia without VSD. Variants often include anomalies of the systemic or pulmonary veins and heterotaxy–asplenia–polysplenia syndromes.

   d. *Clinical signs and symptoms* will vary from CHF in patients with increased pulmonary blood flow to cyanosis in patients with decreased pulmonary blood flow. Associated defects, specifically TAPVR (generally obstructed), create a situation in which repair of the veins is mandatory prior to any further staged reconstruction. Variable degrees of AV valve regurgitation are also encountered and long-term outcomes are related to the degree of regurgitation and ability to repair the valve.

   e. *Diagnostic evaluation* may begin with routine antenatal screening. Postnatal evaluation often includes pulse oximetry, ECG, CXR, echo. Additional imaging with cardiac catheterization or MRI may be needed to fully delineate anatomy.

   f. *Goals and medical patient management* are variable, dependent on all associated cardiac lesions and clinical symptoms. Medications to manage HF or maintain ductal patency may be indicated. Medications and ventilation strategies used to balance systemic pulmonary blood flow and pulmonary blood flow may be required in patients with single-ventricle physiology and ductal-dependent pulmonary blood flow. Use of ECMO support for infants with obstructed total veins at birth may be required for stabilization prior to the operating room. Afterload reduction is required for treatment of patients with moderate to severe AV valve regurgitation.

g. *Goals and surgical patient management* are variable, dependent on the specific constellation of cardiac lesions. Initial surgical/interventional catheterization palliation in a neonate involves interventions to achieve unobstructed systemic blood flow, unrestrictive pulmonary venous return, and stable pulmonary blood flow (shunt, PA band). Complex single-ventricle lesions often result in staged palliation, with the final stage being a Fontan completion.

h. *Complications.* Nerve injury (diaphragmatic paresis or paralysis, vocal cord paresis or paralysis), bleeding, infection, seizures, renal dysfunction, and chylothorax may occur. Endocarditis will remain a lifelong risk (Morgan et al., 2013).

3. *Heterotaxy Syndromes*

a. These syndromes are defined as complex syndromes associated with abnormal arrangement of the thoracic–abdominal organs, often including a congenital heart defect. This may be either right atrial isomerism or left atrial isomerism. May also include conduction abnormalities, dextrocardia, pulmonary vein abnormalities, abnormalities of the spleen, biliary atresia, lung abnormalities, malrotation of the intestines.

b. Their incidence is rare, occurring in 1% of newborns with symptomatic CHD (Park, 2016).

c. The pathophysiology is variable, dependent on the constellation of cardiac lesions. These lesions may present as single ventricle variants with increased, balanced, or decreased pulmonary blood flow.

d. Clinical signs and symptoms are variable. Symptoms may appear at birth (cyanosis, respiratory distress, feeding difficulties, shock) for babies with restricted pulmonary flow, obstructed pulmonary veins, or severe AV valve regurgitation. Some will present at several weeks of age when the PVR falls and there is increased left-to-right shunting and CHF symptoms. Patients may also

be asymptomatic if pulmonary and systemic blood flow is adequately balanced to prevent excessive degrees of cyanosis or CHF.

e. Diagnostic evaluation may begin with routine antenatal screening. Postnatal evaluation often includes pulse oximetry, ECG, CXR, echo, and an abdominal US. Additional imaging with cardiac catheterization or MRI may be needed to adequately image the anatomy.

f. Goals and medical patient management are variable, dependent on cardiac lesions and clinical symptoms. Medications to manage HF or maintain ductal patency may be needed. Antibiotic prophylaxis for spleen abnormalities is generally indicated.

g. Goals and surgical patient management are variable, dependent on the type of cardiac lesions. Complex single-ventricle lesions often result in staged palliation, with the final stage being a Fontan operation.

h. Complications of interventions include nerve injury (diaphragmatic paresis or paralysis, vocal cord paresis or paralysis), bleeding, infection, seizures, renal dysfunction, and chylothorax. These infants are often asplenic and at increased risk of sepsis from encapsulated organisms (Pasternack, 2016). They will require antibiotic prophylaxis at least until 5 years of age and adjustment of their immunizations (Mery et al., 2014).

PEDIATRIC CARDIOMYOPATHY

A. Definition

1. *Pediatric cardiomyopathy (PCM) is a heterogeneous, progressive, chronic disease* of the myocardium associated with cardiac dysfunction and classified by phenotype.

2. *The incidence of PCM* is 1.13/100,000. The most common pediatric cardiomyopathies are dilated (50%) or hypertrophic (42%) CM with highest incidence in infants younger than 1 year of age. It occurs more often in girls, African Americans, and Hispanic children. It is the most common cause of OHT in children older than 1 year of age and the most common cause of HF in children younger than 1 year (Williams & Hammer, 2011).

a. Of these patients, 40% die or require OHT within 2 years of diagnosis.

b. Of these children, 33% have a primary or secondary CM of known etiology (Wilkinson et al., 2010).

3. *Primary myopathy* is a CM confined to the heart muscle and can be genetic, nongenetic, or acquired in origin. *Acquired myopathy* (28%) has multiple etiologies and is not confined to the heart only, but rather it is part of a larger systemic disease state. Myocarditis and other viral infections, cardiovascular conditions (CHD, Kawasaki, hypertension, previous OHT), immunologic disorders (HIV), toxin reactions (drug, alcohol, radiation), obesity or dietary deficiencies, connective tissue or autoimmune diseases, or endocrine diseases may be etiologies of an acquired myopathy (Lipshultz, Cochran, et al., 2013).

    a. Familial inherited *CM* (24%) is defined as a myopathy present in two or more family members (Williams & Hammer, 2011).

    b. Neuromuscular disorders can be associated with CM (22%) and the majority are associated with a genetic basis, including muscular dystrophies, congenital myopathies, metabolic myopathies, and ataxias (Williams & Hammer, 2011).

    c. Metabolic disorders (16%), including inborn errors of metabolism, mitochondrial abnormalities, Pompe disease, Barth syndrome, and fatty acid oxidation defects (carnitine deficiency), may result in CM (Williams & Hammer, 2011).

    d. Malformation syndromes associated with CM (10%) include minor and major physical abnormalities with distinctive facial features that have a primary genetic link, the most common of which is Noonan syndrome (Williams & Hammer, 2011).

    e. Idiopathic CM includes patients without a family history and no specific cause of heart damage that can be identified. Sixty-six percent of CMs are of unknown etiology (Williams & Hammer, 2011).

4. *The pediatric cardiomyopathy registry (PCMR)* was designed to study the epidemiology and clinical course of patients with CM younger than 18 years of age.

    a. Its goal is to promote development of evidence-based etiologic factors specific to prevention and treatment strategies for PCM and to define the incidence, outcome, and outcome predictors for each functional type of PCM.

    b. The retrospective arm (1995–2007) of the registry described clinical outcomes and predictors of disease (Wilkinson et al., 2010).

    c. The prospective arm is ongoing (2005–present) and is examining the effect of OHT on the clinical course of PCM, describes the long-term changes in functional status, examines the relationship to clinical events and outcomes of OHT, and investigates the relationship of blood and cardiac tissue sampling for the study of genetic and viral markers with clinical and functional outcomes (Wilkinson et al., 2010).

B. General Treatment Goals

1. *Symptomatic relief and improved quality of life* are the main treatment goals for any patient with PCM. Generally, these are achieved with medication administration for treatment/control of CHF symptoms (Hong, 2013).

2. *Genetic testing* is obtained, when possible, to better identify an etiology and specify treatment modalities associated with this etiology.

3. *Medical management* to reverse the remodeling process linked to progression of HF is initiated early in the diagnosis.

4. *Improving and maximizing the CO* and matching oxygen delivery to demand and consumption are the key goals in early and ongoing treatment (Schmaltz, 2015).

    a. Transfusion is used to maintain/optimize oxygen-carrying capacity and delivery to tissues.

    b. Decreasing oxygen demand/consumption is achieved through multiple strategies, including sedation and neuromuscular blockade, avoidance of fever and infection. Enteral feeding with a feeding tube to supplement caloric needs or the use of parenteral nutrition in patients with poor bowel perfusion may be needed.

    c. Mechanical ventilation can decrease the oxygen demand by removing the work of breathing, manage preload and systemic venous overload, and it can reduce the afterload to the LV. It is paramount to ventilate at the child's FRC in order to optimize preload, afterload, pulmonary resistance and pulmonary blood flow.

5. *Prevent Thrombus Formation*

    a. Anticoagulation is indicated for patients with severely decreased ventricular function due to the high risk for thrombus formation in the low-flow or low-CO state (Chen, Williams, Chan, & Mondal, 2013).

    b. Preventive anticoagulation is generally indicated for specific PCMs (restrictive and left ventricular noncompaction).

        i. Medications for anticoagulation may be administered by the oral or IV route.

ii. For patients who are acutely ill, compression stockings or compression leg devices may be useful.

6. *OHT* is the only treatment for any PCM progressing to end-stage HF that is not responding to medical therapy.

　　a. HF in a particular patient may require institution of MCS in the form of ECMO or a VAD in order to preserve end-organ function, prevent further development of pulmonary vascular disease and fluid overload, and optimize the patient's overall condition for heart transplantation (Zafar et al., 2015).

C. General Diagnostic Evaluation

1. All patients who present with a possible PCM need to have a thorough family history, detailed dysmorphology, medical evaluation for malformation syndromes, appropriate lab and histologic testing, echo, ECG and, CXR. The results of these tests will vary depending on the type of PCM the patient has. Further testing with cMRI, electrophysiology testing, or cardiac catheterization and/or endomyocardial biopsy will then be conducted depending on PCM classification and the need for further evaluation and data to guide treatment.

2. Signs or symptoms of HF may or may not be present. Murmurs are not always present and can limit the value of the physical exam as a diagnostic tool.

3. CXR may or may not demonstrate cardiomegaly or pulmonary edema.

4. ECG is helpful for arrhythmia detection, chamber enlargement, conduction abnormalities, voltage abnormalities, and the presence of Q waves or ST-T wave changes.

5. Laboratory tests are helpful based on the PCM subtype. A complete blood and platelet count is also warranted as are liver and renal function tests. In some PCM patients, a BNP/N-terminal BNP will reflect a state of worsening ventricular dilation, worsening ventricular function, and volume overload. It may help to differentiate heart disease from respiratory disease, especially when the patient presents to the emergency department. Improvement in serial BNP once a diagnosis is confirmed and treatment initiated suggests a positive response to treatment (Iacob et al., 2017; Şahin, Portakal, Karagöz, Hasçelik, & Özkutlu, 2010).

6. Echocardiography remains the most valuable noninvasive, diagnostic tool to the diagnosis and follow up of PCM. It demonstrates the cardiac anatomy and is able to rule out CHD as an etiology to HF symptoms. It can define the characteristics of a specific PCM such as ventricular function/wall mass/dilation and hypertrophy. It may demonstrate atrial enlargement, valve regurgitation, potential elevations in PAP, and abnormal ventricular relaxation and diastolic function. The cMRI/MRA can visualize LV segments with more accuracy and predict the degree of associated LVH. Both echo and cMRI/MRA can classify, diagnose, and determine the degree of myocardial dysfunction.

D. Dilated Cardiomyopathy

1. *Etiology and Pathophysiology*

　　a. Dilated cardiomyopathy (DCM) is primarily the result of genetic abnormalities in the cardiac myocyte and has multiple identified pathways, including autosomal-dominant, X-linked, autosomal-recessive, and mitochondrial inheritance in 30% to 40% of cases. More than 30 genes have been associated with the DCM phenotype. There is a familial basis in 20% to 34% of patients with DCM. Mutations of genes result in DCM by altering the sarcolemma to sarcomere cytoskeleton within the myocyte. DCM may result from viral myocarditis due to damage to these same protein structures. DCM can also occur as a result of ischemic damage as seen in anomalous LCA, metabolic disorders such a hemochromatosis, carnitine deficiency, or glycogen-storage diseases, and drug toxicity (Kantor, Abraham, Dipchand, Benson, & Redington, 2010).

　　b. It is the most common form of PCM representing approximately 52% of patients with PCM. Forty percent of these patients will fail medical therapy within 2 years of diagnosis. Fifty percent of them will die or require OHT within 5 years of diagnosis. DCM is the leading cause of OHT in children younger than 1 year of age (Harmon et al., 2009).

2. *Phenotypic Expression*

　　a. Classically, DCM is defined as ventricular chamber enlargement and dilation without increasing wall thickening in response to this dilation (Figure 3.106).

　　b. This ventricular dilation will result in progressive systolic ventricular dysfunction.

　　c. These patients present with worsening and often severe symptoms of CHF.

　　d. The highest risk patient groups are children older than 5 years of age at diagnosis, those who present with decompensated HF, those

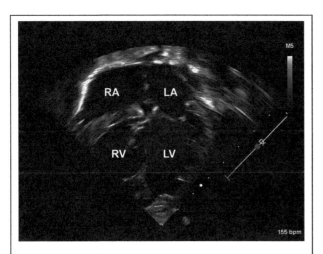

FIGURE 3.106 Dilated cardiomyopathy.

LA, left atrium; RA, right atrium; LV, left ventricle; RV, right ventricle.

Courtesy of CS Mott Children's Hospital, University of Michigan, Congenital Heart Center.

with a lower left ventricular shortening fraction (LVSF) and/or higher LV end-diastolic dimension at diagnosis, those who have moderate to severe MR, patients with PAH, a decreased ejection fraction, or an increased creatinine/serum sodium at diagnosis (Williams & Hammer, 2011).

e. The 1- and 5-year risk of death or OHT in patients with dilated CM is 39% to 53%, the 5-year risk of SCD is 3%. ICD placement for DCM patients is only indicated in patients who develop arrhythmias within 1 month of diagnosis, have moderate or greater MR, have a diminished left ventricular: left ventricular end-diastolic dimension ratio, or have experienced previous aborted SCD. Isolated LV dysfunction is not an indication for ICD placement (Lipshultz, Cochran, et al., 2013; Pahl et al., 2012).

f. DCM patients with poor weight gain (FTT), low body mass index (BMI), and short stature have an increased risk of death (Williams & Hammer, 2011).

g. Better outcomes are associated with higher LVSF at presentation and improvement in the LVSF within 6 months of diagnosis and treatment (Alvarez et al., 2011).

h. Prognosis is dependent on the age at diagnosis and the HF status. Death is secondary to progressive CHF and SCD is rare.

3. *Diagnostic Evaluation*

a. Endomyocardial biopsy and viral serology testing for potential myocarditis are important to define the etiology and guide the therapy for DCM.

b. Clinical symptoms reflect the variable degrees of HF. Tachycardia, tachypnea, increased work of breathing, loss of appetite or poor weight gain, abdominal pain, and exercise intolerance are seen.

c. Physical examination is consistent with the HF symptoms previously described. Pulmonary and or peripheral edema, cool extremities, decreased peripheral pulses, and JVD may also be present depending on the degree of HF and the age of the patient. A murmur of MR may be present as may an S_3 or S_4 gallop.

d. Elevated N-terminal BNP/BNP measurements are associated with cardiac symptoms and are indices of LV dysfunction. These laboratory values are helpful at diagnosis and to guide response to therapy or need for further escalation of treatment (Iacob et al., 2017).

e. Lymphocytopenia, low serum sodium, and higher serum creatinine are markers for the degree of end-organ compromise.

f. ECG demonstrates nonspecific changes, including increased LV forces, flat/inverted T waves, atrial enlargement, and tachycardia.

g. cMRI can assist with confirmation of diagnosis especially if there is consideration of acute myocarditis. cMRI will demonstrate the focal-wall motion abnormalities and delayed enhancement of the dilated ventricle.

h. Cardiac catheterization can evaluate for coronary artery anomalies as an etiology, which could then guide therapy. Hemodynamic data regarding LVEDP and PAP/PVR will help with decision making regarding therapy options.

i. Echo is primarily used for diagnosis and/or follow-up disease progression or regression and can also define underlying anatomic causes of PCM, including outflow tract obstruction, coarctation, primary valvular disease, and coronary artery anomalies. Echo is also used to guide decision making and treatment monitoring. In patients with an EF of less than 20%, evaluation for thrombi or consideration of systemic anticoagulation may be considered.

4. *Goals and Patient Management*

a. Treatment is based on symptoms and the degree of HF at presentation and throughout the course of the disease. Treatment is guided by standardized HF guidelines with escalation of support as needed for patient stabilization. First-line therapy with diuretics and ACE inhibitors will decrease preload and ventricular dilation and will assist with remodeling of the ventricle and afterload reduction. In general, all patients, even those without symptomatic HF, are placed on ACE inhibitors once the diagnosis of DCM is confirmed. ARBs are utilized in patients who are unable to tolerate the side effects of ACE inhibitors. β-Blockers have unknown effectiveness in the pediatric population but are generally utilized in patients with refractory HF symptoms. Aldosterone inhibitors are added for patients with worsening symptoms to block the effects of the renin–angiotensin–aldosterone complex and decrease fluid retention. Digoxin has shown no benefit in patient mortality but has provided symptomatic relief and is utilized based on specific patient symptoms and the rhythm status. It is not recommended for those patients with asymptomatic HF. Anticoagulation with lovenox, aspirin, or warfarin as indicated by the patient's LVSF, thromboembolic history, or echo findings may be necessary. Placement of an ICD is recommended in patients with LV dilation to any z-score greater than 2.6, patients with an arrhythmia history, and those with a diminished thinning of the left ventricular wall in relation to significant ventricular dilation.

b. In patients with decompensated HF, use of vasoactive and inotropic medications, mechanical, and consideration for initiation of MCS is warranted. OHT should be considered as soon as symptoms become refractory or imaging/blood tests indicate worsening of LVSF and LV dilation. Timing of listing for transplant is key to optimize patient outcome and is primarily symptom driven (Mahle, 2015).

c. Progression of DCM associated with worsening of CHF symptoms despite treatment, evidence by echo of increased MR, increasing left ventricular end-diastolic diameter (LVEDD), or decreasing LV systolic function with progression to diastolic dysfunction signal the need to move to more aggressive treatment or listing for OHT (Molina et al., 2013).

5. *Complications* include severe and progressive HF with evidence of respiratory compromise, renal insufficiency, and edema with ascites; thromboembolic events; FTT; arrhythmia development; and SCD.

E. Hypertrophic Cardiomyopathy

1. *Etiology and Pathophysiology*

   a. Hypertrophic cardiomyopathy (HCM) is primarily an autosomal–dominant transmission

(60% of cases; Maron & Olivotto, 2015). All mapped genes encode proteins as part of the sarcomere and are involved in energy production within the cardiac myocyte. There may be a family history of sudden death or HCM. HCM is associated with specific chromosomal syndromes such as Noonan syndrome.

b. HCM is the most common cause of SCD in people younger than 35 years of age, including athletes. It is the second most common PCM occurring in approximately 42% of patients with PCM (Williams & Hammer, 2011).

c. SCD is a common presenting symptom. Thirty-six percent of all pediatric SCD is related to HCM (Bharucha et al., 2015).

   i. The risk of SCD is low in children younger than 1 year of age and rises to peak at 16 years of age, likely related to hormonal shifts of adolescents, then the risk decreases after puberty (Lipshultz, Orav, et al., 2013).

   ii. Besides age, the patients at highest risk for SCD are those with an excessive degree of LV posterior wall thickness, a decreased LVSF, extreme LVOTO, nonsustained VT, and/or syncope.

d. Outcome varies with the etiology of HCM and the age at diagnosis. The prognosis is worse if the child is younger than 1 year of age at diagnosis or when the diagnosis is associated with an inborn error of metabolism or malformation syndromes. The more histologic disarray in the cardiac biopsy, the higher the mortality, development of ventricular arrhythmia, and ischemia at a younger age (Colan, 2015).

e. The 5-year survival for patients with HCM is 82% if diagnosed when younger than 1 year of age and 94% if diagnosed when older than 1 year of age (Colan, 2015).

f. HCM has the most favorable prognosis of all PCM with appropriate treatment and follow up (Lipshultz, Orav, et al., 2013).

g. The highest risk patients are those with two or more risk factors at presentation inclusive of CHF, FTT, or a mixed phenotypic expression (Lipshultz, Orav, et al., 2013).

h. Multiple risk factors at diagnosis are predictive of progression to OHT or death. Progression of HCM indicated by echo or cMRI includes findings of worsening diastolic dysfunction, thickening of the LV cavity with increasing LVOTO, development of MR or PAH, and development of arrhythmia noted in follow-up cardiac monitoring. Prognosis is dependent on the degree of LOVTO, etiology of the HCM, and the age at presentation. Children younger than 1 year of age have the worse outcome and those older than 1 year of age have survival that is independent of age.

2. *Phenotypic Expression*

   a. HCM (Figure 3.107) is the unexplained development of asymmetric ventricular hypertrophy, usually of the septal wall, with excess regional or global wall thickness and a progressive increase in the thickness of the left ventricular posterior wall (LVPW). There is no dilation of the ventricle associated with the hypertrophy. There is abnormal movement of the mitral valve related to the septal hypertrophy (Maron & Olivotto, 2015).

   b. HCM can present with either obstructive or nonobstructive physiology. Presentation is based on the degree of LVOTO and diastolic dysfunction.

   i. Near obliteration of the LVOT during systole may occur in patients with severe obstructive physiology and LVPW thickness. This abrupt decrease in CO predisposes patients to symptoms of chest pain, pulmonary congestion, dyspnea on exertion, palpitations, arrhythmia, syncope/presyncope, abdominal pain, increased work of breathing, and cough (Maron & Olivotto, 2015).

   c. In HCM, there is preserved or possibly hyperdynamic systolic function.

3. *Diagnostic Evaluation*

   a. Metabolic blood and urine testing can assist with the definition of a causal diagnosis and help to guide therapy.

   b. ECG abnormalities are present in 75% to 95% of patients. These include LVH with or without strain and an abnormal QRS axis with the presence of a Q wave.

   c. Echo demonstrates asymmetric hypertrophy with preserved systolic function and volume, decreased diastolic function, and systolic anterior motion of the MV in about 20% of patients. It delineates the degree of LVOTO by gradient and LV wall collapse in systole. In addition, echo is the best tool for following progression of HCM.

   d. cMRI is useful for diagnosis of the degree of fibrosis and LV hypertrophy.

   e. Cardiac catheterization demonstrates an increase in the intraventricular gradient with the Valsalva maneuver.

   f. Physical examination shows a laterally displaced and forceful LV impulse, a loud S_3/S_4, and an systolic ejection murmur at the right upper sternal border. SCD is common as a presenting symptom. Because of this risk factor, any patient, specifically anyone who is young and/or athletic who is experiencing an aborted SCD should be evaluated for HCM and be considered for ICD placement (Gersh et al., 2011).

4. *Goals and Patient Management*

   a. All patients with HCM are encouraged to modify their lifestyle and avoid athletic activities.

   b. Treatment is dependent on the physiology: obstructive versus nonobstructive.

   c. Generally, all patients regardless of physiology will be placed on a lipophilic β-blocker. This medication relieves symptoms with or without improved exercise capacity. In asymptomatic patients, there is some evidence that the use of β-blockers may improve survival and decrease the risk of SCD. Use of calcium channel blockers is generally contraindicated in pediatrics; in adults they may increase subendocardial perfusion, reduce inducible ischemia, decrease dyspnea, and increase exercise

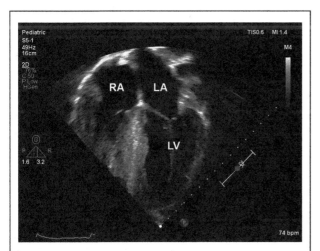

FIGURE 3.107 Hypertrophic cardiopmyopathy

LA, left atrium; LV, left ventricle; RA, right atrium.

Courtesy of CS Mott Children's Hospital, University of Michigan, Congenital Heart Center.

capacity. Both β-blockers and calcium channel blockers prolong diastole and permit a longer LV filling time and can decrease LVOT the gradient (Lipshultz, Orav, et al., 2013; Williams & Hammer, 2011).

d. Digoxin or diuretics are generally contraindicated, as they can increase the LVOTO through increased contractility or decreased preload to the ventricle.

e. The use of antiarrhythmic medications, such as amiodarone, has not shown to be of protective benefit against SCD. Disopyramide may be effective adjunctive therapy for patients with arrhythmia.

f. Avoidance of tachycardia to promote a longer filling time and avoidance of volume depletion with maintenance of preload increases ventricular volume and can protect against LVOT obliteration during systole.

g. Myomectomy/myectomy is offered to patients with severe LVOTO and refractory symptoms. This operation will relieve symptoms but does not alter the risk of SCD or the long-term outcome (Williams & Hammer, 2011).

h. The need for OHT is rare in this myopathy. If indicated, it is primarily in patients younger than 1 year of age, those with a mixed phenotypic expression, those with low weight/FTT or low BMI, or more than one risk factor.

i. Placement of an ICD for secondary prevention of SCD is common. Patients with previous aborted SCD, nonsustained VT on holter, syncope, LVH with an z-score greater than 6, or a first-degree relative with SCD (Lipshultz, Cochran, et al., 2013; Williams & Hammer, 2011).

    i. ICD insertion is the only treatment that is known to prolong life in these patients.

    ii. In prevention of SCD, the risk of SCD must be balanced against the complications of ICD placement, which include inappropriate shock, infection, lead failure, and the psychological and social implications of device placement.

j. Patients with obstructive HCM are best treated with lifestyle modification, lipophilic β-blocker therapy (metoprolol, propranolol), myectomy, and ICD placement.

k. Resynchronization therapy is used in patients with advanced HF and conduction delays. It improves mechanical synchrony, which increases LV filling time, decreases MR, and reduces septal dyskinesis.

5. Complications include chest pain, exercise intolerance, arrhythmia, and SCD.

F. Restrictive Cardiomyopathy

1. *Etiology and Pathophysiology*

a. RCM is a rare form of PCM, with an incidence of 4% to 5% (Park, 2016). The etiology is linked to selected sarcomere contractile protein genes, primarily the troponin I gene, which is most likely responsible for development of RCM. There are some suggestions that RCM may be in part related to desmin accumulation in the cytoplasm. One quarter of these patients have a family history of PCM.

b. Idiopathic RCM is the most common etiology. It can be associated with patients who have amyloidosis, inborn errors of metabolism, sarcoidosis, and scleroderma.

c. Secondary causes include chest radiotherapy, chemotherapy (specifically with anthracyclines), neoplasms, connective tissue disorders, and hemochromatosis.

d. RCM is related to endocardial fibroelastosis from certain types of congenital heart disease and hypereosinophilic syndrome, which is an infiltration of eosinophils with fibrosis and scarring in leukemia patients.

e. Patients presenting at a younger age, with HF symptoms, with a decreased LVSF, or an increased left ventricular end-diastolic posterior wall thickness are at high risk for SCD or acute decompensation.

f. There is only a 20% survival rate at 5 years from diagnosis in patients with RCM and 66% to 100% of patients with RCM have an OHT by 6 years of age. It is the rarest form of PCM, the occurrence rate is less than 5%, with the poorest prognosis of all PCMs. One half of patients die within 2 years of diagnosis and 80% die or need an OHT within 5 years of diagnosis. RCM has the highest risk of SCD, even in patients without symptoms (Webber et al., 2012).

2. *Phenotypic Expression*

a. RCM is a cardiac muscle disease leading to diastolic dysfunction of either or both ventricles, marked by decreased LV compliance and relaxation with impaired filling and increased LVEDP and marked LA enlargement. Impairment occurs when most of the ventricle fills rapidly in early diastole, followed by little to no increase in ventricular volume after the end of early filling. This impairment in LV diastolic filling increases LVEDP and decreases CO. The higher LVEDP results in PA hypertension and, over time, the development of PVOD. Eventually, right-sided HF will ensue as a result of PAH, PVOD (Figure 3.108).

b. Generally, ventricular systolic function and size remain normal until late in the disease. Increased ventricular wall thickness with impaired systolic function heralds the progression of disease.

c. These patients present with symptoms of diastolic HF. FTT, recurrent respiratory infections, chronic congestion, and fatigue may cause the family to seek medical attention. On CXR there may be evidence of pulmonary edema and possibly pleural effusions. On physical examination there is evidence of JVD, ascites, peripheral edema, Kussmaul's sign, pulsus paradoxus, and organomegaly. An audible third heart sound due to abrupt cessation of ventricular filling is a classic auscultatory finding.

d. Syncope, arrhythmias, and palpitations are a frequent complaint of older children. With disease progression, symptoms of decreased CO (fatigue, dyspnea, exercise intolerance) and thromboembolic events are characteristic.

e. Progression of the disease is noted by increased MV inflow variation, enlargement of both atria, increased thickness of the LVPW, and hepatic vein flow reversal on echo.

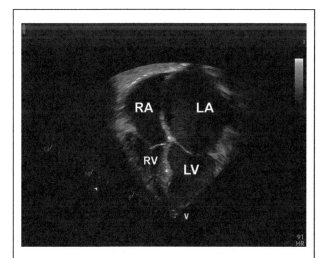

FIGURE 3.108 Restrictive cardiomyopathy

LA, left atrium; RA, right atrium; LV, left ventricle; RV, right ventricle.

Courtesy of CS Mott Children's Hospital, University of Michigan, Congenital Heart Center.

3. *Diagnostic Evaluation*

a. Physical examination shows poor growth, JVD in older children, cough/tachypnea/dyspnea, ascites, and hepatomegaly.

b. Echo shows MV inflow variation and impaired diastolic filling, decreased systolic function, decreased isovolumic relaxation, and hepatic vein flow reversal. It shows amyloid infiltration of the myocardium and valves. Isovolumic relaxation time is decreased and the ratio of early diastolic filling to atrial filling is increased. There is evidence of elevated PAP secondary to LA hypertension (Lipshultz, Cochran, et al., 2013).

c. Increased LVEDP/RVEDP is found at cardiac catheterization. Elevation of atrial pressures and PAH with increased PVR is likely. PVR reactivity testing may show lack of responsiveness to pulmonary vasodilators or oxygen. Further elevation of LVEDP and RVEDP with fluid challenge will show that the LVEDP will increase more and faster than the RV (Lipshultz, Cochran, et al., 2013).

d. ECG may show low voltages in standard leads, biatrial enlargement, ST/T wave changes, and atrial arrhythmias.

e. CXR will show an enlarged atria and variable degrees of pulmonary congestion without cardiomegaly.

f. CT and cMRI provide information about pericardial anatomy to differential RCM from pericardial disease. A pericardium of greater than 4 mm suggests constrictive pericarditis and not RCM, which is key in determining treatment and prognosis (Lipshultz, Cochran, et al., 2013).

g. Cardiac catheterization shows increased end-diastolic pressure and the characteristic square-root sign reflecting rapid filling during early diastole followed by a decrease in ventricular filling. The end-diastolic pressure in both ventricles is elevated, usually the LVEDP is greater than the RVEDP. Elevated diastolic pressure is preload and HR dependent. The high atrial pressures noted from the elevation in RVEDP//LVEDP occur in the presence of low CO (Lipshultz, Cochran, et al., 2013).

4. *Goals and Patient Management*

a. Treatment does not influence outcome for this PCM. Treatment is aimed at relief of symptoms and to optimize patient growth and hemodynamics while evaluating candidacy for transplantation. Treatment approaches include decreasing systemic and pulmonary congestion with careful administration of diuretics in a preload-dependent patient, optimizing diastolic filling by avoiding tachycardia or arrhythmia, and treating arrhythmia if one exists. Early transplantation should be considered in all patients with RCM given the poor prognosis and progressive nature of this disease.

b. Anticoagulation with aspirin or warfarin related to the risk of thromboembolism is recommended. The level of anticoagulation is generally based on the LVSF, evidence of thrombus on imaging studies, and the occurrence of a previous thromboembolic event. Indications for anticoagulation generally agreed upon include dilated atria, tachyarrhythmia, and severely decreased LVSF (Lipshultz, Cochran, et al., 2013).

c. Indications for ICD placement include VT on cardiac monitoring or based on history of syncopal event, atrial fibrillation, and myocardial ischemia. ICD is recommended due to the high incidence of SCD in this population (Bharucha et al., 2015).

d. OHT is the only treatment modality to alter the natural history of the disease process. There is a low wait-list mortality, but to ensure transplant candidacy, listing needs to occur prior to development of pulmonary vascular obstructive disease (PVOD; Williams & Hammer, 2011).

5. *Complications* include severe FTT, SCD, and thromboembolic events.

G. Left Ventricular Noncompaction Cardiomyopathy (LVNC)

1. *Etiology and Pathophysiology*

a. Left ventricular noncompaction cardiomyopathy (LVNC) was established as a distinct form of PCM in 2006. Its increasing incidence is most likely related to the increased recognition of the disease rather than an actual increased occurrence. LVCN represents 9% of PCM (Brescia et al., 2013). Two thirds of cases are transmitted via an X-linked inheritance pattern. There are at least seven phenotypes with variable outcome based on which phenotype is expressed (Lipshultz, Cochran, et al., 2013).

b. LVNC is also associated with various forms of CHD, most specifically, critical AS and HLHS.

c. Metabolic, genetic, chromosomal, neuromuscular, and mitochondrial disease are also associated with LVNC.

d. The outcome for these patients is dependent on the extent of LV diastolic dysfunction. Patients with good function have a better long-term outcome than all PCM except hypertrophic cardiomyopathy. There is a 30% mortality in those diagnosed with LVNC prior to 1 year of age and 70% of infants with VT and CHF die or require OHT by 1 year of age. Six percent of patients die or require an OHT within 5 years of diagnosis (Brescia et al., 2013).

e. Arrhythmia and SCD are the most common risks of LVNC and also major determinants of outcome and prognosis. Half of the patients will sustain SCD with the highest risk patient profile consisting of severe LV diastolic dysfunction, right HF, syncope, and prolongation of the QRS. The onset of VT is an especially poor prognostic sign. LVNC will eventually progress to involve a decrease in the LVSF and this is predictive of death or the need for OHT.

2. *Phenotypic Expression*

a. LVNC is a congenital malformation characterized by abnormal spongy trabeculations of LV, usually the apical portion, as a result of what is theorized to be an arrested development of fetal myocardial compaction at about 5 to 8 weeks gestation. The noncompaction process starts at the base of the heart and advances to the apex. The result is the formation of two distinct myocardial layers: a compacted and noncompacted layer. The noncompacted portion of the ventricular wall does not communicate with the coronary arteries (Figure 3.109; Summers & Mikolich, 2014).

b. The formation of these abnormal trabecules in the apical and midportion of the LV results in intertrabecular recesses, some of which are deep. The end result is abnormal relaxation and restricted ventricular filling with diastolic dysfunction (Jefferies et al., 2015).

c. Symptoms of impaired LV systolic function are the most common, likely resulting from subendocardial hypoperfusion and microcirculatory dysfunction. These symptoms include dyspnea, exercise intolerance, chest pain, atrial arrhythmias, most common are fibrillation, HF, and thromboembolic episodes. Asynchrony between compacted and noncompacted segments leads to global dysfunction of the LV (Lipshultz, Cochran, et al., 2013).

3. *Diagnostic Evaluation*

a. Diagnosis is made after testing for metabolic, genetic, chromosomal, neuromuscular, and mitochondrial diseases.

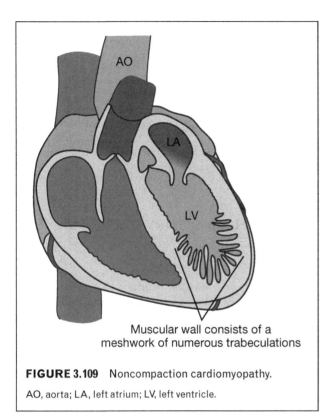

Muscular wall consists of a
meshwork of numerous trabeculations

FIGURE 3.109 Noncompaction cardiomyopathy.

AO, aorta; LA, left atrium; LV, left ventricle.

b. cMRI is the best tool for morphologic evaluation of areas of noncompaction, especially of the deep trabecular recesses and mural thrombi. PET scan is now being utilized for this diagnosis and can best denote subendocardial perfusion (Summers & Mikolich, 2014).

c. Echo demonstrates LV diastolic dysfunction even in the fetus. It defines the areas of noncompaction and is the best tool for following progression of the disease.

4. *Goals and Patient Management*

a. Treatment decisions are based on measures of the LVEF. With an EF greater than 45%, treatment is based on HF symptoms, arrhythmia presentation, or embolic event occurrence. If the EF is less than 45%, aggressive guideline-based HF therapy (AHA Heart Failure Guidelines) with consideration for ICD and anticoagulation. Activity restriction is warranted to prevent SCD, especially in patients with abnormal cardiac dimensions, LV diastolic dysfunction, and arrhythmia. ACE inhibitors or β-blockers are used to treat systolic dysfunction; β-blocker therapy is also recommended for diastolic

dysfunction (Stacey, Caine, & Hundley, 2015; Towbin, Lorts, & Jefferies, 2010).

b. OHT may be the only treatment for patients nonresponsive to medical therapy. For patients with worsening HF, without contraindications to VAD placement, a VAD as a bridge to transplant may be considered. Placement of a VAD as destination therapy may be considered in patients with PVOD that prevents listing for transplantation.

c. For patients with a wide QRS complex and decreased EF, resynchronization therapy may be utilized. ICD placement is considered in all patients based on their risk profile, as SCD occurs in 50% of these patients. Antiarrhythmic medications are recommended for atrial flutter/fibrillation, VT, or patients with a wide QRS complex (Brescia et al., 2013).

d. Anticoagulation with aspirin or warfarin is recommended in patients with LVEF of less than 35%, evidence of thrombus on imaging studies, or a history of a thromboembolic event (Williams & Hammer, 2011).

e. Progression of the disease is characterized by chronic, progressive LV systolic and diastolic dysfunction.

5. Complications include arrhythmia and mural thrombi. SCD is a common complication with progression of disease. FTT and poor weight gain from progressive HF are common.

H. Arrhythmogenic Right Ventricular Myopathy

1. *Etiology and Pathophysiology*

a. ARVM occurs in 2% to 3% of patients with PCM. It belongs to a group of desmosomal complex diseases. Desmosomal gene processes create genetic alterations that affect the intracellular junctions of the cardiac muscle (Gutiérrez, Kamel, & Zimmerman, 2016).

b. Patient survival is associated with progressive HF in older patients and SCD in younger patients.

c. The risk of SCD is highest in younger patients and those with recurrent syncope, previous aborted SCD, LV involvement in the disease process, and specific ARVM gene mutations (Silvano et al., 2013).

2. *Phenotypic Expression*

a. ARVM is a disease that predominantly affects the RV. It is associated with ventricular arrhythmia and an increased risk of SCD in young patients and athletes.

b. It is characterized by myocardial cell loss with fibrofatty infiltration, making the conduction system prone to VT. VT is the result of a reentry mechanism around the myocardial scar that results from healing of the fibrofatty infiltration (Gutiérrez et al., 2016).

c. Presentation of ARVM often follows an episode of aborted SCD.

d. Prognosis is dependent on the ARVM classification and the stage of disease at the time of presentation.

3. *Diagnostic Evaluation*

a. There is no single diagnostic test for this disease. ARVM is diagnosed by a combination of electrophysiology study that demonstrates the area of inducible VT and endomyocardial biopsy for histologic findings consistent with fibrofatty infiltration of RVOT. In addition, familial expression of the disease is considered in evaluation (Silvano et al., 2013).

b. ECG shows a low-voltage RVOT, VT, and LBBB.

c. Radionuclide ventriculography (nuclear isotope scan) may be the best diagnostic tool. It assesses the contraction and filling of the ventricles at rest and with exertion and can demonstrate the abnormal contraction and infiltration by fibrofatty cells of the RVOT.

4. *Goals and Patient Management*

a. Treatment and outcomes are based on the etiology of ARVM and are aimed at suppression of VT and the prevention of SCD. Options for treatment include medication, catheter ablation, and ICD placement. A causal identification in ARVM assists with establishing treatment goals.

b. The most effective medical therapy at this time includes sotalol or β-blockers with amiodarone.

c. Radiofrequency ablation for recurrent VT has a good initial success rate, but has a high recurrence rate due to progression of disease or variable disease substrates. This mode of therapy is generally used in combination with ICD placement.

d. ICD placement is the only treatment that has been associated with increased long-term survival. Indications for placement include syncope/aborted SCD, inducible VT at electrophysiologic testing, nonsustained VT on exercise test or cardiac monitoring, or SCD in one or more first-degree relatives (Silvano et al., 2013).

5. *Complications* are primarily related to arrhythmia and SCD. If an ICD is placed, complications relating to ICD placement can occur. Progression of myocarditis to DCM, once acute infectious phase is completed, can occur. Sudden death from low CO or arrhythmia may occur in the acute phase. Conduction defects may result from inflammation of the conduction system.

ACUTE INFLAMMATORY DISEASES

A. Definition

1. *Myocardial diseases* produce inflammation of cardiac or vascular tissues, including myocarditis, endocarditis, pericarditis, Kawasaki syndrome, and rheumatic heart disease.

B. Myocarditis

1. *Pathophysiology*

a. Myocarditis occurs as focal or diffuse inflammation of the cardiac muscle producing temporary or permanent damage to the myocardium with resultant decrease in cardiac function (Canter & Simpson, 2012).

b. During the acute phase of myocarditis (when the causative organism may be cultured), direct myocardial damage with necrosis of myocardial cells begins, including specialized tissue, such as that of the conduction system. Cellular infiltration of macrophages and natural killer cells results in disintegration of heart muscle, fibrosis, hypertrophy, chamber dilation, mural thrombi, and release of cytokines, such as tumor necrosis factor and interferons, which block viral replication while enhancing negative inflammatory effects. The acute phase of myocarditis lasts several weeks to several months (Towbin, 2016).

c. The chronic phase of myocarditis occurs after several weeks or months, when the acute phase is thought to be treated but new symptoms present. Acute myocarditis does not always progress to chronic myocarditis. If it does progress it is mediated by T cells and natural killer cells that continue to attack the myocardium. The necrotic area of muscle is replaced with scar tissue. Focal hemorrhage, edema, fatty infiltration of the muscle, and fibrosis may also occur. This causes remodeling of the myocardium and a chronic form of myocarditis. It may, but not always, result in DCM and HF (Stendahl, 2015).

d. In individuals who are at genetically increased risk for the development of DCM, there is a persistent activation of T-cells. This causes myosin to be seen as an antigen and auto-antibodies to these antigens are formed and are found in the at-risk individuals.

2. *Etiology*

a. Myocarditis can be caused by any pathogen, including bacteria, viruses, and fungi. Most cases are associated with a viral illness (especially RNA type, e.g., coxsackievirus A and B, influenza A and B), a systemic infection, or active endocarditis.

b. Noninfectious myocarditis may be caused by systemic autoimmune diseases (e.g., systemic lupus erythematosus).

3. *Clinical Signs and Symptoms*

a. Myocarditis involves a history of bacterial or viral illness. Symptoms include fever, tachycardia, lethargy, chest pain, weakness, poor appetite, myalgia, and abdominal pain. Signs may include those of poor systemic perfusion and CHF progressing to shock, a new systolic murmur, tachycardia and/or new arrhythmia, pulsus alternans, and a pericardial or pleural friction rub.

4. *Diagnostic Evaluation*

a. Chest radiographic examination may demonstrate pleural effusion(s) and/or an enlarged cardiac silhouette particularly when a pericardial effusion is present. Lung markings may show pulmonary edema or pulmonary congestion.

b. ECG may show ST changes (elevation or depression), an inverted T wave, a prolonged PR interval, diminished QRS complex and T-wave voltage, or arrhythmias. Most of the ECG changes are nonspecific, however.

c. Echo is used to quantify any effusion, locate and visualize vegetations and abscesses, rule out structural problems, measure end-diastolic pressures, assess ventricular function, and evaluate valve function. A transesophageal echocardiogram may be used to best visualize the presence of vegetations and thrombi to rule out endocarditis.

d. Also included in the laboratory evaluation for myocarditis are titers to assess for elevated IgM to viral illnesses, cardiac enzyme studies, sedimentation rate, and CRP (which may be elevated).

e. Cardiac catheterization is used to identify restrictive pericarditis or CM, evaluate the severity of myocardial constriction, and obtain an endomyocardial biopsy for histologic grading, culture (rarely positive), and polymerase chain reaction (PCR) analysis of tissue for viral genomes.

f. Using needle aspiration to obtain pericardial fluid for analysis and culture and to relieve pericardial effusion or cardiac tamponade, pericardiocentesis may be performed as both a diagnostic tool and intervention.

5. *Goals and Patient Management*

a. Close monitoring for ventricular arrhythmia and supportive care are the main interventions for myocarditis. The goal is to optimize CO and oxygen delivery until the myocarditis resolves. In many cases, this does not occur and support with vasoactive agents, intubation, and, potentially, MCS may be warranted. The use of milrinone is well tolerated and generally beneficial for support of CO and tissue oxygen delivery.

b. If ECMO support is instituted, use of a left atrial cannula for decompression of the left heart is generally indicated, unless the child has an ASD.

c. Careful use of catecholamines is advised, as these may precipitate increased ectopy/arrhythmia and increased myocardial oxygen demand. AV block from the inflammatory process may occur and necessitate cardiac pacing for HR support. The use of isoproterenol or other chronotropic medication may precipitate ventricular ectopy and therefore pacing is the safer method of treating clinically significant AV block in patients not on MCS. For patients with recurrent ventricular ectopy/VT at high risk of SCD, antiarrhythmic therapy, including an amiodarone infusion, may be indicated. Electrolytes and acid–base balance should be maintained within normal limits.

d. The child's activity should be limited and no excessive exercising is permitted in the acute phase of the disease to avoid increasing oxygen demand and consumption on a myocardium that is acutely compromised. In addition, arrhythmias may be precipitated by release of endogenous catecholamines during exercise.

e. Once stable from the acute episode, conversion to oral medication regimens should ensue. Generally, medical management consists of diuretics paired with systemic vasodilators, such as an ACE inhibitor, or ARB if an ACE inhibitor is not tolerated. Use of anticoagulation is not standard treatment unless function is severely compromised or there is evidence of thrombus on echo.

6. *Complications* can include SCD from arrhythmia or low CO in the initial phase of presentation. Once the acute phase is over, conversion to DCM that may progress to need for cardiac transplant is possible. Arrhythmias, including heart block, may occur related to inflammation of conduction tissue. Complete resolution of the disease without sequelae is possible in about 30% of the cases.

C. Endocarditis

1. *Pathophysiology*

a. Endocarditis is an inflammatory process of the inner layer of the heart, the endocardium. Structures included in this diagnosis are cardiac valves, chordae, and the septum. Endocarditis may be classified as infectious or noninfectious, but most often results from a bacteria or fungus in a child with valvular or structural heart disease or an invasive vascular catheter (Baltimore et al., 2015).

b. There is damage to the endothelial lining of the heart, which permits fibrin and platelet deposits and bacterial growth and forms exudative and proliferative material known as a vegetation. Turbulent blood flow or disruption of endothelial tissue from line placement results in mural tissue damage with deposition of platelets and fibrin and thrombus formation with entrapment of circulating organisms. Large colonies of bacteria become encased in masses of fibrin-forming vegetations. Vegetations usually occur at the location of jet lesions. In addition, infection may destroy the valve, invade the myocardium to form an abscess, or result in thrombus formation on valves and eventually deform the valve and cause valve insufficiency. Portions of the lesions may embolize to other organs, resulting in complement activation and inflammatory responses that may contribute to renal dysfunction or affect other organ systems (Figure 3.110).

2. *Etiology*

a. Endocarditis is usually bacterial (*Streptococcus viridans*, *Staphylococcus aureus*) and rarely fungal. It is most likely to affect children with underlying heart disease or intracardiac catheters, especially children with prosthetic valves or those who have

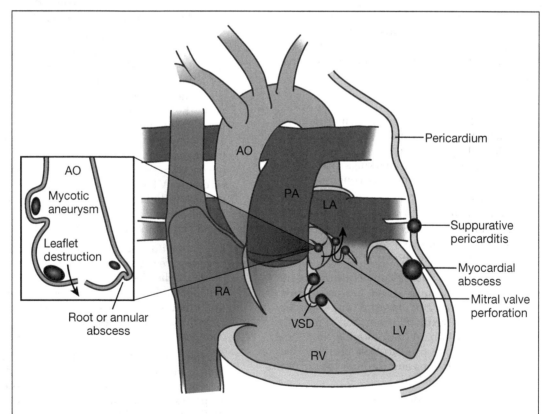

FIGURE 3.110 Common sites of infection in patients requiring surgery for active endocarditis.

AO, aorta; LA, left atrium; LV, left ventricle; PA, pulmonary artery; RA, right atrium; RV, right ventricle; VSD, ventricular septal defect.

undergone surgical interventions (e.g., open heart surgery with foreign patch material, or gastrointestinal tract, genitourinary tract, or dental procedures). Patients at risk for fungal endocarditis are most likely to be infants or immunocompromised children (Baltimore et al., 2015).

3. *Clinical signs and symptoms* are related to the systemic infection. There is general malaise, low-grade persistent fever without response to antipyretics, a new murmur, a rub, or conduction disturbances. CHF symptoms occur if endocarditis progresses to severe valvar regurgitation. CNS symptoms of stroke and headache occur as a result of vegetative emboli (septic emboli) to the brain. Specific to endocarditis, small thrombi may produce splinter hemorrhages under the nail bed or small macular nodules on palms and soles called *Janeway spots*. All end organs may be affected by septic emboli including bowel, spleen, liver, kidney, and lung. Symptoms vary depending on organ involved (Table 3.12).

TABLE 3.12   Terminology Used in the Criteria for Endocarditis

Major Criteria	
Positive blood culture for infective endocarditis	Typical micro-organism for infective endocarditis from two separate blood cultures: HACEK group (haempohilus, actinobacillus, cardiobacterium, eikenella, kingella) *viridans streptococci, Streptococcus bovis* or Community-acquired *Stapylococcus aureus* or Enterococci in the absence of a primary focus or Recovery of a microorganism consistent with infective endocarditis from
Persistent bacteremia	Blood cultures drawn >12 hours apart or All of the three or a majority of four or more separate blood cultures, with first and last more than 1 hour apart Echocardiogram positive for infective endocarditis
Evidence of endocardial involvement	Vegetation or oscillating intracardiac mass, on valve or supporting structures, in the path of regurgitant jets or on implanted material, without an alternative anatomic explanation or Abscess or New dehiscence of prosthetic valve or New valve regurgitation
Minor Criteria	
Predisposition	IV drug use or predisposing heart condition
Fever	Greater than or equal to 38.0°C (100.4°F)
Vascular phenomena	Major septic pulmonary infarcts, arterial emboli, myotic aneurysm, hemorrhage (intracranial, conjunctival), Janeway lesions
Immunologic phenomena	Glomerulonephritis, Osler's nodes, Roth spots, rheumatoid factor
Microbiologic evidence	Positive blood culture without major criterion as noted or Antibodies in blood serum indicating active infection with organism consistent with infective endocarditis
Echocardiogram	Demonstrating evidence of infective endocarditis but not meeting major criterion as noted previously
Diagnosis Requires	
Two major criteria One major and three minor criteria Five minor criteria	

4. *Diagnostic Evaluation*

a. Clinical examination is necessary for neurologic and skin manifestations of endocarditis. Evaluation for CHF symptoms or cardiac tamponade and the presence of a new murmur are classic findings on a clinical examination.

b. CXR demonstrates an enlarged cardiac silhouette when a pericardial effusion or significant AV valve regurgitation is present.

c. ECG may show ST changes (elevation or depression), inverted T wave, prolonged PR interval, diminished QRS complex and T-wave voltage, or arrhythmias.

d. Echo is used to identify the presence and cardiovascular implication of a pericardial effusion, locate and visualize vegetations and abscesses, rule out structural defects, evaluate cardiac function, identify perivalvar leak, and evaluate valve function. A transesophageal view may be used for better visualization.

e. Laboratory studies include cultures (minimum of three blood cultures); WBC and differential (leukocytosis with left shifted differential may be present); titers to assess for elevated IgM; cardiac enzyme studies; and inflammatory markers, including CRP, sedimentation rate, and procalcitonin, which will be elevated. Procalcitonin can assist with differential diagnosis when the cause of the fever is undefined. Trending of all inflammatory markers is key to define the patient's response to therapy. Renal function and liver function tests reflect the degree of CHF, potential presence of septic emboli, and the need for further organ support.

f. Cardiac catheterization is used to identify restrictive pericarditis or CM, evaluate the severity of constriction, and obtain an endomyocardial biopsy for histologic grading, culture (rarely positive), and PCR analysis of tissue for viral genomes.

g. Magnetic resonance imaging/CT for embolic phenomena and for continued evaluation of extension of emboli may be indicated. This is especially indicated if there is evidence of septic emboli to the brain and a need for surgical intervention requiring CPB. This would place the patient at risk of a hemorrhagic conversion in the area of the septic emboli.

h. Pericardiocentesis as both a diagnostic tool and an intervention may be performed using needle aspiration and possibly chest tube placement to obtain pericardial fluid for analysis and culture and to drain a pericardial effusion and relieve tamponade.

5. *Goals and Patient Management*

a. Treatment of CHF and end-organ compromise is vital. Antibiotic therapy is aimed at treatment of identified cultures for a minimum of 6 weeks with suppression therapy based on clinical indications. Requirement for removal (surgical) of infected prosthetic material may be necessary to clear persistently positive blood cultures. In addition, surgical intervention may be indicated if CHF is not manageable, there are recurrent septic emboli, or blood cultures remain positive.

b. Nutritional support is vital, as often appetite is decreased with weight loss prior to diagnosis, combined with persistent poor intake during the course of disease treatment. Confounding variables affecting weight loss may be septic emboli to the bowel or other abdominal organs.

6. *Complications* include irreversible deficits related to septic emboli, inability to clear infection with recurrent bouts of endocarditis despite suppression therapy, heart block requiring pacer insertion, requirement for emergent surgical intervention in the face of infection not completely eradicated, and death (Johnson, Boyce, Cetta, Steckelberg, & Johnson, 2012).

D. Pericarditis

1. *Pathophysiology*

a. Pericarditis is an inflammation of the pericardium that can produce effusions (serous to thick and cheesy exudate) and fibrin deposits within the pericardial sac and/or produce a thickened, scarred pericardium. When present, increasing effusion volume may cause cardiac tamponade due to a rise in extracardiac pressure restricting cardiac inflow and output.

2. *Etiology*

a. Effusive pericarditis is an inflammation of the pericardium that results in the formation of a collection of fluctuant pericardial fluid composed of leukocytes and inflammatory mediators.

b. Constrictive pericarditis is an inflammation of the fibrous and serous pericardium resulting in pericardial thickening and compression of heart.

c. Rarely, pericarditis is both effusive and constrictive.

3. *Clinical signs and symptoms* are dependent on the type of pericarditis.

   a. Effusive pericarditis commonly presents with symptoms of CHF without alteration in cardiac function or with symptoms of cardiac tamponade from untreated and progressive enlargement of a pericardial effusion.

   b. Constrictive pericarditis presents with systolic and diastolic HF symptoms from inability of the heart to fill and empty due to constriction of the pericardium. It may initially be confused with RCM.

4. *Diagnostic Evaluation*

   a. Clinical examination will demonstrate symptoms based on the type of pericarditis. If an effusion is present, symptoms of cardiac tamponade with JVD, cough, low CO, tachycardia, and tachypnea are present. An acute onset of chest pain and the presence of a pericardial rub are also clinical signs and symptoms of pericarditis.

   b. CXR demonstrates an enlarged cardiac silhouette when a pericardial effusion is present.

   c. ECG may show ST changes (elevation or depression), an inverted T wave, a prolonged PR interval, a diminished QRS and T-wave voltage, or arrhythmias.

   d. Echocardiogram is used to determine the size and the degree of cardiac compromise related to the pericardial effusion. This is determined by the presence of atrial-wall collapse and mitral valve inflow variation. The echo will also determine diastolic function and evaluate AV valve function. A transesophageal view may be used for better visualization.

   e. Laboratory studies include cultures to determine whether an infective process is present, renal and liver function tests to determine end-organ function, and inflammatory markers for initial evaluation and trending.

   f. Cardiac catheterization is used to differentiate constrictive pericarditis from other potential disease states, primarily RCM. It will evaluate the severity of constriction and obtain an endomyocardial biopsy for histologic grading, culture (rarely positive), and PCR analysis of tissue for viral genomes. Relief of the effusion with pericardial drainage in effusive disease may alleviate symptoms and improve CO acutely.

   g. MRI is especially helpful in differentiating constrictive pericarditis from RCM and is now the diagnostic test of choice for this differential diagnosis (Lim, 2015).

5. *Goals and patient management* depend on the type of pericarditis.

   a. Effusive pericarditis is treated medically (Lilly, 2013) with anti-inflammatory agents and antibiotics if an infective etiology is found on testing. Surgical drainage, pericardial window, or pericardiocentesis may be indicated for drainage of a symptomatic effusion (Figure 3.111).

   b. Constrictive pericarditis generally requires surgical removal of the pericardium (Lilly, 2013). In some patients, there may be added benefit from the use of NSAIDS, antibiotics, and medical adjunct therapies (Figure 3.112).

6. *Complications* include incomplete relief of symptoms following removal of the pericardium, recurrent effusion, and side effects of the anti-inflammatory medications if prescribed.

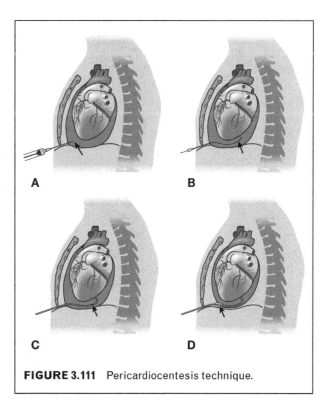

FIGURE 3.111 Pericardiocentesis technique.

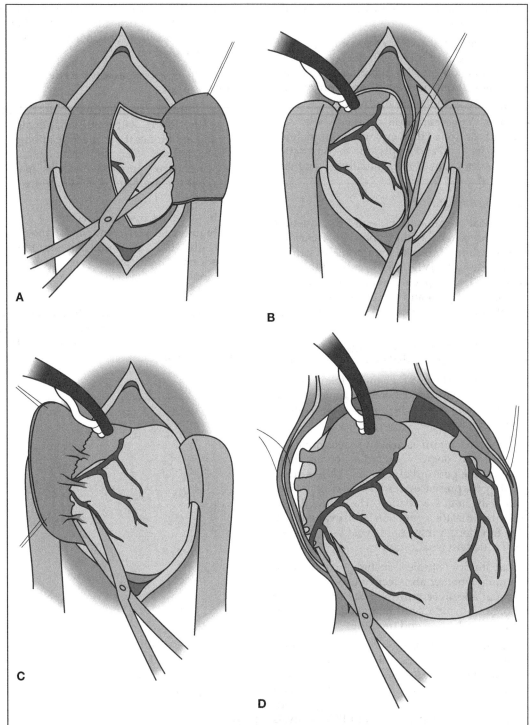

FIGURE 3.112 Total pericardiectomy. (A) Pericardium over left ventricle and left atrium is removed, then the pericardium over right ventricle. (B) Phrenic nerves are preserved but pericardium posterior to the nerves is resected. (C) Pericardium over the right atrium is resected. (D) Pericardium over the pulmonary veins is resected.

E. Rheumatic Heart Disease

1. *Pathophysiology*

   a. This is a postinfectious connective tissue disease caused by rheumatic fever. Group A β-hemolytic streptococcal pharyngitis is the most common bacteria causing acute rheumatic fever. The infection initiates an autoimmune process in a genetically susceptible host that attacks collagen. Streptococcal and myocardial tissues have similar antigenic properties, creating the same antigenic response. The antibodies produced for streptococcal infections react with the host tissue producing antibody-induced tissue damage, generally effecting the mitral valve in the heart (Mayosi, 2015).

2. *Etiology*

   a. Rheumatic fever most often occurs in those aged 6 to 15 years and is rare in children younger than 2 years or older than 15 years. The incidence in the United States decreased after the introduction of antibiotics; it remains common in Third World countries (Mayosi, 2015).

3. *Clinical Signs and Symptoms*

   a. Symptoms include recent pharyngitis or an upper respiratory tract infection, a new murmur, cardiac enlargement on CXR, a friction rub or effusion, and CHF. Arthritis occurs in 70% of patients and may be the presenting symptom. Children experience migratory heat, redness, and joint pain. CNS involvement is characterized by chorea resulting in grimacing, slurred speech, weakness, and purposeless movements (Sydenham chorea or St. Vitus dance). Skin involvement includes painless, firm subcutaneous nodules (0.5–2 cm) over the joints, such as elbows, knuckles, knees, ankles, the scalp, and the spine. Erythema marginatum rheumaticum is a rash characterized by pink, raised, small irregular macules that are nonpruritic. It usually appears on the trunk and limbs but not on the face (Mayosi, 2015).

4. *Diagnostic Evaluation*

   a. Laboratory studies include a throat culture that is usually positive for group A streptococci, WBC, sedimentation rate, CRP, and elevated antistreptolysin O antibody titer.

   b. ECG may show a prolonged PR interval indicating first-degree AV block, diffuse ST–T wave changes, or T-wave inversion.

   c. Echo is used to evaluate for myocarditis, decreased contractility, and valvular insufficiency.

   d. The Jones criteria are used for diagnosis. The patient needs two major or one major and two minor manifestations to make the diagnosis of rheumatic fever (Table 3.13).

5. *Goals and Patient Management*

   a. Streptococcal infection is treated with antibiotics. Cardiac workload is decreased with bed rest in a quiet environment, arrhythmias are controlled with medication as needed, and pain is treated for comfort. Treatment of CHF, if present, follows the standard protocols of diuretics and afterload reduction with close observation for ventricular ectopy.

   b. The use of salicylates for mild carditis and corticosteroids for severe carditis is still somewhat controversial. If these medications are used, they should be tapered slowly over 6 weeks to avoid any rebound phenomena.

   c. Ongoing suppressive therapy with either oral or monthly IM injections of a penicillin agent may be considered due to risk of reinfection.

6. *Complications* include myocardial damage and severe valve regurgitation. Severe decompensated HF requiring vasoactive support may result, especially if there is acute and severe valve regurgitation.

F. Kawasaki Disease

1. *Pathophysiology*

   a. Kawasaki disease (Rowley, 2015) is a microvasculitis of medium-sized muscular arteries. Immunologic activation causes cytokines to make vascular endothelium susceptible to lysis by antibodies. Early fever, multisystem vasculitis, specifically of the coronary arteries, is followed by pancarditis with inflammation of the conduction system, myocardium, pericardium, and endocardium. Myocarditis develops within 3 to 4 weeks and is associated with WBC infiltration, elevated platelet counts, and edema of the conduction system and myocardial muscle. Severe valvulitis can result in the potential development of coronary artery aneurysms, which heal with fibrosis, causing potential thrombus formation and stenosis (Figure 3.113).

TABLE 3.13   Jones Criteria for Diagnosis of Acute Rheumatic Fever

Major manifestations Carditis Polyarthritis Chorea Erythema marginatum Subcutaneous nodules

Minor manifestations
Clinical findings
  Arthralgia
  Fever
  Previous rheumatic fever
Laboratory findings
  Elevated acute phase reactants
    Erythrocyte sedimentation rate
    C-reactive protein
    White blood cell count
  Prolonged PR interval

Supporting evidence or antecedent group A streptococcal infections Positive throat culture Positive rapid streptococcal antigen test Elevated or increasing streptococcal antibody titer

Source: Reprinted with permission from Nichols, D. G., Ungerleider, R. M., Spevak, P. J., Greeley, W. J., Cameron, D. E., Lappe, D. G., & Wetzel, R. C. (2006). *Critical heart disease in infant and children* (2nd ed.). Philadelphia, PA: Elsevier.

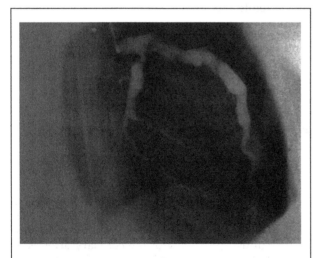

FIGURE 3.113   Cineangiogram photo of aneurysms created by Kawasaki syndrome.

Courtesy of Children's National Medical Center.

2. *Etiology*

  a.   The etiology is unclear, but it is likely a disease of the immune system triggered by an infectious event. It is more prevalent in children of Japanese ancestry and in children younger than 5 years of age. Seasonal outbreaks in winter and spring occur in geographic clusters.

3. *Clinical Signs and Symptoms*

  a.   The acute phase (days 1–10) presents with high fever; conjunctivitis; indurative edema; diffuse red-purple discoloration of palms/soles; cervical lymph node enlargement; skin rash; injected, fissured lips; erythema of the buccal mucosa; and strawberry tongue.

  b.   The subacute phase (days 11–25) presents with desquamation of the tips of the finger and toes; resolution of the rash, fever, and lymphadenopathy; beginning of coronary aneurysm formation; development of a potential pericardial effusion; CHF symptoms; and MI. Thrombocytosis peaks during this phase (Saguil, Fargo, & Grogan, 2015).

  c.   The convalescent phase lasts until the ESR and platelet count return to normal.

4. *Diagnostic Evaluation*

  a.   Laboratory studies are performed to evaluate the myocardial enzymes and to assess for anemia, leukocytosis, thrombocytosis, elevated ESR, elevated serum amylase, liver function, CRP, pyuria, and proteinuria (Table 3.14).

TABLE 3.14   Diagnostic Criteria of Kawasaki Disease

Fever persisting at least 5 days + the presence of four or more of the following five principle features:
• Trunk: Polymorphous exanthema
• Lymph nodes: Swollen lymph nodes
• Lips and oral cavity: Strawberry tongue, diffuse injection of oral mucosa, erythema, and cracking of lips
• Extremities: Edema and erythema of the hands and feet (acute), membranous desquamation of fingertips (convalescent)
• Eyes: Bilateral conjunctival injection without exudate

b. ECG shows nonspecific ST–T wave changes and there may be a prolonged PR interval with various conduction defects.

c. Echo helps in diagnosing coronary aneurysms (may also need arteriography or angiography), pericardial effusions, ventricular dysfunction, and valvular insufficiency. Serial studies are done early and at 6 months to assess for coronary abnormalities.

d. Cardiac catheterization may be used to assess coronary aneurysms and stenosis.

5. *Goals and patient management* are aimed at reducing the risk of coronary artery aneurysm formation and preventing emboli from elevated platelet counts.

a. Anti-inflammatory agents will reduce inflammation and decrease the incidence of coronary abnormalities. High-dose aspirin therapy at doses of 30 to 100 mg/kg daily divided in four doses with intravenous immunoglobulin (IVIG) 2 g/kg over 10 to 12 hours are used for treatment. Repeat doses of IVIG or pulse steroids are used if treatment fails and symptoms persist (McCrindle et al., 2017).

b. Serial ECGs and cardiac isoenzymes are evaluated on a regular basis. Tissue plasminogen activator (tPA) may be indicated if symptoms of an infarction develop. Coronary artery bypass grafting can be used for large aneurysms or significant areas of stenosis.

c. Recovery is usually complete in those who do not develop coronary vasculitis, although second attack may occur. Regression of aneurysms can occur. The long-term impact of coronary vasculitis on future cardiovascular disease is not known.

6. *Complications* include coronary aneurysms with resultant stenosis and infarction. If an aneurysm is larger than 8 mm in size, there is a higher risk of infarct and may require stenting. Systemic emboli to end organs or the coronary arteries may occur due to the proliferation of platelets.

CARDIAC TRANSPLANTATION

A. Definition

1. *Surgical replacement* of the heart is used for end-stage, irreversible cardiac disease in which no other medical or surgical therapy will be successful.

B. Indications for Transplantation

1. *The general indication* (Thrush & Hoffman, 2014) for cardiac transplantation is end-stage HF from systemic ventricular dysfunction not amenable to medical or surgical therapy that causes significant physical limitations or growth failure. The etiologies of this degree of HF include end-stage CM or cardiomyopathies with progressive reversible pulmonary vascular disease, complex CHD not amenable to surgical repair, ischemic myocardial damage with resultant end-stage HF from anomalous LCA, nonmalignant cardiac tumor not amenable to resection, or life-threatening arrhythmias not responsive to medical and surgical therapy (Matsuda, Ichikawa, & Sawa, 2017).

2. *Relative contraindications* to cardiac transplantation include severe and irreversible multiorgan disease; elevated PVR that does not return to normal with medical therapy; severe hypoplasia of the lungs, pulmonary arteries, or pulmonary veins; systemic noncardiac medical conditions, such as active malignancy, that limit the patient's life expectancy.

C. Clinical Signs and Symptoms

1. Signs and symptoms are related to the underlying cardiac condition (see sections "Pediatric Cardiomyopathy," "Congenital Heart Disease," "Heart Failure in Children").

D. Diagnostic Evaluation

1. Cardiac evaluation includes an ECG, echo, and cardiac catheterization to assess function, PVR, and potentially reversible conditions that would negate need for transplantation. A PVR greater than 4 Wood units is of concern, and a PVR greater than 8 Wood units is considered a contraindication for transplant. Additional pulmonary vascular reactivity testing may further determine whether PVR is a contraindication. Exercise stress testing and Holter monitoring can evaluate for arrhythmias as an etiology of or sign of myocardial dysfunction (Table 3.15).

2. *All end-organ systems* are evaluated, including neurologic examination, liver function studies, and renal function analysis by serum laboratory studies, creatinine clearance testing, and glomerular filtration rate renal scan. Serologies determine exposure to viral illnesses and are used as baseline for future exposure as well. Cultures, if indicated, rule out current infection. Because of the risk of superinfection with immunosuppression, active infection is a relative contraindication to transplantation. All organ systems need to have normal function to provide the best possible outcome for transplantation. Relative organ system dysfunction may be acceptable when explained by poor CO and thought to be reversible once transplantation occurs. Recent pulmonary embolism or infarction is a contraindication for transplantation because of the risk of pneumonia after transplantation (Larson et al., 2011).

3. *Immune system* testing includes HLA antigens that determine tissue type that are used to determine the degree of donor–recipient matching. The percentage of reactive antibody (PRA) represents the antibodies within the patient's blood to other human blood that can produce hyperacute rejection during transplant procedure. Other immune markers that may be used to assess function of the immune system cell lines are center specific.

4. *Genetic evaluation* rules out genetic syndromes that might predispose to a disease that would prevent optimum outcome from transplantation.

5. *A financial screening interview* is used to determine insurance plan coverage for transplantation, to assess the family's ability to provide long-term medical care, and to assess drug coverage needed to provide expensive long-term immunosuppressive medications.

6. *Psychosocial evaluation* assesses the patient's and/or family's resources and ability to be successful following cardiac transplantation. This entails screening for circumstances that might prevent positive outcomes of transplantation; identifies concerns that may need to be addressed during the stress of being on a transplant wait-list, during the transplantation, hospitalization, and for the long-term care needs. The evaluation explores prior drug and alcohol history of the patient and/or family, psychiatric disorders, child abuse and neglect history, and prior evidence of the family's inability to care for the child. A formal family conference to discuss transplant process, risk and benefits, and posttransplant regimen is standard of care prior to assigning a transplantation status. Need and candidacy for social assistance are also assessed (Hsu & Lamour, 2015).

E. Transplant Operation

1. *Bicaval left atrial cuff technique* is used by the majority of centers as it limits the required suture lines (Figure 3.114). There are a total of five surgical anastomoses performed in the following order: left atrial cuff, aorta, IVC, SVC, and main PA.

    a. If an ASD is present, it is closed at the time of transplant.

    b. PA or aortic reconstruction may be required at the time of transplant in patients with specific forms of CHD.

    c. Removal of VAD and repair of vessels used for VAD attachment may be required.

F. Goals and Patient Management

1. *Evaluation of cardiovascular function* involves close hemodynamic monitoring. Early postoperative management is highly variable and strongly impacted by factors such as donor heart ischemic time, recipient pretransplant condition, and comorbidities. Close monitoring of atrial pressures

TABLE 3.15   Transplant Evaluation

Laboratories
Aldolase
Amylase
Basic metabolic panel: sodium, potassium, carbon dioxide, chloride, blood urea nitrogen, creatinine, glucose, calcium
Blood type
B-type natriuretic peptide
Complement (C3, C4)
Complete blood count
Creatine kinase
Immunoglobulins (IgG, IgM, IgE)
Iron levels
Lactate dehydrogenase
Lipase
Lipid panel: Total cholesterol, triglyceride level, HDL cholesterol level, LDL cholesterol level
Liver function tests: Albumin, aspartate transferase (AST), alanine transferase (ALT), alkaline phosphate (ALP), total protein
Prealbumin
Reticulocyte count
Sedimentation rate
Thyroid studies (Free T4, TSH, T3)
Uric acid
Urinalysis
Stool sample (culture, ova and parasites, alpha-1 antitrypsin)
Viral hepatitis panel
Human immunodeficiency virus
Cytomegalovirus (CMX IgG, IgM, antigenemia, quantitative PCR, urine)
Epstein-Barr virus (EBV IgG, IgM, EBNA, quantitative PCR)
Respiratory secretions (viral culture, RSV, influenza)
Nasal swab for methicillin-resistant *Staphylococcus aureus*
Purified protein derivative test for tuberculosis
Varicella (IgG)
Toxoplasma (IgG)

Diagnostic Studies (Minimum)	Consulting Services
Cardiac catheterization	Child life
Echocardiogram	Dentistry
Electrocardiogram	Immunology
	Infectious diseases
	Nutrition/Dietician
	Social Work

EBNA, Epstein-Barre nuclear antigen; PCR, polymerase chain reaction; RSV, respiratory syncytial virus.

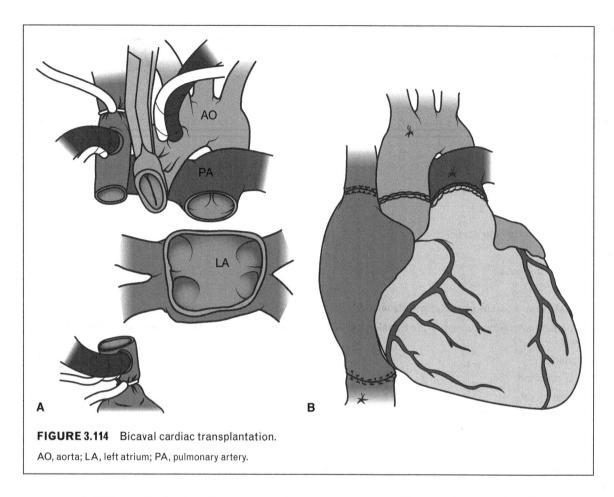

FIGURE 3.114 Bicaval cardiac transplantation.

AO, aorta; LA, left atrium; PA, pulmonary artery.

and use of iNO or afterload reduction may be needed if the PVR remains elevated following transplant. Inotropic agents may be necessary to support right and/or left ventricular function, especially with higher PVR and longer donor ischemic times. Assess for bradycardia resulting from the denervated heart and anticipate the use of chronotropic agents such as isoproterenol (Isuprel) or pacing to support CO. PVCs and short runs of VT may occur due to an irritable myocardium following ischemic stress. Notation of two P waves on ECG is common, reflecting presence of both donor and recipient sinus nodes (Thrush & Hoffman, 2014).

2. *Assess for signs and symptoms of rejection on physical examination, ECG, echo, and endomyocardial biopsy.*

a. Signs and symptoms of rejection vary widely. Patients may be asymptomatic or have nonspecific symptoms such as fatigue, nausea, malaise, emesis, fever, and increased HR from baseline. Symptoms of RV dysfunction, such as edema, abdominal distension, palpitations, AV block, or bradycardia, may be present. Symptoms of LV dysfunction include exceptional dyspnea, orthopnea, and pulmonary edema. As rejection worsens, symptoms of HF/low CO and the end-organ effects are more pronounced, including lethargy, somnolence, oliguria, hypotension, cardiogenic shock, and death.

b. Echo may show decreased systolic or diastolic function, new or worsening AV regurgitation, and the development of a pericardial effusion.

c. The ECG may demonstrate decreased voltages and the presence of a new arrhythmia.

d. Endomyocardial biopsy will grade the degree and type of rejection and is used to guide treatment.

e. Types of rejection include acute cellular rejection (ACR) and antibody-mediated rejection (AMR; Rossano, Cabrera, Shaddy, 2016).

  i. ACR is the most common type of rejection noted in the first 6 months after transplant. The pathology associated with ACR is the presence of lymphocytes in the myocardium found at endomyocardial biopsy. It is a mononuclear inflammatory infiltrate, primarily T-cell-mediated, rejection response aimed against the cardiac allograft.

  ii. AMR occurs when circulating antibodies in the body attack the transplanted heart. The pathology associated with AMR is the presence of capillary endothelial activation and macrophage and/or neutrophil infiltration without edema or hemorrhage accompanied by vascular immunofluorescent deposits of immunoglobulin and complement. This type of rejection is primarily B cell mediated. Specific risk factors associated with acute AMR include a positive crossmatch, presence of donor-specific antibodies, history of elevated panel reactive antibody prior to transplant, and previous cardiac surgeries.

  iii. Treatment of rejection depends on type and severity of rejection, clinical symptoms, and hemodynamic status. For ACR, consider steroids and thymoglobulin. For AMR, consider maximizing current immunosuppression, plasmapheresis, IVIG, and cyclophosphamide.

  iv. In all types of rejection, treatment goals include support of the donor graft and end-organ function.

3. *Provide immunosuppressive medications* (see section "Therapeutic Modalities That Depress the Functions of the Hematologic and Immunologic Systems" in Chapter 8).

a. Induction phase goal (in the immediate postoperative period) is targeted at preventing acute allograft rejection. The current standard is high-dose steroids for multisite immune suppression combined with antilymphocyte antibodies (such as thymoglobulin or ATGAM) and medications to reduce cell-mediated hypersensitivity (such as mycophenolate mofetil or azathioprine; Rossano, Cabrera, Shaddy, 2016).

b. As soon as renal function can tolerate their use, calcineurin inhibitors (CNIs, such as cyclosporine or tacrolimus) will be added. These agents may exacerbate nephrotoxicity in the immediate postoperative phase.

c. Maintenance phase goal (first year after transplant) is to sustain immunosuppression while minimizing CNI exposure and prevent long-term toxicities of all immunosuppressive agents. One approach is triple medication combination of CNI, antimetabolite (mycophenolate mofetil or azathioprine), and glucocorticoids. Newer agents with more selective immunosuppression and fewer side effects are being introduced to cardiac transplant care (Rossano, Cabrera, & Shaddy, 2016).

4. *Assess for signs and symptoms of infection.* Surgical prophylaxis is institutional specific. *Pneumocystis carinii* pneumonia (PCP), cytomegalovirus (CMV), candida, and endocarditis prophylaxis are initiated by all institutions; however, specific medications, timing of initiation, and dosages are institution, patient, and donor specific.

G. Complications

1. *General long-term complications* include rejection, infection, lymphoproliferative disease, accelerated coronary artery disease, hypertension, renal insufficiency or failure, primary organ failure, and death (Thrush & Hoffman, 2014).

2. *Specific early or late complications* include RV dysfunction due to persistent and unresponsive elevations in PVR, biventricular dysfunction from long donor ischemic times and/or long bypass times for the transplant procedure, sinus node dysfunction and/or bradycardia due to denervation of the graft, bleeding in the immediate postoperative period specifically if a second sternotomy with the presence of scar tissue and the need for extensive dissection, and hyperglycemia and fluid retentions as a response to stress or use of high-dose steroids.

CARDIAC TRAUMA

A. Pathophysiology

1. The *pathophysiology* of cardiac trauma depends on the mechanism of injury (Smith, 2016).

    a. *Myocardial contusion* may cause bruising, swelling, muscle dysfunction, internal bleeding, and tamponade.

    b. *Major vessel or cardiac rupture* can occur by narrowing the anteroposterior diameter of the chest. This results in rapid compression and expansion of vessel structures, which produce shearing forces, tearing the aorta, SVC, IVC, or atrial appendage leading to sudden massive blood loss with shock or tamponade (Figure 3.115).

2. *Cardiac tamponade* can occur from a contusion or from penetrating trauma, resulting in blood or fluid accumulation in the pericardial sac. The fluid accumulation impairs ventricular filling and reduces CO (Figure 3.116).

B. Etiology of Cardiac Trauma

1. *Compression* injury results from a direct blow in which the sternum or ribs strike the heart. This impact can cause creation of septal defects, cardiac wall or valve rupture, and coronary artery occlusion. Direct blows to the chest and heart can cause fatal arrhythmias (Holt, 2016).

2. *Acceleration/deceleration* injury may result in avulsion or tears of the aorta, SVC, IVC, or pulmonary veins (Holt, 2016).

3. *Changes in intrachamber pressures* from crush injuries of the abdomen may produce blowout ruptures of cardiac valves, vessels, or septum (Holt, 2016).

4. *Punctures* occur from fractured ribs, bullets, knifes, or other sharp penetrating objects. Another cause of penetrating cardiac trauma involves impaling injuries from falls.

C. Clinical Signs and Symptoms

1. A *high index of suspicion for cardiac trauma* occurs when rib fractures and other chest trauma are diagnosed. A pliable thorax decreases the likelihood of rib fractures in children. With fractures of the first or second rib, assess for aortic arch injury or rupture.

2. *Symptoms of cardiac injury* include widening of the superior mediastinum on chest radiograph, deviation of the nasogastric tube from midline, chest pain, arrhythmias (particularly during transport), bruising on the chest, jugular venous distention, signs of shock and poor systemic perfusion, muffled heart sounds, higher BP in the arms than the legs, and pulsus paradoxus.

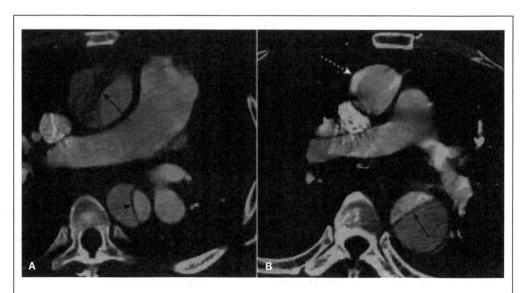

FIGURE 3.115 Aortic dissections.

Source: Reprinted with permission from Herring, W. (2012). *Learning radiology* (2nd ed.). Philadelphia, PA: Elsevier.

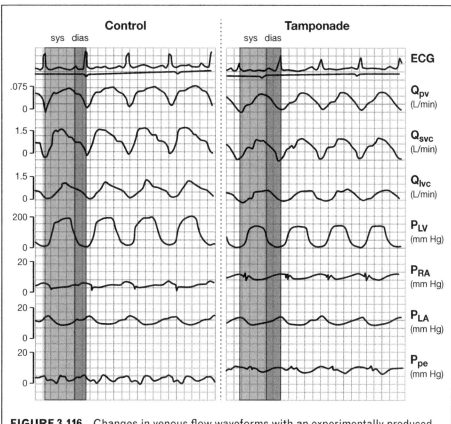

FIGURE 3.116 Changes in venous flow waveforms with an experimentally produced cardiac tamponade in dogs.

dias, diastolic; sys, systolic.

D. Diagnostic Studies

1. *CXR* may demonstrate changes in the cardiac shadow. Blood collection in the pericardium may present on x-ray as an enlarged heart size.

2. *ECG* is relatively insensitive but may show conduction problems, such as RBBB or decreased biventricular forces, if there is bleeding to pericardium and tamponade.

3. *Cardiac enzymes* may help to identify potential cardiac trauma. If the creatine phosphokinase alone is high, it may be from skeletal muscle trauma not cardiac trauma. Enzyme levels may rise slowly if there is no period of compromised myocardial flow or cardiac arrest.

4. *Echo* is used to identify tamponade and show differential ventricular wall motion. A transesophageal echo is used to rule out aortic dissection. Aortogram

or CT angiogram defines aortic injuries, aneurysm, or rupture.

5. *Radionuclide angiography* delineates vascular injuries.

6. *Pericardiocentesis* relieves the pressure from cardiac tamponade resulting from trauma and bleeding. It will not stop the process causing tamponade and often a chest drain is left in place to relieve ongoing fluid buildup until more definitive treatment can occur.

E. Goals and Patient Management

1. *Treat shock* (see "Shock" section).

2. *Surgical intervention* may be required, including pericardiocentesis or emergency thoracotomy/sternotomy.

3. *Endovascular stents* are used for aortic rupture if the risk of CPB or bleeding is prohibitively high.

4. *Minimize shear stress on aortic wall* prior to repair with administration of β-blockers. Support cardiac recovery with the use of inotropic agents and after-load reduction. Maintain preload as necessary to replace volume losses.

5. *Continual assessment and support* of end-organ function is required, especially if there was a period of hypotension or cardiac arrest/hypoxemia prior to surgical repair, if indicated.

F. Complications

1. *Complications* include exsanguination, cardiac arrest (mortality for traumatic cardiac arrest is very high), arrhythmias, and tamponade (see also "Multiple Trauma" in Chapter 9).

CASE STUDIES WITH QUESTIONS, ANSWERS, AND RATIONALES

Case Study 3.1

A 3.4-kg female infant with dysmorphic facial features, cleft palate, and small mouth on initial physical examination is admitted to your care. Referring hospital reports that at 10 hours of age she refused oral feedings, was poorly perfused without palpable pedal pulses, was tachycardic and tachypneic with increased work of breathing. An arterial blood gas demonstrated a lactate of 6.8, a base deficit of 7 with adequate oxygenation, and a normal pH. The infant is urgently transferred to your hospital.

1. Prior to transfer to your hospital what initial intervention(s) should be performed?
   A. Endotracheal intubation
   B. Initiation of PGE₁ despite inability to obtain echocardiogram
   C. Initiation of vasoactive agent to support ventricular function
   D. Placement of invasive monitoring lines, UAC/UVC
   E. All of the above

2. How would you know that your intervention(s) were effective?
   A. Improved pulses and systemic perfusion
   B. Stable lactate, base deficit
   C. Decreased respiratory rate with persistent increased work of breathing and grunting
   D. Narrow pulse pressure

Initial laboratory studies indicate an ionized calcium of 0.7 with a creatinine of 0.9. The CBC, platelets, and remaining electrolytes remain within normal range. Repeat arterial blood gas shows a lactate of 3.4 and a base deficit of 4.

3. What is your differential diagnosis at this time?
   A. Systemic outflow obstruction, possible Turner syndrome
   B. Pulmonary outflow obstruction, possible Noonan's syndrome
   C. Systemic outflow obstruction, possible DiGeorge/velocardiofacial syndrome
   D. Systemic outflow obstruction, possible CHARGE association

The admission chest x-ray demonstrates a narrow mediastinum. A renal ultrasound is obtained due to the period of hypoperfusion and dysmorphism. The renal ultrasound shows hydronephrosis of the left kidney. An echocardiogram demonstrates interrupted aortic arch, ventricular septal defect, and a patent ductus arteriosus. The left ventricular outflow tract is narrowed with posterior deviation of the conal septum.

4. What intervention(s) are important in the overall management of this patient?
   A. Reinstitution of systemic perfusion and maintenance of end-organ function
   B. Obtain chromosomal microanalysis prior to possible transfusion
   C. Close evaluation of electrolytes, particularly hypocalcemia and hypomagnesemia
   D. Screening cranial ultrasound
   E. All of the above

5. In counseling the family, what support and anticipatory guidance discussion might you have?
   A. Palliative care, social work, and genetics referral
   B. Encourage breastfeeding and pumping to maintain supply
   C. Avoid family presence during resuscitative measures and procedures as diagnosis a shock
   D. Ensure the family that the genetic abnormality will not interfere with normal growth and development and future school and sport participation

The infant stabilizes, all organ function is normal, and surgical intervention is scheduled. The planned intervention is VSD closure and aortic arch reconstruction.

6. What specific interventions are required for this patient when going to the operating room?
   A. Perform newborn screen and newborn hearing screen prior to operation

B. Send type and screen for blood for the operating room, ensuring blood bank is aware the infant meets criteria for irradiated blood products
C. Ensure head MRI has been completed
D. Consult with craniofacial surgery for discussion of cleft palate

7. When you are preparing to receive this patient from the operating room what assessments are specific to this infant's diagnosis?
   A. Measurement daily of upper and lower extremity blood pressure
   B. Assessment of neurologic status due to the need for cardiopulmonary bypass/low flow bypass/circulatory arrest
   C. Close monitoring of serum calcium
   D. All of the above

The baby is now back in the ICU following repair. The postoperative echocardiogram shows no residual VSD, no residual arch gradient, but diffusely hypoplastic arch, narrowed subaortic area with gradient of 20 mmHg. The chest tube output is minimal. The CVP and LA pressure are 8 mmHg and 4 mmHg, respectively. The blood pressure is 60/35. The perfusion is adequate and the lactate is 2.8 mmol/L.

8. What potential postoperative complication(s) are you alert to in your care?
   A. Low cardiac output syndrome
   B. Electrolyte abnormalities
   C. Subclinical or clinical seizures
   D. Arrhythmia
   E. All of the above

The blood pressure is now 50/25 mmHg and the CVP and LA pressure are 3 mmHg, the perfusion is decreased with oliguria the past 2 hours and cool extremities. The HR is 220 bpm, increasing slowly over the past 45 minutes. The chest tube output is 30 mL/hr for the last 2 hours. The lactate is now 6.8 mmol/L.

9. What are the potential etiologies for this clinical picture?
   A. Complete heart block from surgical intervention
   B. Residual arch obstruction
   C. Hypovolemia
   D. Tamponade

The baby is given 10 mL/kg of blood and albumin and the blood pressure is marginally improved to 55/28, the HR remains elevated, the CVP/LA are now 6 and 7 mmHg, and the urine output and perfusion remain marginal. The lactate remains 7 mmol/L.

10. What else might you consider?
    A. Evaluation for arrhythmia
    B. Continue to infuse volume replacement

C. Continue increasing vasoactive agents
D. Echocardiogram to rule out tamponade

The HR is unchanged and the infant is found to be in junctional ectopic tachycardia with a HR of 190. Blood pressure remains marginal and lactate is now 8.

11. What intervention(s) should you anticipate?
    A. Hold volume replacement as you know the clinical deterioration is related to the arrhythmia
    B. Atrial overdrive pacing
    C. Ensure maintenance of normothermia to avoid increased afterload on ventricles
    D. Administer a loading dose of amiodarone (5 mg/kg) over 1 hour and initiate amiodarone infusion at 5 mcg/kg/min

You have the rhythm/HR controlled and the blood pressure is improving with lactate reduction to 2.7. About 4 hours later the CVP and LA rise to 13 and the chest tube output stops. The blood pressure is 50/40 mmHg. The lactate is now 6 mmol/L. You give volume without change in blood pressure but with further increase in LA and CVP to 16 mmHg.

12. What may be occurring?
    A. Low cardiac output related to hypovolemia from past chest tube output
    B. Acute left ventricular dysfunction
    C. Dehiscence of VSD patch
    D. Cardiac tamponade

13. Your treatment goal(s) are the following:
    A. Maintain volume and vasoactive support
    B. Ensure replacement of electrolytes, particularly if large volumes of blood products are transfused
    C. Prepare for emergent surgical exploration of the chest for clot or bleeding and prepare the family for sternal exploration and provide explanation of treatment
    D. Ensure patency of chest tube
    E. All of the above

The chest is explored. There is an old clot occluding the chest tube that is removed. The CVP is 8 mmHg and the LA pressure is now 4 mmHg. The blood pressure is now 70/38, and the HR is controlled on amiodarone and atrial pacing at a rate of 150 bpm. She is beginning to increase urine output and the lactate is now 3.2 mmol/L. Diuresis continues well over the next several days and the sternum is closed and progress is made toward extubation. The infant is extubated and immediately demonstrates increased retractions and tachypnea.

A chest x-ray shows both diaphragms in good position, atelectasis, but no collapse of either lung. Respiratory distress is worsening with the presence of inspiratory stridor and no audible cry with agitation.

14. What do you expect as the next step?
   A. Aggressive pulmonary toilet
   B. Respiratory treatments with inhaled albuterol and pulmicort
   C. Decadron and otolaryngology evaluation
   D. Sedation to ease work of breathing

Case Study 3.2

You are working in the pediatric emergency department and an 18-month-old previously healthy toddler is brought in, accompanied by her parents. They report that she has been "under the weather" with a cold for a few days and had the flu about a week ago. She has not had much appetite or energy but they attributed that to the flu and cold. This morning she refuses to get out of bed and her color is "off" and her breathing is hard. You begin to examine the child while waiting for the physicians to arrive.

1. What are you assessing for in particular?
   A. HR, respiratory rate, work of breathing
   B. Temperature and signs of rash or other potentially infectious disease
   C. Hydration status and perfusion
   D. State of consciousness
   E. All of the above

You note edema, a gallop rhythm, tachycardia, tachypnea with retractions and wheezing, hypotension, and decreased peripheral pulses. She is barely responsive to your exam. The physicians order the following studies: serum electrolytes, renal and liver function tests, blood and urine viral and bacterial cultures, a chest x-ray, ECG, and echocardiogram. The chest x-ray demonstrates moderate cardiomegaly with mild pulmonary edema, the laboratory tests demonstrate mildly elevated liver and renal function, decreased serum albumin, her ECG shows left atrial dilation, and the echocardiogram shows a moderately dilated left ventricle without hypertrophy, decreased systolic function, and moderate to severe mitral regurgitation with a severely dilated LA.

2. Which diagnosis is first on your differential diagnosis list?
   A. Hypertrophic cardiomyopathy
   B. Left ventricular noncompaction
   C. Anomalous LCA from the PA
   D. Dilated cardiomyopathy

All serologies are negative. The BNP is markedly elevated at 3,500. She is increasingly obtunded and her blood pressure decreases to 60/40 mmHg with a HR of 180 bpm in sinus rhythm, her respiratory work is markedly increased now with grunting. She is placed on dopamine and milrinone with volume replacement. After a short period of stabilization, you note acute onset of nonperfusing ventricular tachycardia.

3. What is/are your next step(s)?
   A. Page the physician in charge of the patient
   B. Ask the family to step out of the room
   C. Initiate PALS protocols
   D. Page the palliative care team

The child is intubated, intraosseous infusion (IO) inserted, and she is defibrillated three times with eventual conversion to NSR. An arterial and venous line are now in place. She is on dopamine and milrinone with sinus tachycardia and hypotension. Her lactate is 10 and base deficit 15. She is transported to the ICU and upon admission to the ICU her blood pressure falls to 40/20 mmHg per arterial line, her HR is 40 bpm. PALS protocols are initiated again without response to increased vasoactive infusions, vasopressin and epinephrine boluses, and volume resuscitation.

4. Per PALS protocol, what do you expect the next line of therapy to be?
   A. Paging social work and chaplain to discuss end-of-life care and decision making
   B. Aggressive fluid resuscitation
   C. Contact the ECMO team for emergent cannulation to ECMO
   D. Contact the heart failure team and plan for evaluation for transplant

The toddler is now on EMCO with maintenance of adequate perfusion and has weaned from vasoactives with an SVO₂ of 65 and an arterial saturation maintained at 95. Blood and urine cultures remain negative and over the next 5 days her organ function returns to baseline. Her ventilator is at rest settings. She has started enteral trophic feedings and is advancing to full enteral feedings.

5. While on ECMO your nursing care centers on the following:
   A. Avoiding venipunctures or removal of indwelling catheters to prevent bleeding
   B. Maintain neck in neutral position and secure cannulas to prevent dislodgement
   C. Coordinate care with ECMO specialist to prevent complications of ECMO circuit
   D. Perform surveillance cultures for risk of infection
   E. All of the above

6. Considering the cardiac arrest sustained prior to ECMO cannulation, what postresuscitation measures should you consider?
   A. Maintain normothermia to avoid risk of infection
   B. Provide 100% oxygen to maintain saturation greater than 98 for increased organ perfusion
   C. Hypothermia for neuroprotection using the ECMO circuit to maintain temperature
   D. Heavy sedation and analgesia +/− neuromuscular blocking agents

Following a week of ECMO support, repeated attempts at weaning are unsuccessful. Echocardiogram shows severe LA and LV dilation without hypertrophy and severe LV dysfunction. Other organ systems are stable and functioning well, and the patient is neurologically intact.

7. What are the options for this child?
   A. Wean from ECMO to conventional vasoactive and ventilator support with volume resuscitation as needed while preparing the family for the possibility of withdrawal of support
   B. Plan transition to Berlin heart LVAD/RVAD as a destination therapy
   C. Perform a cardiac catheterization and endomyocardial biopsy to rule out active myocarditis and to determine PA pressure and resistance and, if needed, perform pulmonary reactivity testing prior to consideration for transplant listing
   D. Continue current ECMO management strategy with no need for further evaluation at this time

8. If transplantation was to be considered as an option what would this evaluation entail?
   A. Immune evaluation for HLA and PRA to alert the transplant team to possible needed prelisting therapies for elevated antibody activity
   B. Brain MRI or CT for evidence of current or previous stroke, which would preclude listing
   C. Developmental assessment, financial assessment, social assessment as failure of the child or family to meet these criteria would preclude transplant listing
   D. Evaluation of all organ systems via laboratory tests and imaging studies as indicated as evidence of any end-organ dysfunction will preclude transplant

It is now ECMO day 10 and she remains unable to wean from ECMO support. She weighs 10 kg. Mechanical cardiac support with transitioning from ECMO to a ventricular assist device is being considered.

9. Of the patient-specific factors listed, which of the following does not impact decision for transitioning from ECMO to VAD?
   A. Patient size/weight
   B. Organ system function
   C. Cardiac anatomy
   D. Blood type

She survives to transplant. The family is taught about the potential complications of heart transplantation and how to monitor for these.

10. These potential complications include which of the following?
    A. Graft rejection
    B. Infection
    C. Lymphoproliferative disease
    D. Graft atherosclerosis
    E. All of the above

Case Study 3.3

You are caring for a 2-week-old infant presenting with irritability, poor feeding, and tachypnea of 1-day duration. The pregnancy and delivery were uneventful. He has been eating well and gaining weight. No interval illness. On admission, the HR is 220 bpm. Liver is palpated 3 cm below the right costal margin. There is no murmur, rub, or gallop. No fever. Perfusion is diminished with cool extremities and peripheral pulses are 1+ throughout. You take his diaper off and he startles and his HR decreases to 150 bpm. A few minutes later his HR jumps to 220 bpm again.

1. What do you suspect is the most likely cause of the tachycardia?
   A. Sinus tachycardia
   B. Junctional tachycardia
   C. Atrial flutter
   D. Supraventricular tachycardia

Following a 12-lead ECG it is determined the arrhythmia is SVT. His vital signs remain stable while continuing to go in and out of SVT with HRs of up to 240.

2. Possible intervention(s) at this time include which of the following?
   A. Vagal maneuvers, including ice to face, rectal temperature to break the tachycardia
   B. Adenosine as a slow IV infusion to avoid hypotension
   C. Oxygen therapy to support oxygen delivery
   D. Beta-blocker IV push to control the HR

He remains in SVT and his blood pressure and perfusion begin to deteriorate. Vagal maneuvers are no longer breaking the rhythm. His HR is now 260 with a blood pressure of 70/45 mmHg and oxygen saturation of 96%. He is mottled and cool but with palpable peripheral pulses. He is irritable. The decision to administer adenosine is made.

3. Of the following, which is the most unlikely to occur with the injection of adenosine?
   A. Reduction in HR with return to and maintenance of NSR within 5 minutes of the first injection
   B. Possibility of needing repeated and higher doses of adenosine to obtain a sustained reduction in HR

C. Pause/block of the arrhythmia with a brief asystolic period following adenosine administration

D. Startling and crying with injection of adenosine, as the infant will experience chest pain with its administration

Case Study 3.4

A 2-month-old infant with a large VSD is admitted to the hospital in CHF. The parents report she was fine until about 6 weeks of age and then her feedings seemed to be reduced and take longer and she was breathing harder and resting while eating. They said they were concerned because she didn't gain weight between her 4-week checkup and when she went for her immunizations at 6 weeks.

1. What other signs/symptoms of heart failure might you expect to find?

A. Easy respiratory work, clear breath sounds, no increased work of breathing

B. Playful, sleeps well, alert

C. Diaphoresis, poor feeding, and poor weight gain

D. Diaphoresis, frequent emesis, bilateral rales

2. Why did the infant not present with signs and symptoms of CHF until 6 to 8 weeks of life?

A. It takes time for ventricular hypertrophy and dilation to develop and cause CHF symptoms

B. Initial growth in the first weeks of life mask the poor feeding and weight loss at 6 weeks

C. The pulmonary resistance normally decreases at about 6 weeks of age, increasing the left-to-right shunt and pulmonary blood flow causing pulmonary overcirculation and CHF

D. Initial weight loss up to 10% of birth weight is normal in the first 1 to 2 weeks of life and masks poor feeding associated with CHF

3. Nutritional competency was difficult to maintain in this infant. Why? Choose all that apply.

A. Increased caloric expenditure due to increased metabolic demands from CHF

B. Decreased caloric intake due to fatigue, tachypnea with feeding

C. Vitamin D deficiency is common in patients with CHF

D. Potential feeding intolerance due to gastric reflux, bowel edema, and hepatomegaly

4. What intervention(s) can be utilized to support nutritional competence in infants with CHF?

A. Multivitamin and vitamin D supplementation unless receiving only infant formula and then no supplementation is needed

B. Nasogastric tube supplementation to ensure adequate caloric intake and weight gain

C. Increasing caloric density of feedings to support weight gain with intake to as high as 90 to 100 cal/kg/d as tolerated

D. Use parenteral nutrition and lipid infusions only to provide adequate calories in patients with CHF and poor bowel perfusion

Answers and Rationales

Case Study 3.1

1. **E.** Endotracheal intubation is required to support respiratory and cardiovascular function and ensure ventilation during transport as apnea is a side effect of PGE_1. This neonate is demonstrating signs and symptoms of an obstructive congenital heart lesion (i.e., coarctation of the aorta, interrupted aortic arch) with compromised systemic perfusion. Initial stabilization using PGE_1 to maintain ductal patency and prevent and/or correct end-organ dysfunction are required in these neonates. PGE_1 is utilized to maintain patency of the ductus arteriosus and systemic perfusion. Initiation of vasoactive agents is needed to support the ventricle and cardiac output following a shock presentation. Secure IV access for PGE_1, vasoactive medications, and other resuscitative medications should be present prior to transport.

2. **A.** Systemic circulation will be promoted with blood flow through the ductus arteriosus to the descending aorta and systemic circulation. Improved pulses and systemic perfusion indicate that the ductus arteriosus is patent and adequate blood flow achieved. This should improve the lactate and base deficit as perfusion improves and metabolism converts back to aerobic. The respiratory rate may or may not improve, but the work of breathing should improve with improved cardiac output and decreased acidosis. The pulse pressure will be normal, not narrow, as the perfusion increases and cardiogenic shock state is treated.

3. **C.** These findings are consistent with a patient with systemic outflow obstruction, who has improved circulation and systemic perfusion with the institution of PGE_1 to maintain ductal patency. DiGeorge/velocardiofacial syndrome is associated with an increased risk of aortic arch abnormalities, facial dysmorphisms, and cleft lip and palate. Turner's syndrome, which can be associated with coarctation of the aorta, presents with a webbed neck and generally is not associated with cleft lip/palate and a small mouth. Patients with Noonan's syndrome have associated right-sided obstructive lesions, primarily pulmonary stenosis. CHARGE association has anal/recta, renal, abnormalities.

4. E. All of the responses are key to the overall management of the patient. Key to survival and decreased morbidity as well as providing for an optimal operative result is the resumption of systemic perfusion and end-organ function. In view of the dysmorphisms and associated cardiac disease, chromosomal analysis should be performed to determine need for further diagnostic testing and guide specific interventions. Patients with DiGeorge syndrome often exhibit signs of hypocalcemia and hypomagnesaemia. Monitoring and treatment of these and other electrolyte abnormalities is warranted to optimize myocardial function. This infant will require cardiac surgery using cardiopulmonary bypass/low-flow bypass or potentially circulatory arrest. Therefore, a screening cranial US is important to ensure there are no contraindications for the use of cardiopulmonary bypass that would alter the operative plan.

5. B. The neonate may be intubated and will be NPO prior to surgery. In addition, from preoperative shock and postoperative LCOS, bowel function may be at risk and the incidence of NEC is higher in these infants. These infants are also at risk of immunosuppression from age, critical illness, genetic predisposition if DiGeorge syndrome is present, and the use of cardiopulmonary bypass. Breast milk provides an easily digestible feeding that includes antibodies to assist with immune suppression, decrease the risk of NEC, and enhance feeding progression. The infant's mother should be encouraged to pump to maintain supply of breast milk until the infant can tolerate enteral feedings. This may require support from nursing, nutrition, social work, and lactation.

Social work and genetics referral are important. Palliative care is not indicated. Children with DiGeorge syndrome may have learning disabilities, renal anomalies, growth delay, and psychiatric disorders. Although social work, palliative care, and genetics referrals will be important to send at variable points in the infant's hospitalization, a better understanding of the infant's status and initial test results are required. Should resuscitation be required, family presence with appropriate staff support has been shown to increase parental adjustment. If the diagnosis of DiGeorge syndrome is confirmed, learning disabilities of variable degrees will likely be present. Generally, following repair of a VSD and an aortic arch reconstruction, contact competitive sports are restricted. Reassuring the family that future school performance and sports participation will not be altered is a false expectation.

6. B. Blood is required for surgical interventions requiring cardiopulmonary bypass in neonates. This procedure requires cardiopulmonary bypass. Patients with DiGeorge syndrome are at risk for immune deficiency and T cell subset abnormalities due to aplasia/hypoplasia of the thymus. Irradiated blood products should be utilized if the diagnosis of DiGeroge syndrome is suspected to avoid graft versus host reactions. A heart MRI is not indicated at this point, but may be required if there are neurologic complications postoperatively. Craniofacial surgery consult will be obtained after the acute phase of illness to plan intervention and timing for the cleft lip and palate. A newborn screen is performed at 24 hours of age. The hearing screen will not be performed until the infant is off oxygen and out of the ICU.

7. D. This patient is at risk for residual arch obstruction and therefore four limb BP should be obtained. Neurological complications, including stroke, seizure, hemorrhage, are a risk factor for neonates with critical illness and those requiring cardiopulmonary bypass/circulatory arrest for surgery. Close observation for clinical seizures and/or long-term EEG monitoring for subclinical seizures are important. Infants with critical illness and those with DiGeorge syndrome are prone to hypocalcemia. This is particularly important as this presents a risk of seizures and ventricular dysfunction/hypotension postoperatively. Close assessment of serum calcium, magnesium, and albumin are key to optimize electrolytes and myocardial function.

8. E. All of these potential postoperative complications may occur following neonatal cardiac surgery using cardiopulmonary bypass, regardless of the operation. Specific to this infant, electrolyte abnormalities related to DiGeorge syndrome in addition to surgery and diuretic use are common. Arrhythmias, primarily JET and heart block, can occur in the postoperative period.

9. C. Hypotension and tachycardia associated with a low CVP and brisk chest tube output result from hypovolemia regardless of etiology. A residual arch obstruction would not result in a low CVP or high CT output. Tamponade would result in rising CVP and/or LA pressures with hypotension, narrowed pulse pressure, and generally decreased or absent CT drainage. Complete heart block, if present, results in lower HR, even if there is a fast ventricular rate, not tachycardia.

10. A. Volume replacement has resulted in increased CVP/LA pressures but the BP and perfusion remain marginal, and the lactate is elevated. Assessment for an arrhythmia, primarily JET, should be undertaken. The slow rise in HR without response to volume resuscitation is characteristic of JET. Further escalation of vasoactive support may aggravate the HR and arrhythmia further. Continuing to infuse volume is acceptable but the CVP is now in the normal range and the BP has failed to increase. Tamponade is a clinical diagnosis and an echocardiogram can't unequivocally rule this out. Generally, if tamponade is present the filling pressure is elevated and the pulse pressure narrowed.

11. **D.** Intervention is indicated due to the severely compromised condition of the patient. Cool to a temperature of 35°C to 36°C, administer sedative and analgesics to decrease pain and agitation stimulus, vasoactive support using agents such as vasopressin, which have little effect on HR, and medications, such as amiodarone or procainamide, may be used. It would be anticipated that amiodarone load and infusion would be started. Overdrive pacing may be utilized once the HR is lower. Volume replacement as an adjunctive resuscitative effort may be required until the rhythm has been controlled and cardiac output improved.

12. **D.** Abnormally high CVP readings occur as a result of RV, LV, or biventricular dysfunction, TR, tricuspid stenosis, pulmonary hypertension, hypervolemia, and cardiac tamponade. In the postoperative patient with chest tube in place and an abrupt cessation of chest tube output with hypotension, acute rise in CVP with equalization of LA and CVP pressures, acute rise in CVP/LA with infusion of volume, and rising lactate, cardiac tamponade is the most likely etiology. In the presence of acute left ventricular dysfunction, the LA pressure will rise, but the CVP will remain lower. In hypovolemia, the CVP and LA will remain low despite volume replacement.

13. **E.** You would be preparing for emergent surgical bedside exploration of the chest to evacuate clot or control bleeding. You would be preparing the family for the procedure. The chest tube should be milked and the use of a Fogarty catheter to remove clot and stimulate drainage again can be attempted if the patient's condition will tolerate the time required for the procedure. With large volumes of blood transfusion, serum calcium may fall and result in hypotension that is not responsive to volume replacement. Volume replacement and vasoactive support are continued as needed to support the cardiac output until sternal exploration and tamponade are relieved.

14. **C.** Repair of aortic arch obstruction can be associated with laryngeal nerve damage. This presents

once the infant is extubated as inspiratory stridor, a soft/hoarse or inaudible cry, and increasing respiratory distress. Treatment with Decadron and urgent otolaryngology consult to assess airway stability and vocal cord function would be the next step. The use of noninvasive ventilator support may be required. Aggressive pulmonary toilet is excellent for atelectasis but may worsen the respiratory status if the patient is agitated with treatment, therefore, it may need to be modified. Acute treatment with albuterol and use of Pulmicort for long-term therapy of reactive airways are not indicated as this is not a reactive airway issue. The infant should be calm to support respiratory function but sedation may decrease respiratory drive and should be used sparingly.

Case Study 3.2

1. **E.** Assessment of this patient includes gathering data to assist in the differential diagnosis of her illness. Vital signs are key to cardiac and respiratory function. A recent history of a viral illness requires evaluation for ongoing infectious etiology of current state. If she hasn't been feeling well, her hydration may be compromised and therefore perfusion may be diminished from hypovolemia. If she is poorly perfused, hypovolemic, or in shock, she may have an altered state of consciousness. You are trying to differentiate cardiac, respiratory, and infectious etiologies for this presentation.

2. **D.** Classic presentation of a dilated cardiomyopathy is acute cardiac decompensation, evidence of mild end-organ hypoperfusion, cardiomegaly on chest x-ray, and a physical examination consistent with the findings listed. The key is an echocardiogram-demonstrated ventricular dilation and decreased systolic function without ventricular hypertrophy as a response. Mitral regurgitation and LA enlargement result. An anomalous coronary artery will generally present with decreased systolic function with hypertrophy and dilation. Hypertrophic cardiomyopathy and left ventricular noncompaction are not associated with ventricular dilation.

3. **A and C.** Initiate PALS protocols and simultaneously call for help, asking for the physician to be paged. The family should be allowed to remain in the room if they so desire, and the code lead should identify a support person for the family. The palliative care team may need to be paged at some time in the course of this patient's care, but at this time this is not a priority.

4. **C.** The ECMO team should be immediately contacted for initiation of extracorporeal cardiopulmonary resuscitation (eCPR) as there is no response to PALS protocols at this time. Aggressive fluid resuscitation may continue with careful assessment of the dilated ventricle's response to such volume infusions. Paging social work and the chaplain, if not already done, is appropriate, but for family support, not discussions of end-of-life care. Referral to the heart failure/transplant team may also be appropriate; however, not at this time in the patient's care.

5. **E.** While anticoagulated on ECMO, venipunctures and removal of indwelling vascular access lines are contraindicated due to bleeding risk. Removal of temporary pacing wires and chest tubes is generally also contraindicated. Placement of feeding tubes is performed with the assistance of the ECMO team and under controlled circumstances. All care, including turning and suctioning, is performed in coordination with the ECMO specialist. Surveillance cultures are performed every 2 to 3 days as temperature is controlled on the circuit and may inhibit early detection of infection. To avoid kinking of the venous cannula and circuit malfunction and to ensure there is no accidental dislodgement of the cannulas, the head is maintained in the neutral position when the patient is turned or repositioned.

6. **C.** Hypothermia for a period of 24 to 48 hours may provide neuroprotection and will decrease metabolic demand. Normothermia will not decrease the risk of infection. Providing 100% oxygen with saturations greater than 98% may produces free oxygen radical formation and cause further end-organ damage. Heavy sedation/analgesia ± neuromuscular blockade may indeed be warranted, however, if these are utilized in this situation, placement of long-term monitoring EEG is also warranted.

7. **C.** At this time, it is evident that weaning from ECMO support is not imminent and therefore consideration of future therapy should include transplantation. Therefore, cardiac catheterization, biopsy, pulmonary pressure, and resistance testing are warranted with then consideration and evaluation for transplantation and eventual listing. Conversion to a VAD is another realistic option, especially to allow for potential recovery of the myocardium or if needed to provide for transition while awaiting transplant. At this time, use as destination therapy only is premature. Without evidence of a medical condition that would preclude transplantation, weaning from ECMO and preparing the family for end-of-life care is premature. Continuing ECMO without any further plan is not an option

as there has been no myocardial recovery in over a week and the risk of ECMO complications will continue to increase.

8. **A.** A full immunologic evaluation is vital to prevent hyperacute or acute rejection and risk graft loss. If pretransplant testing shows abnormal elevations in antibody activity medications or plasmaphoresis can be utilized and the patients immunology studies retested. Minor degrees of end-organ dysfunction believed to be reversible are not a contraindication to transplant. Previous stroke as identified on MRI/CT is also not an absolute contraindication to transplant. Developmental, social, and financial evaluations are used to guide future assistance decisions for the family and child, not to determine listing status.

9. **D.** The blood type is not relevant to transition to a VAD. Cardiac anatomy, specifically single ventricle anatomy is a consideration. Patient weight/size is important when determining the type of VAD to use. Organ system function is important as if there is evidence of irreversible organ dysfunction; conversion to a VAD is not indicated.

10. **E.** All of these are potential complications of cardiac transplantation.

Case Study 3.3

1. **D.** The most likely etiology of a tachycardia with evidence of CHF that increases quickly and terminates with a vagal maneuver is supraventricular tachycardia. Sinus tachycardia will not increase and terminates quickly. Junctional tachycardia increases slowly in rate and does not abruptly terminate. It would be extremely rare for an infant without previous cardiac history or surgery to present in atrial flutter. Also, atrial flutter does not increase and decrease rates as this infant demonstrated.

2. **A.** The infant is hemodynamically stable at this time; therefore, use of vagal maneuvers to break the tachycardia are indicated at this time. Adenosine should be given as fast IV push with rapid saline flush. Beta-blockers may be used, generally orally, to control recurrent SVT. They are never given IV push. Oxygen therapy in a patient with hemodynamically important SVT is not contraindicated, in a hemodynamically stable patient, it is not necessary and it will not increase oxygen delivery.

3. **A.** Adenosine is given as a fast IV push with a flush to follow this. The first injection often does not terminate the arrhythmia, but multiple injections

with increasing doses may be required. There is chest pain associated with the injection and the infant may startle or cry with its administration. The pain response is of short duration. The family should be prepared for a short pause or even the potential of heart block for several seconds follow administration of adenosine prior to termination of the arrhythmia and return to NSR.

Case Study 3.4

1. **C.** Infants with CHF demonstrate poor weight gain, poor feeding, and diaphoresis with feeding. The infants are usually not playful and happy and do not sleep well. Early in the course of CHF they may not have increased work of breathing, but they will be tachypneic. As the CHF increases the work of breathing also increases. The breath sounds may or may not demonstrate rales.

2. **C.** The normal transition of the neonatal circulation and pressures takes 4 to 6 weeks. Therefore, as the right-sided pressures are initially elevated the VSD does not shunt left to right until the pulmonary resistance falls at 4 to 6 weeks of life. In infants with a large VSD, this drop in pulmonary resistance results in left to right shunting of blood through the VSD. This results in increased pulmonary blood flow, tachypnea, tachycardia, and diaphoresis with feeding, poor feeding, and lack of weight gain. Ventricular dilation and/or hypertrophy may eventually occur depending on how long the VSD is present prior to repair; however, they do not cause the symptoms of heart failure.

3. **A, B, C, and D.** All of these are true for infants with CHF and nutritional incompetence.

4. **B.** Use of a nasogastric tube to supplement oral intake will ensure appropriate caloric and volume intake and can be increased as tolerated if weight gain is not established. Increasing caloric density of the feedings can be utilized to assist with caloric competency while restricting total volume. This may require up to 130 to 140 cal/kg/d. Multivitamins and vitamin D may be required in newborns regardless of breast milk or formula feeding. The use of only TPN and lipids is not indicated unless there is a functional bowel issue.

REFERENCES

Abman, S., Hansmann, G., Archer, S. L., Ivy, D. D., Adatia, I., Chung, W. K., ... Wessel, D. L. (2015). Pediatric pulmonary hypertension. Guidelines from the American Heart Association and American Thoracic Society. *Circulation, 132*, 2037–2099. Retrieved from http://circ.ahajournals.org/content/132/21/2037

Adachi, I., Burki, S., Zafar, F., & Morales, D. L. S. (2015). Pediatric ventricular assist devices. *Journal of Thoracic Disease, 7*(12), 2194–2202.

Adams, F. H., Emmanouilides, G. C., & Riemenschneider, T. A. (2016). *Moss' heart disease in infants, children, and adolescents* (9th ed.). Philadelphia, PA: Elsevier.

Almond, C. (2013). Berlin Heart EXCOR pediatric ventricular assist device for bridge to heart transplantation in US children. *Circulation, 127*(16), 1702–1711.

Alvarez, J. A., Orav, E. J., Wilkinson, J. D., Fleming, L. E., Lee, D. J., Sleeper, L. A, ... Lipshultz, S. E. (2011). Competing risks for death and cardiac transplantation in children with dilated cardiomyopathy: Results from the Pediatric Cardiomyopathy Registry. *Circulation, 124*(7), 814–823. doi:10.1161/CIRCULATIONAHA.110.973826

American Heart Association. (2015). *Pediatric advanced life support provider manual*. Dallas, TX: Author.

Atkins, D., de Caen, A. R., Berger, S., Samson, R. A., Schexnayder, S. M., Joyner, B. L., ... Meaney, P. A. (2018). 2017 American Heart Association focused update on pediatric basic life support and cardiopulmonary resuscitation quality. *Circulation, 137*, e1–e6. doi:10.1161/CIR.0000000000000540

Averin, K. (2012). Postoperative assessment of laryngopharyngeal dysfunction in neonates after norwood operation. *Annals of Thoracic Surgery, 94*(4), 1257–1261.

Backer, C. L., & Mavroudis, C. (2013a). Atrial septal defect, partial anomalous pulmonary venous connection and scimitar syndrome. In C. Mavroudis & K. L. Backer (Eds.), *Pediatric cardiac surgery* (4th ed., pp. 295–310). Hoboken, NJ: Wiley-Blackwell.

Backer, C. L., & Mavroudis, C. (2013b). Atrioventricular canal defects. In C. Mavroudis & C. L. Backer (Eds.), *Pediatric cardiac surgery* (4th ed., pp. 342–360). Hoboken, NJ: Wiley-Blackwell.

Balady, G. J., & Morise, A. P. (2015). Exercise testing. In D. L. Mann, R. O. Bonow, D. P Zipes, & P. Libby (Eds.), *Braunwald's heart disease: A textbook of cardiovascular medicine* (10th ed., pp. 155–174). Philadelphia, PA: Elsevier-Saunders.

Baltimore, R. S., Gewitz, M., Baddour, L. M., Beerman, L. B., Jackson, M. A., Lockhart, P. B., ... Willoughby, R. (2015). Infective endocarditis in childhood: 2015 update: A scientific statement from the American Heart Association. *Circulation, 132*(15), 1487–1515.

Bates, L. S. (2017). *Bate's guide to physical examination and history taking* (12th ed.). Philadelphia, PA: Wolters-Kluwer Health/Lippincott Williams & Wilkins.

Bharucha, R., Lee, K. J., Daubeney, P. E. F., Nugent, A. W., Turner, C., Sholler, G. F., . . . National Australian Childhood Cardiomyopathy Study Investigators (2015). Sudden death in childhood cardiomyopathy. *Journal of the American College of Cardiology, 65*(21), 2302–2310. doi:10.1016/j.jacc.2015.03.552

Brescia, S. T., Rossano, J. W., Pignatelli, R., Jefferies, J. L., Price, J. F., Decker, J. A., ... Kim, J. J. (2013). Mortality and sudden death in pediatric left ventricular noncompaction in a tertiary referral center. *Circulation, 127*(22), 2202–2208.

Bronicki, R. A., & Chang, A. C. (2011). Management of the postoperative pediatric cardiac surgical patient. *Critical Care Medicine, 39*(8), 1974–1984.

Bronicki, R. A., Taylor, M., & Baden, H. (2016). Critical heart failure and shock. *Pediatric Critical Care Medicine, 17*(8), S124–S130.

Brown, D. W., Mangeot, C., Anderson, J. B., Peterson, L. E., King, E. C., Lihn, S. L., ... Lannon, C. M. (2016). Digoxin use is associated with reduced interstage mortality in patients with no history of arrhythmia after stage I palliation for single ventricle heart disease. *Journal of the American Heart Association, 5*(1), e002376. doi:10.1161/JAHA.115.002376

Brugada, J., Blom, N., Sarquella-Brugada, G., Blomstrom-Lundqvist, C., Deanfield, J., Janousek, J., ... Rosenthal, E. (2013). Pharmalogical and non-pharmalogical therapy for arrhythmia in the pediatric population: AHRA and AEPC arrythmia working group joint consensus statement. *Eurospace, 15*(9), 1337–1382.

Burkhardt, B., Rücker, G., & Stiller, R. G. (2015, March 25). Prophylactic milrinone for the prevention of low cardiac output syndrome and mortality in children undergoing surgery for congenital heart disease. *Cochrane Database of Systematic Reviews, 2015*(3), CD009515. doi:10.1002/14651858.CD009515.pub2

Butt, W., Heard, M., & Peek, G. J. (2013). Clinical management of the extracorporeal membrane oxygenation circuit. *Pediatric Critical Care Medicine, 14*(5 Suppl. 1), S13–S19.

Callow, L. B. (1992). Current strategies in the nursing care of infants with hypoplastic left-heart syndrome undergoing first-stage palliation with the Norwood operation. *Heart & Lung, 20*, 463–470.

Canter, C. E., & Simpson, K. P. (2012). Diagnosis and treatment of myocarditis in children in the current era. *Circulation, 129*(1), 115–128.

Castaneda, A. R., Jonas, R. A., Mayer, J. E., & Hanley F. L. (2006). *Cardiac surgery of the neonate and infant* (2nd ed.). Philadelphia, PA: W. B. Saunders.

Chen, K., Williams, S., Chan, A. K., & Mondal, T. K. (2013). Thrombosis and embolism in pediatric cardiomyopathy. *Blood, Coagulation and Fibrinolysis, 24*(3), 221–230. doi:10.1097/MBC.0b013e32835bfd85

Chow, S. L., Maisel, A. S., Anand, I., Bozkurt, B., De Boer, R. A., Felker, G. M., ... Zile, M. R. (2017). Role of biomarkers for the prevention, assessment, and management of heart failure: A scientific state from the American Heart Association. *Circulation, 135*(22), e1054–e1091.

Christiansen, J., Dyck, J. D., Elyas, B. G., Lilley, M., Bamforth, J. S., Hicks, M., ... Somerville, M. J. (2015). Chromosome 1q21.1 contiguous gene deletion is associated with congenital heart disease. *Circulation Research, 94*(11), 1429–1435.

Colan, S. D. (2015). Epidemiology and cause-specific outcome of hypertrophic cardiomyopathy in children: Findings from the pediatric cardiomyopathy registry. *Circulation, 115*, 773–781.

Colucci, W. S., & Chen, H. H. (2017). Natriuretic peptide measurement in heart failure. In S. B. Yeon (Ed.), *UpToDate.* Retrieved from https://www.uptodate.com/contents/natriuretic-peptide-measurement-in-heart-failure

Cooper, B. M., & Ravishankar, C. (2013). Nutrition and growth in congenital heart disease: A challenge in children. *Cardiology, 28*(2), 122–129.

Costello, J., Gellatly, M., Daniel, J., Justo, R. N., & Weir, K. (2014). Growth restriction in infants and young children with congenital heart disease. *Congenital Heart Disease, 10*(5), 447–456.

Curley, M. A. Q., Meyer, E. C., Scoppettuolo, L. A., McGann, E. A., Trainor, B. P., Rachwal, C. M., & Hickey, P. A. (2012). Parent presence during invasive procedures and resuscitation: Evaluation of a clinical practice change. *American Journal Respiratory and Critical Care Medicine, 186*(11), 1133–1139.

Curtis, A. B., Worley, S. J., Adamson, P. B., Chung, E. S., Niazi, I., Sherfesee, L., ... Sutton, M. J. (2013). Biventricular pacing for atrioventricular block and systemic dysfunction. *New England Journal of Medicine, 368*(6), 1588–1593.

Davidson, J. J., Kinley, C., & Bhatt, D. I. (2015). Cardiac catheterization. In D. L. Mann, R. O. Bonow, D. P. Zipes, & P. Libby (Eds.), *Braunwald's heart disease: A textbook of cardiovascular medicine* (10th ed., pp. 364–386). Philadelphia, PA: Elsevier-Saunders.

del Nido, P. J., & Baird C. (2012). Congenital mitral valve stenosis: Anatomic variants and surgical reconstruction. *Seminars in Thoracic and Cardiovascular Surgery and Pediatric Cardiac Surgery Annals, 15*(1), 69–74. doi:10.1053/j.pcsu.2012.01.011

DeMauro, S. B., Millar, D., & Kirpalani, H. (2014). Noninvasive respiratory support for neonates. *Currents Opinions in Pediatrics, 26*(2), 157–162.

Devaney, E. J., & Bove, E. L. (2013). Congenitally corrected transposition of the great arteries. In C. Mavroudis & C. L. Backer (Eds.), *Pediatric cardiac surgery* (4th ed., pp. 530–541). Hoboken, NJ: Wiley-Blackwell.

Dominico, M., & Herrera, M. (2015). Quick references. In M. B. Jones, D. Klugman, R. K. Fitzgeralds, L. M. Kohr, J. T. Berger, J. M. Costello, & R. Bronicki (Eds.), *Pediatric cardiac intensive care handbook* (pp. 1–8). Washington, DC: Pediatric Intensive Care Books.

Duderstadt, K. G. (Ed.). (2014). *Pediatric physical examination* (2nd ed.). St. Louis, MO: Mosby.

Duncan, B. W. (2013). Pediatric mechanical circulatory support. In C. Mavroudis & C. L. Backer (Eds.), *Pediatric cardiac surgery* (4th ed., pp. 856–866). Hoboken, NJ: Wiley-Blackwell.

Durandy, Y., Rubatti, M., & Couturier, R. (2010). Near Infrared Spectroscopy during pediatric cardiac surgery: Errors and pitalls. *Perfusion, 26*(5), 441–446.

Ellesøe, S. G., Johansen, M. M., Bjerre, J. V., Hojortdal, V. E., Brunak, S., & Larsen, L. A. (2016). Familial atrial septal defect and sudden cardiac death: Identification of a novel *NKX2-5* mutation and a review of the literature. *Congenital Heart Disease, 11*, 283–290. doi:10.1111/chd.12317

Engorn, B., & Flerlage, J. (2015). *The Harriet Lane handbook* (12th ed.). Philadelphia, PA: Elsevier, Saunders.

Feinstein, J. A., Benson, D. W., Dubin, A. M., Cohen, M. S., Maxey, D. M., Mahle, W. T., ... Martin, G. R. (2012). Hypoplastic left heart syndrome: Current considerations and expectations. *Journal of the American College of Cardiology, 59*(Suppl. 1), S1–S42.

Fillipps, D. J., & Bucciarelli, R. L.(2015). Cardiac evaluation of the newborn. *Pediatric Clinics of North America, 62*(2), 471–489.

Flori, H. R., Johnson, L. D., Hanley, F. L., & Fineman, J. R. (2000). Transthoracic intracardiac catheters in pediatric patients recovering from congenital heart defect surgery: Associated complications and outcomes. *Critical Care Medicine, 28*(8), 2997–3001.

Fox, D., Stream, A. R., & Bull, T. (2014). Perioperative management of the patient with pulmonary hypertension. *Seminars in Cardiothoracic and Vascular Anesthesia, 18*(4), 310–318.

Fredenburg, T. B., Johnson, T. R., & Cohen, M. D. (2011). The Fontan procedure: Anatomy, complications, and manifestations of failure. *Radiographics, 31*(2), 453–463.

Gallet, R., Lellouche, N., Mitchell-Heggs, L., Bouhemad, B., Bensaid, A., Dubois-Randé, J. L., ... Lim, P. (2012). Prognosis value of central venous oxygen saturation in acute decompensated heart failure. *Archives of Cardiovascular Disease, 105*(1), 5–12. doi:10.1016/j.acvd.2011.10.005

Gersh, B. J., Maron, B. J., Bonow, R. O., Dearani, J. A., Fifer, M. A., Link, M. S., ... Yancy, C. W. (2011). 2011 ACCF/AHA guideline for the diagnosis and treatment of hypertrophic cardiomyopathy: Exectuive summary: A report of the American College of Cardiology Foundation/American Heart Association Task Force on Practice Guidelines. *Journal of the American College of Cardiology,* 58(25), 2703–2738. doi:10.1016/j.jacc.2011.10.825

Giglia, T. M., Massicotte, M. P., Tweddell, J. S., Barst, R. J., Bauman, M., Erickson, C. C., … Webb, C. L. (2013). Prevention and treatment of thrombosis in pediatric and congenital heart disease: A scientific statement from the American Heart Association. *Circulation,* 128(24), 2622–2703.

Gutiérrez, S. L., Kamel, I. R., & Zimmerman, S. L. (2016). Current concepts on diagnosis and prognosis of arrhythmogenic right ventricular cardiomyopathy/dysplasia. *Journal of Thoracic Imaging,* 31(6), 324–335. doi:10.1097/RTI.0000000000000171

Hall, J. E. (Ed.). (2016). *Guyton and Hall textbook of medical physiology* (13th ed.). Philadelphia, PA: Elsevier.

Harmon, W. G., Sleeper, L. A., Cuniberti, L., Messere, J., Colan, S. D., Orav, E. J., … Lipshultz, S. E. (2009). Treating children with idiopathic dilated cardiomyopathy. *American Journal of Cardiology,* 104(2), 281–286. doi:10.1016/j.amjcard.2009.03.033

Hazinski, M. F. (Ed.). (2013). *Nursing care of the critically ill child* (3rd ed.). St. Louis, MO: Mosby.

Heching, H. G., Bacha, E. A., & Liberman, L. (2015). Post pericardiotomy syndrome in pediatric patients following closure of secundum atrial septal defects: Incidence and risk factors. *Pediatric Cardiology,* 36(3), 498–502.

Hermsen, J., & Chen, J. (2015). Surgical considerations in d-transposition of the great arteries. *Seminars in Cardiothoracic and Vascular Anesthesia,* 19(3), 223–232. doi:10.1177/1089253215584195

Herring, W. (2012). *Learning radiology* (2nd ed.). Philadelphia, PA: Elsevier.

Hong, Y. M. (2013). Cardiomyopathies in children. *Korean Journal of Pediatrics,* 56(2), 52–59.

Hornik, C. P., He, X., Jacobs, J. P., Li, J. S., Jaquiss, R. D. B., Jacobs, M. L., … Pasquali, S. K. (2011). Complications after the norwood operation: An analysis of the society of thoracic surgeons congenital heart surgery database. *Annals of Thoracic Surgery,* 92(5), 1734–1740.

Hsu, D. T., & Lamour, J. M. (2015). Changing indications for pediatric heart transplantation: Complex congenital heart disease. *Circulation,* 131(1), 91–99. doi:10.1161/CIRCULATIONAHA.114.001377

Iacob, D., Butnariu, A., Leucuta, D. C., Samaşca, G., Deleanu, D., & Lupan, I. (2017). Evaluation of NT-proBNP in children with heart failure younger than 3 years old. *Romanian Journal of Internal Medicine,* 55(2), 69–74.

Ivy, D., Abman, S. H., Barst, R. J., Berger, R. M., Bonnet, D., Fleming, T. R., … Beghetti, M. (2013). Pediatric pulmonary hypertension. *Journal of the American College of Cardiology,* 62(Suppl. 25), D117–D126.

Jabre, P., Belpomme, V., Azoulay, E., Jacob, L., Bertrand, L., Lapostolle, F., … Adnet, F. (2013). Family presence during cardiopulmonary resuscitation. *New England Journal of Medicine,* 368(11), 1008–1018.

Jacobs, J. P., Mavroudis, C., Quintessenza, J. A., Chai, P. J., Pasquali, S. K., Hill, K. D., … Cameron, D. (2014). Reoperations for pediatric and congenital heart disease: An analysis of the Society of Thoracic Surgeons (STS) congenital heart surgery database. *Thoracic and Cardiovascular Surgery Pediatric Cardiology Annuals,* 17(1), 2–8.

Jacobs, M. L. (2013). The functionally univentricular heart and Fontan operation. In C. Mavroudis & C. L. Backer (Eds.), *Pediatric cardiac surgery* (4th ed., pp. 542–570). Hoboken, NJ: Wiley-Blackwell.

Jefferies, J. L., Hoffman, T. M., & Nelson, D. P. (2010). Heart failure treatment in the intensive care unit in children. *Heart Failure Clinic,* 6(4), 531–558.

Jefferies, J. L., Wilkinson, J. D., Sleeper, L. A., Colan, S. D., Lu, M., Pahl, E., … Pediatric Cardiomyopathy Registry Investigators. (2015). Cardiomyopathy phenotypes and outcomes for children with left ventricular myocardial noncompaction: Results from the Pediatric Cardiomyopathy Registry. *Journal of Cardiac Failure,* 21(11), 877–884. doi:10.1016/j.cardfail.2015.06.381

Jesurum, J. (2001). SVO₂ monitoring. *Critical Care Nures,* 21(1), 79–83.

Johnson, J. A., Boyce, T. G., Cetta, F., Steckelberg, J. M., & Johnson, J. N. (2012). Infective endocarditis in the pediatric patient: A 60-year single-institution review. *Mayo Clinic Proceedings,* 87(7), 629–635. doi:10.1016/j.mayocp.2012.02.023

Jonas, J. A. (2015). Management of interrupted aortic arch. *Seminars in Thoracic and Cardiovascular Surgery,* 27(2), 177–188.

Kaiser, D. W., Tsai, V., Heidenreich, P. A., Goldstein, M. K., Wang, Y., Curtis, J., & Turakhia, M. P. (2015). Defibrillator implantations for primary prevention in the United States: Inappropriate care or inadequate documentation: Insights from the National Cardiovascular Data ICD Registry. *Heart Rhythm,* 12(10), 2086–2093.

Kambam, J. (1994). Atrial septal defect. In J. Kambam (Ed.), *Cardiac anesthesia for infants and children.* St. Louis, MO: Mosby.

Kanter, K. R., Kogon, B. E., Kirshbom, P. M., & Carlock, P. R. (2010). Symptomatic neonatal tetralogy of Fallot: Repair or shunt? *Annals of Thoracic Surgery,* 89(3), 858–863. doi:10.1016/j.athoracsur.2009.12.060

Kantor, P. F., Abraham, J. R., Dipchand, A. I., Benson, L. N., & Redington, A. N. (2010). The impact of changing medical therapy on transplantation-free survival in pediatric dilated cardiomyopathy. *Journal of the American College of Cardiology,* 55(13), 1377–1384. doi:10.1016/j.jacc.2009.11.059

Karamichalis, J. M., Darst, J. R., Mitchell, M. B., & Clarke, D. R. (2013). Isolated right ventricular outflow tract obstruction. In C. Mavroudis & C. L. Backer (Eds.), *Pediatric cardiac surgery* (4th ed., pp. 385–409). Hoboken, NJ: Wiley-Blackwell.

Katz, A. M. (2011). *Physiology of the heart* (5th ed.). Philadelphia, PA, Lippincott Williams & Wilkins.

Kirk, R., Dipchand, A. I., Rosenthal, D. N., Addonizio, L., Burch, M., Chrisant, M., … Weintraub, R. (2014). The International Society for Heart and Lung Transplantation Guidelines for the management of pediatric heart failure: Executive summary. *Journal of Heart and Lung Transplantation,* 33(9), 888–909.

Kirklin, J. K. (2015). Advances in mechanical assist devices and artificial hearts for children. *Current Opinion in Pediatrics,* 27(5), 597–603.

Kugler, J. D. (2016). Electrophysiology studies. In H. D. Allen, D. J. Driscoll, R. E.Shaddy, & T. F. Feltes (Eds.), *Moss and Adams' Heart disease in infants, children, and adolescents* (7th ed., pp. 275–292). Philadelphia, PA: Wolters Kluwer.

Latus, H., Delhaas, T., Schranz, D., & Apitz, C. (2015). Treatment of pulmonary arterial hypertension in children. *National Review Cardiology,* 12(4), 244–254.

Li, J. S., & Newburger, J. W. (2010). Antiplatelet therapy in pediatric cardiovascular patients. *Pediatric Cardiology,* 31(4), 454–461. doi:10.1007/s00246-010-9672-2

Libby, P., Gerszten, R. E., & Ricker, P. M. (2015). Biomarkers, proteomics, metabolomics, and personalized medicine. In D. L. Mann, R. O. Bonow, D. P. Zipes, & P. Libby (Eds.), *Braunwald's heart disease: A textbook of cardiovascular medicine* (10th ed., pp. 84–95). Philadelphia, PA: Elsevier-Saunders.

Lilly, L. S. (2013). Treatment of acute and recurrent idiopathic pericarditis. *Circulation,* 127(16), 1723–1726.

Lim, T. H. (Ed.). (2015). *Practical textbook of cardiac CT and MRI.* Berlin: Springer-Verlag.

Lipshultz, S. E., Cochran, T. R., Briston, D. A., Brown, S. R., Sambatakos, P. J., Miller, T. L., … Wilkinson, J. D. (2013).

Pediatric cardiomyopathies: Causes, epidemiology, clinical course, preventive strategies and therapies. *Future Cardiology, 9*(6), 817–848. doi:10.2217/fca.13.66

Lipshultz, S. E., Orav, E. J., Wilkinson, J. D., Towbin, J. A., Messere, J. E., Lowe, A. M., … Colan, S. D. (2013). Risk stratification at diagnosis for children with hypertrophic cardiomyopathy: An analysis of data from the Pediatric Cardiomyopathy Registry. *Lancet, 382*(9908), 1889–1897. doi:10.1016/S0140-6736(13)61685-2

Mahle, W. T. (2015). Mechanical circulatory support in pediatric cardiomyopathy. *Progress in Cardiology, 39*(7), 29–32.

Mahle, W. T. (2016). Early extubation after repair of tetralogy of Fallot and the Fontan procedure: An analysis of the Society of Thoracic Surgeons congenital heart surgery database. *Annals of Thoracic Surgery, 102*(3), 850–858.

Mahle, W. T., Matthews, E., Kanter, K. R., Kogon, B. E., Hamrick, S. E., Strickland, M. J. (2014). Inflammatory response after neonatal cardiac surgery and its relationship to clinical outcomes. *Annals of Thoracic Surgery, 97*(3), 950–956.

Mahle, W. T., Newburger, J. W., Matherne, G. P., Smith, F. C., Hoke, T. R., Koppel, R., … Grosse, S. D. (2014). Role of pulse oximetry in examining newborns for congenital heart disease: A scientific statement from the AHA and AAP. *Pediatrics, 124*(2), 823–836.

Marino, B. S. (2013). New concepts in predicting, evaluating and managing neurodevelopmental outcomes in children with congenital heart disease. *Current Opinion in Pediatrics, 25*(5), 574–584.

Maron, B. J., & Olivotto, I. (2015). Hypertrophic cardiomyopathy. In D. L. Mann, R. O. Bonow, D. P. Zipes, & P. Libby (Eds.), *Braunwald's heart disease: A textbook of cardiovascular medicine* (10th ed., pp. 1574–1588). Philadelphia, PA: Elsevier-Saunders.

Matsuda, H., Ichikawa, H., & Sawa, Y. (2017). Heart transplantation for adults with congenital heart disease: Current status and future prospects. *General Thoracic and Cardiovascular Surgery, 65*(6), 309–320.

Mavroudis, C., & Backer, C. L. (2013a). *Pediatric cardiac surgery* (4th ed.). St. Louis, MO: Mosby.

Mavroudis, C., & Backer, C. L. (2013b). Transposition of the great arteries. In C. Mavroudis & C. L. Backer (Eds.), *Pediatric cardiac surgery* (4th ed., pp. 492–529). Hoboken, NJ: Wiley-Blackwell.

Mavroudis, C., & Backer, C. L. (2013c). Truncus arteriosus. In C. Mavroudis & C. L. Backer (Eds.), *Pediatric cardiac surgery* (4th ed., pp. 361–375). Hoboken, NJ: Wiley-Blackwell.

Mavroudis, C., Backer, C. L., Jacobs, J. P., & Anderson, R. H. (2013). Ventricular septal defect. In C. Mavroudis & C. L. Backer (Eds.), *Pediatric cardiac surgery* (4th ed., pp. 311–342). Hoboken, NJ: Wiley-Blackwell.

Mavroudis, C., Doge-Khatami, A., Backer, C. L., & Lorber, R. (2013). Coronary artery anomalies. In C. Mavroudis & C. L. Backer (Eds.), *Pediatric cardiac surgery* (4th ed., pp. 715–743). Hoboken, NJ: Wiley-Blackwell.

Mayosi, J. C. (2015). Rheumatic diseases and the cardiovascular system. In D. L. Mann, R. O. Bonow, D. P. Zipes, & P. Libby (Eds.), *Braunwald's heart disease: A textbook of cardiovascular medicine* (10th ed., pp. 1843–1863). Philadelphia, PA: Elsevier-Saunders.

McCrindle, B. W., Rowley, A. H., Newburger, J. W., Burns, J. C., Bolger, A. F., Gewitz, M., … Pahl, E. (2017). Diagnosis, treatment, and long-term management of Kawasaki disease: A scientific statement for health professionals from the American Heart Association. *Circulation, 135*(17), e927–e999. doi:10.1161/CIR.0000000000000484

McElhinnery, D. B., Hedrick, H. L., Bush, D. M., Pereira, G. R., Stafford, P. W., Gaynor, J. W., … Wernovsky, G. (2000). Necrotizing enterocolitis in neonates with congenital heart disease: Risk factors and outcomes. *Pediatrics, 106*(5), 1080–1087. doi:10.1542/peds.106.5.1080

Mery, C., Moffett, B. S., Khan, M. S., Zhang, W., Guzmán-Pruneda, F. A., Fraser, C. D., Jr., & Cabrera, A. G. (2014). Incidence and treatment of chylothorax after cardiac surgery in children: Analysis of a large multi-institution database. *Journal of Thoracic and Cardiovascular Surgery, 147*(2), 678–686.

Mesher, A. L., & McMullan, D. M.(2014). Extracorporeal life support for the neonatal cardiac patient: Outcomes and new directions. *Seminars in Perinatology, 38*(2), 97–103.

Miller, J. W., Vu, D., Chai, P. J., Kreutzer, J., Hossain, M. M., Jacobs, J. P., & Loepke, A. W. (2014). Patient and procedural characteristics for successful and failed immediate tracheal exutbation in the operating room following cardiac surgery in infancy. *Pediatric Anesthesia, 24*(8), 830–839.

Molina, K. M., Shrader, P., Colan, S. D., Mital, S., Margossian, R., Sleeper, L. A., … Tani, L. Y. (2013). Predictors of disease progression in pediatric dilated cardiomyopathy. *Circulation Heart Failure, 6*(6), 1214–1222. doi:10.1161/CIRCHEARTFAILURE.113.000125

Monagle, P., Cochrane, A., Roberts, R., Manlhiot, C., Weintraub, R., Szechtman, B., … McCrindle, B. W. (2011). A multicenter, randomized trial comparing heparin/warfarin and acetylsalicylic acid as primary thromboprophylaxis for 2 years after the Fontan procedure in children. *Journal of the American College of Cardiology, 58*(6), 645–651.

Morgan, C. J., Zappitelli, M., Robertson, C. M., Alton, G. Y., Sauve, R. S., Joffe, A. R., … Rebeyka, I. M. (2013). Risk factors for and outcomes of acute kidney injury in neonates undergoing complex cardiac surgery. *Journal of Pediatrics, 162*(1), 120–127.

Mumtaz, M. A., Qyreshi, A., Mvaroudis, C., & Backer, C. L. (2013). Patent ductus arteriosus. In C. Mavroudis & C. L. Backer (Eds.), *Pediatric cardiac surgery* (4th ed., pp. 225–233). Hoboken, NJ: Wiley-Blackwell.

Murray, J. M., Hellinger, A., Dionne, R., Brown, L., Galvin, R., Griggs, S., … Almond, C. S. (2015). Utility of a dedicated pediatric cardiac anticoagulation program: The Boston Children's Hospital experience. *Pediatric Cardiology, 36*(4), 842–850.

Murtuza, B., Barron, D. J., Stumper, O., Stickley, J., Eaton, D., Jones, T. J., & Brawn, W. J. (2011). Anatomic repair for congenitally corrected transposition of the great arteries: A single institution 19-year experience. *Journal of Thoracic and Cardiovascular Surgery, 142*(6), 1348–1357. doi:10.1016/j.jtcvs.2011.08.016

Neumar, R. W., Shuster, M., Callaway, C. W., Gent, L. M., Atkins, D. L., Bhanji, F., . . . Hazinski, M. F. (2015). American Heart Association response to the 2015 Institute of Medicine report on strategies to improve cardiac arrest survival. *Circulation, 132*(18), 1049–1070. doi:10.1161/CIR.0000000000000252

Nichols, D. G., Ungerleider, R. M., Spevak, P. J., Greeley, W. J., Cameron, D. E., Lappe, D. G., & Wetzel, R. C. (Eds.). (2006). *Critical heart disease in infants and children* (2nd ed.). Philadelphia, PA: Elsevier.

Nieves, J. A., Fosse, G. P., Rummell, M., Whalen, R. L., Fernandes, S. M., Gupta, P., . . . Hazinski, M. F. (2013). Cardiovascular disorders. In M. F. Hazinski (Ed.), *Nursing care of the critically ill child* (pp. 181–461). St. Louis, MO: Elsevier-Mosby.

O'Connor, M. J., & Rossano, J. W. (2014). Ventricular assist devices in children. *Current Opinion in Cardiology, 29*(1), 113–121. doi:10.1097/HCO.0000000000000030

Ohye, R. G., Schonbeck, J. V., Eghtesady, P., Laussen, P. C., Pizarro, C., Shrader, P., … Pearson, G. D. (2012). Cause, timing, and location of death in the single ventricle reconstruction trial. *Journal of Thoracic and Cardiovascular Surgery, 144*(4), 907–914. doi:10.1016/j.jtcvs.2012.04.028

Owens, J. L., & Musa, N. (2009). Nutrition support after neonatal cardiac surgery. *Nutrition in Clinical Practice, 24*(2), 242–249. doi:10.1177/0884533609332086

Pahl, E., Sleeper, L. A., Canter, C. E., Hsu, D. T., Lu, M., Webber, S. A., . . . Pediatric Cardiomyopathy Registry Investigators. (2012). Incidence of and risk factors for sudden cardiac death in children with dilated cardiomyopathy: A report from the Pediatric Cardiomyopathy Registry. *Journal of American College of Cardiology, 59*(6), 607–615. doi:10.1016/j.jacc.2011.10.878

Park, M. K. (2016). *Park's The Pediatric Cardiology Handbook* (5th ed.). Philadelphia, PA: Saunders-Elsevier.

Park, M. K., & Guntheroth, W. G. (2006). *How to read pediatric ECGs* (4th ed.). Philadelphia, PA: Elsevier.

Pasternack, M. S. (2016). Prevention of sepsis in the asplenic patient. In S. Bond (Ed.), *UpToDate*. Retrieved from https://www.uptodate.com/contents/prevention-of-sepsis-in-the-asplenic-patient

Pearl, J. M., Permut, L. C., & Laks, H. (1996). Tricuspid atresia. In A. E. Bauer, A. S. Geha, G. L. Hammond, H. Laks, & K. S. Naunheim (Eds.), *Glenn's thoracic and cardiovascular surgery* (6th ed., pp. 1431–1449). Stamford, CT: Appleton & Lange.

Pomerantz, W. J. & Roback, M. G. (2018). Pathophysiology and calssification of shock in children. In J. F. Wiley (Ed.), *UpToDate*. Retrieved from https://www.uptodate.com/contents/pathophysiology-and-classification-of-shock-in-children

Reddy, V. M., & Hanley, F. L. (2013). Surgical treatment of pulmonary atresia with ventricular septal defect. In C. Mavroudis & C. L. Backer (Eds.), *Pediatric cardiac surgery* (4th ed., pp. 428–442). Hoboken, NJ: Wiley-Blackwell.

Redington, A. (2012). Low cardiac output due to acute right ventricular dysfunction and cardiopulmonary interactions in congenital heart disease. *Pulmonary Circulation, 4*(2), 191–199. doi:10.1086/675982

Reuter-Rice, K., & Bolick, B. N. (2014). Fenoldopam. Retrieved from http://www.wolterskluwercdi.com/lexicomp-online

Rossano, J. W., Cabrera, A. G., & Shaddy, R. E. (2016). Heart transplantation—The pediatric cardiac critical care perspective. *Pediatric Critical Care Medicine, 17*(8), S171–S177.

Rossano, J. W., Cabrera, A. G., Jefferies, J. L., Naim, M. P., & Humlicek, T. (2016). Pediatric Cardiac Intensive Care Society 2014 consensus statement: Pharmacotherapies in cardiac critical care chronic heart failure. *Pediatric Critical Care Medicine, 17*(3 Suppl. 1), S16–S19. doi:10.1097/PCC.0000000000000.624

Rowley, A. H. (2015). The complexities of the diagnosis and management of Kawasaki disease. *Infectious Disease Clinics of North America, 3*(3), 525–537. doi:10.1016/j.idc.2015.05.006

Rummel, M. (2013). Anticoagulation. In M. F. Hazinski (Ed.), *Nursing care of the critically ill child* (3rd ed., pp. 301–305). St. Louis, MO: Mosby-Elsevier.

Saguil, A., Fargo, M., & Grogan, S. (2015). Diagnosis and management of Kawasaki disease. *American Family Physician, 91*(6), 365–371. Retrieved from https://www.aafp.org/afp/2015/0315/p365.html

Şahin, M., Portakal, O., Karagöz, T., Hasçelik, G., & Özkutlu, S. (2010). Diagnostic performance of BNP and NT-ProBNP measurements in children with heart failure based on congenital heart defects and cardiomyopathies. *Clinical Biochemistry, 43*, 1278–1281. doi:10.1016/j.clinbiochem.2010.08.002

Said, J. P., & Kugler, J. D. (2016). Electrophysiology studies and electrophysiologic therapeutic catherization. In H. D. Allen, R. E. Shaddy, D. J. Penny, T. F. Feltes, & F. Cetta (Eds.), *Moss and Adams' heart disease in infants, children, and adolescents* (pp. 579–623). Philadelphia, PA: Wolter Kluwer.

Sanderson, R. G., & Kurth, C. L. (Eds.). (1983). *The cardiac patient: A comprehensive approach* (2nd ed., p. 129). Philadelphia, PA: W. B. Saunders.

Schmaltz, A. A. (2015). Chronic congestive heart failure in infancy and childhood: New aspects of diagnosis and treatment. *Klinik Padiatric, 227*(1), 3–9. doi:10.1055/s-0034-1389974

Silvano, M., Corrado, D., Köbe. J., Mönnig, G., Basso, C., Thiene, G., & Eckardt, L. (2013). Risk stratification in arrhythmogenic right ventricular cardiomyopathy. *Herzshrittmacherther Elektrophysiol, 24*(4), 202–208. doi:10.1007/s00399-013-0291-5

Silvestry, F. E. (2018). Postoperative complications among patients undergoing cardiac surgery. In G. Finlay (Ed.), *UpToDate*. Retrieved from https://www.uptodate.com/contents/Postoperative-complications-among-patients-undergoing-cardiac-surgery

Slicker, J., Hehir, D. A., Horsley, M., Monczka, J., Stern, K. W., Roman, B., ... Anderson, J. B. (2013). Nutrition algorithms for infants with hypoplastic left heart syndrome: Birth through the first interstage period. *Congenital Heart Disease, 8*(2), 89–102. doi:10.1111/j.1747-0803.2012.007.05.x

Smith, G. A. (2016). Cardiac trauma. In H. D. Allen, D. J. Driscoll, R. E. Shaddy, & T. F. Feltes (Eds.), *Moss and Adams' heart disease in infants, children, and adolescents* (7th ed., pp. 502–509). Philadelphia, PA: Wolters Kluwer.

Snider, A. R., & Serwer, G. A. (2001). *Echocardiography in pediatric heart disease*. St. Louis, MO: Mosby.

Solomon, S. D., & Gillia, L. (2015). Echocardiography. In D. L. Mann, R. O. Bonow, D. P. Zipes, & P. Libby (Eds.), *Braunwald's heart disease: A textbook of cardiovascular medicine* (pp. 179–252). Philadelphia, PA: Elsevier Saunders.

Stacey, R. B., Caine, A. J., Jr., & Hundley, W. G. (2015). Evaluation and management of left ventricular noncompaction cardiomyopathy. *Current Heart Failure Reports, 12*(1), 61–67. doi:10.1007/s11897-014-0237-1

Steffen, R. J., Miletic, K. G., Schraufnagel, D. P., Vargo, P. R., Fukamachi, K., Stewart, R. D., & Moazami, N. (2016). Mechanical circulatory support in pediatrics. *Expert Review of Medical Devices, 13*(5), 507–514. doi:10.1586/17434440.2016.1162710

Stewart, R. D., Mavroudis, C., & Backer, C. L. (2013) Tetralogy of fallot. In C. Mavroudis & C. L. Backer (Eds.), *Pediatric cardiac surgery* (pp. 410–427). Hoboken, NJ: Wiley-Blackwell.

Strychowsky, J., Rukholm, G., Gupta, M. K., & Reid, D. (2014). Unilateral vocal fold paralysis after congenital cardiothoracic surgery: A meta-analysis. *Pediatrics, 133*(6), e1708–e1723. doi:10.1542/peds.2013-3939

Summers, J., & Mikolich, B. (2014). Left ventricular noncompaction: A cariomyopathy with distinct characteristics and risks. *Journal of Cardiovascular Nursing, 29*(6), 535–543.

Swerdlow, C. D., Wang, P. J., & Zipes, D. P. (2015). Pacemakers and implantable cardioverter-defibrillators. In D. L. Mann, R. O. Bonow, D. P. Zipes, & P. Libby (Eds.), *Braunwald's heart disease: A textbook of cardiovascular medicine* (pp. 721–747). Philadelphia, PA: Elsevier Saunders.

Tabbutt, S., Ghanayem, N., Ravishankar, C., Sleeper, L. A., Cooper, D. S., Frank, D. U., ... Laussen, P. (2012). Risk factors for hospital morbidity and mortality after the Norwood procedure: A report from the Pediatric Heart Network Single Ventricle Reconstruction trial. *Journal of Thoracic and Cardiovascular Surgery, 144*(4), 882–895. doi:10.1016/j.jtcvs.2012.05.019

Taketomo, C. K. (2016). *Pediatric and neonatal dosage handbook* (23rd ed.). Philadelphia, PA: Lexicomp, Wolters Kluwer. Retrieved from https://online.lexi.com

Tchervenkov, C. I., Bernier, P.-L., Del Duca, D., Hill, S., Ota, N., & Mavroudis, C. (2013). Left ventricular outflow tract obstruction.

In C. Mavroudis & C. L. Backer (Eds.), *Pediatric cardiac surgery* (4th ed., pp. 588–618). Hoboken, NJ: Wiley-Blackwell.

Thiagarajan, R. R. (2016). Extracorporeal membrane oxygenation for cardiac indications in children. *Pediatric Critical Care Medicine, 17*(8), S155–S159.

Thrush, P. T., & Hoffman, T. M. (2014). Pediatric heart transplantation—indications and outcomes in the current era. *Journal of Thoracic Disease, 6*(8), 1080–1096. doi:10.3978/j.issn.2072-1439.2014.06.16

Towbin, J. A. (2016). Myocarditis. In H. D. Allen, D. J. Driscoll, R. E. Shaddy, & T. F. Feltes (Eds.), *Moss and Adams' heart disease in infants, children, and adolescents* (7th ed., pp. 1207–1224). Philadelphia, PA: Wolters Kluwer.

Towbin, J. A., Lorts, A., & Jefferies, J. L. (2010). Left ventricular non-compaction cardiomyopathy. *Lancet, 386*(9995), 813–825. doi:10.1016/S0140-6736(14)61282-4

Udelson, J. E., Diliszian, V., & Bobow, R. (2015). Nuclear cardiology. In D. L. Mann, R. O. Bonow, D. P. Zipes, & P. Libby (Eds.), *Braunwald's heart disease: A textbook of cardiovascular medicine* (10th ed., pp. 271–316). Philadelphia, PA: Elsevier Saunders.

Wagner, G. S. (2008). *Marriot's practical electrocardiography* (11th ed.). Philadelphia, PA: Lippincott Williams & Wilkins.

Webber, S. A., Lipshultz, S. E., Sleeper, L. A., Lu, M., Wilkinson, J. D., Addonizio, L. J., … Towbin, J. A. (2012). Outcomes of restrictive cardiomyopathy in childhood and the influence of phenotype: A report from the pediatric cardiomyopathy registry. *Circulation, 126*(10), 1237–1244.

Weiss, S. L., & Pomerantz, S. L. (2017). Septic shock in children: Ongoing management after resuscitation . In J. F. Wiley (Ed.), *UpToDate*. Retrieved from https://www.uptodate.com/contents/septic-shock-in-children-ongoing-management-after-resuscitation

Wiley, K. A., Demo, E. M., Walker, P., & Shuler, C. O. (2016). Exploring the discussion of risk of sudden cardiac death. *Pediatric Cardiology, 37*(2), 262–270. doi:10.1007/s00246-015-1272-8

Wilkinson, J. D., Landy, D. C., Colan, S. D., Towbin, J. A., Sleeper, L. A., Orav, E. J., … Lipshultz, S. E. (2010). The pediatric cardiomyopathy registry and heart failure: Key results from the first 15 years. *Heart Failure Clinics, 6*(4), 401–413. doi:10.1016/j.hfc.2010.05.002

Williams, G. D., & Hammer, G. B. (2011). Cardiomyopathy in childhood. *Current Opinion in Anesthesiology, 24*(3), 289–300. doi:10.1097/ACO.0b013e3283462257

Winch, P. D., Staudt, A. M., Sebastian, R., Corridore, M., Tumin, D., Simsic, J., … Tobias, J. D. (2016). Learning from experience: Improving early tracheal extubation success after congenital cardiac surgery. *Pediatric Critical Care Medicine, 17*(7), 630–637. doi:10.1097/PCC.0000000000000789

Witherall, C. L. (1994). Cardiac rhythm control devices. *Critical Care Nursing Clinics of North America, 6*, 95–102.

Zafar, F., Castleberry, C., Khan, M. S., Mehta, V., Bryant, R., 3rd, Lorts, A., … Morales, D. L. (2015). Pediatric heart transplant waiting list mortality in the era of ventricular assist devices. *Journal of Heart and Lung Transplantation, 34*(1), 82–88. doi:10.1016/j.healun.2014.09.018

Further Reading

Barnea, O., Santamore, W. P., Rossi, A., Salloum, E., Chien, S., Austin, E. H. (1998). Estimation of oxygen delivery in newborns with a univentricular circulation. *Circulation, 98*(14), 1407–1413.

Benson, D. W. (2000). Advances in cardiovascular genetics and embryology: Role of transcription factors in congenital heart disease. *Current Opinions in Pediatrics, 12*(5), 497–500.

Collins II, R. (2013). Contemporary reviews in cardiovascular medicine: Cardiovascular disease in Williams syndrome. *Circulation, 127*(21), 2125–2134.

Craig, J., Smith, J. B., & Fineman, L. D. (2001). Tissue perfusion. In M. A. Q. Curley, P. A. Moloney-Harmon (Eds.), *Critical care nursing of infants and children* (2nd ed.). Philadelphia, PA: W. B. Saunders.

Dent, C. L., & Schwartz, S. M. (2009). Postoperative care of the pediatric cardiac surgical patient. In D. S. Wheeler, H. R. Wong, & T. P. Shanley (Eds.), *Cardiovascular pediatric critical illness and injury* (2nd ed., pp. 169–182). London, UK: Springer-Verlag.

Dichter, C. H., & Curley, M. A. Q. (2001). Shock. In M. A. Q. Curley & P. A. Moloney-Harmon (Eds.), *Critical care nursing of infants and children* (2nd ed.). Philadelphia, PA: W. B. Saunders.

Franck, L. S., Harris, S., Soetenga, D., Amling, J., & Curley, M. (2008). The withdrawal assessment tool (WAT-1): Measuring iatrogenic withdrawal symptoms in pediatric critical care. *Pediatric Critical Care Medicine, 9*(6), 573–580.

Genizi, J., Miron, D., Spiegel, R., Fink, D., & Horowitz, Y. (2003). Kawasaki disease in very young infants: High prevalence of atypical presentation and coronary arteritis. *Clinical Pediatrics, 42*(3), 263–267.

Goldmuntz, E. (2001). The epidemiology and genetics of congenital heart disease. *Clinics in Perinatology, 28*(1), 1–10. doi:10.1016/S0095-5108(05)70067-1

Hershberger, R. E., Lindenfeld, J., Mestroni, L., Seidman, C. E., Taylor, M. R., & Towbin, J. A. (2009). Genetic evaluation of cardiomyopathy—A heart failure Society of America practice guideline. *Journal of Cardiac Failure, 15*(2), 83–97. doi:10.1016/j.cardfail.2009.01.006

Kaiser, L. R., Kron, I. L., & Spray, T. L. (Eds.). (2006). *Master of cardiothoracic surgery* (2nd ed.). Philadelphia, PA: Lippincott Williams & Wilkins.

Larson, R. L., Canter, C. E., Naftel, D. C., Tressler, M., Rosenthal, D. N., Blume, E. D., … Lipshultz, S. E. (2011). The impact of heart failure severity at time of listing for cardiac transplantation on survival in pediatric cardiomyopathy. *Journal of Heart and Lung Transplantation, 30*(7), 755–760. doi:10.1016/j.healun.2011.01.718

Linder, C. M., Suddaby, E. C., & Mowery, B. D. (2004). Parental presence during resuscitation: Help or hindrance? *Pediatric Nurse, 30*(2), 126–127, 148.

McGahey, P. R. (2002). Family presence during pediatric resuscitation: A focus on staff. *Critical Care Nurse, 22*(6), 29–34.

Prahash, A., & Lynch, T. (2004). B-type natriuretic peptide: A diagnostic, prognostic, and therapeutic tool in heart failure. *American Journal of Critical Care, 13*(1), 46–55.

Rheuban, K. S. (2008). Pericardial diseases. In H. D. Allen, E. B. Clark, H. P. Gutgesell, & D. J. Driscoll (Eds.), *Moss and Adams' heart disease in infants, children, and adolescents* (7th ed., pp. 1281–1290). Philadelphia, PA: Lippincott Williams & Wilkins.

Synbas, P. N. (1978). *Trauma to the heart and great vessels.* Philadelphia, PA: W. B. Saunders.

Takahashi, M. (2008). Kawasaki syndrome (mucocutaneous lymph node syndrome). In H. D. Allen, E. B. Clark, H. P. Gutgesell, & D. J. Driscoll (Eds.), *Moss and Adams' heart disease in infants, children, and adolescents* (7th ed., pp. 1242–1256). Philadelphia, PA: Lippincott Williams & Wilkins.

Vick, G. W. (2003). Recent advances in pediatric cardiovascular MRI. *Current Opinions in Pediatrics, 15*(5), 454–462.

Vizgirda, V. M. (1999). The genetic basis for cardiac dysrhythmias and the long QT syndrome. *Cardiovascular Nurse, 13*(4), 34–45.

Walsh, E. P. (2001). Clinical approach to diagnosis and acute management of tachycardias in children. In E. P. Walsh & J. K. Triendman (Eds.), *Cardiac arrhythmias in children and young adults with congenital heart disease.* Philadelphia, PA: Lippincott Williams & Wilkins.

NEUROLOGIC SYSTEM

Paula Vernon-Levett

CENTRAL NERVOUS SYSTEM

Developmental Anatomy

A. Embryogenesis

The nervous system is one of the first organ systems to develop in the embryo (neurula).

1. All body tissues are derived from three different *germ cell layers*:

    a. The mesoderm forms future muscle, skeleton, connective tissue, and the cardiovascular and urogenital systems; it assists in the early development of neural tissue; and forms the notochord, which is incorporated into the future spinal column.

    b. The endoderm forms the future gut and associated organs.

    c. The surface ectoderm forms future skin, nails, epidermis, hair, and mammary glands, whereas the neuroectoderm forms future neural tissue.

2. *Neurulation* is the process of neural tube formation and cerebrum development (Figure 4.1).

    a. The neural plate is composed of specialized neuroectoderm cells arising from the embryo that thicken on either side of the neural groove (on the dorsal surface), forming a flat plate with distinct lateral edges present at approximately 20 days gestation.

    b. The neural groove is the anteroposterior groove in the ectoderm that appears at 2½ weeks gestation. Development proceeds cranially.

    c. The neural crest contains the specialized cells that originate from the neural plate but separate from it to form a parallel band that extends the length of the neural plate. The neural crest gives rise to the future peripheral nervous system (PNS), spinal and autonomic ganglia, and some nonneural tissue (including the meninges). It is present at 3½ weeks gestation.

    d. The neural tube is formed by the lateral edges (folds) of the neural plate, which fold and grow medially until they meet and form a tube.

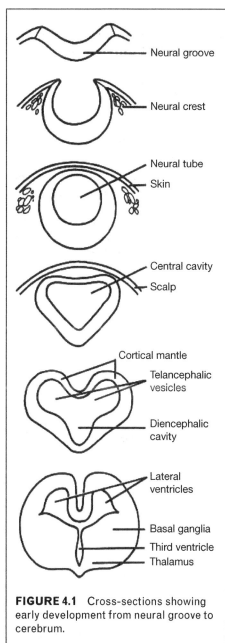

FIGURE 4.1 Cross-sections showing early development from neural groove to cerebrum.

Source: From Waxman, S. G. (1996). *Correlative neuroanatomy* (23rd ed.). Stamford, CT: Appleton & Lange.

The cavity of the neural tube becomes the future ventricular system of the brain and central canal of the spinal cord. It is closed at 4 weeks gestation.

e. Epidermal (sensory) placodes are composed of nine or 10 pairs that arise from separate ectoderm thickening in the head region. Together with the neural crest, they give rise to cranial nerves and cranial sensory organs.

3. *Brain Development.* Further specialization of the neural tube forms three distinct swellings (vesicles) at the rostral end of the tube.

a. The neural tube forms three bulges (primary brain vesicles) at its cephalic end that develop future parts of the brain (represented at 4 weeks gestation): prosencephalon (forebrain), mesencephalon (midbrain), and rhombencephalon (hindbrain; Figure 4.2).

b. Early in the second fetal month, two of the three primary brain vesicles further subdivide to form secondary vesicles. The prosencephalon forms the telencephalon (future preoptic region and paired cerebral hemispheres of the mature brain) and the diencephalon (future hypothalamus and thalamus of the mature brain). The mesencephalon remains the midbrain (future superior and inferior colliculi; red, reticular, and black nuclei; and cerebral peduncles of the mature brain). The rhombencephalon forms the metencephalon (future pons and cerebellum of the mature brain) and the myelencephalon (future medulla of the mature brain).

c. Fissure formation begins in the fourth fetal month with development of the lateral sulcus (of the cerebrum) and the posterolateral sulcus (of the cerebellum). The central sulcus, calcarine sulcus, and parietooccipital sulcus are visible in the fifth fetal month. All main gyri and sulci are present by the seventh fetal month.

d. Myelination of the brain begins at approximately 24 weeks gestation and progresses rapidly during the first 2 years of life with slower maturation into adulthood. Oligodendrocytes and Schwann cells form myelin (primarily composed of lipids and proteins), which wraps around axons to form a sheath. The myelin sheath acts as an insulator of axonal segments and is responsible for high-velocity nerve conduction.

4. *Spinal cord development* begins from the caudal portion of the neural tube. The earliest nerve fiber tracts appear around the fifth gestational week. Long association tracts appear at the third gestational month. Pyramidal tracts appear in the fifth gestational month.

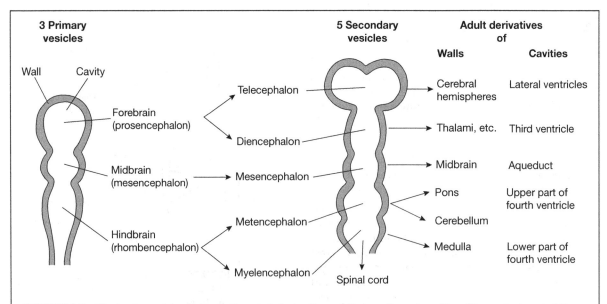

FIGURE 4.2 The brain vesicles indicate the adult derivatives of their walls and cavities. The rostral part of the third ventricle form from the cavity of the telencephalon. Most of the ventricles are derived from the cavity of the diencephalon.

Source: Reprinted with permission from Moore, K. L., & Persaud, T. V. N. (1993). *The developing human: Clinically oriented embryology* (5th ed.). Philadelphia, PA: Elsevier.

5. *Neural Tissue Specialization*

a. Neural tissue further differentiates into four concentric zones around the central canal that develop into specific areas of the mature brain. The ventricular zone is located adjacent to the central canal and is a precursor to neurons and macroglia. The subventricular zone generates certain classes of neurons and macroglia and some deep structures of the cerebrum. The intermediate (mantle) zone evolves into gray matter. The marginal zone has no primary cells of its own but evolves into most of the white matter.

b. Sensory components of the central nervous system (CNS) develop from further divisions of the neural tube. The basal plate is the ventral portion of the neural tube, which contributes to the efferent (motor) system. The alar plate is the dorsal portion of the neural tube that contributes to the afferent (sensory) system.

B. Neuron and Associated Cells

1. The *neuron* is the functional and anatomic unit of the nervous system (Figure 4.3). The cell body (soma) contains the nucleus and comprises most of the gray matter. The perikaryon (neuroplasm) is cytoplasm surrounding the nucleus. The perikaryon contains granular, filamentous, and membranous organelles. Two types of neuronal processes include the dendrites and axons.

a. Each neuron usually contains several dendrites, which conduct impulses toward the cell body (afferent).

b. Each neuron only has one axon. A myelin sheath encases some axons (white matter) and increases transmission of impulses. Nodes of Ranvier are normal interruptions in the myelin sheath that have ion channels required for regenerating an action potential. Axons conduct impulses away from the cell body (efferent).

c. The synapse is the site of contact of one neuron with another neuron. Transmission of electrical or chemical signals occurs between these neurons. The neuron sending the message is the presynaptic cell and the neuron receiving the message is the postsynaptic cell. The *synaptic cleft* is the space between the axonal terminal swelling (bouton) of the presynaptic neuron and the postsynaptic location on another neuron, usually a dendrite. The neuromuscular junction is the termination of a nerve fiber in a muscle cell, and the neuroglandular junction is the termination of a nerve fiber in a glandular cell.

    i. Chemical transmission. The presynaptic axon has a vesicle in the cytoplasm of the bouton that contains an active neurotransmitter agent. Once the neurotransmitter is released into the synaptic cleft, it attaches to a receptor on the postsynaptic membrane;

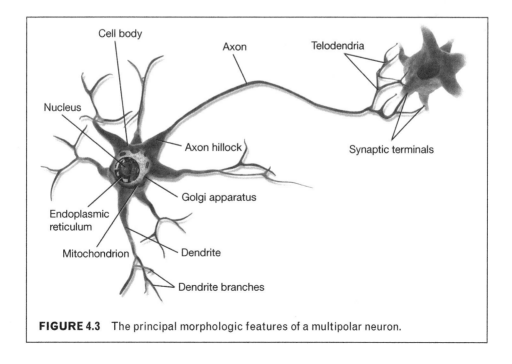

FIGURE 4.3 The principal morphologic features of a multipolar neuron.

the resulting response may be excitatory or inhibitory.

ii. Electrical transmission. The membrane of one cell is closely connected to the membrane of another cell via small pores known as *gap junctions*. The connection is also known as an *electrical synapse*. As the membrane potential of the presynaptic neuron changes, ions travel to the postsynaptic neuron and depolarize the neuron.

2. *Neuroglias* are the supporting and nourishing structures of the nervous system. There are four main types: oligodendrocytes (produce myelin), astrocytes (support, bind, and nourish neurons), microglia (phagocytic properties), and ependyma (line the ventricular system and choroid plexus and produce cerebrospinal fluid [CSF]).

C. Extracerebral Structures

1. The *scalp* is composed of skin, subcutaneous tissue, galea aponeurotica, and pericranium.

2. The *skull* of the infant consists of eight bones: two frontal (one bone after metopic suture fuses), two parietal, two temporal, one occipital, one ethmoid, and one sphenoid.

3. The *sutures* (Figure 4.4) are dense, white, fibrous, connective-tissue membranes that separate the bones. The sagittal suture separates the two parietal bones on top of the skull. The coronal suture (frontoparietal) connects the frontal and parietal bones transversely. The basilar suture is created by the junction of the basilar surface of the occipital bone with the posterior surface of the sphenoid bone. The lambdoid suture connects the parietal and occipital bones transversely.

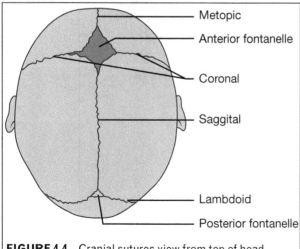

FIGURE 4.4 Cranial sutures view from top of head.

Labels: Metopic, Anterior fontanelle, Coronal, Saggital, Lambdoid, Posterior fontanelle

4. The *fontanelles* are areas where several sutures join together. The posterior fontanelle is formed by the intersection of the sagittal and lambdoid sutures. Two anterolateral fontanelles are formed by the intersection of the frontal, parietal, temporal, and sphenoid bones. The anterior fontanelle is formed by the intersection of the coronal and sagittal sutures. Two posterolateral fontanelles are formed by the intersection of the parietal, occipital, and temporal bones. The posterior and anterolateral fontanelles close at 2 months after birth. The anterior fontanelle closes between 12 and 18 months. The posterolateral closes at 24 months.

5. *Meninges* are three membranous connective-tissue layers that cover the brain. The dura mater is the outermost layer and consists of two layers. The outer periosteum adheres to the inner surface of the skull and vertebrae. The inner layer folds inward as dural reflections, dividing the cerebral hemispheres (falx cerebri), separating the cerebrum from the cerebellum and brainstem (tentorium cerebelli), and dividing the two cerebellar hemispheres (falx cerebelli). The arachnoid is the middle transparent avascular covering with many fine collagen strands (trabeculae). The pia mater is the inner, delicate, clear membrane that adheres directly to the surface of the brain and spinal cord.

6. *Ventricular System and CSF Circulation*

a. The *ventricles* are four interconnecting chambers lined by ependyma. The paired lateral ventricles are contained within the cerebral hemispheres, subdivided into four parts: the anterior horn located in the frontal lobe, the body located in the parietal lobe, the inferior horn located in the temporal lobe, and the occipital horn located in the occipital lobe. The third ventricle is connected to the lateral ventricles via the foramen of Monro and connected to the fourth ventricle via the aqueduct of Sylvius. The fourth ventricle communicates with the third ventricle and subarachnoid space around the brain and spinal cord via three exit points. The foramen of Magendie exits to the cisterna magna (central canal of spinal cord) and the spinal subarachnoid space. The foramina of Luschka exit to the cisterna magna and the subarachnoid space around the brain.

b. The *choroid plexuses* are branched and highly vascular structures and consist of numerous villi. The choroid plexus is a three-layer membrane consisting of the choroid capillary endothelium, pial cells, and the choroid epithelium. It is located in all four ventricles and parenchyma and is responsible for the majority of CSF production.

c. *CSF* is produced from arterial blood by the choroid plexuses located in the ventricles and, to a lesser degree, by ependymal cells lining the ventricles and spinal cord. The hourly rate of CSF production fluctuates and output increases logarithmically with age and body weight. Gender also plays a role with males producing more than females. The rate of CSF production is highest in infants. On average, the rate of production is approximately 0.3 to 0.4 mL/min and the total volume is replaced every 6.5 to 9.0 hours. The total static CSF volume in the ventricular system also varies by age and is approximately 150 mL in adults (Cartwright & Wallace, 2007; Sakka, Coll, & Chazal, 2011) and is proportionately less in infants and children.

d. Historically, the purpose and function of CSF was considered to be for protection of the CNS via mechanical support. Recent data suggest that it also plays an important role in homeostasis of the interstitial fluid, removal of waste products, and regulation of neuronal function (Sakka et al., 2011).

e. The classical hypothesis for circulation of CSF is detailed in Figure 4.5. The four ventricles of the brain are a series of communicating cavities that contain and circulate CSF. From the two lateral ventricles, CSF passes to the third ventricle via the foramina of Monro. It travels from the third ventricle to the fourth ventricle via the aqueduct of Sylvius. The combined CSF volume passes through two lateral foramina of Luschka and the medial foramen of Magendie into the cisterna magna. CSF travels upward around the cerebrum via the subarachnoid space and downward around the spinal cord via the spinal subarachnoid space.

f. *Absorption* occurs primarily through the arachnoid villi. The fingerlike projections from the arachnoid layer extend into the superior sagittal sinus function as one-way valves allowing CSF to exit the sagittal sinus, but the projections prevent blood from entering the subarachnoid space. The rate of absorption depends on CSF pressure (higher pressures result in more absorption to a certain point) and venous pressure (higher venous pressures can impede absorption). With normal physiological conditions, CSF secretion in the ventricles and absorption of CSF in the venous sinuses are balanced (Orešković & Klarica, 2010).

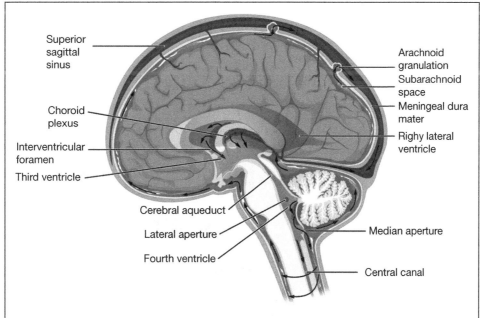

FIGURE 4.5 Location scheme of the choroid plexuses and the distribution of CSF in the human central nervous system. CSF is shown as the gray area and the arrows point the direction of CSF circulation and the sites of CSF absorption.

CSF, cerebrospinal fluid.

g. *Characteristics* of normal CSF include the following: CSF is primarily composed of water. It is clear and odorless; glucose concentration is one half to one third of the serum glucose concentration; protein concentration is 15 to 45 mg/dL (higher in term infants, median 74 mg/dL), white blood cells (WBCs) are usually absent (however, a few may be present, especially in neonates, median 3 cells/μL), and red blood cells (RBCs) are absent except during traumatic lumbar tap (Srinivasan et al., 2012). The opening CSF pressure obtained during a lumbar puncture is dynamic and is related to the patient's body position, age, depth of sedation, activities, and physiologic condition. A CSF opening pressure of <28 cm H_2O (equivalent to 20.5 mmHg) is considered normal for most children. However, it should not be interpreted in isolation, but combined with other clinical assessments (Avery, 2014).

D. The Brain is Divided Into the Cerebrum, Diencephalon, Brainstem, Reticular Formation, and the Cerebellum (Figure 4.6)

1. *Cerebrum (Telencephalon)*

a. The *cerebral hemispheres* consist of four lobes: The frontal lobes hold the primary motor cortex, Broca's motor speech area (written and spoken language), and personality. The temporal lobes are responsible for reception and interpretation of auditory information, emotional and visceral responses, and retention of recent memory. The parietal lobe is responsible for comprehension of language, orientation of spatial relationships, and initial processing of tactile and proprioceptive information. The occipital lobe is responsible for the reception and interpretation of visual stimuli.

b. *Basal ganglia* are located deep in the cerebral hemispheres and are composed of four nuclei providing unconscious control of lower motor neurons. The basal ganglia are processing stations, linking the cerebral cortex to specific thalamic nuclei.

c. The *corpus callosum* is the largest commissural tract and is composed of a bundle of transverse nerve fibers connecting the two cerebral hemispheres. It transfers information between cerebral hemispheres and makes up the roof of the lateral ventricles and the third ventricle.

d. The *limbic system* refers to several structures, including the limbic lobe, hippocampus and connections, amygdala, septal nuclei, hypothalamus, anterior thalamic nuclei, and portions of the basal ganglia. This system is primarily responsible for affective behavior and autonomic control.

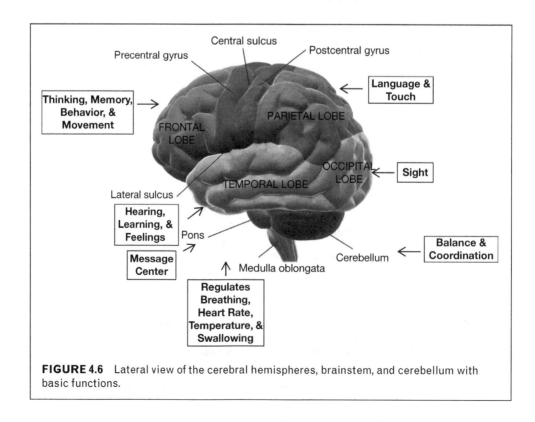

FIGURE 4.6 Lateral view of the cerebral hemispheres, brainstem, and cerebellum with basic functions.

2. The *diencephalon* is the rostral end of the brainstem and is located deep within the cerebrum. Sometimes it is classified as part of the brainstem. Anatomically, it is divided into the following:

    a. The *epithalamus* is a narrow band forming the roof of the diencephalon. It includes the habenula and pineal gland. The epithalamus's exact function is not well understood, but it is associated with the limbic system, optic reflexes, and reproductive activity.

    b. The *thalami* are the largest subdivision of the diencephalon. Two egg-shaped masses are located deep in each cerebral hemisphere, and their primary function is to be a relay station for sensory input.

    c. The *hypothalamus* forms the base of the diencephalon and the floor and inferior lateral walls of the lateral ventricles. It is a very small structure that contains several nuclei that connects the CNS to the endocrine system. The primary function of the hypothalamus is to maintain physiologic homeostasis by regulating a number of visceral responses, as well as more complex behavioral and emotional responses.

    d. The *subthalamus* is located lateral to the hypothalamus and is functionally integrated with the pyramidal pathways.

3. The *brainstem* consists of three continuous structures located beneath the thalamus (Figure 4.7).

    a. The *mesencephalon (midbrain)* is located rostral on the brainstem between the diencephalon and metencephalon and is the origin of cranial nerves III and IV. The primary function of the mesencephalon is to be a relay center for visual and auditory reflexes. It is also the center for postural reflexes and the righting reflex (maintains the head in an upright position).

    b. The *metencephalon (pons)* is located above the medulla and ventral to the cerebellum and serves as the origin of cranial nerves V, VI, VII, and VIII. It contains nerve fibers that form the reticular formation and are continuous with other parts of the brain. The metencephalon also contains the medial longitudinal fasciculus (MLF), which is composed of efferent fibers. The pons helps to regulate respiration.

    c. The *myelencephalon (medulla oblongata)* is continuous with the pons rostrally and the spinal cord caudally, and is the origin of cranial nerves IX through XII. Predominant functions of the myelencephalon include the primary respiratory and cardiac centers and the vasomotor centers.

4. The *reticular formation* is a diffuse network of neurons located in the brainstem. It begins at the

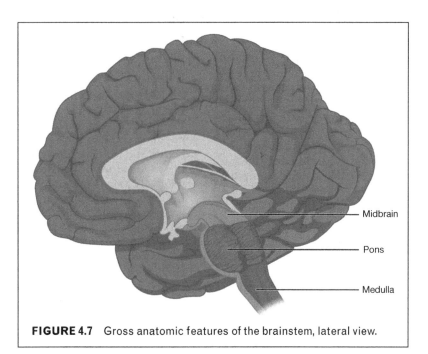

FIGURE 4.7 Gross anatomic features of the brainstem, lateral view.

upper end of the spinal cord and extends upward to the hypothalamus and adjacent areas. This formation contains both sensory and motor neurons, nuclei that interact with the extrapyramidal motor control system. The reticular formation is the site of the reticular activating system (RAS), which assists in regulating awareness (sleep–wake cycles).

5. The *cerebellum* is located superior to the fourth ventricle and contains two lobes. It is connected to the brainstem via three pairs of fiber bundles (cerebellar peduncles). Primary functions of the cerebellum include coordination of voluntary movements, control of muscle tone, and maintenance of equilibrium.

E. Cerebral Circulation

1. *Arterial blood* is supplied by two paired vessels: the common carotid arteries and the vertebral arteries.

   a. The common carotid arteries are located anteriorly; each bifurcates into two vessels. The internal carotid artery enters the cranial cavity and extends to the circle of Willis, where several major vessels meet. The anterior cerebral arteries supply the medial aspect of the cerebral hemispheres and the frontoparietal regions. The middle cerebral artery supplies much of the lateral aspect of the cerebral hemispheres and basal ganglia. The posterior cerebral arteries supply the lateral, medial, and inferior occipital cortex. The posterior communicating arteries connect anterior and posterior circulation.

   b. The external carotid arteries supply arterial circulation to the extracerebral structures (skin and muscle of the face and scalp).

   c. The vertebral arteries are located posteriorly; they originate from the subclavian arteries and join to form the basilar artery. Numerous vessels arise from the vertebral and basilar arteries and include the superior cerebellar artery, anterior inferior cerebellar artery, posterior inferior cerebellar artery, meningeal artery, anterior and posterior spinal arteries, and posterior cerebral arteries. Collectively, all the vessels supply the cerebellum, brainstem, occipital lobe, and inferior and medial surfaces of the temporal lobes.

2. *Venous blood* is supplied by a network composed of valveless, thin-walled cerebral veins. The superficial veins drain the external surfaces of the brain and include the superior cerebral vein, middle cerebral vein, and inferior cerebral vein, which empty into the dural venous sinuses. The deep veins drain internal areas of the brain and include the basal veins, vein of Rosenthal, and the great vein of Galen.

All venous drainage empties at the base of the skull via the internal jugular veins.

3. The *blood–brain barrier (BBB)* is a dynamic component of the neurovascular unit. It is composed of the anatomic structures and physiologic processes that separate the brain and blood compartments. Brain capillaries are characterized by tight junctions between endothelial cells, astrocytes with foot processes that encase capillaries and neurons, and endothelial cells with large numbers of mitochondria (responsible for energy-dependent transport). The BBB is believed to be incompletely developed in the preterm neonate. Physiologic properties of the morphologic barrier prevent rapid transport of blood to the brain and maintain a delicate homeostatic balance within the internal brain environment. Chemical barriers and tight junctions restrict some substances such as large serum protein molecules and some chemotherapeutic agents, but it also responds to nutrient requirements and local chemical signals in both healthy and pathologic conditions (Benarroch, 2012). Substances easily transported across the membrane include water, oxygen, carbon dioxide, glucose, and some lipid-soluble substances such as alcohol and anesthetics.

4. The *blood–CSF barrier* is composed of the anatomic structures and physiologic processes that separate the brain and CSF compartments (functionally similar to BBB). The morphologic barrier is created by high impermeability of choroid epithelial cells to most substances.

F. Spinal Cord and Column

1. The *spinal column* consists of 33 vertebrae: seven cervical, 12 thoracic, five lumbar, five fused sacral, and four fused coccygeal segments (Figure 4.8).

2. *Vertebrae.* The cylinder body is located anteriorly and increases in size as it progresses downward. The posterior arch has two pedicles and two laminae. The pedicles project posterolaterally from the bodies and form part of the transverse foramen. The two laminae are located posteriorly and are thin and relatively long. The spinous processes are formed by fusion of the two laminae and vary in shape, size, and direction depending on location. The transverse process is located on each side of the arch, providing a lever for muscle attachment. The articular processes (two superior and two inferior) form synovial joints with corresponding processes on adjacent vertebrae. The intervertebral foramina are formed by notches on the superior and inferior borders of the pedicles of the adjacent vertebrae, providing a channel for spinal vessels and nerves. The intervertebral

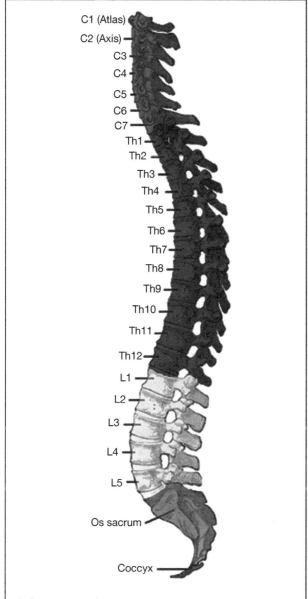

FIGURE 4.8 The vertebral column.

Source: Gray, H. (1918). *Anatomy of the human body* (20th ed.). Phliadelphia, PA: Lea and Febiger.

discs are fibrocartilage tissue interposed between adjacent vertebrae consisting of an outer concentric layer of fibrous tissue (annulus fibrosus) and a central spongy pulp (nucleus pulposus). The discs provide an elastic buffer to absorb mechanical shocks.

3. The *spinal cord* is an extension of the medulla oblongata. It extends downward, tapering (conus medullaris), and terminates at the lower border of the first lumbar vertebra in the adult and at the third lumbar vertebra in the neonate. The filum terminale is a slender, median, fibrous thread that extends from the conus medullaris to the coccyx.

a. Outer coverings are continuous with the corresponding cerebral meninges. The *dura mater* consists of only one layer, does not adhere to vertebrae, and merges with the filum terminale. The spinal cord is suspended from the dura mater via a series of 22 pairs of denticulate ligaments. The epidural space is located between the dura layer and periosteum of the vertebrae. It contains venous plexuses and fat and is the location for injection of anesthetics. The *arachnoid mater* is nonvascular and extends caudally to the second sacral level, where it merges with the filum terminale. The subarachnoid space contains CSF and blood vessels and surrounds the spinal cord (spinal or lumbar cistern). The *pia mater* is directly attached to the spinal cord, its roots, and the filum terminale and is vascular.

b. The inner core of the spinal cord is composed of gray and white matter. Butterfly- or H-shaped *gray matter* consists of cell bodies and unmyelinated fibers. They are anatomically and functionally divided into regions (Figure 4.9). The anterior (ventral) horns contain the neuronal cell bodies of motor neurons supplying the skeletal muscles. The posterior (dorsal) horns contain the neuronal cell bodies involved in sensory input to the spinal cord. The lateral horns contain preganglionic fibers of the autonomic nervous system (ANS).

c. *White matter* surrounds the gray matter and consists of myelinated (predominate) and unmyelinated fibers. They are arranged into three pairs of funiculi (columns): posterior, lateral, and anterior. Funiculi are subdivided into bundles of nerve fibers (tracts or fasciculi) that are functionally distinct. Ascending (sensory) pathways transmit sensory information from peripheral receptors to the cerebral and cerebellar cortex and transmit pain, touch, temperature, spatial relationships, vibration, passive movement, and position sense. Descending (motor) pathways contain upper motor neurons, originate from the cerebrum, and descend to the spinal cord (and brainstem). They play a major role in voluntary motor movement. The central canal is lined with ependymal cells, contains CSF, and is continuous with the fourth ventricle in the medulla oblongata. Tracts are of clinical significance and are named based on the column in which the tract travels, origination of cells, and termination of fibers. Table 4.1 lists the names of ascending and descending spinal tracts and their primary function.

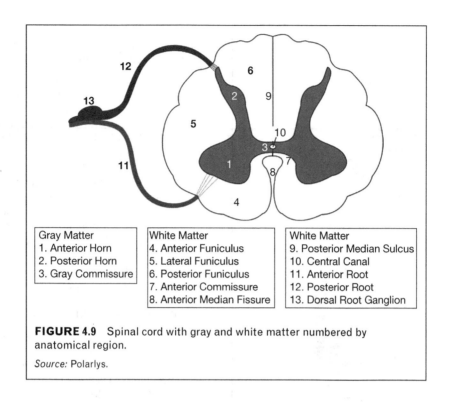

Gray Matter	
1. Anterior Horn	
2. Posterior Horn	
3. Gray Commissure	

White Matter	
4. Anterior Funiculus	
5. Lateral Funiculus	
6. Posterior Funiculus	
7. Anterior Commissure	
8. Anterior Median Fissure	

White Matter	
9. Posterior Median Sulcus	
10. Central Canal	
11. Anterior Root	
12. Posterior Root	
13. Dorsal Root Ganglion	

FIGURE 4.9 Spinal cord with gray and white matter numbered by anatomical region.

Source: Polarlys.

TABLE 4.1   Common Ascending and Descending Spinal Tracts

Tract Name	Function
Ascending (sensory)	
Dorsal (posterior) spinocerebellar	Proprioception
Ventral (anterior) spinocerebellar	Proprioception
Lateral spinothalamic	Pain, temperature
Ventral (anterior) spinothalamic	Touch, pressure
Descending (motor)	
Corticospinal (pyramidal tracts)	
Ventral (anterior) corticospinal	Skilled voluntary movements
Lateral corticospinal	Skilled voluntary movements
Rubrospinal	Fine movements, muscle tone
Vestibulospinal	Aid equilibrium, extensor muscle tone
Reticulospinal	Posture, muscle tone
Tectospinal	Mediates optic and auditory reflex movement

Source: From Curley, M. A., & Patricia, M. A. (2001). *Critical care nursing of infants and children* (2nd ed.). Philadelphia, PA: Mosby Elsevier. Copyright Elsevier (2001).

4. The *reflex arc* is an intrinsic neural circuit that, once activated, follows a specific response without conscious control. The *monosynaptic reflex arc* consists of a sensory end organ (receptor), afferent nerve fibers, one synapse, efferent nerve fibers, and muscle fiber or glandular cell (effector). A classic example is a deep-tendon reflex (DTR; Figure 4.10). The *polysynaptic reflex arc* consists of a sensory end organ, afferent nerve fibers, multiple interneurons and synapses, efferent nerve fibers, and an effector. A classic example is withdrawal of an extremity from pain stimuli.

G. Spinal Column Circulation

Arterial blood is supplied from branches of vertebral arteries and the radicular arteries derived from segmental vessels (i.e., deep cervical, intercostal, lumbar, and sacral arteries). The arteries pass through the intervertebral foramina and divide into two branches: the smaller anterior spinal artery and the larger posterior spinal artery. Venous drainage is via the venous plexus and the veins that parallel arteries.

DEVELOPMENTAL PHYSIOLOGY

A. Impulse Conduction

1. During the *resting membrane potential (RMP;* i.e., the inability to conduct a nerve impulse), the intracellular fluid (neuroplasm) of a neuron has a more negative electrical charge compared to the extracellular fluid, resulting in an imbalance in electrical charge across the cell membrane. Sodium (Na^+) and chloride (Cl^-) are in higher concentration in extracellular fluid. Potassium (K^+) is in higher concentration in intracellular fluid. This electrical imbalance across the cell membrane results from three main processes:

a. There are selective ion channels that allow K^+ ions to pass freely across the cell membrane into the extracellular compartment.

b. A negatively charged protein molecule inside the cell cannot cross the membrane.

c. There is an ionic pump that moves three Na^+ out of the cell for every two K^+ it moves into the cell.

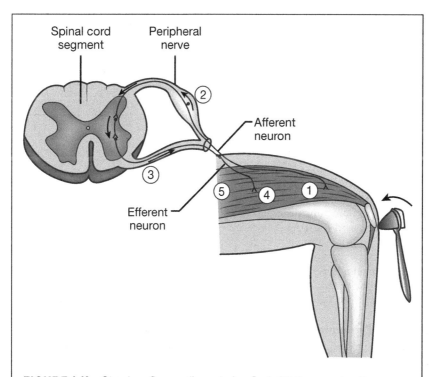

FIGURE 4.10   Simple reflex arc (knee-jerk reflex). (1) the receptor, the sensory nerve fiber that first picks up the impulse as the hammer strikes the tendon; (2) the sensory transmitter, the afferent neuron that passes the impulse to the spinal cord; (3) the motor transmitter, the efferent neuron that passes the impulse to the effector (muscle); (4) the neuroeffector junction, a specialized endplate of motor nerves; (5) the effector, a muscle that carries out the actual response (jerking of knee).

2. As *depolarization* occurs in response to an electrochemical stimulus, the cell membrane becomes more permeable to Na^+. Na^+ enters the cell, and the membrane becomes less negative internally. Initial depolarization must be greater than a certain threshold value for depolarization to continue.

3. The *action potential* is the response of the neuron to depolarization. Impulsive flow of ionic current is produced briefly. After a brief delay, the membrane potential shifts back to negative. Na^+ flow is inactivated, and K^+ permeability increases.

4. *Repolarization* is the reestablishment of negative polarity of the RMP. The cell membrane becomes impermeable to Na^+ and more permeable to K^+. RMP returns to normal via the sodium–potassium pump.

5. The action potential is self-propagating and is an all-or-none phenomenon. The impulse travels as a full-blown force or not at all. The action potential in a myelinated nerve fiber is propagated by saltatory conduction, jumping from one node of Ranvier to the next node of Ranvier. Myelin improves conduction of action potentials.

6. The *presynaptic membrane action potential* activates the release of neurotransmitters contained in vesicles. Neurotransmitters diffuse across the synapse, producing a synaptic delay.

7. The *postsynaptic membrane* contains receptors that combine with neurotransmitters to alter the membrane permeability to specific ions. Excitatory neurotransmitters include glutamate, aspartate, and acetylcholine. The receptor responds with increased permeability for Na^+ and K^+, net influx of Na^+, and cell membrane changes in a depolarizing direction (excitatory postsynaptic potential [EPSP]) and initiates an action potential. Inhibitory neurotransmitters include glycine and γ-aminobutyric acid (GABA). The receptor responds with an increase in permeability for K^+ and Cl^- but not Na^+, an outward flow of K^+, and cell membrane potential shifts in a hypopolarizing direction (inhibitory postsynaptic potential [IPSP]), which decreases excitability and inhibits an action potential.

B. Intracranial Pressure Dynamics

1. *Modified Monro-Kellie Doctrine.* The rigid skull contains three volume compartments: brain tissue (80%–90%), CSF (5%–10%), and blood (5%–10%). The brain tissue, CSF, and blood exist in a state of volume equilibrium. If there is an increase in any one or more of the volume compartments, there must be a reciprocal change in one or more of the other volume compartments to maintain pressure equilibrium:

$$\text{Intracranial volume} = \text{Vol}_{\text{brain}} + \text{Vol}_{\text{CSF}} + \text{Vol}_{\text{blood}}$$

2. *Pressure–Volume Relationships*

a. Intracranial pressure (ICP) is generally measured in mmHg to allow for comparison with mean arterial pressure (MAP) and allows for quick calculation of cerebral perfusion pressure (CPP). Normal ICP varies in different age groups and is lowest during infancy (Welch, 1980).

  i.   Newborn. 0.7 to 1.5 mmHg

  ii. Infants. 1.5 to 6 mmHg

  iii. Children. 3 to 7.5 mmHg

  iv. Adult. Less than 10 mmHg

b. The volume–pressure curve represents the relationship between changes in intracranial volume and the resulting ICP (Figure 4.11). *Elastance* is the change in pressure that occurs with a change in volume ($\Delta P/\Delta V$). *Compliance* is the inverse relationship of elastance ($\Delta V/\Delta P$). The ICP curve is not linear but is a three-phase hyperbolic curve. *Phase 1*, the compensatory phase, is the flat portion of the curve, reflecting good compliance and normal ICP. Temporary increases in ICP are "buffered" by several mechanisms: CSF translocation to the spinal subarachnoid space, venous blood displaced to the extracranial compartment through valveless

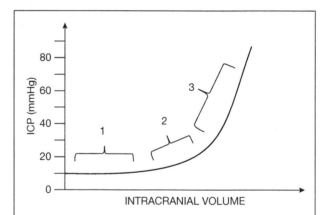

FIGURE 4.11 The relationship between ICP and intracranial volume. The relationship between pressure and volume is not linear. The flat portion of the curve "1" represents normal ICP and good compliance. The exponential portion of the curve "2" represents normal ICP with poor compliance. The steep portion of the curve "3" represents increased ICP with poor compliance, compensatory mechanisms have been exhausted.

ICP, intracranial pressure.

veins, and decreased production or increased reabsorption of CSF. *Phase 2* is the exponential portion of the curve, representing early decompensation with normal ICP but poor compliance (i.e., slight increases in volume are not tolerated). The critical point when compliance is lost varies and depends on several factors: rate of volumetric change (rapid increases in ICP are not tolerated well), age (younger child has less buffering capacity with acute increases in ICP), and medical interventions. *Phase 3* is the steep portion of the curve, representing the failure of compensation with increased ICP and poor compliance.

3. *Brain Metabolism*

   a. *Oxygen.* Twenty percent of cardiac output is delivered to the brain, although the brain comprises only 2% of the total body weight. Brain cells require a constant and consistent delivery of oxygen and are dependent on aerobic metabolism. The cerebral metabolic rate of oxygen ($CMRO_2$) is approximately 3 to 3.5 mL/100 g/min in the adult but is not constant throughout the brain; gray matter consumes more than white matter (Tameem & Krovvidi, 2013). The exact $CMRO_2$ in the neonate and infant is unknown.

   b. *Glucose.* Glucose stores in the brain are minimal; therefore, cells also require a constant and consistent delivery of glucose. Glucose is associated with significant brain cellular processes, including protein synthesis, amino acid metabolism, neurotransmitter release, membrane function, and pH homeostasis. The cerebral metabolic rate of glucose ($CMR_{glucose}$) is 4.0 to 5.0 mg/100 g/min in the adult (Tameem & Krovvidi, 2013). The exact $CMR_{glucose}$ in the neonate and infant is unknown. Hypoglycemia and hyperglycemia can cause neurologic damage.

4. *Cerebral Blood Flow*

   a. *Normal cerebral blood flow* (*CBF*) in the brain of the neonate is widely variable with an unknown lower limit. The actual delivery of oxygen to the tissues is affected by the percentage of circulating fetal hemoglobin. Normal CBF varies throughout the brain; it is highest in gray matter and lowest in white matter. Average (whole brain) CBF in the child is 105 mL/100 g/min (Jensen, 1980). Adolescents and adults have an average CBF of 45 to 55 mL/100 g/min.

   b. *Determinants of CBF* are best described by the following equation for laminar flow:

   $$CBF = \frac{\Delta P \pi r 4}{8 \eta l}$$

where ΔP = cerebral perfusion pressure
r = radius
η = viscosity of blood
l = length of blood vessel
π = constant, 3.14

CBF is directly related to CPP and vessel caliber and inversely related to vessel length and blood viscosity.

   i. The smaller the *arteriolar radius*, the greater the resistance to CBF. Mechanisms that change the caliber of the vessel are cerebral autoregulation and chemical regulation. Autoregulation is a compensatory mechanism that matches CBF to CMR by altering the radius of the cerebral vessels (i.e., vasoconstriction or vasodilation). A constant CBF is maintained when the MAP is between 50 and 150 mmHg. Outside this range, autoregulation may break down with inadequate or excessive cerebral perfusion. Autoregulation may be impaired in patients with neurologic injury and rapid and severe brain swelling may occur. $PacO_2$ (pH) affects the cerebral arteriolar radius: low $PacO_2$ (elevated pH) causes vasoconstriction and high $PacO_2$ (decreased pH) causes vasodilation. PaO_2, to a lesser extent, affects the cerebral arteriolar radius: PaO_2 less than 50 mmHg causes vasodilation and PaO_2 greater than 50 mmHg causes vasoconstriction, but remains constant. Figure 4.12 illustrates autoregulation by showing the effects of CPP, oxygen, and carbon dioxide on CBF. Increased *blood viscosity* (polycythemia) decreases CBF. The *length of the vascular bed* is constant at any point in time. Increased length increases resistance to CBF.

   ii. *CPP* represents the pressure difference between inflow (arterial) pressure and outflow (venous) pressure across the cerebral vascular bed. Clinically, it is most often calculated by the following equation: CPP = MAP – ICP. CPP measurement varies depending on where the arterial and ICP transducers are leveled. There is consensus that external ICP transducers are leveled at a location that approximates the lateral ventricles; for example, the tragus of the ear. There is considerable variation in the literature and clinical practice with respect to leveling the arterial transducer. Some centers level the arterial transducer at the right atrium, whereas other centers level it as they do the ICP transducer. The level of the transducer is not an issue when patients are maintained in a flat position, but there can be significant differences in CPP calculations when the upper

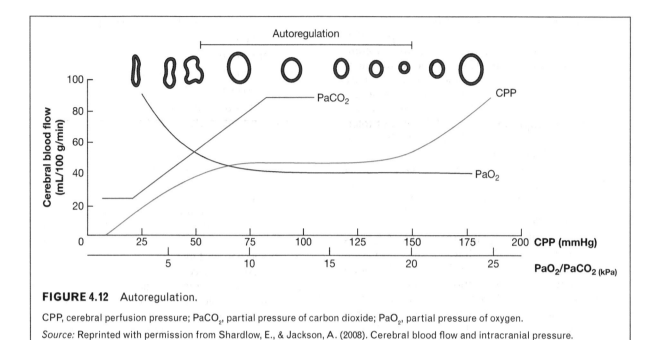

FIGURE 4.12 Autoregulation.

CPP, cerebral perfusion pressure; PaCO$_2$, partial pressure of carbon dioxide; PaO$_2$, partial pressure of oxygen.

Source: Reprinted with permission from Shardlow, E., & Jackson, A. (2008). Cerebral blood flow and intracranial pressure. *Anaesthesia & Intensive Care Medicine, 9*(5), 222–225. doi:10.1016/j.mpaic.2008.03.009 Copyright 2008 with permission from Elsevier.

body and head are elevated. The hydrostatic difference between both transducers increases as the patient's head is elevated. Until a consensus is reached on how to measure CPP, caution is required when interpreting CPP-targeted therapies and consistency in leveling technique should be maintained (Rao, Klepstad, Losvik, & Solheim, 2013).

iii. The optimal CPP in the pediatric patient is unknown. In normal adolescents and adults, CPP is variable and ranges between 70 and 90 mmHg with a constant CBF (Tameem & Krovvidi, 2013). The lower threshold of CPP when targeting therapy is unknown. Current guidelines in children with traumatic brain injury (TBI) recommend a lower threshold of 40 to 50 mmHg, infants at the lower range and adolescents at the upper range (Kochanek et al., 2012).

PERIPHERAL NERVOUS SYSTEM

Developmental Anatomy

A. Sensory and Motor Components

1. *Spinal nerves* are mixed nerves, which carry sensory, motor, and autonomic signals between the spinal cord and the body. They are connected to the spinal cord via two roots.

a. The *dorsal (posterior) root* carries afferent (sensory) fibers that transmit impulses from sensory receptors in the body to the spinal cord. The fibers supply the innervation for a particular segment of the body called a *dermatome* (Figure 4.13). *Afferent fibers* are subdivided according to function. General somatic afferent (GSA) fibers transmit impulses from sensors in the extremities and body wall. General visceral afferent (GVA) fibers transmit impulses from sensors in the viscera.

b. The *ventral (anterior) root* carries efferent (motor) fibers that transmit impulses from the spinal cord. Efferent fibers are subdivided according to function. General somatic efferent (GSE) fibers innervate voluntary striated muscle. General visceral efferent (GVE) fibers innervate involuntary smooth muscles, cardiac muscle, and glands.

c. Fusion of the roots forms 31 spinal nerves: eight pairs of cervical, 12 pairs of thoracic, five pairs of lumbar, five pairs of sacral, and one coccygeal. Cauda equina (horse's tail) is the long root of lumbar and sacral nerves contained within the spinal cistern (the spinal cord is shorter than the vertebral column). Thoracic, lumbar, and sacral nerves are numbered according to the vertebra just rostral to the foramen through which they pass. Cervical nerves are numbered for

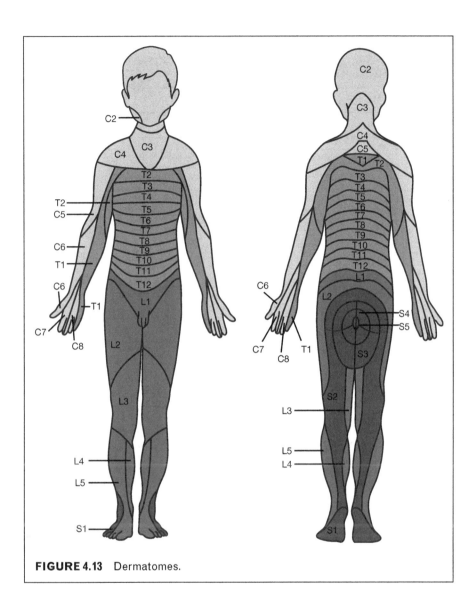

FIGURE 4.13 Dermatomes.

the vertebra just caudal to the foramen through which they pass. Fibers are also classified functionally according to conduction velocity.

2. *Cranial nerves* are the peripheral nerves of the brain. Cranial nerve I fibers originate from the olfactory mucosa in the nasal cavity, cranial nerve II fibers originate in the retina, and cranial nerves III through XII originate from different locations of the brainstem. Classification by type and function is described in Table 4.2.

3. *Autonomic Nervous System*

　a. Components of the ANS are located in the CNS and the PNS. The primary (preganglionic)

neuron originates in the CNS. The axon of the primary neuron travels outside the CNS to synapse on a secondary (postganglionic) neuron found in one of the autonomic ganglia. The postganglionic fiber terminates in an organ or structure.

　b. In the *sympathetic (thoracolumbar) division* (Figure 4.14), preganglionic fibers originate in the intermediolateral cell column of segments T-1 through T-12. Fibers emerge from the spinal cord through the ventral roots and branch into the white rami communicants. White rami communicants send fibers to the paired trunk ganglia (located laterally on each side of the thoracic and

TABLE 4.2   Classification of Cranial Nerves

Cranial Nerve	Name	Type	Function
I	Olfactory	Sensory	Olfaction
II	Optic	Sensory	Vision
III	Oculomotor	Motor	Pupillary constriction and accommodation, extraocular movements, elevation of upper eyelid
IV	Trochlear	Motor	Deviation of the eye (inward on adduction, downward on abduction)
V	Trigeminal	Sensory and motor	Muscles of mastication; sensory innervation of the face, nose, and mouth
VI	Abducens	Motor	Lateral deviation of the eye
VII	Facial	Sensory and motor	Muscles of facial expression; sensory components of taste and salivation
VIII	Acoustic	Sensory	Hearing and balance
IX	Glossopharyngeal	Sensory and motor	Motor to pharyngeal region (swallowing); salivation and taste; thermal sensations from posterior tongue, tonsils, and Eustachian tubes
X	Vagus	Sensory and motor	Sensory innervation of the larynx and pharynx; motor innervation of the palate and pharynx; and parasympathetic functions
XI	Spinal accessory	Motor	Motor innervation of the sternocleidomastoid muscle and the upper portion of the trapezius muscle (shoulder shrug, turning head)
XII	Hypoglossal	Motor	Movement of the tongue

Source: Curley, M. A., & Patricia, M. A. (2001). *Critical care nursing of infants and children* (2nd ed.). Philadelphia, PA: Mosby Elsevier. Copyright Elsevier (2001).

lumbar vertebrae), where they synapse with post-ganglionic fibers. The postganglionic fibers exit the trunk ganglia and innervate different organs and structures. T-1 to T-5 innervates the head and neck. T-1 and T-2 innervates the eye. T-2 to T-6 innervates the heart and lungs. T-6 to L-2 innervates the abdominal viscera. L-1 and L-2 are to the urinary, genital, and lower digestive systems.

c.   In the *parasympathetic (craniosacral) division* (Figure 4.15), preganglionic fibers originate

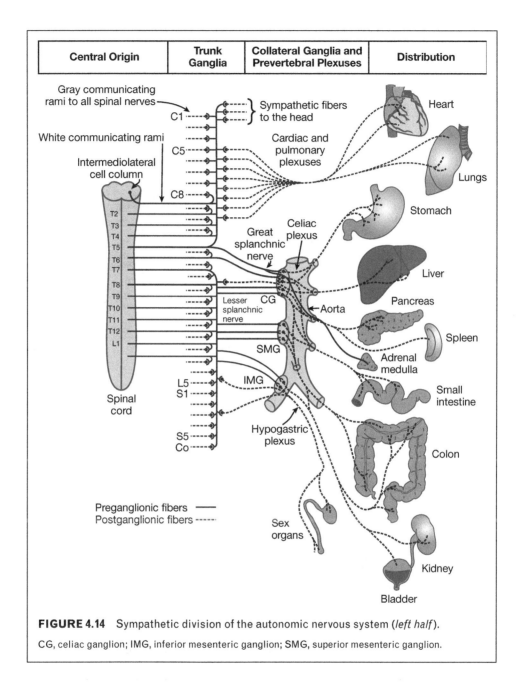

Central Origin	Trunk Ganglia	Collateral Ganglia and Prevertebral Plexuses	Distribution

Gray communicating rami to all spinal nerves

Sympathetic fibers to the head

White communicating rami

Intermediolateral cell column

Cardiac and pulmonary plexuses

Heart

Lungs

Stomach

Great splanchnic nerve

Celiac plexus

Liver

Pancreas

Lesser splanchnic nerve

CG

Aorta

Spleen

SMG

Adrenal medulla

IMG

Small intestine

Spinal cord

Hypogastric plexus

Colon

Preganglionic fibers ——
Postganglionic fibers -----

Sex organs

Kidney

Bladder

FIGURE 4.14 Sympathetic division of the autonomic nervous system (*left half*).

CG, celiac ganglion; IMG, inferior mesenteric ganglion; SMG, superior mesenteric ganglion.

from two areas: brainstem preganglionic fibers (often travel in the cranial nerves, specifically, cranial nerves III, VII, IX, and X) and the middle segments of the sacral region. Nerve fibers are distributed exclusively to visceral organs. Most preganglionic fibers have long axons that synapse with a few postganglionic fibers with short axons. The synapse usually occurs in the end organ. The cranial fibers innervate visceral structures including the head, thoracic cavity, and abdominal cavity. The sacral fibers

give rise to the pelvic nerve, which innervates most of the large intestine, pelvic viscera, and genitalia.

ESSENTIAL PHYSIOLOGY

A. Neural Transmission

Neural transmission in the ANS occurs via neurotransmitters. Sympathetic division preganglionic nerve

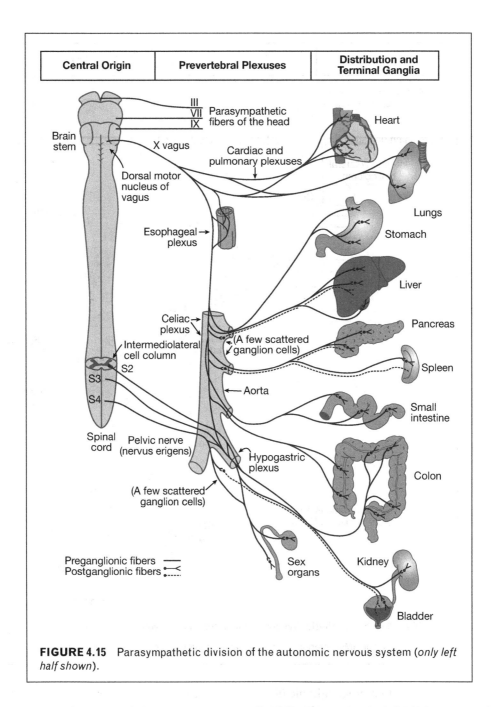

FIGURE 4.15 Parasympathetic division of the autonomic nervous system (*only left half shown*).

terminals secrete acetylcholine (*cholinergic*), postganglionic nerve terminals secrete norepinephrine (*adrenergic*), and the postganglionic nerve terminals to sweat glands secrete acetylcholine. Parasympathetic division preganglionic nerve terminals secrete acetylcholine, and postganglionic nerve terminals secrete acetylcholine. Acetylcholine is deactivated by cholinesterase. Norepinephrine is deactivated by monoamine oxidase (MAO) and catechol O-methyltransferase (COMT).

B. Systemic Effects of ANS Innervation

Systemic effects of ANS innervation (Table 4.3): The sympathetic division is organized to exert influences over widespread body regions. Stimulation prepares the body for the intense muscular activity needed for the "fight-or-flight" response. The parasympathetic division is organized to exert influences in localized discrete areas of the body. Stimulation prepares the body primarily for "resting" bodily functions.

TABLE 4.3 Autonomic Nerve Stimulation

Effector Organ	Sympathetic (Noradrenergic)		Parasympathetic (Cholinergic) Effects[a]
	Effects	Receptor(s)	
Neurotransmitter			
	Usually norepinephrine[b]		Acetylcholine
Eye			
	Pupil dilation	α_1	Pupil constriction
Heart			
Sinoatrial node	Increases heart rate	β_1, β_2	Decreases heart rate; vagal arrest
Atria	Increases contractility	β_1, β_2	Decreases contractility; some increase in conduction velocity
AV node, conduction	Increases conduction velocity	β_1, β_2	Decreases conduction velocity
Ventricles	Increases ventricular rate, contractility, and conduction velocity	β_1, β_2	Decreases contractility
Blood vessels			
Skin	Constriction	α_1, α_2	Dilation, minor effect
Coronary	Dilation; constriction, minor effect	α_1, α_2, β_2	Minor constriction; strong dilation
Cerebral	Constriction, minor effect	α	Dilation, minor effect
Pulmonary	Dilation; constriction, minor effect	α, β	Dilation, minor effect
Abdominal viscera	Constriction (primarily)	α_1, β_2	
Lungs			
Bronchial muscle	Dilation	β_2	Constriction
Bronchial glands			Stimulates secretion
Gastrointestinal tract			
Motility and tone	Inhibits (relaxation) primarily	α_1, α_2 β_1, β_2	Stimulates (contraction)
Sphincters	Stimulates (contraction)	α_1	Inhibits (relaxation)
Secretion	May inhibit (contraction)	α_2	Stimulates (contraction)
Urinary bladder			
Detrusor	Inhibits (relaxation) primarily	β_2	Stimulates (contraction)
Trigone and sphincter	Stimulates (contraction)	α_1	Inhibits (relaxation) primarily

(continued)

TABLE 4.3 Autonomic Nerve Stimulation *(continued)*

Effector Organ	Sympathetic (Noradrenergic)		Parasympathetic (Cholinergic) Effects[a]
	Effects	Receptor(s)	
Pancreas			
Acini	Decreases secretion	α	Increases secretion
Islets	Decreases insulin and glucagon secretion Increases insulin	α_1, α_2 β_2	Increases insulin and glucagon secretion

AV, atrioventricular.

[a]All parasympathetic responses are mediated by activation of muscarinic receptors.
[b]The sympathetic neurotransmitter for sweat glands and adrenal medulla is acetylcholine.

CLINICAL ASSESSMENT OF NEUROLOGIC FUNCTION

The nervous system is incompletely developed at birth and takes several years to mature. Consequently, neurologic assessment of the infant and young child must be individualized to reflect neurodevelopment and temperament of the child.

A. History

1. *Chief Complaint.* Use the parents' own words and description and solicit information from school-aged and older children when their condition permits.

2. *Present Illness.* Describe onset and development, associated symptoms, and factors that relieve or exacerbate symptoms.

3. *Past History.* Infant and toddler history should summarize antenatal, perinatal, and postnatal courses, including maternal infections, medications taken during pregnancy, Apgar scores, gestational age, and birth complications such as meconium aspiration, seizure activity, or respiratory status (oxygen requirements). History should include a chronologic list of developmental milestones, childhood illnesses, immunization status, significant or chronic illnesses (e.g., seizures, diabetes, and head injury), and medications.

4. *Family History.* Some neurologic disorders manifest themselves as disturbances in other body systems; therefore, it is important to review the patient's past history.

a. *Neurologic disorders* may be static or progressive and may be traumatic (acquired) or congenital.

b. *Endocrine disorders* with neurologic implications include diabetic coma and thyroid disease and hormonal imbalances (growth disorders).

c. *Cardiovascular disorders* with neurologic implications include cyanotic heart disease (risk for brain infarcts and abscesses) and aneurysms (may have a higher incidence in families with a known history).

d. *Congenital disorders* with neurologic implications include neural tube defects (NTDs) and metabolic disorders (e.g., phenylketonuria [PKU], cretinism).

e. *Genetic disorders* may have a neurologic origin or may affect the neurologic system. Most neurodegenerative disorders are transmitted as a recessive gene. Epilepsies and migraine headaches tend to be transmitted as a dominant trait.

f. *Renal disorders* may produce metabolic imbalances that affect neurologic functioning (e.g., acute renal failure and the increased risk of cerebral edema).

5. *Social history* should include school performance, types of play activities and recreation, substance abuse, and smoking.

B. Physical Examination

1. *General appearance* evaluation includes behavior, dress, speech and conversation, gait, emotional state, and symmetry of body structures.

2. *Skull Examination*

a. *Inspection* of the skull includes occipito-frontal head circumference, shape and symmetry of head, transillumination (increased with serous fluid [caput succedaneum] and decreased with blood fluid [cephalhematoma]). Extreme downward rotation of the eyes and paralysis of upward gaze (setting sun sign) is often seen with hydrocephalus. Craniofacial malformation may be present with craniosynostosis from premature closure of one or more cranial sutures.

b. *Palpation* of the *fontanelles* should occur while the infant is upright and quiet. Fontanelles that remain open beyond the usual period of closure may be related to disorders that abnormally increase the intracranial contents (e.g., tumors, hydrocephalus). The anterior fontanelle is usually 4 to 6 cm at its largest diameter at birth, and the posterior fontanelle is usually 1 to 2 cm at its largest diameter at birth. The anterior fontanelle may be full and tense with increased ICP, crying, vomiting, or coughing in the infant. Pulsations of the anterior fontanelle reflect the peripheral pulse and are normally barely palpable. Palpation of sutures reveals overriding sutures (common with vaginal deliveries) or premature closure of the sutures. Widely separated sutures may suggest hydrocephalus.

c. *Auscultation* of the skull using a bell stethoscope with the child in an erect position is performed over six areas: the temporal fossae, both globes, and the reticulo auricular or mastoid regions. In all cases, a transmitted cardiac murmur should be excluded. Bruit (spontaneous) in the young child may be normal, but an abnormal bruit is often loud, harsh, and asymmetric or accompanied by a thrill, or both.

d. *Percussion* of the skull is normally dull. A "cracked-pot" sound (Macewen's sign) is heard with separated sutures and increased ICP.

3. *Level of Consciousness*

a. *Consciousness* is a state of awareness of self and environment. There are two major components of consciousness and disease states affect them differently. First, there is the *content* of consciousness, which represents mental function, or higher intellectual activity and is primarily at the level of the cerebral hemispheres. The second component of consciousness is *arousal*, or wakefulness, and its function is primarily located throughout the brainstem, an extensive network of nuclei and interconnecting fibers known as the *RAS*. Maintaining alertness requires intact function of the cerebral hemispheres and arousal mechanisms located in the RAS. Impaired consciousness is from impairment of both cerebral hemispheres or dysfunction of the RAS.

b. Altered states of consciousness are on a continuum and represent varying degrees of neurologic dysfunction. Many terms are used to describe acute altered states of consciousness and several of these terms are used incorrectly or mean different things to different observers. *Clouding of consciousness* is characterized by reduced wakefulness, confusion, and alternating drowsiness and hyperexcitability. In its mildest form, the patient is distracted, has inattention, and judgment is reduced. In more severe states, the patient is more confused and may misinterpret stimuli. *Delirium* is a neurocognitive disorder due to a somatic illness or treatment. Although a child may experience delirium anywhere, it is more likely to occur in the hospital. Many conditions can cause delirium such as fever, infections, medications, or metabolic disorders. It is usually a temporary and reversible state when the underlying condition is identified and treated. It is a disturbance of consciousness and is characterized by disorientation, fear, irritability, visual hallucinations, and agitation. The patient has reduced ability to focus and sustain attention. Memory may be altered with language disturbances. This disturbance usually develops over a short period and may fluctuate throughout the day. There is evidence to suggest that there is a relationship between severity of illness and pediatric delirium (Silver et al., 2015). *Emergence/agitation* delirium is a condition that may occur in children in the immediate postoperative or postprocedure period. It usually resolves in 30 to 45 minutes without intervention. Several bedside tools have been introduced to clinically screen and guide treatment for delirium in pediatric patients, such as the *Pediatric Anesthesia Emergence Delirium Scale (PAED;* Sikich & Lerman, 2004), the *pediatric Confusion Assessment Method for ICU (pCAM-ICU;* Smith et al., 2011), the *Cornell Assessment Pediatric Delirium tool (CAP-D;* Traube et al., 2014), and the *Sophia Observation Withdrawal Symptoms-Pediatric Delirium scale (SOS-PD;* Ista, van Dijk, de Hoog, Tibboel, & Duivenvoorden, 2009).

Several variables (e.g., age, gender, severity of illness) may affect the validity of a tool and should be taken into consideration when using them (Luetz et al. 2016). *Obtundation* is characterized by mild to moderate reduction in alertness, reduced interest in the environment, and increased periods of sleep. Stimuli of mild to moderate intensity fail to arouse the patient. If arousal does occur, the patient is slow to respond. *Stupor* is characterized by unresponsiveness except to vigorous and repeated stimuli. Once the stimulus is removed, the patient drifts back to a deep sleep-like state. *Coma* is indicated by severely reduced or absent verbal or motor response to environmental stimuli. The patient may respond to noxious stimuli with abnormal motor movements, but they lack localization or defensive movements (Posner, Saper, Schiff, & Plum, 2007).

c. *Mental status* assessment in infants and children is more complex than in older patients because of their immature neurologic development. There are also significant normal developmental ranges among infants and toddlers. Establishing the child's preillness baseline is imperative and requires caregiver cooperation and accurate recall. In infants, assess the quality of the cry, alertness and level of activity, feeding patterns, language development, presence or absence of primitive reflexes, patterns of sleep and wakefulness, and responses to caregivers. In children, assess attention, alertness, orientation, cognition, memory, affect, and perception. The mental status of older children and adolescents can be assessed using more traditional methods (e.g., orientation to person, place and time; short-term and long-term memory; and speech and language).

d. The cause of coma may be structural or metabolic. If the cause is structural, brain imaging studies are useful in identifying the extent and location of the brain lesion. If the cause of coma is metabolic, laboratory studies (e.g., metabolic panels or toxic screen) and perfusion scans are useful. Coma scales are used to grade the degree of unresponsiveness by standardized assessments. The Glasgow Coma Scale (GCS) is the most widely used scoring system and assesses arousability in relation to three responses: eye opening (arousal state), verbal response (content of consciousness), and motor response (arousal state and content of consciousness). Each response is given the best number for a given response. The sum of the numbers ranges between 3 (least responsive) and 15 (normal). The GCS cannot be applied directly to children younger than 5 years, particularly the verbal scale. For example, the best response under *Verbal* is "oriented" and the best response under *Motor* is "obeys commands"; these are not realistic responses in young children. A number of coma scales have been developed to accommodate preverbal children and infants, and typically, are scored in a similar fashion to the GCS. When assessing the unconscious state in a child, it is important to note the level of intensity of stimulation necessary to arouse the child and their specific response. Stimuli used to elicit a response should start with voice or touch. If the patient does not respond, the nurse should escalate to a noxious stimulus (e.g., sternal rub or nail bed compression). Careful attention is given to preventing injury, especially in patients with a coagulopathy. Table 4.4 compares the GCS to a modified version that can be used in children less than 5 years of age.

4. *Pain and Sedation Monitoring*

a. Infants and children admitted to the pediatric intensive care unit (PICU) frequently experience discomfort from their preexisting injury or condition. Pain and agitation may continue as they undergo numerous procedures and as a consequence of multidisciplinary management.

b. Assessing pain and agitation in patients with altered states of consciousness is challenging and requires close scrutiny of the patient's physiologic status and clinical response to analgesia and sedation. The goal is maximal comfort without diminishing patient responsiveness. Sedation and analgesia need to be balanced so that meaningful serial neurological assessments can be performed while minimizing pain, agitation, and stress.

c. The use of pain assessment tools and scales is recommended to provide consistency among observers, to recognize and trend pain levels, and to determine the effectiveness of comfort alleviating interventions. Commonly used pain assessment scales in the PICU include the *COMFORT Behavior Scale* (Ambuel, Hamlett, Marx, & Blumer, 1992) *COMFORT-B Scale* (Bai, Hsu, Tang, & van Dijk, 2012), and the *FLACC Scale* (Merkel, Voepel-Lewis, & Malviya, 2002).

d. Optimal sedation level is important to improve patient outcomes (e.g., length of stay

TABLE 4.4   Glasgow Coma Scale and Child's Glasgow Coma Scale

Activity	>5 Years of Age	<5 Years of Age	Score
Verbal response	• No response • Incomprehensible sounds • Inappropriate words • Confused • Oriented	• No response • Moans to pain • Cries to pain • Irritable cry, unusual or diminished baseline level • Alert, babbles, coos, says words, or sentences (normal for age)	1 2 3 4 5
Eye opening	• None • To pain • To speech • Spontaneously	• None • To pain • To speech • Spontaneously	1 2 3 4
Motor response	• None • Abnormal extensor to noxious stimuli • Abnormal flexor to noxious stimuli • Withdraws to noxious stimuli • Localizes to touch • Obeys commands	• None • Abnormal extensor to noxious stimuli • Abnormal flexor to noxious stimuli • Withdraws to noxious stimuli • Localizes (>9 mo) to noxious stimuli • Normal spontaneous movements	1 2 3 4 5 6
Total score[a]			**3–15**

[a]Total score = sum of the score for each of the three components. Score for a fully oriented alert patient = 15. Score for a mute immobile patient with no eye opening = 3; For motor response, score the best response for asymmetrical responses; For children >5 years, responses are similar to adult.

Sources: Adapted from Kirkham, F., Newton, C., & Whitehouse, W. (2008). Pediatric coma scales. *Developmental Medicine & Child Neurology, 50*, 267–274. doi:10.1111/j.1469-8749.2008.02042.x; Teasdale, G., & Jennett, B. (1974). Assessment of coma and impaired consciousness. *Lancet, 304*(7872), 81–84. doi:10.1016/S0140-6736(74)91639-0

and ventilator days) and to minimize patient distress. Commonly used sedation assessment scales in the PICU include the *COMFORT Behavior Scale* (Ambuel et al., 1992), *COMFORT-B scale* (Bai et al., 2012), and the *State Behavior Scale* (Curley, Harris, & Fraser, 2006).

5. *Motor Function.* Assessment of normal motor development proceeds cephalocaudally and proximodistally.

a. Assess *primitive reflexes* in infants and toddlers and determine their presence or absence, time of disappearance, and the symmetry of the reflex. The most commonly evaluated reflexes include the following:

i. Moro: Elicited by a sudden movement of the body that causes a change in equilibrium. The response is extension and abduction of the upper extremities (fingers fan), followed by flexion and adduction. The reflex appears between 28 to 32 weeks gestation and disappears by 3 to 5 months after birth.

ii. Palmar grasp. Elicited by the examiner's placing his or her index finger into the ulnar side of the infant's hand and pressing against the palmar surface. The response is immediate flexion of the infant's fingers around the examiner's finger. The reflex appears at 28 weeks gestation and disappears between 4 and 6 months after birth.

iii. Parachute. Elicited by holding the infant in a ventral position. A sudden plunge downward produces extension and abduction of the infant's arms and fingers. The reflex appears at 4 to 9 months after birth and persists throughout life (the response is usually covered up with voluntary movement in older individuals).

iv. Rooting. Elicited by stroking the perioral skin at the corner of the mouth; moving laterally toward the cheek, upper lip, and lower lip. The infant turns his or her head toward the stimulated side with sucking movements. The reflex appears at 28 weeks gestation and disappears between 3 and 4 months after birth.

v. Placing. Elicited with the infant supported in a vertical position with the dorsum of one foot pressed against a hard surface. The infant's foot will flex and extend, simulating walking. The reflex appears at 35 to 37 weeks gestation and disappears at 1 to 2 months after birth.

vi. Asymmetric tonic neck response. Elicited by rotating the infant's head to the side while the infant's chest is maintained in a flat position. The arm and leg extend on the side to which the infant's face is turned, and the opposite arm and leg flex. The reflex appears at birth to 2 months and disappears between 4 and 6 months.

b. Assess for *developmental milestones* (e.g., sitting, crawling, and walking).

c. If the patient can follow commands, assess *muscle strength and tone, symmetry of movement, and DTRs*. Not all DTRs are present in the infant because of the immaturity of the corticospinal tracts. DTRs are tested based on the segmental level they innervate. The usual reflexes include biceps (segmental levels C-5 and C-6), brachioradialis (segmental levels C-5 and C-6), triceps (segmental levels C-7 and C-8), knee (segmental levels L-2, L-3, and L-4), and ankle (segmental levels S-1 and S-2). The technique for eliciting DTRs is similar to that used for adults; however, the hammer may be replaced with the examiner's semiflexed index finger. The technique includes positioning the limb so that the muscle is slightly stretched, striking the tendon briskly to create an additional sudden tendon stretch, and testing both muscle groups on each side of the body. Reflex responses are usually graded on a scale from 0 (no response) to 4+ (very brisk, hyperactive; may be indicative of disease). Abnormal findings include very brisk or asymmetric responses or deviations from a previous assessment.

d. *Superficial reflexes* include the Babinski, abdominal, and cremasteric reflexes. The technique for eliciting *Babinski's reflex* includes using a sharp object (thumbnail) to stimulate the plantar surface of the foot. Stimulation begins at the heel and travels along the lateral border of the sole, crossing over the base of the metatarsals to the great toe. A normal response in children younger than 1 to 2 years is immediate dorsiflexion of the great toe and subsequent separation (fanning) of the other toes; this response is abnormal in older children and adults. A normal response beyond the second year is plantar flexion of the toes. The *abdominal reflex* is elicited by lightly, but briskly stroking each side of the abdomen, above and below the umbilicus. A normal response is contraction of the abdominal muscles and deviation of the umbilicus toward the stimulus. The reflex may not be present at birth but is consistently present at 6 months of age. An asymmetric response is abnormal. The *cremasteric reflex* (only found in males) is elicited by lightly but briskly stroking the inner aspect of each of the upper thighs. A normal response is elevation of the testicle on the side stimulated. It may not be present at birth but occurs consistently at approximately 6 months of age. An asymmetric response is abnormal.

e. *Abnormal motor responses* in the comatose patient include *decorticate posturing* (consisting of flexion and adduction of the upper extremities and extension of the lower extremities with plantar flexion representing dysfunction of the cerebral hemispheres or upper part of the brainstem), *decerebrate posturing* (extensor posturing consisting of extension, adduction, and hyperpronation of the upper and lower extremities and plantar flexion representing dysfunction at the pontomesencephalic level), and *flaccidity* (no motor response to external stimuli representing severe dysfunction of the lower brainstem and vital centers for which spinal cord injury [SCI] and stroke must be ruled out).

f. All extremities should be assessed independently. Specific stimuli to elicit a motor response should be documented.

6. *Sensory Function*

a. In infants, sensory testing results are variable and less reliable than in the older child. Light touch is assessed by stroking an extremity (the normal response is to withdraw the limb). Vibration sense is assessed with a tuning fork over bony areas (the normal response is cessation of movement and often a look of surprise). Proprioception cannot be tested in infants or comatose patients because it requires participation of the patient. Pain sensation is assessed with nail bed pressure (at the end of examination).

b. Light touch and superficial pain are assessed in older children in all four extremities. If abnormalities are noted, a more detailed segmental assessment is done. Proprioception is tested by asking the child to close his or her eyes and move a finger or toe up or down and then asking the child to identify whether the movement is up or down. Pain sensation is tested at the end of the examination by using a pin to test the various dermatomes (see Figure 4.13).

7. *Cerebellar Function*

a. In infants and toddlers, cerebellar function should be assessed by observing the child during play or usual activities. Abnormal findings include tremors, which are rhythmic alterations in movement and, unlike spontaneous seizures, are usually precipitated by a variety of stimuli (e.g., sudden changes in movement) with no alteration in the level of consciousness. Dysmetria (inability to control the range of movement in muscle action) or gait abnormalities (e.g., wide-based or waddling type of gait) may also be noticed.

b. Maneuvers to assess older children include the finger-to-nose test, the heel–shin test, observation of gait, and toe-to-heel walking. The finger-to-nose test is performed while the child stands erect with arms extended at the sides; the child is then asked to touch his or her nose with alternating index fingers. An abnormal finding is seen if the child completely misses his or her nose. The heel–shin test is done while the child is in a supine position. The child is asked to place one heel rapidly down the shin from the knee to the ankle and repeat on the other side. Movements should be coordinated and accurate. The child can also be instructed to touch each finger to the thumb of the same hand in rapid succession. Each hand is tested, and the response should be symmetric. Observation of gait can be made while the child walks toward and away from the examiner. The child should have good posture and balance. During toe-to-heel walking, the child places the heel of one foot to the toe of the other foot and continues this maneuver for a distance of several feet. The child should have good balance.

8. *Cranial Nerve Function.* The order and specific nerves to be tested depend on the age and condition of the child. Age-specific techniques used to assess cranial nerves in infants and children are included in Table 4.5.

9. *Funduscopic Examination*

a. Normal findings include a red reflex that is orange-red and fairly uniform in color, a creamy pink optic disc with an indented center (physiologic depression) and smooth margins, and veins that are slightly wider than arteries.

TABLE 4.5 Cranial Nerve Evaluation

Cranial Nerve	Functions	Methods of Testing	Comments
Infant[a]			
I	Olfactory Sense of smell	Assess patency of both nostrils. Hold noxious odor near each nostril separately. Observe for generalized body movement or cry.	Unreliable test for infants. Although smell is intact, the immature myelination prohibits an integrated, voluntary motor response.
II	Optic Vision	Inspect the fundus with an ophthalmoscope. Test visual fields by introducing a brightly colored object into each visual field from behind the infant. In the infant with a pincer grasp, observe the visual acuity used in spotting and picking up crumbs and small objects.	The optic disc is pale, gray, and poorly developed in the infant. The macula (area of central vision) is not fully developed until 4 months, at which time the infant will notice light contrast and different colors. Infants are capable of binocular fixation at 3 months and can follow the object for visual field testing.

(continued)

TABLE 4.5 Cranial Nerve Evaluation *(continued)*

Cranial Nerve	Functions	Methods of Testing	Comments
III	Oculomotor Pupillary constriction, elevation of the upper eyelid, and most of the extraocular movements	Check pupillary responses: Shine light directly into each eye from the side and observe the briskness and completeness of the direct pupillary response. Check the consensual response by shining the light into one eye and observing the response in the other eye. Record the size of the pupil in millimeters. Note the shape and equality of the pupils. Note the infant's spontaneous eye opening and any ptosis. Note the presence of doll's eyes (oculocephalic reflex): Turn the head to one side quickly and watch the position of the eyes. A positive response, when the eyes move in the opposite direction as though still gazing in the initial direction, is present with an intact brainstem. Check extraocular movements (cranial nerves III, IV, and IV). Test for accommodation, noting constriction and convergence as a bright object is brought toward the nose.	Early signs of increased ICP include a sluggishly reactive pupil and incomplete constriction. Infants older than the age of 3 months are able to accommodate for near vision. The setting-sun sign (portion of sclera visible between the iris and upper eyelid) can result from hydrocephalus and brainstem irritation. A negative oculocephalic reflex (doll's eyes) can result from a lesion of the midbrain or pons or from a deep coma.
IV VI III	Trochlear Downward inward movement of the eye Abducens lateral deviation of the eye Oculomotor all other extraocular movements	Check the six fields of gaze: Hold a bright object 18 inches from the infant and move it from the midline into each of the six fields of gaze (upward: inward and outward, laterally: inward and outward, downward: inward and outward) for each eye with someone else holding the infant's head steady. Note conjugate movements of the eyes.	Infants should attempt binocular fixation at the age of 3 months and be able to follow the object smoothly by the age of 1 year. Nystagmus is normal in premature infants and neonates. Dysconjugate movements after the age of 6 weeks can be indicative of blindness.
V	Trigeminal Motor: Innervation to the temporal and masseter muscles; responsible for jaw clenching and lateral movement. Sensory: Innervation to the face with three branches: (a) opthalmic, (b) maxillary, and (c) mandibular	Test the strength of the temporal and masseter muscles by assessing the infant's sucking hold on the nipple or finger. Note jaw symmetry while the infant is crying. Test for the rooting reflex by stroking the cheek and watching the infant turn to the stimulated side. Test the corneal reflex with a cotton wisp touched lightly to the cornea only. Note the response of blinking and possible tearing.	Jaw weakness and an impaired suck can be present in infants with trigeminal damage. Infants can blink asymmetrically in response to corneal stimulation. Most infants produce tears by the age of 2–3 months. The sensory component of the corneal reflex is the trigeminal nerve, and the motor component is the facial nerve.

(continued)

TABLE 4.5 Cranial Nerve Evaluation *(continued)*

Cranial Nerve	Functions	Methods of Testing	Comments
VII	Facial Motor: Innervation to the muscles of the face, including the forehead, eyes, and mouth Sensory: Innervation to the anterior two-thirds of the tongue where sweet, sour, and salty sensors predominate	Observe facial symmetry during crying and smiling.	Although taste is intact at birth, taste testing is not reliable in infants and rarely done. Infants will usually wrinkle their foreheads when crying. Central facial damage will result in paralysis from the eye down, and peripheral damage produces paralysis on the entire side of the face.
VIII	Acoustic Cochlear division: Hearing Vestibular division: Balance	Test acoustic blink reflex by creating a loud noise near infant and noting the blink in response. Create loud noise and note appropriate response for age. Test vestibular branch with doll's eye maneuver (see cranial nerve III) and caloric testing; iced saline is injected into the ear canal with a syringe by the physician after assuring that the tympanic membrane is intact. Note the normal response of nystagmus with the eye jerking away from the irrigated ear.	During the neonatal period, there is a generalized response to noise, usually a cry or Moro reflex. At about 8–10 weeks, the infant will stop moving to listen to the sound. At about 3–4 months, the infant will turn his or her head toward the noise. This response is expected by the age of 8 months at the latest. In coma with an intact brainstem, caloric testing can demonstrate deviation of eyes toward the irrigated ear. With brainstem lesions, there is usually no response.
IX	Glossopharyngeal Sensory: Innervation to the pharynx and taste on the posterior one third of the tongue	Stimulate a gag. Note hoarse or stridorous crying. Observe swallowing with feedings, and note excessive drooling.	Some drooling is normal in infants. The autonomic system is intact at birth, but infants are particularly sensitive to parasympathetic stimulation. For example, the infant can readily demonstrate bradycardia during gagging or suctioning.
X	Vagus Sensory: Innervation to the pharynx and larynx Motor: Innervation to palate and pharynx and parasympathetic functions		
XI	Spinal accessory Motor: Innervation to the sternomastoid muscle and the upper portion of the trapezius muscle	Observe the infant's head movement from side to side.	Damage to the nerve can result in difficulty in turning the head from side to side.

(continued)

TABLE 4.5 Cranial Nerve Evaluation *(continued)*

Cranial Nerve	Functions	Methods of Testing	Comments
XII	Hypoglossal Motor: Innervation to the tongue	Gently pinch the infant's nostrils to produce reflex opening of the mouth and raising of the tongue. Note tongue asymmetry, deviation, or atrophy. Observe the tongue movements during sucking.	Damage to the nerve can result in paresis, paralysis, deviation, or fasciculations.
Child[b]			
I	Olfactory Sense of smell	Ensure that both nasal passages are patent and unobstructed. Ask child to close eyes and identify smells, testing each nostril separately. Use familiar odors, such as peanut butter, oranges, and chocolate.	Unreliable test results are common in toddlers and young children. Damage to this nerve results in perversion or loss of smell. Unilateral loss of smell can indicate a tumor of the anterior fossa. Temporary or permanent loss of smell can also be related to trauma to the olfactory bulbs or tracts or an upper respiratory tract infection.
II	Optic Vision	Test visual acuity in the younger child by observing recognition of familiar objects or people at a distance. This nerve can be tested with an eye chart (such as a Snellen chart) when children are about 6–7 years of age. Test color acuity through recognition of colored objects. Determine visual fields through the confrontation method: (a) seat the child at your eye level approximately 2–3 feet away; (b) ask the child to stare at your nose (using a bright sticker on the end of your nose can help); (c) bring a brightly colored object into the child's field of vision from the nasal, lateral, superior, and inferior fields; and (d) compare the child's visual fields to your own. Inspect the fundus with an ophthalmoscope for optic atrophy or papilledema.	Damage to this nerve can result in ipsilateral visual impairment. Homonymous hemianopsia can result from spastic hemiplegia. Bilateral (bitemporal) hemianopsia can result from a tumor of the optic chiasm or craniopharyngioma. The confrontation method is a rough evaluation of visual fields. Specialized testing is required for an accurate evaluation. Specific fundoscopic findings in the pediatric patient include: (a) the child's retina is lighter than the adult's, (b) the macula is not fully differentiated, and (c) papilledema is rare in children before complete closure of the fontanelles and sutures.

(continued)

TABLE 4.5 Cranial Nerve Evaluation *(continued)*

Cranial Nerve	Functions	Methods of Testing	Comments
III	Oculomotor Pupillary constriction, elevation of the upper eyelid, and most of the extraocular movements	Check pupillary responses by shining a light directly into each eye from the side and observing the briskness and completeness of the direct pupillary response. Check the consensual response by shining the light into one eye and observing the briskness in response of the other pupil. Record the size of pupil in millimeters. Note the shape and equality of the pupils. Note the opening of the upper eyelids and ptosis (drooping). Check the extraocular movements.	Compression of the parasympathetic nerve fiber on the third cranial nerve allows sympathetic dominance and pupillary dilatation. Because the third nerve is located at the tentorial notch, increases in ICP can result in ipsilateral, contralateral, or bilateral pupillary dilatation. Early signs of increased ICP include a sluggish response to light or incomplete constriction. Other abnormal findings that should be noted include: (a) anisocoria (unequal pupils), (b) bilaterally pinpoint fixed pupils (damage to sympathetic nerves at brainstem), and (c) hippus (rhythmical dilatation and constriction of pupils in response to light).
IV	Trochlear Downward, inward movement of the eye	Check the six fields of gaze by holding a bright object 18 inches from the child and moving it from the midline into each of the six fields of gaze for each eye.	Damage to the fourth nerve can cause diplopia (double vision) and altered downward eye movement.
VI	Abducens Lateral deviation of the eye	Ask the child to follow the object with his or her eyes but to keep the head steady. Note conjugate movements of the eyes and absence of nystagmus except in the extreme lateral position.	Damage to the sixth nerve can produce deviation of the head toward the weak muscle to avoid diplopia. Dysconjugate gaze can indicate blindness, and a conjugate horizontal gaze palsy suggests a lesion of the brainstem or cerebral hemisphere. Vertical gaze paralysis suggests brainstem dysfunction, and upward gaze paralysis suggests hydrocephalus or a tumor of the pineal region.
III	Oculomotor All other extraocular movements	Check for accommodation by bringing an object from 18 inches away from the child in toward the nose. As the object is brought toward the nose, check for convergence of the eyes and pupillary constriction.	Damage to the third nerve can result in ptosis; outward and downward displacement of the eye; and a large, sluggish pupil (in addition to the changes noted earlier).

(continued)

TABLE 4.5   Cranial Nerve Evaluation *(continued)*

Cranial Nerve	Functions	Methods of Testing	Comments
V	Trigeminal Motor: Innervation to the temporal and masseter muscles; responsible for clenching and lateral movement of the jaw Sensory: Innervation to the face with three branches: ophthalmic, maxillary, and mandibular	Motor: While palpating the temporal and then masseter muscles, ask the child to clench his or her teeth or bite on a safe object. Note the muscle strength. Ask the child to move his or her jaw from side to side and observe the symmetry of jaw movement during laughter, crying, or talking. Sensory: With the child's eyes closed, test the three sensory branches of the nerve by using first a cotton wisp and then a sharp object on the forehead, cheeks, and jaw. Substitute the dull end of the object occasionally to test the child's reliability. If abnormal findings are present, evaluate temperature sensation using test tubes filled with hot and cold water. Test the corneal reflex with a cotton wisp touched lightly to the cornea only. Note the response of blinking and some tearing.	Damage to the motor component of the nerve can result in impaired mastication. A unilateral paralysis can cause deviation of the jaw to the affected side when the child opens his or her mouth. Trauma, infections, or tumors can impair facial sensation or produce paroxysmal facial pain. The sensory component of the corneal reflex is the trigeminal nerve, and the motor component is the facial nerve. Use of contact lenses in the older child can diminish or abolish the corneal reflex. If the child in an intensive care setting is being tested frequently for pain sensation, it may be wise to use a sterile needle for testing.
VII	Facial Motor: Innervation to the muscles of the face, including the forehead, eyes, and mouth Sensory: Innervation to the anterior two thirds of the tongue where sweet, sour, and salty sensors predominate	Motor: Inspect the child's face for asymmetry during rest and while talking or crying. Ask the child to raise his or her eyebrows, to make a "mad" face, to close eyes very tightly, to show teeth, to smile, to puff out cheeks, and to make a "funny" face. In the younger child, watch facial expressions during play. Sensory: Ask the child to hold out his or her tongue. Using an applicator, apply sweet, salty, or sour substances to the child's tongue.	Damage to this nerve can result in facial weakness or paralysis. Central facial damage will result in paralysis from the eye down, while peripheral damage can produce paralysis on the entire side of face. Damage can also result in the loss of taste sensation on the anterior two thirds of the tongue. Younger children may not cooperate or be reliable in responding to taste testing.
VIII	Acoustic Cochlear division: Hearing Vestibular division: Balance	Cochlear: Check fine hearing by holding a ticking watch 1 or 2 inches from one ear while occluding the other ear. Repeat on the opposite side. Check for gross hearing by standing 1–2 feet away from the child and whisper something the child will be able to repeat. Vestibular: Test the vestibular branch using caloric testing. Iced saline (of varying amounts for different ages) is injected into the external ear canal with a syringe. Note the normal response of nystagmus with eye jerking away from the irrigated ear.	Damage to the nerve can result in impaired hearing, tinnitus, vertigo, nystagmus, and unilateral or bilateral deafness. The Rinne and Weber tests can be used for further assessment of this nerve. Deviation of the eyes toward the irrigated ear can occur in coma with an intact brainstem. Caloric testing usually results in no response in brainstem lesions.

(continued)

TABLE 4.5   Cranial Nerve Evaluation *(continued)*

Cranial Nerve	Functions	Methods of Testing	Comments
IX	Glossopharyngeal Sensory: Innervation to the pharynx and taste on the posterior one third of the tongue	Test the two nerves together by asking the child to say "ah" or yawn. During this action, observe the upward motion of the soft palate and uvula and the upward, inward movement of the posterior pharynx.	Damage to these nerves can result in impaired sensation, dysphagia (difficulty swallowing), dysarthria (difficulty talking), dysphonia, excessive drooling, stridor, and autonomic nervous system changes related to the vagus nerve. Adolescent boys can demonstrate hoarseness and voice changes related to normal puberty.
X	Vagus Sensory: Innervation to the pharynx and larynx Motor: Innervation to the palate and pharynx and parasympathetic functions	Touch the side of the uvula with a tongue blade, and note the upward movement and deviation to the stimulated side. Touch the posterior portion of the tongue with a tongue blade to stimulate a gag reflex. Note any hoarseness, and observe the child's ability to swallow without pain or choking. Note excessive drooling or coughing. Test bitter taste on the posterior one third of the tongue.	
XI	Spinal accessory Motor: Innervation to the sternocleidomastoid muscle and the upper portion of the trapezius muscle	Ask the child to turn his or her head from side to side against the pressure of your hands to test for strength. Note the normal ROM of approximately 170 degrees. Ask the child to shrug his or her shoulders against the pressure of your hands. You may need to demonstrate this action to younger children.	Damage to this nerve can produce asymmetrical shoulder posture, drooping shoulders, impaired strength in lifting the shoulders, or difficulty in turning the head to either side.
XII	Hypoglossal Motor: Innervation to the tongue	Inspect the younger child's tongue for fasciculations and symmetrical movement. Ask the older child to stick out his or her tongue, and observe for asymmetry, deviation, or atrophy.	Damage to this nerve can result in atrophy, weakness, deviation, or fasciculations of the tongue. Fine, irregular, occasional tremors of the tongue are normal when holding out the tongue.

ICP, intracranial pressure; ROM, range of motion.

Sources: Adapted from Slota, M. C. (1983a). Neurological assessment of the infant and toddler. *Critical Care Nursing, 3*(5),87–92; Slota, M. C. (1983b). Pediatric neurological assessment. *Critical Care Nursing, 3*(6), 106–112.

b. Abnormal findings include papilledema, which is characterized by blurring of the nasal and upper margins of the optic disc. Papilledema is seen with increased ICP in the older child or in the infant with acute, rapid increased ICP. Retinal hemorrhage may occur with subarachnoid hemorrhage (SAH), severe diabetes, and shaken baby syndrome.

10. *Vital Signs*

a. *Respiratory patterns* are the first of the vital signs to change with neurologic dysfunction.

Respiratory patterns are more informative than is the respiratory rate. Patterns may overlap or change depending on progression of neurologic dysfunction and are difficult to assess in the intubated and ventilated patient.

    i. *Cheyne–Stokes respirations* are described as periodic breathing with phases of hyperpnea alternating with apnea. The location of the lesion is bilateral, hemispheric, or diencephalic.

    ii. *Central neurogenic hyperventilation* is sustained, rapid, and fairly deep hyperpnea. The exact mechanism in the brain (if any) that causes this is unknown.

    iii. An *apneustic respiratory pattern* is characterized by a prolonged inspiration with a pause at full inspiration lasting 2 to 3 seconds. This represents damage to the brainstem near the level of the fifth cranial nerve nucleus.

    iv. *Ataxic respirations* consist of a completely irregular breathing pattern with deep and shallow breaths. They are seen in patients with damage to the respiratory centers in the medulla.

b. Temperature. Temperature changes are nonspecific in most patients with neurologic dysfunction. Hyperthermia may result from abnormalities of the brain itself or from toxic substances that affect the temperature-regulating centers. Patients at risk for hyperthermia include neonates (due to immature development of thermoregulation centers), children with CNS infections (due to the effects of pyrogens on the hypothalamus), and children with status epilepticus (SE; may be due to hypothalamic dysfunction as well as increased total body oxygen consumption). Hypothermia may be seen in neonates (same as mentioned earlier) and in brain death because of loss of hypothalamic function.

c. Pulse and blood pressure. Changes in pulse and blood pressure are very late and ominous signs of neurologic dysfunction. Cushing's reflex is an increase in systolic pressure greater than diastolic pressure (i.e., widened pulse pressure) and bradycardia. Cardiac dysrhythmias are seen with some TBIs. Vasodilation with systemic hypotension may be seen with spinal trauma or sympathetic insufficiency.

C. Brain-Death Determination

1. Most states have adopted guidelines to define death the same way for infants, children, and adults. One of two conditions must exist:

a. Irreversible cessation of breathing and circulation *or*

b. Irreversible cessation of whole-brain function (i.e., cortical and brainstem)

2. The difference in brain-death determination between children and adults is not the legal definition of death but the process of confirming brain death. Several sets of guidelines have been published for the determination of brain death in children. The most widely accepted guidelines are those originally published by the Ad Hoc Task Force for the Determination of Brain Death in Children in 1987 and updated in 2011 (Nakagawa, Ashwal, Mathur, Mysore, & The Committee for Determination of Brain Death in Infants Children, 2012).

a. History. The cause of coma must be known to establish irreversibility. Prerequisites must be met prior to initiating the clinical evaluation. There must be an absence of complicating factors, such as hemodynamic instability, supra-therapeutic levels of sedatives and analgesics, paralyzing agents, severe hypothermia, or metabolic disturbances. Cardiopulmonary resuscitation may interfere with the reliability of the neurologic exam and it should be delayed for ≥24 to 48 hours postresuscitation.

b. To determine brain death, the physical examination should demonstrate that coma and apnea coexist. The clinical examination should demonstrate a lack of function in the entire brain. Clinical signs include flaccidity, absence of movement (except for spinal cord reflexes), and absence of brainstem function. Loss of brainstem function is determined by nonreactive, midposition or fully dilated pupils; absence of oculocephalic (doll's eyes) and oculovestibular (cold calorics) reflexes (refer to Table 4.5); and absence of corneal, gag, cough, sucking, and rooting reflexes.

c. Apnea testing must be performed with the clinical examination and the patient must have complete absence of respiratory effort with standardized apnea testing. Following disconnection from the ventilator several conditions must occur: adequate time (5–10 minutes) to allow $PaCO_2$ to increase to levels sufficient to stimulate respiration, adequate oxygenation, and absence of cardiovascular instability. The $PaCO_2$ must be 20 mmHg above the baseline $PaCO_2$ and ≥60 mmHg.

d. Two examinations with apnea testing separated by an observation period are required. Consistent examination techniques are required throughout the observation period and must be performed by two separate attending physicians; apnea testing may be done by the same physician. The recommended observation periods are

    i. Infants 37 weeks gestational age to 30 days: 24-hour observation

    ii. Children older than 30 days to 18 years: 12-hour observation

e. Ancillary studies (EEG and CBF) are not required to diagnose brain death and should not be used as a substitute for the clinical examination. Ancillary studies may be used when the clinical examination or apnea testing cannot be completed, if there is uncertainty about the results, to reduce the observation period, or if there is a medication that may affect the exam (Nakagawa et al., 2012).

3. There is insufficient evidence in the literature to support recommendations for the preterm newborn. The exact cause of coma is often unknown in the preterm newborn and the accuracy of ancillary tests in this age group is uncertain.

INVASIVE AND NONINVASIVE DIAGNOSTIC STUDIES

A. Assessing Anatomic Integrity

1. *Radiograph*

a. *Description.* Roentgenographic films of skull and spine demonstrate structural deficits only. The radiation penetrates all body tissues and is absorbed to varying degrees, resulting in different shadow intensities.

b. *Clinical use. Skull films* are used to determine fractures, widened sutures, tumors, calcification, and bone erosion. *Spinal films* are used to evaluate the integrity of the vertebral structures, including the vertebral body, disc interspace, lamina, and pedicles. Spinal films are also used to evaluate fractures, dislocations, and degeneration of bone.

c. *Nursing implications.* Immobilize fractures with splints, cervical collars, traction devices, or age-appropriate immobilizers. Provide routine safe transport care, including use of appropriate monitoring devices, elevation of side rails, good alignment of affected body structure(s), securing standby emergency equipment, and serial monitoring of neurovascular status. Explain the procedure to older children or parents, including the length of the procedure, purpose of the procedure, sensations and appearance of the environment, and expectations of the child during the procedure (e.g., to remain quiet without body movement).

2. *CT Scan*

a. *Description.* CT scans use multiple x-ray beams that pass through the brain at different angles. The beams are picked up by receptors that digitally send the information to a computer. The computer formats the information and displays an image for every section of the brain that is studied. Different anatomical structures of the brain absorb various levels of radiation energy depending on tissue density of the structure. CT scan differentiates tissue density relative to water via a computer. Highly dense structures (e.g., bone, fresh blood) appear white, and low-density areas (e.g., air, CSF, fat) appear dark. Contrast may be used with a CT and provides good visualization of vascular structures and leaks in blood vessels. Advances continue to be made in CT technology and include increased patient comfort, faster scanning times, and higher resolution. Disadvantages include radiation exposure and use of contrast.

b. *Interpretation.* CT scans are interpreted sequentially and systematically. The left side of the brain is displayed on the right of the scan as the viewer faces it. Each CT scan section is examined for characteristic anatomical landmarks, some requiring measurement. The first image usually begins with a cut through the posterior fossa followed by sections that advance superiorly. Anatomical structures are viewed in terms of size, location, and symmetry. Sections are then examined for abnormal densities (e.g., blood clots, tumors) and enlarged structures. The basilar cistern is the area of subarachnoid space that surrounds the midbrain. Diffuse brain swelling is recognized on CT scan as a decrease in ventricular size, absence or compression of the basilar cistern, and loss of differentiation between gray and white matter. Visual loss of the third ventricle and loss of sulci indicate an increase in brain bulk (swelling). Asymmetry is almost always an abnormal sign that indicates volume changes between compartments. Figure 4.16 demonstrates four CT scans that show abnormalities.

c. *Clinical use.* Because of cost, speed, and availability, CT scan is used for examination of acute neurologic dysfunction. CT scan is superior to MRI in detecting blood (especially SAH) and in

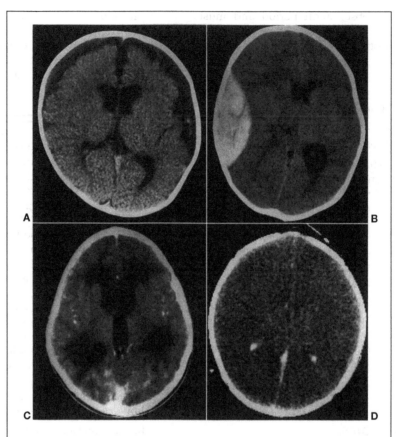

FIGURE 4.16 (A) Nonenhanced CT scan of a 9-month-old infant showing bilateral acute and chronic subdural hematoma. Ventricles are mildly enlarged. (B) CT scan showing a large right-sided epidural hematoma with a characteristic biconvex appearance in a 10-month-old girl. The midline structures are displaced to the left, with effacement of much of the ventricular system on the right, moderate dilatation of the front horns of both lateral ventricles and marked dilatation of the posterior portion of the left lateral ventricle. The basal cisterns are effaced. (C) CT scan demonstrates enlarged lateral and third ventricles caused by obstruction of the aqueduct of Sylvius by a venous angioma. (D) CT scan of a severely asphyxiated term newborn at 3 days of age. Note the generalized decreased densities with total loss of gray matter and white matter differentiation.

Source: Reprinted with permission from Swaiman, K. F., & Ashwal, S. (1999). *Pediatric neurology: Principles and practice* (3rd ed.). St. Louis, MO: Mosby.

evaluating cortical bone structures of skull and spine. Contrast-enhanced CT (CECT) is used to detect lesions that cause BBB breakdown, to visualize blood vessels and well-vascularized lesions, and to rule out cerebral metastases. It is difficult to visualize the posterior fossa because of bone obstruction.

d. *Nursing implications.* Before the procedure, the patient and family should be told that the machine surrounds the body and clicking and whirring noises may be heard. The procedure is painless, except for a venipuncture if contrast medium is used. The child is required to remain still throughout the procedure; sedation may be required. If contrast medium is used, the patient may experience an unusual sensation during the procedure (e.g., a burning or warm sensation for about 20–30 seconds during injection of the contrast medium). The use of contrast media is contraindicated in patients with acute renal failure.

e. *Postprocedure monitoring* includes assessing for an allergic reaction to the contrast medium (e.g., tachycardia, hypotension, fever, and chills) and observing the contrast injection site (if used) for bleeding, swelling, redness, and pain.

3. *MRI*

a. *Description.* MRI differentiates tissues by their response to radiofrequency pulses in a magnetic field; lesions have either a high or low signal (in contrast to x-ray density seen with a CT scan).

b. *Clinical use.* MRI is used to distinguish soft tissues (e.g., SCI and brain tumors) and to identify small infarcts, infections, inflammatory areas, and demyelinating plaques. MRI provides clear sagittal images; therefore, it is the procedure of choice for suspected lesions of the spinal cord or cervicomedullary junction. MRI can delineate between tissue structure (e.g., white and gray matter).

 i. MRI does not use radiation. Other advantages of MRI as compared to CT scan include better definition of normal and pathologic lesions (except for those listed previously for CT scan), better three-dimensional information and relationships, demonstration of blood and CSF flow, and evaluation of tumors in the posterior fossa that are normally obstructed by bone artifact in CT imaging.

 ii. Disadvantages of MRI as compared to CT scan are the requirement of more time and cooperation from the patient and difficulty in continuously monitoring the patient during the procedure because of the magnetic field; however, newer MRI-compatible monitors are becoming increasingly more available. Another disadvantage of MRI is that it is contraindicated in patients with metallic implants (e.g., pacemakers, aneurysm clips). Figures 4.17A and 4.17B compare a CT scan to an MRI in a 3-year-old child with suspected meningitis.

c. *Nursing implications.* When the patient's condition permits, preprocedural education should include the information that the machine turns around the patient and makes a loud noise much like a washing machine. The procedure is long, and the child must lie still. If a contrast medium is used, an unusual sensation may occur (i.e., a warm rushing sensation for approximately

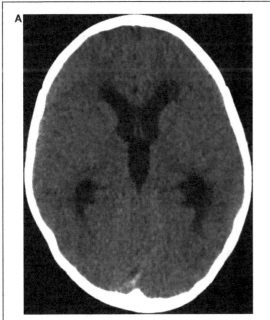 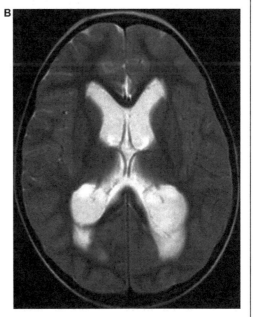

FIGURE 4.17 (A) and (B) A comparison of nonenhanced CT scan with MRI in a 3-year-old with meningitis. (A) CT scan demonstrates stable hydrocephalus of the lateral, third, and fourth ventricles. (B) MRI demonstrates diffuse ventriculomegaly involving lateral, third, and fourth ventricles.

20–30 seconds during injection). The procedure is painless, except for venipuncture when a contrast medium is used. All metallic objects must be removed from the patient, parents, and supportive staff who may accompany the patient. Inquire about implantable metallic objects (e.g., pacemakers, electronic implants, surgical clips, and ferromagnetic items). Sedation is often required for small children. Postprocedure monitoring is the same as for CT scan.

4. *Cerebral Angiogram*

   a. *Description.* Cerebral angiogram requires injection (usually femoral cannulation) of radiopaque dye followed by sequential skull radiographs or digital subtraction technique (intra-arterial digital subtraction angiography [IADSA]). IADSA is the gold standard for definitive assessment of cerebral vasculature and should be considered in children when pathology of small distal arteries is suspected or to identify infarcts or hemorrhage not identified on CT or MRI.

   b. *Clinical use.* Since the advent of CT scan and MRI, angiogram use is more restricted. It is usually reserved for confirmation of lesions and identification of vascular occlusions, recanalization, ulceration and dissection of large arteries, and stenosis of small arteries. It is the procedure of choice for aneurysms and arteriovascular malformations and is used to detect CBF alterations.

   c. *Nursing implications*

   i. Preprocedural education should include describing the purpose of the procedure, the length of the procedure (usually takes several hours), possible sensations the patient may experience during the procedure (e.g., a burning or warm sensation for about 20–30 seconds during injection of the contrast medium), and the possible need for sedation and its expected effects. Contrast medium is excreted by the kidneys; patients are encouraged to drink liberally the day before the procedure or intravenous (IV) fluids may be increased as ordered. Nothing-by-mouth restrictions prior to the test usually apply for 12 hours. All jewelry and hair ornaments must be removed.

   ii. Postprocedure monitoring. Patients should avoid movement of the affected extremity to prevent dislodgment of a clot, bleeding, and hematoma formation. Frequently assess the neurovascular status and pressure dressing of a cannulated extremity; usually every 15 minutes for an hour, then every 30 minutes for an hour, and then every hour until the patient is stable. Assess for bleeding, hematoma, or infection at the cannulation site. Restrict activity initially; usually 12 to 24 hours. Monitor vital signs for signs of shock (e.g., alteration in consciousness, hypotension, diminished pulses, and tachycardia) at the same intervals as the neurovascular assessment. Assess for an allergic reaction to contrast medium (e.g., tachycardia, hypotension, fever, and chills). Encourage hydration with sips of water or IV fluids. Maintain intake and output record for 24 hours.

5. *Radioisotope Scan*

   a. *Description.* A radioisotope, which naturally emits positrons, is injected into the circulation, and a brain-scanning device detects areas of uptake of the isotope (occurs with altered BBB or highly vascularized area). An image is created and indicates the location and relative concentration of the radioactive isotope in different regions of the brain.

   b. *Clinical use.* It measures important metabolic functions, such as blood flow, oxygen use, and sugar metabolism. The use of a radioisotope scan has been limited since the development of the CT scan. A radioisotope scan is effective in identifying isodense lesions such as subdural hematoma, blood clots with the same density as adjacent tissue, intracerebral infection, and inflammation. A radioisotope scan is also effective in the evaluation of patients with epilepsy because it may help to identify epileptic foci prior to excision.

   c. *Nursing implications.* Preprocedural education includes explaining the purpose for and length of the procedure. A small venipuncture is necessary for isotope injection. Time delay may be necessary for adequate uptake of the isotope. There is a small radiation hazard to the patient and staff; however, the half-life of nuclides is extremely short.

B. Assessing Physiologic Alterations

1. *Lumbar Puncture and CSF Analysis*

   a. *Description.* Lumbar puncture is the most frequently performed neurologic diagnostic test to assess CSF composition. Lumbar puncture is performed by inserting a needle into the spinal subarachnoid space distal to the spinal cord (between L-3 and L-4 or L-4 and L-5 vertebral interspace).

b. *Clinical use* is to measure CSF pressure, analyze CSF, inject or remove substances, and deliver spinal anesthesia.

c. *Nursing implications.* Preprocedural education includes a description of the sensations that may be experienced during the procedure (e.g., pressure from gloved hand, warmth from local anesthetic, etc.) Local anesthetic is used requiring a small needle insertion at the site of the lumbar puncture. A topical anesthetic, prilocaine-lidocaine (EMLA) can be used, but requires application 30 minutes prior to the procedure. Burning may be felt for a few seconds at the infiltration site. A side-lying position is used most often with the child's knees flexed to the chest. The child is held in place with the back close to the edge of the examining table. The nurse should avoid placing any weight on the child. An alternative position to use for infants to distend the dural sac slightly, and therefore ease insertion, is the sitting position. The infant's buttocks are placed at the edge of the table, and the infant's neck and hips are flexed and stabilized. Following the procedure, assess the insertion site for bleeding, infection, CSF leak, hematoma, and swelling. Potential complications include brainstem herniation with elevated ICP at the time of the procedure, hematoma, infection, headache, radiculopathy, and spinal, epidural, or subarachnoid bleeding.

2. *Transcranial Doppler Ultrasound*

a. *Description.* Noninvasive calculation of mean velocity and direction of CBF is achieved by means of a 2-MHz ultrasound probe held to thin areas of the skull, called *cranial windows*. There are three main windows (temporal, orbital, and occipital) that allow access to different arteries. The transcranial Doppler ultrasound (TCD) ultrasound beam bounces off erythrocytes in an exposed artery and returns the signal to the transducer. Velocity signals are displayed as pulsatile waveforms that can be recorded through a window with auditory confirmation (swooshing sound) with each cardiac cycle (Harris, 2014). The TCD ultrasound does not directly measure blood flow, but the velocity signals are directly proportional to blood flow and therefore can accurately measure any change in flow.

b. *Clinical uses* are for diagnosis of cranial stenosis, vasospasm, cerebral emboli and vessel occlusion. It is used also for assessing CBF and collateral flow patterns, testing carbon dioxide and blood pressure vasoreactivity, evaluating stroke risk, and detection of changes in ICP (an increase in pulsatility).

c. *Nursing implications.* Ultrasound may be done at the bedside and has no major complications or contraindications. Preprocedural education should include instructing the patient to lie still or provide age-appropriate comfort and distraction. Sedation may be required.

3. *Xenon-Enhanced CT Scan*

a. *Description.* The CT technique uses the high-density form of stable nonradioactive xenon to measure brain tissue buildup of this atom following inhalation of a xenon gas mixture. It is based on the principle that the rate of uptake or clearance of an inert diffusible gas is proportional to blood flow in the tissue. The brain is scanned before, during, and after the procedure, and end-tidal xenon concentration is measured and computer calculated to estimate CBF. The procedure is fast (washout is approximately 3 minutes) and the inhaled xenon has a short physiologic half-life (approximately 30 seconds) and low risk for side effects (Rostami, Engquist, & Enblad, 2014).

b. *Clinical uses* are for diagnosis of ischemic and hemorrhagic stroke, SAH, occlusive vascular disease, vasospasm, arteriovenous malformations (AVMs), cerebral hypertension, global hypoxic–ischemic injury, and of intracranial trauma. It is becoming accepted as the standard for quantitative CBF measurement (Carlson et al., 2011).

c. *Nursing implications.* Preprocedural education includes instructing the patient to lie still and inhale a gas mixture. The CT scanner may frighten patients. There are no known risks with the procedure. Xenon is known to cause vasodilation and should be used with caution in patients with increased ICP. Rare adverse events reported include headache, seizures, nausea and vomiting, and change in neurologic status.

4. *Electroencephalograms*

a. *Description.* An EEG records spontaneous electrical activity across the surface of the brain. Activity is characterized by the frequency (Hertz [Hz]), symmetry, latency (milliseconds [msec]), amplitude (microvolts [mV]) and patterns of electrical signals. Common EEG abnormalities include the following:

   i. Diffuse slowing of background rhythms is a common nonspecific finding seen in patients with diffuse encephalopathies and some structural abnormalities.

ii. Focal slowing of parenchyma indicates localized dysfunction.

iii. Triphasic waves seen in toxic metabolic encephalopathies consist of generalized synchronous waves occurring in brief runs.

iv. Epileptic discharges are associated with seizure disorders.

v. Periodic lateralizing epileptiform discharges (PLEDs) suggest an acute destructive cerebral lesion.

vi. Generalized periodic sharp waves are seen most commonly in patients following cerebral anoxia.

b. *Clinical uses* include the diagnosis of epilepsy, dementia and diffuse encephalopathies, brain lesions, cerebral ischemia, some cerebral infections, and brain death. It is also used to monitor the effects of medications on brain activity, such as barbiturates when inducing a chemical coma. Figure 4.18 illustrates four different EEG patterns commonly seen in infants and children.

c. *Nursing implications.* Preprocedural teaching should include a description of the sensations and setup of scalp leads. Sleep deprivation may be used to precipitate certain types of seizure discharges. It involves keeping the patient awake for all or part of the night before the EEG is to be performed. Depending on specific orders, the patient may be awake or asleep during the EEG. Discontinuation of anticonvulsants may be used prior to an EEG as an activation technique for seizure discharges. Describe the testing procedures to the child or family. Hyperventilation is an activation technique (i.e., induces seizure discharges) that requires voluntary hyperventilation. Photic stimulation is an activation technique (flashing a light in the eyes at various frequencies). Routine monitoring during the procedure includes observation of seizure activity, observation of other activity, and monitoring of vital functions as dictated by the patient's condition. Accurate documentation of the patient's behaviors and nursing interventions with continuous EEG recording is essential. Shampoo the patient's hair after the procedure.

5. *Video-EEG*

a. *Description.* Video-EEG (v-EEG) technology uses scalp electrodes placed on a child according to the international 10-20 system. The child is admitted into a special dedicated room with a camera and microphone. Usually one parent or legal guardian stays with the child in the room during the recording while a trained nurse supervises the procedure. The usual duration of a v-EEG is 48 hours or longer depending on the frequency of the child's seizures. Seizure medications may be withheld during the monitoring.

b. *Clinical use* of v-EEG is to distinguish epileptic from nonepileptic events and is used in the management of some children with epilepsy. It is indicated for the diagnosis of paroxysmal events, to identify seizure type, to evaluate intractable

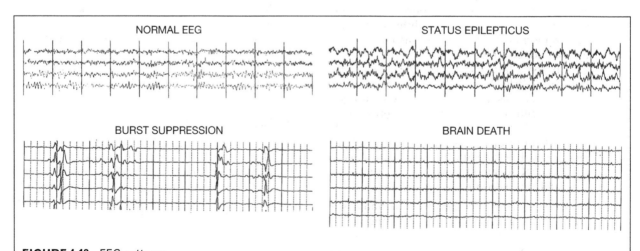

FIGURE 4.18 EEG patterns.

Source: Reprinted with permission from Harris, C. (2014). Neuromonitoring indications and utility in the intensive care unit. *Critical Care Nursing, 34*(3), 30–40. doi:10.4037/ccn2014506

epilepsy, to identify nonepileptic spells and to identify candidates for epileptic surgery (Riquet et al., 2011).

c. *Nursing implications.* Preprocedural preparation should include a description of the monitoring equipment and electrode placement, and how the electrodes are connected to a cord that is connected to a machine (network feed and amplifier) or wall unit. Instruct the parents regarding any personal electronic equipment that may interfere with the EEG recordings. Cell phones or laptop computers may be used when operated by battery power. Parents are asked to help keep their child in a location where the camera is focused, usually the bed or crib. They are instructed to avoid blocking the camera during an event. Standard seizure precautions are implemented.

6. *Evoked Potential Studies*

a. *Description.* Evoked potentials (EPs) are derivatives of an EEG and measure electrical activity produced by a specific neural structure along a sensory pathway. The measurement is called an evoked response (ER). EP electrical activity is generally much slower than spontaneous cortical electrical activity (EEG) and measures minute voltage changes produced in response to a specific stimulus, such as a click, shock, or light pattern. EP studies assess the entire sensory pathway from the peripheral sensory organ all the way to the brain cortex. Neural pathways studied are visual-evoked response (VER), brainstem auditory-evoked response (BAER), somatosensory-evoked response (SSER), and multimodality-evoked response (MMER) depending on the sensory system suspected to be pathologic.

    i. VER uses a visual stimulus to the eye, usually a strobe light, which causes an electrical response in the occipital area. The response is recorded with electrodes placed on the scalp overlying the vertex and occipital area.

    ii. BAER uses a clicking sound applied to either ear to evaluate central auditory pathways of the brainstem. BAERs also use electrodes placed on the scalp. There are five common types of waves recorded by the BAER that correspond to five different anatomic locations in the brainstem. BAERs are more resistant to medications or anesthesia compared to somatosensory-EPs.

    iii. SSERs are used to measure the integrity of an ascending (sensory) spinal cord pathway. Electrodes are attached to the scalp to capture responses generated from peripheral needle electrodes placed in the skin along peripheral nerves. The time it takes the stimulus to travel from the peripheral nerve to the cortex of the brain is measured. A delayed or absent response is abnormal and indicates a loss in the integrity of the nerve.

    iv. MMER uses a combination of the stimuli previously described to evoke multiple responses from different locations of the brain.

b. *Clinical uses* are to identify dysfunction in specific sensory pathways. EP studies do not require voluntary patient response, and therefore, can be used in comatose and nonverbal patients. VER studies are used to detect blindness and eyesight problems in infants. In older patients, it can be used to detect multiple sclerosis, Parkinson's disease, occipital lobe tumor, and cerebrovascular accident (CVA). BAER studies are used primarily to detect hearing disorders in infants. It may also assist with detection of posterior fossa tumors, CVA of the brainstem or temporal lobe cortex, auditory nerve damage, acoustic nerve neuroma, and demyelinating diseases. SSER studies are used to detect SPIs and monitor spinal cord function during surgery.

c. *Nursing implications.* Preprocedural education includes teaching the patient what to expect from stimuli. In visual testing, the patient sees a strobe or alternating checkerboard. In auditory testing, the patient hears clicks. In somatosensory testing, the patient feels an electrical current on the skin. The procedure is lengthy. Sedation may be required for agitation or anxiety. After the test, completely remove the gel and glue from the patient's scalp to prevent skin breakdown.

NEUROLOGIC MONITORING

A. ICP Monitoring

1. *Description.* ICP monitoring is a technique in which a catheter is placed directly within the cranium to measure ICP. Less frequently, a transducer is placed indirectly on the anterior fontanelle to measure ICP.

2. *Clinical uses* include assessment of ICP for the prevention of herniation and the preservation of cerebral perfusion.

3. *Classification of Systems. Type of Transducer*

a. In *fluid-coupled systems*, the compartment that is being monitored is connected to an external strain-gauge transducer via a fluid pathway. Fluid column pulsations are converted into millimeters of mercury. Advantages include the low cost, accuracy (with an intraventricular catheter), and ability to zero and recalibrate after insertion. Disadvantages include that the accuracy depends on the catheter location; artifact is present with movement; the procedure requires transducer leveling with position changes; and the system may become obstructed with tissue, blood, air, or bone.

b. *Fiber-optic catheters* have a transducer tip that is nonfluid filled. A mirrored diaphragm (in the tip of the transducer) moves in response to pressure and is sensed by light fibers. Information is converted into an analog signal and displayed on a pressure monitor. Advantages include the theoretical low risk of infection because of the lack of a fluid column and stopcocks, accurate ICP value, excellent waveform quality with fewer artifacts, placement in brain parenchyma, and the fact that transducer leveling is not required after insertion (Cecil et al., 2011). Disadvantages include a greater cost than the fluid-filled system, requirement for dedicated hardware, special handling of the catheter and cable to avoid breakage, inability to rezero after insertion, and inability to drain CSF as a treatment modality unless a catheter is placed in a lateral ventricle.

c. A *catheter-tip strain-gauge catheter* is a monitoring system that consists of a miniature strain-gauge pressure sensor positioned at the tip of a flexible nylon tube. When the transducer is bent because of ICP, the resistance changes, and an ICP is calculated. It is similar to the fiber-optic system in that several brain locations can be monitored and the microsensor is calibrated prior to insertion. Unlike the fiber-optic system, it is housed in tubing which is resistant to breakage and allows for tunneling under the scalp.

d. A *pneumatic sensor* is a microtransducer ICP monitoring device that uses a small air-pouch that surrounds the distal end of the catheter and is connected to a pressure transducer with tubing. The ICP is transmitted across the thin pouch wall to the air volume in the pouch and transformed into an electric signal by the transducer. The monitor that is used with the system zeroes automatically once per hour. Catheter types include intraventricular, intraparenchymal, subdural, and epidural. Advantages include in-vivo self-zeroing, MRI compatible, and relatively inexpensive.

e. An *external fiber-optic transducer* is applied to the anterior fontanelle and measures ICP indirectly. Fontanelle tonometers are used only rarely in infants. Advantages include its noninvasive nature and lack of complications. Disadvantages include the lack of accurate ICP measurements (amount of external pressure applied to the sensor can alter measurements), the fact that it may underestimate ICP and may not record acute increases in ICP, additional cost, and that compliance testing and CSF drainage are not possible.

4. *Classification of Systems. Anatomic locations* (fluid-coupled, fiber-optic, catheter-tip strain-gauge systems, or pneumatic sensor): ICP can be monitored in several locations, but the most common sites are intraparenchymal and ventricular. Surface monitors, such as subarachnoid, subdural, and epidural catheters, have been shown to be less accurate and used infrequently (Raboel, Bartek, Andresen, Bellander, & Romner, 2012).

a. The *intraventricular* location is the gold standard of ICP monitoring. Ventricular monitoring is located deep within the brain and is therefore considered to be more accurate in reflecting whole-brain pressure. The catheter tip is usually placed in the anterior horn of the lateral ventricle through the nondominant cerebral hemisphere. Waveform quality is excellent. Advantages are that the catheter allows drainage of CSF, is accurate and reliable, permits administration of medications, and permits volume-pressure compliance testing. Disadvantages include higher risk of infection and bleeding, longer insertion time (collapsed or small ventricles make insertion difficult or prohibitive), and risk of CSF leakage. Currently, there are antibiotic-impregnated and coated ventricular catheters available.

b. *Subarachnoid bolts* are inserted into the subarachnoid space via a twist drill hole in the nondominant prefrontal cranium behind the hairline just anterior to the coronal suture. Different types of bolts are available (e.g., Philly bolt, Richmond bolt, Leeds screw). Pediatric bolts are usually shorter and lighter compared to adult bolts. Waveform quality is good initially, but may dampen with time with a fluid-filled system. Advantages are that subarachnoid bolts are quick to insert and useful when ventricles are collapsed and access is impossible. Disadvantages are that tissue may occlude the device, CSF leakage may occur, ICP may be underestimated, and the bolt requires the skull to be intact.

c. *Subdural catheters* are inserted below the dura mater and above the subarachnoid space in the same manner as the subarachnoid bolt. Used primarily after surgery for evacuation of a clot, the catheter is placed at the operative site. Waveform quality is poor and used primarily for trending. Advantages include low risk of hemorrhage, quick and easy insertion, alternate site when the ventricles are collapsed (access is impossible), and lower infection risk compared to an intraventricular catheter. Disadvantages include the potential underestimation of ICP, the inability to drain CSF, and the requirement of an intact skull.

d. *Epidural catheters* are inserted below the skull and above the dura mater. They are considered to be an indirect measure of ICP. Waveform quality is poor and used primarily for trending. Advantages are that epidural catheters have the least invasive placement (dura mater remains intact), there is a low risk of infection, quick and easy insertion, no risk for CSF leakage, and low risk for brain injury. Disadvantages are that epidural catheters provide an indirect measurement that is not as accurate and reliable as measurements made with other catheter systems and that epidural catheters are unable to drain CSF.

e. *Intraparenchymal fiber-optic transduced tipped or strain-gauge tipped catheters* are placed directly into the brain tissue (via a bolt or screw device) approximately 1 cm below the subarachnoid space. Waveform quality is good. Advantages include the low risk of infection, quick and easy insertion, and accuracy and reliability. Disadvantages are the same as for all fiber-optic systems.

5. *Nursing Implications*

a. *Zeroing and calibrating* the fluid-filled systems depends on the manufacturer's recommendation, unit practice, location of the catheter, and the risk of infection.

i. The fluid-coupled ICP transducer connects to the bedside monitor via a pressure cable that is plugged into a pressure module. The transducer should be *level* at the foramen of Monro (e.g., outer canthus of the eye, tragus of the ear). The level should be changed with every position change. Once leveled, the transducer is zeroed (American Association of Neuroscience Nurses, 2011). The transducer is rezeroed according to unit policy or as a troubleshooting technique.

ii. Catheter-tipped transducers are zeroed before insertion and are factory set, no calibration is required. Transducers may be calibrated with the bedside monitor. Leveling for catheter-tipped transducers and pneumatic sensor systems is not required. The transducer is located at the tip of the catheter.

b. *Insertion site care* is basically the same for all systems. Maintain a dry and intact occlusive dressing. Maintain aseptic technique with dressing changes. Notify the physician for leakage on and around the dressing. Evaluate the insertion site for CSF leakage, bleeding, hematoma, and infection. The diagnosis of meningitis or ventriculitis is made on the basis of positive results from CSF cultures; fever and leukocytosis are less predictive. Local signs of catheter infection include redness, swelling, and drainage at the insertion site.

c. *Maintain infection control* by using aseptic technique when handling the system. In fluid-filled systems, minimize the number of connections and stopcocks. Maintain a closed system by covering all entry ports with caps. Minimize the number of times the system is entered. Avoid dislodging or breaking the system by avoiding tension on the tubing or fiber-optic cables. Tape the tubing to the dressing, clip or pin the cable to the patient, avoid kinking the cable, and use caution when repositioning or transporting the patient. Notify the physician of any loose connections at the insertion site.

6. *Waveform Analysis.* ICP monitoring not only measures absolute pressure numerically, it also provides information about intracranial dynamics from waveform analysis. The normal ICP waveform has a pulsatile quality at two different frequencies. One waveform frequency is synchronous with each cardiac cycle and resembles the arterial waveform, and the other waveform frequency is slower and synchronous with the respiratory cycle. The cardiac cycle waveform has three pulse waves with descending peaks that represent arterial pulsations in large cerebral vessels (Figure 4.19).

a. P_1 (*percussion wave*) is the first peak that originates from pulsations of the choroid plexus. It is a sharp peak, consistent in amplitude, and the largest of all waves.

b. P_2 (*rebound or tidal wave*) is more variable in shape and amplitude and smaller than the percussion wave and may become larger than the other two waves with decreased intracranial compliance. It ends in the dicrotic notch (aortic closure), just prior to the P_3.

c. P_3 (*dicrotic wave*) follows P_1 and P_2 and is the smallest of the three waves and has a venous origin. After the dicrotic wave, pressure usually decreases to diastolic baseline.

7. *Abnormal ICP waveforms* (Lundberg waves) may present when ICP is elevated and there is a decrease in intracranial compliance (Figure 4.20).

a. *A waves (plateau)* are spontaneous, rapid, irregular increases in ICP to 50 to 100 mmHg lasting 5 to 20 minutes. A waves are frequently associated with dilated pupil(s), vomiting, abnormal posturing, decreased level of consciousness, widened pulse pressure, dysrhythmias, and decreased respirations. They represent impaired CBF and decreased intracranial compliance. Cerebral blood vessels vasodilate in response to decreased CPP. They should be promptly treated (American Association of Neuroscience Nurses, 2011).

b. *B waves* are sharp rhythmic increases in ICP to 50 mmHg lasting 30 seconds to 2 minutes. B waves are related to respirations. They may precede A waves or seizures or occur during

a headache, posturing, or decreased level of consciousness.

c. *C waves* are small waves that occur every 4 to 8 minutes and result from fluctuations in the systemic pulse and respirations. They are clinically insignificant.

B. Jugular Venous Oxygen Saturation Monitoring

1. *Description.* Blood from the brain primarily drains through the venous sinuses with most of it continuing to the right and left sigmoid sinus. From this point, it continues down through the jugular foramen to the right and left jugular veins. The jugular bulb is the dilatation of the jugular vein as it exits through the base of the skull. Each jugular bulb receives blood from both sides of the brain with approximately 70% from the same-sided hemisphere and 30% from the opposite hemisphere (Bhagat, Bhardwaj, & Grover, 2015). Measuring venous saturation as it drains the brain provides an estimate of cerebral oxygenation, CBF, and cerebral metabolic requirement. Jugular venous oxygen saturation ($SjVO_2$) monitoring may be intermittent or continuous and is used to measure the balance between cerebral oxygen delivery and cerebral oxygen consumption. Jugular venous oximetry requires retrograde cannulation of the internal jugular vein. The catheter is advanced and placed in the jugular venous bulb where there is the least amount of extracerebral venous contamination. No consensus exists as to which jugular vein should be cannulated, that is, right or left. However, the right internal jugular vein is cannulated more often than the left because it is usually larger and it drains a greater proportion of blood from the sagittal sinus. Some clinicians advocate cannulating the jugular vein on the side of injury or the right side for diffuse injury. Normal $SjVO_2$ values are maintained between 55% and 75% (Le Roux et al., 2014). Abnormalities that increase oxygen consumption (e.g., fever or seizures) or that decrease oxygen delivery (e.g., increased ICP, hypotension, hypoxia, hypocapnia, or anemia) can decrease $SjVO_2$. Nonviable brain tissue does not extract oxygen, and therefore, $SjVO_2$ may be abnormally high (>75%). $SjVO_2$ values <50% suggest a relative lack of oxygen delivery compared to demand and is associated with poor outcome in patients (Bhagat et al., 2015).

2. *Clinical use* is to evaluate and manage patients with cerebral ischemia. It is used most often in patients with TBI and in neurosurgical patients, and to a lesser extent in cardiac surgery patients

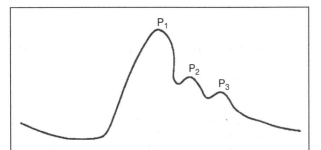

FIGURE 4.19 Components of a normal intracranial pressure waveform.

Source: Reprinted with permission from McQuillan, K. A. (1991). Intracranial pressure monitoring: Technical imperatives. *AACN Advanced Critical Care, 2* (4), 623–636. doi:10.4037/15597768-1991-4003

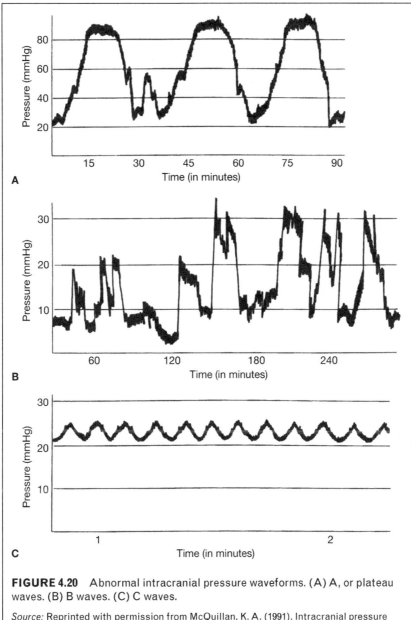

FIGURE 4.20 Abnormal intracranial pressure waveforms. (A) A, or plateau waves. (B) B waves. (C) C waves.

Source: Reprinted with permission from McQuillan, K. A. (1991). Intracranial pressure monitoring: Technical imperatives. *AACN Advanced Critical Care, 2*(4), 623–636. doi:10.4037/15597768-1991-4003

and in patients who have sustained a cardiac arrest. $SjVO_2$ monitoring may be used with ICP monitoring and CPP measurements. Together they can help determine whether a given CPP value is sufficient to supply adequate cerebral oxygenation.

    a. An advantage of $SjVO_2$ monitoring is its more accurate identification of cerebral ischemia versus ICP and CPP monitoring alone.

    b. Disadvantages include reliability of low $SjVO_2$ values; verification with blood sampling is required. $SjVO_2$ values represent more global ischemia; they are less representative of local ischemia. Because of catheter size, continuous $SjVO_2$ monitoring is not suitable for infants and small children usually younger than 8 years of age or 30 kg: It may impede venous drainage or cause obstruction of the internal jugular.

Misplacement of the catheter tip may occur due to anatomic variations and abnormalities of the vein; values may be inaccurate.

3. *Nursing Implications*

a. Verify low levels of $SjVO_2$: check the light intensity indicator on the monitor, send a blood sample for laboratory measurement, reposition the patient's head and neck, and flush the catheter with 2 to 3 mL of normal saline. Recognize $SjVO_2$ desaturation (<50%) and identify possible causes: low SaO_2 (<90%), increased oxygen consumption, hypercarbia, hypotension, increased ICP, and anemia.

b. Anticipate potential complications from catheter cannulation: hematoma formation, catheter sepsis, venous thrombosis, and local infection.

c. Calibrate the oximetry catheter at regular intervals (usually every 8–12 hours) with venous blood gas analysis.

d. Avoid excessive flushing of catheter and medication administration through the catheter.

e. If a percutaneous blood sample is taken from a site close to the jugular bulb (within 2 cm), withdraw the blood sample at a minimum rate of 2 mL/min to avoid extracerebral contamination.

C. Brain Tissue Oxygen Monitoring

1. *Description.* Brain tissue oxygen ($PbtO_2$) monitoring is a technique used to evaluate brain tissue oxygenation, and, in some cases, brain temperature. It is a continuous measurement of local brain tissue oxygen and a useful complement to ICP, $SjVO_2$, and CPP monitoring, particularly in TBI patients. It is used more often in adult neurological critical care. A $PbtO_2$ catheter is inserted through a cranial bolt deep into the subcortical white matter of the brain. Catheters can also be positioned around injured brain tissue or next to brain tissue that is at risk for secondary injury, for example, ischemia or vasospasm (Oddo, Villa, & Citerio, 2012). Precise normal $PbtO_2$ values are not known, but are believed to range between 23 and 35 mmHg depending on the monitoring system used. A lower critical $PbtO_2$ threshold of 20 mmHg represents a severe lack of brain oxygen and should be treated (Le Roux et al., 2014). The TBI guidelines have no Level I or Level II recommendation due to the lack of studies in children.

Their Level III recommendation is to maintain $PbtO_2 \geq 10$ mmHg (Kochanek et al., 2012).

2. *Clinical Use.* Used for patients at risk for cerebral ischemia and/or hypoxia and to evaluate the effectiveness of interventions that alter cerebral oxygenation (e.g., TBI, SAH, ischemia, intraoperative monitoring).

3. *Nursing Implications.* Maintain infection control with sterile dressings over insertion site. Assess and document $PbtO_2$ values in response to changes in clinical status and in response to clinical interventions.

D. Near-Infrared Spectroscopy

1. *Description.* Near-infrared spectroscopy (NIRS) is a continuous noninvasive technique used to assess regional cortical tissue oxygenation. This technology uses near-infrared light at wavelengths that are absorbed by hemoglobin and measures the percentage of oxygenated versus deoxygenated hemoglobin in tissue beds. Near-infrared light penetrates the skull and allows for real-time assessment. Sensors are placed on the patient's forehead to measure cerebral tissue oxygenation (NIRS-C) or on the skin overlying the renal somatic area (NIRS-R). Similar to systemic venous saturation, NIRS readings reflect primarily venous saturation of oxygenation and provide an assessment of oxygen supply and consumption in the tissue beneath the sensor (Marimón, Dockery, Sheridan, & Agarwal, 2012).

2. *Clinical Use.* It assists with detection and correction of oxygenation issues associated with low cardiac output, shock, seizures, and renal injury. It is used most often in cardiovascular surgery to detect cerebral oxygenation changes during surgical cardiac arrest and during cardiopulmonary bypass. More recent uses include the neonatal population to assess hypoxic–ischemic encephalopathy (HIE), hypotension, cerebral autoregulation, respiratory distress syndrome, apnea and bradycardia, and periventricular hemorrhage (Scheeren, Schober, & Schwarte, 2012; Sood, McLaughlin, & Cortez, 2015).

3. *Nursing Implications.* Universal normal values are not established and values should be used for trending and compared with patient baseline data. Clinical decisions should be based on each patient's clinical situation and physiology. Measurements may be erroneous due to body position, circulating blood volume, cardiac function, peripheral vascular resistance, and venous pressure. Cerebral sensors are placed on the right or left side of the forehead avoiding hair. Sensors should be changed according to manufacturer recommendations and institutional polices.

INTRACRANIAL DEVICES

A. External Ventricular Shunt

1. *Description.* An external ventricular drainage (EVD) or ventriculostomy is a temporary closed system with a sterile catheter placed in the lateral

ventricle (usually on the right) through a burr hole. The catheter is externalized through the ventriculostomy site or from a secondary incision after being tunneled under the scalp. It may include an ICP transducer for monitoring or may function just as a drainage system (Figure 4.21). The distal end of the catheter is connected to a simple extraventricular drain.

2. *Indications* include intermittent or continuous drainage of CSF for acute intracranial hypertension, ventricular shunt malfunction, infection, obstructive hydrocephalus (including tumor), and intracranial hemorrhage (ICH).

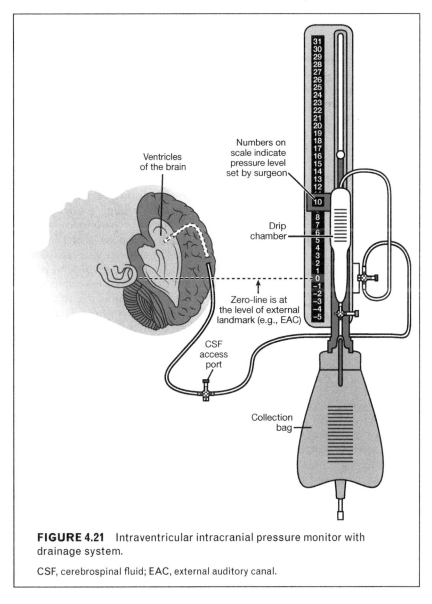

FIGURE 4.21 Intraventricular intracranial pressure monitor with drainage system.

CSF, cerebrospinal fluid; EAC, external auditory canal.

3. *Potential complications* include infection, hemorrhage, collapse of ventricles, leakage of fluid, leakage of air into the ventricular system, and seizures.

4. *Nursing Implications*

   a. Several EVD systems are available but have similar components, including a drip chamber, collection bag, and drainage pressure scale.

   b. Note whether the internal shunt valve was removed. The absence of a valve requires careful leveling of the EVD.

   c. Specific orders are obtained from the physician for care. With the foramen of Monro or lateral ventricles used as the zero reference point, the drip chamber is moved up or down to adjust the amount of CSF drainage. Anatomic location of the zero reference point is usually the external auditory meatus. The height of the drip chamber relative to the reference point controls the rate of CSF drainage. CSF automatically drains when the ICP is greater than the pressure created by the level of the drip chamber (1 mmHg is equal to 1.36 cm H_2O). Specific times when the tubing should be clamped (e.g., too much CSF drainage, during transport, during vigorous activity) or unclamped (e.g., signs and symptoms of increased ICP) and the level of head elevation are ordered by the physician.

   d. Nursing responsibilities include assessing and documenting the amount of CSF drainage. CSF flow is controlled by physician order (i.e., level of the drip chamber), the initial problem, and hydration status. However, normal CSF flow is usually 3 to 5 mL/hr in an infant, 5 to 10 mL/hr in a toddler or child, and 10 to 15 mL/hr in an adolescent. CSF should be clear and colorless. Initially, CSF may be blood tinged but it should turn clear in 1 to 2 hours or longer for ICH.

   i. Assess the system for patency by assessing the ICP waveform if a transducer is being used (i.e., the waveform would be dampened). Assess for fluctuation of the CSF fluid in the tubing with each heartbeat and respiration (if the system does not have a one-way valve). When the system is not draining, lower the collection cylinder until you see drainage (with a physician order); if the system has an external valve, compress the valve several times with the clamp open. Refer to the specific manufacturer's recommendations.

   ii. Assess the system for loose connections.

   iii. Notify the physician for significant changes in the patient's neurologic status or abrupt cessation or too much drainage of CSF (i.e., if beyond the initial evacuation period, CSF drainage exceeds the established norms or exceeds the physician's prescribed amount).

   iv. Document the reference level and maintain the drip chamber or drainage bag at the prescribed level.

   v. Prevent infection of the CSF. Observe the catheter exit site or dressing for drainage. Change the catheter dressing using aseptic technique. Monitor the patient's temperature and other signs of systemic infection (e.g., hypotension, increased WBC count, positive results from blood or CSF cultures).

B. Internal Ventricular Shunt

1. *Description.* A ventricular shunt is an internal catheter system designed to drain the lateral ventricles of CSF by bypassing part of the ventricular system. Many systems are available, but the major components are similar: two catheters and a one-way valve. A ventricular catheter is placed in the anterior horn of the right lateral ventricle. It is inserted through a burr hole usually in the region of the right parietooccipital area; the left side is avoided because of the location of the speech center. The catheter is tunneled under skin to minimize infection. A reservoir and pressure valve are placed directly under the scalp on the skull bones, usually above or behind the ear. There are different types of pressure control valves that regulate CSF drainage usually with a nonmetallic design. Specific features may include a reservoir and pressure setting adjustment. Distal tubing is attached to the valve and may be placed in one of several body cavities. The peritoneum (Figure 4.22) is the most common cavity used. The distal catheter is tunneled subcutaneously to the upper quadrant of the abdomen. A small incision is made in the abdomen, and the catheter is guided into the peritoneum, where CSF is absorbed. Extra tubing is coiled in the abdomen to allow for growth. The right atrium is only used if abdominal problems preclude a peritoneal catheter. The distal catheter is inserted into the right atrium via passage through the subclavian vein, or less frequently, inserted directly into the right atrium. The pleural cavity is used infrequently, only when the above locations are contraindicated.

2. *Clinical Use.* For hydrocephalus (acute and chronic).

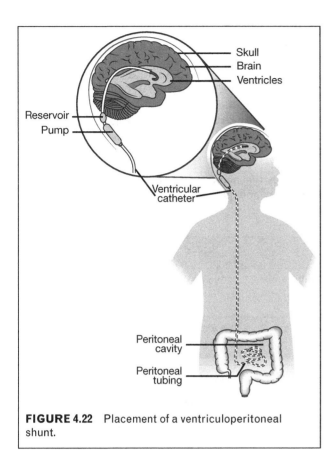

FIGURE 4.22 Placement of a ventriculoperitoneal shunt.

3. *Complications* of the ventriculoperitoneal (VP) shunt include bowel perforation, ascites, and ileus. Complications of the ventriculoatrial (VA) shunt include catheter movement, dysrhythmias, operative risks with more extensive surgery, endocarditis, and congestive heart failure. Complications of the ventriculopleural shunt include pleural effusion, pulmonary infection, and respiratory compromise.

   a. All shunting devices and body cavities that are receptacles are at risk for infection, including ventriculitis, meningitis, and systemic infection.

   b. Mechanical failure, although rare, may occur from valve malfunction and reservoirs that become obstructed with debris or disconnected from the distal catheter. The distal catheter may become disconnected and migrate to other areas (e.g., right ventricle or pulmonary artery from a VA shunt, perforated intestine from a VP shunt). Obstruction from tissue, clots, and debris may occur in the ventricular tip, valves, reservoir, internal catheters, and distal catheter tip.

   c. Clinical manifestations of shunt obstruction and malfunction are similar and generally relate to increased ICP (e.g., a tense and bulging anterior fontanelle, poor feeding, and increase in head circumference in the infant; headaches, blurred vision, vomiting, or papilledema in the toddler and child).

4. *Nursing Implications*

   a. Monitor neurologic status. Rapid evacuation of the ventricles (although rare with newer pressure regulated valves) may cause collapse of the ventricles, shearing of small vessels, and ICH. Obstruction of the system can cause signs and symptoms of increased ICP. Seizures may occur.

   b. Monitor for signs of infection, including redness or drainage at shunt site, hypothermia (more often in the neonate) or hyperthermia, redness, swelling, and tenderness along the subcutaneous tract, and nonspecific signs (e.g., lethargy, irritability, poor feeding, weight loss, pallor).

   c. Monitor for signs of excessive CSF drainage, including a sunken fontanelle and increased sodium loss.

   d. Prevent skin breakdown by elevating the head of the bed as ordered, positioning the patient on the unaffected side of the skull or using pressure reduction devices to protect skin over the shunt when the patient is lying on the affected side, promoting good nutrition, and turning the patient every 2 hours.

   e. Monitor for signs of ileus, including abdominal distention, vomiting, large orogastric residuals (i.e., more than one half of previous hours' intake), and hypoactive or absent bowel sounds.

   f. Newer pressure valves often include a magnet and precaution must be observed around magnetic sources, such as some audio headphones. Common environmental electromagnetic radiation (e.g., security scanners, microwave, metal detectors, computers) will not affect the valve. For patients having an MRI study, the physician will need to check the pressure settings on the valve and adjust if needed.

PHARMACOLOGY

A. Analgesia and Sedation

Analgesia and sedation are widely used in critically ill children. The goals of therapy are to promote natural sleep, decrease pain, minimize anxiety, and manage delirium. In addition to monitoring and assessing pain and sedation with scales, medication selection and monitoring are important. To optimize care in the neurologically impaired child, pharmacologic variables need to be considered. Table 4.6 is a list of sedatives and opioids commonly used for children.

B. Antimicrobial Therapy

1. Specific antimicrobial therapy for CNS infections depends on the pathogen suspected or identified,

patient age, and associated complications. Beyond stabilization of a child with a suspected CNS infection, treatment priority is administration of antimicrobials when indicated, for example, bacterial meningitis and herpes simplex viruses (HSVs). Table 4.7 lists the most common pathogens seen with CNS infections and the antimicrobials used according to age.

2. *Empiric Therapy Immediately Initiated*

   a. *Neonatal.* Empiric antimicrobial therapy in the neonate has traditionally been ampicillin and gentamicin. With increasing resistance

TABLE 4.6. Sedative and Opioid Medications in Children

Drug	Dose (IV)	Comment
Dexmedetomidine	0.5–1 mcg/kg/dose over 10 min 0.2–0.7 mcg/kg/hr infusion	Avoid in patients with heart block, severe ventricular dysfunction, hypovolemia
Etomidate	0.1–0.3 mg/kg/dose over 30–60 sec	Avoid in patients with adrenal suppression; irritating to small vessels
Fentanyl	1–2 mcg/kg/dose IV q 2–4 hr infants; q 30–60 min children Max dose: 300 mcg total 0.5–1 mcg/kg/hr infusion	Skeletal muscle and chest-wall rigidity with rapid administration in infants; less hypotensive effects compared to morphine
Ketamine	Full-term neonate: 0.2–1 mg/kg/dose IV over 2–3 min Infants and children: 0.5–2 mg/kg/dose IV	Bronchodilator, consider with asthma
Lorazepam	0.05–0.1 mg/kg/dose IV q 4–6 hr Max dose: 4 mg	Avoid in hypotensive patients
Midazolam	0.05–0.1 mg/kg/dose 0.06–0.12 mg/kg/hr infusion Higher dose may be used in mechanically ventilated patient; lower doses when used with other CNS depressants	Avoid in hemodynamically unstable patient
Morphine	Neonate: 0.05–0.1 mg/kg/dose IV q 4–6 hr; Continuous: 10–30 mcg/kg/hr Infants and children: 0.05–0.2 mg/kg/dose q 2–4 hr; continuous: 10–40 mcg/kg/hr (ventilated patients may receive larger doses, more frequent intervals)	Avoid in hypotensive patients
Pentobarbital	High-dose coma: Load: 10 mg/kg over 30 min, then 5 mg/kg every hour for 3 hr, maintenance infusion: 1 mg/kg/hr	Avoid in hemodynamically unstable patient; adjust dose to burst suppression on EEG
Propofol	Short-term use only in children Consult local and institutional regulations for policies and procedures	Avoid in hemodynamically unstable patient

CNS, central nervous system; IV, intravenous; q, every.

Source: From Taketomo, C. K., Hodding, J. H., & Kraus, D. M. (2015). *Pediatric & neonatal dosage handbook: A universal resource for clinicians treating pediatric and neonatal patients* (22nd ed.). Hudson, OH: Lexicomp.

TABLE 4.7   Antimicrobial Therapy for Central Nervous System Infections in Children

Bacterial Meningitis			
Age	Predominant Organism(s)	Antibiotic	Duration of Antibiotics[a]
<1 month	GBS, *Escherichia coli*, *Listeria monocytogenes*, *Streptococcus pneumoniae* (less common), *Neisseria meningitidis* (less common)	Ampicillin and gentamicin Cefotaxime may be used in place of gentamicin for resistant gram negative enteric organisms to ampicillin	GBS: 14–21 days; *L. monocytogenes, S. pneumoniae*: 14 days; Gram-negative bacilli: 21 days
1–3 months	GBS, *Streptococcus pneumoniae, Neisseria meningitidis*, Gram-negative bacilli, *Haemophilus influenzae type b* (less common)	Vancomycin and cefotaxime or ceftriaxone; rifampin considered for pneumococcal meningitis; Vancomycin plus rifampin or meropenem used for penicillin allergies	GBS 14–21 days; *S. pneumoniae* 10–14 days; Hib 7–10 days; *N. meningitidis* 5–7 days; *L. monocytogenes* 14–21 days; Gram-negative bacilli 21 days
3–18 years	*Streptococcus pneumoniae, Neisseria meningitidis*, GBS (less common), *Haemophilus influenzae type b* (less common)	Vancomycin and cefotaxime or ceftriaxone; rifampin considered for pneumococcal meningitis; Vancomycin plus rifampin or meropenem used for penicillin allergies	*S. pneumoniae* 10–14 days; Hib 7–10 days; *N. meningitidis* 5–7 days
Viral Meningitis			
	Enteroviruses, La Crosse virus, Western equine virus, St. Louis virus, herpes simplex type 2, varicella zoster, HIV, mumps virus, measles virus, lymphocytic choriomeningitis virus	Acyclovir for HSV controversial	Neonatal HSV: 14–21 days Infants 1–3 months HIV: 21 days 3 months to <12 years: 14–21 days >12 years: 14–21 days
Encephalitis			
	West Nile virus, Cytomegalovirus, Epstein–Barr virus, La Crosse virus, Western equine virus, St. Louis virus, Eastern equine virus, Powassan virus, herpes simplex type 1, influenza virus, HIV, rabies virus	Acyclovir for HSV	Neonatal HSV: 14–21 days Infants 1–3 months HIV: 21 days 3 months to <12 years: 14–21 days >12 years: 14–21 days

GBS, group B *Streptococcus*; HSV, herpes simplex virus.

[a]Uncomplicated meningitis.

Sources: Encephalitis recommendation from Falchek, S. J. (2012). Encephalitis in the pediatric population. *Pediatrics in Review, 33*(3), 122–133. 10.1542/pir.33-3-122; Meningitis recommendations from Swanson, D. (2015). Meningitis. *Pediatrics in Review, 36*(12), 514–526. doi:10.1542/pir.36-12-514; Tan, Y. C., Gill, A. K., & Kim, K. S. (2015). Treatment strategies for central nervous system infections: An update. *Expert Opinion on Pharmacotherapy, 16*(2), 187–203. doi:10.1517/14656566.2015.973851

of *Escherichia coli* and other gram-negative enterococci to ampicillin, a third generation cephalosporin often takes the place of gentamicin.

b. *Older than 1 month of age.* General recommendations often include third-generation cephalosporins (cefotaxime or ceftriaxone) plus vancomycin. Vancomycin is added to cover the emergence of cephalosporin resistant organisms.

3. Specific targeted therapy is started once the pathogen has been identified with antibiotic susceptibilities.

4. *Acyclovir* should be initiated in all suspected cases of encephalitis pending results of diagnostic studies. Treatment with acyclovir continues for HSV encephalitis. Other antiviral medications commonly used to treat some forms of encephalitis include ganciclovir and foscarnet (older patients and adults).

C. Hyperosmolar Therapy Used to Control Cerebral Swelling

1. *Hypertonic saline* is commonly used to treat increased ICP. It may be given as a bolus (range between 6.5 and 10 mL/kg) or as a continuous infusion of 3% normal saline (range between 0.1 and 1.0 mL/kg). The lowest dose needed to maintain the ICP below 20 mmHg is recommended. Potential side effects include rebound increased ICP, hyperchloremic acidosis, renal impairment, SAH, and excessive urinary losses. Serum osmolality should be monitored, and although many practitioners consider 360 mOsm/L the upper threshold of safety, there is no consensus on this value (Kochanek et al., 2012).

2. *Mannitol* is used frequently to control cerebral swelling and reduce ICP, but it has not been studied with controlled clinical trials in children. Its effect on ICP is through two mechanisms. First, it produces an osmotic gradient between the intravascular and extravascular compartments. The net effect is movement of water from the interstitium into the cerebral vasculature, where it can be removed via the kidneys. A secondary effect of mannitol is a compensatory vasoconstriction due to decreased blood viscosity (with intact autoregulation). Total cerebral blood volume decreases, but CBF is maintained. Dosing guidelines for mannitol range between 0.25 and 1.0 mg/kg of body weight. Euvolemia is maintained by fluid replacement. Serum osmolality is monitored and is generally maintained below or at 320 mOsm/L, but there is limited research to confirm this parameter. Potential complications of mannitol when used in high doses and at frequent intervals (i.e., creating hyperosmolality) include acute renal failure, possible rebound intracranial swelling (when mannitol diffuses into the extravascular compartment and reverses the osmotic gradient), electrolyte imbalances from increased diuresis via the kidneys, and fluid shifts.

D. Anticonvulsant Medications Used to Control Seizures

1. *Benzodiazepines* act rapidly and are used in the *initial therapy phase* when the seizure duration reaches 5 minutes and should conclude by 20 minutes (Table 4.8). IV administration is preferred, but intramuscular (IM), rectal, and buccal routes may be used until IV access is obtained. Lorazepam is preferred for IV administration; midazolam for IM (intranasal and buccally) administration; and diazepam for IV or rectal administration (Abend et al., 2014; Brophy et al., 2012; Glauser et al., 2016). A significant number of children will continue to have seizures after receiving benzodiazepines.

2. The *second phase* of therapy begins when the seizure persists for 20 minutes and ends at 40 minutes (Glauser et al., 2016). There are differences in expert opinion and no evidence-based preference exists for anticonvulsant therapy during the second phase of treatment. The choice often depends on patient-specific circumstances and condition. The Neurocritical Care Society guidelines and American Epilepsy Society guidelines consider *fosphenytoin* a good option. Fosphenytoin is a water-soluble prodrug of phenytoin that is quickly converted to phenytoin with higher unbound peak levels. Advantages over phenytoin include that it does not precipitate in commonly used IV solutions, it can be administered IM, and can be infused more quickly (7–10 minutes). Fosphenytoin also has less significant side effects (e.g., extravasation reactions, hypotension, and cardiac dysrhythmias). Both phenytoin and fosphenytoin are not sedating and are useful for assessing patients with an altered mental status. The American Epilepsy Society guidelines also include IV levetiracetam and IV valproic acid as reasonable options during this phase (Glauser et al., 2016).

3. *Phenobarbital* is often used in combination with other anticonvulsants because it is longer acting. It may also be used during the second phase when other medications listed earlier are not available.

4. The *third-phase therapy* begins when the seizure duration is at 40 minutes. There is no evidence to guide therapy during this phase and second-phase medications may be repeated or anesthetic doses of midazolam, thiopental, pentobarbital, or propofol may be administered (Glauser et al., 2016).

TABLE 4.8   Anticonvulsants in Children

Drug	Dose	Comment
Benzodiazepine is the initial therapy of choice (0–5 min)[b]		
Lorazepam	0.05–0.1 mg/kg/dose IV slow over 2–5 min, may repeat dose once, max dose 4 mg[a,b]	Used for IV route
Midazolam	0.1–0.3 mg/kg/dose intranasal or IM[a] Max dose 5 mg 5 mg/dose for 13–40 kg[b] 10 mg/dose for >40 kg[b]	Used for IM or intranasal routes when IV route is not available
Diazepam	Rectal gel not recommended for infants <6 months[a] 6 months to 2 years: dose not established PR Children 2–5 years: 0.5 mg/kg/dose PR Children 6–11 years: 0.3 mg/kg/dose PR Children >12 years: 0.2 mg/kg/dose PR 0.15–0.2 mg/kg/dose IV, may repeat once, max dose 10 mg/dose[b]	Used for rectal route when intravenous route is not available IV diazepam not recommended in infants <30 days[a]
Second therapy of choice, no evidence-based preference (20–40 min)[b]		
Fosphenytoin	20 mg PE/kg IV; Max dose is 1,500 mg[b], Max rate is 1.0–3.0 mg PE/kg/min not to exceed 150 mg PE/min (lower dose for neonates[a] Maintenance dose: 4–8 mg PE/kg/dose in two divided doses, max dose 300 mg PE/dose[a]	Phenobarbital is preferred in neonates[a] Fosphenytoin is preferred over phenytoin due to lower risk of cardiac side effects Dose adjusted per serum levels Compatible in NS and dextrose
Levetiracetam	Neonatal: limited data available[a] 60 mg/kg IV, max dose 4,500 mg[b] infuse over 15 min[a] Maintenance dose: 30–55 mg/kg/dose IV divided twice daily, infuse over 15 min[a]	
Valproic acid	Loading dose: 20–40 mg/kg/dose IV[a,b] Max dose 3,000 mg[b] Maintenance dose: 5 mg/kg/hr IV infusion[a]	Not recommended in neonates due to hepatotoxicity[a] Limited data available for infants and children May be considered for refractory SE[a]
Phenobarbital	Neonatal patients[a]: Loading dose: 15–20 mg/kg IV, may repeat 5–10 mg/kg dose q 15–20 min, maintenance dose: 3–4 mg/kg/dose Infants and children[a]: Loading dose: 15–20 mg/kg IV, max dose 1,000 mg, may repeat once after 10–15 min (Max total dose 40 mg/kg) Maintenance dose: Infants to ≤ 5 years: 3–5 mg/kg/dose Children >5 years: 2–3 mg/kg/dose Adolescents: 1–3 mg/kg/dose	Use for infants and children when other primary and secondary therapies are not available[b] Preferred over phenytoin and fosphenytoin for neonates[a] Dose adjusted per serum levels May cause hypotension

IM, intramuscular; IV, intravenous; NS, normal saline; PR, rectal route; q, every; SE, status epilepticus.

Note: Fosphenytoin dose, concentration, and infusion rates are expressed as PE, phenytoin equivalent.

Sources: [a]Adapted from Taketomo, C. K., Hodding, J. H., & Kraus, D. M. (2015). *Pediatric & neonatal dosage handbook: A universal resource for clinicians treating pediatric and neonatal patients* (22nd ed.). Hudson, OH: Lexicomp; [b]Glauser, T., Shinnar, S., Gloss, D., Alldredge, B., Arya, R., Bainbridge, J., . . . Treiman, D. (2016). Evidence-based guidelines: Treatment of convulsive status epilepticus in children and adults: Report of the guideline committee of the American Epilepsy Society. *Epilepsy Currents, 16*(1), 48–61. doi:10.5698/1535-7597-16.1.48

NEUROLOGIC DISORDERS

Intracranial Hypertension

A. Definition and Etiology

A sustained elevation of ICP above 20 mmHg is considered pathologic. Increased ICP, or intracranial hypertension, is not a disease state but is a final common pathway for a number of neurologic pathologies. Specific occurrence rates are unknown.

1. Neurologic pathologies that produce increased ICP are broadly classified into those that increase cerebral blood volume, CSF, or brain tissue (specific pathologies are discussed in later sections).

    a. *Cerebral edema* may increase ICP and results from a number of different pathologies. It is defined as an increase in the fluid content of brain tissue. It is not a single entity and occurs in several different forms.

    b. *Cellular (cytotoxic) edema* is characterized by neuronal swelling and often brain swelling. It may result from a number of brain insults, including trauma, infarction, or neoplasm. When a brain insult results in hypoxia or ischemia, it produces a failure of intracellular adenosine triphosphate (ATP)-dependent transport systems. Depletion of ATP with uncontrolled influx of extracellular ions, particularly Na^+ and later Cl^-, causes ionic shifts with an increase in intracellular osmoles. Intracellular osmolarity drives inflow of water into the cell. Intracellular volume increases and there is alteration of the cell membrane. When the ionic pumps in the plasma membrane fail completely, the swollen cell dies (Rungta et al., 2015).

    c. *Vasogenic edema* is characterized by increased permeability of the capillary endothelium to macromolecules. Large plasma molecules move from the vascular compartment into the extracellular spaces, pulling water with them. Vasogenic edema occurs after vascular injury (e.g., abscess, hemorrhage, infarction, and contusion), tumors, or disruption of the BBB and accumulation of extracellular fluid.

    d. *Interstitial edema* is characterized by transependymal movement of CSF fluid from the ventricles into the extracellular spaces of brain tissue. It results from increased CSF hydrostatic pressure associated with noncommunicating hydrocephalus. This edema is most prominent in the white matter around ventricles.

B. Pathophysiology

1. Regardless of the cause, when intracranial volume exceeds the buffering capacity of the brain, *ICP increases* (see "Intracranial Pressure Dynamics" section).

2. Increased ICP causes a number of interrelated pathologic processes, resulting in distortion and *herniation* of brain tissue (Figure 4.23). Intracranial contents are separated or compartmentalized via anatomical structures (e.g., falx cerebri, tentorium cerebelli). When there is a significant pressure gradient between two brain compartments, brain tissue may be displaced (herniates) from its normal location into adjacent space. There are several types of herniations.

    a. *Transentorial herniation* occurs when ICP is increased significantly above the tentorium, that is, supratentorial. One of the most common types is a *subfalcine herniation*. This represents displacement of the cingulate gyrus under the falx cerebri into the opposite hemisphere,

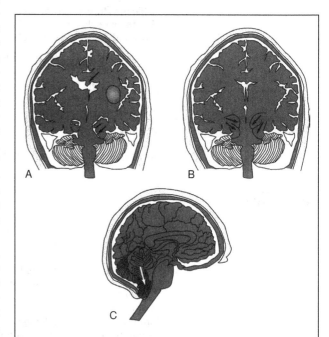

FIGURE 4.23 Herniation syndromes. (A) Midline shift indicating cingulate herniation. (B) Protrusion of uncus through the tentorial notch. Downward displacement of supratentorial region through the tentorial notch as seen in central herniation. (C) Herniation of cerebellar tonsils into the foramen magnum.

Source: Published with permission of the American Association of Critical-Care Nurses, from Morrison, C. A. (1987). Brain herniation syndromes. *Critical Care Nursing, 7*(5), 35–38. Permission conveyed through Copyright Clearance Center, Inc.

causing compression of the internal cerebral vein. Progression of the herniation may occur with unilateral displacement of the uncus on the medial temporal lobe through the tentorial notch. *Central herniation* is a symmetric downward displacement of the cerebral hemispheres, basal ganglia, diencephalon, and midbrain through the tentorial notch.

b. *Infratentorial herniation* occurs with an increase in intracranial volume and ICP in the brain structures below the tentorial membrane. Downward displacement of one or both of the cerebellar tonsils (*downward tonsillar herniation*) occurs through the foramen magnum. Less common is upward displacement of the cerebellar tonsils through the tentorial notch.

3. Increased ICP also results in a *reduction in CBF* from compression of major vessels; brain ischemia, anoxia, and neuronal cell death may occur.

C. Clinical Presentation

1. *History.* Increased ICP may occur from a variety of brain insults that are acute or chronic and congenital or acquired. The diagnosis of increased ICP can be challenging. Early symptoms may be nonspecific, especially in infants. An alteration in level of consciousness can also delay diagnosis. Historical features that suggest nontraumatic etiologies of increased ICP include growth abnormalities, lethargy, personality change, persistent vomiting (especially in the morning), and a focal deficit.

2. *Physical examination* may confirm the presence of increased ICP, but a normal examination may not rule it out.

a. *Chronic symptoms in infants* are usually nonspecific and include irritability, poor feeding, and lethargy. An abnormal increase in head circumference is noted; patients in the 95th percentile require further evaluation. The normal rate of head growth in the first year of life is approximately 2 cm/month for first 3 months, 1 cm/month for 3 to 6 months, and 0.5 cm/month for the remaining 6 months. The setting-sun sign is a classic "sunset" appearance of the eyes (i.e., the sclera are visible above the iris, and the infant is unable to look upward with the head facing forward). Vomiting, a large and full anterior fontanelle, the "cracked-pot" sound when the skull is percussed, and separation of cranial sutures also occur.

b. *Chronic symptoms in children* include headache (local or generalized), vomiting in the absence of nausea, especially on rising in the morning, blurred vision and decreased acuity, altered mental status (e.g., confusion, memory loss, fatigue, irritability), papilledema, and gait disturbances.

c. With *acute changes*, age becomes less of a factor in differentiating clinical manifestations. Vital sign changes include a change in the respiratory pattern, progressing from irregular to absent respirations. The constellation of systolic pressure increases relative to diastolic pressure (widened pulse pressure), bradycardia, and respiratory depression (Cushing's triad) is another late and preterminal sign. The pupils are dilated and fixed because of cranial nerve III compression. The patient's level of consciousness progresses from restlessness to unresponsiveness. Motor function progresses from hemiparesis, hemiplegia, or decorticate posturing to flaccid paralysis or decerebrate posturing.

d. *Herniation symptoms* depend on the location and type of herniation. There are few signs specific to subfalcine herniation. Changes in the patient's mental status and level of consciousness may be the only clue. Uncal herniation first presses against the midbrain with disruption of the parasympathetic fibers that run along the third cranial nerve, resulting in unilateral pupil dilation on the same side as the lesion and contralateral hemiplegia. Later signs include paralysis of extraocular eye movements, coma, and, if left untreated, death. Early signs of central herniation include alteration in the level of consciousness, alteration of the respiratory pattern (e.g., yawning and sighs), small reactive pupils, and bilateral Babinski reflexes. Later signs include Cheyne–Stokes breathing, decorticate posturing, oculocephalic reflex, and coma. Downward tonsillar herniation symptoms occur very rapidly (e.g., cardiorespiratory failure). Other clinical signs of upward tonsillar herniation include developing hydrocephalus and coma. Midbrain compression produces downward deviation of the eyes, and pontine compression produces small reactive pupils and decerebrate posturing.

3. *Diagnostic Tests.* Selection of specific studies depends on the cause of the increased ICP. For acute changes, CT scan without contrast is the radiographic study of choice in children with suspected increased ICP. The primary objective of the emergent CT scan is to identify a cause of increased ICP that requires immediate neurosurgical intervention. CT scan with contrast is useful to identify a brain abscess or meningeal enhancement. MRI is the imaging modality of choice in less emergent situations or if the CT scan is normal, but the patient has neurological symptoms. MRI is more diagnostic than CT for early stroke, venous thromboses, posterior fossa tumors, and demyelinating lesions. CBF studies are used to confirm brain death, especially if the clinical examination is equivocal.

4. *Clinical Course.* The patient's clinical course depends on the etiology of the increased ICP. Some brain lesions or injuries (e.g., brain tumor or epidural hematoma) may respond to surgical treatment and ICP can be restored to normal levels. On the other hand, increased ICP from cytotoxic edema and neuronal death may be irreversible.

D. Patient Care Management

1. *Preventive Care.* Beyond screening for potential neurological injuries that have the potential to increase ICP, preventive strategies are directed at early recognition of increased ICP and early interventions. Once the etiology of increased ICP is identified, corrective measures are implemented (e.g., insert a shunting device for hydrocephalus, excise tumors, and remove extradural hematomas). An ICP catheter is inserted for monitoring ICP, and a ventriculostomy is established for CSF drainage. SjO_2 and $PbtO_2$ monitoring may be used to identify and treat cerebral ischemia. Medications to reduce cerebral swelling (e.g., diuretics and hyperosmolar agents) are administered. Decompressive craniectomy (removal of part of the skull) may be considered to treat patients with uncontrolled ICP following TBI (Kochanek et al., 2012).

2. *Direct Care*

    a. Restore circulation, airway, and breathing.

    b. The cornerstone of increased ICP management is to reduce ICP while maintaining adequate CBF. The goal is to prevent secondary brain injury. Neurosurgery is recommended for brain lesions and injuries that can be surgically corrected (e.g., brain tumor or epidural hematoma) or to implant devices to control ICP (e.g., ventricular shunt).

    c. Medical management for sustained increases in ICP ≥20 mmHg should be considered (Kochanek et al., 2012).

3. *Supportive Care*

    a. Perform baseline and serial *neurologic assessments*. When indicated, monitor serum medication levels, urine and serum osmolality, electrolytes, ICP, CPP, SjO_2, $PbtO_2$, arterial blood gases (ABGs), end-tidal CO_2 ($ETCO_2$), and arterial saturation.

    b. *Prophylactic hyperventilation* ($PaCO_2$ <30 mmHg) is avoided in the initial 48 hours following a TBI. If hyperventilation is used beyond this time period to treat refractory ICP, neuromonitoring for cerebral ischemia is recommended (Kochanek et al., 2012). Hyperventilation decreases ICP by reducing $PaCO_2$, which, in turn, causes vasoconstriction of cerebral arterioles. Low $PaCO_2$ causes pH to increase (decreased H^+ concentration), and initially, decreases cerebral tissue acidosis. Precapillary arterioles constrict in response to decreased H^+ concentration. If autoregulation is intact, CBF, cerebral blood volume, and ICP decrease. However, prolonged use of hyperventilation may produce ischemic injury, especially adjacent to injured tissue. Monitor and trend, CPP, ICP, SjO_2, $PbtO_2$ with $ETCO_2$ to prevent ischemia.

    c. Neuromuscular blockade may be used to control ventilation and improve cerebral venous outflow: it reduces shivering, posturing, and airway and intrathoracic pressures. It prevents increases in metabolic demand by eliminating skeletal muscle contraction.

    d. Maintain oxygenation and normal PaO_2. Hypoxemia (PaO_2 below 50 mmHg) produces cerebral vasodilation and an increase in cerebral blood volume. Individualize the endotracheal tube suctioning procedure based on the patient's response. Lidocaine may be given prior to suctioning to blunt increases in ICP during suctioning. Perform serial respiratory assessments and continuously monitor arterial oxygen saturation.

    e. Promote cerebral venous drainage. Elevate the head of the bed 30 degrees to promote displacement of venous blood volume to extracranial vessels. Prevent increased intraabdominal pressure by using stool softeners, decompressing the stomach, and minimizing gastric residuals. Prevent increased intrathoracic pressure by individualizing the use of positive end-expiratory pressure (PEEP) and avoiding chest physiotherapy during periods of poor cerebral compliance. Maintain body alignment (e.g., avoid flexion of the hips and neck) to prevent cerebral venous drainage obstruction.

    f. Reduce environmental stimuli by minimizing noxious procedures, individualizing nursing activities to control ICP, avoiding cluster care, and maintaining effective pain control.

    g. Control cerebral metabolism. An increase causes increased CBF and cerebral blood volume. Treat hyperthermia aggressively with antipyretics and cooling devices. Moderate hypothermia

(32°C–33°C) beginning within 8 hours after a severe TBI and lasting up to 48 hours should be considered to control cerebral hypertension. Rewarming should be gradual and should be at a rate of <0.5°C per hour (Kochanek et al., 2012). Control seizures quickly with anticonvulsants. Prophylactic administration of phenytoin may be considered for children with severe TBI to prevent posttraumatic seizures. Barbiturate coma is generally used when all other conventional therapies have been exhausted in hemodynamically stable patients with salvageable head injury (Kochanek et al., 2012). An induced barbiturate coma reduces cerebral metabolism and therefore decreases CBF and cerebral blood volume. It is associated with significant negative cardiac effects (e.g., decreased contractility, dysrhythmias, vasodilation, and hypotension). Continuous arterial monitoring is recommended and inotropic agents are used concomitantly or are on standby.

h. Administer hyperosmolar therapy. Hypertonic saline is effective for lowering cerebral hypertension. Mannitol is a widely used agent to control ICP in patients, but there are fewer studies in children to demonstrate its efficacy (see "Pharmacology" section).

i. Administer diuretics that can be used alone or, more frequently, in combination with mannitol. The proposed effects are total body fluid reduction and decreased CSF production. Monitor fluids and serum and urine electrolytes and osmolalities. Fluid restriction must be individualized and hypovolemia avoided.

j. Steroids are used in children with some neurologic conditions (e.g., brain tumors); however, their use is not recommended in patients with a TBI (Kochanek et al., 2012).

k. Increase CSF drainage and lower cerebral blood volume by elevating the head of the bed to promote displacement of CSF to the spinal subarachnoid space. Maintain ventricular CSF drainage (see "Intracranial Devices" section).

l. Treat hypotension with fluid resuscitation using crystalloids, colloids, and blood products. When patient is euvolemic, vasopressors may be used to increase MAP and CPP.

m. Correct sodium disturbances due to diabetes insipidus (DI), syndrome of inappropriate antidiuretic hormone (SIADH), or cerebral salt wasting syndrome (CSW). The most common form of DI is central, meaning there is a deficiency of antidiuretic hormone (ADH) due to either failure of synthesis in the hypothalamus or failure of secretion from the posterior pituitary. Hallmark signs of DI include large quantity of dilute urine output, hypernatremia, serum osmolality, and low urine osmolality. SIADH and CSW are both associated with intracranial diseases and have overlapping clinical findings: hyponatremia, concentrated urine, and high urine sodium (usually >20 mEq/L). Unlike SIADH, where there is retention of free water (euvolemia or hypervolemia) and hyponatremia due to elevated ADH, CSW syndrome is associated with hyponatremia with hypovolemia (Maesaka et al., 2014). See Chapter 6 for an expanded discussion on assessment and treatment of these endocrine disorders.

E. Outcomes

Patient outcomes depend on the cause of increased ICP and how well CBF can be maintained. Regardless of the cause, outcomes are poor in patients with sustained elevations in ICP >20 mmHg and compromised CBF due to secondary brain injury. Herniation syndromes that are not immediately corrected may cause irreversible neurologic damage.

SEIZURES

A. Definition and Etiology

1. A *seizure* is an uncontrolled, time-limited alteration in behavior that results from abnormal electrical discharge from cortical neurons in any part of the brain. A brief seizure lasts less than 5 minutes and is most common.

2. Historically, *SE* is defined as a prolonged seizure (usually defined as 30 minutes or longer) or multiple consecutive seizures without regaining consciousness. Current evidence recognizes that most seizures are brief, lasting less than 5 minutes. If a seizure does last longer than 5 minutes, it most likely will be prolonged. The most recent Neurocritical Care Society guidelines now defines SE as "5 minutes or more of (i) continuous clinical and/or electrographic seizure activity or (ii) recurrent seizure activity without recovery (returning to baseline) between seizures" (Brophy et al., 2012, p. 5). Current guidelines from the American Epilepsy Society use a 5-minute seizure duration as the treatment threshold to minimize the development of SE and improve patient outcomes (Glauser et al., 2016).

3. *Refractory status epilepticus (RSE)* refers to patients who do not respond to standard treatment for SE.

4. *Epilepsy* is a term used to define a chronic disorder characterized by recurrent and unprovoked seizures. It is commonly referred to as a *seizure disorder*.

5. *Classification of seizures* varies among experts, but the International League Against Epilepsy (ILAE) Commission on Classification and Terminology devides seizures into two broad classifications: focal and generalized (Berg et al., 2010).

    a. *Focal seizures* start in one part of the brain. They may stay local or spread to other areas of the brain. The terms *simple* and *complex* are no longer recommended; these terms were often misused or misunderstood. The ILAE Commission stated there was inadequate information to create a scientific classification for focal seizure. Therefore, it is recommended that focal seizures be described by major types of symptoms and by the degree of impairment or change in consciousness (e.g., without impairment of consciousness with observable motor or autonomic symptoms; without impairment of consciousness evolving to a bilateral convulsive seizure; Berg et al., 2010).

    b. *Generalized seizures (convulsive or nonconvulsive)* originate in cortical or subcortical areas in the brain and quickly involve networks that spread bilaterally. Generalized seizures include

        i. Absence seizures (typical, atypical, absence with special features)

        ii. Myoclonic seizures (myoclonic, myoclonic tonic, myoclonic atonic)

        iii. Clonic seizures

        iv. Tonic seizures

        v. Atonic seizures

6. *Etiology*

    a. Seizures are the most common neurologic disorder seen in children. The estimated lifetime prevalence of epilepsy/seizure disorder is 1% (Russ, Larson, & Halfon, 2012).

    b. The underlying types (etiology) of seizures are *genetic, structural/metabolic,* and *unknown* (Berg et al., 2010).

        i. Genetic epilepsy is the direct result of a known or presumed genetic defect in which seizures are a prominent feature.

        ii. Structural/metabolic seizures result from a distinct structural or metabolic condition, for example, a CNS infection, brain tumor, trauma, stroke, electrolyte imbalance, or low anticonvulsant level (Abend et al., 2014).

        iii. *Unknown* is a term used to designate the cause of the seizure as currently unknown, although it may be related to an unrecognized disorder. They are poorly understood and account for one third of all epilepsies.

    c. A *febrile seizure* is defined as a seizure accompanied by a fever (temperature ≥100.4°F or 38°C) without a CNS infection in children 6 to 60 months of age. This is the most common form of childhood seizure, with an occurrence rate of 2% to 5% of all children (American Academy of Pediatrics, 2011).

    d. Risk factors include age (more common in the young and elderly), family history of previous seizure, neurologic disease, head trauma, and neurodevelopmental abnormalities.

B. Pathophysiology

1. The precise pathophysiologic mechanism underlying seizures is unknown. Seizures are believed to be heterogeneous, and, at a basic level, they represent an imbalance between excitatory and inhibitory neurotransmission in the brain.

2. In the absence of a compromised CNS, the brain is usually protected from a seizure by compensatory mechanisms. However, after approximately 20 to 30 minutes, severe alterations in brain function occur. Seizures increase the metabolic demand and CBF requirements of the parts of the cortex with repeated neuronal discharges. Prolonged seizures cause an uncoupling of CBF supply and metabolic demand, resulting in regional hypoxia, which may lead to cell death.

3. *Systemic effects* may also occur in patients, especially in patients with RSE. During SE, the hypothalamus and brainstem are stimulated with an almost immediate release of catecholamines into the systemic circulation. Cardiovascular effects include alterations in heart rate and blood pressure (early) and cardiac failure and shock (late). Respiratory dysfunction may also occur and includes apnea, tachypnea, aspiration, respiratory acidosis, and airway obstruction. Renal effects include oliguria, uremia, and acute tubular necrosis. ANS effects include hyperpyrexia, diaphoresis, vomiting, and hypersecretion. Metabolic or biochemical effects include metabolic acidosis, hypoglycemia, hyperkalemia, and elevated creatine phosphokinase (CPK).

Early systemic changes with a seizure are usually self-limiting, but systemic changes that occur late in an episode of RSE pose more of a threat to neurologic function and integrity.

C. Clinical Presentation

1. *History*

a. Defining characteristics vary with the type of seizure. The most common type of seizure requiring admission to the ICU is *generalized tonic–clonic* (GTC) status epilepticus (formerly known as a *grand mal seizure*).

b. The majority of children who have a seizure have a normal (other than EEG findings) neurologic examination and neuroimaging studies. Therefore, the history is important to diagnosis the underlying cause of the seizure. A detailed account of the child's behavior prior to, during, and after the seizure is critical. Observations and questions to ask to clarify the type of seizure include:

    i. Were there any warning signs before the seizure?

    ii. What was the patient's behavior during seizure?

    iii. How long did the seizure last?

    iv. How did the patient feel after the seizure?

    v. How long did it take to get back to baseline?

c. If the patient has a known history of seizures, it is important to ask patients and families about previous therapies that were successful or unsuccessful in managing the seizure.

d. There are several major phases of a seizure:

    i. A *prodromal (preictal) period* may precede a seizure. The prodrome may occur days to hours before the seizure. Symptoms include headache, irritability, loss of appetite, insomnia, and change in mood. The physiologic basis is unknown.

    ii. *The ictal period* is the time during the actual seizure when physical changes occur in the body. An *aura* is often the first symptom of a seizure. It represents an abnormal focal electrical discharge from the brain and is sometimes an indescribable feeling. Clinical manifestations of an aura vary considerably among patients and may include focal motor symptoms such as finger movement and clonic movement of an extremity; focal sensory symptoms such as

a "needles-and-pins" sensation or numbness; autonomic symptoms such as vomiting, pallor, flushing, sweating, dizziness, erection of body hairs, pupillary dilation, tachycardia, and incontinence; and psychic symptoms such as visual, auditory, and olfactory hallucinations and fear. Motor symptoms of a generalized seizure are easily recognized. The tonic phase is characterized by rigid extension of the arms and legs. The clonic phase follows and is characterized by relaxation of the muscles alternating with contractions (rhythmic jerks). Following the clonic phase the bladder and bowel sphincters relax, and urinary and bowel incontinence may occur.

    iii. The *postictal* period is the recovery period after the seizure. Some children recover quickly and others may take minutes to hours to return to their baseline. Several factors determine how quickly a child recovers and include the location of brain the seizure impacted, duration of the seizure, and anticonvulsants used. Patients may experience sensory/emotional symptoms (e.g., confused, lethargic, amnesic, scared, anxious) and have physical changes (e.g., headache, nausea, bruising).

2. *Physical Examination*

a. Airway, breathing, and circulation are assessed in the initial physical examination. Patients may not be able to maintain their own airway and ventilation, especially with prolonged seizures.

b. Life-threatening injuries may occur during a seizure and need to be identified quickly.

c. The physical examination assists in the diagnosis of specific epileptic syndromes and in identifying any injuries that may have occurred during a generalized seizure.

    i. Abdominal examination with hepatomegaly may suggest a storage disease.

    ii. Cardiac examination with ECG may reveal a cardiogenic cause, for example, a disorder that decreases cardiac output.

    iii. Skin examination may suggest a neurocutaneous disorder associated with seizures.

3. *Diagnostic Tests*

a. Specific studies used to identify the underlying cause of the seizure vary depending on the suspected neuropathology. The diagnostic workup should be started immediately and simultaneously with treatment.

b. Routine laboratory tests include serum glucose (finger-stick glucose immediately); complete blood count (CBC); basic metabolic panel; calcium, magnesium, and anticonvulsant medication levels.

c. Structural abnormalities that may be the cause of the seizure need to be investigated and neuroimaging is recommended (e.g., an MRI or CT scan).

d. EEG provides adjunctive data for diagnosing a seizure. In most patients, the incidence of epileptiform discharges is highest in the first 24 hours; however, in some children the EEG immediately after a seizure may be normal or with nonspecific findings. Specific EEG patterns vary depending on the type and location of seizure (Table 4.9).

e. If the history and physical examination and neuroimaging do not reveal a cause for the seizure, the child should be further evaluated with tests and laboratory screening (e.g., lumbar puncture and CSF analysis, toxicology screen, liver function tests, ABG, and chromosomal karyotype).

4. *Clinical Course*

a. Most seizures in children last less than 5 minutes. Seizures that last longer than 5 minutes often do not stop spontaneously (Brophy et al., 2012).

b. Some patients recover from a seizure quickly and spontaneously, whereas others develop SE or RSE.

D. Patient Care Management

1. *Preventive Care*

a. Monitor anticonvulsant medication levels in patients with a history of seizures.

TABLE 4.9 EEG Epileptiform Patterns

Generalized Epileptiform Patterns		
Pattern	**Description**	**Significance**
Spike (Polyspike)-and-wave pattern	Most common type is bilaterally synchronous single or polyspike discharge	Associated with generalized seizure disorder. Photic stimulation may cause spike-and-wave discharge.
Sharp-and-slow-wave complex	Pattern consists of sharp wave of negative polarity and slow waves. Diffusely distributed, but may be asymmetric or confined to an area (quadrant).	Highest incidence is in children between 1 and 5 years of age. Most clinical seizures are tonic.
Hypsarrhythmia	Chaotic mixture of high-amplitude slow waves, multifocal spikes, and intrahemispheric/interhemispheric asynchrony. May be preceded by burst suppression or low-voltage invariant pattern in newborn.	Most common interictal EEG pattern with infantile spasms.
Generalized periodic discharges	Broader waveforms compared to bilateral synchronous spike-and-wave discharges.	Seen in subacute sclerosing encephalitis in children.
Focal Epileptiform Patterns		
Rolandic spikes	High-amplitude spike-and-slow wavers are prominent as single or occur in runs in the central and midtemporal regions.	Most commonly associated with genetic epilepsy. Some patients only have spikes during sleep.
Occipital spikes	Repetitive occipital spike discharges on eye closure.	Benign childhood epilepsy. Clinical presentation may have visual alterations with hallucinations.

Source: Adapted from Scher, M. S., & Ashwal, S. (1999). Pediatric neurophysiologic evaluation. In K. F. Swaiman (Ed.), *Pediatric neurology* (3rd ed., pp. 142–181). St. Louis, MO: Mosby.

b. When indicated, identify patient-specific seizure triggers and try to avoid.

c. Wearing protective helmets may be indicated for some patients at risk for seizure-related injuries.

2. *Direct Care*

a. The management goals for a patient with a seizure are to emergently stop both clinical and electrographic seizure activity; prevent patient injury; and maintain airway, breathing, and circulation.

b. For an unexpected seizure, immediately clear the environment of potentially hazardous materials. In anticipation of seizure activity, maintain seizure precautions (e.g., standby oxygen, padded side rails, suction equipment). The patient should not be restrained during seizures.

c. Maintain an open and unobstructed airway using caution not to inflict oral trauma. Provide supplemental oxygen. Provide support ventilation as needed, including bag-valve-mask ventilation or tracheal intubation for apnea or prolonged seizure.

d. Secure venous access and administer dextrose if hypoglycemia is suspected or confirmed by rapid test.

e. Document seizure activity, including information about the prodromal period, aura, and duration of the seizure, characteristics of motor behaviors, and characteristics of the postictal phase. Assess mental status following the seizure.

f. Treatment of SE with anticonvulsant medications usually occurs in phases (Glauser et al., 2016):

   i. Stabilization phase: 0 to 5 minutes

   ii. Initial therapy phase: 5 to 20 minutes

   iii. Secondary therapy phase: 20 to 40 minutes

   iv. Third therapy phase: 40 to 60 minutes

g. Definitive control of SE should occur within 60 minutes (Brophy et al., 2012; see Table 4.6).

h. For patients with RSE, additional interventions may be required, including an increased dosage and frequency of the medications mentioned previously. There is no specific anticonvulsant recommendation or standard and therapy should be individualized for each patient. Continuous infusions may be started and alternated depending on effectiveness and the patient's hemodynamic status.

i. *Alternative therapies* may be used if SE does not respond to anticonvulsant therapy. Alternative therapies include induced coma and inhaled anesthetics. However, specific guidelines do not exist to manage patients with induced coma and inhaled anesthetics. General anesthesia is not used as often as IV anesthesia (e.g., barbiturates, ketamine) because it requires gas-scavenging equipment and operating room facilities. Nonpharmacological alternative therapies include ketogenic diet, hypothermia, and electroconvulsive therapy.

j. *Surgery* is an alternative therapy and is especially helpful when seizures are caused by a structural defect in the CNS (e.g., brain tumor). Surgery may also be considered in children whose seizures are not from a structural defect and cannot be controlled with medications and aggressive treatment. When surgery is recommended, there are two main types: resection of the area of the brain that causes seizures and disconnection of nerve pathways (e.g., corpus callosotomy) to prevent the spread of seizure activity.

k. A *vagus nerve stimulator (VNS)* is a pacemaker-like device that delivers pulses of electricity to the vagus nerve. It is placed surgically under the skin in the upper chest. The patient has a handheld magnet that is used to activate the VNS to abort or shorten the seizure. If the patient has an aura or seizure, the magnet is moved over the generator (swiping motion). Functional MRI is contraindicated in patients with VNS. This is considered adjunctive treatment for children with partial or generalized epilepsy, especially in children resistant to anticonvulsant therapy and when they are poor candidates for surgery. It may also be considered in children with Lennox–Gastaut syndrome (Morris et al., 2013).

3. *Supportive Care*

a. Assess for a patent airway, ventilatory effort, and adequate oxygenation via skin color, ABGs, and pulse oximetry.

b. Support circulation with fluids, vasopressors, and inotropes.

c. Monitor electrolytes, calcium, glucose, toxic screen, and renal panel. Correct electrolyte imbalance and hypoglycemia.

d. Perform serial neurologic examinations.

e. Discuss potential long-term effects of anticonvulsive therapy with the patient and family. Phenytoin can cause gingival hyperplasia, lymphadenopathy, hirsutism, acromegaloid facies, ataxia, nystagmus, rickets, and folate deficiency. Phenobarbital can cause hyperkinesis, drowsiness, and rash. Carbamazepine can cause drowsiness and abdominal distress. Valproate sodium can cause drowsiness, alopecia, and abdominal discomfort.

E. Outcomes

1. *Morbidity and mortality* are highest among patients with RSE.

2. Outcome in patients with acute symptomatic SE is related to the etiology.

3. Because seizures are heterogenous, outcomes in patients with SE are variable and are related to numerous factors, for example, underlying epilepsy, genetics, response to treatment, and previous episodes.

STROKE OR CVA

Stroke is a neurologic injury that results from an interruption in CBF from two main causes: occlusion of blood vessels (*acute ischemic stroke [AIS]*) or rupture of blood vessels (*hemorrhagic stroke*). Stroke is relatively rare in children. The annual *incidence* of pediatric stroke varies depending on cause and risk factors and the child's age. The estimated incidence of all forms of stroke in children in the United States, ages 0 to 15 years, is 6.4/100,000 (Roger et al., 2011).

Acute Ischemic Stroke

A. Definition and Etiology

1. *AIS* represents impaired CBF to a part of the brain from occlusion of a cerebral blood vessel. It is most often due to arterial occlusion, but it may also be caused by occlusion of cerebral veins and sinuses, for example, cerebral venous sinus thrombosis (CVST).

2. There are subtypes of AIS according to the Pediatric Stroke Classification: sickle cell, cardioembolic, Moyamoya syndrome, cervical arterial dissection, steno-occlusive cerebral arteriopathy, other determined etiology, multiple probable/possible etiologies, and undetermined (Lanni et al., 2011).

3. The majority of AIS in children occurs in the distribution of the middle cerebral artery (Rosa et al., 2015).

4. The etiology and risk factors for AIS are many and include disorders related to vasculopathy, congenital heart disease, coagulopathy, infection, genetic disease, metabolism, iron deficiency anemia, and sickle cell anemia (Simma, Höliner, & Luetschg, 2012).

5. Unlike adults, AIS in children accounts for about half of all strokes; in adults 80% to 85% of all strokes are ischemic (Tsze & Valente, 2011).

B. Pathophysiology

1. Regardless of the cause of ischemic stroke, the final common pathway is reduced CBF. The brain has little to no energy stores and neurons require a constant and consistent level of nutrients and oxygen. Short periods of ischemia can produce irreversible damage. The extent of neurologic damage depends on the location, size, and duration of vascular occlusion and whether collateral circulation is present.

2. With CVST, abnormal clots form in veins or sinuses and block venous drainage. Impaired drainage results in back pressure in the venous system, and the pressure subsequently reduces arterial blood supply to a region of the brain.

3. Focal ischemia is more common in children. The exception is cardiopulmonary arrest or low cardiac output states in which global ischemia is a more common pattern.

C. Clinical Presentation

1. *History*

   a. There can be significant differences in the clinical presentation of children with AIS and it varies with age, extent of ischemia, and etiology. Children with embolic stroke usually present more suddenly, while those with thrombosis have more of a gradual presentation (Lanni et al., 2011).

   b. It is important to identify risk factors for AIS that would prompt further historical questioning with the parents and child. Many children with AIS have more than one risk factor.

      i. Cardiac disease is the most common cause of AIS in children, accounting for one third of all cases.

      ii. Hematologic disorders (e.g., sickle cell disease) contribute to AIS from occlusion of small vessels.

iii. CNS infections can cause AIS from local vasculitis and thrombosis.

iv. *Moyamoya* syndrome has a genetic basis and is characterized by progressive stenosis of the internal carotid arteries and formation of collateral vessels.

v. Trauma of the head and neck is associated with dissection of the carotid or vertebral arteries.

vi. Certain medications (e.g., amphetamines, ecstasy, cocaine) and glue sniffing may cause cerebral infarcts and stimulant drugs may cause vasculopathies leading to infarcts (Lanni et al., 2011; Tsze & Valente, 2011).

2. *Physical Examination*

a. AIS presents most often with a focal neurologic deficit, predominantly hemiplegia. Seizures may occur, and are not restricted to age or type.

b. The younger the child, the more nonspecific the findings. For example, symptoms may include

i. Newborns. Focal seizures or lethargy

ii. Infants. Lethargy, apnea spells, hypotonia

iii. Toddlers. Increased crying and sleepiness, irritability, feeding difficulties, vomiting, and sepsis-like symptoms

iv. Older children. More specific neurologic deficits similar to adults (e.g., hemiparesis, aphasia, speech difficulties, visual deficits, facial "droop," and headache)

c. Symptoms will vary depending on the vessel occluded.

i. Anterior cerebral artery. Lower extremity weakness

ii. Middle cerebral artery. Hemiplegia with upper limb predominance, hemianopsia, dysphasia

iii. Posterior circulation. Vertigo, ataxia, nystagmus (Tsze & Valente, 2011)

3. *Diagnostic Tests*

a. Differential diagnosis of AIS is challenging, as there are many other conditions that have a similar presentation and neurologic deficits. Rapid diagnosis is important to minimize or prevent neurologic injury.

b. Laboratory studies in the acute phase include routine chemistry, electrolytes, hematology, and coagulation studies. For differential diagnosis, more specific tests are ordered, for example, to identify infectious or metabolic causes of AIS.

c. Neuroimaging is often the first step in diagnosing a child who is acutely ill and AIS is suspected. For emergent diagnosis, the two imaging modalities most often used are CT scan and MRI. For patients who are cooperative or comatose, MRI should be considered as first choice neuroimaging. When MRI is not available or in an uncooperative child, CT scan should be considered. IADSA should be used in children when suspected infarcts are not recognized by CT or MRI (Lanni et al., 2011). The following are descriptions of neuroimaging modalities used to identify AIS:

i. CT scan without contrast can be performed quickly and can exclude hemorrhage in the acute phase if MRI is not available. It has low sensitivity for detecting AIS.

ii. CT angiography (CTA) is a noninvasive method for evaluating intra- and extracranial circulation, and provides critical information in early stages AIS.

iii. MRI identifies the cause of hemorrhage, and identifies vascular malformations eligible for surgery or interventional therapy.

iv. MRI with diffusion-weighted imaging (DWI) is most sensitive in diagnosing cytotoxic edema, common with DWI. It can exclude hemorrhage and it can determine the volume of tissue at risk and the vascular distribution of ischemia.

v. MR angiography (MRA) defines vascular anatomy of the circle of Willis and neck vessels.

vi. MR venography (MRV) can exclude CVST.

d. An electrocardiogram and echocardiogram are used in patients with known or suspected cardiac disease.

4. *Clinical Course*

a. AIS is variable and depends on the extent and duration of the ischemic event.

b. A second stroke occurs in 10% to 25% of all children (Roach et al., 2008).

D. Patient Care Management

1. *Preventive Care*

a. Because the ischemic event is usually the first sign of neurologic injury in the child, prevention strategies are difficult.

b. Children with one or more risk factors (e.g., sickle cell anemia, cardiovascular disease) should have a higher level of surveillance and medical plans to reduce the likelihood of cerebral vessel occlusion.

2. *Direct Care*

a. Evidence-based treatment is lacking in the pediatric research literature. However, several specialty groups have practice guidelines that have been extrapolated from adult and pediatric populations.

b. Other than prevention, there is no direct care for AIS; all treatment is supportive.

3. *Supportive Care*

a. Treatment of pediatric AIS involves two phases: initial treatment to preserve neurologic function and long-term care to prevent a second stroke.

    i. The initial phase includes assessment of airway, ventilation, and circulation.

    ii. Perform serial neurologic assessments.

b. Once hemorrhagic stroke has been excluded, most guidelines recommend antithrombotic treatment; however, there is not consensus on specific treatment indications.

    i. For acute and short-term anticoagulation, unfractioned heparin (UFH) or low-molecular-weight heparins (LMWHs) are sometimes initiated until the cause of the stroke can be identified (Roach et al., 2008).

    ii. Aspirin is sometimes used for initial treatment until there is a clear indication for anticoagulation. There is more agreement among experts to use aspirin for secondary stroke prevention (Rosa et al., 2015). The optimum duration of aspirin therapy is not well defined.

c. Long-term anticoagulation treatment to prevent secondary stroke includes aspirin, warfarin, and LMWH injections.

d. Currently, thrombolytic therapy with tissue plasminogen activator (tPA) may be considered in a select group with CVST, but generally is not recommended in children outside of a clinical protocol (Roach et al., 2008; Rosa et al., 2015; Tsze & Valente, 2011).

e. Endovascular mechanical thrombectomy has been used in children, but there are no safety guidelines or recommendations to follow.

f. Additional supportive interventions include control of fever, normalize oxygenation, control systemic hypertension, and normalize serum glucose levels. Patients are restricted to bedrest with the bed flat; they should not ambulate or sit upright.

g. Treat seizures with antiepileptic medications, but prophylactic treatment for seizures in not recommended (Roach et al., 2008).

h. Induced hypothermia is not recommended outside of a clinical trial.

E. Outcomes

1. Reported deaths for AIS range from 7% to 28%. Unlike hemorrhagic stroke, AIS mortality rates are not declining and may be due to underlying causes or risk factors that are not modifiable (Greenham, Gordon, Anderson, & Mackay, 2016).

2. Long-term outcomes for pediatric AIS are uncertain and depend on stroke severity and timing of interventions.

3. The *Pediatric Stroke Outcome Measure (PSOM)* is a tool designed to measure outcomes for pediatric stroke (Kitchen et al., 2012).

Intracranial Hemorrhage

A. Definition and Etiology

1. There are several causes of hemorrhagic stroke in children, including intracerebral hemorrhage and SAH.

2. The etiologies for hemorrhagic stroke are primarily from vascular malformations (e.g., aneurysm or AVM), but underlying disease or trauma may also cause an acute ICH (Simma et al., 2012).

a. *AVM* is the most common cause of hemorrhagic stroke beyond infancy (Tsze & Valente, 2011). It is an abnormal connection between arteries and veins, called a *nidus*, without an interposed capillary bed. AVMs can occur in any part of the brain and can vary in size from a few millimeters to large formations. Characteristically, they are cone shaped and thin walled and may involve parenchymal or meningeal tissue. The majority of cases are supratentorial.

b. An *aneurysm* represents a weakening in the arterial wall. The size may vary from a few millimeters to 2 to 3 cm. Most aneurysms are saccular and are located at bifurcations of major cerebral arteries. Approximately 5% of children have greater than one aneurysm (Roach et al., 2008). Aneurysms may be congenital (majority), traumatic, arteriosclerotic, or septic in origin. A high percentage of aneurysms are found in the posterior circulation, and, compared to adults, they have a greater incidence of giant aneurysms. They may be associated with unrepaired coarctation of the aorta and subacute bacterial endocarditis (SBE). Aneurysms in children are more distal in origin, are more likely giant or mycotic aneurysms, are less likely to be atherosclerotic, and are located more peripherally (e.g., distal branches of the middle cerebral artery) than in adults.

c. Hematologic disorders, genetic vasculopathies, and hypertension are other causes or risk factors for ICH.

B. Pathophysiology

1. AVMs occur early in fetal development from failure of the capillaries to develop. Supply of blood to adjacent brain tissue is diminished or absent (ischemia) because of the diversion of arterial blood flow through the nidus without the benefit of capillaries to allow diffusion of oxygen and glucose (i.e., there is a vascular "steal"). Without the inherent resistance to blood flow through a capillary bed, blood flow through the vascular malformation is increased. A pressure gradient develops, and the malformation continues to grow; collateral vessels develop, which adds to the mass. Because there are no capillaries, high pressure arterial blood empties directly into thin-walled veins. Veins are at risk for rupturing with hemorrhage. Neurologic dysfunction can occur from compression of surrounding tissue, ischemia of surrounding tissue and gliosis, hemorrhage, and hydrocephalus from obstruction of CSF.

2. Abnormalities exist in the arterial wall of aneurysms, especially in the elastica and media layers. There are four main types of aneurysms:

a. A *saccular (berry) aneurysm* is rare in childhood. The sac gradually grows over time, usually rupturing between the third to sixth decades of life.

b. A *fusiform (giant) aneurysm* results from diffuse atherosclerotic changes. It is commonly found in basilar arteries or terminal ends of internal carotids.

c. A *mycotic aneurysm* is relatively common in children compared to adults. It results from arteritis due to bacterial emboli.

d. A *traumatic aneurysm* is a weakening of the arterial wall that occurs from a bone fracture or penetrating missile. It is rare in childhood.

3. An aneurysm is significant when it ruptures and hemorrhages. Patients usually have acute symptoms, with bleeding into the subarachnoid space. A clot forms following rupture of an aneurysm. Seven to 10 days later the clot dissolves, and the patient is at risk for rebleeding. A rapid injection of blood into the brain may produce an acute increase in ICP. Cerebral hypertension may also result from obstruction of CSF circulation. Hypothalamic disturbances may occur from close proximity of hemorrhage to the hypothalamus. Vasospasm may be seen early following hemorrhage, however, the incidence is far less than in the adult population

C. Clinical Presentation

1. *History*

a. The vast majority of children with vascular malformations present with hemorrhagic stroke and the incidence increases with age (Lanni et al., 2011).

b. Similar to AIS, the clinical presentation of ICH varies and depends on the child's age and size and location of the hemorrhage.

c. Newborns present most often with focal seizures, apnea, or lethargy.

d. Infants may have similar symptoms to newborns with a history poor feeding or respiratory distress.

e. In older children, the most common signs include headache, alteration in consciousness, seizures, and vomiting. Focal signs may be present and relate to the location of the hemorrhage (Lanni et al., 2011).

f. Meningeal irritation occurs with SAH. Rapid neurologic deterioration ensues with rupture and bleeding into the ventricles.

g. Congestive heart failure may occur in neonates with a large AVM because of the increased cardiac output necessary to support the AVM blood flow (often seen in vein of Galen aneurysms).

h. Some congenital and hereditary disorders are associated with aneurysms, especially coarctation of the aorta.

i. With aneurysms, children may be asymptomatic for many years. Nonspecific findings include nausea, back pain, lethargy, and photophobia. A giant aneurysm may present as a mass effect (increased ICP).

2. *Physical Examination*

a. The physical examination is similar to children with AIS; all body systems are examined with emphasis on neurologic function.

b. Specific clinical findings may include a bulging fontanelle (infants), hemiplegia, hemianopsia, or dysphasia. Veins may be enlarged on the scalp or face. A cranial systolic bruit is heard over the carotid arteries, mastoid bone, or eyes.

c. Localized periorbital pain and diplopia or ptosis may indicate third cranial nerve compression from an aneurysm.

3. *Diagnostic Tests*

a. Neuroimaging is similar to AIS.

b. Laboratory testing is similar to AIS; there are no specific testing guidelines for pediatric stroke.

4. *Clinical Course*

a. AVMs are present at birth, but the patient may not become symptomatic until 10 to 20 years of age. The exception is an infant with a large AVM producing high cardiac output failure.

b. Children with a known AVM have an annual hemorrhage risk of 2% to 4% (Roach et al., 2008).

c. Aneurysms may be congenital or acquired later in childhood. The progression of the disease depends on many variables (e.g., size, location, and etiology).

d. The likelihood of a child developing a second aneurysm later in life is unknown.

D. Patient Care Management

1. *Preventive Care*

a. There is no known way to prevent an aneurysm or AVM from forming.

b. Once a hemorrhagic stroke has occurred, treatment is supportive and directed at reducing the risk of rebleeding and preserving neurologic function.

c. If a vascular lesion has been identified prior to rupture, interventions are directed at preventing hemorrhage.

　　i. Asymptomatic children with conditions that place them at risk for intracranial aneurysms may have cranial MRAs at prescribed intervals (1–5 years).

　　ii. Some vascular lesions should be corrected if clinically feasible.

　　iii. Age-appropriate instructions are given to patients to control blood pressure, avoid smoking, and avoid stimulant drugs. The risks and benefits of taking aspirin and antithrombin medications are discussed.

2. *Direct Care*

a. Surgical management of hemorrhagic strokes is controversial and is individualized for each child.

b. For AVM, treatment varies and depends on size and location of the AVM, age of the patient, cerebral dominance, technical support, condition of the patient, and characteristics of feeder vessels. Often treatment options are used in combination.

　　i. Total surgical resection is ideal, but some vascular abnormalities are inoperable.

　　ii. Inoperable or small AVMs (<3 cm in diameter) may use stereotactic radiosurgery (SRS). It is minimally invasive and uses computer guidance to concentrate radiation to the AVM. Advantages include the ability to coagulate small, fragile, vessels; provide hemostasis following surgical resection; and clearly define the AVM.

　　iii. Embolization is performed by inserting a catheter into the cerebral circulation (e.g., carotid or vertebral arteries) and depositing a substance (e.g., Silastic sphere, Gelfoam, metallic pellet) to block blood vessels within the lesion. The use of transarterial embolization alone rarely obliterates an AVM in its entirety and is most often used as adjunctive therapy (i.e., staged embolizations can reduce the size of an AVM for surgical resection).

c. Surgical options for an aneurysm include occluding the aneurysm at its neck with clips (most common), occluding the parent vessel on either side of the aneurysm (dependent on collateral circulation), coating the aneurysm with a material after wrapping it in muslin, or embolization of the aneurysm.

d. Treatment following rupture of an intracranial aneurysm is to prevent rebleeding of the aneurysm and control cerebral vasospasm. Controversy exists as to when an operation is of benefit. Early surgery (i.e., within the first hours or days) carries a high risk because of the critical condition of the patient, and cerebral vasospasm, which may occur between 4 and 12 days after the hemorrhage. Postponing surgery until the patient is more stable (e.g., CPP normal, MAP normal, ICP <20 mmHg, neurologic status unchanged or improved from baseline) and cerebral vasospasm has been relieved carries a risk of a second bleed (the first 48 hours are associated with the highest incidence of rebleeding). Although cerebral vasospasm may occur, the incidence is low in children. Routine nimodipine prophylaxis for the prevention of cerebral vasospasm is not recommended in children and a recent study found no benefit for nimodipine use in children with SAH (Heffren, McIntosh, & Reiter, 2015). Evidence-based monitoring and treatment guidelines for nimodipine require additional research in children.

e. Surgical evacuation of supratentorial hematomas is not recommended for most patients. There are exceptions for children who are at risk for herniation syndromes or to control increased ICP (Roach et al., 2008).

3. *Supportive Care*

a. With the exception of antithrombotic therapy, supportive care is similar to AIS: optimize respiratory function, control systemic hypertension, control ICP, and control seizures.

b. Patients with SAH may need vasospasm management.

E. Outcomes

1. Similar to AIS, outcome following an ICH depends on location on the hemorrhage, extent of the bleeding, time between rupture and treatment, and general baseline health of the child. Most children will experience long-term neurological, motor, and cognitive impairments (Greenham et al., 2016).

2. When the vascular malformation can be completely removed or obliterated and hemorrhage is minimized or absent, outcomes are best.

3. Mortality range for hemorrhagic stroke is 6% to 54%. Mortality rates have been declining, presumably from better critical care management (Greenham et al., 2016).

Intraventricular Hemorrhage

A. Definition and Etiology

1. Intraventricular hemorrhage (IVH; also known as *germinal matrix hemorrhage*) is a major complication

of prematurity and the incidence increases with decreasing gestational age and birth weight.

2. It involves bleeding into the subependymal germinal matrix (also known as *ganglionic eminence*) at the level of the foramen of Monro (periventricular). The bleeding may disrupt the lining of the ependymal and extend into the lateral ventricles and throughout the ventricular system (intraventricular; Volpe, 2015).

3. The etiology of IVH is multifactorial, but is related to two major conditions of prematurity: immaturity and fragility of germinal matrix and immaturity of CBF autoregulation.

4. ICH is relatively uncommon in the term newborn, and when it is present, it has a different etiology compared to premature newborns (Bano, Chaudhary, Garga, Yadav, & Singh, 2014).

a. Unlike premature newborns, ICH in term newborns may be subdural, subarachnoid, intraventricular, parenchymal, or rarely, epidural.

b. It is not unusual for ICH to involve multiple brain compartments.

c. Subdural and SAHs are commonly associated with birth trauma (e.g., forceps delivery).

d. Intraparenchymal hemorrhage is less common than subdural and subarachnoid hemorrhage.

5. The incidence of IVH in the term newborn is significantly less common than the premature newborn, presumably due to greater maturity of the brain.

6. *Risk factors* that increase IVH and ICH in the preterm and term newborn include hypoxia, placental abruption, infections that alter CBF in the periventricular region, respiratory complications such as pneumothorax (or any condition that increases venous pressure and impedes cerebral venous return), and rapid infusion of hyperosmolar infusions.

B. Pathophysiology

1. The pathogenesis of IVH in the premature newborn is related to brain immaturity.

a. Presence of subependymal germinal matrix (periventricular region) is characteristic of prematurity. The matrix is a highly vascular, gelatinous area with vessels that lack supporting structure. Glial and neuronal precursor cells are perfused by numerous fragile capillaries that predispose the premature newborn to hemorrhage. The periventricular region is highly vulnerable to hemorrhage in the first 48 hours of life, especially in preterm neonates (Ballabh, 2010).

b. It is believed that preterm infants are vulnerable to fluctuations in CBF due to immaturity of autoregulation. Impaired autoregulation results in pressure-passive circulation, and the newborn cannot maintain constant CBF with changes in systemic blood pressure. Impaired autoregulation makes the premature newborn susceptible to hypoperfusion and ischemia at the border of the germinal matrix.

2. The pathogenesis of ICH in the term newborn is related more to birth trauma or vascular malformations (Bano et al., 2014).

a. Moulding of the skull may stretch and tear blood vessels around the dura and produce subdural bleeding.

b. Tearing of blood vessels in the dural sinuses produces subarachnoid bleeding.

c. Infections, vascular malformations, asphyxia, and clotting abnormalities may cause intraparenchymal bleeding in the cerebral cortex and cerebellum.

3. Blood clots within the ventricular system may obstruct the flow and absorption of CSF, resulting in progressive hydrocephalus.

4. A classification system to determine the severity and grading of IVH was originally developed by Knake (1978) and is based on the presence and amount of blood in the germinal matrix and lateral ventricles. Although it has been modified over the years with expanded definitions, the basic grades are still used clinically.

a. Grade I. Germinal matrix hemorrhage only

b. Grade II. IVH without ventricular dilation

c. Grade III. IVH with ventricular dilation

d. Grade IV. Intraventricular and parenchymal hemorrhage

C. Clinical Presentation

1. *History*

a. *Maternal* history is important in identifying medication therapy (e.g., steroids, indomethacin), genetic disorders, previous birth history, and preexisting clinical conditions.

b. *Perinatal* history is important in identifying risk factors for the development of IVH and ICH in the newborn.

i. Prenatal factors. Maternal chorioamnionitis, maternal preeclampsia, prenatal asphyxia

ii. Labor and delivery. Mode of delivery, breech presentation, delayed cord clamping, and intrapartal asphyxia

iii. Neonatal factors. Prematurity, respiratory distress, patent ductus arteriosus, hypotension, metabolic acidosis, neonatal resuscitation, anemia

2. *Physical Examination*

a. Three basic clinical syndromes may be seen.

i. A *saltatory syndrome* is a subtle deterioration that progresses over hours to days. Clinical features include depressed level of consciousness, hypotonia, irritability, low hematocrit, abnormal eye movements and position, and alteration in spontaneous movements. Respiratory dysfunction is sometimes observed.

ii. A *silent syndrome* is clinically undetected and is usually diagnosed on routine ultrasound examinations of the head.

iii. The least common presentation is *catastrophic* deterioration progressing in minutes to hours. Clinical features include coma, apnea, generalized seizures, abnormal posturing, unreactive pupils, drop in hematocrit, and alteration in vital signs (e.g., hypotension, bradycardia) and endocrine function.

b. Physical findings associated with posthemorrhagic hydrocephalus (PHH) may include bulging fontanel, apnea, pupillary changes, and seizures.

3. *Diagnostic Tests*

a. Neuroimaging

i. Cranial ultrasound (CUS) is the study of choice. It identifies the degree and location of the hemorrhage. Advantages include its portability, low cost, and noninvasive nature.

ii. Doppler ultrasound may be used for imaging and flow-velocity measurements.

iii. CT scan and MRI identify structures as listed earlier. Disadvantages include transporting the patient to another location, maintaining patient stability during the procedure, and the difficulty of doing serial examinations. CT scans, especially with serial exams, has the added adverse effects of radiation. MRI is superior to CUS when detecting white matter abnormalities is important.

iv.   Once IVH is diagnosed, follow-up CUS examinations are necessary to follow progression or resolution of IVH and to detect complications of IVH (Ment et al., 2002).

4. *Clinical Course*

a.   The majority of premature newborns with IVH are diagnosed within the first week of life.

b.   The clinical course depends on the severity of IVH, hemodynamic stability of the neonate, and the presence of complications. Mild cases are self-limiting and bleeding resolves over weeks to months. Severe cases may have significant neurologic sequelae.

D. Patient Care Management

1. *Preventive Care*

a.   Prevention of IVH is primarily directed at reducing premature delivery, for example, special care for high-risk pregnancies, treatment of maternal infections, and treatment to halt premature labor.

b.   For premature newborns, hemodynamic stabilization is critical, especially in the first week of life. Hypotension, hypercarbia and hypoxia are important to prevent; they indirectly affect cerebral autoregulation.

c.   When IVH is present, prevention is directed at halting the progression of bleeding and reducing complications.

d.   Because a significant number of premature infants with IVH are clinically silent, routine CUS screening is recommended for neonates <30 weeks gestation or weighing <1,500 g at birth (Ment et al., 2002). The timing of the first routine screening CUS varies widely ranging from the first 6 to 12 hours of life to the second week of life (Al-Abdi & Al-Aamri, 2014).

e.   For term newborns, ICH prevention is focused on normal vaginal delivery with or without obstetric instrument. Forced vaginal delivery should be avoided.

2. *Direct Care*

a.   No specific surgical treatment is required for nonprogressive hydrocephalus.

b.   In communicating hydrocephalus, *serial lumbar puncture* for CSF removal is associated with a lower need for a permanent ventricular shunt.

c.   A *VP shunt* may be required for PHH that does not resolve spontaneously or respond to CSF removal with lumbar punctures.

d.   In noncommunicating hydrocephalus, *endoscopic third ventriculostomy* is an option.

3. *Supportive Care*

a.   Beyond routine critical care of the newborn, optimize respiratory and cardiovascular function.

b.   Avoid hypotension and extreme fluctuations in blood pressure.

c.   Avoid hypercarbia and hypoxia; they increase cerebral vasodilation.

E. Outcomes

1.   Most premature neonates with IVH (Grades I–II) have spontaneous resolution of bleeding and minimal complications. However, there are a few studies that suggest neonates with mild IVH (Grades I–II) may be at greater risk of impaired neurodevelopmental than originally reported (Volpe, 2015).

2.   Premature neonates with more severe IVH (Grades III–IV) have more complications and neurologic sequelae, for example, PHH, periventricular hemorrhagic infarction (PVHI), cerebellar hemorrhagic injury (CHI), and periventricular leukomalacia (PVL).

3.   In neonates with IVH, approximately 35% will develop posthemorrhagic ventricular dilatation and 22% of these patients will progress to PHH (Piro, 2015).

CNS INFECTIONS

A. Definition and Etiology

1.   *Meningitis* is an inflammation of the meninges, the outer covering of the brain and spinal cord.

a.   *Bacterial* meningitis is diagnosed with evidence of a bacterial pathogen in the CSF. Since the introduction of hemophilus b conjugate vaccine and pneumococcal conjugate vaccine, the incidence of invasive *Haemophilus influenzae* and pneumococcal disease have decreased significantly. Currently, the most common causative agents of bacterial meningitis in the United States are *Neisseria meningitidis*, group B *Streptococcus*,

Streptococcus pneumoniae, Haemophilus influenzae, and *Listeria monocytogenes*. Despite a significant decrease in bacterial meningitis among children over the last three decades, the incidence among infants less than 2 months has not declined. The major pathogen for this age is group B *Streptococcus* and *Escherichia coli* (Swanson, 2015; Thigpen et al., 2011).

b. *Viral* (aseptic) meningitis is defined as inflammation of the meninges without evidence of bacterial pathogen in the CSF (by usual laboratory testing). Because of widespread use of conjugate vaccines, the incidence of viral meningitis has surpassed bacterial meningitis (Nigrovic, Fine, Monuteaux, Shah, & Neuman, 2013). The most common pathogen for viral meningitis in the United States is Non-polio enteroviruses (Richard & Lepe, 2013). Less common viruses that can cause meningitis include mumps virus, herpesviruses, measles virus, influenza virus, arboviruses, adenoviruses, and lymphocytic choriomeningitis virus. Children less than 5 and children with compromised immune systems are at greatest risk for the disease.

2. *Encephalitis* is an acute inflammation of brain parenchyma and occasionally the meninges in association with clinical signs of neurologic dysfunction. The etiology in most children is unknown; however, children who are immunosuppressed are at greater risk. Encephalitis pathogens include arthropod-borne viruses and HSV. It may also occur from systemic viral infections. Neonatal HSV is commonly acquired during vaginal delivery with an infected maternal tract; HSV type 2 causes more cases than type 1.

B. Pathophysiology

1. *Bacterial Meningitis*. Pathogens usually arise from a distant site (usually nasal mucosa) and colonize. They enter the bloodstream, producing septicemia, and then invade the meninges. Less frequently, pathogens infect the meninges via a direct route (e.g., depressed skull fracture, penetrating missile). Pathogens proliferate and spread into CSF and then invade parenchyma and blood vessel walls, producing vasculitis or cerebral edema. Purulent exudate may obstruct CSF pathways, producing hydrocephalus. Cell necrosis may also occur. Increased ICP may be seen in advanced or untreated disease from loss of cerebral autoregulation, cerebral edema, and hydrocephalus.

2. *Viral Meningitis*. Pathogenesis remains unclear. It is believed that the port of entry is the nasal pharynx,

where the viral pathogen colonizes and spreads to the CNS via the bloodstream.

3. *Encephalitis*. Viral invasion begins in extraneural tissue (e.g., mastoid) and travels to the CNS via the bloodstream. Once in the CNS, pathogens may enter the CSF circulation through the choroid plexus or through passive transfer through the BBB. Less frequently, pathogens may enter the CNS along peripheral nerves or via the olfactory system. Widespread nerve cell degeneration may occur, as well as vascular occlusion (leading to infarction), cerebral edema, cell necrosis, and increased ICP (Falchek, 2012).

C. Clinical Presentation

1. *History*

    a. Meningitis

       i. Initial symptoms and history are similar between *viral* and *bacterial meningitis*; however, symptoms are age related. Infants usually have very nonspecific or vague symptoms (e.g., lethargy, irritable, poor feeding, seizures, apnea, or vomiting). Children usually have a history of fever, headache and "stiff neck."

       ii. The presentation of symptoms may evolve over a few days or more acutely occurring over a few hours.

    b. Prodromal symptoms of encephalitis are "flu-like" and include fever, malaise, myalgia, upper respiratory symptoms, nausea, and vomiting. Symptoms may progress to headache, "stiff neck," seizures, behavioral changes, sensory disturbances, and altered level of consciousness.

    c. Suspicion of encephalitis is considered when the above acute symptoms present without an identifiable external cause (Falchek, 2012).

    d. Historical questioning includes recent illness, antibiotic use, recent travel, animal exposure, drug allergies, exposure to infection, immune status, and vaccinations.

    e. Maternal history (especially group B *Streptococcus* HSV status or presence or premature rupture of membranes) is important.

2. *Physical Examination*

    a. *Bacterial meningitis*

       i. In children, the three classic signs of meningitis are nuchal rigidity (stiff neck), Brudzinski's sign (flexion of the hips and knees with passive flexion of the neck), and Kernig's sign (back pain and resistance after passive extension of the lower legs). Although these signs may be present, they do not reliably occur in all children and cannot be used to diagnose or exclude meningitis (Amarilyo, Alper, Ben-Tov, & Grisaru-Soen, 2011; Bilavsky et al., 2013).

ii. Other signs and symptoms that may be present in children with meningitis include photophobia (abnormal intolerance of light), fever, vomiting, lethargy, headache, and alteration in consciousness. Petechial rash may occur with *Neisseria meningitidis*.

iii. Late stages may produce increased ICP and cardiovascular collapse.

iv. Symptoms in infants are less specific and include vomiting, lethargy, bulging fontanelle, hypothermia or hyperthermia, diarrhea, seizure, and poor feeding.

b. *Viral meningitis* has physical findings similar to bacterial meningitis, but they are usually milder. Most infants younger than 12 months have minimal physical findings.

c. Clinical findings in encephalitis include lethargy, drowsiness, stupor that may progress to coma, seizures, and localized symptoms. Compared to bacterial meningitis, encephalitis has more focal neurologic signs. Severe cases may have signs and symptoms of increased ICP. Meningeal signs may be present and depend on the degree of meningeal involvement (vs. cerebral involvement).

3. *Diagnostic Tests*

a. Baseline studies should include CBC with differential, electrolytes with renal function, glucose, prothrombin time (PT)/partial thromboplastin time (PTT), metabolic panel, and cultures. Elevated serum procalcitonin and C-reactive protein are suggestive of meningitis, but cannot reliably distinguish between bacterial and viral pathogens (Swanson, 2015).

b. CSF analysis is the gold standard for diagnosing bacterial meningitis and should be performed on any child suspected of having meningitis. Obstructive hydrocephalus or risk of herniation must be ruled out before an LP can be performed.

c. No single CSF test parameter reliably distinguishes bacterial from nonbacterial meningitis. CSF analysis in bacterial meningitis usually demonstrates the following:

i. Elevated white blood count (WBC); polymorphonuclear cells predominate

ii. Elevated protein content (normal 10–30 mg/dL)

iii. Decreased glucose content (normal 40–80 mg/dL)

iv. Positive results from Gram stain

v. Positive results from culture for organism

vi. Color. Turbid or cloudy

vii. In rare instances, no or few CSF WBCs may be seen early in the course of meningitis

viii. Results are variable in the neonate, as the WBC count may be normal, glucose content may be normal (it should be compared to serum), and protein levels are normally higher in neonates (20–170 mg/dL)

d. CSF results in viral meningitis demonstrate the following:

i. Slightly elevated WBC count; lymphocytes predominate

ii. Normal or slightly increased protein content

iii. Normal glucose content

iv. Negative results from Gram stain or culture for bacteria

e. CSF results in encephalitis are variable but may be similar to viral meningitis. Viral antibodies immunoglobulin M (IgM) may be found. Large amounts of RBCs may be seen with HSV.

f. *Neuroimaging.* CT scan and MRI are not commonly used in the diagnosis of meningitis. CT scan may be used prior to LP to rule out conditions that may lead to brain herniation, but delay in treatment is avoided. If a CT scan is needed before the LP, blood cultures are obtained followed immediately with antibiotics. Clinically stable children with suspected bacterial meningitis and no signs of brain herniation should have an immediate LP (Swanson, 2015). Neuroimaging may demonstrate abnormal findings in children with meningitis but do not predict outcome or the degree of brain swelling. MRI is most often used for encephalitis and may suggest specific etiologic agents. CT scan is used when MRI is not available.

g. *Adjunctive tests*

i. CSF should be sent for *polymerase chain reaction (PCR)* analysis for enterovirus, and for some cases of HSV and West Nile viruses (Richard & Lepe, 2013). For encephalitis, serology testing for Epstein–Barr virus, cytomegalovirus, and mycoplasma is indicated.

   ii. EEG is used as an adjunctive study, particularly for encephalitis. It is helpful in identifying cerebral dysfunction, focal abnormalities, and seizures. Epileptic discharges from the temporal lobe may suggest HSV encephalitis (Thompson, Kneen, Riordan, Kelly, & Pollard, 2012).

   h. *Brain biopsy* is the definitive diagnostic study for encephalitis but is rarely performed because the procedure poses risks to the patient and treatment would remain the same (i.e., supportive). Biopsy may be considered in patients with unknown etiology whose condition deteriorates despite treatment with an antiviral agent.

  4. *Clinical Course*

   a. *Bacterial infection.* Course of illness varies considerably, it may resolve over weeks with therapy or the course can be protracted with shock states or increased ICP.

   b. *Viral infection.* Clinical course is usually self-limiting with improvement seen in 7 to 14 days. Infants less than 1 month and immunocompromised children are more likely to have severe disease.

   c. *Encephalitis.* Course of illness varies considerably (mild to elevated ICP and death) and depends somewhat on the infectious agent and the specific CNS structures involved. California, Herpes, and La Crosse encephalitis may be severe, whereas St. Louis encephalitis tends to be mild.

D. Patient Care Management

  1. *Preventive Care*

   a. Vaccinations are available for *Streptococcus pneumoniae*, *Neisseria meningitidis*, and *Haemophilus influenzae* and should be given to patients as recommended. Chemoprophylaxis is given to close contacts (e.g., family members, day-care contacts, and primary caregivers in the hospital) of patients with *Haemophilus influenzae* and *Neisseria meningitidis*.

   b. There are no vaccines to protect against enteroviruses, but there are vaccines for some viral diseases (e.g., measles, mumps, rubella, varicella). Immunizations should be current.

   c. Many types of encephalitis are transmitted by an infected mosquito and vaccines for encephalitis are limited. Prevention measures include using insect repellent, wearing protective clothing, and staying indoors when mosquitos are most active.

  2. *Direct Care*

   a. Ensure adequate circulation, oxygenation, and ventilation.

   b. Antimicrobial therapy is the mainstay of bacterial meningitis treatment and should be started promptly following an LP and cultures. Antiviral treatment is used for some types of viral infections, but supportive care is all that is usually available for encephalitis and viral meningitis. ICP monitoring is not routinely used for CNS infections.

   c. Empiric therapy is directed at the most likely bacteria based on patient's age, as well as local resistance patterns (see Table 4.7).

   d. Administration of dexamethasone is controversial for pneumococcal meningitis (Swanson, 2015). It has been shown to reduce hearing loss in children with *Haemophilus influenzae* meningitis, but not in meningitis from other pathogens. Current dosing guidelines are 0.6 mg/kg/d in four divided doses given intravenously for the first 2 days of antimicrobial therapy. Dexamethasone should be administered at the time of the first antimicrobial dose. It is not used for aseptic meningitis.

  3. *Supportive Care*

   a. Respiratory isolation may be used for 24 hours for patients with bacterial meningitis caused by or suspected to be caused by *Haemophilus influenzae* or *Neisseria meningitidis*. Maintain enteric precautions for aseptic meningitis for 7 days from the onset of disease.

   b. Provide serial neurologic assessment, including head circumference in infants, assess for increased ICP, and monitor fluid and electrolyte status.

   c. Prevent or manage seizures.

   d. Monitor urine output, hemodynamic parameters, and serum and urine electrolytes and osmolality.

   e. Maintain body temperature in the normal range using antipyretics and sponging with tepid water.

   f. Maintain a quiet environment by dimming lights and controlling noise.

   g. Alleviate nausea and vomiting by administering oral care and antiemetics.

h. Control increased ICP.

i. Administer analgesics for complaints of headache, arthralgia, and neck pain.

E. Outcomes

1. Outcome and prognosis for bacterial meningitis vary and are related to age, pathogen, clinical status at time of treatment, and time of initiation of therapy. Alteration in level of consciousness at time of presentation is associated with higher mortality. Hearing loss is significant, especially in children with pneumococcal meningitis. Other neurologic sequelae (e.g., neurocognitive disorders, seizures, paresis, cranial nerve palsies, hypothalamic dysfunction) have also been reported in infants and children (Swanson, 2015).

2. Long-term studies on outcome and prognosis following encephalitis are limited. HSV in neonates and children has been studied the most and continues to show poor outcomes (Thompson et al., 2012).

SPACE-OCCUPYING LESIONS (TUMORS)

A. Definition and Etiology

1. CNS tumors are an abnormal proliferation of cells in the brain or spinal cord; they may be benign or malignant. Brain tumors represent 20% of all childhood cancers. They are the most common solid tumor and the second most common cancer (leukemia is first) in children.

2. The cause of primary brain tumors is unknown. There are two risk factors associated with brain tumors: history of significant doses of radiation to the CNS and presence of a genetic syndrome that is associated with brain tumors (e.g., neurofibromatosis, tuberous sclerosis, and Von Hippel-Lindau syndrome; Fleming & Chi, 2012).

3. Historically, the *classification of brain tumors* has been based primarily on histogenesis from light microscopic features. Recently, the World Health Organization (WHO) completed a major revision of the classification of CNS tumors to integrate molecular genetic parameters with histology (Louis et al., 2016).

4. The most common types of brain tumors in young children are broadly classified as *gliomas* and account for 75% of all brain tumors. The three most common glial subtypes are defined by glial tissue: astrocytes, ependymal cells, and oligodendrocytes.

a. *Astrocytomas* are the most common type of brain tumors in children and can be found throughout the CNS. The infratentorial area of the brain has the highest incidence (cerebellum, brainstem, and hypothalamus).

b. *Anaplastic astrocytoma* and *glioblastoma* are other types of diffuse astrocytomas and are highly malignant with a poor prognosis.

c. *Ependymomas* typically arise from the ependymal lining of the ventricles, most commonly the fourth ventricle in children.

5. *Embryonal tumors* represent a significant number of CNS tumors in children and are from poorly differentiated neuroepithelia cells. The two main types are primitive neuroectodermal tumor (PNET) and atypical teratoid/rhabdoid tumor.

a. *Medulloblastoma* is a PNET and generally develops in the midline of the vermis and growth may extend into the fourth ventricle.

b. It represents approximately 25% of all pediatric brain tumors and is the most common primary malignant CNS tumor.

6. Less common are tumors found in ventricles (e.g., choroid plexus papillomas and carcinomas), from nonneuroepithelial tissue (e.g., craniopharyngioma and pineal-region tumors), and from the outer membranes of the brain (e.g., meningeal tumors).

B. Pathophysiology

1. The majority of CNS tumors in children originate from neural elements within the brain or spinal cord (*primary*) and less frequently from a distant cancer (*metastatic*).

2. CNS tumors represent abnormal cell growth and differentiation and have lethal effects on normal neural tissues through several mechanisms:

a. Tumor cells invade, infiltrate, or supplant normal parenchymal tissue, disrupting normal neural function.

b. Abnormal growth and edema may cause increased ICP with distortion and herniation of normal brain structures and compression of blood vessels (ischemia).

c. Compression of neural pathways with diminished transmission of neural impulses.

d. Infratentorial tumors, especially located by the third and fourth ventricle, can cause obstructive hydrocephalus.

e. Tumors may generate new blood vessels (*angiogenesis*) and disrupt the BBB and cause edema.

C. Clinical Presentation

1. *History*

   a. Presenting complaints of children with a brain tumor vary and often mimic other childhood illnesses.

   b. Symptoms on initial presentation will generally relate to age, location, and rate of growth of the tumor.

   i. Infants and toddlers usually present with nonspecific symptoms (e.g., vomiting, lethargy, unsteadiness, failure to thrive, and irritability). Weakness and seizures are less common.

   ii. Children and adolescents may have a pattern of headaches and vomiting that initially may have been diagnosed as a migraine.

   iii. School-age children may have a history of personality changes or a change in school performance.

2. *Physical Examination*

   a. Infants with *obstructive hydrocephalus* may have enlarged fontanels, enlarged head circumference, and cranial suture diastasis.

   b. *Localized symptoms of supratentorial tumors:*

   i. Tumors located near the *cortical surface* cause seizures and focal cerebral dysfunction. Symptoms depend on the area affected, but may include motor dysfunction, irritability, and speech dysfunction.

   ii. *Deep cerebral hemispheric tumors* cause hemiplegia and visual field defects.

   iii. *Frontal lobe tumors* provoke behavioral changes, language dysfunction, motor weakness, and seizures with focal motor onset or tonic–clonic movements.

   iv. *Occipital lobe tumors* cause visual field dysfunction (e.g., homonymous hemianopsia, which describes a defect in the right or left halves of the visual fields of the two eyes) and visual hallucinations.

   v. *Temporal lobe tumors* produce auditory and speech dysfunction such as receptive aphasia, olfactory dysfunction such as involuntary smacking or licking of the lips, and psychomotor seizures.

   vi. *Sella turcica area tumors* produce eating dysfunction, metabolic dysfunction, and autonomic seizures.

   vii. *Parietal lobe tumors* cause reading dysfunction and dysfunction in awareness of contralateral extremities.

   c. Localized symptoms of infratentorial tumors:

   i. *Cerebellar tumors* cause impaired coordination and balance, truncal ataxia (irregular muscular coordination of the upper body), and nystagmus.

   ii. *Brainstem tumors* cause cranial nerve dysfunction, ataxia, and corticospinal tract dysfunction. Patients may also present in cardiorespiratory failure with disruption of vital functioning centers.

3. *Diagnostic Tests*

   a. Routine laboratory studies may include CBC with differential, coagulation studies, metabolic panel, electrolytes.

   b. *Neuroimaging*

   i. CT scan is performed in a child who presents with nonspecific neurological symptoms in the emergency room; it is useful in making an initial diagnosis of brain tumor.

   ii. MRI is the preferred diagnostic study for nonemergent presentations and is performed with and without contrast. It provides a better definition of tumor than a CT scan and identifies small tumors not seen on CT scan. MRI demonstrates the tumor in all planes and it is useful for developing a treatment plan that uses image-guided therapies. Craniospinal MRI with gadolinium is used to determine the extent of tumor spread in the CSF pathways. MRI is frequently used to evaluate tumor response to therapy and progression (Poussaint, Panigrahy, & Huisman, 2015).

   c. The presence or absence of specific protein markers secreted from some tumor cells is important in the diagnosis of germ cell tumors. Serum or spinal fluid tumor markers of human chorionic gonadotropin (HCG) and alpha-fetoprotein (AFP) may be elevated in a child with a pineal-region tumor. Elevated levels of HCG and AFP usually indicate nongerminomatous germ cell tumor.

   d. CSF polyamines may be elevated in several types of brain tumors and hydrocephalus.

   e. Brain biopsy is required to make a tissue diagnosis for specific treatment protocols and is usually done during surgical tumor debulking.

4. *Clinical Course*

a. The clinical course depends on type of tumor, location, rate of growth, and age of patient.

b. In general, brain tumors do not metastasize outside the brain or spinal cord.

c. A malignant tumor compared to a benign tumor generally signifies a poorer outcome. However, a child with a benign brain tumor may have a poor prognosis if the tumor is in an unresectable location.

D. Patient Care Management

1. *Preventive Care.* There are no specific interventions to follow to prevent brain cancer.

2. *Direct care* for most brain tumors uses a combination of surgery, radiation, and chemotherapy.

a. *Surgery* is used to obtain tissue for histologic examination, reduce tumor size (debulk), remove tumor, and insert VP shunts for patients with surgically uncorrectable hydrocephalus.

   i. The goal of "debulking" is to remove as much tumor as possible to relieve symptoms and to improve the effectiveness of complimentary treatments.

   ii. Total resection is rarely possible, but is the only option for survival in some tumor subtypes. Surgeons balance life-saving resection with morbidity. Intraoperative MRI has improved the safety and effectiveness of brain tumor resections with minimal damage to surrounding normal tissue.

   iii. CSF diversion may be accomplished with a VP shunt, or more recently with an endoscopic third ventriculostomy.

   iv. Radioactive implants may be inserted surgically for localized treatment of a tumor.

b. *Radiation therapy* uses high-energy beams to suspected or known areas of the tumor.

   i. Standard photon energy (x-ray) is delivered to a localized area or to the entire brain and spinal cord. It is delayed as long as possible in infants and toddlers to avoid damage to normal developing brain tissue. Stereotactic techniques have improved effectiveness of irradiation and have limited damage to normal tissue.

   ii. Proton beam therapy is a more highly targeted therapy than conventional photon radiotherapy. Proton radiation can use stereotactic procedures that consist of a basic frame that attaches to the patient's skull. Side arms (Y-axis) and vertical (Z-axis) and horizontal (X-axis) bars and an arc are attached to the frame. With the use of a CT scan or MRI and the prior coordinates, instruments are precisely directed to a specific tumor area. Proton beam therapy is used for tumors when less radiation is warranted because of location or age of the patient. The advantage is less damage to surrounding normal tissue.

   iii. 3-D conformal radiotherapy integrates many beams and precisely directs radiotherapy to the desired site. This minimizes toxicity to surrounding normal tissue.

c. Traditional *chemotherapy* has been less effective in treating brain tumors, in part because the BBB limits many systemic drugs from entering the CNS. However, chemotherapy's effectiveness has increased over the last two decades.

   i. As with most other childhood cancers, combination chemotherapy is more effective than single-agent therapy.

   ii. A surgically placed chemotherapy wafer is another option for localized medication delivery. It is placed in the area where a tumor was removed surgically.

   iii. Commonly used chemotherapeutic agents include vincristine, cyclophosphamide, cisplatin, carboplatin, etoposide, lomustine, and carmustine.

   iv. Chemotherapeutic agents are most effective with treating astrocytomas, medulloblastomas, and chiasmal gliomas.

   v. Children younger than 3 years of age are usually treated with radical surgical resection and chemotherapy to delay irradiation for 1 to 2 years to allow brain tissue development (Spennato et al., 2015). Another option to delay radiation therapy is to use high doses of multiagent chemotherapy with autologous stem cell rescue (Fleming & Chi, 2012).

d. Newer medications are being designed as *targeted therapy*; specific tumor cell signaling is targeted versus using nonspecific medications that are toxic to the entire cell. This type of therapy stops the growth and spread of tumor cells while limiting damage to normal cells.

3. *Supportive Care*

a. Provide serial neurologic assessment, including head circumference in infants; assess for increased ICP; and monitor fluid and electrolyte status.

b. Maintain cardiorespiratory functioning.

c. Care is directed at minimizing the side-effects of treatment.

    i. Routine postoperative surgical care for craniotomy

    ii. Fluid, nutrition, and antiemetics for chemotherapy

    iii. Blood product transfusions for support of hematologic function

    iv. Skin care for radiotherapy

d. *Steroids* may be used to control cerebral swelling, reduce nausea, reduce allergic reactions, and destroy cancer cells.

e. *Antiseizure* medication is used to control or prevent seizures.

E. Outcomes

1. The prognosis depends on multiple factors: type of tumor, extent of disease, size and location of the tumor, tumor response to therapy, and age and baseline health of child.

2. The best prognosis occurs with complete surgical resection.

3. More than 60% of children will be cured.

HYDROCEPHALUS

A. Definition and Etiology

1. *Hydrocephalus* is not a disease, but is a pathological condition characterized by progressive accumulation of CSF under pressure within the ventricular system, spinal central canal, or subarachnoid spaces of the CNS. It develops from a variety of conditions and diseases.

2. *Developmental hydrocephalus* is present when an extrinsic cause for CSF accumulation is not evident. Hydrocephalus may be present at birth and results from a congenital condition or it may progress over time. The most common conditions that cause developmental hydrocephalus are myelomeningocele, aqueductal obstruction, posterior fossa crowding, presence of cysts or cephaloceles, or communicating hydrocephalus (Tully et al., 2015).

    a. Most cases of hydrocephalus from a myelomeningocele have classic *Chiari II malformations*.

    b. Aqueductal obstructions are seen with midline brainstem and cerebellar malformations.

    c. Posterior fossa crowding is commonly associated with *Chiari I malformations*.

    d. Cysts and cephaloceles that produce hydrocephalus tend to be midline (as seen with agenesis of the corpus callosum), or less frequent, Dandy–Walker malformations.

    e. With communicating hydrocephalus, brain malformations are uncommon.

3. *Acquired hydrocephalus* results from a known extrinsic event, including hemorrhage, neoplasm, infection, and trauma.

4. Hydrocephalus is also commonly described as noncommunicating (obstructive) or communicating.

    a. *Noncommunicating hydrocephalus* refers to an obstruction within the ventricular system that prevents circulation and reabsorption of CSF.

    b. *Communicating hydrocephalus* refers to a blockage to CSF circulation outside of the ventricular system in subarachnoid space or poor CSF absorption at the Pacchionian granulations. Increased venous sinus pressure from a venous thrombosis or occlusion of venous sinuses from hemorrhage may inhibit reabsorption of CSF.

5. Two other descriptions of hydrocephalus that may be seen are:

    a. *Normal-pressure hydrocephalus* (NPH; low pressure, adult, or occult hydrocephalus) occurs usually in middle age from arachnoid adhesions, SAH, infection, tumor, or complication of surgery.

    b. *Hydrocephalus ex vacuo* refers to ventricular enlargement from loss of brain parenchyma rather than an overproduction of CSF. Brain tissue may shrink or atrophy allowing for the lateral ventricles to expand and fill the vacated brain tissue.

B. Pathophysiology

1. Historically, the pathophysiology of hydrocephalus is based on CSF circulation theory with three premises:

    a. CSF is actively produced, primarily from the choroid plexus.

    b. CSF is passively reabsorbed by the arachnoid villi inside the dural venous sinuses.

    c. CSF flow is unidirectional from the site of secretion to the site of reabsorption.

    d. Based on the circulation theory, any obstruction that prevents CSF flow and reabsorption will produce hydrocephalus.

2. Although the circulation theory is widely accepted, there are alterative theories that describe the pathophysiology of hydrocephalus. Some believe that fluid shifts in the CNS are similar to other parts of the body, and factors, such as osmotic and hydrostatic pressures, influence CSF and interstitial fluid volumes between the ventricular compartment and the surrounding tissue (Bulat & Klarica, 2011; Krishnamurthy & Li, 2014; Orešković & Klarica, 2011).

3. If the ventricles continue to enlarge, thinning and stretching of the cortical mantle will occur. Edema may be present in the periventricular white matter in the early phase, but, if left untreated, edema will be replaced with fibrosis, demyelination, axonal degeneration, and loss of cerebral cortical neurons.

C. Clinical Presentation

1. *History*

   a. Hydrocephalus may be diagnosed in utero.

   b. Clinical presentation depends on the child's age, cause of hydrocephalus, location of obstruction, duration of condition, and rapidity of onset.

     i. Slowly progressing hydrocephalus in an infant may have a history of poor feeding, irritability, lethargy, and vomiting. Children may have arrested growth or symptoms of increased ICP (e.g., headache, vomiting, blurred vision, drowsiness).

     ii. Acute hydrocephalus with increased ICP may present with rapid deterioration.

2. *Physical Examination*

   a. Presumptive diagnosis is based on clinical examination and presenting signs.

   b. Physical findings in infants may include increased head circumference, setting-sun sign (sclera of the eyes are visible above the iris), Macewen's sign or "cracked-pot" sound when the skull is percussed, tense or bulging fontanelles, prominent scalp veins, thin and shiny scalp skin, spasticity of lower limbs, and high-pitched cry with increased ICP.

   c. Physical findings in older children include macrocephaly, unsteady broad-based gait with history of falling, deterioration in school performance, urinary incontinence, papilledema, diplopia, seizures, and behavioral changes such as irritability, lethargy, and personality changes.

3. *Diagnostic Tests*

   a. There is no specific routine laboratory test that is diagnostic for hydrocephalus.

   b. Neuroimaging

     i. CT scan can assess the size of the ventricles and other structures that may be obstructing the ventricular system.

     ii. MRI has better imaging of the posterior fossa than CT scan. It can evaluate Chiari malformation and tumors and can differentiate NPH from cerebral atrophy.

     iii. Ultrasonography through the anterior fontanelle can evaluate intraventricular and subependymal hemorrhage and the progression of hydrocephalus.

     iv. Skull radiograph demonstrates separated sutures or widened sutures, a "beaten silver" appearance from thinning of the skull, widened or split sutures, and the size of the cranial vault. It can also recognize erosion of the sella turcica.

   c. CSF analysis may demonstrate the presence of infection or inflammatory process and to evaluate posthemorrhagic or postmeningitic hydrocephalus.

4. *Clinical Course*

   a. Depending on the cause of hydrocephalus, it may resolve spontaneously or with temporary CSF diversion therapy.

   b. Developmental hydrocephalus usually progresses without intervention.

   c. The majority of patients without treatment for hydrocephalus will die.

D. Patient Care Management

1. *Preventative Care*

   a. If hydrocephalus is acquired and the condition that caused it is treatable, temporary CSF diversion may control and arrest the CSF accumulation.

   b. Minimize the risk of acquired hydrocephalus through prevention measures:

     i. Meningitis. Keep vaccinations current and restrict travel to known infectious regions.

     ii. TBI. Wear seatbelts and helmets and use appropriate safety equipment.

2. *Direct Care*

   a. For rapid-onset hydrocephalus with symptomatic increased ICP, emergent procedures include a ventricular tap (infant) or open ventricular drainage through a ventriculostomy.

b. An LP may be used for conditions that produce hydrocephalus, but it is expected resolve spontaneously (e.g., IVH).

c. Ventricular shunts are used in the majority of patients with hydrocephalus (see section on "Intracranial Devices"). Shunt technology has improved significantly over the last several decades; however, they are not without flaws. Complications may include infection, mechanical failure, and obstructions, and the distal catheter will most likely need lengthening as the child grows.

d. Alternatives to shunting are less common and include cerebral aqueductoplasty, tumor removal, and endoscopic fenestration of the third ventricle.

3. *Supportive Care*

a. Provide serial neurologic assessment, including head circumference in infants; assess for increased ICP; and monitor fluid and electrolyte status.

b. Maintain cardiorespiratory functioning.

c. Shunt systems need to be monitored for complications.

d. Provide routine postoperative care following surgical insertion of shunt (e.g., pain control, incision care, infection).

E. Outcomes

1. Because hydrocephalus is not a disease, but a final common pathway for a number of disorders, it is difficult to predict outcome.

2. Children with well-controlled hydrocephalus have the best outcomes.

3. Children with chronic hydrocephalus have increased risk for cognitive and physical developmental abnormalities.

TRAUMATIC BRAIN INJURY

A. Definition and Etiology

1. *TBI* has been defined inconsistently in the past, but there are key elements that all current definitions have in common: There is an alteration in brain function or evidence of brain pathology, and it is caused by an external force. The alterations in brain function may be temporary or permanent.

2. Beyond the first year of life, multiple trauma is the leading cause of death and disability among children. Approximately 500,000 children are admitted to an emergency department annually. Boys are victims almost twice as often as girls.

3. The most common causes of TBI are related to falls and motor vehicle-related accidents (Faul, Xu, Wald, Coronado, & Dellinger, 2010). Children younger than 2 years of age who sustain a TBI are usually occupants of motor vehicles and are often not restrained or improperly restrained. Infants sustain TBIs in falls, walker-related injuries, and non-accidental injuries. Older children and adolescents are injured in bicycle-related or motorcycle-related accidents, with firearms and assaults, and during recreational activities. Risk factors include young age, substance abuse, and lack of protective devices (e.g., helmets; see discussion on multiple trauma in Chapter 9).

B. Pathophysiology

1. *Primary injuries* occur at the time of or within seconds of traumatic impact.

a. *Skull fractures* are usually linear in infants and occur along a suture line or perpendicular to a suture line. Diastasis (separation of cranial sutures) may occur in infants and small children; the separation may progress to growing fractures (i.e., a gradual erosion and separation of the fracture line) when accompanied by dural tears. Depressed fractures may represent depressed bone fragments or indentation of pliable skull bone without loss of bone integrity ("ping pong" depression in an infant). *Basilar fractures* are a break in the basilar portions of the frontal, ethmoid, sphenoid, temporal, or occipital bones.

b. A *concussion* is defined by the Third International Conference on Concussion in Sport as (McCrory et al., 2009):

a complex pathophysiological process affecting the brain, induced by traumatic biomechanical forces. Several common features that incorporate clinical, pathologic and biomechanical injury constructs that may be utilized in defining the nature of a concussive head injury include

- External force transmitted to head

- Short-term neurologic impairment

- Functional disturbance without structural disturbance

- Results in clinical symptoms that resolve; post-concussion symptoms may persist
- Neuroimaging is negative

2. *Secondary injuries* develop after the traumatic event and are a consequence of the primary injury.

   a. *Cerebral lacerations* are tears in the brain tissue often associated with skull fractures. They are less common in children because the smoother inner table of the skull offers less resistance between bone and brain tissue.

   b. *Cerebral contusions* are heterogeneous areas of hemorrhage and edema within the brain tissue. They begin as primary injuries, but swelling, hemorrhage, and subsequent increased ICP produce secondary injuries. These are less common in young children compared to adolescents and adults.

   c. Extradural hematomas. Subdural hematoma represents bleeding into the dural space, usually venous in origin from bilateral bridging of cerebral veins. They are more common than epidural hematomas in children. Epidural hematoma represents a collection of blood (usually arterial in origin) in the extradural space. The most common location is under the temporal bone from the middle meningeal artery. These are less common in children compared to adults.

   d. *Diffuse generalized cerebral swelling* following a severe TBI is more common in children than adults. Edema is classified into two main categories: cytotoxic (cellular) and vasogenic. Early studies proposed that the cerebral swelling seen following TBI was predominantly from a vasogenic cause. Newer studies propose that TBI swelling is from a combination of vasogenic and cytotoxic mechanisms. Donkin and Vink (2010) state that early cerebral swelling is vasogenic from opening of the BBB and cytotoxic edema progresses more slowly with a peak of 48 to 72 hours. Despite the cause, when swelling is extensive, there is a rapid increase in ICP, which results in compression and herniation of brain structures.

C. Clinical Presentation

1. *History*

   a. Falls are responsible for the majority of TBI in children younger than 9 years old. Infants and toddlers are more likely to fall from furniture, beds, or parents' arms while older children are more likely to fall from playground equipment.

   b. Children older than 9 years with a TBI are most likely to have a history of a motor vehicle-related accident (Tracy et al., 2013).

2. Physical examination findings depend on the type and severity of the injury.

   a. Simple *linear fractures* usually are asymptomatic.

   b. *Basilar fractures* present with specific physical findings.

      i. Battle's sign represents postauricular hematoma and swelling from damage to the sigmoid sinus temporal bone.

      ii. The raccoon or panda sign represents a periorbital blood collection from an anterior skull base fracture (there is absence of a subconjunctival hemorrhage).

      iii. Rhinorrhea represents CSF leakage into the middle ear cavity with drainage through the Eustachian tube into the nose. Anosmia is the lack of smell from damage to the olfactory nerve. Both are usually related to middle fossa basilar fracture.

      iv. Hemotympanum represents a blood collection behind the tympanic membrane from a temporal bone fracture. If the dura mater is torn at the same time, CSF may leak out of the ear canal (otorrhea).

      v. Vertigo may occur with damage to the inner ear.

      vi. Acute deterioration with associated hemorrhage and increased ICP is most often seen with occipital transverse fractures because of the close proximity to the vital centers of the brainstem.

   c. *Cerebral contusion* findings depend on location of the injury. Most injuries occur on the cortical surface of the temporal and frontal lobes from acceleration–deceleration forces, placing the patient at risk for focal seizures. The size of the injury and the shift in brain structures also affect presentation. Large contusions can produce a significant mass effect with shifting of intracranial structures and increased ICP. Clinical signs of increased ICP and herniation may present. Symptoms also depend on the degree of associated swelling. Swelling occurs around the contusion 3 to 4 days following the injury. Significant swelling can also cause shifting of brain structures and increased ICP.

d. *Concussion* may present with loss of consciousness, retrograde amnesia, headaches, vomiting, fatigue, and posttraumatic seizures. Diaphoresis, pallor, and lethargy may occur in infants.

e. Physical findings of *epidural hematoma* vary. Infants may present with a bulging fontanelle, anemia with significant bleeding, and separation of cranial sutures. Older children demonstrate hemiparesis or hemiplegia and anisocoria (*anisocoria* is an inequality of the pupils, usually greater than 1 mm difference; some individuals normally have unequal pupils, usually less than 1 mm difference). All ages may have symptoms of increased ICP in severe epidural hematoma.

f. Physical findings of *subdural hematoma* are usually nonspecific and may include drowsiness, lethargy, and irritability. Retinal hemorrhages and seizures may occur especially in children younger than 3 years of age. Significant bleeding produces tense, bulging, and pulseless fontanelles. Retinal hemorrhages in a child younger than 3 years old are highly suggestive of intentional injury.

g. Physical findings of *generalized cerebral swelling* are associated with increased ICP; however, significant swelling may not peak for 2 to 3 days.

3. *Diagnostic Tests*

a. Routine laboratory studies include CBC with differential, metabolic panel, coagulation studies, electrolytes, urine and serum osmolalities, and serum glucose.

b. Neuroimaging

   i. CT scan remains the gold standard for acute evaluation of a TBI. Mass lesions are identified with and without shifts in brain structures. Bone windows identify basilar fractures. Epidural hematoma demonstrates a double-convex (lentiform), hyperdense area, and does not cross cranial suture lines (Figure 4.16B). Subdural hematoma demonstrates a more diffuse blood collection crossing cranial suture lines. The acute phase is usually hyperdense and crescent shaped (Figure 4.16A). Cerebral swelling and edema results in changes in density.

   ii. MRI is indicated in acute TBI when the clinical examination is not consistent with CT scan findings. It is superior to the CT scan in imaging nonhemorrhagic contusions, white matter abnormalities, and posterior fossa and small vascular lesions.

   iii. Advanced neuroimaging techniques (e.g., diffuse-weighted imaging and diffusion-tensor imaging) are beneficial in identifying abnormalities in the brain that have implications for long-term sequelae. They are not available in most centers, and are used primarily in research studies.

   iv. Routine skull radiographs are no longer used to evaluate acute TBI and have been supplanted by the CT scan. However, skull radiographs are useful in identifying missile injuries and some depressed skull fractures.

4. *Clinical Course*

a. The clinical course depends on the type of TBI and the presence of increased ICP.

b. Patients with brain lesions that can be surgically evacuated or do not have increased ICP usually respond to supportive care with a good recovery.

c. TBIs that result in uncontrolled ICP usually progress to brain herniation, ischemic injury and death.

D. Patient Care Management

1. *Preventive Care*

a. Beyond safety measures to prevent a TBI, prevention is directed at minimizing secondary brain injury.

b. The cervical spine should be immobilized until the cervical spine has been cleared of injury.

2. *Direct Care*

a. In 2012, *Guidelines for the Acute Medical Management of Severe Traumatic Brain Injury in Infants, Children, and Adolescents* were revised (Kochanek et al., 2012). These guidelines provide a foundation for how children are managed with a TBI.

b. Initiate immediate resuscitation and support of airway, breathing, and circulation.

c. Initiate neuromonitoring. *ICP monitoring* is usually recommended for patients with severe injury, including those with a Glasgow Coma Score (GCS) <8, abnormal CT findings with potential for increased ICP, and comatose patients with or without an abnormal CT scan. Advanced neuromonitoring may include transcranial Doppler, NIRS, and jugular oximetry (see "Neurologic Monitoring" section).

d. Surgical management depends on the type of lesion. In general, children require surgery less often. Extradural hematomas are evacuated.

Large intracerebral hemorrhages producing midline shifts may be removed. Growing fractures are repaired with cranioplasty. Decompressive craniectomy with duraplasty may be considered for children with acute deterioration from herniation or uncontrolled ICP elevation.

3. *Supportive Care*

a. Medical management is supportive and directed toward preventing secondary injury, including hypoxia and ischemia, increased ICP, and complications (e.g., seizures, obstructive hydrocephalus, hypotension).

b. Maintain ventilation and oxygenation by controlling ventilation (e.g., intubation and manual ventilation) and administering supplemental oxygen. Support the cardiovascular system (e.g., cardiac compressions, inotropic agents, fluids).

c. Provide baseline and serial cardiovascular, respiratory, and neurologic assessments.

d. Administer oxygen to maintain SaO_2 >95%. Maintain good pulmonary toilet and PEEP when a patient is receiving manual ventilation. Preoxygenate and sedate patient prior to suctioning. Administer fluids as ordered while maintaining adequate perfusion. Administer diuretics as ordered. (A complete description of ICP and CPP management is discussed in the section "Intracranial Hypertension: Patient Care Management").

E. Outcomes

1. Morbidity and mortality from a TBI vary considerably and depend on severity of injury, presence of comorbidities, age of patient, and location of injury.

2. Diffuse cerebral swelling with increased ICP is responsible for significant morbidity and mortality in children.

ENCEPHALOPATHY

A. Definition and Etiology

1. *Encephalopathy* is a broad term used to describe any condition that produces a generalized disturbance in brain cellular metabolism resulting in an alteration of consciousness. In infants and children, the list of potential etiologies is endless; causes may be chronic or acute, static or progressive, and inherited or acquired. The prototypic encephalopathy seen in critically ill infants and children is HIE.

2. *HIE* is a final common pathway for a number of pathologies that produce brain injury from two physiologic abnormalities: damage to brain tissue from ischemia (reduction in CBF) and damage to brain tissue from hypoxia (decreased oxygen) or anoxia (absence of oxygen).

3. In neonates, HIE is the most common type of neonatal encephalopathy and results from hypoxia and ischemia during the prenatal, intranatal, or postnatal periods.

4. In older infants and children, a common cause of encephalopathy is HIE from cardiac arrest or low perfusion states (e.g., heart disease).

B. Pathophysiology

1. The pathophysiology of HIE is complex, multifactorial, interrelated, and not completely understood. Several mechanisms may be activated during and after an hypoxic–ischemic event and include brain energy failure, calcium-mediated injury, excitotoxic injury, activation of intracellular proteases, release of free fatty acids, activation of nitric oxide synthesis, formation of oxygen radicals, reperfusion injury, and inflammatory injury. The progression of damage starts with alteration in the cell membrane, then cellular metabolism ceases, and finally neurons die. Shortly after a hypoxic–ischemic insult, brain damage may not be apparent. If the patient survives and perfusion is restored, changes to brain tissue appear within hours. Some cells of the brain are more sensitive to hypoxic–ischemic insults and sustain more injury. For example, neurons are more vulnerable compared to glial cells due to their high energy requirements. Gray matter uses more than twice the ATP compared to white matter; consequently, the cerebral cortex is damaged more often than other areas of the brain with a hypoxic–ischemic insult (Perkin & Ashwal, 2012).

2. With severe HIE, cytotoxic edema develops in the initial phase of injury followed by vasogenic edema. Both types edema can increase ICP, which compounds the effects with compression of blood vessels and further ischemia.

C. Clinical Presentation

1. *History*

a. Because HIE is not a disease entity, the clinical history is as varied as the number of disorders that cause it.

b. Important interview questions include length of hypoxic–ischemic event, precipitating events, presence of cardiac or respiratory arrest, neurologic symptoms during event, and interventions used to restore perfusion.

c. Newborns presumed to have HIE have a history of fetal heart rate abnormalities, fetal distress, or acute sentinel event.

2. *Physical Examination*

a. Physical findings may be minor (e.g., amnesia) or severe (e.g., coma or death) and relate to the severity of injury.

b. In newborns, a significant number of hypoxic–ischemic events occur before birth. The newborn is presumed to have HIE with nonspecific clinical findings: fetal heart rate abnormalities, fetal distress, cord arterial acidemia, low Apgar scores, and need for respiratory support. Other physical findings that have been categorized to reflect the severity of HIE in newborns (Horn et al., 2013; Sarnat & Sarnat, 1976):

  i. Mild HIE. Hyperalert, normal tone and activity, exaggerated Moro reflex, and normal autonomic function

  ii. Moderate HIE. Lethargic, decreased activity; distal flexion; hypotonia; primitive reflexes sluggish; constricted pupils; bradycardia; and periods of apnea

  iii. Severe HIE. Coma, decerebrate posturing, absent spontaneous activity, flaccid, apnea, nonreactive pupils, and absent neonatal reflexes

3. *Diagnostic Tests*

a. Routine laboratory studies include CBC with differential, serum electrolytes with renal function, metabolic panel, blood gas, and coagulation studies.

b. Neuroimaging for HIE is with a head MRI. It is considered to be the best neuroimaging study to identify the presence and pattern of injury, and to predict long-term outcome in term infants. DWI MRI is better at identifying early insults.

c. EEG findings depend on the extent of cortical damage. In newborns, characteristic patterns were originally described by Sarnat and Sarnat (1976):

  i. Mild HIE may have a normal EEG.

  ii. Moderate HIE may show early low voltage and continuous delta and theta waves. Later changes show periodic pattern (awake) and seizures.

  iii. Severe HIE may show early periodic pattern with isopotential phases and later all isopotential.

d. Older children may have EEG patterns that are more variable and relate to severity and etiology. Slight to moderate insults demonstrate changes in peak frequency or asymmetric rhythms from homotopic regions in each hemisphere. Severe insults demonstrate progressive slowing of electrical activity. EEG is used for seizure monitoring.

4. *Clinical Course*

a. Patients with short episodes (1–2 minutes or mild newborn HIE) of hypoxic–ischemic events usually recover fully.

b. Patients with longer episodes of hypoxic–ischemic have a more protracted course with increased mortality.

D. Patient Care Management

1. *Preventive Care*

a. Initiate resuscitation immediately to restore oxygenation and perfusion to minimize hypoxic–ischemic insult or secondary reperfusion injury.

b. *Neuroprotective* measures to prevent secondary brain injury include

  i. *Therapeutic hypothermia* (33°C–35°C depending on type of cooling) for 72 hours with selective head cooling or systemic cooling is recommended for newborns with HIE. The inclusion criteria include (Committee on Fetus and Newborn et al., 2014):

  • ≥36 weeks gestation and <6 hours

  • Apgar ≤5 at 10 minutes

  • Continued need for resuscitation at 10 minutes after birth or

  • pH <7.0 or base deficit ≥16 mmol/L and

  • Moderate or severe encephalopathy on clinical examination

  ii. Therapeutic hypothermia for children with HIE has not been studied extensively and recommendations do not exist (Imataka & Arisaka, 2015).

2. *Direct Care*

a. Immediate care is directed at resuscitation and stabilization of the child.

b. There is no specific treatment for HIE that is widely accepted. Interventions are supportive and directed at the cause of the hypoxic–ischemic event.

3. *Supportive Care*

a. Support normal hemodynamics for adequate CBF.

b. ICP monitoring is not recommended. NIRS may be used for trending brain tissue oxygenation.

c. Maintain normothermia in the child; therapeutic hypothermia is recommended for neonatal HIE.

d. Maintain normal serum glucose levels.

e. Prevent and control seizures.

E. Outcomes

1. Outcomes vary and depend on the characteristics of the hypoxic–ischemic event, age of patient, and interventions.

2. Neurologic signs on admission are not always predictive of neurologic outcome.

3. Although the data are inconsistent, several predictors associated with poor outcome include

a. In normothermic children, absence of motor and pupillary (Abend et al., 2012)

b. Presence of seizures

c. Cardiopulmonary arrest

d. Severe MRI and EEG abnormalities

SPINAL CORD INJURY

A. Definition and Etiology

1. *Complete cord injury* is the complete loss of motor and sensory function due to interruption of nerve pathways below the level of the injury. *Quadriplegia* is the complete loss of leg function and loss or limited use of arms from cervical injury. *Paraplegia* is the loss of leg function alone from high lumbar injury.

2. *Incomplete cord injury* causes some loss of motor and sensory function with some sparing of function below the level of the injury.

a. *Posterior cord syndrome* is caused by injury to the dorsal columns. There is loss of proprioception but other sensory and motor function is preserved.

b. *Anterior cord syndrome* from injury to the anterior cord results in loss of motor function below the level of the injury. Sensory function is lost except for proprioception and vibration sense.

c. *Central cord syndrome* is caused by injury or edema to the central spinal cord in the cervical area. Greater motor deficits occur in the upper extremities compared with the lower extremities. Sensory deficits are variable but are usually greater in the upper extremities. Bowel and bladder dysfunction is common.

d. *Partial spinal cord syndrome* (Brown–Séquard's syndrome) results from injury to one side of the spinal cord, resulting in loss of voluntary motor function on the same side as the injury. Loss of pain, temperature, and touch occurs on the contralateral side.

e. *Conus medullaris* is an injury to the sacral cord and lumbar nerve roots, resulting in an areflexic bladder, bowel, and lower limb.

3. SCI is rare in children compared to adults, but when it does occur, the upper cervical spine is more commonly injured in small children than in adolescents and adults (J. R. Leonard, Jaffe, Kuppermann, Olsen, & Leonard, 2014).

4. Children have a higher incidence of *spinal cord injury without radiographic abnormality (SCIWORA)*. This condition occurs predominantly in younger children and is thought to result from severe subluxation and trauma of the vertebral column. Infants and young children (usually <8–10 years of age) have ligamentous flexibility and elasticity of the immature spine. The spinal column can withstand significant stretching without disruption. In contrast, the spinal cord cannot withstand significant stretch. The mismatch between the spinal column and the spinal cord predisposes the young child to SCI. Young children are also more prone to dislocation without fracture. When fractures do occur, the characteristics of the fracture vary with skeletal maturation.

5. Adolescents have a higher incidence of SCI and the mechanisms and patterns of injury closely resemble those of adults. Unlike young children, fractures are more common and soft tissue injury is less common. Subaxial cervical spine injuries (C5 and C6) are more common than axial injuries.

6. Mechanisms of SCI differ between children and adults. In children younger than 8 years old, the most common cause of SCI is motor vehicle related followed by falls. Motor vehicle and sports-related injuries are more common in older children and adolescents. "Seat belt"–type injuries (flexion–distraction) are almost exclusively seen in children younger than 13 years. Flexion–distraction injuries occur when children are restrained in an automobile with only a lap belt. Intestinal and lumbar spine injuries occur as a result of flexion of the upper body against a fixed lap belt with a high-impact motor vehicle accident.

7. Nontraumatic causes include tumor, disc herniation, infection, spinal stenosis, and congenital abnormalities.

B. Pathophysiology

1. Infants and young children predominantly have *SCIWORA*. In older children and adults, SCI most often occurs from vertebral injury, usually from acceleration–deceleration or deformation forces. Hyperextension causes fracture and dislocation of the posterior elements. Hyperflexion causes fracture or dislocation of the vertebral bodies, discs, or ligaments. Vertical compression causes shattering fractures. Rotational forces cause rupture of the supporting ligaments and fractures.

2. Similar to TBIs, the pathophysiology of SCI involves primary injury from the direct impact and subsequent secondary injury.

3. *Primary SCIs and Consequences*

　　a. *Concussion of the cord* is caused by stretching and shearing of the spinal cord without tissue trauma. It causes a temporary disruption of cord-mediated functions.

　　b. *Contusion of the cord* is a bruising and swelling of the cord, causing a temporary or permanent loss of cord-mediated function.

　　c. *Laceration* is a tearing of neural tissue. The condition is reversible with minimal injury but may result in permanent dysfunction of cord-mediated functions.

　　d. *Transection of the cord* is severing of the cord, causing permanent loss of cord-mediated function.

　　e. *Hemorrhage of the cord* is blood vessel damage with bleeding into neural tissue. There is no major loss of function, depending on the extent of injury.

　　f. *Damage to the blood vessels* that supply the cord results in decreased perfusion of the spinal cord with local ischemia. Alteration in function depends on the severity of ischemia.

4. *Secondary SCI* usually follows a severe primary SCI; the process is complex, interrelated, and not completely understood. Intracellular and extracellular changes cause an increase in excitatory amino acids, increase in free oxygen radical formation, alteration in calcium homeostasis, and increase in platelet-activating factor (PAF). Cellular alterations produce edema, damage to cell membranes, ischemia, and cellular death at the level of injury and approximately two segments above and below it. Normal activity is lost at and below the level of the injury.

5. *Spinal shock* (complete loss of reflex function) may result from acute SCI. It can occur within 60 minutes of the injury and may last for 7 to 20 days. It results from loss of integrity of the ANS below the level of injury, producing venous pooling, bradycardia, and hypotension.

6. *Autonomic dysreflexia* is a life-threatening complication in SCI. It is rare during the acute phase, but it may occur any time after an SCI. Autonomic dysreflexia results from an uncontrolled, paroxysmal, continuous lower motor neuron reflex arc due to stimulation of the sympathetic nervous system. The response typically occurs from stimulation of sensory receptors (e.g., distended bladder or bowel) below the level of the cord injury. The ANS responds with arteriolar vasospasm resulting in increased blood pressure. Carotid sinus baroreceptors are stimulated and respond with activation of the vasomotor centers in the brainstem via the ninth and tenth cranial nerves. The parasympathetic nervous system (vagus nerve) sends a stimulus to the heart, causing bradycardia and vasodilation. The peripheral vessels and viscera do not respond because the efferent pulse cannot pass through the spinal cord. The vagus nerve is not "turned off," and profound bradycardia may occur.

7. *Temperature regulation* is impaired in patients with injuries above T-1 because of the loss of connection between temperature centers in the hypothalamus and sympathetic outflow of the spinal cord. Body temperature is regulated by the ambient temperature.

C. Clinical Presentation

1. *History*

　　a. Questions about patient history should focus on symptoms related to the vertebral column and motor and sensory deficits. Pain is a common complaint.

　　b. Mechanism of injury that may predict an SCI include:

i. Infants with a history of falling, TBI, blunt trauma, or motor vehicle-related accident

ii. Older children with a history of a motor vehicle–related accident, sports injury, or collision or fall from a bicycle

iii. Adolescents with a history of motor vehicle accident, sporting injury, or diving or swimming accident

2. *Physical Examination*

a. Several physical findings are highly predictive of cervical spine injury following blunt injury: altered mental status, focal neurologic deficits, neck pain, torticollis, injury to the torso, predisposing condition, motor vehicle crash, and diving (J. C. Leonard et al., 2011). A GCS of <14 is predictive of SCI in children younger than 3 years old (Tilt, Babineau, Fenster, Ahmad, & Roskind, 2012).

b. Sensory and motor dysfunction depend on the type and level of SCI (Kirshblum et al., 2011).

i. Sensory examination is completed in each of the 28 dermatomes on the right and left sides of the body. In each dermatome (both sides of the body), light touch and pinprick sensations are scored on a three-point scale.

   1) 0 = absent

   2) 1 = altered

   3) 2 = normal

ii. Motor examination is completed by testing key muscle functions corresponding to 10 paired myotomes (C5-T1 and L2-S1). The strength of each muscle function is graded on a six-point scale.

   1) 0 = total paralysis

   2) 1 = palpable or visible contraction

   3) 2 = active movement, full range of motion (ROM) without gravity

   4) 3 = active movement, full ROM against gravity

   5) 4 = active movement, full ROM against gravity and moderate resistance in a muscle specific position

   6) 5 = normal, active movement, full ROM and full resistance in a muscle specific position

   7) 5* = normal

c. Injuries are broadly classified as being neurologically complete or incomplete based on whether or not sensory and motor function is spared in the sacral segments. The American Spinal Injury Association (ASIA) developed an Impairment Scale (AIS) to grade SCIs according to spinal cord level and severity (Kirshblum et al., 2011).

i. Grade A. Complete. No motor and sensory function is preserved in sacral segments S4 to S5.

ii. Grade B. Sensory incomplete. Sensory, but no motor function is preserved below the neurological level of the injury (NLI) (including S4–S5), and no motor function more than three levels below the motor level on either side of the body.

iii. Grade C. Motor incomplete. Motor function is preserved below the NLI and more than 50% of key muscle functions below the single NLI have muscle grade <3.

iv. Grade D. Motor incomplete. Motor function is preserved below the NLI and at least 50% muscle functions below the NLI have a muscle grade of ≥3.

v. Grade E. Normal. All neurologic function has returned.

d. *Complete transection* results in loss of voluntary movement of body parts, loss of sensation to body parts, and loss of autonomic and spinal reflexes below the level of the injury. Reflex activity may return in 1 to 2 weeks.

e. *Incomplete transection* causes variable levels of vasomotor instability and bowel and bladder dysfunction; and asymmetric flaccid paralysis, asymmetric loss of reflexes, variable sensory function (e.g., pain, temperature, touch, pressure, proprioception), and variable visceral and somatic responses below the level of injury.

f. *Spinal shock in the acute period* results in loss of vasomotor tone with complete transection causing hypotension, poor venous circulation, and bradycardia; loss of perspiration below the level of the injury; and loss of bladder and rectal control.

g. *Autonomic hyperreflexia* is a complication that usually occurs after the acute phase of an SCI with findings of hypertension, diaphoresis, change in heart rate, muscle spasms, headache, blurred vision, and skin color changes.

3. *Diagnostic Tests*

a. Routine laboratory studies include CBC with differential, metabolic panel, coagulation studies, electrolytes, and serum glucose. An ABG is useful when ventilation or oxygenation is compromised.

b. Neuroimaging traditionally begins with standard radiographs of the affected region of the spine. Other imaging studies are included when indicated.

   i. Radiographic spine films are examined carefully to determine the integrity of each component of each vertebra and alignment of each segment. Frequently, spinal cord trauma occurs without radiographic findings in children because of their cartilaginous spine. Several normal variants occur in the pediatric cervical spine that may be confused with pathologic conditions (Schöneberg, Schweiger, Lendemans, & Waydhas, 2013).

   ii. CT scan is used when radiographs do not adequately explain the clinical picture or show suspicious findings (Schöneberg , Schweiger, Hussmann, et al., 2013). It may also be indicated when a head CT is already ordered.

   iii. MRI is the best imaging technique for evaluation of soft tissue injury of the spine. It clearly identifies the relationship of the spinal cord and surrounding vertebral elements and readily identifies cord compression. Approximately half of all children with SCI fail to demonstrate radiographic abnormalities on plain films, CT scans, or myelograms. MRI can usually identify spinal cord pathology with SCIWORA. Clinical assessment should be considered when evaluating SCI. It may be used in patients with neurologic symptoms, especially if the CT scan and radiograph are negative. It may also be considered in children who have an inconsistent physical examination or who are planned to be intubated and sedated for a period of time. MRI is not routinely used in unstable patients but is an excellent study for follow-up care.

   iv. Myelography is used when pathology is unclear and is helpful in identifying spinal cord abnormalities, including cord hematoma, epidural hematoma, swelling, and preexisting disease.

4. *Clinical course* depends on the type and location of SCI.

   a. Incomplete SCI has the best outlook for neurologic recovery.

b. Neurologic deficits of the spinal cord often increase in the immediate hours following the injury. An early sign is the extension of a sensory-deficit cephalad.

c. Neurologic recovery usually plateaus in the first 3 to 6 months, but may be later in some patients.

D. Patient Care Management

1. *Preventive care* is directed at protecting the spinal cord from injury or the progression of injury. *Immobilization* of the spine until it can be surgically stabilized is imperative. During transport, a semirigid cervical collar and spine backboard (ideally with a head well to keep the head in a neutral position) should be used. Foam blocks or linen rolls and tape help to further stabilize the head and shoulders on a backboard.

2. *Direct Care*

   a. *Spinal canal decompression* is used to prevent secondary injury to the spinal cord. Cervical traction is used to stabilize fractures or when subluxation has occurred. Muscle relaxants are frequently used with traction. *Surgical decompression* with posterior laminectomy and debridement may be indicated once the patient has stabilized and bleeding and swelling have stopped (usually after 7–10 days).

   b. Stabilization of the spine with *surgical fixation* is accomplished by the fusion of two or more vertebrae with the insertion of bone grafts, metal rods, or wires. A halo jacket involves the placement of a halo ring around the skull fixated with screws to the skull. The ring is attached to a padded jacket or cast made into a vest via vertical rods and a horizontal articulation device. Traction is adjusted to stabilize cervical fractures.

3. *Supportive Care*

   a. Beyond resuscitation and stabilization of the spine, careful serial neurologic examinations are performed to check for injury progression and improvement.

   b. Assess the patient immediately for *bladder distension* (palpation or ultrasound) and insert a urinary catheter.

   c. *Oxygenation and ventilation* may be impaired, especially with high SCI. Assess for spontaneous or effective ventilations; monitor oxygenation (e.g., ABGs, SaO$_2$); assess effectiveness of cough and ability to mobilize secretions, respiratory rate, pattern, and work of breathing (note acute changes), and breath sounds. Decompress the stomach with an indwelling orogastric tube.

d. Support *circulation* as needed using fluids plus inotropic and vasopressor agents. Maintain functioning of invasive lines. Correct bradycardia with atropine, an anticholinergic drug used to increase the rate of cardiac conduction. Eliminate the precipitating cause of bradycardia (e.g., hypothermia, distended bladder).

e. Pharmacologic prevention of a secondary injury with *high-dose steroids* has been suggested in adult clinical trials as a neuroprotective treatment. In 2013, the American Association of Neurological Surgeons and Congress of Neurological Surgeons stated that glucocorticoids are not recommended for acute SCI (Hurlbert et al., 2013). In children, the beneficial role of high-dose steroids remains unclear and is not recommended (Pettiford et al., 2011).

f. *Deep vein thrombosis (DVT)* is a significant concern in patients with altered mobility. Assess respiratory status for acute deterioration, perform serial measurements of the legs, and assess for signs of venous thrombosis (pain, swelling, redness, and tenderness in the lower extremities). Apply antiembolism stockings or mechanical devices designed to improve venous return from the lower extremities. Consult with physical or occupational therapy to plan appropriate ROM and positioning therapy. Maintain good hydration. Administer subcutaneous heparin or warfarin when indicated.

g. Children with an SCI are at risk for loss of *skin integrity* and require serial skin assessments. Change the patient's position frequently and use a pressure reduction surface if available; maintain dry and clean bed linens and clothing; provide meticulous skin care; and consult with physical or occupational therapy to plan appropriate ROM and positioning therapy.

h. *Thermal regulation* may be impaired in children with a SCI. Adjust the environmental temperature to maintain normal temperature range, adjust clothing and bed linens, correct hypothermia (e.g., warming blanket, heating lamps, warm linens), and correct hyperthermia (e.g., remove excessive clothing, sponge with tepid water).

i. *Bowel and bladder elimination* may be impaired. Assess for bladder or abdominal distention, monitor intake and output, assess stools for frequency, consistency, and color, and monitor urine cultures. Maintain urinary drainage with intermittent or indwelling catheterization, obtain routine urine cultures and renal studies, maintain good hydration, and administer stool softeners and bulk-forming agents.

E. Outcomes

1. Spinal cord level and extent (completeness) of the injury are predictive of neurologic recovery. The child's age, comorbidities, TBI, and systemic injuries increase mortality.

2. *High cervical injuries* may cause immediate death. Infants have the highest rate of axial injury and the highest mortality.

3. Children with the greatest degree of improvement have incomplete SCI and most improvement is seen in the first 6 months post injury.

SCOLIOSIS AND SPINAL FUSIONS

A. Description and Etiology

1. *Scoliosis* is musculoskeletal disorder defined as a lateral curvature of the spine greater than 10 degrees. The major types of scoliosis are syndromic, congenital, neuromuscular (resulting from abnormalities of myoneural pathways), and idiopathic (infantile, juvenile, adolescent). Related are secondary or pathologic causes from tumors, Chiari, and spondylolisthesis.

2. *Syndromic scoliosis* is recognized as scoliosis associated with a systemic disease, including Down syndrome, Marfan syndrome, neurofibromatosis, Rett syndrome, Prader–Willi syndrome, and osteogenesis imperfecta. There is limited research that discusses these conditions as one entity.

3. *Congenital scoliosis* is an embryologic malformation during the fifth and eighth weeks of embryonic development. Most cases are spontaneous, but may also be related to maternal diabetes, alcohol, and some medications. There may be associated anomalies, especially genitourinary, respiratory (hypoplastic lung) and cardiac. The vertebral malformations may be due to failure of formation (e.g., hemivertebrae, wedged vertebrae) or failure of segmentation (e.g., block vertebrae) or a combination of both (Kaspiris, Grivas, Weiss, & Turnbull, 2011).

4. *Neuromuscular scoliosis* occurs secondary to neuropathic or myopathic diseases that are classified as abnormalities with central motor neuron (e.g., cerebral palsy, hereditary ataxia), peripheral motor neuron (e.g., acute anterior poliomyelitis, infantile spinal amyotrophy, hereditary sensory, and motor neuropathy), mixed, neuromuscular junction (e.g., myasthenia), and muscular (e.g., Duchenne myopathy, arthrogryposis; Vialle, Thévenin-Lemoine, & Mary, 2013). In general, nerves and muscles do not maintain balance and alignment of the spine.

5. *Idiopathic* scoliosis is the most common spinal deformity and it can occur at any age. There are three subgroups of idiopathic scoliosis and are based on age of appearance.

    a. *Infantile scoliosis* onset occurs in the first 3 years of life with no known cause. Effects males and females equally.

    b. *Juvenile scoliosis* onset occurs between 4 and 10 years and represents 10% to 15% of all idiopathic scoliosis. The lateral curve is usually to the right in the thoracic region. The cause of idiopathic juvenile scoliosis is unknown.

    c. *Adolescent idiopathic scoliosis (AIS)* onset occurs in patients older than 10 years. It is the most common form of idiopathic scoliosis representing 90% of all cases (Wajchenberg, Astur, Kanas, & Martins, 2016). Curves of 10 degrees have an equal prevalence between females and males. However, as the curves get larger, the ratio of females to males increases dramatically, with approximately a 10:1 ratio for curves greater than 30 degrees (Miyanji, 2014). Although the etiology is unknown, approximately 30% of AIS patients have a family history of scoliosis. Current consensus maintains that AIS has a multifactorial etiology with a genetic predisposition.

B. Pathophysiology

1. Scoliosis is an abnormal lateral curvature of the spine that results from a variety of causes. In most cases, the lateral curvature progresses gradually, but often worsens during growth spurts.

2. Initial *pathologic changes* begin in the soft tissues, which shorten on the concave side of the curve. Vertebral deformity occurs as a result of unequal forces applied to the epiphyseal center of the ossification (growth plates). Curves progress during growth spurts. A large curve can be physically disabling and may compromise respiratory function.

Thoracic insufficiency syndrome (TIS) is the inability of the thorax to support normal breathing and lung growth. The lungs need adequate thoracic volume to grow and ventilate. With scoliosis, the curve rotates the spine into the chest on the convexity of the curve, flattening the chest with loss of thoracic volume. The deformity prevents the ribs from assisting with thoracic expansion during breathing and ventilation becomes totally dependent on the diaphragm.

C. Clinical Presentation

    1. *History*

        a. Questions are directed at causes of progressive spinal curvature (e.g., birth defects, trauma, and neuromuscular disorders, genetic and nongenetic syndromes). Age of onset is important in identifying the type of scoliosis.

        b. History includes menstrual history, birth and developmental history, and family history of scoliosis and back pain.

        c. Patients with neuromuscular scoliosis tend to be pain free, but have poor balance and coordination of their trunk, neck, and head. Sitting is often difficult.

    2. *Physical Examination*

        a. A common finding of neuromuscular scoliosis is pelvic obliquity, a condition in which the child's pelvis is unevenly tilted; one side is higher than the other. Kyphosis is frequently present, too.

        b. Physical findings in syndromic scoliosis are highly variable and are based on the underlying syndrome and degree of curvature.

        c. The first sign in idiopathic scoliosis is often uneven hips and shoulders. Physical changes are most noticeable when the child bends forward and may include one more prominent breast or scapula and posterior humping of ribs or hips. A "torso" lean, shift of the body to the right or left, can occur. An inclinometer is often used to quantify the spinal abnormality.

        d. Gait may be abnormal in all forms of scoliosis.

    3. *Diagnostic Tests*

        a. A radiograph of the spine confirms the diagnosis of scoliosis. A standing posterior–anterior radiograph using the Cobb angle measurement in the frontal plane is the gold standard for scoliosis evaluation. Serial radiographs are used to assess and document the progression of the curve. Radiation is not without risks and, as a result, newer imaging modalities that limit ionizing radiation are under investigation.

b. Serial pulmonary function tests may be used to trend lung capacity.

c. Echocardiograms may be used to trend cardiac function.

4. *Clinical Course*

a. Syndromic scoliosis has an unpredictable course due to the varied causal syndromes and generally has a higher incidence of surgical complications (Levy, Schulz, Fornari, & Wollowick, 2015).

b. Neuromuscular scoliosis is more likely to progress to the spinal curve, which may continue into adulthood. TIS may develop.

c. Congenital scoliosis. Curve may progress and some patients require treatment.

d. Infantile idiopathic scoliosis resolves without treatment in >90% of cases.

e. Juvenile idiopathic scoliosis. Curves that reach 30 degrees tend to progress and 70% of cases require surgery.

f. AIS. Curves less than 30 degrees at skeletal maturity usually do not progress. Thoracic curves of 50 to 75 degrees usually continue to progress. Lumbar curves greater than 30 degrees tend to progress, especially if there is significant rotational abnormality (Miyanji, 2014).

D. Patient Care Management

1. *Preventive Care.* Scoliosis cannot be prevented. Treatment is aimed at preventing progression of the spinal curve.

2. *Direct Care*

a. In 90% of cases, scoliotic curves are mild and no active treatment is necessary.

b. There are three treatment options for scoliosis that are based on the risk of curve progression, etiology, pattern of curve, and age of the patient: observation, bracing, and surgery.

c. Observation. Mild curves (in a prepubescent patient) or moderate curves (<40°–45°) in patients who have completed their growth require observation. Infantile scoliosis is observed with curves less than 20 degrees. The young child is evaluated every 3 to 12 months and older children and adolescents are evaluated every 3 to 4 months. Curves usually progress during growth spurts.

d. Rigid bracing (thoracolumbosacral orthosis) is the most common nonoperative treatment for prevention of curve progression and is used most often for AIS. It is usually recommended in growing children with 20 to 40 **degrees** curves. Infantile idiopathic scoliosis is usually for curves greater than 25 degrees and juvenile idiopathic scoliosis for curves greater than 20 degrees. Bracing significantly decreases the progression of high-risk curves in adolescents waiting for skeletal maturity and surgery. The longer the brace is worn each day, the greater the benefit (Weinstein, Dolan, Wright, & Dobbs, 2013).

e. Surgery is indicated in patients with skeletal immaturity with curves of 40 to 50 degrees or in patients with a skeletal maturity and curves greater than 50 degrees. The goal of surgery is to achieve solid arthrodesis, balanced three-dimensional correction, and limited size of surgical fusion. The surgical options include open posterior instrumentation and fusion, open anterior instrumentation and fusion, and thoracoscopic techniques.

i. The *posterior approach* with segmental instrumentation is used most often for idiopathic scoliosis. There have been surgical advances with posterior systems and the use of thoracic pedicle screws and rods is routine. Pedicle screws traverse all three areas of the vertebra (anterior, middle, posterior) and, with malleable rods, the surgeon can exert more force in the fixation system to correct the spinal deformity.

ii. If the patient has significant hypokyphosis, lordosis, or lower curves (thoracolumbar and lumber), the *anterior approach* is considered. The primary advantage of anterior spinal instrumentation and fusion in AIS is the ability to restore thoracic kyphosis. The anterior approach is associated with more postoperative complications and increased length of stay.

iii. Anterior approach with *video-assisted thoracoscopic surgery (VATS)* is a newer option for treating AIS that is used with an anterior approach. It compares favorably with the posterior approach in terms of coronal plane curve correction and balance, complications, and pulmonary function. It is associated with fewer transfusions, smaller incisions, and less operative loss. Disadvantages include single-lung ventilation and risk of bleeding. Long-term follow-up studies are needed to demonstrate clinical benefits.

iv. Surgical correction is a challenge in juvenile idiopathic scoliosis and in young children with scoliosis. Ideally, definitive surgery is delayed for skeletal maturity. However, in children with severe curves or rapidly progressing curves, bracing or casting alone may be inadequate and surgery is indicated. Traditionally, growing rods are implanted above and below the curve and then lengthened surgically every 6 to 12 months. The disadvantage is multiple surgeries with potential complications are required. A newer technique to avoid multiple surgeries is the use of *magnetic expansion control (MAGEC)* rods. MAGEC rods are implanted once and spinal lengthening is accomplished noninvasively with magnets and an external remote controller. The lengthening procedure is done every 3 to 4 months without surgery.

v. Children who develop TIS require monitoring and treatment. A surgical technique to improve or correct thoracic insufficiency is with a vertical expandable prosthetic titanium rib (VEPTR). The titanium prosthesis is inserted on the posterior part of the rib cage with one end attached to a superior rib and the distal end attached to an inferior rib. The device is then used to expand the ribs every 2 to 3 months while the child continues to skeletal maturity (Watts, 2016).

3. *Supportive Care*

a. Management of patients with scoliosis varies with the etiology, age of patient, severity of curve, comorbidities, and phase of treatment.

b. During the observation phase, maintaining good nutrition, bowel and bladder elimination, cardiac function, and respiratory function are important. Serial imaging is required to monitor the progression of the spinal curve and TIS.

c. During the bracing phase, monitoring as described is continued. Compliance with wearing a brace may be an issue with adolescents and continued support and education are required.

d. During the surgery phase, routine postoperative critical care is initiated. Neurovascular assessment of lower extremities is used to identify abnormal changes from baseline (e.g., hematoma compressing spinal cord).

i. Inadequate ventilation. Support ventilation as needed by administering supplemental oxygen to maintain SaO_2 >95%, maintaining pain control, assisting with airway clearance (suctioning, position changes, and cough and deep breathing), and administering bronchodilators as needed. Monitor chest tube drainage (for anterior fusions).

ii. Bleeding. Monitor intake and output, vital signs and hemodynamic pressures, thoracostomy tube drainage for amount and color, hemoglobin and hematocrit, surgical drains for amount and color, and surgical dressing for drainage amount and color.

iii. Pain. Use nonpharmacologic measures individualized to age, culture, and past experiences, including distractors, imagery, and controlled breathing. Encourage parental involvement. Administer analgesics by continuous infusion or patient-controlled analgesia. Position the child for comfort.

e. Psychological support is required at all phases of treatment.

E. OUTCOMES

1. Outcomes vary and depend on etiology of scoliosis, age of onset, severity of curve, and comorbidities.

2. Children with idiopathic early-onset scoliosis with curves greater than 30 to 35 degrees will usually have progression of their curve.

3. Children younger than 2 years of age with infantile idiopathic scoliosis and curves less than 35 degrees usually require no treatment.

4. Surgery can halt the progression of the lateral curve and, in most cases, improve the curve.

5. Most surgeries for routine AIS have low morbidity and mortality rates. Typically, children may return to school in 3 to 4 weeks with gradual return to activities over weeks and months.

CONGENITAL NEUROLOGIC ABNORMALITIES

A. Description and Etiology

1. *Myelodysplasia, spinal dysraphism,* and *spina bifida* are terms that are used interchangeably to describe a collection of disorders characterized by vertebral arch fusion defects and abnormalities of the spinal cord and coverings. These defects, as well as all disorders of the neural tube, are collectively referred to as *NTDs.* The two most common NTDs are spina bifida and anencephaly.

2. *Spina bifida cystica,* incomplete fusion of one or more vertebral laminae, results in external protrusion of the spinal tissue. Two classifications include *myelomeningocele,* a protruding saclike structure containing meninges, spinal fluid, and neural tissue, and *meningocele*, a protruding sac containing only meninges and CSF.

3. *Spina bifida occulta* is incomplete fusion at one level without a protrusion of neural structures. The defect is not apparent to the naked eye.

4. *Anencephaly* is a serious NTD in which parts of the brain and skull never develop. Almost universally, all anencehphalous newborns die shortly after birth.

5. The etiology of congenital neurologic abnormalities is unknown and possibly multifactorial. A deficiency in maternal folic acid is highly associated with NTDs. The abnormality occurs early in embryonic development.

B. Pathophysiology

1. NTDs result from failure of differentiation and closure of the embryonic neural tube. Defects occur early in gestational development, by the 17th to 30th day. The most common defects are anencephaly and myelomeningocele. Anencephaly results from failed closure of the rostral end of the neural tube and myelomeningocele from failed closure of the caudal end of the neural tube.

2. In spina bifida, the most common parts of the spine affected are the lower thoracic lumbar and sacral areas. The anterior aspects of the spinal cord are frequently intact with varying degrees of destruction to the dorsal columns. Sometimes it is associated with brain abnormalities, including cellular migration, agenesis of the corpus callosum, arachnoid cysts, and Arnold–Chiari malformations. The degree of functional impairment depends on the extent of the defect and associated neural tissue.

3. Some patients with NTDs develop progressive tethering (tethered cord syndrome) in which the spinal cord becomes fastened to a fixed structure (e.g., bone). Over time, with linear growth the spinal cord becomes abnormally stretched. This stretching can cause lower limb dysfunction and impairment of bowel and bladder elimination.

C. Clinical Presentation

1. *History*

    a. Most open NTDs are readily apparent at birth.

    b. Closed NTDs have a more varied presentation and may present without any sacral or cutaneous marker. Infants may have a history of asymmetry of legs or foot or hammering or clawing of the toes. Other historical findings may include weakness or sensory loss in a leg, and bowel or bladder dysfunction. Symptoms of spinal cord compression may be seen with a congenital dermal sinus or intraspinal cyst.

2. *Physical Examination*

    a. A complete neurological examination of the newborn with an open NTD is performed to identify and document structural and functional abnormalities. It is the baseline for future assessments.

    b. *Spina bifida occulta* often goes undetected. Possible signs (over the midline of the lumbosacral area) include a palpable mass, dermal sinus, skin discoloration, and a tuft of hair. Spinal cord or nerve involvement may demonstrate asymmetry of the lower extremities, persistent enuresis (late onset), and progressive weakness of one or both legs.

    c. *Meningocele* is a visible defect of the cord and covering. It may have minimal to no involvement of the lower extremities.

    d. *Myelomeningocele* dysfunction ranges from minimal impairment to total paralysis of the lower extremities. Lumbosacral lesions usually result in some hip, knee, or ankle flexion. Sensory involvement is usually symmetric but patchy. Usually, some degree of bowel and bladder dysfunction exists. *Arnold–Chiari type II* deformity is present in the majority of cases. It consists of elongation and herniation of the cerebellar vermis through the foramen magnum, displacement and distortion of the medulla (including the fourth ventricle), impeded CSF flow and hydrocephalus, and possibly lower bulbar dysfunction producing apnea, vocal cord paralysis, and stridor.

3. *Diagnostic Tests*

    a. Screen patient for latex allergies.

    b. Maternal *serum AFP* levels are used as a screening tool for open NTDs during the 16th and 18th weeks of gestation. Any level above the normal range is further evaluated. *Amniotic fluid AFP* levels can also be used to screen for NTDs.

    c. Neuroimaging

        i. *Radiographs* may be taken of the entire spine to identify the precise level of deformity and to rule out deformities at other levels.

ii. *CT scan* allows direct visualization of the bony defect and anatomy. It also helps to identify hydrocephalus. Risk of radiation exposure needs to be considered.

iii. *MRI* is the study of choice for imaging neural tissue and contents of the sac or defect. It can visualize both intracranial and intraspinal defects.

iv. *Ultrasound* technology is frequently used during pregnancy and it may identify an NTD.

4. *Clinical Course*

   a. Newborns with anencephaly usually die shortly after birth.

   b. Mild closed NTDs may go unrecognized or have subtle neurologic findings.

   c. Open NTDs have a varied course and it depends on the level of the defect and the amount of neural tissue involvement and presence of hydrocephalus.

D. Patient Care Management

1. *Preventive Care*

   a. *Folic acid* administered to women prior to the beginning of pregnancy through the first trimester has been shown to reduce the occurrence of NTDs.

   b. The American Academy of Pediatrics recommends daily administration of folic acid to all childbearing females (American Academy of Pediatrics. Committee on Genetics, 1999).

2. *Direct Care*

   a. There is no cure for NTDs. The nerve tissue that is damaged or fails to develop cannot be repaired or replaced. The priorities for treating myelomeningocele are prevention of infection and to protect the exposed nerves and structures from trauma.

   b. In recent years, immediate closure of the protruding sac is indicated. The goals of surgery are to preserve all neural tissue, provide a physiologic skin barrier, and control progressive hydrocephalus. Surgical closure involves several steps, including dissection of the exposed sac, closure of the dura over preserved neural tissue, and closure of the skin covering the repair. Skin grafting may be necessary.

   c. If hydrocephalus is present, a CSF shunting device is inserted, or the foramen magnum is enlarged.

   d. Surgical release of a tethered cord may be indicated for some patients with tethered cord syndrome. Early surgery may reverse neurologic symptoms.

3. *Supportive Care*

   a. Management depends on the type of NTD the patient has and the severity of neurologic impairment.

   b. Newborns with myelomeningocele present challenges during vaginal delivery (protecting the sac from trauma) and during the resuscitation phase. Newborns often need positive pressure ventilation and positioning the newborn for bag-valve-mask ventilation and intubation requires a team approach (da Silva et al., 2014).

   c. For open NTDs, protect the sac with a sterile saline moist dressing preoperatively and maintain the child in a prone or side-lying position before and immediately after the operation to promote wound healing.

   d. Provide routine postoperative care, maintain sterile dry wound dressings, administer antibiotics as ordered, and prevent contamination of the wound from feces and urine. Monitor vital signs, WBC count, cultures, and urine studies; assess the sac's protective barrier (before and after the operation) for drainage, odor, and color; assess neurologic functioning, including head circumference and fontanelles and signs of increased ICP; and assess for bladder distention and monitoring urinary output.

   e. Patients with ventricular shunts need routine postoperative management and follow-up (see section on intracranial devices).

   f. Children with NTDs often have latex allergies. Provide a latex-free environment: label room "latex safe," remove all latex products from patient's immediate environment, check all products for latex content, notify ancillary departments; and disseminate latex allergy protocol.

   g. Some children require assistive devices (e.g., wheelchairs, walkers, braces) for their daily activities.

   h. Bowel and bladder elimination is altered for many children requiring intermittent catheterizations and bowel management regimen.

E. Outcomes

1. Outcomes depend on the etiology, severity of defect, and associated environmental factors.

2. Generally, children with spina bifida can have active lives, but some may require assist devices. Intelligence and learning are often normal.

CASE STUDIES WITH QUESTIONS, ANSWERS, AND RATIONALES

Case Study 4.1

A 5-year-old female (unrestrained) was ejected from the back seat of a car during a motor vehicle collision. At the scene, the child was responsive to pain, moaning, and becoming progressively more agitated. Her GCS was 11. On admission to the emergency department, she underwent routine trauma screening and had a CT scan of her head and cervical spine. The radiologist read the brain CT and identified a biconvex-shaped (lenticular) hyperdense area with a significant midline shift. The CT scan of the cervical spine was negative. During the CT scan, the child's GCS decreased to 9.

1. Based on the CT scan report and clinical presentation, the child most likely has the following traumatic brain injury:
   A. Diffuse cerebral swelling
   B. Subdural hematoma
   C. Brainstem hemorrhage
   D. Epidural hematoma

2. Once the patient was diagnosed by CT scan with a neurologic injury, the most important next intervention would be to
   A. Transfer the patient to the PICU
   B. Transfer the patient to the operating room
   C. Transfer the patient to the general floor
   D. Transfer the patient back to the emergency department

3. Twelve hours postinjury, the child is in the PICU, intubated, ventilated with monitoring of central venous pressure, peripheral arterial pressure, and ICP. The ICP is 18 mmHg, and the arterial pressure is 110/73 mmHg with a mean of 86. The CPP is best described as
   A. Normal
   B. Too low for her age
   C. Too high for her age
   D. Cannot be determined from information

4. Two days postinjury, the patient is diagnosed with tetraplegia (all four limbs). The diagnostic test that should be performed at this point in time is
   A. Repeat CT of the cervical spine
   B. Brainstem auditory evoked potential response

   C. MRI of the cervical spine
   D. Cerebral arterial angiogram

Case Study 4.2

A 5-month-old male is admitted to the PICU with a 3-day history of fever, upper respiratory symptoms, and irritability. Currently, the infant's vital signs are temperature 40°C, heart rate 100 bpm, respiratory rate 32 breaths/min, blood pressure 110/85 mmHg, and pulse oximetry 94%. He is lethargic and only responds to painful stimuli. His anterior fontanel is full and tense, pupils are reactive, and GCS is 12. His perfusion and color are good and he moves all extremities, albeit weakly. Intravenous access is secured and fluids started. A CBC, blood cultures, and metabolic panel are drawn. Bedside glucose is 98 mg/dL. Increased ICP is suspected.

1. The next interventions should be
   A. Lumbar puncture, then administer ceftriaxone
   B. CT scan, then administer ceftriaxone
   C. Administer ceftriaxone, then get CT scan
   D. CT scan, then lumbar puncture

2. A lumbar puncture with CSF analysis is performed. The CSF analysis shows clear fluid, total WBC of 475 cells/mcL, 80% lymphocytes, glucose 60 mg% (serum glucose 90 mg/dL, and protein 55 mg/dL. Gram stain is negative.

   The CSF analysis best describes which of the following central nervous system infections?
   A. Viral meningitis
   B. Bacterial meningitis
   C. Viral encephalitis
   D. Bacterial encephalitis

3. Based on the CSF results, the nurse should anticipate which intervention:
   A. Administer acyclovir
   B. Discontinue antibiotic
   C. Adding vancomycin to ceftriaxone
   D. Administer immunoglobulin (IVIG)

Answers and Rationales

Case Study 4.1

1. **D.** The CT scan identified a common feature of epidural hematoma; biconvex hyperdense area with a midline shift. An acute deterioration in her GCS also is highly suspicious of a rapidly expanding lesion that can occur from arterial bleeding. Epidural bleeding is frequently from the middle meningeal artery.

2. B. The patient requires immediate evacuation of the epidural hematoma and control of bleeding.

3. A. CPP is calculated; MAP minus mean ICP equals 68 mmHg, which is normal for this patient.

4. C. Because of the malleability of the pediatric cervical spine, it is possible to have significant spinal cord damage without obvious injury to the vertebrae. The condition is known as *spinal cord injury without radiographic abnormality (SCIWORA)*. An MRI is needed to identify cervical tissue injury.

Case Study 4.2

1. C. If increased ICP is suspected, the lumbar puncture should be delayed until confirmation of a normal ICP. However, antibiotic administration should not be delayed while getting a CT scan.

2. A. Viral meningitis (aseptic meningitis) is characterized by WBC less than 1000 cells/mcL, lymphocytic predominance, glucose greater than 60% of serum glucose, elevated protein, negative Gram stain, and clear appearance.

3. B. The meningitis is viral and antibiotics are not indicated.

REFERENCES

Abels, L. (1986). *Critical care nursing: A physiologic approach.* St. Louis, MO: Mosby.

Abend, N. S., Bearden, D., Helbig, I., McGuire, J., Narula, S., Panzer, J. A., . . . Dlugos, D. J. (2014). Status epilepticus and refractory status epilepticus management. *Seminars in Pediatric Neurology, 21*(4), 263–274. doi:10.1016/j.spen.2014.12.006

Abend, N. S., Topjian, A. A., Kessler, S. K., Gutierrez-Colina, A. M., Berg, R. A., Nadkarni, V., . . . Ichord, R. N. (2012). Outcome prediction by motor and pupillary responses in children treated with therapeutic hypothermia after cardiac arrest. *Pediatric Critical Care Medicine, 13*(1), 32–38. doi:10.1097/pcc.0b013e3182196a7b

Al-Abdi, S., & Al-Aamri, M. (2014). A systematic review and meta-analysis of the timing of early intraventricular hemorrhage in preterm neonates: Clinical and research implications. *Journal of Clinical Neonatology, 3*(2), 76–88. doi:10.4103/2249-4847.134674

Amarilyo, G., Alper, A., Ben-Tov, A., & Grisaru-Soen, G. (2011). Diagnostic accuracy of clinical symptoms and signs in children with meningitis. *Pediatric Emergency Care, 27*(3), 196–199. doi:10.1097/pec.0b013e31820d6543

Ambuel, B., Hamlett, K. W., Marx, C. M., & Blumer, J. L. (1992). Assessing distress in pediatric intensive care environments: The COMFORT Scale. *Journal of Pediatric Psychology, 17*(1), 95–109. doi:10.1093/jpepsy/17.1.95

American Academy of Pediatrics. (2011). Febrile seizures: Guideline for the neurodiagnostic evaluation of the child with a simple febrile seizure. *Pediatrics, 127*(2), 389–394. doi:10.1542/peds.2010-3318

American Academy of Pediatrics Committee on Genetics. (1999). Folic acid for the prevention of neural tube defects. *Pediatrics, 104*(2), 325–327. doi:10.1542/peds.104.2.325

American Association of Neuroscience Nurses. (2011). Care of the patient undergoing intracranial pressure monitoring/external ventricular drainage or lumbar drainage. Retrieved from http://apps.aann.org/Default.aspx?TabID=251&productId=192054487

Avery, R. A. (2014). Interpretation of lumbar puncture opening pressure measurements in children. *Journal of Neuro-Ophthalmology, 34*(3), 284–287. doi:10.1097/wno.0000000000000154

Bai, J., Hsu, L., Tang, Y., & van Dijk, M. (2012). Validation of the COMFORT behavior scale and the FLACC scale for pain assessment in Chinese children after cardiac surgery. *Pain Management Nursing, 13*(1), 18–26. doi:10.1016/j.pmn.2010.07.002

Ballabh, P. (2010). Intraventricular hemorrhage in premature infants: Mechanism of disease. *Pediatric Research, 67*(1), 1–8. doi:10.1203/pdr.0b013e3181c1b176

Bano, S., Chaudhary, V., Garga, U. C., Yadav, S., & Singh, S. K. (2014). Intracranial hemorrhage in the newborn. In V. Chaudhary (Ed.), Intracerebral hemorrhage (pp. 1–10). London, United Kingdom: IntechOpen. doi:10.5772/58476

Benarroch, E. E. (2012). Blood–brain barrier: Recent developments and clinical correlations. *Neurology, 78*, 1268–1276. doi:10.1212/WNL.0b013e318250d8bc

Berg, A. T., Berkovic, S. F., Brodie, M. J., Buchhalter, J., Cross, J. H., van Emde Boas, W., . . . Scheffer, I. E. (2010). Revised terminology and concepts for organization of seizures and epilepsies: Report of the ILAE Commission on Classification and Terminology, 2005–2009. *Epilepsia, 51*(4), 676–685. doi:10.1111/j.1528-1167.2010.02522.x

Betz, C. L., Hunsberger, M. M., & Wright, S. (1994). *Family-centered nursing care of children* (2nd ed.). Philadelphia, PA: W. B. Saunders.

Bhagat, H., Bhardwaj, A., & Grover, V. (2015). Jugular venous oximetry. *Journal of Neuroanaesthesiology and Critical Care, 2*(3), 225. doi:10.4103/2348-0548.165046

Bilavsky, E., Leibovitz, E., Elkon-Tamir, E., Fruchtman, Y., Ifergan, G., & Greenberg, D. (2013). The diagnostic accuracy of the 'classic meningeal signs' in children with suspected bacterial meningitis. *European Journal of Emergency Medicine, 20*(5), 361–363. doi:10.1097/mej.0b013e3283585f20

Brophy, G. M., Bell, R., Claassen, J., Alldredge, B., Bleck, T. P., Glauser, T., . . . Vespa, P. M. (2012). Guidelines for the evaluation and management of status epilepticus. *Neurocritical Care, 17*(1), 3–23. doi:10.1007/s12028-012-9695-z

Bulat, M., & Klarica, M. (2011). Recent insights into a new hydrodynamics of the cerebrospinal fluid. *Brain Research Reviews, 65*(2), 99–112. doi:10.1016/j.brainresrev.2010.08.002

Carlson, A. P., Brown, A. M., Zager, E., Uchino, K., Marks, M. P., Robertson, C., . . . Yonas, H. (2011). Xenon-enhanced cerebral blood flow at 28% xenon provides uniquely safe access to quantitative, clinically useful cerebral blood flow information: A multicenter study. *American Journal of Neuroradiology, 32*(7), 1315–1320. doi:10.3174/ajnr.a2522

Cartwright, C. C., & Wallace, D. C. (Eds.). (2007). *Nursing care of the pediatric neurosurgery patient.* Berlin, Germany: Springer-Verlag

Cecil, S., Chen, P. M., Callaway, S. E., Rowland, S. M., Adler, D. E., & Chen, J. W. (2011). Traumatic brain injury: Advanced multimodal neuromonitoring from theory to clinical practice. *Critical Care Nurse*, 31(2), 25–37. doi:10.4037/ccn2010226

Committee on Fetus and Newborn, Papile LA, Baley JE, Benitz W, Cummings J, Carlo WA, . . . Wang KS. (2014). Hypothermia and neonatal encephalopathy. *Pediatrics*, 133(6), 1146–1150. doi:10.1542/peds.2014-0899

Curley, M. A., Harris, S. K., & Fraser, K. (2006). State behavioral scale (SBS) a sedation assessment instrument for infants and young children supported on mechanical ventilation. *Pediatric Critical Care Medicine*, 7(2), 195. doi:10.1097/00130478-200603000-00039

Curley, M. A., & Patricia, M. A. (2001). *Critical care nursing of infants and children* (2nd ed.). Philadelphia, PA: W. B. Saunders.

Donkin, J. J., & Vink, R. (2010). Mechanisms of cerebral edema in traumatic brain injury: Therapeutic developments. *Current Opinion in Neurology*, 23(3), 293–299. doi:10.1097/wco.0b013e328337f451

Falchek, S. J. (2012). Encephalitis in the pediatric population. *Pediatrics in Review*, 33(3), 122–133. doi:10.1542/pir.33-3-122

Faul, M., Xu, L., Wald, M. M., Coronado, V., & Dellinger, A. M. (2010). Traumatic brain injury in the United States: National estimates of prevalence and incidence, 2002–2006. *Injury Prevention*, 16(Suppl. 1), A268. doi:10.1136/ip.2010.029215.951

Fleming, A. J., & Chi, S. N. (2012). Brain tumors in children. *Current Problems in Pediatric and Adolescent Health Care*, 42(4), 80–103. doi:10.1016/j.cppeds.2011.12.002

Fuhrman, B. P., & Zimmerman, J. J. (1992). *Pediatric critical care*. St. Louis, MO: Mosby-Year Book.

Glauser, T., Shinnar, S., Gloss, D., Alldredge, B., Arya, R., Bainbridge, J., . . . Treiman, D. (2016). Evidence-based guideline: Treatment of convulsive status epilepticus in children and adults: Report of the guideline committee on the American Epilepsy Society. *Epilepsy Currents*, 16(1), 48–61. doi:10.5698/1535-7597-16.1.48

Greenham, M., Gordon, A., Anderson, V., & Mackay, M. T. (2016). Outcome in childhood stroke. *Stroke*, 47(4), 1159–1164. doi:10.1161/strokeaha.115.011622

Harris, C. (2014). Neuromonitoring indications and utility in the intensive care unit. *Critical Care Nurse*, 34(3), 30–40. doi:10.4037/ccn2014506

Heffren, J., McIntosh, A. M., & Reiter, P. D. (2015). Nimodipine for the prevention of cerebral vasospasm after subarachnoid hemorrhage in 12 children. *Pediatric Neurology*, 52, 356–360. doi:10.1016/j.pediatrneurol.2014.11.003

Horn, A. R., Swingler, G. H., Myer, L., Linley, L. L., Raban, M. S., Joolay, Y., . . . Robertson, N. J. (2013). Early clinical signs in neonates with hypoxic ischemic encephalopathy predict an abnormal amplitude-integrated electroencephalogram at age 6 hours. *BMC Pediatrics*, 13(1), 52. doi:10.1186/1471-2431-13-52

Hurlbert, R. J., Hadley, M. N., Walters, B. C., Aarabi, B., Dhall, S. S., Gelb, D. E., . . . Theodore, N. (2013). Pharmacological therapy for acute spinal cord injury. *Neurosurgery*, 72, 93–105. doi:10.1227/neu.0b013e31827765c6

Imataka, G., & Arisaka, O. (2015). Brain hypothermia therapy for childhood acute encephalopathy based on clinical evidence (Review). *Experimental and Therapeutic Medicine*, 10, 1624–1626. doi:10.3892/etm.2015.2760

Ista, E., van Dijk, M., de Hoog, M., Tibboel, D., & Duivenvoorden, H. (2009). Construction of the Sophia Observation withdrawal Symptoms-scale (SOS) for critically ill children. *Intensive Care Medicine*, 35, 1075–1081. doi:10.1007/s00134-009-1487-3

Jensen, D. (1980). *The human nervous system*. New York, NY: Appleton-Century-Crofts.

Kaspiris, A., Grivas, T. B., Weiss, H., & Turnbull, D. (2011). Surgical and conservative treatment of patients with congenital scoliosis: α search for long-term results. *Scoliosis*, 6(1), 12. doi:10.1186/1748-7161-6-12

Kirkham, F. J., Newton, C. R., & Whitehouse, W. (2008). Paediatric coma scales. *Developmental Medicine & Child Neurology*, 50, 267–274. doi:10.1111/j.1469-8749.2008.02042.x

Kirshblum, S. C., Burns, S. P., Biering-Sorensen, F., Donovan, W., Graves, D. E., Jha, A., . . . Waring, W. (2011). International standards for neurological classification of spinal cord injury (Revised 2011). *Journal of Spinal Cord Medicine*, 34(6), 535–546. doi:10.1179/204577211X13207446293695

Kitchen, L., Westmacott, R., Friefeld, S., MacGregor, D., Curtis, R., Allen, A., . . . deVeber, G. (2012). The pediatric stroke outcome measure: A validation and reliability study. *Stroke*, 43(6), 1602–1608. doi:10.1161/strokeaha.111.639583

Knake, J. E. (1978). Incidence and evolution of subependymal and intraventricular hemorrhage. *Journal of Computer Assisted Tomography*, 2(5), 667. doi:10.1097/00004728-197811000-00063

Kochanek, P. M., Carney, N., Adelson, P. D., Ashwal, S., Bell, M. J., Bratton, S., . . . Warden, C. R. (2012). Guidelines for the acute medical management of severe traumatic brain injury in infants, children, and adolescents—Second edition. *Pediatric Critical Care Medicine*, 13(Suppl. 1), S1–S2. doi:10.1097/pcc.0b013e31823f435c

Krishnamurthy, S., & Li, J. (2014). New concepts in the pathogenesis of hydrocephalus. *Translational Pediatrics*, 3(3), 185–194. doi:10.3978/j.issn.2224-4336.2014.07.02

Lanni, G., Catalucci, A., Conti, L., Di Sibio, A., Paonessa, A., & Gallucci, M. (2011). Pediatric stroke: Clinical findings and radiological approach. *Stroke Research and Treatment*, 2011, 1–11. doi:10.4061/2011/172168

Leonard, J. C., Kuppermann, N., Olsen, C., Babcock-Cimpello, L., Brown, K., Mahajan, P., . . . Jaffe, D. M. (2011). Factors associated with cervical spine injury in children after blunt trauma. *Annals of Emergency Medicine*, 58(2), 145–155. doi:10.1016/j.annemergmed.2010.08.038

Leonard, J. R., Jaffe, D. M., Kuppermann, N., Olsen, C. S., & Leonard, J. C. (2014). Cervical spine injury patterns in children. *Pediatrics*, 133(5), e1179–e1188. doi:10.1542/peds.2013-3505

Le Roux, P., Menon, D. K., Citerio, G., Vespa, P., Bader, M. K., Brophy, G. M., . . . Taccone, F. (2014). Consensus summary statement of the International Multidisciplinary Consensus Conference on multimodality monitoring in neurocritical care. *Neurocritical Care*, 21(S2), 1–26. doi:10.1007/s12028-014-0041-5

Levy, B. J., Schulz, J. F., Fornari, E. D., & Wollowick, A. L. (2015). Complications associated with surgical repair of syndromic scoliosis. *Scoliosis*, 10(1), 14. doi:10.1186/s13013-015-0035-x

Louis, D. N., Perry, A., Reifenberger, G., Deimling, A. V., Figarella-Branger, D., Cavenee, W. K., . . . Ellison, D. W. (2016). The 2016 World Health Organization classification of tumors of the central nervous system: A summary. *Acta Neuropathologica*, 131(6), 803–820. doi:10.1007/s00401-016-1545-1

Luetz, A., Gensel, D., Müller, J., Weiss, B., Martiny, V., Heinz, A., . . . Spies, C. (2016). Validity of different delirium assessment tools for critically ill children: Covariates matter. *Critical Care Medicine*, 44(11), 2060–2069. doi:10.1097/CCM.0000000000001840

Maesaka, J., Imbriano, L., Mattana, J., Gallagher, D., Bade, N., & Sharif, S. (2014). Differentiating SIADH from cerebral/renal salt wasting: Failure of the volume approach and need for a new approach to hyponatremia. *Journal of Clinical Medicine*, 3(4), 1373–1385. doi:10.3390/jcm3041373

Marimón, G. A., Dockery, W. K., Sheridan, M. J., & Agarwal, S. (2012). Near-infrared spectroscopy cerebral and somatic (renal) oxygen saturation correlation to continuous venous oxygen saturation via intravenous oximetry catheter. *Journal of Critical Care, 27*(3), 314.e13–314.e18. doi:10.1016/j.jcrc.2011.10.002

McCrory, P., Meeuwisse, W., Johnston, K., Dvorak, J., Aubry, M., Molloy, M., & Cantu, R. (2009). Consensus statement on concussion in sport 3rd international conference on concussion in sport held in Zurich, November 2008. *Clinical Journal of Sport Medicine, 19*(3), 185–200. doi:10.1097/jsm.0b013e3181a501db

McQuillan, K. A. (1991). Intracranial pressure monitoring: Technical imperatives. *AACN Advanced Critical Care, 2*(4), 623–636. doi:10.4037/15597768-1991-4003

Ment, L. R., Bada, H. S., Barnes, P., Grant, P. E., Hirtz, D., Papile, L. A., . . . Slovis, T. L. (2002). Practice parameter: Neuroimaging of the neonate: [RETIRED] Report of the Quality Standards Subcommittee of the American Academy of Neurology and the Practice Committee of the Child Neurology Society. *Neurology, 58*(12), 1726–1738. doi:10.1212/wnl.58.12.1726

Merkel, S., Voepel-Lewis, T., & Malviya, S. (2002). Pain assessment in infants and young children: The FLACC scale. *American Journal of Nursing, 102*(10), 55–58. doi:10.1097/00000446-200210000-00024

Miyanji, F. (2014). Adolescent idiopathic scoliosis: Current perspectives. *Orthopedic Research and Reviews, 2014,* (6) 17–26. doi:10.2147/orr.s37321

Moore, K. L., & Persaud, T. V. N. (1993). *The developing human: Clinically oriented embryology* (5th ed.). Philadelphia, PA: Elsevier.

Morris, G. L., Gloss, D., Buchhalter, J., Mack, K. J., Nickels, K., & Harden, C. (2013). Evidence-based guideline update: Vagus nerve stimulation for the treatment of epilepsy. *Epilepsy Currents, 13*(6), 297–303. doi:10.5698/1535-7597-13.6.297

Morrison, C. A. M. (1987). Brain herniation syndromes. *Critical Care Nursing, 7*(5), 35–38.

Nakagawa, T. A., Ashwal, S., Mathur, M., Mysore, M., & The Committee for Determination of Brain Death in Infants Children (2012). Guidelines for the determination of brain death in infants and children: An update of the 1987 task force recommendations—Executive summary. *Annals of Neurology, 71*(4), 573–585. doi:10.1002/ana.23552

Nigrovic, L. E., Fine, A. M., Monuteaux, M. C., Shah, S. S., & Neuman, M. I. (2013). Trends in the management of viral meningitis at United States children's hospitals. *Pediatrics, 131*(4), 670–676. doi:10.1542/peds.2012-3077

Oddo, M., Villa, F., & Citerio, G. (2012). Brain multimodality monitoring. *Current Opinion in Critical Care, 18*(2), 111–118. doi:10.1097/mcc.0b013e32835132a5

Orešković, D., & Klarica, M. (2010). The formation of cerebrospinal fluid: Nearly a hundred years of interpretations and misinterpretations. *Brain Research Reviews, 64,* 241–262. doi:10.1016/j.brainresrev.2010.04.006

Orešković, D., & Klarica, M. (2011). Development of hydrocephalus and classical hypothesis of cerebrospinal fluid hydrodynamics: Facts and illusions. *Progress in Neurobiology, 94*(3), 238–258. doi:10.1016/j.pneurobio.2011.05.005

Perkin, R. M., & Ashwal, S. (2012). Hypoxic-ischemic encephalopathy in infants and older children. *Swaiman's Pediatric Neurology, 2,* 1149–1184. doi:10.1016/b978-1-4377-0435-8.00076-7

Pettiford, J. N., Bikhchandani, J., Ostlie, D. J., St. Peter, S. D., Sharp, R. J., & Juang, D. (2011). A review: The role of high dose methylprednisolone in spinal cord trauma in children. *Pediatric Surgery International, 28*(3), 287–294. doi:10.1007/s00383-011-3012-3

Piro, E. (2015). Germinal matrix hemorrhage-intraventricular hemorrhage: Pathogenesis and outcomes. *Italian Journal of Pediatrics, 41*(Suppl. 1), A31. doi:10.1186/1824-7288-41-s1-a31

Posner, J. B., Saper, C. B., Schiff, N. D., & Plum, F. (2007). *Plum and Posner's diagnosis of stupor and coma* (4th ed.). New York, NY: Oxford University Press.

Poussaint, T. Y., Panigrahy, A., & Huisman, T. A. (2015). Pediatric brain tumors. *Pediatric Radiology, 45*(Suppl. 3), 443–453. doi:10.1007/s00247-015-3326-8

Raboel, P. H., Bartek, J., Jr., Andresen, M., Bellander, B. M., & Romner, B. (2012). Intracranial pressure monitoring: Invasive versus non-invasive methods—A review. *Critical Care Research and Practice, 2012,* 1–14. doi:10.1155/2012/950393

Rao, V., Klepstad, P., Losvik, O. K., & Solheim, O. (2013). Confusion with cerebral perfusion pressure in a literature review of current guidelines and survey of clinical practice. *Scandinavian Journal of Trauma, Resuscitation & Emergency Medicine, 21*(1), 78–82. doi:10.1186/1757-7241-21-78

Richard, G. C., & Lepe, M. (2013). Meningitis in children: Diagnosis and treatment for the emergency clinician. *Clinical Pediatric Emergency Medicine, 14*(2), 146–156. doi:10.1016/j.cpem.2013.04.008

Riquet, A., Lamblin, M., Bastos, M., Bulteau, C., Derambure, P., Vallée, L., & Auvin, S. (2011). Usefulness of video-EEG monitoring in children. *Seizure, 20*(1), 18–22. doi:10.1016/j.seizure.2010.09.011

Roach, E. S., Golomb, M. R., Adams, R., Biller, J., Daniels, S., deVeber, G., . . . Smith, E. R. (2008). Management of stroke in infants and children: A scientific statement from a special writing group of the American Heart Association Stroke Council and the Council on Cardiovascular Disease in the Young. *Stroke, 39*(9), 2644–2691. doi:10.1161/strokeaha.108.189696

Roger, V. L., Go, A. S., Lloyd-Jones, D. M., Benjamin, E. J., Berry, J. D., Borden, W. B., . . . Turner, M. B. (2011). Heart disease and stroke statistics—2012 update: A report from the American Heart Association. *Circulation, 125*(1), e2–e220. doi:10.1161/cir.0b013e31823ac046

Rosa, M., De Lucia, S., Rinaldi, V. E., Gal, J. L., Desmarest, M., Veropalumbo, C., . . . Titomanlio, L. (2015). Paediatric arterial ischemic stroke: Acute management, recent advances and remaining issues. *Italian Journal of Pediatrics, 41*(1), 95. doi:10.1186/s13052-015-0174-y

Rostami, E., Engquist, H., & Enblad, P. (2014). Imaging of cerebral blood flow in patients with severe traumatic brain injury in the neurointensive care. *Frontiers in Neurology, 5,* 114. doi:10.3389/fneur.2014.00114

Rungta, R., Choi, H., Tyson, J., Malik, A., Dissing-Olesen, L., Lin, P., . . . MacVicar, B. (2015). The cellular mechanisms of neuronal swelling underlying cytotoxic edema. *Cell, 161*(3), 610–621. doi:10.1016/j.cell.2015.03.029

Russ, S. A., Larson, K., & Halfon, N. (2012). A national profile of childhood epilepsy and seizure disorder. *Pediatrics, 129*(2), 256–264. doi:10.1542/peds.2010-1371

Sakka, L., Coll, G., & Chazal, J. (2011). Anatomy and physiology of cerebrospinal fluid. *European Annals of Otorhinolaryngology, Head and Neck Diseases, 128*(6), 309–316. doi:10.1016/j.anorl.2011.03.002

Sarnat, H. B., & Sarnat, M. S. (1976). Neonatal encephalopathy following fetal distress. *Archives of Neurology, 33*(10), 696-705. doi:10.1001/archneur.1976.00500100030012

Scheeren, T. W., Schober, P., & Schwarte, L. A. (2012). Monitoring tissue oxygenation by near infrared spectroscopy (NIRS):

Background and current applications. *Journal of Clinical Monitoring and Computing, 26*(4), 279–287. doi:10.1007/s10877-012-9348-y

Scher, M. S., & Ashwal, S. (1999). Pediatric neurophysiologic evaluation. In K. F. Swaiman (Ed.), *Pediatric neurology* (3rd ed., pp. 142–181). St. Louis, MO: Mosby.

Schöneberg, C., Schweiger, B., Hussmann, B., Kauther, M. D., Lendemans, S., & Waydhas, C. (2013). Diagnosis of cervical spine injuries in children: A systematic review. *European Journal of Trauma and Emergency Surgery, 39*(6), 653–665. doi:10.1007/s00068-013-0295-1

Schöneberg, C., Schweiger, B., Lendemans, S., & Waydhas, C. (2013b). Special considerations in the interpretation of plain radiographs of the cervical spine in children. A review of the literature. *European Journal of Trauma and Emergency Surgery, 39*(6), 647–652. doi:10.1007/s00068-013-0305-3

Shardlow, E., & Jackson, A. (2008). Cerebral blood flow and intracranial pressure. *Anaesthesia & Intensive Care Medicine, 9*(5), 222–225. doi:10.1016/j.mpaic.2008.03.009

Sikich, N., & Lerman, J. (2004). Development and psychometric evaluation of the pediatric anesthesia emergence delirium scale. *Anesthesiology, 100*, 1138–1145. Retrieved from http://anesthesiology.pubs.asahq.org/article.aspx?articleid=1942731

da Silva, S. A., de Almeida, M. F., Moron, A. F., Cavalheiro, S., Dastoli, P. A., & Guinsburg, R. (2014). Resuscitation at birth in neonates with meningomyelocele. *Journal of Perinatal Medicine, 42*(1), 113–119. doi:10.1515/jpm-2013-0021

Silver, G., Traube, C., Gerber, L. M., Sun, X., Kearney, J., Patel, A., & Greenwald, B. (2015). Pediatric delirium and associated risk factors. *Pediatric Critical Care Medicine, 16*(4), 303–309. doi:10.1097/pcc.0000000000000356

Simma, B., Höliner, I., & Luetschg, J. (2012). Therapy in pediatric stroke. *European Journal of Pediatrics, 172*(7), 867–875. doi:10.1007/s00431-012-1863-9

Slota, M. C. (1983a). Neurological assessment of the infant and toddler. *Critical Care Nursing, 3*(5), 87–94.

Slota, M. C. (1983b). Pediatric neurological assessment. *Critical Care Nursing, 3*(6), 106–112.

Smith, H., Boyd, J., Fuchs, D., Melvin, K., Berry, P., Shintani, A., . . . Ely, E. (2011). Diagnosing delirium in critically ill children: Validity and reliability of Pediatric Confusion Assessment Method for the intensive care unit. *Critical Care Medicine, 39*(1), 150–157. doi:10.1097/CCM.0b013e3181feb489

Sood, B. G., McLaughlin, K., & Cortez, J. (2015). Near-infrared spectroscopy: Applications in neonates. *Seminars in Fetal and Neonatal Medicine, 20*(3), 164–172. doi:10.1016/j.siny.2015.03.008

Spennato, P., Nicosia, G., Quaglietta, L., Donofrio, V., Mirone, G., Martino, G. D., . . . Cinalli, G. (2015). Posterior fossa tumors in infants and neonates. *Child's Nervous System, 31*(10), 1751–1772. doi:10.1007/s00381-015-2783-6

Srinivasan, L., Shah, S. S., Padula, M. A., Abbasi, S., McGowan, K. L., & Harris, M. C. (2012, October). Cerebrospinal fluid reference ranges in term and preterm infants in the neonatal intensive care unit. *Journal of Pediatrics, 161*(4), 729–734 doi:10.1016/j.jpeds.2012.03.051.

Swaiman, K. F., & Ashwal, S. (1999). *Pediatric neurology: Principles & practice* (3rd ed.). Philadelphia, PA: Mosby.

Swanson, D. (2015). Meningitis. *Pediatrics in Review, 36*(12), 514–526. doi:10.1542/pir.36-12-514

Taketomo, C. K., Hodding, J. H., & Kraus, D. M. (2015). *Pediatric & neonatal dosage handbook: A universal resource for clinicians treating pediatric and neonatal patients* (22nd ed.). Hudson, OH: Lexicomp.

Tameem, A., & Krovvidi, H. (2013). Cerebral physiology. *Continuing Education in Anaesthesia Critical Care & Pain, 13*(4), 113–118. doi:10.1093/bjaceaccp/mkt001

Tan, Y. C., Gill, A. K., & Kim, K. S. (2015). Treatment strategies for central nervous system infections: An update. *Expert Opinion on Pharmacotherapy, 16*(2), 187–203. doi:10.1517/14656566.2015.973851

Teasdale, G., & Jennett, B. (1974). Assessment of coma and impaired consciousness. *Lancet, 304*(7872), 81–84 doi:10.1016/S0140-6736(74)91639-0.

Thigpen, M. C., Whitney, C. G., Messonnier, N. E., Zell, E. R., Lynfield, R., Hadler, J. L., . . . Schuchat, A. (2011). Bacterial meningitis in the United States, 1998–2007. *New England Journal of Medicine, 364*(21), 2016–2025. doi:10.1056/nejmoa1005384

Thompson, C., Kneen, R., Riordan, A., Kelly, D., & Pollard, A. J. (2012). Encephalitis in children. *Archives of Disease in Childhood, 97*(2), 150–161. doi:10.1136/archdischild-2011-300100

Tilt, L., Babineau, J., Fenster, D., Ahmad, F., & Roskind, C. G. (2012). Blunt cervical spine injury in children. *Current Opinion in Pediatrics, 24*(3), 301–306. doi:10.1097/mop.0b013e3283527035

Tracy, E. T., Englum, B. R., Barbas, A. S., Foley, C., Rice, H. E., & Shapiro, M. L. (2013). Pediatric injury patterns by year of age. *Journal of Pediatric Surgery, 48*(6), 1384–1388. doi:10.1016/j.jpedsurg.2013.03.041

Traube, C., Silver, G., Kearney, J., Patel, A., Atkinson, T. M., Yoon, M. J., . . . Greenwald, B. (2014). Cornell Assessment of Pediatric Delirium: A valid, rapid, observational tool for screening delirium in the PICU. *Critical Care Medicine, 42*(3), 656–663. doi:10.1097/CCM.0b013e3182a66b76

Tsze, D. S., & Valente, J. H. (2011). Pediatric stroke: A review. *Emergency Medicine International, 2011*, 1–10. doi:10.1155/2011/734506

Tully, H. M., Ishak, G. E., Rue, T. C., Dempsey, J. C., Browd, S. R., Millen, K. J., . . . Dobyns, W. B. (2015). Two hundred thirty-six children with developmental hydrocephalus: Causes and clinical consequences. *Journal of Child Neurology, 31*(3), 309–320. doi:10.1177/0883073815592222

Vialle, R., Thévenin-Lemoine, C., & Mary, P. (2013). Neuromuscular scoliosis. *Orthopaedics & Traumatology: Surgery & Research, 99*(1 Suppl.), S124–S139. doi:10.1016/j.otsr.2012.11.002

Volpe, J. J. (2015). Impaired neurodevelopmental outcome after mild germinal matrix-intraventricular hemorrhage. *Pediatrics, 136*(6), 1185–1187. doi:10.1542/peds.2015-3553

Wajchenberg, M., Astur, N., Kanas, M., & Martins, D. E. (2016). Adolescent idiopathic scoliosis: Current concepts on neurological and muscular etiologies. *Scoliosis and Spinal Disorders Scoliosis, 11*(1), 4. doi:10.1186/s13013-016-0066-y

Watts, S. L. (2016). Use of a vertical expandable prosthetic titanium rib in children with thoracic insufficiency syndrome and scoliosis. *Critical Care Nurse, 36*(2), 52–61. doi:10.4037/ccn2016230

Waxman, S. G. (1996). *Correlative neuroanatomy* (23rd ed.). Stamford, CT: Appleton & Lange.

Weinstein, S. L., Dolan, L. A., Wright, J. G., & Dobbs, M. B. (2013). Effects of bracing in adolescents with idiopathic scoliosis. *New England Journal of Medicine, 369*(16), 1512–1521. doi:10.1056/nejmoa1307337

Welch, K. (1980). The intracranial pressure in infants. *Journal of Neurosurgery, 52*, 693–699. doi:10.3171/jns.1980.52.5.0693

5 RENAL SYSTEM
Michelle A. Dokas

DEVELOPMENTAL ANATOMY OF THE RENAL SYSTEM

A. Anatomic Location

The kidneys are positioned within the retroperitoneal space and are surrounded by adipose tissue and loose connective tissue. The kidneys lie along the lower two thoracic vertebrae and the first four lumbar vertebrae. They are not fixed but move with the diaphragm and are supported by the surrounding vascular system, adipose tissue, and fibrous tissue called the *renal fascia*. The right kidney lies slightly lower than the left.

B. Anatomic Structure

1. *Development.* All nephrons are formed by 28 weeks gestation. Kidney weight doubles in the first month of life. Filtration and absorption capabilities are not developed until the epithelial cells of the nephrons mature. As the loop of Henle matures and elongates, the ability to concentrate urine improves. Infants are more vulnerable to dehydration and fluid overload because of their inability to concentrate or to excrete urine in response to changes in fluid status. Bladder capacity is age dependent: infants, 15 to 20 mL; adults, 600 to 800 mL. The kidneys of infants and children are relatively large for their body size and age, making them more susceptible to trauma.

2. *Gross Structures* (Figure 5.1)

    a. The *capsule* is the thin, fibrous, tough outer covering of the kidney.

    b. The structural unit of the kidney is the lobe. Each lobe is composed of a pyramid and the overlying cortex. On average, there are 14 lobes in each kidney.

    c. The outer portion of the kidney is the *cortex.* It contains all the glomeruli, the proximal and distal convoluted tubules, the first portions of the loop of Henle, and the collecting ducts.

    d. The inner region contains the *medulla* and the *pelvis*. The medulla has a pyramidal shape and contains primarily the collecting ducts and loops of Henle. The pelvis forms the upper end of the ureter. It is formed by the merging of the collecting ducts and tubular structures. It provides the pathway of urine from the kidney to the ureter. The fluid in the pelvis is identical to urine.

3. *Gross Renal Vasculature.* About 20% to 25% of the total cardiac output is delivered to the kidneys. Two renal arteries branch from the descending aorta, and each renal artery branches repeatedly into arterioles.

4. *Microscopic Structure*

    a. The *nephron* is the functional unit of the kidney. Each mature kidney has about 1 million nephrons. Formation of nephrons is completed at birth, new ones cannot be formed. The *nephron wall* is composed of a single layer of epithelial cells. The top end (origin) of the nephron is called *Bowman's capsule*, which is found in the cortex of the kidney. The fluid in Bowman's capsule is a filtrate of blood plasma.

    b. There are two types of nephrons. *Cortical* nephrons (85% of nephrons) originate in the outer portion of the cortex and have short loops of Henle that reach only the outer region of the medulla. *Juxtaglomerular* nephrons originate closer to the medulla, have very long loops of Henle that reach deep into the medulla, and are important for water conservation in the body.

    c. The nephron can be divided into three parts: vascular components, tubular components, and collecting ducts.

        i. Vascular components of the nephron. Afferent arterioles originate from the medulla and cortex and leads to the capillary bed, which is called the glomerulus (Bowman's capsule and the *glomerulus* may be referred to collectively as the *glomerulus*). Afferent arterioles bring blood to the glomerulus. Efferent arterioles take blood as it exits the glomerulus to the second capillary bed of peritubular capillaries, which supply the proximal and distal tubules in the cortex. Efferent arterioles of juxtaglomerular nephrons send off branches to create the *vasa recta*, a loop of straight vessels that stretch deep down to supply the medulla, extending alongside the descending limbs

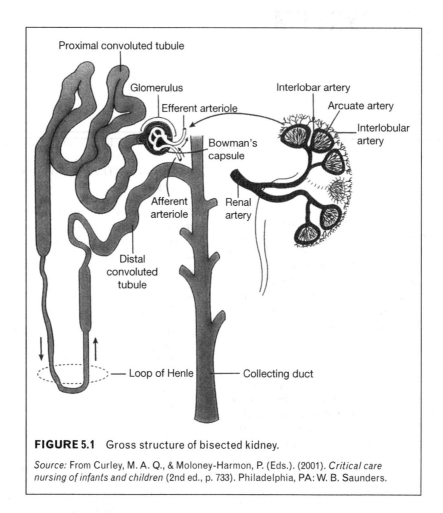

FIGURE 5.1   Gross structure of bisected kidney.

Source: From Curley, M. A. Q., & Moloney-Harmon, P. (Eds.). (2001). *Critical care nursing of infants and children* (2nd ed., p. 733). Philadelphia, PA: W. B. Saunders.

of the loop of Henle and back up toward the cortex.

ii. Tubular components of the nephron (Figure 5.2). The proximal tubule leads to Bowman's capsule. The tubule begins as coiled and convoluted (proximal convoluted tubule) and then straightens as it extends into the medulla. The descending limb of the loop of Henle is a long, thin tubule that extends deep into the medulla. At its deepest point in the medulla, it turns sharply upward toward the cortex. The ascending limb of the loop of Henle is considerably thicker than the descending limb. It becomes continuous with the distal tubule. The distal tubule is a coiled, convoluted structure responsible for final adjustments of filtrate.

iii.   Collecting ducts gather fluid from several nephrons and drain into larger ducts, which drain into the minor calyces, then into the renal pelvis, then to the ureter.

DEVELOPMENTAL PHYSIOLOGY AND CLINICAL ASSESSMENT OF KIDNEY FUNCTION

A. Basic Transport Mechanisms

The following concepts are integral to the formation of urine in the kidney:

1. *During active transport,* substances combine with a carrier and diffuse against the concentration gradient through the tubular membrane with the help of adenosine triphosphate (ATP). Sodium, glucose, amino acids, calcium, potassium, chloride, bicarbonate, and phosphate are reabsorbed from the tubule by active transport.

2. *Passive transport* involves movement of substances in response to changes in the concentration gradient, without the assistance of ATP or a carrier. *Diffusion* is the spontaneous movement of solutes across a semipermeable membrane from a high concentration to

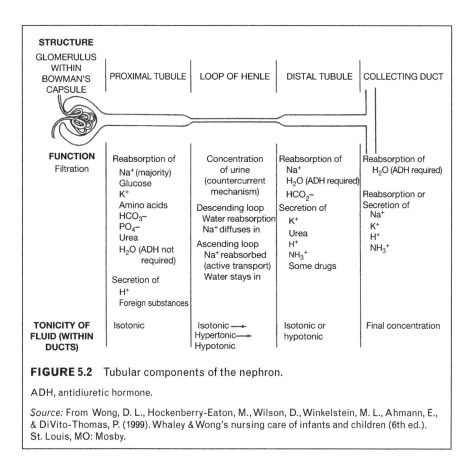

FIGURE 5.2 Tubular components of the nephron.

ADH, antidiuretic hormone.

Source: From Wong, D. L., Hockenberry-Eaton, M., Wilson, D., Winkelstein, M. L., Ahmann, E., & DiVito-Thomas, P. (1999). Whaley & Wong's nursing care of infants and children (6th ed.). St. Louis, MO: Mosby.

a lesser concentration. For example, as water reabsorbs out of the tubule and the urea concentration in the tubule increases, urea diffuses out of the tubule. *Osmosis* is the spontaneous movement of water across a semipermeable membrane from an area of lesser solute concentration to an area of greater solute concentration. For example, as sodium is reabsorbed from the tubule and its concentration increases outside the tubule, water moves out of the tubule to balance the concentration gradient. Serum colloid osmotic pressure is the opposing pressure preventing free water from moving out of the vascular space.

B. Urine Formation

Urine formation involves the following physiologic processes: filtration, reabsorption, and secretion.

1. *Filtration*

a. Fluid and various substances, known as the *glomerular filtrate*, are filtered from the plasma through the porous walls of the glomerular capillaries into Bowman's capsule and on to the renal tubules. Glomerular filtrate is primarily composed of water; it is essentially the same substance as blood plasma except for the larger protein molecules, such as albumin, because they are largely unable to move through the filtration barrier.

b. The pathway for filtration is through capillary fenestrations across the basement membrane and through slit passages. The ability to resist passing and to pass through filtration pathways depend on size, shape, and electrical charge of the molecules. Albumin (protein) molecules are too large to permeate the glomerular membrane, creating a high osmotic pressure that opposes orthostatic filtration from the vascular space.

c. The "forcing" pressure, or filtration pressure, is the net pressure acting to force substances out of the glomerulus.

   i. The primary force is the hydrostatic pressure of the blood inside the capillaries generated by the pumping action of the heart.

   ii. The secondary forces are the oncotic pressure of the plasma in the glomerular capillaries and the hydrostatic pressure in Bowman's capsule.

d. *Regulation of glomerular filtration rate* (GFR)

   i.   Renal blood flow (RBF) and GFR must remain relatively constant over a wide range of perfusion pressures and in various physiological states such as disease. This is referred to as *autoregulation*. Numerous neural and hormonal factors can alter RBF, such as renal vasoconstrictors that decrease RBF, including endothelin, angiotensin II, thromboxane, alpha-adrenergic receptor stimulators, vasopressin, and catecholamines. Vasodilators that may relax renal vascular smooth muscle include prostaglandins, atrial peptides, bradykinin, fenoldopam, and nitric oxide. Failure of these mechanisms can lead to renal dysfunction in all of the disease states discussed in this chaper.

   ii.   Changes in filtration pressure can directly affect GFR. Factors affecting filtration pressure, and thus the GFR, include vasoconstriction or vasodilation of afferent and efferent arterioles, blood flow rate, tubule obstruction, and changes in serum osmotic pressure. RBF is controlled by sympathetic nerve impulses that constrict arterioles. The effect on GFR depends on which arteriole (afferent or efferent) is constricted (Table 5.1).

   iii.   Vasodilation and vasoconstriction are autoregulatory responses to changes in systemic arterial pressure. They occur to maintain constant RBF and a stable GFR. A distal tubular feedback mechanism ensures constant delivery of filtrate to the distal tubule. Failure of this autoregulatory response can be due to obstruction, trauma, dehydration, or disease.

   iv.   The effect of shock on GFR and renal function is detailed in Figure 5.3.

e. *Measuring filtration.* Clearance is the volume of a specific substance filtered from the plasma over a designated time, generally:

$$\text{Clearance (mL/min/1.73m)} = \text{Concentration of substance in urine} \times \text{Volume of urine collected/plasma concentration of that substance}$$

   i.   Substances used to assess GFR include creatinine, inulin (nonmetabolizable sugar), radioisotopes, radiocontrast agents, and cystatin-C.

   ii.   GFR as estimated by creatinine clearance alone is less accurate. *Creatinine* is an endogenous waste product that is produced by the muscles and excreted by the kidneys. Estimates of GFR using creatinine clearance and cystatin-C together are more accurate, especially in children (Traynor, Mactier, Geddes, & Fox, 2006).

TABLE 5.1   Factors Affecting GFR

Factors	Physiologic Response	Net Effect on GFR
Afferent arteriole vasoconstriction, efferent arteriole vasodilation, or both	Decreased blood flow Decreased glomerular hydration pressure	Decrease
Afferent arteriole vasodilation or efferent arteriole vasoconstriction	Blood backs up in the glomerulus Increased hydrostatic pressure	Increase
Decrease in plasma protein concentration	Decreased plasma osmotic pressure	Increase
Slow blood flow	Larger proportions of the plasma filter out of the glomerulus Plasma osmotic pressure rises	Decrease
Rapid blood flow	Less change in plasma osmotic pressure	Increase
Tubular obstruction	Fluid backs up in the renal tubules Hydrostatic pressure increases in Bowman's capsule	Decrease

GFR, glomerular filtration rate.

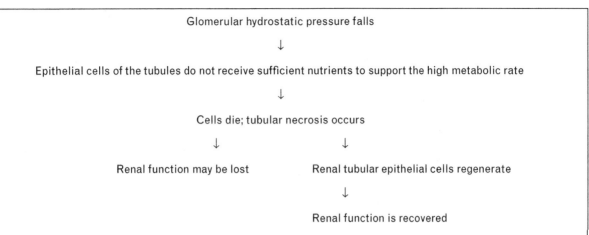

Glomerular hydrostatic pressure falls

↓

Epithelial cells of the tubules do not receive sufficient nutrients to support the high metabolic rate

↓

Cells die; tubular necrosis occurs

↓   ↓

Renal function may be lost   Renal tubular epithelial cells regenerate

↓

Renal function is recovered

FIGURE 5.3   Renal response to shock.

iii. GFR as measured by creatinine clearance

1) First week of life. GFR = 15 to 20 mL/min/1.73 m^2

2) At the second week of life. GFR = 35 to 40 mL/min/1.73 m^2

3) At 6 months. GFR = 60 mL/min/1.73 m^2

4) At 1 year. GFR = 80 to 120 mL/min/1.73 m^2

iv. The filtration fraction (FF) is the percentage of fluid filtered into Bowman's capsule by the glomerulus in relationship to the total renal plasma flow (normal = 20%).

v. Alteration in GFR occurs with decreased renal perfusion, changes in glomerular perfusion pressures (e.g., shock, glomerular nephritis), and decreases in plasma oncotic pressure (e.g., nephrotic syndrome).

2. *Tubular Reabsorption.* As fluid flows along the nephron, past the cells of the tubular wall, substances are reabsorbed from the renal tubule and returned to the blood via the peritubular capillaries.

a. Most of tubular reabsorption occurs in the proximal tubule. By the time the filtrate reaches the end of the proximal tubule, two thirds of the water and virtually all the nutrients have been reabsorbed and returned to the blood. The proximal tubules play a role in acid–base balance and regulation of calcium, magnesium, and phosphorus. The proximal tubules have active transport systems for secretion of organic acids and bases from blood to tubule lumen.

b. The tubular cells lining the walls of the proximal tubules are surrounded by two different membranes that aid in water and solute reabsorption. The convoluted portion of the proximal tubule has a brush-like border of microvilli that greatly increases surface area exposed to glomerular filtrate and enhances reabsorption. The basolateral membrane has no microvilli but has an abundance of sodium and potassium pumps and other diffusion transport systems for glucose and amino acids.

c. Segments of the renal tubule use particular modes of transport to reabsorb certain substances. Substances reabsorbed by active transport depend on carriers. If the amount of substance exceeds the number of carriers (renal tubular threshold), the remaining substance will remain in the filtrate and be excreted in urine (e.g., glucosuria). Glucosuria only occurs when plasma glucose levels exceed 180 mg/dL.

d. Fluid reabsorption is determined by the net sodium reabsorption. If the GFR decreases, net sodium reabsorption decreases and fluid reabsorption decreases. If the GFR increases, net sodium reabsorption increases and fluid reabsorption increases.

e. Several factors enhance the rate of fluid reabsorption from the renal tubule. The efferent arteriole is narrower than the peritubular capillary; therefore, blood flowing from the efferent arteriole to the peritubular capillary is under relatively low pressure. The wall of the renal capillary is more permeable than other capillaries.

f. The prime "mover" for most of the proximal tubular transport is the active transport of sodium. Water is reabsorbed by osmosis in response to the reabsorption of sodium ions by active transport. Amino acids and glucose are cotransported (reabsorbed) with sodium into the interstitial fluid and eventually to capillaries. When sodium is reabsorbed from the tubule, it takes chloride with it, changing the osmotic gradient and favoring the reabsorption of water into the interstitium and eventually to the capillaries. When water is absorbed from the tubule, the concentration of the remaining solutes increases, therefore increasing the diffusion of other solutes into the interstitial space and eventually to the capillaries.

g. *Measuring reabsorption.* The amount of solute reabsorbed is the difference between the amount of solute filtered into the glomerulus and the amount of solute excreted in the urine (assuming the amount filtered is greater than the amount excreted).

3. *Tubular secretion* is the process by which certain substances are removed from the blood or plasma of the peritubular capillary and added to the fluid of the renal tubule through active or passive transport.

a. Certain organic compounds (such as penicillin, creatinine, and histamine) are actively secreted into tubular fluid by the epithelium of the proximal convoluted segment.

b. Hydrogen ions are secreted by the distal segment and the collecting ducts. Hydrogen ion secretion plays an important role in acid–base balance.

c. Potassium ions are secreted into tubular fluid because of the electrochemical attraction created by sodium reabsorption.

d. *Measuring secretion.* The amount of solute secreted is the difference between the amount of solute filtered into the glomerulus and the amount of solute excreted in the urine (assuming the amount filtered is less than the amount excreted).

C. Water and Sodium Balance

1. *Measuring Water Balance and Regulation of Urine Concentration.* Normal serum osmolarity is 272 to 290 mOsm/L. The calculation for serum osmolarity is (2 × serum NA) + (serum glucose/18) + (blood urea nitrogen [BUN]/2.8). Normal urine osmolarity is approximately 300 mOsm/L. This usually correlates with a urine-specific gravity of 1.010 to 1.015.

2. *Role of Countercurrent Mechanism in Concentrating and Diluting*

a. *Filtrate concentration* changes as it flows from the proximal tubule to the collecting ducts. Filtrate becomes increasingly concentrated as it moves from the proximal tubule through the descending limb to the loop of Henle. Maximum concentration occurs at the tip of the loop of Henle. Filtrate becomes less concentrated as it moves up the ascending limb of the loop and on to the collecting duct.

b. *Juxtamedullary nephrons* and the medullary portion of the kidney play a major role in this countercurrent mechanism. Sodium and chloride are actively reabsorbed out of the thick portion of the ascending limb into the interstitial space and peritubular capillaries, creating an osmotic gradient between the interstitium and the tubule. This segment of the tubule is impermeable to water, and water cannot be reabsorbed with sodium. In response to this osmotic gradient, water is passively reabsorbed out of the descending limb into the interstitium and peritubular capillaries. A concentration gradient is created, and filtrate is more dilute as it enters the collecting duct. As this dilute urine enters the distal tubule and collecting ducts, antidiuretic hormone (ADH) controls the amount of water reabsorption according to the need for dilute or concentrated urine. ADH is released from the hypothalamus. If dilute urine is needed, ADH is inhibited. If water conservation or concentrated urine is needed, ADH is secreted.

3. *Hormonal Control of Water Balance*

a. Vasopressin, or ADH, plays a role in water balance. The distal convoluted tubule and collecting duct are impermeable to water; so water may be excreted as dilute urine. If ADH is present, the distal tubule and collecting ducts become permeable, water is reabsorbed, and urine is more concentrated. A rise in the solute concentration of the extracellular fluids and blood plasma stimulates cells in the hypothalamus to increase production of ADH and to cause release of ADH from the posterior pituitary. In the kidney, ADH initiates retention of water and decrease in solute concentration. Decreased solute concentration causes decreased ADH release, which causes dilute urine. Increased solute concentration causes increased ADH release, which causes concentrated urine.

b. Aldosterone is responsible for virtually all sodium and water reabsorption in the collecting duct. This region of the renal tubule fine-tunes sodium excretion. The adrenal cortex releases aldosterone in response to angiotensin II, hyperkalemia, hyponatremia, decreased pulse pressure, or decreased right atrial distention. Aldosterone increases sodium reabsorption by increasing the number of sodium channels in the apical plasma membrane of the principal cell. Aldosterone stimulates the secretion of potassium and hydrogen and decreases potassium reabsorption.

c. Other factors also control renal sodium excretion. Hormones that lead to retention of sodium include growth hormone, cortisol, insulin, and estrogen. These act at the tubular level. Parathyroid hormone (PTH), progesterone, and glycogen inhibit tubular reabsorption of sodium. Atrial natriuretic peptide, a 28-amino peptide produced and secreted in the atria of the heart, is released in response to atrial stretch, for example, in response to expansion of central blood volume. This peptide then enhances sodium excretion in part by inhibiting sodium reabsorption on the collecting duct.

4. *Sodium and Water Reabsorption*

a. Sodium concentration is higher in the lumen of the tubule than in the cells lining the tubule, so sodium moves into the tubular cells. Because the proximal tubule's brush border has no sodium pump, the sodium cannot be pumped back into the lumen. Only the basolateral membrane can pump out sodium into the interstitial spaces and then diffuse into the peritubular capillaries. When sodium (positively charged) is reabsorbed, it leaves the tubule and moves into the tubular wall, which is followed by negatively charged ions, such as, chloride, phosphate, and bicarbonate.

b. Every sodium or chloride ion that leaves the tubule means the loss of osmotically active particles from the tubule to the interstitium. The movement of particles creates a change in osmotic gradient favoring water reabsorption, and water follows the sodium and chloride into the interstitium. With less sodium in the tubule, the concentration of solutes in the tubule increases, thereby increasing diffusion of other solutes out of the tubule and into the interstitial space. As water is reabsorbed from the filtrate into the peritubular capillaries, substances remaining in the tubule become more concentrated. As a result, water moves into the tubules. As sodium reabsorption increases, water reabsorption increases and vice versa.

c. Alteration in the GFR influences the amount of sodium reabsorbed or secreted. When the GFR decreases (e.g., dehydration, sepsis), sodium and water reabsorption increases. Decreased volume decreases venous, atrial, and arterial pressures. Pressoreceptors decrease the number of impulses to the brainstem, which activates sympathetic impulses to stimulate renin release from the juxtaglomerular cells in the afferent arterioles. Renin is converted to angiotensin I, which is converted to angiotensin II, which causes vasoconstriction and secretion of aldosterone. This creates "thirst" in an effort to increase volume. As water volume increases, ADH is secreted to maintain water and solute balance.

D. Electrolyte Balance

1. *Potassium Ion (K^+)*

a. The kidney is chiefly responsible for maintaining potassium homeostasis. Potassium has a normal serum value of approximately 3.5 to 5 mEq/L. It is the most abundant solute inside cells (145 mEq/L); a very small amount is present in the serum. Potassium is an important factor in the performance of many enzyme systems, playing a role in the maintenance of cell volume, pH, and cell excitability (*membrane potentials*). Decreasing serum potassium depolarizes membranes and raises excitability (e.g., cardiac rhythm deterioration leading to fibrillation). Increasing serum potassium hyperpolarizes membranes and decreases excitability (e.g., skeletal and smooth-muscle weakness and decreased reflexes). Acid–base balance changes; hormone imbalance and pharmacologic agents frequently cause postassium shifts.

b. Potassium excretion is regulated mainly by the collecting duct, but is a complex regulating mechanism that is intertwined with sodium and hydrogen transport. The secretion and excretion of potassium are also influenced by plasma concentration of postassium, dietary potassium, aldosterone, angiontensin II, and delivery of sodium to prinicpal cells (Eaton & Pooler, 2013). Most potassium is reabsorbed in the proximal tubule and the loop of Henle. The distal tubule and collecting ducts have a high concentration of intracellular potassium owing to the action of the sodium–potassium pumps. Changes in renal regulation of potassium are due to changes in potassium secretion in the distal tubule and collecting duct. Increases in intracellular potassium increase the secretion and excretion of potassium. Increases in plasma potassium stimulate the adrenal cortex to secrete aldosterone, which promotes secretion and excretion of potassium.

c. Any drug that interferes with aldosterone activity (e.g., angiotensin-converting enzyme [ACE] inhibitors, angiotensin II receptor blockers, spironolactone, heparin, and beta-blockers) will inhibit potassium secretion and increase serum potassium levels.

d. Drugs that block the principal cell sodium channel also inhibit potassium secretion (e.g., trimethoprim, pentamidime, amiloride) and may lead to increased serum potassium levels (Daly & Farrington, 2013).

e. In acidosis, potassium excretion decreases. Distal tubular and collecting-duct cells lose potassium to the plasma, leakage and secretion of potassium into tubules decrease, and potassium shifts from the cells into the plasma. In alkalosis, potassium excretion increases. Potassium increases in the distal tubule and collecting duct. Leakage and secretion of potassium increase. Potassium shifts into the cells. With a shift from acidosis to alkalosis, serum potassium decreases because of the shift into the cells.

2. *Sodium*

a. The normal serum value is approximately 135 to 145 mEq/L. Hyponatremia may lead to seizure activity. Excess of sodium leads to edema and hypertension. Dilutional hyponatremia occurs secondary to hypotonic fluid intake and impaired free water excretion. The hyponatremia corrects slowly with free water diuresis.

b. Management may include dialysis or continuous renal replacement therapy (CRRT) for severe or symptomatic hyponatremia (serum Na^+ <125 mEq/L) in the oliguric, hypervolemic patient or oliguric, hypernatremic patient (Na^+ >150 mEq/L). Hyponatremic metabolic acidosis may be treated with administration of sodium, partly in the form of sodium bicarbonate. Administration of isotonic saline 0.9% is indicated for fluid loss and dehydration, whereas administration of hypertonic 3% saline is indicated if the patient is fluid overloaded and has significant hyponatremia. Hypertonic saline is used until the serum sodium is corrected to a "safe" level, often considered to be greater than 125 mEq/L, and then transitioned to a less hypertonic intravenous (IV) solution.

3. *Phosphate (Phosphorus, Inorganic)*

a. Normal serum values in the newborn are 4.2 to 6.5 mg/dL. Normal values in children aged 1 to 5 years are 3.5 to 6.5 mg/dL and in older children range from 2.5 to 4.5 mg/dL. Renal excretion of phosphate is the body's primary mechanism for regulation of phosphate; therefore, patients in renal failure are at high risk for hyperphosphatemia.

b. PTH indirectly affects serum phosphate levels by affecting calcium. Phosphate and calcium are reabsorbed from bone. Tubular reabsorption of phosphate is decreased as tubular reabsorption of sodium increases. PTH enhances intestinal absorption of calcium and phosphate. Vitamin D is converted to its active form by the liver and kidneys, thereby regulating phosphate and calcium balance. Active absorption of phosphate (and calcium) by the intestine is stimulated by vitamin D. Reabsorption of phosphate and calcium from bone to extracellular fluid is facilitated by vitamin D. Vitamin D stimulates renal tubular reabsorption of phosphate and calcium.

4. *Calcium*

a. The normal serum value is 9 to 11 mg/dL (total calcium) and 1.00 to 1.4 mmol/dL (ionized calcium). Calcium exists in two forms: ionized and nonionized. About 45% to 50% is ionized, meaning "free" and not bound to albumin. Ionized calcium is the physiologically active form of calcium. Albumin-bound calcium is not filtered at the glomerulus. Decreased serum albumin levels may affect serum calcium levels.

b. PTH is the most important regulator of calcium. Hypocalcemia stimulates the release of PTH, which decreases renal excretion of calcium and increases urinary excretion of phosphorus. Hypercalcemia inhibits the release of PTH.

5. *Magnesium.* The normal serum values are 1.8 to 2.3 mEq/L. Magnesium is an essential cofactor for many metabolic enzymatic processes in the body. Eighty percent of plasma magnesium is filtered at the glomerulus, and only a small amount of this filtrate is excreted.

E. Regulation of Acid–Base Balance

1. *Definitions.* An *acid* is a source of hydrogen ions. A *base* takes up or absorbs hydrogen ions. A *buffer* combines with an acid or base to maintain a stable pH.

2. In an effort to achieve an acid–base balance, the lungs regulate carbon dioxide and the kidneys regulate bicarbonate. With normal digestion, metabolic acids (hydrogen ions) are produced. Metabolic hydrogen ions are picked up by serum bicarbonate and form carbon dioxide. An increased level of carbon dioxide and hydrogen ions stimulates increased respiration, which helps to eliminate carbon dioxide and reverse acidosis. Respiratory regulation of acid–base balance is generally inadequate in severe metabolic acidosis and alkalosis.

3. The kidney regulates acid–base balance through hydrogen secretion and bicarbonate reabsorption. Hydrogen ions are secreted (removed from the blood and plasma of the peritubular capillary and added to the fluid of the renal tubule) at the distal tubule and the collecting duct. Bicarbonate is filtered at the glomerulus and is not readily reabsorbed because the peritubular capillary membrane is not highly permeable to the molecule. HCO_3^- combines with H^+ in the tubular cell to form carbonic acid (H_2CO_3). The carbonic acid rapily dissociates and is diffused into the tubular cell where carbonic anhydrase catalyzes the reaction between CO_2 and H_2O to form HCO_3^- and H^+. In the distal tubule, hydrogen also combines with nonbicarbonate buffers for the elimination of excess acids in the urine. The end effect is alkalinity of the plasma (McCance & Huether, 2010).

a. *Renal response in alkalotic conditions.* Potassium excretion increases, chloride is reabsorbed with sodium, and bicarbonate is excreted. If an increase in filtrate bicarbonate is secondary to increased serum concentration, bicarbonate excretion increases. If an increase in filtrate bicarbonate is secondary to hypovolemia (e.g., in persistent vomiting), hydrogen ion secretion and bicarbonate reabsorption from the tubules increase, preventing excretion of excess bicarbonate. Alkalosis is corrected as volume status is restored.

b. *Renal response in acidotic conditions.* Potassium excretion decreases. Bicarbonate is reabsorbed with sodium, and chloride is excreted. Bicarbonate diffuses into the extracellular compartment and ultimately into the plasma (via the renal vein), resulting in reabsorption of hydrogen ions. Renal excretion of acid (ammonium excretion) increases.

F. Regulation of Arterial Blood Pressure

1. *Maintenance of Circulating Blood Volume.* Circulating blood volume is maintained by sodium and water balance. A countercurrent mechanism plays a role in concentrating and diluting. Hormonal control of water balance is mediated by ADH and aldosterone, initiated by hypothalamic

osmoreceptors and cardiopulmonary baroreceptors. Large decreases in plasma volume elicit significant concentrations of ADH to exert direct vasoconstrictor effects on arteriolar smooth muscle to increase total peripheral resistance. Renal arterioles and mesangial cells also respond to a high plasma concentration of ADH, prompting retention of both sodium and water by lowering GFR (Eaton & Pooler, 2013).

2. *Regulation of peripheral vascular resistance* is via the renin–angiotensin–aldosterone system and the central nervous system (CNS) (Figure 5.4). Juxtaglomerular cells release renin in response to a decrease in glomerular pressure (*kidney perfusion pressure*), an increase in sympathetic nervous system stimulation, decreased sodium in the distal tubule, or

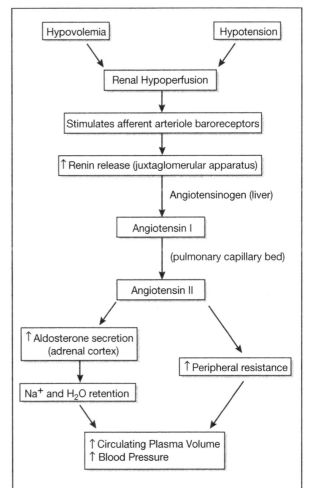

FIGURE 5.4 Renin–angiotensin aldosterone cascade to maintain systemic perfusion pressure.

Source: From Curley, M. A. Q., & Moloney-Harmon, P. (Eds.). (2001). *Critical care nursing of infants and children* (2nd ed., p. 735). Philadelphia, PA: W. B. Saunders.

vasoconstrictive agents. Renin diffuses into the circulatory system and converts angiotensinogen into angiotensin I. As angiotensin I circulates to the lungs, it converts to angiotensin II (and also produces aldosterone). Angiotensin II is a powerful vasoconstrictor of the peripheral vascular system. Angiotensin II stimulates aldosterone secretion, which causes an increase in water and sodium reabsorption. The sympathetic nervous system also regulates peripheral vascular resistance by causing vasoconstriction.

G. Regulation of RBF

1. Prostaglandins are vasoactive substances that act by either dilating or constricting renal vessels. Their effect is limited to the renal vasculature.

2. Three prostaglandins are produced by cells in the kidney's cortical and medullary structures. Thromboxane A_2 is a vasoconstrictor. Prostacyclin (PGI_2) and prostaglandin E_2 (PGE_2) are vasodilators. PGI_2 and PGE_2 produce direct vasodilation of afferent arterioles, which helps to maintain RBF and glomerular perfusion. PGE_2 increases urine output by counteracting the actions of ADH. PGE_2 increases sodium excretion by inhibiting its reabsorption from the renal tubules.

H. Elimination of Toxins and Metabolic Wastes

1. Urea is produced in the liver as a by-product of amino acid metabolism. Amino acids and proteins are metabolized in the liver and yield ammonia, which is very toxic until the liver rapidly detoxifies it into urea. Urea production proceeds continuously and constitutes about half of the usual solute content of urine. It is freely filtered by the kidney; about 50% of urea is passively reabsorbed, and 50% is excreted in the urine.

2. Uric acid is a by-product of metabolism of certain organic bases in nucleic acids. Ninety percent is reabsorbed in the glomerular filtrate, and 10% is secreted into the renal tubule.

3. Creatinine is the end product of protein metabolism. Under normal conditions, creatinine is completely filtered by the proximal tubules and excreted in the urine. Its complete elimination makes it an excellent marker of renal function. The creatinine level is proportional to the BUN level. The normal BUN-to-creatinine ratio is 10:1 to 15:1. An increase in both BUN and creatinine signals renal dysfunction. An increase in BUN without an increase in creatinine may be an indication of dehydration, decreased renal perfusion, or catabolism.

I. Stimulation of Bone Marrow Erythrocyte Production

1. Erythropoietin is a hormone produced in the kidneys that stimulates red blood cell (RBC) production from the bone marrow, and a deficiency of production leads to anemia. The anemia associated with chronic kidney disease (CKD) is due mainly to a deficiency of erythropoietin. In renal failure, production of erythropoietin is insufficient. However, often the anemia of CKD can be improved with iron supplementation. Some children with CKD have iron depletion even when taking iron supplements.

2. IV and subcutaneous recombinant human erythropoietin are available for treatment of anemia secondary to CKD. Side effects include hypertension, seizures, and vascular access thrombus formation. This is often administered at the time of dialysis if the patient is receiving intermittent dialysis therapy.

3. Uremia shortens the life span of RBCs and is a significant contributor to anemia. It also decreases platelet function.

4. Transfusions should be avoided as much as possible, not only because of risks, such as communicable disease and fluid overload, but also to avoid further decrease of the significantly inhibited positive feedback loop stimulating erythropoeitin production.

5. Other possible deficiencies should be assessed before therapy is initiated, including vitamin B_{12} deficiency, folate deficiency, or aluminum intoxication (the latter leading to microcytic anemia). Throughout the course of therapy, iron stores (serum iron, ferritin, and total iron-binding capacity [TIBC]) should be evaluated frequently because the rapid proliferative response may not be accompanied by an adequate availability of iron. If iron stores prove insufficient during the course of therapy, replacement should be implemented (Table 5.2).

INVASIVE AND NONINVASIVE DIAGNOSTIC STUDIES

A. Imaging

1. *Renal ultrasound with doppler (RUS)* is readily available, accurate, reliable, and noninvasive. It can show size, shape, and anatomical variants. Asymmetry indicates unilateral disease process. RUS avoids radiation and contrast media, which may be nephrotoxic. Increased echogenicity of the renal parenchyma is a common nonspecific indicator of intrinsic renal disease. In some cases of acute tubular

TABLE 5.2   Pediatric Iron Studies

TIBC	Transferrin	Iron	Tsat	Ferritin
Direct, quantitative measurement of transferrin	Iron is bound to this globulin protein Carried to the bone marrow for incorporation into hemoglobin Produced in liver	Measurement of the quantity of iron bound to transferrin	Percent saturation of iron bound to transferrin Calculated: Tsat (%) = $\dfrac{Iron}{TIBC} \times 100$	Good indicator of available iron stores The major iron storage protein
Normal: 25–420 µg/dL or 43–73 µmol/L	Normal: 200–400 µg/dL	Normal: 60–190 µg/dL or 13–31 µmol/L	Normal: 30%–40%	Normal: Newborn: 25–200 ng/mL 1 month: 200–600 ng/mL 2–5 months: 50–200 ng/mL 6 months–15 years: 7–142 ng/mL
Elevated in iron deficiency Decreased in chronic illness Varies minimally with intake More a reflection of hepatic function (transferrin produced in liver) and nutrition than iron metabolism		Decreased level in iron deficiency Decreased in chronic illness Elevated after massive blood product transfusion	Decreased in iron deficiency Normal in chronic illness	Interfering factors: Recent transfusion Ingestion of meal high in iron Disorders of excessive iron storage Hemolytic diseases transfusion

TIBC, total iron-binding capacity; Tsat, transferrin saturation.

necrosis (ATN), renal parenchymal echogenicity may be normal. RBF is generally reduced in ARF, and Doppler flow ultrasound can detect low blood flow. Low RBF or abnormal blood flow associated with renal artery stenosis can also be detected. Low RBF can also be indicative of pyelonephritis and may show small renal calculi (Wu, Bellah, & Snyder, 2016). Complete absence of flow suggests complete thrombosis of the renal circulation (Toto, 2004).

2. *Voiding cystourethorography (VCUG)* is the most sensitive and effective way to assess for the presence of urinary reflux.

3. *Dimercaptosuccinic acid scanning (DMSA)* is the critical test for renal scarring associated with reflux as well as detection of urinary obstruction and urine leak. It is more sensitive than intravenous pyelogram (IVP) and is noninvasive.

4. A *MAG3 renal scan* looks at functional renal function and the collecting system. It is useful in assessing for hydronephrosis and can distinguish ATN from prerenal or other intrinsic renal disease.

5. *CT and helical CT* show more detailed anatomy than ultrasound. Helical CT is the gold standard for diagnosing renal calculi. Evaluation of cystic structures is more precise with CT (Lerma, 2009). It is also preferred in any child with abdominal trauma. Most currently, the use of CT angiography (CTA) can evaluate for renal hypertension, vasculitis, vascular malformations, and renal trauma (Wu et al., 2016).

6. *MRI and magnetic renal angiography (MRA)* are useful tests for patients with a contrast allergy. MRI shows more specific anatomic details. MRA is now the standard of care for renal vessels and thrombotic disorders. Use of contrast is not recommended when estimated GFR is ≤30 mL/min (Lerma, 2009).

7. *Kidney angiogram* is helpful in patients with acute kidney injury (AKI) caused by vascular disorders, including renal artery stenosis and renal artery emboli, but should be used cautiously in patients with compromised renal function.

B. Laboratory Evaluation

1. *Urinalysis* is the most important noninvasive test and is easily obtainable. It shows:

a. *pH.* Normal 6 to 8. pH <6.0 is suggestive of metabolic acidosis. pH >8 is suspicious for renal tubular acidosis.

b. *Specific gravity.* Demonstrates hydration status.

c. *Leukocyte esterase.* Tests for the prescence of white blood cells (WBCs) and is indicitative of infection.

d. *Red cells.* May indicate trauma, glomerulonephritis, nephrolithiasis.

e. *Protein.* Is specific for albumin and should not be present. More than 1+ protein is consistent with nephrotic syndrome.

f. *Ketones and glucose.* Ketones in the presence of normal serum glucose would suggest renal tubular dysfunction as well as presence of poorly controlled diabetes (although not reliable for the diagnosis of diabetes) or Fanconi syndrome.

2. *Complete blood count (CBC)* assesses for anemia (see Table 5.2).

3. *Serum chemistries with BUN and creatinine.* Normal creatinine varies with age (Table 5.3).

4. *Urine electrolyte measurement* in AKI is performed to test functional integrity of the renal tubules.

5. *The most informative urine test* is the fractional excretion of sodium (FENa); results are inaccurate if the patient is on diuretics or prior infusion of saline (Lerma, 2009).

$$FENa = \frac{Urine\ Na \times Plasma\ Cr}{Urine\ Cr \times Plasma\ Na} \times 100$$

a. *Results.* Less than 1%—prerenal renal failure such as intravascular volume depletion due to fluid losses or sequestration, hypotension, sepsis, and so on; greater than 2%—intrinsic or chronic renal failure.

C. Kidney biopsy should be performed only when clinical, biochemical, and noninvasive imaging studies are insufficient for diagnosis and there is reasonable belief that the test results will alter therapy.

ACUTE KIDNEY INJURY

A. Definitions

1. *AKI* is the sudden loss of renal capacity for filtration and tubular reabsorption, resulting in accumulation of wastes, fluid and electrolyte imbalance, and acid–base imbalances. AKI had previously been termed *acute renal failure*, however, with advancements in understanding that kidney injury is an independant risk factor for mortality, develeopment of standardized definitions, and discovery of AKI biomarkers, the nomenclature has changed. Several nephrology groups developed the RIFLE critiera for AKI. RIFLE stratifies for risk, injury, failure, and outcomes of loss and end-stage kidney disease.

a. Risk is defined as 50% rise in serum creatinine over baseline or less than 0.5 mL/kg/hr of urine output for 6 hours.

b. Injury is defined as two- to three-times rise in baseline creatinine or urine output <0.5 mL/kg/hr for 16 hours

c. Failure is defined as rise in serum creatinine more than three times baseline or urine output <0.5 mL/kg/hr for 24 hours or <0.3 mL/kg/hr for 12 hours (Fortenberry, Paden, & Goldstein, 2013).

TABLE 5.3 Normal Serum Creatinine Based on Age

Age	Normal Creatinine Levels (mg/dL)
1 month and younger	1
Second month of life	<0.5
3 months–6 years	<0.6
6–15 years	<1.0

B. Causes

1. There are many causes of AKI in children, including prerenal causes, intrinsic renal failure, (also known as ATN), and postrenal failure.

2. Prerenal causes, the most common cause of AKI, are usually caused by poor perfusion (Table 5.4). A decrease in renal perfusion causes decreased glomerular perfusion and GFR. Prerenal causes, by definition, are not associated with any intrinsic parenchymal disease. Impaired RBF may be secondary to impaired cardiac performance, intravascular volume depletion, renal vasoconstriction, or renal artery thrombosis. When reduction of RBF is mild to moderate, kidney blood flow and GFR are maintained by autoregulatory response. This is accomplished by autoregulation of afferent arteriolar dilation and efferent arteriolar vasoconstriction. Prerenal AKI will occur when adaptive mechanisms fail and GFR falls. There is a good prognosis for kidney function if prompt recognition and restoration of adequate RBF is achieved. Two common classes of medications, nonsteroidal anti-inflammatory drugs (NSAIDs) and ACE inhibitors, can cause prerenal AKI by impairing renal autoregulation. Hypoxic/ischemic and nephrotoxic acute kidney failure are the most common causes of hospital-acquired kidney failure. In more current studies, cardiopulmonary bypass has been associated with a 20% to 40% AKI rate (Fortenberry et al., 2013).

3. Intrinsic renal failure is also known as ATN and is related to decreased perfusion to the renal parenchyma as in hemolytic uremic syndrome (HUS), acute glomerulonephritis, or acute interstitial nephritis. The condition is typically reversible except when ischemia is severe enough to cause cortical necrosis producing oliguria (rare). *ATN* is the death of tubular cells, which may result when tubular cells are deprived of oxygen (*ischemic ATN*) or when they have been exposed to a toxic drug or molecule (*nephrotoxic ATN*). When mean arterial blood pressure drops significantly, renal autoregulatory processes are no longer functional, often leading to development of ATN and uremic syndrome. Multiple factors, including systemic maldistribution of volume and decrease in blood flow secondary to circulating mediators, affect blood and oxygen delivery to the kidneys. Fortunately, new tubular cells usually replace those that have died. The tubular cells of the kidneys undergo a continuous cycle of cell death and renewal, much like the cells of the skin (Lerma, 2009).

   a. *Etiology*

      i. *Nephrotoxic* ATN is a toxic insult to the renal tubules secondary to nephrotoxic drugs, radiographic contrast dye, organic solvents, or inappropriate levels of hemoglobin or myoglobin. Tubular epithelium necrosis occurs. The healing process and prognosis are better than that for ischemic ATN because the supporting basement membrane is not affected. The most frequently used nephrotoxic medications that have been associated with ATN in the pediatric population include lasix, gentamycin, vancomycin, and gancyclovir (Slater et al., 2017).

TABLE 5.4   Causes of Prerenal Acute Kidney Injury

Volume Depletion	Cardiac Dysfunction	Peripheral Vasodilation	Afferent Arteriolar Constriction	Efferent Arteriolar Vasodilation
Inadequate intake	Acute myocardial infarction	Sepsis	Hypercalcemia	ACE inhibitors
Hemorrhage	Cardiomyopathy	Cirrhosis	Sepsis	ARBs
Gastrointestinal losses	Valvular disease	Chronic anemia	Hepatorenal syndrome	
Renal losses	Arrhythmias	Medications (e.g., NSAIDs, amphotericin B, cyclosporine)		
Skin losses	Cardiopulmonary bypass			
Third spacing				

ACE, angiotensin-converting enzyme; ARBs, angiotensin II receptor blockers; NSAIDs, nonsteroidal anti-inflammatory drugs.

ii. *Ischemic* ATN (hemodynamically mediated renal failure) is a sudden and sustained decline of GFR and necrosis of the tubule cells secondary to nephrotoxic injury. Compensatory and autoregulatory mechanisms are exhausted. Renal oxygen delivery is critically impaired, causing tubular and cellular damage. The body attempts to compensate and maintain adequate RBF and GFR by sodium and water retention, which results in decreased urine output. Oliguric ATN has a much worse prognosis than nonoliguric ATN. Common complications of AKI are noted in Table 5.5.

b. *Pathophysiology*

i. Vasoactive factors. Arteriolar vasoconstriction is induced.

ii. Tubular factors. As the hydrostatic pressure increases, there is back leak from the tubular lumen to the vasa recta. Cellular sloughing and casts cause tubular obstruction.

iii. Vascular factors. In low blood flow states, nephrotoxins are concentrated in the renal tubular cells. Glomerular capillary permeability increases for proteins and decreases for potassium.

iv. Metabolic factors. Damage to the cell membrane and impaired cellular function occur as the calcium flux is altered and oxygen free radicals are formed.

c. *The clinical course of ATN can be divided into four phases*

i. The *onset*, or *initiating phase*, is the time from the precipitating event until cell injury occurs. The duration is hours to days. It may correspond with prerenal failure. Renal failure is reversible at this point. The time course may be *hours* for postischemic ATN compared with *days* for nephrotoxic ATN.

ii. The *oliguric phase* is the time from cell injury to the development of uremia. Duration is 1 to 2 weeks. Oliguria (urine output of less than 1 mL/kg/hr) is more common in postischemic ATN. *Anuria* (no urine output) is uncommon in ATN, which is more common in postrenal obstruction. The following events characterize development of severe nephron dysfunction and uremia or uremic syndrome during this phase:

- GFR is significantly decreased.
- Hypervolemia occurs.
- BUN and plasma creatinine increase.

TABLE 5.5 Common Complications of Acute Kidney Failure

Metabolic	Cardiovascular	Gastrointestinal	Neurologic	Hematologic	Infectious	Other
Hyperkalemia	Pulmonary edema	Nausea	Neuromuscular irritability	Anemia	Pneumonia	Hiccups
Metabolic acidosis	Arrhythmias	Vomiting	Asterixis	Bleeding	Septicemia	Increased parathyroid hormone
Hyponatremia	Pericarditis	Malnutrition	Seizures		Urinary tract infection	Low total triiodothyronine
Hypocalcemia	Pericardial effusion	Gastrointestinal hemorrhage	Mental status changes			Low thyroxine
Hyperphosphatemia	Pulmonary embolism					Normal free thyroxine
Hypermagnesemia	Hypertension					
Hyperuricemia	Myocardial infarction					

Source: Adapted from Toto, R. D. (2004). Approach to patient with kidney disease. In B. M. Brenner (Ed.), Brenner & Rector's: The kidney (7th ed., pp. 1079–1086). Philadelphia, PA: Elsevier.

- Electrolyte imbalances occur.
- Metabolic acidosis is present.
- Side effects of the accumulation of uremic toxins are evident (sluggishness, insomnia, itching, slurring of speech, anorexia, nausea, vomiting, confusion, asterixis, seizures, coma).

iii. The *diuretic phase* is the beginning of recovery characterized by improved urine output, increased urea excretion, and solute excretion. Duration is 7 to 14 days. Signs of gradual improvement of overall renal function are seen. In the early part of the phase, urine output dramatically increases each day. In the beginning of the diuretic phase, "dumb" urine is excreted; "dumb" urine is similar to filtrate and shows little function of reabsorption or secretion. Throughout the diuretic phase, urea excretion and solute reabsorption and secretion improve. By the end of this phase, the BUN has fallen and stabilized, electrolyte balance and acidosis are improved, and GFR begins to return to normal. Renal replacement therapy may be indicated during this phase until kidney function has returned enough to control fluid and electrolyte balance. Administration of fluid to replace urine output may be necessary if the patient's volume status and assessment indicate.

iv. During the *recovery phase*, renal function slowly reoccurs. It may take years for renal function to return to normal. There may be residual damage and a certain percentage of unrecoverable renal function. Children may have some degree of chronic renal failure for months or years after the insult but generally have steadily improving renal function as months and years pass. Intermittent monitoring of renal function will be required (Lerma, 2009).

4. Postrenal failure is usually associated with obstruction of urine flow at any point in the ureters, bladder, or urethral meatus and is caused by such conditions as Wilms' tumor, renal calculi, blood clots, or edema. AKI secondary to postrenal failure is a relatively small percentage of the cases of AKI, but it is an important cause of renal failure in newborn males with posterior urethral valve. Hydronephrosis is a key finding indicating the presence of obstruction.

C. Laboratory Findings in AKI

1. *Urinalysis.* Common findings in AKI. Diagnostic laboratory values (urine and serum) are detailed in Table 5.6.

- **a.** *Urinary sediment*
  - i. Intrinsic kidney failure
- **b.** *Color*
  - i. "Dirty" brown. Intrinsic kidney failure
  - ii. Reddish brown. Acute glomerulonephritis
  - iii. Bilious tinge. Mixed hepatic and renal failure

TABLE 5.6　Diagnostic Laboratory Values (Urine and Serum)

Diagnostic Labs	Prerenal	ATN
Urine output	Decreased	Decreased or normal
Urine sediment	Normal	Red blood cell casts, cellular debris
Specific gravity	High (>1.020)	Low (≤1.010)
Osmolality (urine-to-plasma ratio)	>1.5 (>1.2 in neonates)	<1.2
Urine sodium	Low (<10 mEq/L)	High (>30 mEq/L) (>25 mEq/L in neonates)
Creatinine (urine-to-plasma ratio)	>15:1	<10:1
FENa (%)	<1 (<2.5 in neonates)	>2 (>3 in neonates)
Creatinine	Normal or slowly increasing	High and increasing
BUN	High	High and increasing

ATN, acute tubular necrosis; BUN, blood urea nitrogen; FENa, excreted fraction of filtered sodium.

Note: Diuretic administration may affect results or measurement of urine sodium.

   c. *Proteinuria*

     i. Glomerulonephritis

     ii. Interstitial nephritis

     iii. Toxic and infectious causes

   d. *Casts*

     i. RBC casts. Glomerulonephritis or vasculitis

     ii. WBC casts. Interstitial nephritis

     iii. Granular casts. Glomerulonephritis

     iv. Uric acid crystals. Tumor lysis syndrome (TLS)

     v. Calcium oxylate crystals. Ethylene glycol ingestion

     vi. Acetaminophen crystals. Acetaminophen toxicity (acute)

2. *Serum Chemistries*

   a. *Hyperkalemia*

     i. Hyperkalemia occurs secondary to decreased renal excretion. Oliguric patients do not excrete sufficient potassium to maintain a normal balance. Hyperkalemia may be exacerbated by metabolic acidosis, which causes a shift of potassium from the intracellular space. Continued acid production occurs from catabolic cellular metabolism, despite loss of renal excretory function. Multiple blood transfusions and RBC hemolysis release potassium. The longer the blood is stored, the higher the potassium content of the blood as a result of cell lysis and potassium release. Blood banks generally release the oldest unit of blood first. In an infant or child with hyperkalemia requiring blood transfusion, a specific request should be made for a fresh unit of blood.

     ii. ECG changes secondary to hyperkalemia can range from peaked T waves, prolonged PR interval, and complete heart block to ventricular fibrillation as the potassium level increases.

     iii. Other clinical manifestations may include muscle cramps, muscle weakness, muscle twitching, abdominal cramps, diarrhea, and ileus.

     iv. Management of hyperkalemia depends on the severity of electrolyte imbalance. Patients with a serum potassium level greater than 7 mEq/L and evidence of myocardial toxicity are at an extremely high risk for lethal arrhythmias. Prompt, aggressive intervention is critical for survival.

1) Treatment measures include the administration of insulin (0.1 units/kg regular insulin) and hypertonic glucose (0.5 to 1 mL/kg 50% dextrose) to promote cellular uptake of potassium. These medications essentially "move" the potassium around in the body and are *not* causing true potassium excretion. The effects of cellular shifts on serum potassium are short lived and require frequent monitoring of serum sodium and potassium. These medications may need to be redosed until potassium excretion occurs.

2) Albuterol is another pharmacologic strategy used to shift serum potassium into the cellular space, although it is not as potent as IV strategies. Its peak action is 90 to 120 minutes. Patients with hyperkalemia may be placed on continuous inhaled albuterol.

3) Movement of the potassium into the cells can be facilitated by administration of sodium bicarbonate (1–3 mEq/kg) in the absense of acidosis. (*Caution:* Do not mix calcium and bicarbonate in IV solutions because precipitation will occur.)

4) Stabilize the myocardium with IV calcium (10–20 mg/kg per dose calcium chloride [infants and children] or 50–100 mg/kg per dose calcium gluconate [infants and children]).

5) Eliminate exogenous sources of potassium (potassium-free hydration).

6) Remove potassium from the patient using resin exchange via the gastrointestinal tract with a sodium polystyrene sulfonate (Kayexalate) enema (1 g/kg per dose). (*Note*: Repeat the enema two or three times per 24-hour period if necessary.) Sodium polystyrene sulfonate (Kayexalate) exchanges sodium for potassium in the gastrointestinal tract. It must be retained in the gastrointestinal tract to cause the renin exchange and ultimate removal of potassium. If it is not retained, the dose should be repeated. It may be instilled high in the rectum using a red rubber tube. Full effect is usually seen in 4 hours.

7) If kidney function is absent or severely impaired, or if hyperkalemia is severe, consider hemodialysis. Hemodialysis against a potassium-free dialysate can decrease serum potassium as rapidly as 1.5 mEq/hr. CRRT without potassium in the

replacement fluid or dialysate is also an option if the patient is too hemodynamically unstable to tolerate hemodialysis.

b. *Hyperphosphatemia*

i. Hyperphosphatemia occurs primarily as a result of the kidney's inability to excrete phosphate in mild to moderate renal insufficiency. Phosphorus homeostasis is maintained by an increase in phosphorus excretion per nephron through the action of PTH. As renal failure progresses and GFR is less than 30 mL per minute, elevated phosphorus level will ensue. Hyperphosphatemia may also be secondary to TLS, rhabdomyolysis, bowel infarction, ileus, or the use of oral phosphates and/or sodium phosphate enemas in the presence of gastrointestinal tract abnormalities.

ii. Hyperphosphatemia may not produce signs and symptoms until levels are very high (>10 mEq/L); however, a secondary hypocalcemia may develop as an attempt to compensate. See clinical manifestations in the discussion of hypocalcemia.

iii. Management of hyperphosphatemia may include IV fluid therapy to increase phosphorus excretion or administration of IV calcium. Use of enteral calcium-based phosphate binders should be considered. Administration of phosphorus-containing agents and dietary phosphorus intake should be minimized. Acute situations can be managed initially with the administration of insulin and glucose by shifting phosphorus from the extracellular space to the intracellular space. Management of severe hyperphosphatemia (greater than 10–12 mEq/L) may include hemodialysis or renal replacement therapy to decrease phosphate levels.

iv. Long-term sequelae include increased risk of mortality, cardiovascular disease, bone disease, and extraskeletal calcification of soft tissues, including blood vessels, lungs, kidneys, and joints.

c. *Hypocalcemia*

i. Pathophysiology. Serum calcium declines reciprocally as phosphorus rises. Alterations in calcium most often occur secondary to hyperphosphatemia. Other reasons for hypocalcemia include induced resistance to the action of PTH, crush injury (occurs early), severe muscle damage, large transfusions of citrate-containing blood products, sepsis, and hypomagnesemia.

ii. Clinical manifestations of calcium or phosphate imbalance include CNS changes (anxiety, tetany, and seizures), muscle cramps, hypotension, and Trousseau's and Chvostek's signs.

iii. Management of hypocalcemia includes decreasing the serum phosphate levels and replacing magnesium, if indicated, to increase PTH release. If the patient is symptomatic, administer IV 10% calcium gluconate (50–100 mg/kg per dose; maximum dose, 2 g). If a more rapid response is required, use calcium chloride (10–20 mg/kg per dose [infants and children] and 37–74 mg/kg per dose [neonates]; maximum dose, 1 g). Infuse slowly (do not exceed 1 mL/min), and monitor for bradycardia and asystole with IV calcium infusion. Because of high osmolar content, extravasation with IV administration can cause severe tissue damage.

iv. In AKI, PTH's ability to serve as a regulator of phosphorus and calcium balance is compromised because of the alteration in the renal absorption of calcium and excretion of phosphate. Decreased synthesis of the active form of vitamin D results in hypocalcemia.

d. *Hypermagnesemia*

i. Mild hypermagnesemia may occur in AKI secondary to decreased renal excretion of magnesium. It may be secondary to the use of magnesium-containing antacids (Maalox) or total parenteral nutrition (TPN).

ii. Clinical manifestations. Acute elevations may depress the CNS, peripheral neuromuscular junction, and deep-tendon reflexes. There is an increased potential for hypotension, hypoventilation, and cardiac arrhythmias.

iii. Management of hypermagnesemia usually does not require intervention other than discontinuing magnesium-containing substances (e.g., Maalox). Calcium acts as a direct antagonist to magnesium. In life-threatening situations, IV calcium may be administered. Dialysis may be used for removal of magnesium because loop diuretics in particular enhance magnesium excretion. PTH stimulates reabsorption of magnesium from the tubules.

e. Glucose intolerance may develop secondary to decreased peripheral sensitivity to insulin when renal excretion is decreased. Renal replacement therapy can remove glucose.

f. Uremia is related to the accumulation of toxins and waste products normally excreted in the urine and is measured as BUN.

   i. Azotemia refers to a high serum concentration of nitrogenous wastes. Buildup of creatinine is not harmful to the body; however, uremia can have deleterious effects. Uremic pericarditis occurs only in the presence of prolonged severe renal failure and results from chemical irritation of the pericardium secondary to the metabolic abnormalities. It may culminate in cardiac tamponade or cause recurrent hypotension during hemodialysis. If adequate relief of uremic pericarditis does not occur with hemodialysis, pericardiectomy is recommended.

   ii. Clinical manifestations are due to toxic effects of substances such as urea and ammonia. Neurologic symptoms include lethargy, confusion, seizures, and coma. Gastrointestinal tract symptoms include anorexia, nausea, vomiting, diarrhea, and gastrointestinal tract bleeding. Cardiovascular symptoms include hypervolemia and hypotension secondary to shifts of fluid into the extracellular space. Hematologic compromise involves normochromic, normocytic anemia, thrombocytopenia, platelet dysfunction, and increased bleeding time. Skin symptoms include pruritus and discoloration. Immunosuppression may result. Bone manifestations include osteodystrophies such as osteomalacia, adynamic bone disease, and growth retardation in children. Endocrine manifestations include sexual dysfunction, hyperprolactinemia contributing to amenorrhea and galactorrhea in women, low total T4 and T3 and free T3, but normal free T4, reverse T3, and thyroid-stimulating hormone (TSH), suggesting a normal thyroid state. In early CKD, increased insulin resistance and glucose intolerance (azotemic pseudodiabetes), elevated triglycerides and very low-density lipoprotein (VLDL) and decreased high-density lipoprotein (HDL), and decreased protein synthesis and increased catabolism (Lerma, 2009).

   iii. Initial management includes conservative therapies related to diet and medications. The goals of conservative treatment are to treat the cause of CKD if possible and detect/treat any reversible cause of decreased kidney function, prevent/slow progression of CKD, prevent/treat complications of CKD, prevent/treat complications associated with other comorbid conditions such as diabetes and cardiovascular disease, and prepare for replacement therapy. Referral to a nephrologist should occur when estimated GFR is less than 30 mL/min (Stage IV; Lerma, 2009). *Management* for symptomatic patients may include renal replacement therapy (either dialysis or transplantation).

g. *Acid–Base Imbalance*

   i. Metabolic acidosis occurs in AKI because of alterations in renal function, including a decrease in GFR, decreased hydrogen ion secretion, decreased bicarbonate reabsorption, decreased ammonia (NH_3) synthesis, and ammonium (NH_4) excretion. Acidosis in ARF results in an increase in the anion gap.

Anion gap = Sodium – (Chloride + Bicarbonate)

   ii. Clinical manifestations of acidosis secondary to AKI include increased minute ventilation, a change in mental status as ammonium excretion decreases, and hyperkalemia as potassium excretion decreases, causing an increased potential for lethal dysrhythmias. Other manifestations can include decreased cardiac output, decreased tissue perfusion, and altered oxygen delivery.

   iii. Management involves the correction of metabolic acidosis. Minor adjustments may be made by hyperventilation. IV administration of bicarbonate in the form of sodium bicarbonate or THAM may be necessary for significant correction (Table 5.7).

h. Hematologic changes include anemia and abnormal platelet function. Anemia is related to decreased erythrocyte production, changes secondary to volume status (i.e., hemoconcentration or hemodilution), frequent blood sampling, and bleeding. Patients with chronic renal failure require erythropoietin supplementation because of decreased erythrocyte production. Although platelet number is generally normal in uremia, the bleeding time is prolonged because of defective platelet activation and adhesiveness. Coagulation tests are normal in AKI. Skin bleeding time is the best predictor of clinical bleeding. Uremic bleeding is usually mild mucocutaneous bleeding. If a uremic patient bleeds, consider a structural or other hemostatic abnormality. If the hemostatic defect is thought to be related solely to the renal failure, peritoneal or hemodialysis can usually reverse the hemostatic disorder. Uremic patients who undergo surgery are always at risk for bleeding. Consider administration of desmopressin (DDAVP) before surgery.

TABLE 5.7 Renal Response to Changes in Acid–Base Balance

Change in Acid–Base Balance	Renal Response
Respiratory Acidosis	
Carbon dioxide and bicarbonate are retained	Increase bicarbonate in plasma to take up hydrogen ions
Plasma hydrogen ions rise	Acid excreted in urine
Respiratory Alkalosis	
Elimination or blowing off of carbon dioxide increases	Increase excretion of bicarbonate to conserve dioxide hydrogen ions
Plasma hydrogen ion concentration decreases	
Metabolic Acidosis	
Plasma bicarbonate decreases and plasma hydrogen ion concentration increases	Replenish bicarbonate
Metabolic Alkalosis	
Plasma bicarbonate increases	Fewer intracellular hydrogen ions available for secretion
Plasma and intracellular hydrogen ion concentration decreases	Some bicarbonate escapes into the urine (alkaline urine)
Chronic Acidosis	
	Increase production of ammonia (NH_3) to bind with hydrogen ions and excrete ammonium (NH_4^+) in urine

TABLE 5.8 Clinical Manifestations of Potential Multisystem Complications Secondary to AKI

System	Clinical Manifestations
Cardiovascular	ECG changes secondary to hyperkalemia
Respiratory	Pneumonia, pulmonary edema
Gastrointestinal	Hemorrhage, abdominal cramping, nausea and vomiting, diarrhea, malnutrition
Neurologic	Altered mental status
Metabolic	Acidosis, hypercalcemia, hyperkalemia, uremia, hypermagnesemia, hyperphosphatemia, hyperuricemia
Hematologic	Anemia, coagulopathy
Infection	Sepsis, pneumonia

AKI, acute kidney injury.

i. Infection is a risk for AKI patients, who have an altered immune response secondary to the suppression of macrophages by uremic toxins. Invasive lines increase the risk. Prophylactic antibiotic therapy is generally not indicated.

j. Complications include potential multisystem complications (Table 5.8).

D. **Management of AKI**

1. Response to treatment is related to the extent of nephron damage and ATN.

a. In *prerenal failure*, there is no actual nephron damage and the kidneys respond well to treatment for symptoms of decreased urine output, electrolyte abnormalities, or both.

b. In *true intrinsic ATN*, actual nephron damage has occurred and response to therapy to treat the underlying problem of renal dysfunction is variable. Some function may return, or it may not.

2. The plan of care to support renal function includes eliminating the cause of AKI, if known, and discontinuing or altering the dose of potentially nephrotoxic medications. All drugs excreted by the kidneys require an alteration of the dosage based on the level of renal function. Serum concentrations of potentially toxic drugs should be closely monitored. Creatinine clearance and serum creatinine should be monitored when using potentially nephrotoxic agents. Drug-dosage alteration is indicated with increased levels of serum creatinine. If a patient is receiving renal replacement therapy, drug supplementation may be necessary to restore the drug that is removed or filtrated.

3. Maintain adequate intravascular volume and maintain adequate blood pressure. Administer inotropic agents as needed to support cardiac output and perfusion to the kidneys.

4. Pharmacologic support includes diuretics and other agents. Common indications for diuretic therapy include pulmonary edema, hypertension, hypercalcemia, hyperkalemia, generalized edema, hypervolemia, and increased intracranial pressure. Diuretics promote renal excretion of water, either directly or indirectly by acting on different segments of the tubules.

a. *Loop diuretics* inhibit reabsorption of sodium and chloride in the ascending loop of Henle and distal renal tubule, interfering with the chloride-binding cotransport system. This leads to increased excretion of water, potassium, sodium, chloride, magnesium, and calcium. Furosemide (Lasix) and bumetanide (Bumex) are two of the most potent loop diuretics. Lasix can be given as bolus doses of 1 mg/kg/dose or as a continuous drip with a starting dose of 0.05–0.1 mg/kg/hr. Potential complications include hypovolemia, hypokalemia, hyponatremia, metabolic alkalosis, hypercalciuria, hypomagnesemia, hyperglycemia, ototoxicity, renal calculi, and thrombocytopenia.

b. *Thiazide diuretics* inhibit sodium reabsorption in the distal tubules, leading to excretion of sodium, chloride, potassium, bicarbonate, magnesium, phosphate, calcium, and water. Chlorothiazide (Diuril; dose is 2 mg/kg/dose IV every 8–12 hours) or hydrochlorothiazide (HydroDIURIL) is frequently used as a secondary or adjunct agent in diuretic therapy. Potential complications are similar to loop diuretics. Potassium supplemental therapy may be indicated.

c. *Nonthiazide, sulfonamide diuretics* inhibit sodium reabsorption in the cortical diluting site and proximal tubules, leading to increased excretion of sodium and water as well as potassium and hydrogen ions. Metolazone (Zaroxolyn) is frequently used as a secondary agent in conjunction with loop diuretics.

d. *Potassium-sparing diuretics* compete with aldosterone for binding sites in the distal tubule, increasing sodium chloride and water excretion while conserving potassium and hydrogen ions. Spironolactone (aldosterone antagonist) is the most commonly used agent. Potassium-sparing diuretics are used in conjunction with a potassium-depleting diuretic agent to decrease the occurrence of hypokalemia. They also have minimal side effects but may block the effect of aldosterone on arteriolar smooth muscle.

e. *Osmotic diuretics* increase the osmotic pressure in the glomerular filtrate, which inhibits tubular reabsorption of water and electrolytes, thus increasing urinary output. Mannitol is a sugar that is relatively inert and freely filtered by the glomerulus; however, it is not greatly reabsorbed by the renal tubule. The transient pulling of fluid into the intravascular space can increase the intravascular volume significantly; therefore, mannitol should not be used with patients in congestive heart failure and hypervolemia or in those with renal failure.

f. *Acetazolamide (Diamox)* acts by competitively inhibiting carbonic anhydrase, resulting in increased excretion of sodium, potassium, bicarbonate, and water. It also results in a decrease in the formation of aqueous humor. Metabolic acidosis can result secondary to the limitation of secretion of hydrogen ions from the tubule and subsequent decreased reabsorption of bicarbonate and sodium.

g. *Fenoldopam* is a continuous infusion that is a dopamine 1 receptor agonist. It contains both renal vasodilatory and naturetic properties secondary to tubular sodium excretion (Moffett, Mott, Nelson, Goldstein, & Jeffries, 2008). Dose is 0.3 to 0.5 mcg/kg/min. Therefore, in critically ill children, it can both improve urine output and decrease blood pressure in hypertensive patients at higher doses.

E. Replacement Therapy

Consider renal replacement therapy if function cannot be adequately supported using the preceding measures.

F. Complications

Complications of end-stage renal disease (ESRD) include hypertensive disease, hyperlipidemia, and hyperparathyroidism because of poor control of calcium and phosphate levels.

HEMOLYTIC UREMIC SYNDROME

A. Definition

HUS is the simultaneous occurrence of hemolytic anemia, thrombocytopenia, and renal failure. It is the most common cause of acute renal failure in young children (Kliegman, Stanton, St. Geme, & Schor, 2016).

B. Pathophysiology

Pathophysiology is characterized by microangiopathy with platelet aggregation and fibrin deposition in small vessels in the kidney, gut, and CNS. Hemolytic anemia is believed to be a result of the shearing of red cells as they pass through narrowed vessels.

C. Types of HUS

1. Typical HUS peaks from June to September with gastrointestinal prodromes (vomiting, diarrhea, abdominal pain) during the days to weeks preceding onset. HUS is characteristically a disease of young children. *Escherichia coli* 0157:H7 causes a large number of cases of typical HUS.

2. Atypical HUS is an extremely rare group of disorders of the kidneys and is distinctly different from the HUS syndrome caused by *E. coli* 0157:H7. It occurs year round and there is generally no gastrointestinal prodrome. It is rare in children younger than 2 years. Relapses can occur, and these cases may evolve to terminal renal failure. Children with atypical HUS are much more likely to develop chronic complications such as kidney failure and severe high blood pressure. Familial occurrence is possible. There is substantial evidence that atypical HUS is a genetic disorder.

D. Clinical Symptoms

Clinical symptoms of HUS include bloody diarrhea (more common in typical HUS), mild to moderate hypertension, fever, lethargy, decreased urine output, and paleness, petechia, dehydration.

E. Laboratory Findings

Laboratory findings reveal increased schistocyte number on peripheral smear, anemia (age specific), and an elevated reticulocyte count. Other indicators of intravascular hemolysis include elevated lactate dehydrogenase (LDH), increased indirect bilirubin level, and low haptoglobin level. The Coomb's test is negative. Mild leukocytosis may accompany hemolytic anemia. Thrombocytopenia is uniformly present, and the platelet count is generally less than $60,000/mm^3$. Prothrombin time, partial thromboplastin time, fibrinogen level, and coagulation factors are normal (Swartz, 2008).

F. Management and Treatment

Management and treatment are primarily focused on general supportive care and treatment of complications such as AKI, anemia, CNS symptoms, and abdominal symptoms. Platelet transfusion is warranted if the patient is actively bleeding. Peritoneal dialysis (PD) is the treatment of choice until renal function returns.

G. Outcomes

1. Prognosis—Mortality is less than 10% with typical HUS. Hypertension, proteinuria, and low GFR effects 25% of patients. Prognosis is worse with patients who have neurological involvement.

2. Significant renal failure is seen in more than 90% of patients with HUS. Dialysis is required for many of these patients.

NEPHROTIC SYNDROME

A. Nephrotic syndrome is a pediatric disorder that is characterized by proteinuria greater than 40 mg/m²/hr, hypoalbuminemia, edema, and hyperlipidemia that occurs secondary to glomerular damage. It can be a primary or secondary disease.

1. *Nephrotic syndrome* in children is primarily "idiopathic" (90%), and its presentation and relapses are often associated with a recent upper respiratory infection. It usually presents between 2 and 6 years of age and affects males more often than females. Idiopathic nephrotic syndrome can be divided into three morphologic patterns: (1) minimal-change disease (85%), (2) mesangial proliferation (5%), or (3) focal sclerosis (10%). Presenting signs and symptoms include periorbital edema, dependent edema, ascites, foamy appearance of the urine, weight gain, irritability, pleural effusions, and decreased appetite.

2. *Secondary nephrotic syndrome* can be induced by membranous nephropathy, glomerulonephritis, lupus nephritis, malaria, hepatitis B, and HIV. It has also been associated with malignancy and can occur as a result of exposure to numerous renal toxic drugs and chemicals.

3. *Diagnosis.* Urinalysis that reveals +3 or +4 protein with occasional microscopic hematuria, decreased creatinine clearance, low serum albumin, elevated cholesterol, and triglycerides.

4. *Treatment* includes diuretics, antihypertensive medications, and dietary salt restriction to manage symptoms. Patients with minimal-change disease may be responsive to corticosteroid therapy; however, if the proteinuria persists for longer than a month, a renal biopsy may be indicated to determine the precise cause of the disease. Many patients require low-dose steroid therapy for 3 to 6 months and if a relapse occurs. Patients who are resistant to steroids or have frequent relapse may be treated with cyclophosphamide.

OTHER DISEASES CAUSING AKI

A. Acute Glomerulonephritis

Acute glomerulonephritis refers to a specific set of renal diseases (such as lupus nephritis and poststreptococcal nephritis) that result from immunologic mechanisms triggering inflammation and proliferation of glomerular tissue.

1. Acute glomerulonephritis is currently described as a clinical syndrome that frequently manifests as a sudden onset of hematuria, proteinuria, and red cell casts. With the exception of poststreptococcal glomerulonephritis, the exact triggers for the formation of the immune complexes are unclear. In streptococcal infection, involvement of derivatives of streptococcal proteins has been reported. A streptococcal neuraminidase may alter host immunoglobulin G (IgG). IgG combines with host antibodies. IgG/anti-IgG immune complexes are formed and then collect in the glomeruli. In addition, antibody titers to other antigens, such as antistreptolysin O or antihyaluronidase, DNAase-B, and streptokinase, provide evidence of a recent streptococcal infection and may be elevated. Antigen–antibody complexes mediate glomerular injury. Hypofiltration occurs as a result of decreased glomerular blood flow. Glomerular blood flow decreases as a result of arteriolar vasoconstriction, capillary obstruction by thrombi, and endothelial cell edema from proliferation of endothelial cells and WBC infiltration.

2. Clinical signs and symptoms include salt and water retention secondary to decreased GFR, RBC, or granular casts in the urine, declining renal function, hypertension, hematuria, oliguria, and other nonspecific symptoms such as fever, malaise, abdominal discomfort, nausea, or vomiting.

3. Management includes sodium and water restriction and treatment of underlying disease as well as management of declining renal function.

4. *Outcome.* Sporadic cases of acute nephritis progress to a chronic form. This progression occurs in as many as 30% of adult and 10% of pediatric patients. The mortality rate of acute glomerulonephritis has been reported at 0% to 7%. The male-to-female ratio is 2:1. Most cases of acute glomerulonephritis occur in patients aged 5 to 15 years.

B. Hepatorenal Syndrome

Hepatorenal syndrome is renal failure that develops in the presence of end-stage liver disease in absence of intrinsic kidney disease. Hepatorenal failure may accompany liver failure related to fulminant hepatic failure, hepatic malignancy, liver resection, hepatitis, or biliary tract obstruction.

1. Kidney dysfunction results from renal hypoperfusion characterized by intense constriction of the renal cortical vasculature resulting in decreased GFR leading to oliguria and avid sodium retention. Portal hypertension and resultant splanchnic sequestration increase cardiac output and decrease peripheral vascular resistance, termed *hyperdynamic circulation*. In response, vasoconstrictor systems (including the renin-angiotensin system) are activated and direct the kidneys to retain water and sodium in order to maintain hemodynamic stability. As cirrhosis worsens, increased systemic vasodilation and accompanying compensatory vasoconstriction further compromise renal perfusion leading to renal failure.

2. Signs and symptoms include increased renal vascular resistance, decreased glomerular filtration, increased sodium and water retention (secondary to hyperaldosteronism), decreased urine output, and electrolyte and coagulation abnormalities. Symptoms are marked by rapid and progressive deterioration of renal function and the patient typically demonstrates severely decompensated liver cirrhosis, jaundice, and hyponatremia. Oliguria and rising creatinine develop over a few days. In approximately 50% of patients, it is difficult to pinpoint a cause triggering the event. For the remainder, onset of hepatrorenal syndrome follows a readily apparent precipitating event such as infection, significant gastrointestinal hemorrhage, overaggressive diuresis, or large volume paracentesis (>5 L) without replacement of the intravascular volume (Lerma, 2009).

3. After exclusion of other causes of renal disease, management includes treatment of the hepatic failure and support of renal function. Intravascular volume depletion and nephrotoxic agents should also be avoided. Sepsis should be considered in the patient with cirrhosis with acute renal deterioration and a full septic workup should be completed even in the absence of symptoms such as leukocytosis and fever. Pharmacological interventions are aimed at improving systemic hemodynamics by increasing systemic or splanchnic vasoconstriction in order to improve renal perfusion pressure and glomerular filtration (Lerma, 2009).

4. Prognosis is poor for patients without subsequent liver transplant as it is the only established therapy that improves renal failure.

C. Tumor Lysis Syndrome

TLS typically occurs after effective chemotherapy or radiation, but it may occur after treatment with glucocorticoids, antiestrogen tamoxifen, and interferon. It is most likely to occur in patients with poorly differentiated leukemias and lymphomas, a high WBC count, or bulky lymphoma. During tumor lysis, rapid release of intracellular metabolites exceeds the excretory capacity of the kidneys.

1. Potential effects of tumor lysis include hyperuricemia, hypocalcemia, hyperphosphatemia, hyperkalemia, and hyperxanthinemia. These electrolyte imbalances lead to crystallization, tubular obstruction, decreased urine output, and renal failure. The severity of the condition is proportional to the tumor burden, rapid proliferation kinetics (such as Burkitt's lymphoma or acute lymphocytic leukemia), extensive bone marrow involvement, LDH levels above 1,500 IU/mL, and with tumors highly sensitive to chemotherapy or radiation. Patients are at increased risk of developing TLS when there is a previous history of renal impairment, volume depletion, concomitant nephrotoxic medication use, and an acidic urine pH that can facilitate uric acid crystal formation (Lerma, 2009). Prevention of complications from cell breakdown is the optimal goal.

2. *Prevention is paramount.* At-risk patients should receive vigorous hydration and allopurinol before cancer treatment is begun. Urate oxidases and urinary alkalinization should be considered. Electrolyte imbalances should be treated promptly. Hypocalcemia should not be treated unless the patient is symptomatic because administration of calcium may precipitate metastatic calcifications in a patient with hyperphosphatemia. PD is not as effective as hemodialysis because the clearance rates for phosphate and uric acid are significantly lower. Severe electrolyte disturbances may require hemodialysis or CRRT and may be required in up to 30% of patients of AKI associated with TLS. Left untreated, TLS may lead to severe, life-threatening cardiac arrhythmias, seizures, muscle paralysis, and death (Lerma, 2009).

D. Cardiac Failure and Cardiopulmonary Bypass

Changes in renal function may be attributed to hypovolemia or hypervolemia, hypotension, and electrolyte imbalance. Worsening cardiac function in patients with heart failure leads to decreased cardiac output, which may lead to decreased renal flow and decreased GFR, decreased flow to the parenchyma, and ATN. AKI incidence ranges from 1% to 82% in ICU and postoperative cardiopulmonary bypass patients admitted to the ICU (Fortenberry et al., 2013).

E. Rhabdomyolysis

Rhabdomyolysis can be caused directly by muscle injury or indirectly by several medical conditions (Table 5.9). It results in lysis of the cell membrane and leakage of its contents, including myoglobin, potassium, phosphorus, and enzymes, into the bloodstream.

1. *Diagnosis.* Myoglobin is a small, bright-red protein that is common in muscle cells. It gives the muscle much of its red coloration. Myoglobin stores oxygen for use when muscles are exercised. The cellular release of myoglobin is often accompanied by an increase of creatine kinase (CK). Myoglobin is readily filtered by the kidney and, when excreted into the urine, it is called *myoglobinuria*. Myoglobin can precipitate, causing tubular obstruction and acute renal insufficiency. Myoglobinuria is often minimally present in most individuals after intense exertion. Factors, such as volume depletion, exercising in the heat, eccentric muscle contractions, and fasting, are potentiating factors. Increased mortality is associated with rhabdolyolysis caused by severe trauma and crush injuries. Other causes of rhabdomylysis include metablolic myopathies, hypoxia/ischemia, certain licit and illicit drugs, congestive heart failure, malignant hyperthermia, and snake bites. Clinical features of myoglobinuria are typically suffucient to recognize the condition and include weakness, discomfort, pain, tenderness, swelling, tea-colored urine, kidney dysfunction, fever, and leukocytosis. It can be recognized clinically by urinalysis with a dipstick strongly positive for heme and urine sediment with few or no red cells. A more sensitive and diagnostic finding is an elevated creatine phosphokinase (CPK). CK peaks at 12 to 36 hours after muscle injury and acute rhabdomyolysis is seen with levels exceeding 5,000 IU/L. Although transient elevations of serum creatinine disproportionate to elevation of BUN is often seen in early acute rhabdmyolysis, ARF seldom occurs until CPK levels exceed 15,000 to 20,000. Hypoalbuminuria, hyperkalemia, hyperphosphatemia, hypocalcemia, and hyperuricemia may also be observed (Lerma, 2009).

TABLE 5.9   Causes of Rhabdomyolsis and Myoglobinuria

Trauma	Infections	Fluid and Electrolyte Disorders	Drug Abuse	Medications	Thermoregulatory
Crush syndrome	Bacterial	Hypophosphatemia	Cocaine	Statins	Hyperthermia
Compression injury	Viral, most commonly influenza	Hypokalemia	Heroin	Clofibrate	Heat stroke
Compartment syndrome	Fungal (e.g., Candida, aspergillus)	Hypo/hypernatremia	Alcohol		Malignant hyperthermia (anesthesia induced)
Vascular occlusion	Malaria	Ketoacidosis	Amphetamines		
		Hyperosmolar coma	Ecstasy		

2. Renal failure may ensue from myoglobinuria resulting from ferrihemate toxicity, tubular obstruction, altered GFR, hypotension, and crystal formations. Aspartate aminotransferase and alanine aminotransferase may also be elevated as they are released from necrotic muscle.

3. Prevention of renal failure hinges on prompt and aggressive treatment that includes volume depletion and maintenance of high urine output. Mannitol and alkalinization of the urine may also be considered. Hyperkalemic cardiotoxicity may occur in patients with hypocalcemia and should be monitored for electrocardiographic changes associated with hyperkalemia despite observing modest serum hyperkalemia. Calcium infusions, as well as frequent or near constant hemodialysis, may be necessary if cardiotoxicity is observed.

RENAL REPLACEMENT THERAPIES

Renal replacement therapies for infants and children include PD, hemodialysis, and CRRT.

A. Methods of Solute Clearance and Water Removal: Convection, Diffusion, Ultrafiltration

1. Convective transport occurs when water and small particles are carried through membrane pores into ultrafiltrate by the hydrostatic pressure created by a moving stream of fluid containing large protein molecules. The important determinants of convective transport are the direction and rate of the solvent flux across the membrane. Unlike diffusion, it is not influenced by any solute concentration gradient.

2. Diffusion is the removal of a solute from a higher concentration to a lower concentration to establish equilibrium. If adequate clearance is not obtained by convection alone, it may be necessary to influence clearance by diffusion as well.

3. Ultrafiltration is the removal of extracellular fluid via convection. The rate of removal is determined by the surface area of the filter membrane, the permeability coefficient of the membrane to water, and the transmembrane pressure gradient.

B. Peritoneal Dialysis

1. *Indications for PD* include an inability to tolerate anticoagulation, ATN, renal cortical necrosis, renal agenesis, bilateral renal dysplasia, and other renal dysfunction requiring long-term, nonemergent therapy. PD is often used for infants and children in either AKI or chronic renal failure. Selection of this modality is influenced by considerations such as availability, convenience, medical factors, and socioeconomic factors. One absolute contraindication is an unsuitable peritoneum secondary to adhesions, fibrosis, or malignancy.

2. *Types of PD* include continuous ambulatory PD (CAPD), manual PD, or continuous-cycling PD using a computerized cycler device. Access is via a soft catheter placed in the peritoneal space. Catheter placement can be performed in the operating room or at the bedside.

   a. *Process.* An ordered amount of dialysate is instilled via a catheter into the peritoneal cavity. The removal of water and solutes (*ultrafiltrate*) is adjusted by raising the osmolarity of the dialysate (increasing the glucose concentration) or increasing the dwell time. Dwell times impact waste and fluid removal. Long dwell times may achieve good waste and solute clearance but poor fluid removal. Short dwell times have poor waste and solute clearance but remove a significant amount of fluid. Solutes are transported by diffusion and ultrafiltration. Smaller solutes, such as creatinine, urea, and potassium, diffuse down a concentration gradient into the peritoneal dialysate and removal is maximal at the start of the dwell. Glucose, lactate, and calcium diffuse in the opposite direction into the blood. The amount of dialysate placed into the peritoneal space (*inflow volume*) is determined by gradually increasing volumes from 15 to 50 mL/kg of body weight as tolerated. Standard dialysate solution contains dextrose, sodium, calcium, magnesium, chloride, and lactate (which is metabolized to produce bicarbonate). Potassium, heparin, or antimicrobial medications can be added to the dialysate fluid as needed. CAPD or manual PD may be needed in infants and small children when inflow volumes are less than 50 mL. Excessive inflow volume can be assessed by monitoring for signs of pain, discomfort, or respiratory compromise on inflow. The dialysate solution must be warmed to or near body temperature to prevent hypothermia.

b. *Manual PD* is more time-consuming than the cycler method. It involves manual timing of fluid dwell within the abdomen, exact measurement of inflow and outflow volumes, calculation of net ultrafiltration after each dwell time, and cumulative ultrafiltrate tabulation. Inflow is initiated, the catheter is clamped, and a timer is set to mark dwell time completion. Clots, kinks, and catheter position can affect the ability to inflow adequately. Dwell cycles generally range from 30 to 120 minutes and include fill, dwell, and drain times. On completion of the dwell time, the catheter is unclamped and the outflow drains to a urine collection bag to be measured. Drain times are dependent on catheter patency. The net ultrafiltrate is calculated (outflow volume minus inflow volume). The cycle is repeated at ordered intervals.

c. *CAPD* via a cycler utilizes the same principles as manual PD, but it requires less hands-on nursing time, has a decreased incidence of infection because of having a closed system, provides a programmable automated ultrafiltrate calculation, and has a built-in mechanism for dialysate warming.

3. *Potential complications of PD* include peritonitis, which can be indicated by cloudy dialysate, abdominal pain, tenderness, or sepsis. Mechanical and iatrogenic catheter problems may also occur and include leakage at the insertion site, bowel perforation, retroperitoneal hemorrhage, increased intraabdominal pressure resulting from obstruction of the catheter, and hernia. Ultrafiltration failure may occur as the result of the failure of PD fluid removal to match the volume balance needs of the patient. Patients present with signs and symptoms of volume overload and reversible causes should be addresed before considering alteration in peritoneal membrane function. Other complications include impaired pulmonary function related to abdominal distention or fluid overload, decreased cardiac output and stroke volume related to fluid status, hypoproteinemia resulting from protein losses in the dialysate, and hyperglycemia related to absorption of dextrose from the dialysate. Hyperglycemia may require treatment with insulin. Delayed growth and development have also been shown in children undergoing PD (Zaritsky & Warady, 2011).

C. Hemodialysis

1. *Indications for hemodialysis* may include symptomatic electrolyte imbalance, hypervolemia, pulmonary edema, severe acidosis, anuria not responsive to other therapy, severely elevated BUN and creatinine, cardiac failure, TLS, hepatic failure, hyperammonemia, drug intoxication, and other conditions that require rapid, efficient correction of the abnormality. Hemodiaysis effectively removes small-molecular-weight molecules and is relatively ineffective in removing large-sized molecules and protein-bound substances.

2. *Process.* An extracorporeal circuit carries blood from the patient via a large-bore venous catheter through a filter or artificial kidney and back to the patient. The filter is a semipermeable membrane through which water, solutes, and other substances are filtered (ultrafiltrate). Removal of small solutes is a function of the membrane surface area. Larger molecular-weight solutes are removed by membranes with larger membrane pores. Removal of solutes occurs through the filter by diffusion, which is created by infusion of the dialysate into the filter (the opposite side of the semipermeable membrane) countercurrent to the flow of blood. Negative pressure is added to the dialysate side of the circuit to increase the fluid and solute removal from the blood. Positive pressure is generated via a roller pump on the venous side of the blood circuit, increasing removal of excess fluid. Blood access is obtained via a double-lumen central venous catheter via two single-lumen central venous catheters or via an arterial-venous fistula. It is important to consider the extracorporeal circuit volume in relation to the child's circulating blood volume to prevent hypovolemia. If the extracorporeal circuit volume is greater than 10% of the child's circulating blood volume or if the child weighs less than 10 kg, the circuit may be primed with a colloid substance. Small-volume artificial kidneys and circuit sizes have enabled hemodialysis to be an option for small infants.

3. *Potential complications* include hypotension (most common), muscle cramping, nausea and vomiting, hypovolemia, hypervolemia, systemic bleeding, filter rupture or circuit disconnection, infection, and transfusion reaction.

4. *Nursing Implications.* Vital signs, oxygenation, hemodynamic parameters, fluid status, electrolyte balance, and physiologic response to treatment must be closely monitored. Inadequately treated intravascular hypovolemia, rapid electrolyte and pH changes, and hypoxemia will significantly affect cardiac function and lead to severe compromise. Volume expanders, such as albumin or isotonic crystalloid products, should be readily available during treatment. Rapid decrease in the patient's nitrogenous waste load may also result in osmotic changes that lead to an altered level of consciousness known as *disequilibrium syndrome*. Hemodialysis removes drugs along with the solutes, water, and toxins; therefore drug dosing must be adjusted for the patient receiving hemodialysis. A hemodynamically unstable child may not tolerate the rapid fluid removal associated with hemodialysis and may require a more gentle therapy such as PD or CRRT.

D. Continuous Renal Replacement Therapy

1. *Indications for CRRT* include ARF with hemodynamic instability, azotemia, severe electrolyte imbalance, hypervolemia, and symptomatic metabolic abnormalities. CRRT may also be initiated in patients who would otherwise not be able to receive adequate nutrition owing to fluid restriction. CRRT is appropriate for hemodynamically unstable patients who are unable to tolerate hemodialysis and patients who are not candidates for PD. Other indications include sepsis for removal of inflammatory cytokines and those patients with acute renal failure in conjuction with brain injury and cerebral edema to avoid large fluctuations in cerebral perfusion pressure (Garzotto, Zanella, & Ronco, 2014).

2. *Process*

    a. *CRRT* uses a double-lumen venous catheter or two single-lumen venous catheters. It offers a highly efficient circuit that is driven by a roller-head pump and is the preferred method of renal replacement therapy for the hemodynamically unstable patient in many neonatal and pediatric intensive care units (PICUs) because it minimizes large shifts in metabolic and fluid status. A number of different pumps are commercially available for hemofiltration, but they all work in a similar fashion. A roller-head pump drives the blood through the hemofilter, and one or more other roller-head pumps control the ultrafiltration rate, replacement fluid, and dialysis rate. Several methods of CRRT can be used to accomplish the goal of fluid or solute removal. The method used is dictated by the patient's condition as well as the institutional policies and preferences.

    b. *Continuous venovenous hemofiltration (CVVH)* uses the principles of ultrafiltration and convection to allow for fluid and solute removal. It is the most widely used method of CRRT (Lerma, 2009). Blood is drawn from one port of a venous catheter, propelled through a hemofilter using a roller-head pump, and returned to the other port of the venous catheter. Ultrafiltration and convection are accomplished as the blood moves through the semipermeable membrane of the hemofilter. The ultrafiltration rate is controlled by programming the hemofiltration pump's fluid controller for an ordered amount each hour. To obtain adequate clearance, large volumes of ultrafiltrate are removed and replacement fluid is infused to maintain the desired fluid balance. The replacement rate is also controlled via the hemofiltration pump's fluid-control module.

    c. *Continuous venovenous hemofiltration with dialysis (CVVH-D)* is similar to CVVH but uses a diffusion gradient instead of convection to provide clearance. The process of blood removal is the same as with CVVH, but a dialysate solution is infused into the outside compartment of the hemofilter, countercurrent to the blood, to provide diffusive transport of solutes and water. As with CVVH, the ultrafiltration rate and the dialysate rate are both controlled by the hemofiltration pump's fluid controller or additional infusion pumps. Little or no replacement fluid is used.

    d. *Continuous venovenous hemodiafiltration (CVVH-DF)* uses the principles of ultrafiltration, convection, and diffusion to remove fluid and solutes. The process is similar to CVVH-D, but it also utilizes high ultrafiltration rates with replacement fluid, as in CVVH. This method of CRRT may be used for patients in whom one of the other methods is not providing adequate clearance (Sutherland & Alexander, 2012).

e. *Slow continuous ultrafiltration (SCUF)* may be used to remove a set amount of fluid from a patient each hour. This method of CRRT utilizes the principles of ultrafiltration and convection. It is effective for fluid removal, but it does not utilize a high ultrafiltration rate or replacement fluid and therefore will not provide adequate clearance of solutes.

3. *Methods for Measuring Filtration Capability or Performance of the Filter and Circuit*

a. *Clearance* is removal of solutes from the plasma and is dependent on the filter's capability for removing individual molecules, the size of the solute, the solute's protein-binding capacity, and the rate of blood flow through the hemofilter. Clearance for a particular molecule can be expressed by the ultrafiltrate-to-plasma ratio, known as the *sieving coefficient*

$$\text{Sieving coefficient} = \frac{\text{Concentration of } x \text{ in ultrafiltrate} \left[(x) \text{UF} \right]}{\text{Concentration of } x \text{ in plasma} \left[(x) \text{ plasma} \right]}$$

$$(1 = 100\% \text{ Clearance})$$

b. Another indicator of the efficiency of the system is the *FF*. The FF is reflective of the fraction of plasma water being removed by ultrafiltration. Optimum FF is a percentage that is high enough to provide adequate solute and fluid removal needs but not so high that blood viscosity and increased oncotic pressure impact filter performance.

$$\text{Filtration fraction}(\%) = \frac{(\text{QF})\text{Ultrafiltration rate}(\text{mL}/\text{min})}{(\text{QP})\text{Plasma flow rate at the inlet}(\text{mL}/\text{min})}$$

4. Nursing implications for the hemodynamically unstable infant or child during CRRT

a. *Limited vascular access sites and catheter diameter* often limit blood pump speed and therefore impact circuit efficiency and solute clearance. The challenges of vascular access are greatest in infants and small children because of the small size of the vessels in relation to the catheter. Access may also be difficult in patients with an underlying coagulopathy because of concerns of bleeding during placement of these large-bore catheters. It may be necessary to attempt to correct the coagulopathy before access placement. Optimal placement in an infant or small child would be an internal jugular or subclavian catheter with the tip at the junction of the right atrium, thus preventing "pulling of the vessel wall" and subsequent obstruction to flow. A femoral catheter may be used, however, and the pump speed is adjusted accordingly. As with all indwelling lines, infection is also a risk factor.

b. *Thermoregulation* is a significant issue with infants and small children. Depending on the extracorporeal volume of the circuit compared with the child's size, a significant amount of heat may be lost via the circuit. Fluid- and blood-warmer systems or external heat sources should be used to maintain normothermia. Many of the hemofiltration pumps now available have a blood- or fluid-warming device incorporated in them. Small-volume extracorporeal tubing sets are ideal if they are available for the pump that is being used.

c. *Anticoagulation* is often necessary to maintain patency of the circuit. Heparinization or citrate regional anticoagulation are the two most commonly used methods of anticoagulation.

i. Heparinization involves infusing a heparin solution into the prefilter side of the circuit with the goal of maintaining activated clotting times (ACTs) at 1.5 to two times normal. In the absence of a coagulopathy, a heparin bolus is given to the patient before initiation of therapy. In the presence of coagulopathy, heparin administration may be contraindicated, and the life span of the circuit may be decreased (Sutherland & Alexander, 2012). Heparinization is an effective method of anticoagulating the circuit, but precautions must be taken as the patient is also systemically anticoagulated.

ii. Citrate regional anticoagulation is gaining popularity as the circuit may be anticoagulated without systemic effects. Sodium citrate is infused via the "arterial limb" of the circuit to chelate calcium and prevent clotting. The goal of the therapy is to keep the ionized calcium level of the circuit below 0.5 mmol/L. A calcium infusion is given to the patient via a separate line or via the distal "venous return limb" to maintain the patient's ionized calcium in the normal range (1.1–1.3 mmol/L). Citrate anticoagulation has certain inherent concerns in the pediatric population, the most common of which are the development of a metabolic alkalosis, hypocalcemia, hyperglycemia, and "citrate lock." These problems are seen because the blood flow rate per weight of the pediatric patient is greater than in adults; thus the citrate load is often significantly higher. *Citrate lock* is a phenomenon in which the patient's total calcium level rises as the ionized calcium level decreases. This is the result of infusing the citrate solution at a rate that exceeds the hepatic metabolism and CRRT clearance of citrate. Stopping the citrate infusion for a number of hours and restarting at a lower rate should remedy the situation. Metabolic alkalosis results from the breakdown of citrate to bicarbonate at a rate greater than it can be cleared. Hypocalcemia results from inadequate repletion of calcium to the patient and should be treated by increasing the calcium infusion. Hyperglycemia may result from the large infusion of citrate, which is in a glucose-based solution, or from the high flow of glucose containing dialysate solutions. Prompt recognition of these potential complications can prevent untoward effects to the patient. Citrate regional anticoagulation has generally been performed with diffusive clearance using a calcium-free dialysate solution to allow for the removal of the large citrate load; however, recent information in the literature suggests that ultrafiltration and convection alone might be adequate to clear citrate by-products (Davis, Neumayr, Geile, Doctor, & Hmeil, 2014).

iii.   The benefit of routine flushes of normal saline, lactated Ringer's, or filter replacement solution to maintain circuit patency and decrease clotting is debatable.

d.   *Hemodynamic stability.* The CRRT circuit volume should be considered in relationship to the child's circulating blood volume. In small infants and children, it may be necessary to prime the circuit with whole blood or another colloid substance. If the circuit is primed with a blood product preserved with citrate, assess the serum calcium level before CRRT initiation and treat if necessary to decrease the risk of hypotension secondary to hypocalcemia. Because of drug clearance by the hemofilter, it may be necessary to titrate the infusion of vasoactive agents just before or in the first few minutes after initiation of CRRT. If the preceding precautions are taken, the incidence of hemodynamic instability during initiation of CRRT is rare.

e.   *Fluid balance.* Fluid management is an integral component of management for the critically ill patient. In the presence of shock and multiorgan failure, replacment therapies are essential. Fluid overload may be an important independent factor associated with increased morbidity and mortality as it results in vital organ dysfunction and ischemia, especially if fluid overload is greater than 10% to 20% of baseline. The goal of fluid management would therefore be to remove excess fluid while maintaining cardiac output, hemodynamic stability, and optimizing pharmacological and nutritional support. Setting targets is vital in fluid management with CRRT (Lerma, 2009). It may be necessary to begin at an ordered zero fluid balance and slowly adjust the fluid removal as tolerated in order to minimize over- or underestimation of the patient's need, which may result in worsening volume overload or hypotension from intravascular volume depletion. Strict fluid intake and output are recorded hourly. In a child receiving multiple blood products or fluid boluses, it is important to determine what is to be included in the formula as fluid to be removed. The formula for determining the hourly fluid balance is:

(Total intake) − (Total output) ± (Desired hourly change) = Fluid to be removed

f.   All pumps now available have slightly different calculations for fluid removal and manufacturer recommendations should be followed. Example:

(Total intake) − (Total output) − (Desired hourly change) = Fluid to be removed

(100) − (10) − (−20) = 110mL to be removed

g.   *The extracorporeal circuit.* Plasma-free hemoglobin levels may be measured before initiation of CRRT and daily to monitor RBC destruction. Elevated plasma-free hemoglobin levels indicate the necessity to change the circuit.

h.   *CRRT used in conjuction with extracorporeal membrane oxygenation* (ECMO). Renal failure in patients on ECMO for respiratory or cardiac support is a challenge. CRRT has been used through the ECMO circuit to mediate the fluid overload and renal compromise that often occurs with this therapy. CRRT is attached to the ECMO circuit before the oxygenator, often at the venous bladder. This reduces the risk of air embolism reaching the patient. Anticoagulation of the ECMO circuit mitigates the need for anticoagultion in the CRRT circuit. This is a developing area of research in a very vulnerable population and further study is needed (Askenazi et al., 2012).

RENAL TRANSPLANTATION

A. Criteria for Transplantation

1. All candidates must have ESRD or rapidly approaching ESRD. Preemptive transplants, that is, those performed before dialysis is needed, have better long-term outcomes. CKD is stratified into five catagories, based on GFR. Stage 3b has a GFR 30 to 44 and is classified as moderate to severe kidney failure. Stage 4 has a GFR of 15 to 29 with severely decreased function, and Stage 5 has a GFR of <15 and kidney failure (Inker et al., 2014).

2. Common causes of ESRD requiring transplantation include congenital renal disorder, glomerulonephritis, and ESRD secondary to other disease states or treatment.

3. *Pretransplantation Evaluation Criteria.* Transplant is considered at the time of ESRD diagnosis. Urologic issues should be addressed before transplantation, and the patient should be free of any major multisystem complications (malignancy, advanced cardiopulmonary disease) and active infection. Nutritional status should be optimized, and psychiatric and socioeconomic parameters should be viewed as appropriate (Chaudhuri, Gallo, & Grimm, 2015).

4. Donor considerations include a full health history of the donor with emphasis on diabetes and hypertension; drug use; HIV exposure; malignancies; evaluation of infectious markers, including urine culture and urinalysis; renal mass size; human leukocyte antigen (HLA) matching; dose of vasopressors; and time of resuscitation if donor is deceased. Exclusion criteria include intrinsic renal disease or parenchymal trauma (Chaudhuri et al., 2015).

5. *Postoperative Management*

   a. *Minimize the risk for infection* by observing strict handwashing and other institutional infection-control guidelines and by using strict aseptic techniques with all dressing changes.

   b. *Maintain pulmonary toilet.*

   c. *Closely monitor urinary output* and observe for signs and symptoms of infection.

   d. *Monitor and maintain metabolic and electrolyte balance* (BUN, creatinine, ionized calcium, phosphorus [low], magnesium, glucose, serum albumin [low if recurrence of disease], urinary protein–creatinine ratio).

   e. *Maintain comfort for the patient*, and administer medications as needed to decrease pain or anxiety.

   f. *Administer the daily immunosuppressive* medication regimen as ordered, and monitor serum drug levels as necessary.

   g. *Potential complications* include ATN, rejection, infection, obstruction to urinary flow, hypovolemia, renal artery stenosis, renal vein thrombosis, and ureteral leaks.

   h. *Intermediate-term follow-up* consists of monitoring for hyperparathyroid hormone and hypercalcemia. Parathyroid may still be "revved up" from pretransplant and parathyroid resection may be required.

   i. *Long-term complications.* Posttransplant lymphoproliferative disease and infections (particularly Epstein–Barr virus [EBV], cytomegalovirus [CMV], herpes simplex virus [HSV], BK virus, varicella, and *Pneumocystis carinii* pneumonia [PCP]).

   j. *Outcomes.* Long-term outcomes are better with living donated kidneys than with cadaveric kidneys. Kidney transplants in general have a 90% to 95% success rate at 5 years. However, graft-failure rates increase starting at 13 years of age and peak between 17 and 24 years of age. Two factors that effect graft loss at this age are transition to adult care and noncompliance with medication regimens (Bertram et al., 2016).

RENAL TRAUMA

A. Etiology and Risk Factors

1. Renal trauma is the most common traumatic genitourinary injury in the pediatric population. Contusion or laceration constitute the majority of renal injuries and are often seen in association with other more life-threatening injuries.

2. The most common source of renal trauma is blunt trauma, primarily from motor-vehicle crashes. The two types of blunt trauma causing most renal injuries are direct compression from external force or deceleration injury. With deceleration injury, there is a concern for laceration of the renal artery. In addition, acute renal trauma may occur as a result of decreased perfusion. Lumbar scoliosis and fracture of the body or transverse processes of the spine transmit significant injury to the retroperitoneal region. Penetrating trauma is a rare but increasing cause of renal injury in children.

3. Children are at greater risk than adults for blunt force renal trauma because of the larger size of a child's kidney in relation to abdomen size, underdevelopment of a child's abdominal wall muscles, and lack of protection from the lower ribs. Children with underlying renal abnormalities are at greater risk of injury from mild blunt force trauma than those with normal kidneys (Chong, Cherry-Bukowiec, Willatt, & Kielar, 2016).

B. Clinical Manifestations

1. Signs and symptoms of genitourinary trauma include blood at the urethral meatus; high-riding prostate; gross hematuria; and labial, scrotal, or perianal ecchymosis or hematoma. Hematuria occurs in 90% of cases. If the patient is hypovolemic, hematuria may not manifest until after fluid replacement. There is no correlation between the magnitude of injury and the degree of hematuria. These signs and symptoms are contraindications to bladder catheterization.

2. In penetrating trauma, proximity of the wound to the genitourinary area increases suspicion of renal trauma.

3. In blunt trauma, the child may be asymptomatic or complain of abdominal or flank pain.

C. Interpretations From Diagnostic Studies

1. CT is the gold standard imaging study for renal trauma in children (Wu et al., 2016). Advantages include more accurate demonstration of renal injury, visualization of nonvascularized regions, and simultaneous visualization of the other intraabdominal organs. Abdominal or kidney, ureter, and bladder (KUB) film demonstrating obliteration of the renal shadow is suggestive of renal trauma. Up to 85% of plain abdominal films demonstrate normal findings despite proven renal trauma.

2. IVP may be done if an isolated urogenital injury is suspected. This examination allows evaluation of all genitourinary structures.

3. Ultrasonography has limited application in evaluation of renal trauma, but may have utility in a rapid initial screen. Doppler-enhanced ultrasound gives information related to renal perfusion and the integrity of vascular pedicles of the kidney.

4. Arteriography may assist in planning surgical intervention if vascular disruption has occurred.

5. Radionucleotide renal scan demonstrates renal function, perfusion, and urinary extravasation. It is useful if there is a contraindication to contrast dye.

6. Use of MRI is limited because of the technique and the amount of information gained.

D. Classification

Renal injuries are classified as grade I to V and range in severity from a Grade I, contusion with microscopic or gross hematuria, to the most severe Grade V, which can involve a laceration with a completely shattered kidney and an avulsion of the renal hilum, with devascularization of the kidney. For more details, please refer to *Organ Injury Scaling: Kidney* (http://www.trauma.org/archive/scores/ois-renal.htm). This scale has been validated and increasing severity of renal classifictions correlates with the need for surgery (Santucci et al., 2001).

E. Desired Patient Outcomes

1. Absence of hematuria

2. Adequate urine output

3. Absence of hypertension

4. Negative results from radiographic studies

F. Treatment

1. Most penetrating renal injuries require surgical exploration and potential intervention.

2. Management of blunt trauma is dependent on the stability of the child and the extent of injury. Eighty-five percent of blunt-trauma cases are minor injuries (grades I–III), requiring only observation and bed rest until gross hematuria resolves. If results from initial radiographic studies are abnormal, continued follow-up for a year or longer might be necessary.

3. Management of major renal trauma can be divided into two groups: operative or nonoperative. Patients who are hemodynamically unstable despite transfusion must be managed surgically. However, controversy remains about whether to treat patients with major injury involving urinary extravasation or renal fracture conservatively (nonoperatively) or aggressively (operatively). Data exist to support both approaches.

4. Long-term follow-up (i.e., 6 months–1 year) is important because hypertension is subtle yet frequently associated with vascular trauma.

PREVENTION OF CATHETER-ASSOCIATED URINARY TRACT INFECTIONS

A. Background

Catheter-associated urinary tract infections (CAUTIs) account fot 12% of hospital infections and are the fourth most common type of in-hospital infection. They can lead to complications such as pyelonephritis, gram-negative bacteremia, endocarditits, and meningitis. They translate to prolonged hospital stays and increased costs and mortality (Centers for Disease Control and Prevention [CDC], 2016). CAUTI guidelines were first established by the CDC in 1981 and were revised in 2017, in conjuction with the Healthcare Infection Control Practices Advisory Committee (Gould, Umscheid, Agarwal, Kuntz, Pegues, & Healthcare Infection Control Practices Advisory Committee, 2017). Many institutions are now using these guidelines to develop infection-control bundles to reduce complications and reduce costs.

B. Summary of Guidelines

1. Indications for catheter use (see Tables 5.10 and 5.11). Reccomendations also include leaving catheter in place only as long as necessary and removing as soon as possible.

2. Use proper techniques for catheter insertion, including hand hygiene and properly trained personnel, appropriate equipment, proper drainage, and bladder scanning as available.

3. Proper techniques for catheter maintenance include the use of closed drainage systems and unobstructed flow. If closed system is compromised, then replacement of the catheter and the system is recommended.

4. Quality-improvement programs should be instituted at each institution to assess adherence to policies, educate staff, and monitor risk assessment.

5. Administration infrastructure provides guidelines and bundles, education and training, supplies, a system of documentation, and resources.

6. Surveillance via risk-assessment, documenting number of CAUTI per 1,000 catheter-days, number of bloodstream infections related to catheter days, and rate of catheter use. Nurses are intrinsic and extremely valuable in preventing these infections.

C. Effectiveness

CAUTI bundles, implemented and maintained by nurses, have been shown to greatly reduce the incidence of infections in the pediatric population. In Düzkaya, Bozkurt, Uysal, and Yakut (2016), the colonization rate of urinary catheters dropped from 2.2% to 0.8% and the contamination rate declined by almost half after the implementation of CAUTI bundles.

TABLE 5.10   Examples of Appropriate Indications for Indwelling Urethral Catheter Use

Patient has acute urinary retention or bladder outlet obstruction
Need for accurate measurements of urinary output in critically ill patients
Perioperative use for selected surgical procedures: • Patients undergoing urologic surgery or other surgery on contiguous structures of the genitourinary tract • Anticipated prolonged duration of surgery (catheters inserted for this reason should be removed in PACU) • Patients anticipated to receive large-volume infusions or diuretics during surgery • Need for intraoperative monitoring of urinary output
To assist in healing of open sacral or perineal wounds in incontinent patients
Patient requires prolonged immobilization (e.g., potentially unstable thoracic or lumbar spine, multiple traumatic injuries such as pelvic fractures)
To improve comfort for end-of-life care if needed

PACU, postanesthesia care unit.

Note: These indications are based primarily on expert consensus.

Source: Gould, C., Umscheid, C., Agarwal, R., Kuntz, G., Pegues, D., & Healthcare Infection Control Practices Advisory Committee (2017, February 15). *Guideline for prevention of catheter-associated urinary tract infections 2009.* Retrieved from https://www.cdc.gov/infectioncontrol/pdf/guidelines/cauti-guidelines.pdf

TABLE 5.11   Examples of Inappropriate Uses of Indwelling Catheters

As a substitute for nursing care of the patient or resident with incontinence
As a means of obtaining urine for culture or other diagnostic tests when the patient can voluntarily void
For prolonged postoperative duration without appropriate indications (e.g., structural repair of urethra or contiguous structures, prolonged effect of epidural anesthesia, etc.)

Note: These indications are based primarily on expert consensus.

Source: Gould, C., Umscheid, C., Agarwal, R., Kuntz, G., Pegues, D., & Healthcare Infection Control Practices Advisory Committee (2017, February 15). *Guideline for prevention of catheter-associated urinary tract infections 2009.* Retrieved from https://www.cdc.gov/infectioncontrol/pdf/guidelines/cauti-guidelines.pdf

CASE STUDIES WITH QUESTIONS, ANSWERS, AND RATIONALES

Case Study 5.1

A 3-year-old girl is admitted to the PICU with abdominal pain, vomiting, diarrhea, and altered level of consciousness. Vital signs are temperature 38.9°C, HR 158 bpm, RR 40 breaths/min, BP 82/45 mmHg. Mucous membranes are dry, no tears when crying. Her mother states she has been sick for 3 days. No wet diapers in the past 12 hours. Her labs show Na 148 mEq/L, K 5.5 mEq/L, Cl 102 mEq/L, CO_2 20 mEq/L, BUN 96 mg/dL, creatinine 1.9 mg/dL, glucose 103 mg/dL, calcium 9 mg/dL, Mg 1.8 mg/dL, Phos 5 mg/dL. CBC shows HGB 7.8 g/dL, HCT 27%, WBC 17 K/uL, PLTS 83 K/uL. CBG shows pH 7.23, CO_2 29 mmHg, PO_2 92 mmHg, oxygen saturation 98%, HCO_3 18 mmol/L. Shistocytes are noted on smear. Her mother states that she and the girl's father had mild nausea and vomiting last week after eating at a fast-food restaurant.

1. Your first intervention would include:
   A. Administer a 10 mL/kg fluid bolus and reassess fluid status.
   B. Prepare for transport to CT scan for head CT for neurologic status.
   C. Prepare for immediate intubation due to altered mental status.
   D. Draw blood cultures and administer antibiotics immediately.

2. After initial intervention, the patient's mental status improves but she continues to be aneuric. The preferred mode of dialysis in this patient is:
   A. CRRT
   B. Hemodialysis
   C. Peritoneal dialysis

Case Study 5.2

A 6-month-old girl is admitted to the PICU with a 3-day history of nausea and vomiting. Her physical exam and laboratory results are consistent with moderate to severe dehydration. While providing adequate fluid resuscitation, the physician orders a Foley catheter to be placed. Your institution has a CAUTI bundle in place to prevent infection.

1. The most appropriate actions in this bundle include:
   A. Refuse to place the catheter as this patient does not meet criteria for a Foley according to the guidelines.
   B. Place the Foley with clean technique.
   C. Allow the medical assistant who is not trained on Foley placement to give it a try.
   D. As the RN caring for the child, place the Foley with sterile technique and maintain a closed drainage system with no dependent loops.

Case Study 5.3

You are caring for a 5-year-old boy who has sustained third-degree burns over 50% of his body. He is critically ill and has acute renal failure with a BUN of 98 mg/dL and Cr of 3.4 mg/dL. He is on CRRT with citrate as the anticoagulant. This hour, the labs results are as follows: ABG: pH 7.59, pCO_2 34 mmHg, PO_2 99 mmHg, oxygen saturation 100%, HCO_3 41 mmol/L, Ionized calcium 0.9 mmol/L, serum calcium 11 mg/dL.

1. Your first actions should be:
   A. Redraw labs in 1 hour.
   B. Notify the medical staff, stop the citrate infusion, and anticipate redrawing labs in an hour and restarting citrate at a slower rate when appropriate.
   C. Notify the medical staff and anticipate increasing the rate calcium infusion.
   D. Notify the medical staff and anticipate decreasing the rate on the ventilator for the alkalosis.

Case Study 5.4

You are caring for a 12-year old who underwent open-heart surgery for removal of a subaortic membrane. His postoperative labs show: Na 140 mEq/L, K 2.8 mEq/L, Cl 109 mEq/L, CO_2 25 mEq/L, BUN 27 mg/dL, Cr 1.8 mg/dL, Mg 2 mg/dL, Ca 8.5 mg/dL. He is having occasional premature ventricular contractions that are becoming more frequent. You have standing electrolyte replacement orders in EMR.

1. You should:
    A. Administer IV calcium gluconate at a dose of 100 mg/kg over 1 hour in a central line.
    B. Administer IV potassium chloride at a dose of 1 mEq/kg over 5 minutes in a central line.
    C. Administer IV potassium chloride at a dose of 1 mEq/kg over 1 hour in a central line.
    D. Administer IV potassium chloride at a dose of 1 mEq/kg over 1 hour in a peripheral line.

Answers and Rationales

Case Study 5.1

1. **A.** Her history, physical exam, vital signs, and laboratory results are consistent with fluid loss and dehydration. Judicious fluid resuscitation is the first goal of therapy. Neurologic improvement mitigates the need for neurologic imaging or intubation. Blood cultures and antibiotics are necessary and would occur after fluid resuscitation is started. The presence of shistocytes on the blood smear is consistent with a diagnosis of HUS.

2. **C.** Peritoneal dialysis is the preferred mode of dialysis for this diagnosis at this time.

Case Study 5.2

1. **D.** Per Healthcare Infection Control Practices Advisory Committee (HICPAC) guidelines, this patient meets criteria for indwelling catheter placement as she is acutely critically ill and needs accurate measurements of urinary output. Foleys must always be placed with sterile technique by staff who have been formally trained.

Case Study 5.3

1. **B.** These labs are consistent with citrate lock and immediate action needs to be taken. Treatment for citrate lock is to stop the citrate infusion and restart at a lower rate when appropriate. Increasing the calcium infusion is not appropriate as the serum calcium level is already high. Adjusting the rate on the ventilator is not appropriate as this arterial blood gas shows a metabolic alkalosis with mild respiratory compensation, not a respiratory alkalosis.

Case Study 5.4

1. **C.** A potassium level of 2.8 is low. The presence of ectopy is alarming, likely a symptom of the hypokalemia. Potassium should always be given in a central line over 1 hour. Ususal dose is 0.5 to 1 mEq/kg/dose. The serum calcium level is normal, so this option is not appropriate. Hypocalcemia does not usually manifest with ectopy.

REFERENCES

Askenazi, D. J., Selewski, D. T., Paden, M. L., Cooper, D. S., Bridges, B. C., Zappitelli, M., & Fleming, G. M. (2012). Renal replacement therapy in critically ill patients receiving extracorporeal membrane oxygenation. *Clinical Journal of the American Society of Nephrology*, 7(8), 1328–1336. doi:10.2215/CJN.12731211

Bertram, J. F., Goldstein, S. L., Pape, L., Schaefer, F., Shroff, R. C., & Warady, B. A. (2016). Kidney disease in children: Latest advances and remaining challenges. *Nature Reviews: Nephrology*, 12(3), 182–191. doi:10.1038/nrneph.2015.219

Chaudhuri, A., Gallo, A., & Grimm, P. (2015). Pediatric deceased donor renal transplantation: An approach to decision making 1. Pediatric kidney allocation in the USA: The old and the new. *Pediatric Transplantation*, 19(7), 776–784. doi:10.1111/petr.12569

Chong, S. T., Cherry-Bukowiec, J. R., Willatt, J. M., & Kielar, A. Z. (2016). Renal trauma: Imaging evaluation and implications for clinical management. *Abdominal Radiology*, 41(8), 1565–1579. doi:10.1007/s00261-016-0731-x

Curley, M. A. Q., & Moloney-Harmon, P. (Eds.). (2001). *Critical care nursing of infants and children* (p. 733). Philadelphia, PA: W. B. Saunders.

Daly, K., & Farrington, E. (2013). Hypokalemia and hyperkalemia in infants and children: Pathophysiology and treatment. *Journal of Pediatric Health Care*, 27(6), 486–496. doi:10.1016/j.pedhc.2013.08.003

Davis, T. K., Neumayr, T., Geile, K., Doctor, A., & Hmeil, P. (2014). Citrate anticoagulation during continuous renal replacement therapy in pediatric critical care. *Pediatric Critical Care Medicine*, 15(5), 471–485. doi:10.1097/PCC.0000000000000148

Düzkaya, D., Bozkurt, G., Uysal, G., & Yakut, T. (2016). The effects of bundles on catheter-associated urinary tract infections in the pediatric intensive care unit. *Clinical Nurse Specialist*, 30(6), 341–346. doi:10.1097/NUR.0000000000000246

Eaton, D. C., & Pooler, J. P. (2013). *Vander's renal physiology* (8th ed. pp. 1–19). New York, NY: McGraw-Hill.

Fortenberry, J. D., Paden, M. L., & Goldstein, S. L. (2013). Acute kidney injury in children: An update on diagnosis and treatment. *Pediatric Clinics of North America*, 60(3), 669–688. doi:10.1016/j.pcl.2013.02.006

Garzotto, F., Zanella, M., & Ronco, C. (2014). The evolution of pediatric continuous renal replacement therapy. *Nephron Clinical Practice*, 127(1–4), 172–175. doi:10.1159/000363204

Gould, C. V., Umscheid, C. A., Agarwal, R. K., Kuntz, G., Pegues, D. A., Healthcare Infection Control Practices Advisory Committee. (2017). *Guideline for prevention of catheter-associated urinary tract infections*. Retrieved from https://www.cdc.gov/hicpac/pdf/CAUTI/CAUTIguideline2009final.pdf

Inker, L., Astor, B., Fox, C., Isakova, T., Lash, J., Peralta, C., ... Feldman, H. (2014). KDOQI US Commentary on the 2012 KDIGO clinical practice guideline for the evaluation and management of CKD. *American Journal of Kidney Diseases*, *63*(5), 713–735. doi:10.1053/j.ajkd.2014.01.416

Kliegman, R. M., Stanton, B., St. Geme, J., & Schor, N. F. (2016). *Nelson textbook of pediatrics* (20th ed.). Philadelphia, PA: Elsevier.

Lerma, E. V. (2009). Approach to the patient with renal disease. In E. V. Lerma, J. S. Berns, & A. R. Nissenson (Eds.), *Current diagnosis & treatment: Nephrology & hypertension* (pp. 1–6). New York, NY: McGraw-Hill.

McCance, K. L., & Huether, S. E. (Eds.). (2010). *Pathophysiology: The biologic basis for disease in adults and children* (6th ed.). Maryland Heights, MO: Mosby Elsevier.

Moffett, B. S., Mott, A. R., Nelson, D. P., Goldstein, S. L., & Jeffries, J. L. (2008). Renal effects of fenoldopam in critically ill pediatric patients: A retrospective review. *Pediatric Critical Care Medicine*, *9*(4), 403–406. doi:10.1097/PCC.0b013e3181728c25

Organ injury scaling: Kidney. (n.d.). Retrieved from http://www.trauma.org/archive/scores/ois-renal.html

Perkin, R. M., Swift, J. D., Newton, D. A., & Anas, N. G. (Eds.). (2008). *Pediatric hospital medicine* (2nd ed.). Philadelphia, PA: Lippincott Williams & Wilkins.

Santucci, R. A., McAnnich, J. W., Safir, M., Mario, L. A., Service, S., & Segal, M. R. (2001). Validation of the American Association for the Surgery of Trauma organ injury severity scale for the kidney. *Journal of J Trauma*, *50*(2), 195–200. Retrieved from https://journals.lww.com/jtrauma/Abstract/2001/02000/Validation_of_the_American_Association_for_the.2.aspx

Slater, M., Gruneir, A., Rochon, P., Howard, A., Koren, G., & Parshuram, S. (2017). Identifying high-risk medications associated with acute kidney injury in critically ill patients: A pharmacoepidemiologic evaluation. *Paediatric Drugs*, *19*(1), 59–67. doi:10.1007/s40272-016-0205-1

Sutherland, S. M., & Alexander, S. R. (2012). Continuous renal replacement therapy in children. *Pediatric Nephrology*, *27*, 2007–2016. doi:10.1007/s00467-011-2080-x

Swartz, M. W. (Ed.). (2008). *The 5-minute pediatric consult*. Philadelphia, PA: Lippincott Williams & Wilkins.

Toto, R. D. (2004). Approach to patient with kidney disease. In B. M. Brenner (Ed.), *Brenner & Rector's: The kidney* (7th ed., pp. 1079–1086). Philadelphia, PA: Elsevier.

Traynor, J., Mactier, R., Geddes, C. C., & Fox, J. G. (2006). How to measure renal function in clinical practice. *British Medical Journal*, *33*(7571), 733–737. doi:10.1136/bmj.38975.390370.7C

Wong, D. L., Hockenberry-Eaton, M., Wilson, D., Winkelstein, M. L., Ahmann, E., & DiVito-Thomas, P. (1999). *Whaley & Wong's nursing care of infants and children* (6th ed.). St. Louis, MO: Mosby.

Wu, H.-Y., Bellah, R., & Snyder, H. M. (2016). Radiographic evaluation of pediatric urinary tract. In M. Cendron (Ed.), *Medscape*. Retrieved from http://emedicine.medscape.com/article/1016549-overview

Zaritsky, J., & Warady, B. A. (2011). Peritoneal dialysis in Infants and young children. *Seminars in Nephrology, 31*(2), 213–224. doi:10.1016/j.semnephrol.2011.01.009

6 ENDOCRINE SYSTEM

Jennifer LaMie Joiner

Two types of endocrine problems are seen in pediatric critical care: (a) specific endocrine abnormalities (diabetes mellitus [DM], panhypopituitarism) and (b) endocrine dysfunction secondary to critical illness (sick euthyroid or syndrome of inappropriate antidiuretic hormone [SIADH]).

ENDOCRINOLOGY CONCEPTS

A. Role of the Endocrine System

1. The endocrine system maintains homeostasis, including fluid and electrolyte balance, blood pressure, intravascular volume and maintenance of fat, muscle, and bone.

2. Functions of the endocrine system involve control and regulation of metabolism, maintenance of energy stores, growth and development, reproduction and sex differentiation, growth and coordination of the body's response to stress (e.g., trauma, critical illness, infection, major surgery) via the secretion of counterregulatory hormones (Buzby, 2012; Molina, 2013).

3. Integrated functions include central nervous system (CNS) input to the endocrine system via the hypothalamic–pituitary complex. The immune system contributes to endocrine regulation via activation of proinflammatory mediators (interleukin-1, tumor necrosis factor; von Saint Andre-von Arnim et al., 2013).

4. Most diseases from the endocrine system occur as a result of hypersecretion, hyposecretion, altered response at the tissue level, or tumors in an endocrine gland (Buzby, 2012).

5. Many of the most powerful therapies used in the pediatric intensive care unit (PICU) are mediators of the neuroendocrine system and include epinephrine, norepinephrine, vasopressin, insulin, and steroids.

B. Endocrine Glands

These glands or organs consist of specialized cells that synthesize and secrete biochemical messengers (hormones) in response to specific signals (e.g., hyperglycemia, hyperosmolality, hypocalcemia).

1. Endocrine glands secrete hormones directly into the bloodstream (e.g., adrenal glands, endocrine pancreas, thyroid gland).

2. Exocrine glands secrete biochemical substances that are released into ducts to be delivered to target organs (e.g., salivary glands, sebaceous glands, exocrine pancreas, sweat glands).

3. *Major Glands*

   a. Hypothalamus–pituitary complex (anterior and posterior pituitary gland)

   b. Thyroid gland

   c. Parathyroid glands

   d. Adrenal glands

   e. Islets of Langerhans in the pancreas

   f. Gonads

   g. Other sources. Cells that are normally considered outside the endocrine system can manufacture and secrete hormones in response to certain circumstances (e.g., pneumocytes may secrete adrenocorticotropic hormone [ACTH]). Cardiac myocytes secrete atrial natriuretic peptide (ANP), dendroaspis natriuretic peptide (DNP), and brain or B-type natriuretic peptide (BNP) in response to myocardial stretch and overload (Yee, Burns, & Wijdicks, 2010). ANP and BNP cause natriuresis (salt loss) and diuresis. An elevated BNP level serves as a biomarker when left ventricle dysfunction and heart failure exist (Rossano & Shaddy, 2014).

C. Hormones

1. Hormones (Table 6.1) are chemical messengers that are released directly into the bloodstream from endocrine glands in response to specific stimuli or signals that cause:

   a. Hormones bind with the specific receptor, target cell, or organ, which initiates specific cell response. Cells that do not possess this specific receptor do not respond (Hall, 2016). Receptors are located on the cell membrane,

TABLE 6.1   Summary of the Endocrine System

Gland/Hormone	Effect	Hypofunction	Hyperfunction
Adenohypophysis (Anterior Pituitary)[a]			
STH or (GH) Target tissue: Bones	Promotes growth of bone and soft tissues Has main effect on linear growth Maintains a normal rate of protein synthesis Conserves carbohydrate utilization and promotes fat mobilization Is essential for proliferation of cartilage cells at epiphyseal plate Is ineffective for linear growth after epiphyseal closure Has hyperglycemic effect (antiinsulin action)	Epiphyseal fusion with cessation of growth Prepubertal dwarfism Pituitary cachexia (Simmonds' disease) Generalized growth retardation Hypoglycemia	Prepubertal gigantism Acromegaly (after full growth is attained) Diabetes mellitus Postpubertal hypoproteinemia
Thyrotopin (TSH) Target tissue: Thyroid hormone	Promotes and maintains growth and development of thyroid gland Stimulates thyroid hormone secretion	Hypothyroidism Marked delay of puberty Juvenile myxedema	Hyperthyroidism Thyrotoxicosis Graves' disease
ACTH Target tissue: Adrenal cortex	Promotes and maintains growth and development of adrenal cortex Stimulates adrenal cortex to secrete glucocorticoids and androgens	Acute adrenocortical insufficiency (Addison disease) Hypoglycemia Increased skin pigmentation	Cushing's syndrome
Gonadotropins Target tissue: Gonads	Stimulate gonads to mature and produce sex hormones and germ cells	Absent or incomplete spontaneous puberty	Precocious puberty Early epiphyseal closure
FSH Target tissue: Ovaries, testes	Male: Stimulates development of seminiferous tubules Initiates spermatogenesis Female: Stimulates Graafian follicles to mature and secrete estrogen	Hypogonadism Sterility Absence or loss of secondary sex characteristics Amenorrhea	Precocious puberty Primary gonadal failure Hirsutism Polycystic ovary Early epiphyseal closure
LH[b] Target tissue: Ovaries, testes	Male: Stimulates differentiation of Leydig cells, which secrete androgens, principally testosterone Female: Produces rupture of follicle with discharge of mature ovum Stimulates secretion of progesterone by corpus luteum	Hypogonadism Sterility Impotence Absence or loss of secondary sex characteristics Ovarian failure Eunuchism	Precocius puberty Primary gonadal failure Hirsutism Polycystic ovary Early epiphyseal closure
Prolactin (luteotropic hormone) Target tissue: Ovaries, breasts MSH Target tissue: skin	Stimulates milk secretion Maintains corpus luteum and progesterone secretion during pregnancy Promotes pigmentation of skin	Inability to lactate Amenorrhea Diminished or absent skin pigmentation	Galactorrhea Functional hypogonadism Increased skin pigmentation

(continued)

TABLE 6.1   Summary of the Endocrine System *(continued)*

Gland/Hormone	Effect	Hypofunction	Hyperfunction
Neurohypophysis (Posterior Pituitary)			
ADH (vasopressin) Target tissue: Renal tubules Oxytocin Target tissue: Uterus, breasts	Acts on distal and collecting tubules, making them more permeable to water, thus increasing reabsorption and decreasing excretion of urine Stimulates powerful contractions of uterus Causes ejection of milk from alveoli into breast ducts (letdown reflex)	Diabetes insipidus	Syndrome of inappropriate secretion of ADH Fluid retention Hyponatremia
Thyroid			
T_4 and T_3	Regulates metabolic rate; controls rate of growth of body cells Especially important for growth of bones, teeth, and brain Promotes mobilization of fats and gluconeogenesis	Hypothyroidism Myxedema Hashimoto thyroiditis General growth is greatly reduced; extent depends on age at which deficiency occurs Mental retardation in infant	Exophthalmic goiter (Graves' disease) Accelerated linear growth Early epiphyseal closure
Thyrocalcitonin	Regulates calcium and phosphorus metabolism Influences ossification and development of bone		
Parathyroid Glands			
PTH	Promotes calcium reabsorption from blood, bone, and intestines Promotes excretion of phosphorus in kidney tubules	Hypocalcemia (tetany)	Hypercalcemia (bone demineralization) Hypophosphatemia
Adrenal Cortex			
Mineralocorticoids Aldosterone	Stimulate renal tubules to reabsorb sodium, thus promoting water retention but potassium loss	Adrenocortical insufficiency	Electrolyte imbalance Hyperaldosteronism
Sex hormones (androgens, estrogens, progesterone)	Influence development of bone, reproductive organs, and secondary sexual characteristics	Male: Feminization	Adrenogenital syndrome
Glucocorticoids Cortisol (hydrocortisone and compound F) Corticosterone (compound B)	Promote normal fat, protein, and carbohydrate metabolism In excess, tend to accelerate gluconeogenesis and protein and fat catabolism Mobilize body defenses during periods of stress Suppress inflammatory reaction	Addison disease Acute adrenocortical insufficiency Impaired growth and sexual function	Cushing's syndrome Severe impairment of growth with slowing in skeletal maturation

(continued)

TABLE 6.1   Summary of the Endocrine System *(continued)*

Gland/Hormone	Effect	Hypofunction	Hyperfunction
Adrenal Medulla			
Epinephrine (adrenaline), norepinephrine (noradrenaline)	Produces vasoconstriction of heart and smooth muscles (raises blood pressure) Increases blood sugar via glycolysis Inhibits gastrointestinal activity Activates sweat glands		Hyperfunction caused by: pheochromocytoma neuroblastoma ganglioneuroma
Islets of Langerhans of Pancreas			
Insulin (beta cells)	Promotes glucose transport into the cells Increases glucose utilization, glycogenesis, and glycolysis Promotes fatty acid transport into cells and lipogenesis Promotes amino acid transport into cells and protein synthesis Diabetes mellitus	Hyperinsulinism	
Glucagon (alpha cells)	Acts as antagonist to insulin, thereby increasing blood glucose concentration by accelerating glycogenolysis Able to inhibit secretion of both insulin and glycogen		Hyperglycemia May be instrumental in genesis of DKA in diabetes mellitus
Somatostatin (delta cells)	Able to inhibit secretion of both insulin and glycogen		
Ovaries			
Estrogen	Accelerates growth of epithelial cells, especially in uterus following menses Promotes protein anabolism Promotes epiphyseal closure of bones Promotes breast development during puberty and pregnancy Plays role in sexual function Stimulates water and sodium reabsorption in renal tubules Stimulates ripening of ova	Lack of or repression of sexual development	Precocious puberty: Early epiphyseal closure
Progesterone	Prepares uterus for nidation of fertilized ovum and aids in maintenance of pregnancy Aids in development of alveolar system of breasts during pregnancy Inhibits myometrial contractions Has effect on protein catabolism Promotes salt and water retention, especially in endometrium		

(continued)

TABLE 6.1 Summary of the Endocrine System *(continued)*

Gland/Hormone	Effect	Hypofunction	Hyperfunction
Testes			
Testosterone	Accelerates protein anabolism for growth Promotes epiphyseal closure Promotes development of secondary sex characteristics Plays role in sexual function Stimulates testes to produce spermatozoa	Delayed sexual development, or eunuchoidism	Precocious puberty: Early epiphyseal closure

ACTH, adrenocorticotropic hormone; ADH, antidiuretic hormone; DKA, diabetic ketoacidosis; FSH, follicle-stimulating hormone; GH, growth hormone; LH, luteinizing hormone; MSH, melanocyte-stimulating hormone; PTH, parathyroid hormone; STH, somatotropic hormone; TSH, thyroid-stimulating hormone; T_3, triiodothyronine; T_4, thyroxine.

[a]For each anterior pituitary hormone, there is a corresponding hypothalamic-releasing factor. A deficiency in these factors caused by inhibiting anterior pituitary hormone synthesis produces the same effects.

[b]In the male, LH is sometimes known as interstitial cell-stimulating hormone.

Source: From Hockenberry, M. J., & Wilson, D. (Eds.). (2015). *Wong's nursing care of infants and children* (10th ed.). St. Louis, MO: Elsevier.

in cell cytoplasm, or in the nucleus of the cell and activity varies based on cell signaling (Hall, 2016).

b. Facilitation of communication between cells, both locally and distally.

2. *Chemical Structures of Hormones* (Hall, 2016)

a. *Proteins and polypeptides* (water-soluble) are synthesized from amino acids. They bind to cell surface membranes. Examples are anterior and posterior pituitary hormones.

b. *Steroids* (lipid soluble) are synthesized from cholesterol. They diffuse through the plasma membrane and enter the cytoplasm. Examples are cortisol, aldosterone, estrogen, progesterone, and testosterone.

c. *Derivatives of the amino acid tyrosine* are synthesized and stored until needed then released based on mechanism of action. Thyroxine (T_4) and triiodothyronine (T_3) from the thyroid gland are synthesized by adding iodine to tyrosine and can take months for full effect. Epinephrine and norepinephrine from the adrenal medulla are modified from tyrosine and can be ready for action within seconds to minutes.

3. Information about hormones, interactions with each other, and their interactions with the

nervous system and immune system continue to be investigated. Several second messenger systems exist that are important in the activation of hormones that maintain intracellular functions on cell membranes and include the cyclic adenosine monophosphate, phospholipase, and calcium–calmodulin systems.

4. Hormones can be exogenously administered to critically ill patients.

D. Feedback Mechanism

1. Feedback loops are used to regulate secretion of hormones in the hypothalmic-pituitary loop (Figure 6.1).

2. Negative feedback (Figure 6.2) is the primary mechanism in controlling hormonal regulation and prevents overproduction of hormones to their target tissues (Hall, 2016; McCance & Huether, 2015). Negative feedback occurs when the specific cell response has been achieved or exceeded and the information is relayed to the secreting gland to inhibit secretion. The feedback can be short or long looped.

3. Negative feedback in hormonal release is responsible for maintaining homeostasis and inhibition of this system could result in a pathologic condition (Brashers, Jones, & Huether, 2014).

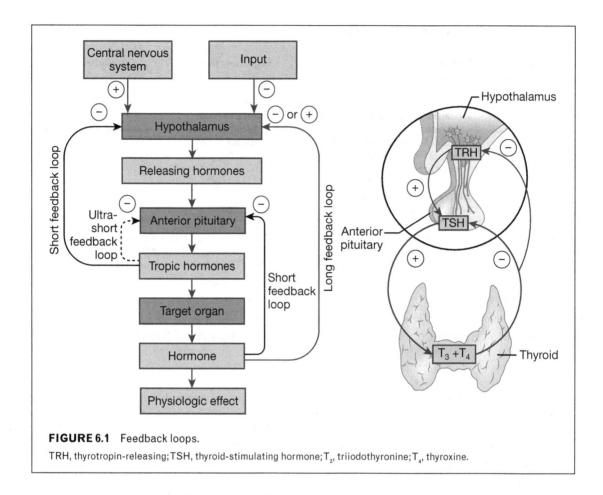

FIGURE 6.1 Feedback loops.

TRH, thyrotropin-releasing; TSH, thyroid-stimulating hormone; T$_3$, triiodothyronine; T$_4$, thyroxine.

DEVELOPMENTAL ANATOMY AND PHYSIOLOGY

A. Hypothalamic–Pituitary Complex (Neuroendocrine System)

1. *Embryology*

a. The *hypothalamus* arises from the diencephalon after a proliferation of neuroblasts. The fibers of the supraoptic tract are present by 12 weeks gestation with maturation of the neurons by 30 weeks (Schoenwolf, Bleyl, Brauer, & Francis-West, 2015).

    i. Antidiuretic hormone (ADH) and oxytocin production begin at about 12 weeks gestation.

b. The *pituitary gland* has a double embryonic origin, which contributes to the differentiation of the anterior and posterior lobes. Pituitary development begins around 4 weeks of gestation

(Schoenwolf et al., 2015). Pituitary hormone secretion begins by 8 to 10 weeks gestation (Dattani & Gevers, 2016).

c. *Anterior pituitary* is recognizable by 3 to 4 weeks gestation and appears fully functional by 17 weeks. It originates from Rathke's pouch, which is ectodermal tissue from the oropharynx that migrates to join the posterior pituitary. By week 5 of gestation, a connection between Rathke's pouch and the infundibulum is present (Dattani & Gevers, 2016).

    i. Secretory granules are found by 10 to 12 weeks gestation and production of ACTH occurs by 8 weeks gestation, somatotropin by 10 or 11 weeks gestation, follicle-stimulating hormone (FSH) and luteinizing hormone (LH) by 11 weeks gestation, prolactin by 12 weeks gestation, and TSH by 15 weeks'gestation (Dattani & Gevers, 2016).

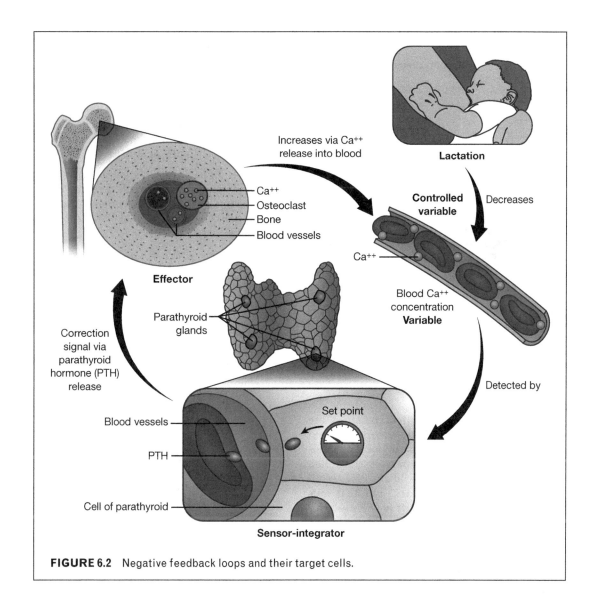

FIGURE 6.2 Negative feedback loops and their target cells.

d. *Posterior pituitary* originates from the neuro-ectoderm of the diencephalon (hypothalamus). It develops during week 5 or 6 of gestation (Schoenwolf et al., 2015).

   i. The fetal posterior pituitary is capable of maintaining fetal osmolality and blood volume. In the fetus and newborn, increased levels of ADH are found secondary to hypoxia and stress. Serum levels of ADH in the newborn correlate with the length of labor. Data indicate that ADH secretion is fully mature in the newborn; however, renal responsiveness may be decreased.

2. *Role of the Hypothalamus.* The hypothalamus functions as a center to integrate incoming stimuli from the CNS and the peripheral nervous system (PNS). It translates neurotransmitter hormonal signals into appropriate endocrine responses (Hall, 2016). Secretion of pituitary hormones is controlled through either hormonal or nervous system signals from the hypothalamus that terminate in the posterior pituitary (Hall, 2016). The stimulating and

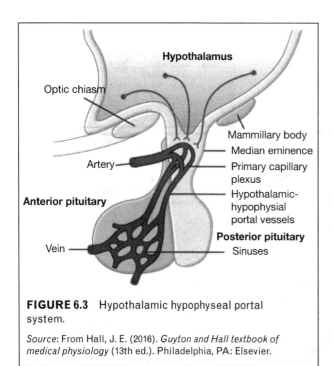

FIGURE 6.3 Hypothalamic hypophyseal portal system.

Source: From Hall, J. E. (2016). *Guyton and Hall textbook of medical physiology* (13th ed.). Philadelphia, PA: Elsevier.

inhibiting hormones from the hypothalamus are carried to the anterior lobe of the pituitary gland via the hypothalamic–hypophyseal portal vessels (Figure 6.3). The posterior pituitary is controlled by the hypothalamus via nerve fibers that terminate in the posterior pituitary. The hypothalamus synthesizes ADH and transports it to the posterior pituitary.

3. *Anatomic Location* (Figure 6.4). The *hypothalamus* is anterior and below the thalamus. It forms the floor and the walls of the third ventricle. The pituitary gland (also called the *hypophysis*) is located in the sella turcica below the optic chiasm, on the superior surface of the sphenoid bone, and covered by dura. The pituitary gland is connected to the hypothalamus by the pituitary stalk or *infundibulum*. The pituitary gland can be accessed surgically through the back of the nose. The pituitary gland has two distinct lobes that produce different hormones (Figure 6.4).

    a. *Anterior pituitary (adenohypophysis)* constitutes 75% of the weight of the pituitary gland (Brashers et al., 2014). Hypothalamic-releasing hormones control hormone secretion. The anterior pituitary secretes growth hormone, ACTH, TSH, prolactin, FSH, and LH.

    b. *Posterior pituitary (neurohypophysis)* hormones are controlled by nerve fibers in the hypothalamus called the *hypothalamohypophysia tract* (which contains approximately 100,000 nerve fibers). The posterior pituitary secretes ADH and oxytocin. These hormones are synthesized in the hypothalamus, transported via nerve tracts in the pituitary stalk, and stored in the posterior pituitary (Robinson & Verbalis, 2016).

    c. *Pituitary stalk* serves as a communication and connection between the brain and the pituitary gland. The stalk contains axons and neuronal cells that originate in the hypothalamus (Brashers et al., 2014).

4. *Cell Types of the Hypothalamus, Neurohypophysis, and Adenohypophysis*

    a. The *supraoptic and paraventricular nuclei* originate in the hypothalamus. *Thirst receptors* and *osmoreceptors* are located in the hypothalamus close to the supraoptic nucleus. ADH is formed primarily in the supraoptic nucleus, but small amounts of ADH are produced in the paraventricular nucleus. Oxytocin is formed primarily in the paraventricular nucleus (Hall, 2016).

    b. The *posterior pituitary* is composed of pituicytes. Pituicytes do not secrete hormones but rather provide support structures for the nerve fibers that come from the hypothalamus (Hall, 2016). These nerve-like endings contain secretory granules that lie on the surface of the capillaries where they release ADH and oxytocin.

    c. The *anterior pituitary* consists of six different types of secretory cells (Brashers et al., 2014).

        i. Somatotrophs secrete growth hormone (GH) and play a key role in metabolic processes for growth.

        ii. Lactotrophs secrete prolactin and proliferate during pregnancy secondary to elevated estrogen levels to aid in milk production.

        iii. Corticotrophs secrete ACTH, which stimulates steroid production in the adrenals, beta-lipotropin and beta-endorphins in adipose cells for release of fatty acids, regulation of body temperature, and analgesia in brain receptors.

        iv. Gonadotrophs secrete LH and FSH, which are necessary for ovulation, follicle maturation, and spermatogenesis.

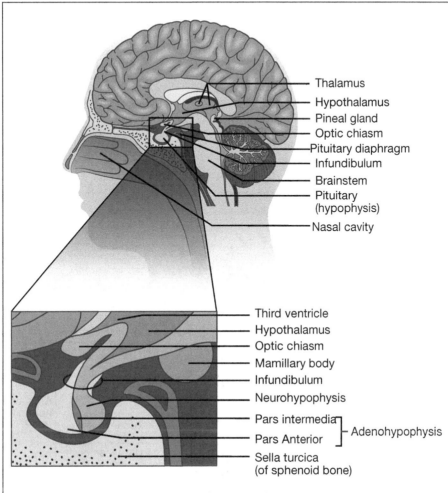

Thalamus
Hypothalamus
Pineal gland
Optic chiasm
Pituitary diaphragm
Infundibulum
Brainstem
Pituitary (hypophysis)
Nasal cavity

Third ventricle
Hypothalamus
Optic chiasm
Mamillary body
Infundibulum
Neurohypophysis
Pars intermedia
Pars Anterior — Adenohypophysis
Sella turcica (of sphenoid bone)

FIGURE 6.4 Location and structure of pituitary gland and hypothalamic–pituitary–adrenal complex.

v. Thyrotrophs secrete TSH, which stimulates thyroid hormone production, iodide uptake, and hyperplasia of thymocytes.

vi. Melanotrophs secrete melanocyte-stimulating hormone (MSH), which promotes secretion of melanin.

5. *Hypothalamic Hormones*

a. *Growth hormone-releasing hormone (GHRH)* stimulates release of GH.

b. *Thyrotropin-releasing hormone (TRH)* stimulates release of TSH.

c. *Corticotropin-releasing hormone (CRH)* stimulates release of ACTH and beta-endorphin.

d. *Gonadotropin-releasing hormone (GnRH)* stimulates release of LH and FSH.

e. *Somatostatin* inhibits release of GH, renin, and parathyroid hormone (PTH) and decreases secretion of TSH, glucagon, and insulin.

f. *Dopamine (prolactin inhibitory hormone)* inhibits synthesis and secretion of prolactin.

g. *Prolactin-releasing factor (PRF)* stimulates the secretion of prolactin.

h. *Substance P* inhibits synthesis and secretion of ACTH and stimulates secretion of GH, FSH, LH, and prolactin.

i. These hormones are transported to the *anterior pituitary* by the hypophyseal portal vessels. The releasing/inhibitory hormones regulate the stimulation and secretion of the anterior pituitary hormones (Brashers et al., 2014; Hall, 2016).

6. *Anterior Pituitary Hormones* (Figures 6.5 and 6.6)

a. *Growth hormone*

i. Biosynthesis. GH is a polypeptide hormone secreted by the somatotroph cells.

ii. Regulation. The strongest stimulus for release is GHRH, but it can also be stimulated by apomorphine, levodopa, and norepinephrine (Kaiser & Ho, 2016). Endorphins will also cause a release during times of severe stress or exercise (Kaiser & Ho,

2016). GHRH is transported to the anterior pituitary via the hypothalamic–hypophyseal portal vessels. Starvation, hypoglycemia, stress, exercise, and low fatty acid levels can stimulate GH release.

iii. The inhibition of GH release occurs secondary to somatostatin, hyperglycemia, exogenous GH, obesity, and corticosteroids. Somatostatin is secreted by cells in the periventricular region (located above the optic chiasm) in the hypothalamus and

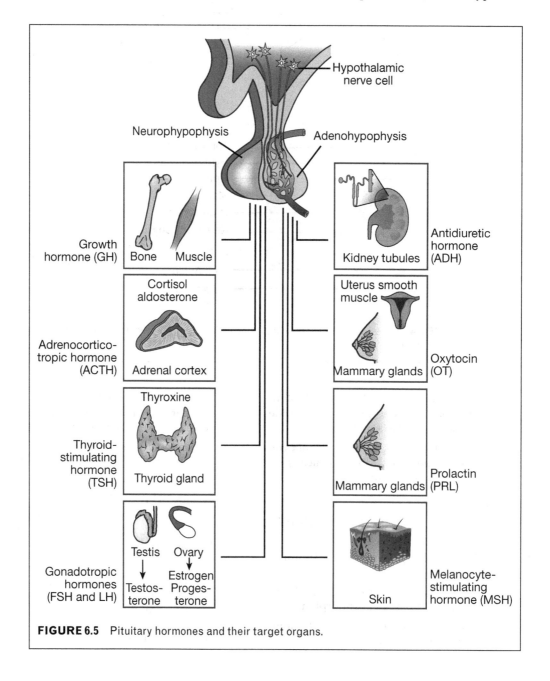

FIGURE 6.5 Pituitary hormones and their target organs.

in the delta cells of the pancreas (Hall, 2016). The peptide Gherlin, which is synthesized in gastric mucosa and in the hypothalamus, evokes the release of GH secretion, which induces food intake and is being widely studied in gastric bypass patients (Kaiser & Ho, 2016).

iv.   Secretion. GH is released in a pulsatile fashion with increased levels occurring during slow wave deep sleep (70% of daily secretion) and during adolescence (Kaiser & Ho, 2016).

v.   Effects. GH is an anabolic hormone that facilitates linear growth in all tissues of the body with mediation from insulin-like growth factor 1 (IGF-1). GH increases the mobilization of fatty acids from adipose tissue and enhances their conversion to acetyl coenzyme A to be utilized for energy, which spares protein usage. GH offers protection against hypoglycemia as it decreases carbohydrate utilization and increases blood glucose levels (Kaiser & Ho, 2016). GH stimulates bone, cartilage, and tissue growth with the stimulation of osteoclast and osteoblasts which increase bone mass (Brashers et al., 2014).

vi.   Abnormalities of GH secretion. In growth hormone deficiency (GHD), the anterior pituitary fails to produce enough GH; consequently, stature is less than genetic determination would indicate. Most GHD is idiopathic, however, it is important to rule out intracranial tumor. An excessive level of GH produces gigantism, usually caused by pituitary adenoma. Acromegaly is due to excessive GH secretion after the epiphyses of the long bones have closed, which results in excessive growth of the jaw, hands, and feet.

vii.   Role in critical illness. Catabolic states induced by acute illness, including surgery, burns, multiple organ dysfunction, and trauma, produce a state of GH resistance as well as decreased production and action of IGF-1 (Kaiser & Ho, 2016). Surgeries or disease states that affect the hypothalamic–pituitary system will also cause a state of low GH production. There is widespread interest in the use of GH in elevating sport performance and treating osteoporosis and malnutrition states.

b.   *Adrenocorticotropic hormone*

i.   Biosynthesis. ACTH is a polypeptide hormone secreted by corticotroph cells.

ii.   Regulation. The stimulation for the release of ACTH is CRH, which is secreted by the hypothalamus. Pain, stress (cytokines and catecholamines), trauma, hypoxia, low cortisol levels, and vasopressin administration also stimulate release of ACTH (Kaiser & Ho, 2016).

iii.   Inhibition to release of ACTH occurs primarily through negative feedback loops in response to an integrated neuroendocrine process to control the stress response. The response will in turn decrease the formation of CRF, vasopressin, and dopamine. Exogenous steroids decrease ACTH secretion and can lead to adrenal insufficiency (AI; Kaiser & Ho, 2016).

iv.   Secretion. ACTH has a 24-hour circadian pattern with ultradian pulsality that is controlled peripherally by corticosteroids (Kaiser & Ho, 2016). However, this circadian rhythm is not established in newborns. Highest levels occur in the early morning and decrease throughout the day and reach the lowest point between 11 p.m. and 3 a.m. The rhythm is affected by the light/dark cycle and is lost during times of stress. ACTH has melanocyte-stimulating abilities, which determine the concentration of melanin in the skin (Hall, 2016).

v.   Effects. ACTH stimulates the secretion of the adrenocortical hormones (glucocorticoids, mineralocorticoids, and androgens to produce and secrete cortisol and aldosterone [refer to text on cortisol and aldosterone in "Adrenal Glands"]).

vi.   Abnormalities of ACTH secretion. Long-term ACTH oversecretion stimulates hypertrophy, proliferation, and hyperfunction of the adrenal cortex (Hall, 2016). Undersecretion of ACTH leads to AI.

vii.   Role in critical illness. Relative AI is seen in critical illness, especially in sepsis. Hydrocortisone therapy is used for treatment. Treatment is reserved for children with catecholamine resistance (more than two vasoactive agents), sepsis, and those refractory to fluid resuscitation (Carcillo & Fields, 2002). Children on chronic steroids require stress doses of steroids when undergoing surgery or they are critically ill (see "Critical Illness-Related Corticosteroid Insufficiency").

c. *Thyroid-stimulating hormone*

i.   Biosynthesis. TSH, also known as *thyrotropin*, is a glycoprotein hormone secreted by the thyrotroph cells.

ii.   Regulation. Stimulations for the release of TSH include TRH, exposure to severe cold, and decreased level of thyroid hormone. Somatostatin and negative feedback from increased blood levels of thyroid hormones inhibit TSH. Dopamine inhibits TSH secretion and other catecholamines raise levels (Brashers et al., 2014).

iii.   Effects. TSH stimulates the thyroid gland to release T_3 and T_4, increase glucose uptake and oxidation, stimulate iodide metabolism, and increase thyroid cell size and vascularity (Brashers et al., 2014).

iv.   Abnormalities of TSH secretion. Hypersecretion of TSH induces hyperthyroidism. Hyposecretion of TSH induces hypothyroidism.

v.   Role in critical illness. Nonthyroidal illness syndrome, or *sick euthyroid syndrome*, is the most common thyroid abnormality in acute care. This abnormality occurs in patients with critical illness, postsurgery, or when fasting (not caused by pituitary dysfunction) and can be acute or chronic (von Saint Andre-von Arnim et al., 2013). The situation can be compounded when the child is receiving steroids, amiodarone, iodine dyes, propylthiouracil (PTU), or high-dose propranolol. T_3 levels are low, T_4 levels are normal or low, and TSH may be normal or reduced secondary to a decreased response to TRH. It is unclear whether these changes reflect a protective response or a maladaptive process, but studies have shown an association between sick euthyroid and severity of illness and clinical outcomes (von Saint Andre-von Arnim et al., 2013). There is debate regarding thyroid supplementation and most authors agree that supplementation is not necessary as a normal TSH reflects a euthyroid state. Thyroid testing should be repeated once the illness has resolved as hypothyroidism and sick euthyroid can be difficult to distinguish; however, true hypothyroid patients will have low T_4 and increased TSH, whereas an elevation in reverse T_3 level is indicative of sick euthyroid state (von Saint Andre-von Arnim et al., 2013). In premature infants, *hypothyroxinemia of prematurity* can also result in abnormal thyroid function studies, but this is typically transient.

d. *Follicle-stimulating hormone*

i.   Biosynthesis. FSH is a glycoprotein hormone that is secreted by the gonadotroph cells.

ii.   Regulation. The stimulus for FSH release is GnRH secreted by the hypothalamus. FSH secretion is inhibited through negative feedback secondary to increased levels of estrogen secreted by the ovaries and increased levels of inhibin secreted by the testes.

iii.   Effects. In males, FSH stimulates testicular growth; following puberty, FSH promotes spermatogenesis. In females, FSH stimulates the growth of the ovarian follicles and the secretion of estrogen.

iv.   Role in critical illness is unknown.

e. *Luteinizing hormone*

i.   Biosynthesis. LH is a glycoprotein hormone that is secreted by the gonadotroph cells.

ii.   Regulation. The stimulus for release of LH is GnRH secreted by the hypothalamus. Inhibition for the release of LH is negative feedback secondary to increased levels of estrogen, progesterone, and testosterone.

iii.   Effects. In males, LH stimulates the production of testosterone from the Leydig cells and maturation of spermatozoa. In females, LH stimulates estrogen and progesterone production. LH is responsible for ovulation and maintenance of the corpus luteum.

iv.   Role in critical illness is unknown.

f. *Prolactin*

i.   Biosynthesis. Prolactin is a polypeptide hormone that is secreted by the lactotroph cells.

ii.   Regulation. The stimulus for the release of prolactin is oxytocin, which is secreted by the posterior pituitary, TRH, and prolactin-releasing hormone (PRH) from the hypothalamus (Brashers et al., 2014). Immune-derived cytokines and stress also stimulate prolactin release. Inhibition of the release of prolactin is dopamine, which is secreted by the hypothalamus.

iii.   Effects. Prolactin stimulates lactation and during pregnancy increases the growth of the ductal system in the breast and the production of breast milk. It maintains the corpus luteum and progesterone production during pregnancy. Prolactin stimulates immune function by supporting the growth and survival of lymphocytes (Brashers et al., 2014).

iv.   Role in critical illness. Exogenous dopamine blocks prolactin production and may be associated with clinically significant effects on the immune system. Prolactin acts as a second messenger in the IL-2 and B-cell activation and differentiation and on several types of lymphocytes that can directly affect the immune system (Clayton & McCance, 2014). These relationships are under investigation for possible immune therapy.

7. *Posterior Pituitary Hormones (Figure 6.5)*

   a.   *ADH,* or arginine vasopressin (AVP)

      i.   Biosynthesis. ADH is a polypeptide. The prohormone is carried in vesicles through the axons to the posterior pituitary. Final synthesis of the prohormone to ADH occurs in the vesicles during axonal transport.

      ii.   Regulation. Osmoreceptors in the anterior hypothalamus are in close proximity to the supraoptic nucleus. When serum osmolality increases, the cells in this area begin to shrink, stimulating the release of ADH. Nonosmotic regulation occurs with pain, nausea, medications, cardiac failure, and any volume loss (von Saint Andre-von Arnim et al., 2013).

      iii.   The most potent stimulus for ADH release is arise in serum osmolality. Osmotic changes as small as 1% stimulate the release of ADH with normal set point of 280 mOsm/kg (Brashers et al., 2014; Robinson & Verbalis, 2016). These small changes in osmolality also stimulate the thirst mechanism, a protective mechanism to maintain water balance and prevent dehydration. A decrease in circulating blood volume perceived by the baroreceptors in the carotid sinus of the aortic arch also stimulates ADH release

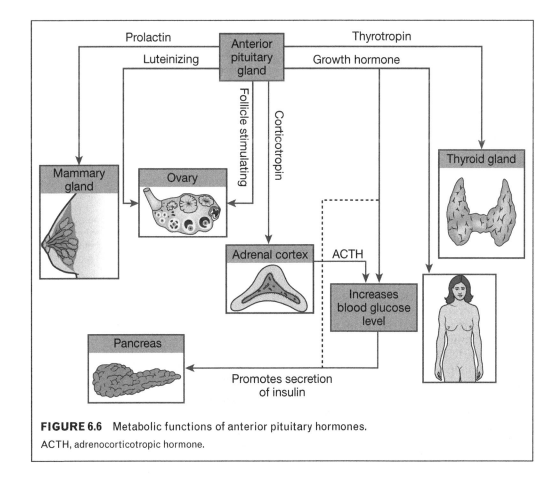

FIGURE 6.6 Metabolic functions of anterior pituitary hormones.
ACTH, adrenocorticotropic hormone.

(Robinson & Verbalis, 2016). Infants, small children, patients who are comatose or disoriented, or individuals who have abnormal thirst response are not able to meet these physiologic demands; therefore, they are dependent on others to ensure an adequate intake of water. Hemorrhage (10%–20% circulating blood loss), hypotension, nausea, hypercapnia, morphine, nicotine, and hypoxemia can activate the release of ADH (Hall, 2016; Robinson & Verbalis, 2016). Catecholamines and angiotensin II can modulate the release of ADH, which is a powerful stimulus to ACTH and prolactin release.

iv. ADH release is inhibited by a serum osmolality below 275 mOsm/kg (Robinson & Verbalis, 2016). The baroreceptors in the carotid sinus and the volume receptors in the left atrium send signals to the brainstem via the vagus and glossopharyngeal nerves. The stimulus is then carried to the hypothalamus. This pathway is primarily inhibitory; however, a fall in pressure or volume decreases the amount of inhibition, facilitating the release of ADH. Vincristine, cyclophosphamide, alcohol, and glucocorticoids inhibit ADH release (Brashers et al., 2014). Atrial natriuretic factor (ANF) inhibits ADH release and its effects on the kidney.

v. Effects. Three receptors mediated by binding to G proteins are responsive to ADH: V_1, V_2, and V_3. V_1 receptors are located in the liver, adrenals, brain, and smooth muscle. When stimulated, they produce smooth-muscle contraction, which leads to powerful *vasoconstriction*. V_2 receptors are located in renal tubular cells, primarily in the collecting tubule and the ascending loop of Henle causing increased permeability leading to increased water reabsorption, increased circulating blood volume leading to an antidiuresis. V_3 receptors have a concentrated location in the anterior pituitary as cortotroph cells but are also found in kidney, thymus, heart, lung, spleen, uterus, and breast tissue. These receptors stimulate the activity of phospholipase C, which raises intracellular calcium levels and aids in the release of ACTH (Brashers et al., 2014; Molina, 2013). ADH enhances sodium chloride (NaCl) transport out of the ascending limb of the loop of Henle. This serves to maximize the interstitial osmotic gradient in the

renal medulla, facilitating water reabsorption and urine concentration (Figure 6.7).

vi. Abnormalities of ADH. Deficiency results in diabetes insipidus (DI). Excess ADH results in SIADH (Yee et al., 2010).

vii. Role in critical illness. Vasopressin is administered to patients who have refractory hypotension with vasodilatory shock states or after cardiac bypass to increase systemic vascular resistance (Brashers et al., 2014). Vasopressin is also administered to patients with acute or chronic ADH deficiency secondary to surgery. The following disorders are associated with ADH: SIADH, cerebral salt wasting (CSW), and DI and are discussed later in this chapter.

b. *Oxytocin*

i. Biosynthesis. Oxytocin is a polypeptide that is almost identical to ADH except for the placement of two of the amino acids in the peptide chain. Like ADH, the prohormone for oxytocin is carried in vesicles through axons from the hypothalamus to the posterior pituitary, where the final

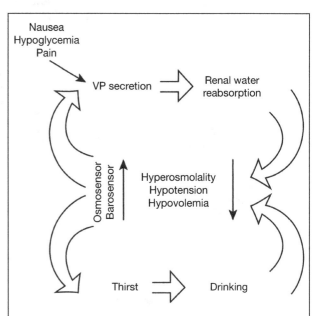

FIGURE 6.7 Regulation of vasopressin, secretion, and serum osmolality.

VP, vasopressin.

Source: From Majzoub, J. A., Muglia, L. J., & Srivatsa, A. (2014). Disorders of the posterior pituitary. In M. Sperling (Ed.), *Pediatric endocrinology* (4th ed., pp. 405–443). Philadelphia, PA: Elsevier.

synthesis of oxytocin occurs during neuronal transport.

ii. Regulation. The stimulus for oxytocin release is an increase in estrogen, the onset of labor from stretch receptors, and stimulation of the cervix and vagina (labor can occur in women with oxytocin deficiency, although the duration is prolonged), suckling stimuli on the nipple, hemorrhage, or psychologic stress. Oxytocin is inhibited by pain, heat, or loud noises (Brashers et al., 2014; Molina, 2013).

iii. Effects. Rhythmic contraction of the smooth muscle of the uterus occurs to induce labor and help with the involution of the uterus to prevent bleeding postpartum. Additional effects: causes release of ACTH with AVP to produce vasoconstriction with prolactin release that is associated with maternal amnesia (Molina, 2013). Also, causes the myoepithelial cells in the alveoli of the mammary gland to stimulate the release of breast milk and may have a role in sperm motility.

B. Thyroid Gland

1. *Embryology.* The thyroid gland is the first fetal endocrine gland to develop. It is recognizable by embryonic day 16 to 17. The gland can form thyroglobulin by the 28th day of gestation and can concentrate iodide and synthesize T_4 by the 11th week of gestation. The development of the thyroid gland begins from the endodermal floor of the primitive pharynx. As the embryo grows, the thyroid gland descends into the neck, passing the laryngeal cartilages. Fetal brain development is dependent on thyroid hormones and lack of it will cause severe disabilities. TSH concentration increases between 18 to 26 weeks gestation. Thyroxine-binding globulin (TBG) levels can be detected by 10 weeks, and progressively increase until term. This causes an elevation of T_4 for the second and third trimesters. Thyroid hormone levels peak at 24 hours of postnatal life and slowly decrease over the next few weeks (Brashers et al., 2014; Molina, 2013; Salvatore, Davies, Schlumberger, Hay, & Larsen, 2016).

2. *Location.* The thyroid gland consists of two lobes located on each side of the trachea below the larynx. A band of tissue called the *isthmus*, which lies over the second to fourth tracheal cartilages, connects the lobes.

3. *Cell Types.* The thyroid gland consists of a large number of follicles filled with colloid. The main constituent of colloid is thyroglobulin, a glycoprotein containing the thyroid hormones. Follicular cells and a basal membrane constitute the outer boundary of the follicle. Cuboidal epithelioid cells secrete colloid. Between the follicular cells are parafollicular cells that secrete calcitonin. The thyroid gland is highly vascular; follicles are in close contact with blood and lymphatic vessels (Brashers et al., 2014; Hall, 2016).

4. *Regulation of Thyroid Hormone.* The thyroid gland secretes T_3, T_4, and calcitonin. The negative feedback mechanism involves the hypothalamus, anterior pituitary gland, and the thyroid gland. TRH initiates the process with release from the hypothalamus, where it circulates and stimulates the release of TSH by the pituitary. Catecholamines and acetylcholine directly affect the secretory action of the follicular cells and regulate its blood flow (Brashers et al., 2014).

5. *Synthesis of Thyroid Hormone.* Synthesis of the thyroid hormones is complex and dependent on iodine and tyrosine. Tyrosine is an amino acid present in the body and iodine must be ingested and absorbed by the GI tract into the blood. The thyroid iodide pump actively transports iodide across the follicular cell membrane to be oxidized into iodine then bind with tyrosine in the thyroglobulin molecule. TSH stimulates the iodide pump. The coupling of iodinated tyrosine forms T_3 (triiodothyronine) or tetraiodothyronine (thyroxine, T_4). The thyroid gland is unique in its ability to store hormones in the follicular colloid for several months until released into the bloodstream; therefore, when synthesis stops, the physiological effects of hyposecretion are not seen for several months. Thyroglobulin is not released into circulating blood; the thyroid hormones must split from the thyroglobulin molecule before its release (Brashers et al., 2014; Molina, 2013; von Saint Andre-von Arnim et al., 2013).

6. *Thyroxine (T_4)*

  a. *Biosynthesis.* In total, 90% of the thyroid hormone production is T_4, and 10% is T_3. They are circulated bound by one of the three carrier proteins (Brashers et al., 2014).

  b. *Regulation.* TSH, low iodide levels, and extreme cold stimulate the release of T_4. Release of T_4 is inhibited by excess iodide and negative feedback resulting from increased levels of thyroid hormones that decrease the anterior pituitary secretion of TSH. Stimulation of the sympathetic nervous system causes a decrease in the secretion of TSH with a subsequent decrease in thyroid hormone secretion.

c. *Effects.* T_4 is a prohormone necessary for the production of T_3. The effects of T_4 are similar to the effects of T_3, although these effects are less potent and have a longer duration of action (half-life 7 days for T_4 and 1 day for T_3; Molina, 2013).

d. *Factors that impair peripheral conversion of T_4 to T_3* are propranolol, amiodarone, glucocorticoids (at anti-inflammatory doses), salicylates, liver failure or fatty liver disease, renal insufficiency, malnutrition, pregnancy, and major illness (sick euthyroid; Molina, 2013; Plumpton, Anderson, & Beca, 2010).

e. *Role in critical illness.* Dopamine administration decreases the response of TSH to TRH and suppresses TSH secretion (Plumpton et al., 2010). Sick euthyroid syndrome is discussed in the Thyroid-stimulating hormone section, Role in critical illness.

7. *Triiodothyronine (T_3)*

a. *Biosynthesis.* T_3 constitutes 10% of the hormones released by the thyroid gland, and the remaining are produced by extrathyroidal deiodination of T_4 (Molina, 2013).

b. Regulation of T_3 is the same as for T_4.

c. *Effects.* On release into the bloodstream, the thyroid hormones bind with plasma proteins. Because of their high affinity for the plasma-binding proteins, the thyroid hormones are released into the peripheral cells very slowly. Once they enter the cell, these hormones bind with intracellular proteins and are stored. Intracellular activity may last days or weeks. T_3 maintains basal metabolic rate and promotes tissue growth through the stimulation of almost all aspects of carbohydrate and fat metabolism. T_3 promotes protein synthesis, regulates body temperature, and stimulates oxygen consumption through an increase in metabolic rate. In addition, T_3 maintains cardiac output, heart rate, and strength of myocardial contraction through increased metabolism and direct effect on the heart. T_3 increases the rate and depth of respiration secondary to increased metabolism and increased carbon dioxide production. An increase in gastrointestinal (GI) tract motility and secretion of digestive enzymes occurs with T_3 (Molina, 2013; Salvatore et al., 2016).

d. *Role in critical illness.* Controversy exists on the treatment of abnormalities in thyroid hormone levels in infants who undergo cardiopulmonary bypass (CPB). It has been documented in the literature that this dysfunction is significant enough to affect myocardial function, even in the absence of primary thyroid disease (Talwar, Kumar, Choudhary, & Airan, 2016). This state of hypothyroidism has been associated with prolonged vent support, low cardiac output state, and left ventricular dysfunction. Thyroid supplementation in the early postoperative period has been given as an adjunct to improve cardiac function in neonates after cardiac surgery and enables a smoother recovery, but duration of therapy remains unclear (Talwar et al., 2016). *Sick euthyroid syndrome* is discussed in the Thyroid-stimulating hormone section, Role in critical illness.

8. *Abnormalities of T_3 and T_4 Secretion (Table 6.2)*

a. *Primary hypothyroidism* can be congenital or acquired and is caused by low levels of thyroid hormones (T_3 or T_4) and an elevated TSH level (von Saint Andre-von Arnim et al., 2013). Worldwide, the leading cause of hypothyroidism is iodine deficiency, but in the United States in children older than 6 years, it is most commonly caused by autoimmune dysfunction (*Hashimoto thyroiditis*). Symptoms may include lowered metabolic rate with lethargy, hypothermia, bradycardia, growth failure, hypotension, weight gain, fatigue, and constipation. Infants left untreated beyond 6 weeks for congenital hypothyroidism develop profound cognitive defects (Ganeson, Kazmi, & Levy, 2012). Newborn screens in all 50 states now include TSH and T_4 (Babler et al., 2013). Severe cases can progress to *myxedema coma* with symptoms of congestive heart failure, hypotension, hypoglycemia, and hypothermia (Jones, Brashers, & Huether, 2010; von Saint Andre-von Arnim et al., 2013). Treatment is provided with age-based supplementation of levothyroxine sodium in doses to normalize TSH and maintain free T_4. Levels must be monitored closely during times of growth and with dose changes (Babler et al., 2013).

b. *Hyperthyroidism* is caused by high levels of thyroid hormones and results in a hypermetabolic state with weight loss, tachycardia, hypertension, wide pulse pressure, irritability with restlessness, diarrhea, and tremor (Babler et al., 2013). The most common type in childhood is Graves' disease, which occurs most frequently in

TABLE 6.2   Clinical Features of Thyroid Dysfunction

Clinical Features of Hyperthyroidism	Clinical Features of Hypothyroidism
Tachycardia	Bradycardia
Anxiety	Lethargy
Hyperactivity	Depression
Fatigue	Somnolence
Diarrhea	Constipation
Heat intolerance	Cold intolerance
Weight loss and increased appetite	Weight gain and decreased appetite

Source: Adapted from Babler, E., Betts, K., Courtney, J., Flores, B., Flynn, C., Laerson, M., . . . Wroley, D. (2013). *Clinical handbook of pediatric endocrinology* (2nd ed.). St Louis, MO: Quality Medical Publishing.

early-adolescent females following an infection (Ganeson et al., 2012). Critical hyperthyroidism or *thyroid storm*, is rarely seen in the pediatric population, but when present can be life threatening with mortality rates of 20% to 30% (S. Srinivasan & Misra, 2015). Symptoms can escalate to the point of cardiovascular collapse with coma and severe hyperthermia. Immediate treatment with volume resuscitation and beta-blocker infusion (halts T_3 activity) is critical. Care must be taken with the use of beta-blockers in this hypermetabolic state if pulmonary artery hypertension or a low cardiac output state are present as these can worsen with their use (Chantra, Limsuwan, & Mahachoklertwattana, 2016). Other treatments are directed at limiting T_4 production by blocking thyroid hormone synthesis with methimiazole or propylthiuracil (PTU). Many providers have stopped using PTU due to dangerous effects on the liver and may also limit the use of methimazole due to its teratogenic affects (Clark, Preissig, Rigby, & Bowyer, 2008; Ganeson et al., 2012; von Saint Andre-von Arnim et al., 2013). Glucocorticoids are used in some instances to block the conversion of T_4 to T_3. Surgery or radioactive iodine treatment is used in many recalcitrant cases and will stop production of thyroid hormone but requires children to be on supplementation for the remainder of their lives (Ganeson et al., 2012).

9. *Calcitonin*

a. *Biosynthesis.* Calcitonin or thyrocalcitonin is a polypeptide produced by the parafollicular or C cells of the thyroid gland. Serum calcitonin is high at birth and slowly decreases over the first week of life, possibly contributing to neonatal hypocalcemia (Molina, 2013).

b. *Regulation.* The stimulus for release of calcitonin is an increase in serum calcium and gastrin. A low serum calcium level inhibits release of calcitonin.

c. *Effects.* Calcitonin plays a minor role in calcium and phosphorus regulation. It opposes the action of PTH and stimulates osteoblasts to deposit calcium for new bone formation. It also enhances renal excretion of calcium, decreases active vitamin D formation to lower serum calcium, and enhances renal excretion of calcium (Brashers et al., 2014).

C. Parathyroid Glands

1. *Embryology.* The third and fourth pharyngeal pouches differentiate into the thymus and parathyroid glands during the fourth to sixth week of gestation occurring synchronously with thyroid development (Dattani & Gevers, 2016). The fourth pouch eventually takes position at the upper poles of the thyroid as the superior parathyroid glands and increases in size to 1 to 2 mm by birth. During gestation, the placenta is impermeable to PTH and calcitonin, but 25-hydroxyvitamin D and calcitriol are transported across the placenta, and the mother remains the sole source of those minerals for the fetus. During the third trimester, active calcium transport occurs across the placenta maintaining fetal calcium concentrations. This system is dependent upon the activity of parathyroid hormone-related protein (PTHrP). Following birth, the newborn must rapidly adapt to this loss of support. Ionized calcium and PTH levels remain low for 48 hours after birth but appropriate

PTH response to hypocalcemia slowly develops in infants during the first weeks of life (Brashers et al., 2014; Dattani & Gevers, 2016).

2. *Location.* Two pairs are usually present (can number from two to six) behind the upper pole of the thyroid gland on each side of the trachea (Brashers et al., 2014).

3. *Cell Types.* The parathyroid gland contains mostly chief cells, which secrete most of the PTH. A small to moderate amount of the poorly understood oxyphil cells are present as well. It is speculated that they might be chief cells that are modified but no longer secrete PTH. The oxyphil cells are absent in infants and children (Hall, 2016).

4. *Parathyroid Hormone* (Figure 6.8)

a. *Biosynthesis.* PTH is a polypeptide composed of many amino acids synthesized on the ribosomes and cleaved to form PTH. It is stored in the secretory granules in the cytoplasm of the chief cells (Brashers et al., 2014).

b. *Regulation.* The stimulus for release of PTH is hypocalcemia, low levels of vitamin D, and mild hypomagnesemia. Release of PTH is inhibited by increased ionized calcium and hypermagnesemia (Molina, 2013).

c. *Effects* (Figure 6.8). PTH is the major hormone in the regulation of serum calcium. In the kidney, PTH increases calcium reabsorption and phosphorus excretion (there is an inverse relationship between calcium and phosphorus). PTH stimulates the conversion of vitamin D to its active form, increases GI tract calcium and phosphate absorption, and promotes bone resorption of calcium (movement out of the bone into the extracellular fluid).

5. *Abnormalities of Parathyroid Function*

a. *Primary hyperparathyroidism* occurs when negative feedback loops fail to inhibit the release of PTH and hypercalcemia results. The hypercalcemia is caused primarily by hyperplasia or adenomas of the gland or, secondarily, as part of a chronic disease state with either malabsorption or deficiency of essential vitamins, such as vitamin D, or hyperphosphatemia from renal disease. Other secondary causes include such drugs as phenytoin, phenobarbital, or laxatives (Brashers et al., 2014).

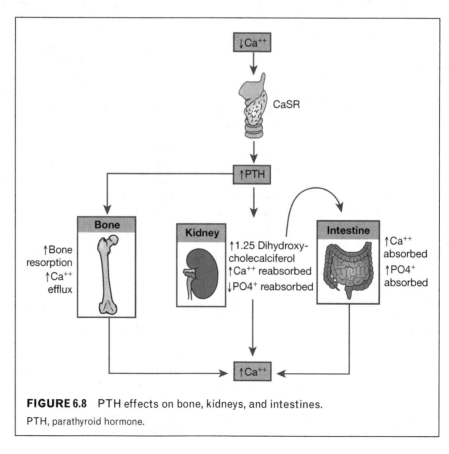

FIGURE 6.8 PTH effects on bone, kidneys, and intestines.

PTH, parathyroid hormone.

b. *Hypoparathyroidism* is the absence of PTH, resulting in hypocalcemia and hyperphosphatemia. This can occur as a result of surgery near the glands, hypomagnesemia, genetic syndromes (DiGeorge), or from an autoimmune/idiopathic diagnosis.

c. *Role in critical illness.* Impaired calcium metabolism resulting from abnormalities of parathyroid function may be seen in infants and lead to profound hypocalcemia with seizures, tetany, and shock (Babler et al., 2013; Molina, 2013). Treatment is with calcium and the active form of vitamin D (Brashers et al., 2014).

D. Pancreas

1. *Embryology*

a. *Dorsal and ventral pancreatic buds* arise from the primitive endoderm and the gland is identifiable by week 4 of gestation (Dattani & Gevers, 2016). Acini (secretory cells) develop from cells around the primitive ducts in the pancreatic buds. The islets of Langerhans develop from cell groups that separate from the primitive buds and form next to the acini. The islets of Langerhans appear at 12 to 16 weeks gestation and are clearly differentiated by 31 weeks (Dattani & Gevers, 2016).

b. *Insulin and glucagon secretion* are identifiable by 8 to 10 weeks gestation. The main determinant of fetal glucose uptake is maternal blood glucose level. Glucose is the main substrate utilized by the fetus and it passes through the placenta through facilitated diffusion. Glucose supply is usually constant, but if autoregulation is necessary it occurs in the liver. The placenta is relatively impermeable to insulin and there are higher numbers of insulin receptors present in fetal cells when compared to adults but downregulation does not occur. Insulin is the major hormone that drives fetal growth. Glucagon levels are high in fetal plasma but receptors are decreased in number. In the last trimester of gestation, hyperglycemia does not get blunted by glucagon levels, thereby promoting the period of rapid growth that occurs. Glucagon levels rise sharply after birth, remain stable during the first 48 hours of life, and then rise progressively throughout the next days of life (Dattani & Gevers, 2016).

c. *Alpha and beta cells* can be recognized by 8 to 10 weeks with alpha cells being the most numerous in number early in gestation, but this becomes equal to beta cells by term (Dattani & Gevers, 2016).

d. *Glucose homeostasis* in the term newborn is essential but supply must be constant and becomes rapidly depleted due to large glucose requirements for brain development. Premature or small-for-gestational-age (SGA) infants have less body fat, low glycogen stores, and therefore less reserves than term infants. The neonate and young child also exhibit hypoglycemia when fasting for shorter periods than the older child or adult. Counterregulatory hormonal responses to hypoglycemia are blunted in this population as well (De León, Thornton, Stanley, & Sperling, 2014).

e. *External sources* of glucose are more important in the neonate because of limited glycogen stores. Hepatic glycogenolysis must be initiated once fasting occurs. Gluconeogenesis will also begin and muscle proteins will be used as an alternate source of glucose. Glycogenolysis will decline within 8 to 12 hours and the transition to inefficient use of fat as a source of energy will begin. Once glucose levels fall to <50 mg/dL, all of these alternate energy resource systems have been initiated and critical hypoglycemic labs should be obtained (De León et al., 2014).

2. *Location.* The pancreas is shaped like a tadpole, with a head, body, and tail, and it lies across the posterior abdominal wall between the spleen and duodenum.

3. *Cell Types*

a. *Exocrine function* includes the acini cells who secrete enzymes important in the digestive process into the duodenum via a network of ducts (Doig & Huether, 2014).

b. *Endocrine function* uses a ductless system that directly secretes insulin, glucagon, and somatostatin into the portal circulation. It constitutes less than 2% of the total pancreatic volume. The islets of Langerhans have four cell types:

    i. Alpha cells, which secrete glucagon, constitute 25% of islet cells.

    ii. Beta cells, which secrete both insulin and amylin, constitute 60% of islet cells.

    iii. Delta cells, which secrete somatostatin, constitute 10% of islet cells.

    iv. Polypeptide cells, which secrete pancreatic polypeptide and gastrin, constitute 5% of islet cells (Brashers et al., 2014).

4. *Insulin*

a. *Biosynthesis.* Insulin is an anabolic hormone stored in secretory granules in the beta cells of the pancreas as proinsulin with a connecting C peptide that has a circulating half-life of 6 minutes (Hall, 2016). It is synthesized on the ribosomes of the beta cells and converted to insulin when the signal comes for its secretion (Brashers et al., 2014; De León et al., 2014).

b. *Secretion.* Beta cells are secreted parasympathetically in response to hormonal, neural, and chemical input when the blood glucose rises (Brashers et al., 2014).

c. *Regulation.* Release of insulin is predominantly stimulated by an increase in blood glucose and amino acid levels (arginine and lysine). Other factors promoting the release of insulin are GI tract hormones (gastrin, cholecystokinin, and secretin), cortisol, GH, proinflammatory cytokines, and glucagon (Hall, 2016; V. Srinivasan & Agus, 2014). The following will inhibit the release of insulin: hypoglycemia, catecholamines, somatostatin, and prostaglandins (Brashers et al., 2014; Hall, 2016). Once blood glucose levels fall to fasting levels, insulin secretion halts.

d. *Effects*

i. Carbohydrate metabolism. Insulin increases glucose uptake by the liver, muscle, and adipose tissue and stimulates glycogen storage in the liver and muscle (*glycogenesis*). Insulin inhibits gluconeogenesis (formation of glucose from noncarbohydrate sources) and glycogenolysis (breakdown of glycogen to glucose). Insulin is not necessary for glucose uptake by the brain and most of the cells are impermeable to glucose (Hall, 2016).

ii. Fat metabolism. Insulin stimulates triglyceride synthesis, transport of fatty acids across the cell membrane, and storage in adipose tissue. Insulin inhibits lipolysis (fat breakdown) and ketogenesis (formation of ketones from fat; Hall, 2016).

iii. Protein metabolism. Insulin facilitates transport of amino acids into the cells, works synergistically with GH to promote growth, and stimulates protein synthesis. Insulin inhibits proteolysis (protein breakdown; Hall, 2016).

iv. Secondary effects of insulin. Insulin assists with the transport of potassium, magnesium, and phosphate into the cell, helping to maintain cellular homeostasis.

e. *Hypoinsulinemia.* Hypoinsulinemia occurs when an abnormally low level of insulin is present in the body. This lack of insulin markedly reduces the rate of transport of glucose across the cell membrane. Reduced insulin secretion also increases the amount of stored triglycerides in the liver, causing increased serum triglycerides, fatty acids, and cholesterol (Brashers et al., 2014). Falling insulin levels also increase serum levels of acetoacetic acid, acetone, and ketone bodies because of increased oxidation of fat (*lipolysis*). Liver and muscle glycogen is converted to glucose and released into the blood (*glycogenolysis*). Gluconeogenesis includes the breakdown of proteins (*proteolysis*) to form glucose (Brashers et al., 2014; Hall, 2016).

f. *Role in critical illness.* Tight control of serum glucose (80–110) utilizing insulin infusions has shown improved outcomes in adult trauma patients but remains debatable in children. The Heart and Lung Failure–Pediatric Insulin Titration (HALF-PINT) study hopes to ascertain whether tight glucose control with intensive insulin therapy can improve outcomes in critically ill children without the deleterious effect of hypoglycemia, as seen in previous studies with tight glucose control (V. Srinivasan & Agus, 2014). Insulin is also used to treat hyperkalemia with concurrent glucose administration.

5. *Glucagon*

a. *Biosynthesis.* Glucagon is a large peptide that is synthesized and secreted by the alpha cells of the islet cells and by cells that line the GI tract.

b. *Regulation.* Hypoglycemia, amino acids (alanine, asparagine, and glycine), ingestion of proteins, sympathetic stimulation, and vigorous exercise are stimulants for the release of glucagon. Hyperglycemia, high levels of circulating fatty acids, and somatostatin suppress release of glucagon (Brashers et al., 2014).

c. *Effects.* Glucagon is a catabolic hormone; a hormone of fuel mobilization. It is an insulin antagonistic hormone that directs the breakdown of liver glycogen (glycogenolysis), increases gluconeogenesis in the liver, and increases the availability of fatty acid to make energy available to the tissues (Brashers et al., 2014).

d. *Role in critical illness.* Glucagon is used as treatment in calcium channel blocker toxicity and for severe hypoglycemia. A relatively high glucagon level is seen in every type of diabetes and is thought to propagate the metabolic problems seen in the disease and may be an important component in its pathogenesis (Brashers et al., 2014).

6. *Somatostatin*

  a. *Biosynthesis.* Somatostatin is a polypeptide synthesized from the islet cells and secreted by the delta cells of the pancreas (Brashers et al., 2014). It is present in the hypothalamus, pancreas, and GI tract.

  b. *Regulation.* Glucose, amino acids, fatty acids, and GI tract hormones stimulate the release of somatostatin, which is essential for their metabolism.

  c. *Effects.* Somatostatin inhibits the secretion of insulin, glucagon, GH, and TSH. It decreases the production of gastric acid and gastrin and prevents excess insulin from being released. It decreases GI tract motility and absorption and helps with regulation of alpha and beta cell function (Brashers et al., 2014).

  d. *Role in critical illness.* Octreotide, which is a somatostatin analog, is used to decrease variceal bleeding seen with portal hypertension and hepatorenal syndrome. Octreotide is being used in the management of chylothorax and hypoglycemia seen in sulfa drug overdose (Chan, Chan, Mengshol, Fish, & Chan, 2013).

7. *Amylin*

  a. *Biosynthesis.* Amylin is an islet amyloid cosecreted with insulin in response to intake of food (Brashers et al., 2014).

  b. *Regulation.* Stimulated in response to high glucose.

  c. *Effects.* Serves as an antihyperglycemic by regulating uptake of nutrients, providing the sensation of saity, and delaying the release of glucagon (Brashers et al., 2014).

  d. *Role in critical illness.* Aggregated amylin is cytotoxic and is suspected of contributing to the loss of beta cells in type 2 diabetes. Amylin is also being used in the treatment of diabetes as an agent for glycemic control and it may play a factor in gastric emptying. Ongoing research is looking at the role amylin may have in development of obesity (Brashers et al., 2014).

E. Adrenal Glands

1. *Embryology*

  a. The adrenal glands develop from two different origins: the cortex, arising from the mesoderm, and the medulla, arising from the neuroectoderm and is found above the much smaller kidney by 8 weeks of gestation. Differentiation of the adrenal medulla occurs late in development. The zona reticularis is not developed until the end of the third year of life and is not fully developed until around 15 years of age. The mesoderm is involved in the development of the gonads (Miller & Flück, 2014).

  b. Fetal cortisol is necessary as a fetus prepares for extrauterine transition. An increase in fetal cortisol occurs in the last 10 weeks of gestation and prepares several systems that are critical for survival. As delivery approaches, cortisone, the active form that would be detrimental in early fetal development, is converted by the liver and lung tissues to cortisol (Dattani & Gevers, 2016). Cortisol progressively decreases during the first 2 months of life.

  c. Early in the fetus's development, there is no *epinephrine*. Norepinephrine is the dominant catecholamine at birth (Miller & Flück, 2014).

2. *Location.* The adrenal glands are small glands that lie atop the kidneys. Each gland has two distinct parts, the cortex, constituting 80% of the gland, and the medulla, constituting 20% of the gland (Babler et al., 2013).

3. *Anatomic Structure.* The adrenal gland is surrounded by a fibrous capsule. The adrenal cortex has three histologically different zones: *zona glomerulosa*, the outermost layer, which constitutes 15% of the cortex; *zona fasciculate*, the middle layer, which constitutes 75% of the cortex; and the zona reticularis, the innermost layer, constituting 10% of the cortex. The adrenal medulla has sympathetic and parasympathetic innervation but the adrenal cortex does not. The adrenal circulation unlike other organs does not run in parallel. Arterial blood supplied by smaller arteries and flows toward the medulla, so medullary chromaffin cells see high steroid concentration in their circulation. The more conventional veins drain into the left renal vein and the vena cava (Miller & Flück, 2014).

4. *Cell Types* (Miller & Flück, 2014)

  a. The *adrenal cortex* is responsible for the secretion of corticosteroids, which are synthesized from cholesterol. These hormones are released from three separate zones in the adrenal cortex. The three zones each secrete unique hormones and from the outside to inside they are often remembered by saying salt, sugar, and sex.

    i. The *zona glomerulosa* is responsible for the secretion of mineralocorticoid and aldosterone.

ii. The *zona fasciculata* is responsible for secreting glucocorticoids, mainly cortisol and a small amount of androgen secretion.

iii. The *zona reticularis* is responsible for secreting androgen, estrogen, and small amounts of glucocorticoid.

b. The *chromaffin cells* are the major cells of the adrenal medulla and they store the catecholamines epinephrine and norepinephrine as secretory granules. They are synthesized from phenylalanine with innervation from the parasympathetic and sympathetic nervous systems. In times of stress, exocytosis occurs after depolarization from acetylcholine, and enhanced amounts of hormones are released (Brashers et al., 2014).

5. *Aldosterone* (Figure 6.9)

a. *Biosynthesis*. Aldosterone is the most potent mineralcorticoid and it is imperative for life functions due to its sodium-retaining properties. It is a steroid compound synthesized from cholesterol absorbed from the blood. Synthesis begins in the zona fasciculata and reticularis with final conversion to active form in the zona glomerulosa (Brashers et al., 2014).

b. *Regulation*. It occurs primarily by angiotensin II via the renin–angiotensin system, but it is

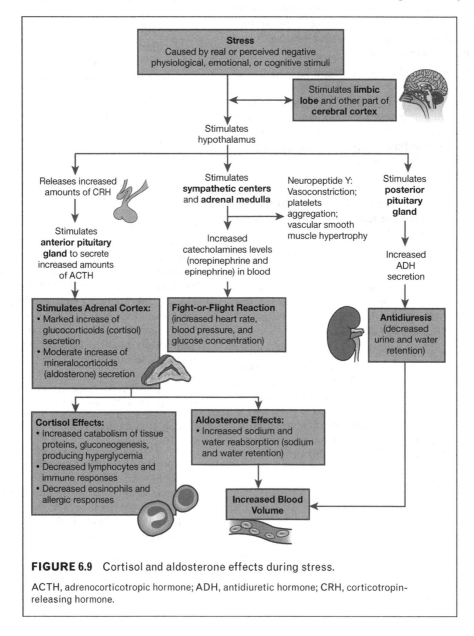

FIGURE 6.9 Cortisol and aldosterone effects during stress.

ACTH, adrenocorticotropic hormone; ADH, antidiuretic hormone; CRH, corticotropin-releasing hormone.

also activated for release by volume depletion, decreased renal perfusion, ACTH and sodium levels, and hyperkalemia. A small increase in serum potassium will triple aldosterone release. This response is imperative for the prevention of the serious cardiotoxic effects brought about by hyperkalemia. Inhibition of aldosterone release occurs secondary to volume expansion, hypokalemia, and low angiotensin levels (Brashers et al., 2014; Hall, 2016).

c. *Effects.* Aldosterone is responsible for 90% of mineralocorticoid activity (Hall, 2016). It acts on the distal tubule, collecting tubule, and collecting duct of the kidney to promote sodium reabsorption and potassium excretion. Along with renal reabsorption of sodium, there is a concurrent movement of water into the vascular bed. The net effect is an increase in extracellular sodium, an increase in extracellular volume, and a decrease in extracellular potassium. Aldosterone promotes reabsorption of sodium and excretion of potassium by the sweat and salivary glands, which promotes hydrogen ion excretion by the kidney and sodium absorption by the intestines. If aldosterone is low or absent, bowel absorption of sodium and water will not occur and diarrhea will result (Brashers et al., 2014; Hall, 2016).

d. *Role in critical illness.* Aldosterone is key to maintenance of extracellular volume. Excess release can have lasting effects of more than 1 to 2 days with notable increase in arterial blood pressure. A subsequent *natriuresis* occurs, which increases the excretion of both water and sodium, and once it normalizes the pressure will return to the previous level (volume rise of 5%–15% causes blood pressure rise of 15–25 mmHg; Hall, 2016).

6. *Cortisol* (Figure 6.9)

a. *Biosynthesis.* Cortisol is a steroid compound derived mostly from cholesterol and is the main product excreted by the adrenal cortex (Miller & Flück, 2014). It is the most potent of the glucocorticoids and has a half-life of 90 minutes (Brashers et al., 2014).

b. *Regulation.* The primary stimulus for secretion of cortisol is ACTH, but *stress* is another strong stimulus. Release of cortisol is inhibited by negative feedback to either the hypothalamus or the anterior pituitary secondary to increased cortisol levels, which produces a decrease in CRH release in the hypothalamus or decrease in ACTH release in the anterior pituitary (Brashers et al., 2014).

c. *Secretion.* Secretion is regulated by the hypothalamus and anterior pituitary. It is released immediately after stimulation from ACTH. It has a diurnal rhythm release with ACTH and peaks in the hours just before awakening. It circulates bound to albumin, the glycoprotein *cortisol-binding globulin* (*CBG*; also known as *transcortin*) or in the unbound active form (Brashers et al., 2014). *Transcortin* serves an important role in the negative feedback loop for cortisol and is elevated when estrogen levels are high (Clayton & McCance, 2014).

d. *Effects.* Cortisol is responsible for 95% of glucocorticoid activity and is necessary in life for stress protection (Hall, 2016). Cortisol increases gluconeogenesis and glycogenolysis to provide a substrate for this stressful time, often leading to hyperglycemia. Protein synthesis decreases, and catabolism of protein increases. Cortisol promotes mobilization of fatty acids from the tissues. An anti-inflammatory cascade occurs with its release that counteracts and modulates the body's immune response and endothelial integrity. Cortisol is potentiated by nitric oxide and it also provides vascular tone to increase blood pressure and prevent capillary leak (Brashers et al., 2014; Levy-Shraga & Pinhas-Hamiel, 2013).

e. *Role in critical illness.* Absolute AI is rare. Relative AI, in which cortisol production is inadequate to the level of stressful stimuli, can be seen in sepsis, trauma, or surgery (Levy-Shraga & Pinhas-Hamiel, 2013). *Critical illness-related corticosteroid insufficiency (CIRCI)* will be discussed later in the chapter.

7. *Abnormalities of Adrenal Cortical Function*

a. AI results in insufficient glucocorticoid and mineralocorticoid release or production and will require the child to have lifelong administration of exogenous hormones. It presents in childhood primarily as congenital adrenal hyperplasia (CAH) or Addison's disease. *CAH* is an autosomal recessive congenital disorder and is the leading cause of AI in childhood (Webb & Krone, 2015). It usually presents in the newborn period with symptoms of shock, ambiguous genitalia, and the very diagnostic electrolyte abnormalities of hyponatremia and hyperkalemia. It has many variants that explain the specific presenting symptoms and is now part of the newborn screen with a 17-hydroxy progesterone level (White, 2016). *Addison's disease* is a rare autoimmune or infectious process in children. It results from an absent or damaged adrenal gland. The deficiency produces initial weakness with weight loss, hyperpigmentation, dehydration, electrolyte imbalances, and altered metabolism (Brashers et al., 2014). The presentation may progress and lead to *adrenal crisis* with hypotension and cardiovascular collapse. Children present in shock due to the acute depletion of adrenal cortical hormones. It is precipitated by vomiting, diarrhea, convulsions, coma, hypotension, hyperpyrexia, tachycardia, and cyanosis. AI can also result from exogenous suppression of hormones with oral or intravenous (IV) steroids, as well as an abrupt withdrawal of steroids after chronic use (White, 2016). Children who suffer from severe sepsis, are premature or less than 6 months of age, and those who have had etomidate administration are at higher risk for adrenal sufficiency.

b. Hyperfunction of the adrenal cortex, or *Cushing syndrome*, is a rare disorder in children resulting in excess cortisol. Excess cortisol can be rarely caused by a pituitary adenoma but more common causes include administration of high dose of exogenous steroids or chronic use of steroids (Brashers et al., 2014). The very typical *"Cushingoid"* effects include weight gain, moon facies, truncal striae, atropy of skin or bruising, emotional lability, hyperglycemia, and high blood pressure (Brashers et al., 2014). With long-term steroid excess, children will have problems with bone demineralization and stunted growth.

8. *Epinephrine*

a. *Biosynthesis.* Epinephrine is a catecholamine derived from the amino acid tyrosine, which is then converted to dopamine in the sympathetic nerve endings. Dopamine is converted to norepinephrine, which is converted to epinephrine in the adrenal medulla. Epinephrine secretion is 80% of the total catecholamine secreted by the adrenal medulla and at rest it is released at 0.2 mcg/kg/min (Hall, 2016).

b. *Regulation.* Neuroendocrine (stress, fear, illness) stimulation causes epinephrine and norepinephrine to be directly released into the blood. Any stimulus that produces a sympathetic response stimulates secretion of epinephrine. The effects are rapid but only seen for seconds to minutes (Brashers et al., 2014). ACTH and glucocorticoids also stimulate release of epinephrine. Inhibition of epinephrine is through negative feedback loops; high levels of circulating catecholamines will produce downregulation of sympathetic receptors.

c. *Effects.* Epinephrine stimulates the beta-adrenergic receptors in the end organs. The greatest effect is due to stimulation of the sympathetic beta-1-adrenergic receptors in the heart, resulting in increased cardiac contractility, conduction velocity, and heart rate. The net result is an increase in cardiac output and blood pressure. In isolation, stimulation of the beta-2-adrenergic receptors of the vascular bed promotes relaxation; however, during stress the vasoconstricting effects of norepinephrine counteract significant vasodilation. Other effects of stimulation of the beta-2-adrenergic receptors are intestinal, bladder and uterine relaxation, and bronchial dilation. Epinephrine increases metabolic activity to a much greater degree than norepinephrine. It increases glycogenolysis and glucose release, resulting in elevations of blood glucose to supply fuel substrates. Circulating epinephrine accounts for 10% of the sympathetic activity during the stress response (Hall, 2016).

d. *Role in critical illness.* Epinephrine is used for hypotension, cold shock, bradycardia, and asystole (Chameides, Samson, Schexnayder, & Hazinski, 2011). Cold shock states are characterized by the presence of cold extremities, delayed capillary refill, and low cardiac output. The actions of epinephrine are dose dependent. At lower doses, epinephrine will have greater beta-2 adrenergic effect and SVR may fall whereas at higher doses alpha-adrenergic effects will be seen and SVR will rise (Davis et al., 2017).

9. *Norepinephrine*

a. *Biosynthesis.* Norepinephrine is synthesized from its precursor dopamine in the nerve endings of the sympathetic nervous system with only minor sources from the medulla.

b. Regulation is the same as for epinephrine.

c. Effects are secondary to stimulation of the alpha-adrenergic receptors in the end organs. The most significant effect during stress is peripheral vasoconstriction supporting blood pressure. Stimulation of the alpha-adrenergic receptors also produces dilation of the iris, contraction of the bladder and intestinal sphincters, and pilomotor contraction.

d. *Role in critical illness.* Norepinephrine is used in hypotensive, vasodilated, warm shock states (Chameides et al., 2011). Children with warm shock will have flash capillary refill; warm, pink extremities; and bounding pulses. Norepinephrine is used to reverse this low SVR state, which is characterized by a wide pulse pressure (when the diastolic pressure is half of the systolic; Davis et al., 2017).

10. *Hyperfunction* of adrenal medulla is rare, and is most often caused by a catecholamine-secreting tumor called *pheochromocytoma*. This tumor arises when the chromaffin cells of the adrenal gland fail to involute and the excess production can cause life-threatening hypertension, tachycardia, diaphoresis, tremors, and headaches (Kline-Tilford, 2016). Diagnosis is made through measurements of metanephrine and catecholamine levels and urine vanillylmandelic acid (VMA). Hypertension control is imperative and is often initially done with alpha- and beta-blocker infusions with subsequent tumor resection. Care must be taken, however, to avoid using beta-blockers alone as unopposed alpha activity could occur.

CLINICAL ASSESSMENT OF ENDOCRINE FUNCTION

Many endocrine disorders develop slowly over time and often go unrecognized by those (parents and caregivers) with daily contact with the child. Assessment through careful history, documentation of past medical conditions, growth patterns, developmental milestones, physical exam findings, and family history are critical to the accurate diagnosis of specific endocrine disorders.

A. History

1. Prenatal history includes prenatal care; complications of pregnancy (i.e., hypertension or preeclampsia); exposure to infections; use of drugs, tobacco, and alcohol; maternal gestational diabetes; or other endocrine disorders such as thyroid disease.

2. Neonatal history includes gestational age, birth weight, complications of labor and delivery, method of delivery, Apgar scores, hospitalization as a newborn, oxygen use, jaundice, neonatal hypoglycemia, newborn screen results, congenital anomalies, and postnatal complications or maladaptions to extra-uterine life such as poor weight gain or feeding difficulties (Babler et al., 2013).

3. Growth and development factors used for evaluation include longitudinal height and weight, recent changes in weight, achievement in developmental milestones, and growth patterns.

   a. *Diet* is assessed, including food preferences, allergies and aversions, content and time of typical meals, snacking behaviors, changes in appetite, and anorexia. Problems with digestion, such as nausea, bloating, food intolerances, abnormal stool patterns, diarrhea, or constipation, are noted.

   b. *School performance and problems* or recent changes in performance are discussed. Assessment of personality and behavioral traits includes recent changes in behavior, irritability, sluggishness, disinterest, lethargy, emotional lability, attention deficits, increased aggressiveness, altered self-esteem, perceptions of body image, family roles, and socialization issues.

   c. *Sleep and rest patterns* are noted, including normal bedtimes, incidence of insomnia, ease of falling asleep, restlessness, snoring, nocturnal enuresis, and night terrors. Also, note activity and exercise patterns, including the types of exercise normally engaged in, stamina, strength, outside interests, and hobbies.

   d. *Sexual maturation*, including the age of development, abnormalities, timing and character of menarche, and sexual activity are recorded.

4. Past medical history includes known endocrine disorders, neurosurgery, trauma or stress, and previous hospitalizations or frequent illnesses.

   a. *Medication history.* Many medications can alter normal endocrine function. Examples of this include:

      i. High-dose steroids can induce hyperglycemia, inhibit normal physiologic release of steroids from the adrenal cortex from, suppressed ACTH release (causing AI during the withdrawal phase causing profound shock), and alter serum electrolytes.

      ii. Antipsychotics can change levels of prolactin and can result in obesity and metabolic abnormalities.

      iii. Propranolol, amiodarone, and glucocorticoids (at anti-inflammatory doses) impair conversion of T_4 to T_3.

      iv. Lithium may induce hypothyroidism, diminish renal concentrating ability (nephrogenic DI), or cause elevations in PTH levels resulting in hypercalcemia.

      v. Antiepileptics like phenytoin and phenobarbital can cause rickets through effects on vitamin D metabolism.

      vi. Attention deficit hyperactivity disorder (ADHD) medications can affect appetite and growth.

vii. Nonsteroidal anti-inflammatory drugs (NSAIDs) enhance renal responsiveness to ADH.

viii. Sedatives, narcotics, and anesthetics can stimulate the thirst mechanism and alter ADH release.

ix. Chemotherapy alters ADH release.

x. Ethanol stimulates the thirst mechanism, alters serum osmolality and ADH release, and alters glucose metabolism.

xi. Tricyclic antidepressants stimulate the thirst mechanism and alter ADH release.

b. Other diseases can have a relationship with endocrine disorders. Cystic fibrosis can be an underlying cause of DM. Renal disease can be an underlying cause of DI and part of the differential diagnosis for ADH abnormalities. Lung disease, including pneumonia, can be an underlying cause of SIADH. Pheochromocytoma is a catecholamine-secreting tumor that can produce life-threatening hypertension, hyperthermia, and cardiovascular collapse.

5. Family history includes parents' ages; height, weight, and body proportions of family members; the parents' age at puberty; familial and genetic diseases; health of parents and siblings; presence of known endocrine and other chronic disorders in other family members to include grandparents, aunts, uncles, and cousins (Babler et al., 2013).

B. Physical Assessment

1. Height and weight, body mass index, and body surface area are measured. Growth velocity and target height are estimated.

2. Body size and proportion, fat distribution, upper and lower body ratios, chest circumference, and arm span are compared with previous measurements, if available.

3. Temperature, blood pressure, and heart rate are recorded.

4. Head circumference and percentiles on age- and sex-related growth charts are plotted.

5. Intake and output are monitored.

6. The head, eyes, ears, nose, and throat (HEENT) survey includes anterior and posterior fontanel, head shape and suture lines, forehead and hair patterns. Observe for sunken or protruding eyes, periorbital edema, gaze, sclera color, pupil symmetry and response, fundus exam, and visual acuity. Examine nose for discharge and patency. Examine ears for pinna placement (low high, posterior), gross hearing, and examination of the tympanic membranes. Palpate the thyroid gland and neck for masses or thrills, lymphadenopathy, and auscultate for the presence of bruits. Assess mucous membranes for moisture and color, and inspect the oral cavity for abnormalities of the lips and palate, presence of caries, and abnormalities in dentition or gum disease.

7. *Skin Assessment.* Evaluate skin turgor and moisture, skin color (including hyperpigmentation, hypopigmentation, nevi, and café au lait spots), texture (including the presence of excess oil, rough or dry skin, acne, and temperature), and hair and nail texture.

8. Neurologic assessment includes the level of consciousness with general demeanor, irritability, lethargy, hyperactivity, or lack of interaction. Function of cranial nerves, pupil responses, fine and gross motor movement, abnormal gait or stance, abnormal movement disorders or rhythmic tics, the presence of tremors, reflexes, abnormal deep tendon reflexes, and the presence of seizure activity or clonus should be noted.

9. Cardiovascular evaluation includes rate, rhythm, and character of heart tones; peripheral pulses; perfusion, capillary fill time, warmth, and mottling of skin; palpation for thrills, heaves, and point of maximal impulse (PMI); edema; and any blood pressure abnormalities, including hypertension, hypotension or orthostatic hypotension, or syncopal events.

10. Respiratory assessment includes the rate and depth of respiration, any alterations of breath odor, chest excursion, chest symmetry and deformities, and characteristics of adventitious breath sounds with differentiation of upper or lower airway abnormal sounds.

11. Abdominal assessment notes the presence of bowel sounds, tenderness or pain, with notice of adiposity. Includes palpation for organomegaly or presence of masses.

12. Genitourinary assessment includes palpation of the kidneys; examination of external genitalia and assessment of secondary sexual characteristics and Tanner staging of breast, pubic hair, testicular volume, and phallus size.

13. Musculoskeletal assessment includes evaluation for disproportionate growth or body habitus with notice of discrepancies of limb length. The presence of genu valgum or genu varum, short or unusually long metacarpals, and palpation of muscles for strength and range-of-motion deficits or scoliosis should be noted.

14. Check general appearance for cleanliness, alertness level, responsiveness to directions, and ability to follow commands. Determine basic short- and long-term memory per developmental level (Babler et al., 2013; Brashers et al., 2014).

C. Diagnostic Studies

1. *Laboratory* (Babler et al., 2013; Brashers et al., 2014)

a. *Blood chemistries* for basic electrolyte screening to include magnesium, phosphorus, calcium and glucose, blood urea nitrogen (BUN), and creatinine (Babler et al., 2013; Brashers et al., 2014). Further important studies include pH, osmolality, and cortisol levels to assess the pituitary–adrenal axis (plasma levels vary with age and time of day). Screening is done for inborn errors of metabolism as age appropriate as inborn errors of metabolism alter fat and glucose metabolism and normal growth. Screening is done for enzyme deficiencies, especially in steroid metabolism through measures of pathway intermediates. Hormone levels are sent to evaluate glands responsiveness to hormones and the target cell or organ. Glycosylated hemoglobin is measured to assess blood glucose control. Vasopressin levels can determine the type of DI.

b. *Urine* is tested for electrolytes, fractional excretion of sodium (FENa), specific gravity, osmolality, glucose, ketones, and pH.

c. Dynamic tests of endocrine function

i. The *water-deprivation test* is used to differentiate causes of polyuria and is described in detail later within the section "Diabetes Insipidus."

ii. An *oral glucose tolerance test* is used to assess for abnormalities in glucose tolerance, to assist in diagnosis of impaired glucose tolerance or diabetes. Following an overnight fast, oral glucose load is administered, and serial blood glucose and determinations are made. A glucose level of 140 mg/dL or less at 2 hours postadministration of glucose is considered normal.

iii. An *insulin tolerance test* is used to assess the hypothalamic–pituitary–adrenal axis and GH response. Following an overnight fast, regular insulin is administered via IV to produce hypoglycemia. Serial blood sampling is performed to determine cortisol, blood glucose, and GH levels. This test requires continuous patient monitoring.

iv. *TRH stimulation* is used to assess TSH reserve and prolactin reserve and secretion. TRH is administered via IV, and serial blood determinations of T_3, T_4, and TSH are obtained to diagnose thyroid dysfunction. This test is not commonly used at the present time.

v. An *ACTH stimulation test* is used to assess the hypothalamic–pituitary–adrenal axis. After obtaining a baseline cortisol level, an IV dose of cortrosyn (synthetic ACTH) is administered and samples are collected for serial timed cortisol levels to diagnose AI. A rise of 9 mcg/dL above baseline level or a cortisol level greater than 18 mcg/dL at 60 minutes demonstrates normal function.

vi. *GH stimulation* is used to diagnose GHD. Various physiologic and pharmacologic stimuli are administered to stimulate the release of GH. A level of 10 ng/mL or more is considered evidence of sufficient GH production.

2. *Pitfalls in the Interpretation of Endocrine Function Tests.* Many hormones are secreted according to specific triggers, diurnal rhythm, oscillating pulses, or following an inciting event. Plasma hormone levels are dependent on the time and circumstances of measurement. A single measurement may not accurately reflect the actual levels of many hormones. In addition, the hormone levels that are labeled "normal" may be appropriate for the healthy person or for an adult but not necessarily for a child in a certain state of critical illness, age, or pubertal level. Other factors that may interfere with endocrine tests include drug therapy, nutritional status, stress, and pathology.

3. *Radiologic Tests*

a. Chest radiographs are used to evaluate for pleural effusions, chest masses, or cardiomegaly.

b. CT scan of the head and neck determines the presence of cerebral edema (CE), tumors, or midline defects. CT scan of the abdomen is used to determine the presence of pancreatic, adrenal, or renal tumors.

c. MRI of the head is used to determine the presence of tumors.

d. Ultrasound of the neck and abdomen is used to determine renal and pancreatic function, to evaluate for thyroid, adrenal, and pancreatic tumors and to determine function.

e. Bone age evaluates growth patterns.

4. An ECG is used to evaluate myocardial function and the presence of dysrhythmias.

CRITICAL ILLNESS-RELATED CORTICOSTEROID INSUFFICIENCY

CIRCI is a relatively new diagnosis in adult critical care and its presence is quickly gaining ground in pediatric critical care literature. At this time, pediatric research is ongoing, but guidelines for adult management for CIRCI (made by the International Task Force of Acute Care) were released in 2008 (Marik et al., 2008). Pediatric research is directed at obtaining rapid and accurate diagnosis and the best treatment algorithm. This section presents the latest literature available and possible pathways for diagnosis and treatment.

A. Pathophysiology

CIRCI occurs when inadequate corticosteroid activity is seen relative to the severity of a patient's illness (Levy-Shraga & Pinhas-Hamiel, 2013). This weak response occurs when there is a decrease in adrenal steroid production due to dysfunction in the HPA axis or when tissue resistance to glucocorticoids exists. The most supported theory for this development is that critical illness causes peptide signals in the body to release *proinflammatory cytokines* (IL-1, IL-2, IL-6, TNF-alpha, interferon gamma; Kwon et al., 2010; von Saint Andre-von Arnim et al., 2013). The cytokines elicit the release of CRH from the hypothalamus stimulating the anterior pituitary to release ACTH, which causes the adrenal gland to produce cortisol (von Saint Andre-von Arnim et al., 2013). Concurrently, the body has a sympathetic response initiated in the brainstem (locus cerulus), which stimulates the release of norepinephrine and epinephrine (Clark et al., 2008). Cortisol levels become depleted due to overwhelming stress and 4 to 7 days into the illness insufficient levels are present (Kwon et al., 2010). Other factors that trigger the development of CIRCI include diminished receptors or receptor sensitivity, low free (unbound) cortisol, low CBG, and hypoalbuminemia as cortisol is bound to albumin (Clark et al., 2008).

B. Etiology and Risk Factors

1. Although a state of homeostasis exists, cortisol production has diurnal variation with a highest level in the early morning, with total cortisol level of 5 to 10 mcg/dL. During times of stress that level rises to 25 to 60 mcg/dL (over 6 months in age) and the body loses its ability for diurnal variation (von Saint Andre-von Arnim et al., 2013). Controversy exists in the literature as some research supports the idea that exogenous steroid administration blunts the protective, natural inflammatory response of the immune system in critical illness, and worse outcomes may be seen with its use (von Saint Andre-von Arnim et al., 2013).

2. *Conditions Associated With CIRCI*

a. Sepsis. Overwhelms the immune system, hypoalbuminemia results

b. Burns. Massive fluid shifts, hypoalbunemia, and hypotension occur

c. Surgery. Stress response

d. Trauma. Traumatic brain injury, multiple organ injury, and hemorrhage

e. Hypoglycemia. High substrate needs exist during times of stress

f. Adrenal insufficiency at baseline. Panhypopituitary, steroid dependence, HPA axis disruption

g. Etomidate. Inhibits steroidogenesis

C. Signs and Symptoms

Signs of CIRCI are vague and can be difficult to diagnose. Some presenting symptoms include abdominal pain, mental status changes, hyponatremia, hypoglycemia, hyperkalemia, neutropenia, fever, and eosinophilia (Levy-Shraga & Pinhas-Hamiel, 2013). Symptoms can be found when sepsis is present or following a traumatic event or surgery. Critically ill children will have hypotension that is unresponsive to fluid and may need multiple vasopressor support (Chameides et al., 2011). There could be hypoglycemia or hyperglycemia. Children will have altered mental status due to an overwhelming illness state and may require intubation for airway protection. Tachycardia or bradycardia may be present with some evidence of cardiac insufficiency (diminished left ventricular function). Children with chronic illness often have inadequate adrenal reserves and during times of stress and sepsis have organ dysfunction sooner (von Saint Andre-von Arnim et al., 2013). Some evidence supports that a baseline level of free cortisol less than 2 mcg/dL and total cortisol of less than 10 mcg/dL may reflect CIRCI (Levy-Shraga & Pinhas-Hamiel, 2013; von Saint Andre-von Arnim et al., 2013).

D. Lab Data

1. *Low Free Cortisol Levels.* Cortisol is depleted under state of persistent stress.

2. *Cytokine Levels (IL-1, 2, and 6, TNF-alpha).* May be elevated.

3. *Random Cortisol Levels.* May be altered in critical illness.

4. *ACTH Levels Increase.* Correlates with high severity of illness scores.

5. *Hyperglycemia or Hypoglycemia.* Low at presentation, elevates with steroid dosing.

6. *Hyponatremia or Hyperkalemia.* May be present due to mineralcorticoid deficiency.

7. *Hypoalbuminemia.* Exists in the face of critical illness.

E. Interpretation of Diagnostic Studies

A great deal of debate exists in the literature on which diagnostic and laboratory studies are the most useful in diagnosing the presence of cortisol deficiency and resistance in critical illness. Random cortisol levels or early-morning levels have been used with great frequency as well as corticotrophin stimulation tests (von Saint Andre-von Arnim et al., 2013). More recent evidence has shown that routine testing may not be necessary and when clinical triggers are reached, hydrocortisone should be initiated. It has also been shown that routine testing has proven to be uninformative and may not identify the more critically ill patients (von Saint Andre-von Arnim et al., 2013).

1. *Random cortisol levels* lack prospective data and support on use in defining adrenal insufficiency but Pediatric Advanced Life Support (PALS) recommends giving hydrocortisone if the random level is less than 18 mcg/dL (Chameides et al., 2011). Many observational studies looking at total cortisol and critically ill children found that as illness worsens IL-6, TNF-alpha, and ACTH levels increase and total cortisol levels drop (von Saint Andre-von Arnim et al., 2013).

2. *Corticotrophin-stimulation tests* begin with a random cortisol level followed by obtaining two more levels, 30 and 60 minutes after administering a dose of corticotrophin 250 mcg IV. An adequate response would be a rise of serum cortisol greater than 18 to 20 mcg/dL (Levy-Shraga & Pinhas-Hamiel, 2013). In the adult literature, baseline cortisol levels greater than 34 mcg/dL and a response of less than 9 mcg/dL from a stimulation test were associated with higher mortality.

3. *Salivary cortisol* can be obtained from the oral cavity and tested by liquid chromatography/tandem mass spectrometry. This level has been shown in the literature to correlate well with serum free cortisol (Gunnala et al., 2015). Rapid bedside testing in real time remains a challenge and unavailable at many institutions.

F. Diagnoses

1. Differential diagnoses may include Addison's disease, CAH, Waterhouse–Friderichsen syndrome, adrenal hemorrhage or thrombosis, chronic steroid usage, systemic inflammatory response associated with sepsis, and medication use (etomidate and ketoconazole; von Saint Andre-von Arnim et al., 2013). Less common causes of adrenal insufficiency can include cellular level depression of receptor sites or alteration in function of signaling peptides.

2. *Collaborative Diagnoses and Comorbidities*

   a. Potential for immunologic compromise related to steroid use

   b. Potential for impaired wound healing and hyperglycemia with steroid use

   c. Potential for cardiovascular collapse secondary to hypotension

   d. Potential for long-term sequelae from overwhelming stress and shock state

G. Treatment Goals

1. Replenish intravascular volume

2. Normalize cardiovascular parameters

3. Prevent periods of hypotension that can lead to end-organ damage

4. Normalize blood glucose levels

5. Initiate antibiotics timely in sepsis

6. Treat the underlying disease state

H. Management

When CIRCI has been established in a patient, corticosteroid supplementation should be implemented with hydrocortisone 2 mg/kg bolus dose with maximum dosing of 100 mg (Chameides et al., 2011). No clear evidence has been identified for duration and dosing of continued therapy, but many authors have used 50 to 100 mg/m²/d divided every 4 to 6 hours. More trials are needed in pediatrics to elucidate information on this subject. With steroids, most providers consider the lowest dose for the shortest duration possible to be the most prudent and weaning should be initiated when vasopressor support is no longer warranted (Davis et al., 2017; von Saint Andre-von Arnim et al., 2013). Caution should be made to taper steroids used for longer than 5 days or from large doses. Studies completed on children with CIRCI showed a reduction of vasopressor use within 4 hours of steroid dosing (Levy-Shraga & Pinhas-Hamiel, 2013). Studies have also shown that concomitant administration of fludrocortisone (Florinef), a mineralcorticoid agent, was associated with shorter duration of norepinephrine support (Levy-Shraga & Pinhas-Hamiel, 2013).

I. Complications

There are many adverse effects that should be considered when administering corticosteroids. Steroids place the body into a catabolic state with resultant hyperglycemia. Research indicates that prolonged hyperglycemia results in poor survival in critically ill children (Hazinski, Mondozzi, & Uridales Baker, 2014). This catabolism results in immunodeficiency, which may lead to poor wound healing and can raise the risks of hospital-acquired infections (von Saint Andre-von Arnim et al., 2013). When steroids are administered with neuromuscular blockade, children have an increased risk of myopathy. Infants who receive steroids can have lasting effects on neurodevelopment outcomes and somatic growth (von Saint Andre-von Arnim et al., 2013).

DIABETES MELLITUS

A. Definitions

DM is a constellation of diseases characterized by an absolute or relative insulin deficiency that causes fasting and postprandial hyperglycemia along with disturbances in the metabolism of protein and fat. Lack of insulin or insulin responsiveness leads to clinical consequences due to alterations in carbohydrate, fat, and protein metabolism (Brashers et al., 2014; Sperling, Tamborlane, Battelino, Weinzimer, & Phillip, 2014).

1. *Type 1a. Autoimmune-mediated disease* is the attributable cause of more than 90% of cases of childhood diabetes. This type results in the T-cell-mediated destruction of the beta cells triggered by either environmental or genetic factors (Brashers et al., 2014). The process may be slow, as some children maintain a limited ability to secrete insulin for a few years after diagnosis. Clinical symptoms manifest when beta cells secretion is 20% or less, causing hyperglycemia

to develop (Sperling et al., 2014). This process occurs in genetically susceptible children in response to an environmental agent (likely viral) that triggers an autoimmune response. This type of diabetes in infants and children requires insulin replacement therapy and is associated with the development of ketoacidosis (Brashers et al., 2014; Sperling et al., 2014).

2. *Type 1b. Idiopathic disease* is less common and is often more fulminant than autoimmune disease. It usually develops in people of Asian or African descent and can be a result of other diseases such as pancreatitis (Brashers et al., 2014). Insulin replacement therapy is needed with the inconsistent insulin deficiency seen with this disease. In 17% to 30% of type 1b patients, autoimmune thyroid disease is also present and in an additional 25% of those children thyroid antibodies are present (American Diabetes Association, 2016).

3. *Type 2. Typical or atypical type 2 DM (T2DM)* constitutes approximately 10% of the DM population in children. Previously referred to as *adult-onset diabetes* or *noninsulin-dependent diabetes*, this disease is associated with obesity, a strong family history of DM, and older age. In the pediatric population, the numbers are rising due to the epidemic of obesity in children and in those with Native American descent (Brashers et al., 2014). This disease occurs as a result of insulin resistance and has an insidious onset. It could be treated with oral agents, diet modification, and exercise.

4. *Maturity-Onset Diabetes of Youth (MODY)*. MODY accounts, for only 1% to 2% of diagnosed cases of diabetes, but should be considered in children with strong family history (two generations) of diabetes, and in children who do not have the phenotype of classic T2DM such as obesity or acanthosis nigricans. Six specific types of autosomal dominant mutations can occur and evaluation should be made at the onset of diabetes symptoms (Brashers et al., 2014). MODY 2 and 3 are the most prevalent, and MODY 1 and 3 are likely to require insulin therapy. In each of the six types (except for MODY 2), there are secondary mutations in the factors required for beta-cell differentiation and the expression of insulin genes (Babler et al., 2013).

B. Diabetic Ketoacidosis

1. *Definition. Diabetic ketoacidosis (DKA)* is an emergency condition that, if left untreated, can have life-threatening consequences. DKA occurs as a result of relative or absolute insulin deficiency and is diagnosed when blood glucose is greater than 200 mg/dL, venous pH is less than 7.3, or bicarbonate is less than 15 mmol/L, and ketonemia/ketonuria are present (von Saint Andre-von Armin et al., 2013). DKA remains the leading cause of morbidity and mortality in children with type 1 diabetes and is the leading cause of hospital admissions. DKA events most often occur when there is nonadherence to insulin regimen or intercurrent illness, stress, or surgery (Brashers et al., 2014).

2. *Pathophysiology*

   a. When the balance of insulin and counter-regulatory hormones are disrupted in the body, DKA occurs. In the absence of insulin, hyperglycemia occurs as tissue uptake of glucose is inhibited and glucose production by the liver is increased. Glycogenolysis (breakdown of glycogen), gluconeogenesis (synthesis of glucose from noncarbohydrate sources), proteolysis, and lipolysis contribute to the metabolic changes in DKA (Brashers et al., 2014; Sperling et al., 2014). Insulin deficiency leads to lipolysis and overproduction of ketone bodies such as beta-hydroxybutyrate and acetoacetates. Bicarbonate buffering does not happen and there is a resultant metabolic acidosis. Counterregulatory hormones (glucagon, cortisol, catecholamines, and GH) are released in times of stress, and they also contribute to hyperglycemia. Glycosuria occurs with osmotic diuresis once the renal threshold for glucose is exceeded (usually around 180 mg/dL; von Saint Andre-von Arnim et al., 2013). Passive electrolyte losses (magnesium, phosphorus, sodium) occur secondary to diuresis, but most concerning is the total body loss of potassium, which can reach up to 3 to 5 mEq/kg (Brashers et al., 2014). Hyperosmolality results secondary to hyperglycemia and free water loss with diuresis. Dehydration occurs secondary to osmotic diuresis and vomiting (Brashers et al., 2014; Sperling et al., 2014). There is a total body fluid shift from the intracellular space to the extracellular space to help compensate for the dehydration. Nausea and vomiting occur secondary to ketoacidosis and this worsens the electrolyte imbalances. Serum osmolarity can become very high, putting patients at risk for the development of CE and stroke.

3. Etiology is related to inadequate endogenous insulin secretion or inadvertent omission of insulin.

Initial presentation is often precipitated by nonadherence to insulin, stress, emotional or psychological problems, infection, surgery, or trauma (Sperling et al., 2014). Often, adolescents do not comply with their treatment plan and are repeatedly admitted in DKA due to familial or personal stress and inability to cope with their chronic illness.

4. Risk factors include a previous history of diabetes with poor control or compliance, young or adolescent age, ethnic minority, lack of health coverage, delayed treatment, lower body mass index, and infection (Brashers et al., 2014).

5. Signs and symptoms (Table 6.3) include polyuria, polydipsia, polyphagia, and hyperglycemia, generally with a serum glucose level greater than 200 mg/dL, and presence of ketones in urine. Other symptoms include weight loss, weakness and lethargy, nausea and vomiting, abdominal pain, dehydration, tachycardia, hypovolemia, poor perfusion, shock, glycosuria, ketonuria, rapid deep respirations (Kussmaul's respirations), and stupor that can lead to coma. However, DKA can occur with normoglycemia or hypoglycemia if severe vomiting is present. Also, indicative of DKA is the presence of acidosis demonstrated by a pH less than 7.30, and serum bicarbonate less than 15 mmol/L (Klein, Sathasivam, Novoa, & Rapaport, 2011). Serum sodium levels may be high, low, or normal with total body sodium depletion secondary to urinary losses or dilutional hyponatremia (fluid shifts from intracellular space to extracellular space) secondary to hyperglycemia. Serum potassium may be high, low, or normal with total body potassium depletion. In acidosis with increased osmolality, potassium shifts from intracellular space to extr cellular space creating more available potassium for use by the body. Insulin and acidosis correction shifts potassium back into the intracellular space and levels may fall. Elevated serum triglycerides are present. The white blood cell (WBC) count is elevated with a shift to the left (Sperling et al., 2014).

6. Classification of the presentation of DKA is based on the degree of acidosis (Klein et al., 2011)

   a. *Mild.* Venous pH less than 7.30 and bicarbonate less than 15 mmol/L

   b. *Moderate.* Venous pH less than 7.20 and bicarbonate less than 10 mmol/L

   c. *Severe.* pH less than 7.10 and bicarbonate less than 5 mmol/L

TABLE 6.3 Signs and Symptoms of Diabetic Ketoacidosis

Symptoms	Underlying Mechanisms
Hyperglycemia	Relative or absolute insulin deficiency
Metabolic acidosis (gap acidosis)	Build up of B-hydroxybutyrate, acetoacetic acids, and acetone in the serum from incomplete oxidization of fatty acids
Dehydration, shock	Osmotic diuresis secondary to hyperglycemia, vomiting
Kussmaul breathing	Deep, rapid breathing; a compensatory mechanism to blow off carbon dioxide and normalize pH
Cardiac arrhythmia	Hypokalemia, hyperkalemia
Sodium imbalance	Total body sodium depleted secondary to sodium loss from osmotic diuresis
	Dilutional hyponatremia secondary to hyperglycemia, fluid drawn into extracellular space, decreases sodium content
Potassium imbalance	Acidosis causes potassium to shift from the intracellular space into extracellular space
	Insulin and acidosis correction returns potassium to intracellular space
	Total body potassium depletion secondary to losses from osmotic diuresis
Mental status changes	Cerebral edema, level of acidosis, degree of dehydration
Hyperosmolality	Hyperglycemia, osmotic diuresis
Ketonuria	Lipolysis causes elevated ketone levels to rise above the renal threshold and spill into the urine
Glucosuria	Glucose spills into the urine when blood glucose exceeds renal threshold

7. *Interpretation of Diagnostic Studies*

a. *Hyperglycemia* is due to insulin deficiency, decreased glucose uptake, gluconeogenesis, and an increase in the counterregulatory hormones.

b. *Glycosuria* occurs secondary to hyperglycemia.

c. *pH* level less than 7.30 and bicarbonate less than 15 mmol/L are due to acetoacetic acid and beta-hydroxybutyrate dehydrogenase (ketones) production. Acidosis could also be due to poor perfusion and accumulation of lactic acid (lactic acidosis).

d. *Ketonuria* is the presence of ketones in the urine. *Ketonemia* is the presence of high serum ketone levels.

e. *Serum osmolality* is greater than 300 mOsm/kg because of hyperglycemia and osmotic diuresis, which leads to *dehydration*.

f. *Electrolyte disturbances* are related to electrolyte loss with osmotic diuresis, shifts between extracellular and intracellular spaces, and metabolic acidosis.

g. *Islet cell antibodies and insulin autoantibodies* are not diagnostic for DKA but may offer a screening tool for detecting patients with autoimmunity.

h. *A glucose tolerance test* has no role in the diagnosis of DKA but can be used to diagnose glucose intolerance in a child with glucosuria and normal or mildly elevated serum glucose.

i. *Glycosylated hemoglobin* (HbA_1) reflects blood glucose control over the last 120 days, or the life of red blood cells. Elevated levels are correlated with high serum glucose concentrations and a level of greater than or equal to 6.5% is diagnostic for diabetes (Babler et al., 2013).

j. *CT scan* is used to diagnose CE, an uncommon but ominous manifestation of DKA that clinically occurs in only about 1% of all cases (von Saint Andre-von Arnim et al., 2013).

8. *Diagnoses*

a. *Differential diagnoses* at presentation include adrenocortical dysfunction, high-dose steroid usage, uremia or lactic acidosis, gastroenteritis with metabolic acidosis, pancreatitis, cystic fibrosis, exogenous catecholamines, stress response (CIRCI), DI, encephalitis, alcoholic ketoacidosis, starvation, hyperosmolar syndrome, and inborn errors of metabolism.

b. *Collaborative diagnoses and comorbidities*

i. Fluid-volume deficit related to osmotic diuresis secondary to hyperglycemia

ii. Low cardiac output related to fluid-volume deficit

iii. Potential for CE related to treatment and hyperosmolar state

iv. Potential for arrhythmias related to electrolyte imbalances

v. Acid–base imbalance related to ketoacidosis

vi. Electrolyte imbalances related to both osmotic diuresis and treatment

vii. Potential for hypoglycemia related to treatment

viii. Potential for self-care deficits related to lifelong treatment and monitoring with possible noncompliance

ix. Alteration in body image related to chronic illness and future complications

x. Alteration in healing related to chronic hyperglycemia

xi. Potential for infection related to inflammatory response from chronic hyperglycemia

xii. Knowledge deficit regarding home management

xiii. Potential for depression related to chronic disease state

9. *Treatment Goals*

a. Correct fluid and electrolyte imbalances slowly

b. Correct metabolic acidosis

c. Infuse insulin to treat hyperglycemia and ketosis

d. Prevent neurologic complications

e. Maintain good glycemic control (long term)

f. Treat underlying disorders

g. Educate and prevent recurrence

10. *Management*

a. *Fluid.* Cautious rehydration in DKA is imperative to prevent CE. For accurate rehydration, knowledge of preillness weight must be known. To calculate the percentage of dehydration present, subtract illness weight from preillness weight and divide this number by preillness weight then multiply by 100% (Taketomo, Hodding, & Kraus, 2015). In most cases, the preillness weight is unknown, and fluid management is based upon estimation of mild, moderate, or severe dehydration. Hyperosmolality is present and in order to prevent CE, replacement should be done over 48 hours. Moderate DKA has an estimated dehydration of 7% to 10% and severe DKA has more than 10% dehydration. In most cases, dehydration is estimated to be 10% in all patients with DKA (von Saint Andre-von Arnim et al., 2013). When shock is present, it is necessary to administer normal saline (NS) 10 mL/kg for volume expansion. Frequent reassessment is necessary and additional boluses may be required if poor perfusion persists. NS is an isotonic fluid but because children in DKA are hyperosmolar, NS is a hypotonic fluid.

b. *Electrolytes.* Potassium and phosphate replacement is imperative in DKA. If hyperkalemia is present initially, an ECG should be performed and it is necessary to wait until urine output is achieved before potassium replacement is initiated. If a normal potassium level is present, initiate replacement with a combination of potassium chloride and potassium phosphate as insulin will drive potassium and phosphate back into the cell, thus decreasing serum levels of potassium and phosphorous (Sperling et al., 2014). Attention should be paid to calcium levels during treatment as rising phosphorus levels will cause hypocalcemia. A hyperchloremic metabolic acidosis can occur during treatment with high chloride-containing fluids, and can be offset with the addition of potassium phosphate (K Phos) to fluid bags. Sodium bicarbonate administration is not routinely recommended and it should never be administered as a bolus as it can precipitate cardiac arrhythmias (Sperling et al., 2014; von Saint Andre-von Arnim et al., 2013).

c. *Insulin.* Rehydration will cause serum glucose to decrease and improve perfusion and acidosis, but an insulin infusion will always be required in DKA. Insulin is needed to normalize serum glucose levels, to suppress ketogenesis and lipolysis, and to resolve ketoacidosis (Sperling et al., 2014). Insulin infusion should begin within an hour of initial fluid replacement at 0.1 units per kilogram of body weight per hour, and should continue until there is a resolution of DKA or a closure in the anion gap. Blood glucose should drop at a rate of 80 to 100 mg/dL per hour, and will occur faster than the resolution of acidosis (Sperling et al., 2014). When the blood glucose falls to near 300 mg/dL with continued acidosis, the addition of 5% or 10% dextrose fluid should be administered via IV and titrated based on hourly glucose parameters to keep blood glucose near 200 mg/dL (von Saint von-Andre Ornim et al., 2013). Insulin dosing may be decreased to 0.05 units/kg/hr if the blood glucose continues to fall despite the addition of 10% dextrose to the IV fluids and acidosis persists. IV insulin should continue until the pH is greater than 7.3, bicarbonate is greater than 15 mmol/L, and the child is tolerating oral intake (von Saint von-Andre Arnim et al., 2013). When transitioning to subcutaneous insulin, give subcutaneous insulin 30 to 60 minutes before discontinuing the continuous infusion.

d. The goal of insulin replacement therapy is to match the normal pattern of secretion by the body as closely as possible through basal dose therapy and to avoid wide shifts in glucose. It is done with a basal/bolus insulin regimen either through insulin pump or through multiple daily subcutaneous injections. There are more than 10 varieties of insulin formularies, which are most often categorized on the duration of action. There are rapid-acting insulins that have high and sharp peaks of effects with a short duration of therapy. The intermediate-acting insulin, neutral protamine Hagedorn (NPH), which has delayed peaks of action, was previously used in new-onset type 1 diabetes to help cover hyperglycemia (Sperling et al., 2014). Long-acting insulin medications were developed to meet the demands for basal insulin needs, and they help patients and families better manage their diabetes (Sperling et al., 2014). During the initial diagnosis time of type 1 diabetes, there is a honeymoon period that can last several months during which there is residual beta-cell function with minimal insulin requirements to maintain euglycemia and prevent ketoacidosis (Sperling et al., 2014).

e. *Monitoring.* Vital signs, blood pressure, intake and output, cardiovascular assessment with continuous ECG monitoring, and neurologic checks are done hourly. Hourly glucometer determination of blood glucose is done at the bedside. Initial laboratory tests should include complete blood count (CBC), chemistry panel, urinalysis, beta-hydroxybutyrate, hemoglobin A1-C, and a blood gas. Electrolytes, beta-hydroxybutyrate, and pH are monitored every 2 to 4 hours until stable, then every 4 to 6 hours until acidosis is resolved. A gradual rise in serum sodium as the glucose levels fall helps prevent rapid changes in serum osmolality and may prevent alteration in mental state. Intake and output, weights, and urine ketones are monitored daily.

11. *Complications*

   a. *Acute*

   i. Hypoglycemia can occur during the treatment of DKA and should be treated with dextrose-containing fluids as described earlier. Persistent acidosis can be related to inadequate fluid replacement, inadequate insulin dosing, insulin resistance, ineffective method of delivery, or a malfunctioning insulin delivery system.

   ii. Hypokalemia can occur because of inadequate potassium replacement and rapid fluid shifts.

   iii. CE occurs in about 1% of episodes of DKA, but continues to have significant mortality and morbidity. It can be apparent on presentation, 4 to 12 hours after treatment has been initiated, or even up to 22 to 48 hours into treatment (von Saint Andre-von Arnim et al., 2013). Mounting evidence supports that many patients in DKA have subclinical CE visible only on CT scans. Symptoms include severe headache, altered mental status, hypertension, bradycardia, and vomiting (Sperling et al., 2014). Risk factors for CE (Table 6.4) include first presentation, high serum BUN and CO_2 (reflective of the degree of dehydration and acidosis), administration of insulin bolus doses, bicarbonate treatment, rapid glucose correction, aggressive fluid administration, and younger age at diagnosis. Treatment at recognition of CE should begin with administration of hypertonic saline or mannitol, elevate the head of the bed, and performing an emergent CT scan of the brain to evaluate CE (Klein et al., 2011). Fluid administration should

TABLE 6.4   Risk Factors in DKA for Cerebral Edema

First presentation
Younger age at diagnosis
Increased BUN
Decreased CO_2
Insulin bolus dosing
Precipitous drops in blood glucose
Aggressive fluid administration
Administration of sodium bicarbonate

BUN, blood urea nitrogen; DKA, diabetic ketoacidosis.

Source: Adapted from Klein, M., Sathasivam, A., Novoa, Y., & Rapaport, R. (2011). Recent consensus statements in pediatric endocrinology: A selective review. *Pediatrics Clinic of North America*, *58*, 1301–1315. doi:10.1016/j.pcl.2011.07.014

be lowered and support of respiratory and neurologic status may become necessary with intubation for Glasgow Coma Scale less than 9.

  iv. Fluid overload and congestive heart failure can occur as a result of aggressive fluid management during treatment.

  v. Aspiration is possible if the level of consciousness is depressed.

  b. *Chronic*

  i. Chronic complications of repeated episodes of DKA can have life-altering ramifications for children with diabetes. Hyperglycemia with poor metabolic control can lead to a chronic state of proinflammation, which leads to further insulin resistance. This state leads to harmful release of cytokines and impairment of the coagulation pathways (V. Srinivasan & Agus, 2014). The Diabetes Control and Complications Trial study revealed that intense glycemic control (which led to nearly normal glucose levels) significantly lowered the risk of serious long-term consequences of diabetes and had low risks of hypoglycemia (Sperling et al., 2014). Other significant chronic problems include repeat episodes of hypoglycemia and hyperglycemia, poor growth, hypertrophy and lipoatrophy of injection sites, limited joint mobility, candidiasis (opportunistic infections), retinopathy, nephropathy, neuropathy (rare in childhood), and macrovascular disease (Sperling et al., 2014).

HYPERGLYCEMIC HYPEROSMOLAR SYNDROME

A. Pathophysiology

The incidence of hyperglycemic hyperosmolar syndrome (HHS) continues to be infrequent in children, but the numbers are increasing. These escalating numbers are associated with a high mortality rate and delayed diagnosis. In HHS, insulin secretion is adequate enough to prevent lipolysis, but not substantial enough to prevent hyperglycemia, thereby producing a state of relative insulin deficiency. The stress response, which includes the release of glucagon, catecholamines, cortisol, and GH, worsen hyperglycemia by increasing gluconeogenesis and glyconeolysis (Zeitler, Haqq, Rosenbloom, & Glaser, 2011). Marked hyperosmolality with significant dehydration and electrolyte losses subsequently occurs. The degree of hyperglycemia, hyperosmolality, and dehydration is much greater in HHS than in DKA and can cause significant sequelae. The absence of ketoacidosis and typical associated physical symptoms seen in DKA may reflect the delay in treatment. This delay can lead to profound shock, kidney dysfunction, altered mental status or coma, rhabdomyolysis, hyperthermia, and ventricular arrhythmias (Price, Losek, & Jackson, 2016; Zeitler et al., 2011).

B. Precipitating Factors

In adults, the most common coexisting condition associated with HHS is type 2 diabetes. In the pediatric population, rising numbers of children with type 2 diabetes may explain the increasing numbers of HHS being seen. Recent literature reveals that children who are affected are often previously healthy, obese African American males with undiagnosed or uncontrolled type 2 diabetes. In infants, HHS is seen in those affected by transient neonatal DM (Wolfsdorf et al., 2014). It is also seen in children with preexisting cardiovascular or renal disease, infections, trauma, burns, pancreatitis, thyrotoxicosis, pneumonia, heat stroke, dialysis, IV hyperalimentation, or children with poor glucose control. Use of medications, such as phenytoin, corticosteroids, beta-blockers, and thiazide diuretics, have been associated with increased risk of HHS (Price et al., 2016; Wolfsdorf et al., 2014; Zeitler et al., 2011).

C. Signs and Symptoms (Table 6.5)

Signs and symptoms can be vague initially and can include headache, abdominal pain, and mild signs of dehydration. Polyuria and polydipsia slowly worsen, and caregivers may fail to recognize them, resulting in delay in seeking care. Abnormal labs include serum

---

TABLE 6.5 Differentiation Between DKA and HHS

Signs and Symptoms	DKA	HHS
Nausea and vomiting	Present	Absent
Neurologic changes	Present	Present
Polyuria	Present	Present
Respiratory rate	Kussmaul respirations	Normal
Blood glucose	Usually >200 mg/dL	>600 mg/dL
Blood ketones	Elevated	Normal
Urine ketones	Present	Absent to mild
Blood HCO$_{3(-)}$	<18 mmol/L	>18 mmol/L
Arterial blood pH	<7.30	>7.30
Serum osmolality	>300 mOsm/kg	>330 mOsm/kg
Sodium deficits	4–11 mEq/kg	2–8 mEq/kg
Potassium deficits	1–10 mEq/kg	0.5–3 mEq/kg
Water deficits	50–100 mL/kg	60–170 mL/kg

DKA, diabetic ketoacidosis; HHS, hyperglycemic hyperosmolar syndrome.

glucose greater than 600 mg/dL, serum osmolality greater than 330 mOsm/kg, normal pH or mild metabolic acidosis, and serum bicarbonate of 18 to 24 mmol/L. Serum sodium levels may be high, low, or normal with total body sodium depletion secondary to urinary losses or dilutional hyponatremia secondary to hyperglycemia. Serum potassium levels may be high, low, or normal with total body depletion. Tachycardia, hypotension, low central venous pressure, shock, and glycosuria without ketonuria may occur. Lethargy, stupor, or coma also may occur. Neurologic impairment is significantly higher in children with HHS than in those with DKA due to hyperosmolality and its consequences. Mortality rate also increases with high osmolality levels (Price et al., 2016; Wolfsdorf et al., 2014; Zeitler et al., 2011).

D. Interpretation of Diagnostic Studies (Table 6.5)

1. Hyperglycemia is due to relative deficiency of insulin. Insulin levels are adequate to prevent ketosis.

2. Glycosuria is secondary to hyperglycemia.

3. Hyperosmolality is secondary to hyperglycemia and loss of free water with osmotic diuresis.

4. Mild metabolic acidosis is secondary to dehydration, low cardiac output, renal insufficiency, and lactic acidosis.

5. Electrolyte deficits are due to urinary losses.

E. Diagnoses

1. Differential diagnoses include sepsis, pancreatitis, renal insufficiency, and adrenocortical dysfunction.

2. *Collaborative Diagnoses and Comorbidities*

    a. Fluid-volume deficit related to osmotic diuresis

    b. Low cardiac output related to fluid-volume deficit

    c. Potential for arrhythmias related to electrolyte disturbances

    d. Acid–base imbalance related to low cardiac output and lactic acidosis

e. Electrolyte imbalances related to osmotic diuresis and treatment

f. Potential for CE and coma related to treatment

g. Potential for hypoglycemia related to treatment

h. Potential for renal failure related to rhabdomyolysis

i. Potential for cardiovascular collapse related to hyperkalemia and hypocalcemia

F. Treatment Goals

1. Correct fluid and electrolyte deficits

2. Correct hyperglycemia and hyperosmolality

3. Prevent neurologic complications

4. Educate about symptoms to prevent recurrence

G. Management

1. *Fluid and electrolyte therapy* involves volume resuscitation of poorly perfused, hypovolemic, or hypotensive patients with isotonic fluid via bolus. Choice of fluids would depend on the osmolality, because low osmolality fluids can lead to significant fluid shifts. Fluid-volume deficit can be calculated or assumed to be near 12% to 15% and should be replaced over 48 hours in addition to daily maintenance fluid. Due to the frequency of renal insufficiency with HHS, potassium is not added until renal function is known and urine output is adequate. Potassium levels decrease rapidly when insulin therapy is initiated secondary to potassium and glucose shifts intracellularly. Both of these imbalances will often correct adequately with fluid volume alone. Phosphorus levels are more severely affected in HHS. Potassium and phosphate replacement can be added to the IV fluids as an equal combination of KCl and KPO_4 at 40 mEq/L. Once serum glucose reaches 300 mg/dL, dextrose should be added to the IV fluids. If hypomagnesemia is present with hypocalcemia, it should be corrected with dosing of 25 to 50 mg/kg/dose every 4 to 6 hours with a maximum infusion rate of 150 mg/min. Bicarbonate therapy is contraindicated due to increased risk of hypokalemia and poor tissue oxygen uptake (Zeitler et al., 2011).

2. *Insulin Therapy.* Often, hyperglycemia is corrected with fluid therapy alone, but insulin may be needed in cases in which more severe ketosis and acidosis is present. Insulin therapy should be used if the drop in glucose is less than 50 mg/dL/hr with fluid therapy. Insulin should be used with caution in HHS and should never be given as a bolus dose. Low-dose insulin therapy at 0.025 to 0.05 units/kg/hr can be used to achieve a gradual decline in hyperglycemia and osmolality, with a goal of a drop of ≤100 mg/dL/hr (Zeitler et al., 2011).

3. *Monitoring.* Physical assessment of cardiovascular system, vital signs, blood pressure, and neurologic checks are done at minimum every 30 to 60 minutes, with continuous cardiac monitoring. Hourly determination of blood glucose is performed at the bedside. Initial laboratory studies include CBC, electrolytes, BUN, creatinine, glucose, and pH. Serum electrolytes, BUN, creatinine, osmolality, creatine kinase, and strict input/output (I/O) are monitored every 2 hours until they become stable. Every 3 to 4 hours, serum calcium, phosphorus, and magnesium should be checked. Daily weights are also monitored (Zeitler et al., 2011).

H. Complications

Complications include thromboembolic phenomenon, malignant hyperthermia, rhabdomyolysis, and infrequently CE or death. If DKA is coexistent, hypoglycemia and CE risks are greater (Zeitler et al., 2011). Neurologic deficits from hyperosmolality generally occur once levels greater than 330 mOsm/kg are reached but are unlikely to cause long-term morbidity. CE or death can occur as a result of rapid correction of the hyperosmolar state. Mortality is caused most frequently by severe dehydration, electrolyte disturbances, and hyperosmolality (Zeitler et al., 2011).

ACUTE HYPOGLYCEMIA

A. Pathophysiology

Hypoglycemia is defined as a serum glucose level less than 50 mg/dL in all ages. Recent consensus recommendations from the Pediatric Endocrine Society define *hypoglycemia* using *Whipple's triad* (Thornton et al., 2015). This triad includes the presence of signs and symptoms of hypoglycemia, low-plasma glucose, and resolution of the symptoms when the glucose level is raised (De León et al., 2014; Thornton et al., 2015). Glucose control in the body is balanced by dietary intake, tissue glucose uptake, and hepatic glucose production that is tightly regulated by insulin. When hypoglycemia occurs, counterregulatory hormones (glucagon, cortisol, catecholamines, and GH) are released. These hormones inhibit storage of glucose, the formation of glycogen, glycolysis, and lipogenesis. In addition, they stimulate glycogenolysis (stored glycogen transforms into glucose), activate lipolysis, increase gluconeogenesis, and ketogenesis to provide alternate energy sources (De León et al., 2014). Hypoglycemia inhibits release of insulin as the body shifts focus to supplying the brain with the limited glucose supply.

B. Etiology

1. Neonatal hypoglycemia can be transient (days to weeks) or persistent (beyond neonatal period) and is caused by immature fasting adaptation, lack of or depletion of glycogen stores, hyperinsulinemia (e.g., infants of diabetic mothers), or lack of exogenous supply. Transient cases are the most common, occurring in four per 1,000 infants and six per 1,000 premature infants (Goel & Choudhury, 2012). Transient cases often resolve within 24 to 48 hours after birth. This short-term hypoglycemia can be normal, but if it persists prompt evaluation and management must be completed to avoid long-term neurologic consequences. Infants who demonstrate persistent hypoglycemia may suffer from hypopituitarism, inborn errors of metabolism (fatty acid oxidation defects or glycogen storage diseases), congenital hyperinsulinism, or adrenocortical deficiency (Thornton et al., 2015). Persistent episodes of hypoglycemia pose significant long-term neurodevelopmental sequelae and occur in 25% to 50% of these infants (Thornton et al., 2015). Prompt recognition, intervention, and prevention are vital to avoid repeat hypoglycemic episodes and neurologic problems in these infants.

2. Childhood hypoglycemia can be caused by inborn errors of metabolism, GHD, cortisol deficiency, hepatic dysfunction, severe malnutrition, infection, or drugs. Congenital sources of hypoglycemia are unlikely after the age of 2.

3. *Hypoglycemia in Diabetes.* Hypoglycemia is one of the most acute problems that children with diabetes can encounter (Ly et al., 2014). These population of children are at particular risk due to use of medications such as exogenous insulin and oral glucose control medications (sulfonylureas). In these children, a blood glucose less than 65 mg/dL serves as a definition for hypoglycemia, while in clinical situations a blood glucose of less than 70 mg/dL is used as a guideline to treat as glucose can fall further (Ly et al., 2014). Unfortunately, repeated episodes of hypoglycemia can cause blunting of the body's response and many children will be asymptomatic until they are severely hypoglycemic. Severe hypoglycemic episodes in the diabetic child pose a significant risk to life.

C. Risk Factors

1. Infants of diabetic mothers (large for gestational age with macrosomia)

2. SGA infants or infants with intrauterine growth retardation

3. Stress or acute infectious illness

4. Children with insulin infusion pumps or children on other exogenous insulin support

5. Infants or children with compromised IV access and nothing-by-mouth (NPO) status

6. Increased metabolism or catabolic state

7. Poor nutrition or feeding habits

8. *Medications.* Beta-blockers (block the response or release of epinephrine), angiotensin-converting enzyme (ACE) inhibitors, sulfonylureas, salicylates, or alcohol ingestion

9. Liver disease or inborn errors of metabolism, including fatty acid oxidative disorders

10. Congenital hyperinsulinism

D. Signs and Symptoms

1. *Associated With Counterregulatory Hormone Stimulation.* Shakiness or trembling, tachycardia, sweating, anxiety, weakness, hunger, nausea, vomiting (Thornton et al., 2015)

2. Neurologic responses to severe hypoglycemia in *infants* can be more subtle and difficult to detect and are seen once infants reach a plasma glucose of 50 to 55 mg/dL (Thornton et al., 2015). Symptoms include a high-pitched cry, hypothermia, tremors, poor feeding, pallor, diaphoresis, seizures, abnormal eye movements, or apnea. Every infant with seizures as a presenting complaint should have his or her glucose checked promptly. Many infants will have no symptoms and with repeat episodes of hypoglycemia all children become less responsive to the effects (Babler et al., 2013).

3. Neurologic responses to severe hypoglycemia in *children* include lethargy, confusion, headache, weakness, anxiety, irritability with personality and visual changes, diaphoresis, twitches, or tremors that can lead to seizure or coma (Babler et al., 2013). Older children with intact cognitive function can verbalize their symptoms, are able to seek out sources of substrates, and correct hypoglycemia before it progresses to severe levels. Special care is needed in children with developmental delays who may be nonverbal or immobile.

E. Interpretation of Diagnostic Studies

1. Low blood glucose is a glucose level of less than 50 mg/dL. If glucose is measured by a glucometer, confirm the results with a serum laboratory sample. When low glucose is obtained, in new-onset hypoglycemia, send critical labs before correction is done to help differentiate causes of hypoglycemia (Figure 6.10; Babler et al., 2013). Critical labs include free fatty acids (FFAs), insulin, serum beta-hydroxybutyrate, cortisol, acylcarnitine profile, lactate, pyruvate, ammonia, GH, and urine ketones (Sarafoglou, Hoffmann, & Roth, 2017). Additional labs that are helpful in diagnosis of certain metabolic abnormalities are serum bicarbonate, plasma amino acids, carnitine levels, and C-peptide. Additional urine tests should be sent with the first void after the hypoglycemic event and can be a bagged sample. These urine tests include organic acids, reducing substances and toxicology screen (Sarafoglou et al., 2017).

2. Low plasma carnitine levels can indicate medium-chain acyl-CoA deficiency (rare).

3. Low plasma levels of GH indicate GH deficiency could have associated adrenal insufficiency.

4. Low cortisol levels may indicate adrenal insufficiency, and could be associated with GH deficiency.

5. Elevated blood insulin levels in the context of hypoglycemia indicate hyperinsulinemia.

6. Urine-reducing substances and hepatomegaly indicate fructose intolerance or galactosemia.

7. Urinary and serum ketones can differentiate between ketotic and nonketotic hypoglycemia. Urine ketones are negative in conditions of hyperinsulinism.

8. FFAs are lower in hyperinsulinism.

9. Metabolic acidosis, ketoacidosis, elevated lactate, and ammonia levels indicate organic acidemia.

10. Hepatomegaly and lactic acidosis suggests glycogen storage diseases or defects in gluconeogenesis.

11. Low GH and cortisol levels indicate hypopituitarism.

12. Abdominal CT scan is rarely used to determine the presence of a pancreatic tumor or other anomalies.

13. Abdominal ultrasound can identify location and presence of an insulinoma. Insulinoma can be confirmed in specialized centers with PET-CT.

F. Diagnoses

1. Differential diagnoses include hyperinsulinism, endocrine deficiencies, inborn errors of metabolism, sepsis, hepatic failure, pancreatic tumors, cardiovascular disease, and neurologic disease (meningitis, seizures).

2. *Collaborative Diagnoses and Comorbidities*
  a. Potential for seizures due to hypoglycemia
  b. Potential for neurologic compromise resulting from decreased amounts of substrate

G. Treatment Goals

1. Correct and maintain normal blood glucose.

2. Prevent further episodes of hypoglycemia.

3. Support metabolic requirements.

H. Management

1. Mild to moderate hypoglycemia can be safely managed in the home or school environment and should be a part of every child with diabetes or persistent hypoglycemia's emergency plan. Once a glucose level of less than 70 mg/dL is reached or a child is symptomatic, immediate oral ingestion of carbohydrates should raise glucose sufficiently, if

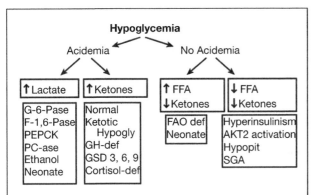

FIGURE 6.10 Hypoglycemia algorithm.

FAO, fatty acid oxidation; FFA, free fatty acids; GH, growth hormone; PEPCK, phosphoenolpyruvate carboxykinase, SGA, small for gestational age.

Source: From De León, D. D., Thornton, P. S., Stanley, C. A., & Sperling, M. A. (2014). Hypoglycemia in the newborn and infant. In Sperling, M. (Ed.), *Pediatric endocrinology* (4th ed., pp. 157–183). Philadelphia, PA: Elsevier.

there is no vomiting present. In *severe hypoglycemia* or if the child is unable to take anything by mouth, glucagon should be administered IM 0.5 mg for those under 12 years of age, 1 mg for ages greater than 12 years, or 10 to 30 mcg/kg (Ly et al., 2014). If the child becomes unconscious or has seizures, it becomes a medical emergency and intravenous or buccal glucose will be needed. Glucose concentration via a peripheral IV should never exceed 12.5% and ideally should be 10% in reliable access.

2. *IV Boluses.* Administer 10% or 25% glucose (0.5–1 g/kg over 1–3 minutes; Chameides et al., 2011).

[M] $0.5-1 g/kg = 5-10$ mL/kg of D_{10} or $2-4$ mL/kg of D_{25}

3. Administer a continuous infusion of 10% dextrose at 8 mg/kg/min with titration up by 25% to 50% for repeat episodes (Babler et al., 2013)

4. Identifiy and treat underlying cause

5. Maintain normothermia

6. Monitor glucose levels

7. In patients with DKA, add dextrose or decrease insulin infusion

8. Treat underlying metabolic disorders

I. Complications

Complications include coma, seizures, acute and long-term neurologic deficits, and death. Rapid administration or highly concentrated fluids may result in too great of an osmotic change and risk of CE exists (Ly et al., 2014). Care must also be taken to prevent the *Somogyi* *effect*, which occurs after hypoglycemia with a rebound hyperglycemia due to the release of counterregulatory hormones (Brashers et al., 2014).

SYNDROME OF INAPPROPRIATE ANTIDIURETIC HORMONE

A. Pathophysiology

SIADH is a common disorder in pediatric critical care and occurs when ADH release in not able to be suppressed. This excess of antidiuretic hormone will result in hyponatremia and impaired water excretion. When the body senses hypernatremia or a rising osmolality, ADH is released to cause water retention or volume expansion (von Saint Andre-von Arnim et al., 2013). In SIADH, excess ADH will act on the renal collecting ducts to become more permeable to water causing a dilutional hyponatremia and hypoosmolar state (Brashers et al., 2014). The urine will have a high osmolality when compared to the serum with urine sodium levels reaching greater than 20 mEq/L (von Saint Andre-von Arnim et al., 2013). Transient cases are common after pituitary surgery and can last for as long as 5 to 7 days after an inciting event (Table 6.6; Brashers et al., 2014).

B. Etiology and Risk Factors

1. *Conditions Associated With SIADH (Table 6.6)*

a. *Meningitis or central nervous system infections.* Guillain–Barré syndrome, encephalitis

b. *Head trauma or cerebral hemorrhage.* Subarachnoid or subdural hemorrhage

TABLE 6.6 Causes of Syndrome of Inappropriate Secretion of Antidiuretic Hormone (Vasopressin)

Central Nervous System	Cancer	Infections	Pulmonary
Head trauma	Small cell of lung	Herpes zoster	Viral pneumonia
Subarachnoid hemorrhage	Duodenum	Respiratory syncytial virus	Bacterial pneumonia
Brain abscess	Pancreas	Tuberculosis	Abscess
Guillain-Barré syndrome	Thymoma	Aspergillosis	
Hydrocephalus	Bladder	Botulism	
Meningitis	Ureter Lymphoma Ewing sarcoma		

Source: From Majzoub, J. A., Muglia, L. J., & Srivatsa, A. (2014). Disorders of the posterior pituitary. In M. Sperling (Ed.). *Pediatric endocrinology* (4th ed., pp. 405–443). Philadelphia, PA: Elsevier.

c. *Cerebral neoplasms.* For example, germ cell tumors, craniopharyngiomas, pituitary tumors, and hypothalamic gliomas

d. *Malignancy.* For example, lymphoma, sarcoma

e. *Pulmonary disease.* Tuberculosis, pneumonia, cystic fibrosis, or asthma

f. *Chronically ill or malnourished* children may develop chronic increased ADH secretion because of a downward resetting of the osmotic receptor; hyponatremia is chronic, and ADH secretion occurs at a lower serum osmolality

g. *Spinal surgery or neurosurgery.* Spinal fusions or ventriculoperitoneal shunts and brain tumors

2. Medications associated with SIADH include opiates, salicylates, antipsychotics, NSAIDs, vincristine, cyclophosphamide, carbamazepine, antidepressants (serotonin reuptake inhibitor, tricyclics), quinolone antibiotics, and barbiturates (von Saint Andre-von Arnim et al., 2013).

3. Other precipitating conditions include severe pain, temperature changes, nausea, cardiac failure, and positive pressure ventilation. Osmoreceptors, such as ANP, stimulate ADH release based on stimulus received from the hypothalamus (von Saint Andre-von Arnim et al., 2013).

C. Signs and Symptoms

1. The severity of clinical presentation depends on the degree and rapidity with which hyponatremia occurs (von Saint Andre-von Arnim et al., 2013). The body can adapt to a slow decrease in sodium level and can remain relatively asymptomatic. Once the sodium level falls less than 120 mEq/L, many children will develop seizures (von Saint Andre-von Arnim et al., 2013).

a. The first symptoms to develop are low urine output, anorexia and fatigue with euvolemia, or hypervolemia.

b. Nausea and vomiting can occur.

c. Headache, confusion, lethargy, altered level of consciousness, or seizures may develop.

d. Weight gain without peripheral edema may occur with elevated central venous pressure (CVP; 6–10 cm H_2O).

e. Hypertension, tachycardia, and coma are late signs.

D. Laboratory Data

1. *Serum osmolality* is less than 275 mOsm/kg. *Urine osmolality* is elevated inappropriately relative to serum osmolality at over 200 mOsm/kg.

TABLE 6.7   Clinical and Laboratory Findings in Diabetes Insipidus

Finding	Result
Serum sodium	>145 mEq/L
Urine output	>4 mL/kg/hr
Serum osmolality	>300 mOsmo/kg
Urine sodium	<30 mEq/L
Urine osmolality	<200 mOsmo/kg
Urine specific gravity	<1.005
Polydipsia	Present
Polyuria	Present
Altered mental status	Present

2. *Serum sodium* is less than 135 mEq/L. Continued renal excretion of sodium occurs with *urine sodium* greater than 20 mEq/L.

3. *Urine specific gravity* is greater than 1.020 in the absence of hypovolemia.

E. Interpretation of Diagnostic Studies (Brashers et al., 2014)

1. Hyponatremia and hypoosmolality occur secondary to water retention and hemodilution.

2. A relative increase in concentration of urine occurs with high specific gravity and increased osmolality because of ADH's effect on the renal tubules, resulting in increased water reabsorption by the kidney.

3. Patient should be clinically euvolemic. If hypovolemic, be concerned about cerebral salt wasting (CSW).

4. Renal, thyroid, and adrenal function tests are normal.

F. Diagnoses

1. Differential diagnoses include other processes that can cause hyponatremia and include pseudohyponatremia, congestive heart failure, water intoxication, glucocorticoid or mineralcorticoid deficiency, hypothyroidism, renal failure, nephrotic syndrome, heat exhaustion (increased sweating), GI-tract losses, laboratory error, and CSW.

2. *Collaborative Diagnoses and Comorbidities*

a. Fluid and volume excess and congestive heart failure related to excessive ADH secretion and water retention

b. Alteration in mental state related to underlying conditions (e.g., meningitis, brain tumors), rapid development of hyponatremia, or acute changes in serum osmolality

c. Potential for seizures related to hyponatremia

d. Potential for cerebral hemorrhage that results from too rapid correction of hypoosmolar state

G. Treatment Goals

1. Normalize serum sodium over 48 to 72 hours.

2. Normalize serum osmolality over 48 to 72 hours.

3. Decrease extravascular fluid volume.

4. Treat underlying disorder or stop medications contributing to effects.

5. Prevent neurologic sequelae.

6. Prevent reoccurrence with careful management.

H. Management

1. Fluid and sodium levels should be normalized slowly over 48 to 72 hours to prevent the development of *central pontine myelinolysis* (see complications). Treatment is based on the degree of hyponatremia and hypoosmolality but the mainstay of therapy includes fluid restriction. Fluid restriction is a combination of insensible fluid losses and urine output, which usually ends up near 750 to 1,000 L/m² per day (von Saint Andre-von Arnim et al., 2013). Sodium correction should be no faster than 0.5 mEq/L/hr, but if serious side effects are present 3% NaCl can be administered via IV push or at a rate of 1 to 2 mL/kg/hr to correct serum sodium to 125 mEq/L. To calculate *sodium correction*: sodium in mEq = [desired sodium (mEq/L) − patient's actual sodium (mEq/L)] × 0.6 × weight (in kilograms; Engorn & Flerlage, 2015). If hypervolemia remains, a loop diuretic may be judiciously used (von Saint Andre-von Arnim et al., 2013). Once serum sodium level is greater than 135 mmol/L, fluid restriction may be liberalized to a maintenance fluid rate.

2. *Location.* A newer medication emerging in the adult literature named *conivaptan*, a nonselective antagonist of the V1a and V2 vasopressor receptor subtypes, acts on the collecting duct to secrete water without electrolytes or "aquauresis" (Yee et al., 2010). This medication helps raise serum sodium levels when euvolemia or hypervolemia is present. The safety and effectiveness of this medication has not been studied in pediatrics.

3. Monitoring includes checking sodium level every 2 hours during the acute phase, and every 4 to 6 hours thereafter. Determine precise intake and output each hour, specific gravity with each void, serum electrolytes, and osmolality (every 4–6 hours until normal) with daily weights. Urine electrolytes and osmolality are obtained at initial diagnosis; however, frequent monitoring is not necessary. Central venous pressure is measured until the goal of a normal level of 6 to 10 cm H₂O is achieved. Heart rate, blood pressure, and neurologic status are closely monitored.

I. Complications

Complications include seizures, CE (can progress to herniation), muscle cramps or weakness, and pulmonary edema or hypertension associated with fluid overload. *Central pontine myelinolysis* can develop if hyponatremia and hypoosmolality are corrected too quickly. This shift causes brain cells to shrink, precipitating cerebral hemorrhage and subsequent brain injury with herniation. Symptoms include tremor, obtundation, amnesia, coma, and seizures (von Saint Andre-von Arnim et al., 2013).

DIABETES INSIPIDUS

A. Pathophysiology

1. DI is a clinical condition that is characterized by inability to concentrate urine, leading to *high volumes of dilute urine* with *high serum osmolality* and *hypernatremia*. There is a loss of water reabsorption in the face of high osmolality and fluid contraction (Simone, 2012). This condition is caused by either an insufficient secretion of ADH (central) or failure of the kidneys to respond to ADH (nephrogenic; Brashers et al., 2014).

2. Central DI is the most common form of DI in critically ill children. Deficiency of ADH is due to failure of the hypothalamus to synthesize, or failure of the posterior pituitary to secrete ADH, or both.

3. Nephrogenic DI is characterized by normal secretion of ADH by the posterior pituitary, but the distal tubule and the collecting duct in the kidney are resistant to its effects. Although nephrogenic DI is a less common type of DI, it is the most difficult form to treat.

B. Etiologies and Risk Factors

1. Central DI can be acquired, genetic (rare), or congenital. *Acquired* forms result from pituitary or suprasellar surgery, traumatic brain injury, brain tumors, CNS infections or malformations, leukemias or lymphomas, CE or brain death, and cerebral vascular anomalies (von Saint Andre-von Arnim et al., 2013). *Congenital* forms could occur with defects of the midline brain (septo-optic dysplasia, holoprosencephaly, or agenesis of the corpus callosum; Simone, 2012).

2. Nephrogenic DI is rare. It can be either congenital or acquired and is associated with *renal disease* (polycystic kidney disease, pyelonephritis, sickle cell nephropathy), *metabolic disturbances* (hypokalemia, chronic hypercalcemia), or caused by *medications* (lithium, amphotericin B, phenytoin, diuretics, and rifampin; Simone, 2012). Another less common acquired reason for the development of DI is *psychogenic DI*, which results from excessive water intake (Thompson, 2016). In most instances, stopping the medication, correcting the metabolic disturbance, or ceasing the excessive water intake could resolve the episode of DI. Other causes may result in chronic DI (Thompson, 2016).

C. Signs and Symptoms (see Table 6.7)

1. Damage to the posterior pituitary from surgery, disease, or trauma causes central DI and results in the very classic *triphasic response* (von Saint Andre-von Arnim et al., 2013).

    a. Stage 1. Polyuric phase–high urine output results from blunted release of ADH (Clark et al., 2008), and may last hours to several days.

    b. Stage 2. Unregulated phase-damaged pituitary and neurons attempt to release ADH stores in an unregulated fashion without negative feedback. This stage may last up to 6 to12 days and often leads to SIADH (von Saint Andre-von Arnim et al., 2013).

    c. Stage 3. Depleted phase-damaged pituitary and neurons are depleted of all stores of ADH and fail to function. This phase may be permanent or transient and supplemental ADH or vasopressin will be required.

2. A large quantity of dilute or clear urine is the first sign of DI (>4 mL/kg/hr).

3. Hypernatremia occurs with serum sodium >145 mEq/L.

4. Serum hyperosmolality occurs with osmolality >300 mOsm/kg.

5. Polyuria occurs with dilute urine and specific gravity less than 1.005.

6. Urine osmolality is less than 200 mOsm/kg.

7. If able, children may report polydipsia, an unrelenting thirst.

8. Signs of dehydration include low central venous pressure, tachycardia, hypotension, poor skin turgor, dry mucous membranes, and weight loss.

9. Altered mental status may occur with lethargy, confusion, and coma.

D. Interpretation of Diagnostic Studies

1. *Hypernatremia and hyperosmolality* are due to water loss with dehydration.

2. *Low specific gravity and urine osmolality* are due to the kidney's inability to reabsorb water and concentrate urine.

3. *Vasopressin levels* are low or unmeasurable in central DI. Vasopressin levels are normal or high in nephrogenic DI as the kidney is unresponsive to ADH being delivered.

4. *MRI or CT scan* is used for the diagnosis of CE or underlying conditions such as cerebral tumors or edema, calcifications, pituitary disorders or tumors, or midline defects. MRI exams are superior as they are more sensitive and provide details regarding the posterior fossa (Simone, 2012).

5. *Pituitary function* tests will determine ACTH, TSH, or GH defects.

6. A *water-deprivation test* can be used to diagnose DI, but it is not typically done in critically ill children. However, during water-deprivation testing many children will require critical care monitoring due to the effects of severe extracellular volume depletion (Babler et al., 2013). The test is completed after an overnight fast; and a baseline weight, serum, and urine osmolality are recorded. Over the next 6 to 8 hours, all fluids and foods are withheld. The child is weighed every hour, and urine and serum osmolality are checked as well as volume and osmolality of every void. At the end of the study, serum laboratory specimens are redrawn. The test is terminated if body weight falls 3% to 5% or ill effects of hypovolemia are seen. DI is diagnosed if urine osmolality is not greater than 300 mOsm/kg before plasma osmolality is greater than 295 mOsm/kg or if serum sodium becomes greater that 145 mmol/L. To differentiate between nephrogenic and neurogenic DI, a subsequent *ADH test* is completed.

A dose of vasopressin (1 unit/m² subcutaneously [SQ]) is given; if the urine osmolality doubles or is greater than 300 mOsm/kg, the patient has central DI, and, if there is no response, it is nephrogenic DI (Babler et al., 2013).

E. Diagnoses

1. Differential diagnoses include DM, excess sodium ingestion (iatrogenic or improperly mixed formula), overuse of diuretics, thirst abnormalities, urinary tract infection, postobstructive uropathy, increased insensible water loss, and primary polydipsia (Simone, 2012).

2. *Collaborative Diagnoses and Comorbidities*

    a. Potential for acute or chronic neurologic insult related to underlying disease process or too rapid a rise of serum osmolality

    b. Potential for low cardiac output secondary to hypovolemia related to diuresis and intravascular volume loss

    c. Potential for the development of CE related to rapid correction of hyperosmolar state

    d. Fluid and electrolyte imbalance related to excessive diuresis

F. Treatment Goals

1. Correct dehydration and fluid deficits.

2. Correct hypernatremia slowly.

3. Control free water loss by the kidney.

4. Prevent neurologic sequelae.

G. Management

1. In central DI, the decision to use fluid, or ADH replacement therapy, or both is often based on severity of the illness, chronicity of hypernatremia, and underlying cause. In many instances, careful fluid replacement is done initially in anticipation of the triphasic response when sodium levels will drop quickly and ADH surges will be present (Clark et al., 2008). Fluid is given as maintenance IV fluids plus urine replacement 1 mL per 1 mL for all urine output greater than 2 mL/kg/hr (Thompson, 2016). In severe presentations with shock or seizures, airway management, fluid resuscitation, and seizure control must take priority. If dehydration is present, NS bolus should be given at 20 mL/kg (Simone, 2012). Anticonvulsant therapy with lorazepam or valium should be administered. Airway stability and seizure control should be ensured prior to attaining diagnostic studies. Hypernatremia is corrected slowly as rapid

correction of osmolality can result in CE. Sodium levels should fall no faster than 0.5 mEq/L per hour over 48 to 72 hours (Chung & Zimmerman, 2009). Patients who are dehydrated will need fluid-volume deficits replaced with NS (relatively hypotonic in hypernatremic patients) or more hypotonic fluids of 0.45% saline based on fluid-volume deficits. ADH replacement therapy is titrated for a urine-output goal less than 4 mL/kg per hour with normal serum sodium (Thompson, 2016). ADH replacement may be administered intranasally, IV, intramuscularly (IM), SQ, orally, or by continuous infusion. During the critical period, vasopressin IV should be initiated at 0.5 mU/kg/hr with the goal of antidiuresis (von Saint Andre-von Arnim et al., 2013) and titrated further based on urine output. Children with an intact thirst mechanism are allowed access to oral fluids with careful monitoring of intake and output, and DDAVP intranasally or SQ is initiated with endocrinology consultation. Infants, comatose patients, or children with an abnormal thirst response require careful monitoring of their fluid intake as they do not act on their thirst.

2. Nephrogenic DI is difficult to treat as it is resistant to vasopressin administration (Thompson, 2016). If it is caused by medications or metabolic disturbances, those must be corrected. A combination of a sodium-restricted diet and a thiazide diuretic (hydrochlorothiazide) has been shown to lower urine output in 40% of infants with nephrogenic DI (Simone, 2012). Decreased oral intake lowers the solute load to the kidneys and the diuretic paradoxically reduces polyuria by causing excessive sodium reabsorption in the proximal tubule. Lower volume delivered to the distal tubule will result in less urine formation and a lower glomerular filtration rate (Simone, 2012). Thiazide diuretics are often used in combination with amiloride or indomethacin in the management of nephrogenic DI. Indomethacin, a prostaglandin inhibitor, works similarly to NSAIDs to inhibit renal production of prostaglandin, thereby enhancing renal responsiveness to ADH (Brashers et al., 2014).

3. Monitoring includes hourly hemodynamic and neurologic assessments while critical, with precise intake and output, daily weights, urine-specific gravity, urine osmolality, serum sodium, and osmolality. In severe cases, serum sodium may need to be monitored every 1 to 2 hours.

H. Complications

Complications include cardiac collapse and shock from rapid diuresis. Neurologic sequelae occur from a rapid rise in serum osmolality, which can lead to seizures, cerebral thrombosis or hemorrhage, and long-term developmental delay. In this hyperosmolar state, CE, herniation, and possible death can also occur. In rare cases, disseminated intravascular coagulopathy (DIC) and acute kidney injury (AKI) have also occurred (Chung & Zimmerman, 2009). Severe electrolyte imbalances can occur secondary to inadequate monitoring of serum electrolytes during therapy, or water intoxication and fluid overload are seen with rehydration or aggressive ADH replacement therapy.

CEREBRAL SALT WASTING

A. Pathophysiology (Figure 6.11)

CSW is a hyponatremic, hypovolemic condition caused by an acute neurologic insult, surgery, or infection (Simone, 2012). The validity of CSW as a disease process has been debated in the literature since its description in 1950. There are two major theories for the development of CSW. The *first theory* involves the inhibition of sympathetic nervous system. Activation of the sympathetic nervous system in conditions of intravascular contraction would increase secretion of renin from the kidneys and a rise in aldosterone (Yee et al., 2010), causing a retention of both sodium and water. If this response is inhibited,

there will be sodium losses in the urine. The *second theory* involves the natriuretic peptides (ANP, DNP, BNP, and C-type natriuretic peptide), which occur in the body to defend during periods of hypervolemia and sodium retention by promoting vascular relaxation. These peptides have unique tissue-specific sites of production, which have potent effects on the regulation of vascular tone. Natriuretic peptides act upon the renal tubules and cause inhibition of water and sodium reabsorption (Yee et al., 2010). These peptides have also been linked to the suppression of aldosterone and renin in the medulla leading to further sodium and water losses. Studies linking cerebral vasospasm and elevated BNP levels indicate a causal link between cerebral injury and the development of this hypovolemic, hyponatremic state (Yee et al., 2010).

B. Etiology and Risk Factors

1. *Conditions Associated With CSW*

   a. Meningitis and encephalitis

   b. Traumatic brain injury and cerebral hemorrhage

   c. Cerebral tumors. Germ cell tumors, craniopharyngiomas, pituitary tumors, hypothalamic gliomas, and third-ventricle tumors are tumors of the

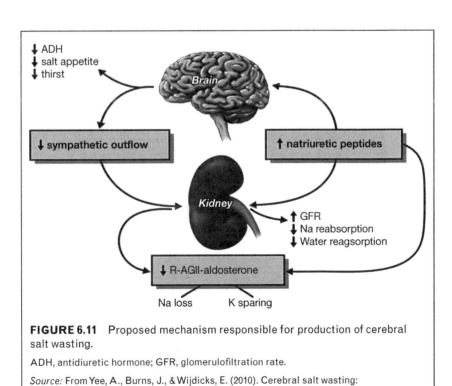

FIGURE 6.11 Proposed mechanism responsible for production of cerebral salt wasting.

ADH, antidiuretic hormone; GFR, glomerulofiltration rate.

Source: From Yee, A., Burns, J., & Wijdicks, E. (2010). Cerebral salt wasting: Pathophysiology, diagnosis, and treatment. *Neurosurgery Clinics of North America, 21,* 339–352. doi:10.1016/j.nec.2009.10.011

cerebrum. Often children who have tumors can have fluctuating states of SIADH, CSW, and DI.

d. *Hydrocephalus* may be chronic or acute.

C. Signs and Symptoms (Table 6.8)

1. CSW is a transient condition that presents within the first 10 days of diagnosis of an acute neurologic condition. The highest risk occurs in the first 48 hours of an inciting event with a mean duration of 6.3 ± 5.4 days (Simone, 2012). Physical signs of volume depletion and dehydration are the defining parameters used to differentiate CSW and SIADH (von Saint Andre-von Arnim et al., 2013). Actual prevalence of CSW is unknown as it often goes unrecognized, but it can be near 10% to 12% in patients with brain tumors or hydrocephalus (Simone, 2012). The severity of presenting symptoms reflects the rapidity of the onset of hyponatremia (Simone, 2012).

a. Signs of dehydration include low central venous pressure (<6 cm H_2O), tachycardia, hypotension, poor skin turgor, dry mucous membranes, delayed capillary refill, and weight loss.

b. Altered mental status can be difficult to recognize in children with neurologic compromise and may include agitation, lethargy, seizures, and ultimately coma.

D. Lab Data

1. Hyponatremia equals serum sodium less than 135 mmol/L

2. Serum osmolality less than 280 mOsm/kg

3. Normal to slightly high urine output—2 to 3 mL/kg/hr with specific gravity near 1.010

4. Urine osmolality measures greater than 200 mOsm/kg

5. Urine sodium greater than 40 mEq/L

6. Low serum uric acid

TABLE 6.8 Differential Diagnosis for CSW and SIADH

Variable	CSW	SIADH
Urine osmolality	↑ (>100 mOsm/kg)	↑ (>100 mOsm/kg)
Urine sodium concentration	↑ (>40 mmol/L)	↑ (>40 mmol/L)
Extracellular fluid volume	↓	↑
Body weight	↓	↔ or ↓
Fluid balance	Negative	Neutral to slightly +
Urine volume	↔ or ↑	↔ or ↓
Heart rate	↔ or ↑	↔
Hematocrit	↑	↔
Albumin	↑	↔
Serum bicarbonate	↑	↔ or ↓
Blood urea nitrogen	↑	↔ or ↓
Serum uric acid	↔ or ↓	↓
Sodium balance	Negative	Neutral or +
Central venous pressure	↓ (<6 cm H_2O)	↔ or slightly + (6–10 cm H_2O)
Wedge pressure	↓	↔ or slightly ↑

CSW, cerebral salt wasting; SIADH, sick euthyroid, or syndrome of inappropriate antidiuretic hormone.

Source: From Yee, A., Burns, J., & Wijdicks, E. (2010), Cerebral salt wasting: Pathophysiology, diagnosis, and treatment. *Neurosurgery Clinics of North America, 21,* 339–352. doi:10.1016/j.nec.2009.10.011

E. Interpretation of Diagnostic Studies

Head CT or brain MRI are useful in establishing what structural abnormalities may have caused the neurologic event that has led to the development of CSW, but they will not provide diagnosis. Lumbar puncture is useful in diagnosing meningitis, which may lead to CSW development (Simone, 2012).

F. Diagnoses

1. *Differential Diagnoses. SIADH* is the most commonly confused differential diagnosis when CSW is suspected. The presentation of hyponatremia and hypoosmolarity can initially cause confusion between the two entities. The defining difference between the two disease states is that in SIADH there will be *euvolemia* and in CSW there will be *hypovolemia* (Yee et al., 2010). CSW can have life-threatening effects secondary to hypovolemia if not differentiated from other disease states, making prompt recognition vital. Other possible differentials would include water intoxication, pseudohyponatremia, adrenal insufficiency, hypothyroidism, congestive heart failure, and liver or kidney disease (Simone, 2012). Further, but less likely diagnoses, would include inborn errors of metabolism, renal tubular dysfunction, and diuretic use (more common in hospitalized patients).

2. *Collaborative Diagnoses and Comorbidities*

   a. Fluid and volume loss related to water depletion

   b. Alteration in mental state related to underlying neurologic processes and rapid development of hyponatremia with low serum osmolality

   c. Potential for cardiovascular collapse and shock secondary to hypovolemia

   d. Potential for seizures related to hyponatremia and neurologic compromise

   e. Potential for cerebral hemorrhage from rapid correction of hypoosmolar state

G. Treatment Goals

1. Replace intravascular volume.

2. Normalize sodium with replacement intravenously or enterally.

3. Prevent neurologic sequelae.

4. Correct serum osmolality and sodium slowly.

5. Treat underlying disorder.

H. Management

1. Fluid should be given in CSW to replete the hypovolemic state caused by natriuresis and diuresis (Yee et al., 2010). If shock is present, an intravenous bolus of 20 mL/kg of isotonic NS should be given. Once euvolemia is reached, fluid type and rate should be near maintenance, and composition should reflect urine sodium losses. Caution should be used during this time, however, as acute increases in serum sodium and osmolality can cause the brain cells to shrink, precipitating cerebral hemorrhage and subsequent brain injury.

2. Sodium should be normalized slowly over 48 to 72 hours and no faster than 0.5 to 1 mEq/hr with a goal to increase no more than 10 mEq/d. *Hypertonic saline* is often used in the treatment of CSW in varying concentrations. When concentrated to 3%, fluid hypertonicity can cause untoward phlebitis or burns to peripheral veins and must be administered via a central venous line. It is often used in less concentrated forms (1%–1.5% NaCl) when it must be administered peripherally via a larger bore needle with good blood return. However, due to large sodium losses in the urine, it is often extremely challenging to attain better sodium levels with less concentrated formulations. When severe hyponatremia presents (<125 mEq/L) or with worsening neurologic exam, 3% saline is given with a goal of 130 mEq/L. There are different opinions on bolus dosing of 3% saline. In general, the accepted dose is 1 to 2 mL/kg/hr and a bolus dose of 12 mL/kg is expected to raise the Na by about 10 mEq/L (Chung & Zimmerman, 2009; Sperling et al., 2014). During correction, hyperchloremic metabolic acidosis could result, necessitating changes to fluid composition. Once children are tolerating enteral feeds, transition to oral sodium supplements could be made until resolution of CSW.

3. Adjunctive medication, such as *fludrocortisone (Florinef)*, has been used successfully to help with the salt losing seen in CSW at dosing of 0.1 to 0.2 mg orally twice daily for up to 3 to 5 days or until the sodium level normalizes (Taketomo et al., 2015; Yee et al., 2010). Close monitoring must be done during treatment when using Florinef, as it can cause hypokalemia and hypertension.

4. Monitoring includes precise intake and output with serum sodium level every 2 to 4 hours during the acute phase then every 4 to 6 hours once the sodium nears normal levels. Urine sodium levels are helpful in directing care and should be monitored with serum Na levels. For example, a urine sodium of 75 mEq/L is equal to replacement fluid of 0.45% NS (Simone, 2012). If the urine sodium is over 75 mEq/L, then higher sodium concentrations in the IV fluids will be needed. Specific gravity should be done with each void, serum electrolytes and osmolality should be done every 4 to 6 hours until normal with daily weights. Urine electrolytes and osmolality are obtained at initial diagnosis; however, frequent monitoring is not necessary. Central venous pressure is obtained with goal of 6 cm water. Heart rate, blood pressure, and neurologic status are monitored every hour.

I. Complications

Complications include seizures and CE, which can progress to herniation. Cerebral hemorrhage can occur if fluid replacement is achieved too quickly. *Central pontine demyelination* can occur when there is too rapid of a correction of hyponatremia and can cause irreversible damage to the white matter (Simone, 2012). Cerebral vasospasm can occur secondarily in patients with aneurysmal subarachnoid hemorrhage who are hypovolemic and can have catastrophic effects (Yee et al., 2010).

SUMMARY

Endocrine disorders in pediatric critical care can be difficult to diagnose and treat. They can have profound effects and are often confused with other disorders. Providers must be diligent in directing their care and pay great attention to detail in the management of these children. If careful and judicious fluid administration and hormone management are done from the beginning of these illnesses, outcomes will improve. Prompt treatment of endocrine disorders return critically ill children to their baseline function and can prevent untoward debilitations in long-term health.

CASE STUDIES WITH QUESTIONS, ANSWERS, AND RATIONALES

Case Study 6.1

A 5-year-old boy was an unrestrained passenger in a motor vehicle collision and suffered traumatic brain injury 2 days previously. He has had elevated intracranial pressures (ICPs) and hypotension with low urine output and a mean arterial pressure (MAP) of 50. He has had hypertonic saline therapy and his sodium level is now 155 with a serum osmolality of 320 and ICP of 22. The night shift reported urine output of 5 mL/kg/hr.

1. What disease process is most likely?
   A. Diabetes mellitus (DM)
   B. Diabetes insipidus (DI)
   C. Cerebral salt wasting (CSW)
   D. Syndrome of inappropriate antidiuretic hormone (SIADH)

2. What is the cerebral perfusion pressure (CPP) of this patient?
   A. 38
   B. 72
   C. 77
   D. 28

Case Study 6.2

A 10-year-old boy with a previous diagnosis of astrocytoma arrives at the emergency room tachycardic with altered mental status, cool extremities, and seizures with a respiratory rate of 8. He is emergently intubated, and after a head CT is completed, he is transferred to the pediatric intensive care unit (PICU). Laboratory results are significant for a serum sodium level of 133 mEq/L, normal serum osmolarity, glucose, and urine output with urine sodium greater than 80 mEq/L.

1. What is the most likely diagnosis?
   A. Diabetes mellitus (DM)
   B. Diabetes insipidus (DI)
   C. Cerebral salt wasting (CSW)
   D. Syndrome of inappropriate antidiuretic hormone (SIADH)

2. What treatment should be promptly initiated?
   A. Urine replacement with normal saline
   B. Fluid restriction for insensible fluid losses
   C. Fluid bolus 20 mL/kg
   D. Administer loop diuretics

Case Study 6.3

A 12-year-old boy arrives at the emergency department with altered mental status, vomiting, and dehydration. He is started on fluid hydration of normal saline (NS) 20 mL/kg and initial chemistry results are significant for a glucose level of 422 mg/dL, serum bicarbonate of 8 mEq/L, pH of 7.22, and ketones in the urine.

1. What is the most likely diagnosis?
   A. Hyperglycemic hyperosmolar syndrome (HHS)
   B. Diabetic ketoacidosis (DKA)
   C. Diabetes insipidus (DI)
   D. Critical illness–related corticosteroid insufficiency (CIRCI)

2. The pediatric intensive care unit (PICU) accepts the patient with diabetic ketoacidosis (DKA) and upon arrival he complains of an excruciating headache with decreased mentation and Kussmaul respirations. What is the most likely complication that is occurring?
   A. Hyperglycemic hyperosmolar syndrome (HHS)
   B. Cerebral edema
   C. Hypoglycemia
   D. Hyponatremia

3. What is the next best treatment?
   A. Notify the neurosurgeon on call
   B. Administration of normal saline (NS) bolus 20 mL/kg
   C. Elevate the head of bed
   D. Administration of sodium bicarbonate

Case Study 6.4

1. A 1-week-old infant presents to the emergency department with poor feeding, hypothermia, and constipation. Initial labs reveal a sodium level of 138, potassium of 4.2, and an elevated thyroid-stimulating hormone (TSH).
   What is the most likely diagnosis?
   A. Congenital adrenal hyperplasia
   B. Hypothyroidism
   C. Adrenal Insufficiency
   D. Hyperthyroidism

Answers and Rationales

Case Study 6.1

1. **B**. DI occurs frequently in severe traumatic brain injury (TBI). DI has a triphasic presentation with initial polyuria hours to days post injury where you will see elevated sodium, high dilute urine output, elevated serum osmolality, specific gravity less than 1.005, urine osmolality less than 200 mOsm/kg, and urine sodium less than 30. The second phase occurs as a result of unregulated antidiuretic hormone (ADH) release from a degenerating pituitary causing symptoms of SIADH. Once ADH stores are depleted, DI symptoms will return and become transient or permanent.

2. **D**. CPP is measured by MAP-ICP (50-22) and helps give an indication of brain perfusion. During ICP spikes and periods of hypotension, the CPP falls dramatically and is associated with poor outcomes. Hypotension and low CPP cause secondary injury to an already edematous and injured brain. CPP

goals are age-directed: infant greater than 40 mmHg, children greater than 50 mmHg, and adults greater than 60 mmHg. Persistently, high ICP can lead to brain herniation and death.

Case Study 6.2

1. **C**. CSW is a hypovolemic, hyponatremic disorder. CSW is often seen in children with neurologic and neurosurgical injuries, infections, or oncologic processes and can be difficult to distinguish from SIADH. SIADH is associated with low urine output (<1 mL/kg/hr) and euvolemia with urine sodium less than 30 mEq/L. Since there is no central venous pressure to monitor, other parameters of hypovolemia should be assessed including skin turgor, temperature, capillary refill, and peripheral pulses.

2. **C**. If shock is present, a fluid bolus of 20 mL/kg should be given with isotonic normal saline until a state of euvolemia is reached; then it should reflect urinary losses. Sodium should be normalized slowly over 24 to 48 hours, no faster than 0.5 to 1 mEq/hr, or no more than 10 mEq/day.

Case Study 6.3

1. **B**. DKA is characterized by glucose greater than 200 mg/dL and venous pH less than 7.3 with ketonuria and serum bicarbonate less than 15 mmol. Children with new onset diabetes will often present in DKA. The episode is usually preceded by a very typical history of polyuria, polydipsia, polyphagia, and hyperglycemia with weight loss.

2. **B**. Cerebral edema is a rare but life-threatening complication that can occur in DKA. Symptoms include severe headache, altered mental status, hypertension, bradycardia, and vomiting.

3. **C**. Treatment of cerebral edema should begin at recognition: administering hypertonic saline or mannitol, elevating the head of the bed, and performing an emergent CT scan of the brain to evaluate degree of edema. Fluid administration should be decreased. If the Glasgow Coma Scale score is less than 9, support of respiratory and neurologic status is necessary. Risk factors for cerebral edema include first presentation, high serum blood urea nitrogen (BUN) and CO_2 (reflective of the degree of dehydration and acidosis), administration of insulin bolus doses, bicarbonate administration, rapid glucose correction, aggressive fluid administration, and younger age at diagnosis.

Case Study 6.4

1. B. Hypothyroidism in the neonate is characterized by poor feeding, hypotonia, constipation, weight loss and decreased activity with weak cry. Lab results seen in hypothyroidism will reveal an elevated TSH and low free T4. Treatment with levothyroxine should be initiated in conjunction with pediatric endocrinology as lack of treatment can lead to significant cognitive impairment.

REFERENCES

American Diabetes Association. (2016). Children and adolescents. *Diabetes Care, 39*(Suppl. 1), S86–S93. doi:10.2337/dc16-S014

Babler, E., Betts, K., Courtney, J., Flores, B., Flynn, C., Laerson, M., . . . Wroley, D. (2013). *Clinical handbook of pediatric endocrinology* (2nd ed.). St Louis, MO: Quality Medical Publishing.

Brashers, V., Jones, R., & Huether, K. (2014). Mechanisms of hormonal regulation. In K. McCance & S. Huether (Eds.), *Pathophysiology: The biologic basis for disease in adults and children* (7th ed., pp. 689–716). St. Louis, MO: Mosby/Elsevier.

Buzby, M. (2012). Endocrine disorders: Physiology and diagnostics. In K. Reuter-Rice & B. Bolick (Eds.), *Pediatric acute care: A guide for interprofessional practice* (pp. 369–376). Burlington, MA: Jones & Bartlett.

Carcillo, J., & Fields, A. (2002). Clinical practice parameters for hemodynamic support of pediatric and neonatal patients in septic shock. *Critical Care Medicine, 30*, 1365–1378. Retrieved from https://journals.lww.com/ccmjournal/Abstract/2002/06000/Clinical_practice_parameters_for_hemodynamic.40.aspx

Chameides, L., Samson, R., Schexnayder, S., & Hazinski, M. (2011). *Pediatric advanced life support provider manual.* Dallas, TX: American Heart Association.

Chan, M., Chan, M., Mengshol, J., Fish, D., & Chan, E. (2013). Octreotide: A drug often used in the critical care setting but not well understood. *Chest, 144*(6), 1937–1945. doi:10.1378/chest.13-0382

Chantra, M., Limsuwan, A., & Mahachoklertwattana, P. (2016). Low cardiac output thyroid storm in a girl with grave's disease. *Pediatrics International, 58*(10), 1080–1083. doi:10.1111/ped.13102

Chung, C., & Zimmerman, D. (2009). Hypernatremia and hyponatremia: Current understanding and management. *Clinical Pediatric Emergency Medicine, 10*(4), 272–278. doi:10.1016/j.cpem.2009.11.002

Clark, L., Preissig, C., Rigby, M., & Bowyer, F. (2008). Endocrine issues in the pediatric intensive care unit. *Pediatric Clinics of North America, 55*, 805–833. doi:10.1016/j.pcl.2008.03.001

Clayton, M., & McCance, K. (2014). Stress and disease. In K. McCance & S. Huether (Eds.), *Pathophysiology: The biologic basis for disease in adults and children* (7th ed., pp. 338–362). St. Louis, MO: Mosby/Elsevier.

Dattani, M., & Gevers, E. (2016). Endocrinology of fetal development. In S. Melmed, K. S. Polonsky, P. R. Larsen, & H. M. Kronenberg (Eds.), *Williams textbook of endocrinology* (13th ed., pp. 849–892). Philadelphia, PA: Elsevier.

Davis, A., Carcillo, J., Aneja, R., Deymann, A., Lin, J., Nguyen, T., . . . Zuckerberg, A. (2017). American College of Critical Care Medicine clinical practice parameters for hemodynamic support of pediatric and neonatal septic shock. *Critical Care Medicine, 45*(6), 1061–1093. doi:10.1097/CCM.0000000000002425

De León, D., Thornton, P., Stanley, C., & Sperling, M. (2014). Hypoglycemia in the newborn and infant. In M. Sperling (Ed.), *Pediatric endocrinology* (4th ed., pp. 157–183). Philadelphia, PA: Elsevier.

Doig, A., & Huether, S. (2014). Structure and function of the digestive system. In K. McCance & S. Huether (Eds.), *Pathophysiology: The biologic basis for disease in adults and children* (7th ed., pp. 1393–1422). St. Louis, MO: Mosby/Elsevier.

Engorn, B., & Flerlage, J. (Eds.). (2015). *The Harriet Lane handbook* (20th ed.). Philadelphia, PA: Elsevier/Saunders.

Ganeson, R., Kazmi, Y., & Levy, R. (2012). Endocrine disorders: Thyroid and parathyroid disorders. In K. Reuter-Rice & B. Bolick (Eds.), *Pediatric acute care: A guide for interprofessional practice* (pp. 394–399). Burlington, MA: Jones & Bartlett.

Goel, P., & Choudhury, S. (2012). Persistent hyperinsulinemic hypoglycemia of infancy: An overview of current concepts. *Journal of Indian Association of Pediatric Surgeons, 17*(3), 99–103. doi:10.4103/0971-9261.98119

Gunnala, V., Guo, R., Minutti, C., Durazo-Arvizu, R., Laporte, C., Matthews, H., . . . Bhatia, R. (2015). Measurement of salivary cortisol level for the diagnosis of critical illness related corticosteroid insufficiency in children. *Pediatrics Critical Care Medicine, 16*(4), e101–e106. doi:10.1097/pcc.0000000000000361

Hall, J. (2016). *Guyton and Hall textbook of medical physiology.* (13th ed.). Philadelphia, PA: Elsevier.

Hazinski, M., Mondozzi, M., & Uridales Baker, R. (2014). Shock, multiple organ dysfunction syndrome, and burns in children. In K. McCance & S. Huether (Eds.), *Pathophysiology: The biologic basis for disease in adults and children* (7th ed., pp. 1699–1727). St. Louis, MO: Mosby/Elsevier.

Hockenberry, M. J., & Wilson, D. (Eds.). (2015). *Wong's nursing care of infants and children* (10th ed.). St. Louis, MO: Elsevier.

Jones, R., Brashers, V., & Huether, S. (2010) Alterations of hormonal regulation. In K. McCance & S. Huether (Eds.), *Pathophysiology: The biologic basis for disease in adults and children* (6th ed., pp. 737–780). Maryland Heights, MO: Mosby/Elsevier.

Kaiser, U., & Ho, K. K. Y. (2016). Pituitary physiology and diagnostic evaluation. In S. Melmed, K. S. Polonsky, P. R. Larsen, & H. M. Kronenberg (Eds.), *Williams textbook of endocrinology* (13th ed., pp. 176–231). Philadelphia, PA: Elsevier.

Klein, M., Sathasivam, A., Novoa, Y., & Rapaport, R. (2011). Recent consensus statements in pediatric endocrinology: A selective review. *Pediatric Clinics of North America, 58*, 1301–1315. doi:10.1016/j.pcl.2011.07.014

Kline-Tilford, A. (2016). Pheochromocytomas. In A. Kline-Tilford, & C. Haut (Eds.), *Lippincott certification review: Pediatric acute care nurse practitioner.* Philadelphia, PA: Wolters Kluwer.

Kwon, Y., Suh, G., Jeon, K., Park, S., Lim, S., Koh, W., . . . Kwon, O. (2010). Serum cytokines and critical illness-related corticosteroid insufficiency. *Intensive Care Medicine, 36*, 1845–1851. doi:10.1007/s00134-010-1971-9

Levy-Shraga, Y., & Pinhas-Hamiel, O. (2013). Critical illness-related corticosteroid insufficiency in children. *Hormone Research Paediatrics, 80*, 309–317. doi:10.1159/000354759

Ly, T. T., Maahs, D. M., Rewers, A., Dunger, D., Oduwole, A., & Jones, T. W. (2014). ISPAD clinical practice consensus guidelines—Hypoglycemia: Assessment and management of hypoglycemia in children and adolescents with diabetes. *Pediatric Diabetes, 15*(Suppl. 20), 180–192. doi:10.1111/pedi.12174

Majzoub, J. A., Muglia, L. J., & Srivatsa, A. (2014). Disorders of the posterior pituitary. In M. Sperling (Ed.). *Pediatric endocrinology* (4th ed. pp. 405–443). Philadelphia, PA: Elsevier.

Marik, P. E., Pastores, S. M., Annane, D., Meduri, G. U., Sprung, C. L., Arlt, W., . . . Vogeser, M. (2008). Recommendations for the diagnosis and management of corticosteroid insufficiency in critically ill adult patients: Consensus statements from an international task force by the American College of Critical Care Medicine. *Critical Care Medicine, 36*(6), 1937–1949. doi:10.1097/CCM.0b013e31817603ba

McCance, K., & Huether, S. (Eds.). (2015). *Pathophysiology: The biologic basis for disease in adults and children* (7th ed.). St. Louis, MO: Mosby/Elsevier.

Miller, W., & Flück, C. (2014). Adrenal cortex and its disorders. In M. Sperling (Ed.). *Pediatric endocrinology* (4th ed., pp. 471–532). Philadelphia, PA: Elsevier.

Molina, P. (2013). *Endocrine physiology* (4th ed.). New York, NY: McGraw-Hill.

Plumpton, K., Anderson, B. J., & Beca, J. (2010). Thyroid hormone and cortisol concentrations after congenital heart surgery in infants younger than 3 months of age. *Intensive Care Medicine, 36*, 321–328. doi:10.1007/s00134-009-1648-4

Price, A., Losek, J., & Jackson, B. (2016). Hyperglycaemic hyperosmolar syndrome in children: Patient characteristics, diagnostic delays and associated complications. *Journal of Paediatrics and Child Health, 52*(1), 80–84. doi:10.1111/jpc.12980

Robinson, A., & Verbalis, J. (2016). Posterior pituitary. In S. Melmed, K. S. Polonsky, P. R. Larsen, & H. M. Kronenberg (Eds.), *Williams textbook of endocrinology* (13th ed., pp. 300–333). Philadelphia, PA: Elsevier.

Rossano, J., & Shaddy, R. (2014). Heart failure in children: Etiology and treatment. *Journal of Pediatrics, 165*(2), 228–233. doi:10.1016/j.jpeds.2014.04.055

Salvatore, D., Davies, T., Schlumberger, M.-J., Hay, I., & Larsen, P. (2016). Thyroid physiology and diagnostic evaluation of patients with thyroid disorders. In S. Melmed, K. S. Polonsky, P. R. Larsen, & H. M. Kronenberg (Eds.), *Williams textbook of endocrinology* (13th ed.). New York, NY: Elsevier.

Sarafoglou, K., Hoffmann, G., & Roth, K. (2017). *Pediatric endocrinology and inborn errors of metabolism* (2nd ed.). New York, NY: McGraw-Hill.

Schoenwolf, G., Bleyl, S., & Brauer, P., & Francis-West, P. (2015). *Larsen's human embryology* (5th ed.). New York, NY: Churchill Livingstone.

Simone, S. (2012). Endocrine disorders: Diabetes insipidus, syndrome of inappropriate antidiuretic homone, and cerebral salt wasting. In K. Reuter-Rice & B. Bolick (Eds.). *Pediatric acute care: A guide for interprofessional practice* (pp. 376–384). Burlington, MA: Jones & Bartlett.

Sperling, M., Tamborlane, W., Battelino, T., Weinzimer, S., & Phillip, M. (2014). Diabetes mellitus. In M. Sperling (Ed.), *Pediatric endocrinology* (4th ed., pp. 846–900). Philadelphia, PA: Elsevier.

Srinivasan, S., & Misra, M. (2015). Hyperthyroidism in children. *Pediatrics in Review, 36*(6), 239–248. doi:10.1542/pir.36-6-239

Srinivasan, V., & Agus, M. (2014). Tight glucose control in critically ill children—A systematic review and meta-analysis. *Pediatric Diabetes, 15*, 75–83. doi:10.1111/pedi.12134

Taketomo, C. K., Hodding, J. H., & Kraus, D. (2015). *Pediatric and neonatal dose handbook* (22nd ed.). Cleveland, OH: Lexi-Comp.

Talwar, S., Kumar, M., Choudhary, S., & Airan, B. (2016). Thyroid hormone supplementation following open-heart surgery in children. *Indian Journal of Thoracic and Cardiovascular Surgery, 32*(1), 17–22. doi:10.1007/s12055-015-0411-4

Templin, D. (2006). Endocrine system. In M. C. Slota (Ed.), *Core curriculum for pediatric critical care nurses* (2nd ed., pp. 446–496). St. Louis, MO: Elsevier.

Thompson, A. (2016). Endocrine disorders: Diabetes insipidus. In A. Kline-Tilford & C. Haut (Eds.), *Lippincott certification review: Pediatric acute care nurse practitioner*. Philadelphia, PA: Wolters Kluwer.

Thornton, P., Stanley, C. A., De León, D., Harris, D., Haymond, M., Hussain, K., . . . Wolfsdorf, J. (2015). Recommendations from the Pediatric Endocrine Society for evaluation and management of persistent hypoglycemia in neonates, infants, and children. *Journal of Pediatrics, 167*(2), 238–245. doi:10.1016/j.jpeds.2015.03.057

von Saint Andre-von Arnim, A., Farris, R., Roberts, J., Yanay, O., Brogan, T., & Zimmerman, J. (2013). Common endocrine issues in the pediatric intensive care unit. *Critical Care Clinics, 29*(2), 335–358. doi:10.1016/j.ccc.2012.11.006

Webb, E., & Krone, N. (2015). Current and novel approaches to children and young people with congenital adrenal insufficiency. *Best Practice & Research Clinical Endocrinology and Metabolism, 29*, 449–468. doi:10.1016/j.beem.2015.04.002

White, M. (2016). Endocrine disorders: Adrenal insufficiency. In A. Kline-Tilford & C. Haut (Eds.), *Lippincott certification review: Pediatric acute care nurse practitioner*. Philadelphia, PA: Wolters Kluwer.

Wolfsdorf, J., Allgrove, J., Craig, M., Edge, J., Glaser, N., Jain, V., . . . Hanas, R. (2014). Diabetic ketoacidosis and hyperglycemic hyperosmolar state. *Pediatric Diabetes, 15*(Suppl. 20), 154–179. doi:10.1111/pedi.12165

Yee, A., Burns, J., & Wijdicks, E. (2010). Cerebral salt wasting: Pathophysiology, diagnosis, and treatment. *Neurosurgery Clinics of North America, 21*, 339–352. doi:10.1016/j.nec.2009.10.011

Zeitler, P., Haqq, A., Rosenbloom, A., & Glaser, N. (2011). Hyperglycemic hyperosmolar syndrome in children: Pathophysiological considerations and suggested guidelines for treatment. *Journal of Pediatrics, 158*(1), 9–14.e2. doi:10.1016/j.jpeds.2010.09.048

7 GASTROINTESTINAL SYSTEM

Sarah A. Martin

DEVELOPMENTAL ANATOMY OF THE GASTROINTESTINAL SYSTEM

A. Embryologic Development of the Digestive Tract (Figure 7.1)

1. The digestive tract develops from the primitive gut, which differentiates into the foregut, midgut, and hindgut by the fourth week of gestation (Little, 2015).

  a. *Foregut.* The foregut consists of the pharynx, esophagus, stomach, proximal duodenum, liver, pancreas, gallbladder, and extrahepatic bile ducts.

  b. *Midgut.* The midgut consists of the distal duodenum, jejunum, ileum, cecum, appendix, ascending colon, and proximal part of transverse colon.

  c. *Hindgut.* The hindgut consists of the remainder of the colon and rectum.

2. The esophagus and trachea are a single tube until the fourth week of gestation, at which time the

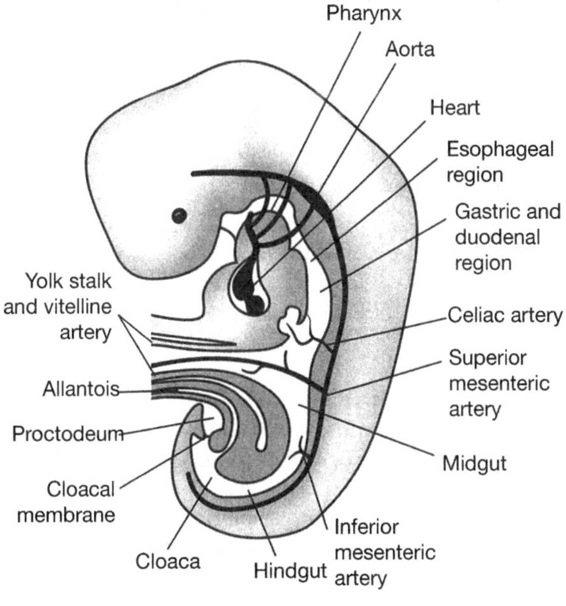

FIGURE 7.1 Primitive gut.

Source: From Kenner, C., & Lott, J. W. (Eds.). (2014). *Comprehensive neonatal nursing* (5th ed., p. 18). New York, NY: Springer Publishing.

tracheoesophageal septum begins to separate the structures.

3. Development of the gut is nearly complete by week 20 of gestation.

DEVELOPMENTAL PHYSIOLOGY OF THE GASTROINTESTINAL SYSTEM

A. Gastric Activity

1. Gastric motility in infants is decreased and somewhat irregular compared with the adult due to delayed maturation of feedback control mechanisms, delayed gastric emptying, and immature coordination of contractions between the antrum of the stomach and the duodenum.

2. Gastroesophageal reflux (GER) is common during the first year because of a complex set of factors, including pressure–volume changes and anatomic relationships causing inappropriate relaxation of the lower esophageal sphincter (LES).

B. Immature Neonatal Liver

The liver matures in function during the first year of life. Toxic substances are inefficiently detoxified.

ANATOMY AND PHYSIOLOGY OF THE GASTROINTESTINAL SYSTEM

A. Structure and Function (Figure 7.2)

1. *Oral Cavity.* The oral cavity serves as a reservoir for chewing and mixing food with saliva. *Salivary glands* include the submandibular, sublingual, and parotid glands. Saliva is composed of water, small amounts of mucus, sodium bicarbonate, chloride, potassium, and amylase. Amylase begins carbohydrate digestion.

2. The *esophagus* propels swallowed food to the stomach. The upper esophageal sphincter prevents air from entering the esophagus during respiration.

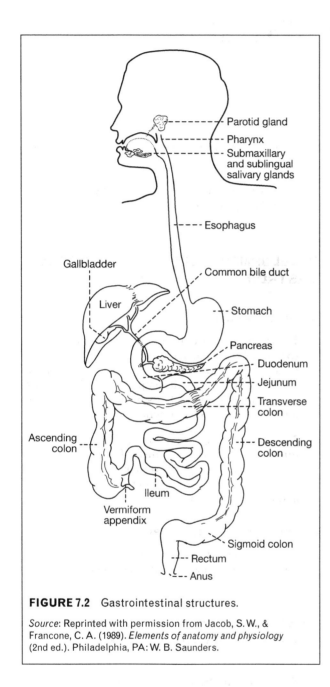

FIGURE 7.2 Gastrointestinal structures.

Source: Reprinted with permission from Jacob, S. W., & Francone, C. A. (1989). *Elements of anatomy and physiology* (2nd ed.). Philadelphia, PA: W. B. Saunders.

The LES closes after swallowing to prevent reflux of gastric contents into the esophagus.

3. *Stomach*

    a. The stomach is a hollow, muscular organ that acts as a reservoir for ingested food. It secretes digestive juices that mix with digested food (chyme). *Parietal cells* secrete hydrochloric acid and intrinsic factor. Intrinsic factor is a glycoprotein that is required for vitamin B_{12} absorption. The secretion is regulated by stimuli (i.e., H_2-histamine receptors). *Chief cells* secrete pepsinogen, which combines with hydrochloric acid to break down protein.

    b. *Gastric emptying* is affected by the volume of food, osmotic pressure, and chemical composition of the contents. Emptying is controlled by the pyloric sphincter. Delayed emptying is caused by foods with high fat content, solid foods, sedatives, sleep, and specific hormones (i.e., secretin and cholecystokinin). Accelerated emptying is caused by foods with high carbohydrate content, liquids, increased volume, and medications (e.g., metoclopramide, erythromycin ethylsuccinate [EES], and azithromycin [zithromax]).

4. The *small intestine* is the primary site for digestion and absorption of fats, amino acids, proteins, carbohydrates, and vitamins. The small intestine is anatomically adapted to increase surface digestion and absorption due to folds of mucosa lined with villi and the brush-border membrane. The brush border contains digestive enzymes and contributes to the transfer of nutrients and electrolytes. The epithelial absorptive cells are called *enterocytes*. Glutamine (amino acid) stimulates the proliferation of enterocytes. The gastrointestinal (GI) tract continuously renews the cells lining its surface.

    a. The *duodenum* is the primary site for the absorption of iron, trace metals, and water-soluble vitamins.

    b. The *jejunum* is the principal absorption site for proteins and sugar carbohydrates. Ninety percent of nutrients and 50% of water and electrolytes are absorbed here.

    c. The *ileum* is responsible for absorption of bile salts and vitamin B_{12}. The ileocecal valve controls the entry of digested material from the ileum into the large intestine and prevents reflux into the small intestine. Digestion in the ileum continues by the action of pancreatic enzymes, intestinal enzymes, and bile salts. Carbohydrates are broken down into monosaccharides and disaccharides and are absorbed by villous capillaries. Proteins are degraded to peptides and amino acids and are absorbed by villous capillaries. Fats are emulsified and reduced to fatty acids and monoglycerides.

5. *Large Intestine.* The anatomic segments of the colon or large intestine include the cecum, ascending colon, transverse colon, descending colon, sigmoid colon, and rectum. Water and electrolytes are reabsorbed in the descending colon. Feces are stored in the rectum. The greatest growth of anaerobic and gram-negative aerobic bacteria is in the ascending colon. *Bacteroides fragilis* (anaerobic) and *Escherichia coli* (aerobic) play a role in metabolizing bile salts and synthesizing vitamins.

6. *Pancreas.* The pancreas's exocrine function is to secrete bicarbonate and enzymes (e.g., amylase, lipase) for digestion and absorption of fats, carbohydrates, and proteins. The pancreas's endocrine function involves islet cells, which function in glucose homeostasis by synthesizing and secreting insulin.

7. *Liver*

  a. *Liver functions* include the following:

    i. Formation of clotting (coagulation) factors I, II, V, VII, IX, X, and XI

    ii. Synthesis of plasma proteins (albumin, fibrinogen, and 60%–80% of globulins)

    iii. Synthesis and transportation of bile (bile salts, pigment, and cholesterol)

    iv. Storage of glycogen, fat, and fat-soluble vitamins

    v. Metabolism of fats, carbohydrates, and proteins

    vi. Metabolism and deactivation of bilirubin, ammonia, and many toxins by oxidation or conjugation reactions

  b. Three fourths of the blood supply to the liver is supplied by the *portal venous system* (blood rich in nutrients) and one fourth by the hepatic artery (blood rich in oxygen).

  c. *Nutrients* are absorbed from the GI tract and transported by either the portal or lymphatic circulation. The lymphatic system plays a pivotal role in transporting lipid-soluble substances.

8. *Biliary Tree and Gallbladder.* The biliary tree serves as the conduit for bile flow from the liver to the duodenum. The gallbladder provides a storage and concentration site for bile.

9. *Splanchnic Circulation.* The splanchnic circulation supplies blood to the stomach, small intestine, and colon. It receives one fourth of the body's cardiac output. The major arterial branches are the celiac, superior mesenteric, and inferior mesenteric. Venous drainage from the stomach, pancreas, small intestine, and colon flows to the portal vein to the liver and then to the heart through the hepatic vein and inferior vena cava.

B. Regulation of Fluid and Electrolyte Movement

  1. Large volumes of water, electrolytes, proteins, and bile salts are secreted and reabsorbed throughout the GI tract, resulting in massive fluid and electrolyte shifts.

  2. Fluid and electrolyte movement occur concurrently with digestion and absorption of nutrients.

CLINICAL ASSESSMENT OF THE GI SYSTEM

A. General Principles of Abdominal Assessment

Examination of the abdomen can be difficult in a child. A frightened child will not cooperate with the examination. A child suffering from multisystem trauma will be unable to localize pain. The preferred order of assessment is inspection, auscultation, palpation, and percussion.

B. Abdominal Examination Assessment Techniques

  1. *Inspection.* Evaluate for size, contour, symmetry, integrity, visible peristalsis, umbilicus, masses, and wounds. Underdeveloped abdominal musculature in children allows easier visualization of masses and fluid waves. Abdominal distention (the abdomen is normally rounded in infants and toddlers) is the hallmark sign of obstruction.

  2. *Auscultation*

    a. Determine the absence, presence, and character of peristalsis or bowel sounds (borborygmi). Bowel sounds are absent in paralytic ileus and peritonitis. A venous hum heard over the upper area of the abdomen suggests portal obstruction. A bruit (caused by turbulent blood flow through a partially occluded artery) suggests abnormal blood flow caused by an arteriovenous malformation (AVM) or aneurysm. High-pitched or hyperactive bowel sounds suggest an obstruction.

    b. Bowel sounds should be heard every 5 to 30 seconds. Listen to all four quadrants for a few minutes to confirm the presence or absence of bowel sounds.

  3. *Palpation.* Begin with light palpation and assess for guarding and tenderness. Consider using the diaphragm of your stethoscope with a focus on the child's face when palpating to asses for pain. With deep palpation, assess for abdominal tone, masses, pulsations, fluid, and organ enlargement. The liver is normally palpated at the right costal margin (RCM) or is nonpalpable. Palpation should be started by the iliac crest to ensure hepatomegaly is appreciated. The spleen is not normally palpable.

4. *Percussion.* Percussion is used to estimate the size of organs and aids in the diagnosis of ascites, obstruction, and peritonitis. Assess for abdominal distention, fluid, masses, or organ enlargement. Percussion of solid organs (liver and spleen) and ascites elicits dullness. Absence of dullness over the liver may be found with free air in the abdomen secondary to perforation. The stomach is tympanic when empty. Depending on contents, the intestines' tone is hyperresonant to tympanic.

C. Developmental Considerations

1. The abdominal wall is less muscular in the infant and toddler, making the abdominal organs easier

to palpate. In the infant, the liver can be palpated 1 to 2 cm below the RCM at the midclavicular line.

2. In younger children, the contour of the abdomen is protuberant because of immature abdominal musculature. After 4 years of age, the abdomen is no longer protuberant when the child is in a supine position; but, because of lumbar lordosis, the abdomen remains protuberant when the child stands.

INVASIVE AND NONINVASIVE DIAGNOSTIC STUDIES

There are numerous laboratory and radiologic diagnostic studies that are obtained for children with a GI disorder. Common laboratory abnormalities for liver disease are summarized in Table 7.1. Diagnostic studies commonly used to determine GI disease are summarized in Table 7.2.

TABLE 7.1 Liver Function Tests

LFT	Function	Pediatric Reference Value	Changes With Liver Failure
ALT	ALT catalyzes the reversible transfer of an amino group between the amino acid alanine and α-glutamic acid.	<37 IU/L	ALT initially increases with cell destruction. Following cell necrosis, enzyme level peaks and then decreases. It may be an ominous sign if the enzyme level peaks and falls rapidly. ALT is more hepatic specific as compared to AST. Isolated increases are characteristic of hepatitis.
AST	AST catalyzes the reversible transfer of the amino group between the amino acid aspartate and α-ketoglutamic acid.	<34 IU/L	AST initially increases with cell destruction. Following cell necrosis, enzyme level peaks and then decreases. It is an ominous sign if the enzyme level peaks and falls rapidly. Isolated increases are characteristic of hepatitis.
ALP	ALP cleaves phosphates from compounds with a single phosphate group. The hepatic isoenzymes are believed to be largely derived from the epithelium of the intrahepatic bile ducts, rather than from hepatocytes.	Newborn: <310 IU/L 1 mo–1 y: <360 IU/L 1–10 y: <290 IU/L 10–15 y: <400 IU/L >15 y: <110 IU/L	ALP levels increase with inflammation or obstruction of the hepatobiliary tract.

(continued)

TABLE 7.1   Liver Function Tests *(continued)*

LFT	Function	Pediatric Reference Value	Changes With Liver Failure
GGTP	GGTP is an isoenzyme of ALP. GGTP catalyzes the transfer of glutamyl groups among peptidase and amino acids.	<120 IU/L	Hepatobiliary causes should be considered with increased levels. Significantly increased levels reflect hepatobiliary obstruction, whereas moderately elevated levels may suggest hepatocellular destruction.
Bilirubin	Bilirubin is a by-product of the heme portion of the breakdown of the hemoglobin molecule. Fat-soluble bilirubin binds to albumin as indirect bilirubin for transport to the liver. In the liver, fat-soluble bilirubin is detached from the albumin and conjugated with glucuronic acid, rendering it water soluble. Direct bilirubin is excreted into the hepatic ducts and eventually into the intestinal tract.	Total bilirubin Newborn: 1–12 mg/dL; Child: 0.2–1.3 mg/dL Direct: 0.1–1.3 mg/dL Indirect: 0.1–1.3 mg/dL	Increased indirect bilirubin levels occur as the liver is unable to conjugate the bilirubin with impaired synthetic function or in the presence of an excessive load of bilirubin in cases of hemolysis. Impaired excretion of direct bilirubin into the bile ducts or biliary tract results in increased levels of direct bilirubin with increased amounts absorbed into the blood. Impaired synthetic function and obstruction increase total bilirubin levels.
PT	PT is the laboratory measure of the time for a fibrin clot to form after tissue thromboplastin (factor III) and calcium are added to the sample. PT allows for clinical evaluation of the extrinsic clotting cascade.	10.5–13.5 sec	A prolonged PT reflects poor utilization of vitamin K due to parenchymal disease or low levels of vitamin K due to obstructive jaundice. With clinical hepatic failure, the failure of the PT to respond after the administration of IV vitamin K reflects significant parenchymal injury.
Albumin	Albumin is the major circulating plasma protein responsible for maintaining plasma oncotic pressure. Albumin levels reflect a component of liver synthetic function.	3.8–5.4 mg/dL	The half-life of albumin is 21 days; therefore, hypoalbuminemia is present with chronic hepatic failure. Interpret with caution, as protein intake and albumin administration may alter the albumin level.
Ammonia	Ammonia is formed from the deamination of amino acids during protein metabolism and is a by-product of the breakdown of colonic bacteria proteins.	Newborn: 50–84 mcg/dL Child: 12–38 mcg/dL	Increased ammonia levels reflect decreased synthetic function. Elevated ammonia levels can occur in the presence of acute or chronic hepatic failure. Elevated ammonia levels may alter neurologic status.

ALP, alkaline phosphatase; ALT, alanine aminotransferase; AST, aspartate aminotransferase; GGTP, γ-glutamyl transpeptidase; LFT, liver function test; PT, prothrombin time.

Source: Adapted from Martin, S. A. (1992). The ABCs of pediatric LFTs. *Journal of Pediatric Nursing, 18*(5), 445–449.

TABLE 7.2   Common Diagnostic Studies for GI Disorders

Procedure	Purpose	Disorder
Abdominal x-ray		
Flat plate Cross table lateral Lateral decubitus	Evaluate organ size, position, gas patterns, air–fluid levels, presence of free air, position of NG or NJ tube	Bowel obstruction, perforation, ileus, NEC
Fluoroscopy		
Barium swallow	Examine the integrity of the esophagus, diagnoses structural abnormalities	Esophageal or strictures, GE reflux
Upper GI series	Examine the esophagus, stomach, and duodenum; diagnose structural abnormalities; delayed gastric emptying	
Upper GI with small bowel follow-through	Same as upper GI with follow-up films of esophagus to small intestine	Small bowel disorders, malrotation, small bowel structure
Endoscopy		
Flexible upper endoscopy	Directly visualize upper GI mucosa, diagnose lesions, determine source of bleeding	Esophageal varices, severe gastritis
Endoscopic retrograde cholangiopancreatography	Directly visualize the biliary and pancreatic ducts	Pseudocyst, gallstones, pancreatitis
Flexible colonoscopy	Directly visualize mucosa of large intestine, diagnose mucosal injury, bleeding source	Polyp, inflammatory bowel disease
Biopsy		
Percutaneous liver biopsy	Obtain liver specimens	Biliary atresia, hepatitis
Nuclear scans		
HIDA scan	Determine liver excretory function	Biliary atresia
Meckel scan	Evaluate location of bleeding (radioactive isotope is taken up by parietal cells)	Meckel's diverticulum
Other scans		
Abdominal ultrasound	Visualize organ structure, suspected appendicitis, intussusception, pyloric stenosis	Liver disease, trauma in unstable child (FAST scan), pancreatitis
Abdominal CT scan with contrast	Evaluate for vascular disorders; definitive imaging of solid organs; evaluate for infection, abscess, traumatic injury, appendicitis	Organ trauma, liver disease, pancreatitis, pseudocyst
MRI	Definitively image abdominal organs in stable child	Hepatic hemangioma, hepatic AVM, appendicitis

AVM, arteriovenous malformation; FAST, focused abdominal sonography for trauma; GE, gastroesophageal; GI, gastrointestinal; HIDA, hepatobilliary iminodiacetic acid; NEC, necrotizing enterocolitis; NG, nasogastric; NJ, nasojejunal.

Source: Modified from Simone, S. (2001). Gastrointestinal critical care problems. In M. A. Q. Curley & P. A. Moloney-Harmon (Eds.), *Critical care nursing of infants and children* (2nd ed., pp. 765–804). Philadelphia, PA: WB Saunders.

PHARMACOLOGY

A. Antibleeding Agents

1. *Vasopressin* (Pitressin; Taketomo, Hodding, & Kraus, 2015)

   a. *Action.* Vasopressin is a nonselective, short-acting vasoconstrictor. It decreases splanchnic blood flow and portal hypertension.

   b. *Uses.* Used to treat acute massive GI hemorrhage.

   c. *Dosage.* Continuous intravenous (IV) infusion. Initial 0.002 to 0.005 units/kg/min; double as needed every 30 minutes to a maximum of 0.01 units/kg/min. If bleeding stops for 12 hours, taper the infusion off over 24 to 48 hours.

   d. *Side effects* include hypertension, bradycardia, arrhythmias, wheezing, bronchospasm, abdominal cramping, vomiting, water intoxication, decreased urine output, hyponatremia, decreased platelet count, and hemorrhage.

2. *Octreotide Acetate* (Sandostatin; Taketomo et al., 2015)

   a. *Action.* Decreases splanchnic blood flow; inhibits gastrin synthesis and gastric acid output.

   b. *Uses.* Used to treat GI hemorrhage and intractable diarrhea. This agent has been used for the treatment of chylothorax. Sandostatin is used when conservative treatment fails.

   c. *Dosage.* Administer 1 to 2 mcg/kg IV bolus; infusion rate 1 to 2 mcg/kg/hr IV for GI hemorrhage, titrating the rate to response. Continuous IV infusion following a bolus dose of 1 mcg/kg followed by 1 mcg/kg/hr. Dosage of 1 to 10 mcg/kg every 12 hours (IV, subcutaneous [SC] administration) is used for intractable diarrhea. Dose reductions are recommended for patients with renal failure.

   d. *Side effects* include bradycardia, chest pain, hypertension, abdominal pain, nausea, diarrhea, headache, fat malabsorption, hypoglycemia or hyperglycemia, hypothyroidism, and possible anaphylactic shock. The incidence of gallstones and biliary sludge is approximately 33% in children receiving the medication for more than 12 months.

3. *Vitamin K1, Phytonadione* (AquaMEPHYTON, mephyton; Taketomo et al., 2015)

   a. *Action.* Provides vitamin K activity and can be used as a cofactor in the liver synthesis of clotting factors II, VII, IX, and X; however, the mechanism of stimulation is unknown.

   b. *Uses.* Prevents and treats hypoprothrombinemia caused by malabsorption, drug- or anticoagulant-induced vitamin K deficiency.

   c. *Dosage.* Note: Dosing presented is for GI-specific diseases for which supplementation is needed and is based on international normalized ratio (INR).

     i. Biliary atresia. Infants 1 to 6 months old: INR more than 1.2 to 1.5: 2.5 mg PO QD (orally every day). INR more than 1.5 to 1.8 initial 2 to 5 mg intramuscular (IM) once followed by 2.5 mg PO once daily. INR more than 1.8 initial 2 to 5 mg IM followed by 5 mg PO once daily.

     ii. Cholestasis. Infants, child, and adolescents: administer 2.4 to 15 mg/d PO.

     iii. Liver disease. Infants, child and adolescents: administer 2.5 to 5 mg/d PO.

   d. *Side effects* include a transient flushing reaction, rare hypotension, hypertension, rare dizziness, rash, and urticaria. U.S. boxed warning: Severe reactions resembling anaphylaxis have occurred during and immediately after IV administration. IV administration should be used when other routes of administration are not feasible and the benefits outweigh the risks.

B. Antiulcer/Gastroesophageal Reflux Disease Agents

1. *Cimetidine* (Tagamet; Slaughter, Stenger, Reagan, & Jadcherla, 2016; Stark & Nylund, 2016; Taketomo et al., 2015)

   a. *Action.* A histamine-2 receptor antagonist (H_2 blocker) that decreases the secretion of acid.

   b. *Uses.* Used for short-term treatment of active duodenal ulcers and gastric ulcers, gastroesophageal reflux disease (GERD), or for long-term prophylaxis and prevention of upper GI tract bleeding.

   c. *Dosage.* Neonate: administer 5 to 10 mg/kg daily PO in divided doses every 6 to 12 hours. Infant: administer 10 to 20 mg/kg daily PO in divided doses every 6 to 12 hours. Child: administer 20 to 40 mg/kg daily PO in divided doses every 6 hours. Dose reductions are recommended for patients with renal impairment.

   d. *Side effects* include bradycardia, tachycardia, hypotension, diarrhea, nausea, vomiting, dizziness, headache, agitation, gynecomastia, elevated serum creatinine, elevated aspartate aminotransferase (AST) and alanine aminotransferase (ALT), neutropenia, pancytopenia, and thrombocytopenia.

e. *Additional warnings.* The use of H$_2$ blockers and proton-pump inhibitors (PPIs) has been associated with increased incidence of gastroenteritis and community-acquired pneumonia in children (Stark & Nylund, 2016). In neonates, there is an associated increased incidence of infectious complications and necrotizing enterocolitis (NEC; Slaughter et al., 2016).

2. *Ranitidine* (Zantac; Slaughter et al., 2016; Stark & Nylund, 2016; Taketomo et al., 2015)

a. *Action.* A histamine-2 receptor antagonist that decreases the secretion of acid.

b. *Uses.* Used for short-term treatment of active peptic ulcer disease, GERD, or long-term prophylaxis and prevention of hypersecretory states and bleeding.

c. *Dosage.* GI bleed or stress ulcer prophylaxis. Infant: administer 2 to 6 mg/kg daily via IV divided every 8 hours. Child and adolescents: administer 3 to 6 mg/kg daily via IV, divided every 6 hours, for a maximum of 300 mg daily; 0.15 to 0.5 mg/kg/dose for one dose followed by 0.08 to 0.2 mg/kg/hr continuous IV infusion. GERD dosing is 5 to 10 mg kg/d divided twice daily; maximum daily dose is 300 mg daily. Dose reduction is recommended for patients with renal impairment.

d. *Side effects* include bradycardia (rapid IV administration), tachycardia, agitation, headache, dizziness, nausea, vomiting, elevated serum creatinine, hepatitis, arthralgia, leukopenia, and thrombocytopenia.

e. *Additional warnings.* The use of H$_2$ blockers and PPIs has been associated with increased incidence of gastroenteritis and community-acquired pneumonia in children (Stark & Nylund, 2016). In neonates, there is an associated increased incidence of infectious complications and NEC (Slaughter et al., 2016).

3. *Famotidine* (Pepcid; Slaughter et al., 2016; Stark & Nylund, 2016; Taketomo et al., 2015)

a. *Action.* A histamine-2 receptor antagonist that decreases the secretion of acid.

b. *Uses.* Used in therapy and treatment of peptic ulcer disease, GERD, and hypersecretory states.

c. *Dosage.* GERD: In infants, administer 0.5 to 1 mg/kg daily PO up to 8 weeks or 0.25 to 0.5 mg/

kg daily via IV. In children and adolescent dosing is 0.25 to 0.5 mg/kg/dose every 12 hours up to 20 mg/dose. Stress ulcer prophylaxis: In infants, children, and adolescents, administer 0.5 to 1 mg/kg/dose every 12 hours, with a maximum dose of 20 mg/dose. Dose reductions are recommended for patients with renal impairment.

d. *Side effects* include arrhythmias, tachycardia, headache, dizziness, constipation, diarrhea, thrombocytopenia, and pancytopenia.

e. *Additional warnings.* The use of H$_2$ blockers and PPIs has been associated with increased incidence of gastroenteritis and community-acquired pneumonia in children (Stark & Nylund, 2016). In neonates, there is an associated increased incidence of infectious complications and NEC (Slaughter et al., 2016).

4. *Omeprazole* (Prilosec; Slaughter et al., 2016; Stark & Nylund, 2016; Taketomo et al., 2015)

a. *Action.* PPI; direct inhibitor of hydrochloric acid secretions at the cellular level. It demonstrates antimicrobial activity against *Helicobacter pylori*.

b. *Uses.* Used for short-term treatment (4–8 weeks) of severe erosive esophagitis and severe GERD and duodenal ulcer disease associated with *H. pylori*.

c. *Dosage.* GERD: In infants, administer 0.7 mg/kg/dose daily PO; for children greater than or equal to 1 year and adolescents 5 kg to less than 10 kg, administer 5 mg Q day PO; 10 kg to less than 20 kg, 10 mg Q day PO; greater than or equal to 20 kg, 20 mg Q day PO; Erosive esophagitis: 5 kg to less than 10 kg, administer 5 mg Q day PO; 10 kg to less than 20 kg, 10 mg Q day PO; greater than or equal to 20 kg, 20 mg Q day PO. *H. pylori* eradication: administer 1 to 2 mg/kg/d divided into two doses; maximum single dose of 20 mg. The capsule form of the medication is a sustained-release capsule. The capsule can be opened and the beads mixed with an acidic medium such as 1 tablespoon of applesauce. The tablets of medication should *not* be crushed. The manufacturer suggests using the suspension for administration in a nasogastric (NG) tube.

d. *Side effects* include bradycardia, tachycardia, nausea, diarrhea, abdominal cramps, headache, dizziness, skin rash, elevated liver enzymes, hypomagnesemia, proteinuria, skin rash, and thrombocytopenia.

e. *Additional warnings.* The use of H$_2$ blockers and PPIs has been associated with increased incidence of gastroenteritis and community-acquired pneumonia in children (Stark & Nylund, 2016). In neonates, there is an associated increased incidence of infectious complications and NEC (Slaughter et al., 2016).

5. *Pantoprazole* (Protonix; Slaughter et al., 2016; Stark & Nylund, 2016; Taketomo et al., 2015)

a. *Action.* In PPI, pantoprazole is a direct inhibitor of hydrochloric acid secretions at the cellular level. This PPI more directly inhibits acid secretion compared with other PPIs. It demonstrates antimicrobial activity against *H. pylori.*

b. *Uses.* Used to treat GERD (Food and Drug Administration [FDA] approved in ages ≥5 years), pathological hypersecretory conditions, and as an adjunct to duodenal ulcer treatment associated with *H. pylori.*

c. *Dosage.* GERD: Infants and children younger than 5 years, administer 1.2 mg/kg/d daily for 4 weeks; children 5 to 11 years, 20 or 40 mg PO daily; children and adolescents, 20 or 40 mg once daily. For gastric acid suppression when PO administration is not appropriate or tolerated, the dose is 0.8 or 1.6 mg IV once daily, maximum dose 80 mg.

d. *Side effects* include hypotension, hypertension, headache, urticaria, pruritus, hyperglycemia, hypermagnesemia, nausea, vomiting, diarrhea, constipation, urinary frequency, elevated liver enzymes, elevated triglyceride levels, cough, and dyspnea. Anaphylaxis has been reported with IV administration.

e. *Additional warnings.* The use of H_2 blockers and PPIs has been associated with increased incidence of gastroenteritis and community-acquired pneumonia in children (Stark & Nylund, 2016). In neonates, there is an associated increased incidence of infectious complications and NEC (Slaughter et al., 2016).

6. *Lansoprazole* (FIRST-Lansoprazole; Slaughter et al., 2016; Stark & Nylund, 2016; Taketomo et al., 2015)

a. *Action.* PPI; acts as a direct inhibitor of hydrochloric acid secretion at the cellular level.

b. *Uses.* For short-term treatment of symptomatic GERD (up to 8 weeks; FDA approved for ≥1 year); for duodenal ulcer treatment associated with *H. pylori*, erosive esophagitis, and hypersecretory conditions.

c. *Dosage.* GERD: Infants 1 to 2 mg/kg/d for weight-based dosing; for fixed dosing in infants older than 3 months, administer 7.5 mg twice a day or 15 mg daily; children 1 to 11 years

who weigh less than or equal to 30 kg, 15 mg daily for up to 12 weeks; children greater than 30 kg, 30 mg daily for up to 12 weeks; children 12 years or older, 15 mg once daily for up to 8 weeks.

d. *Side effects* include hypertension, hypotension, nausea, dyspepsia, abdominal pain, diarrhea, constipation, elevated liver enzymes, dizziness, and headache.

e. *Additional warnings.* The use of H_2 blockers and PPIs has been associated with increased incidence of gastroenteritis and community-acquired pneumonia in children (Stark & Nylund, 2016). In neonates, there is an associated increased incidence of infectious complications and NEC (Slaughter et al., 2016).

7. *Sucralfate* (Carafate; Taketomo et al., 2015)

a. *Action.* Gastric protectant; paste formation and ulcer adhesion occur within 1 to 2 hours of administration and last up to 6 hours.

b. *Uses.* Used for short-term management of duodenal ulcers and gastritis; typically may be used for esophageal, gastric, and rectal erosions.

c. *Dosage.* Dose is not established; administer 40 to 80 mg/kg/d PO in divided doses every 6 hours. Administer 1 hour before meals or on an empty stomach.

d. *Side effects* include constipation and rarely, anaphylaxis, bezoar formation, and hypersensitivity. Decreased absorption of concurrently administered drugs may occur. Safety and efficacy in children have not been established.

8. *Calcium Carbonate* (Maalox; Taketomo et al., 2015)

a. *Action.* Maalox is an antacid that neutralizes gastric acid.

b. *Uses.* Provides symptomatic relief for peptic ulcer, gastritis, esophagitis, hiatal hernia, and treatment of hyperphosphatemia in end-stage renal failure.

c. *Dosage.* In children 2 to 5 years, administer one tablet (400 mg calcium carbonate) as symptoms occur (not to exceed 3 tablets/d); children older than 5 years to 11 years, two tablets (800 mg) as symptoms occur (not to exceed 6 tablets/d); children older than 11 years, two to four tablets as symptoms occur (not to exceed 15 tablets/d).

d. *Side effects* include headache, laxative effect, hypercalcemia, and hypophosphatemia.

C. Prokinetics

1. *Metoclopramide* (Reglan; Taketomo et al., 2015)

   a. *Action.* A potent dopamine receptor antagonist that blocks dopamine receptors in the chemoreceptor trigger zone, preventing emesis; accelerates gastric emptying and intestinal transit time.

   b. *Uses.* For GERD, prevention of postoperative and chemotherapy-related nausea and vomiting, assist with postpyloric feeding tube placement, and diabetic gastroparesis.

   c. *Dosage.* Postpyloric feeding tube placement: In children younger than 6 years, administer 0.1 mg/kg once; 6 to 14 years, give 2.5 to 5 mg as a single dose; and older than 14 years, administer 10 mg as a single dose. GERD: In infants, children, and adolescents, administer 0.1 to 0.2 mg/kg/dose every 6 to 8 hours with a maximum dose of 10 mg.

   d. *Side effects* include extrapyramidal reactions, seizures, hypertension, hypotension, atrioventricular block, constipation, diarrhea, neutropenia, and leukopenia.

2. *Erythromycin* (E.E.S.; Taketomo et al., 2015)

   a. *Action.* Works as a motilin receptor agonist and increases LES tone.

   b. *Uses.* A macrolide antibiotic that can be used as a prokinetic agent.

   c. *Dosage.* In children, an initial dose of 3 mg/kg QID (four times a day) PO.

   d. *Side effects* include QTc prolongation, ventricular arrhythmias, bradycardia, skin rash, abdominal pain, nausea, vomiting, diarrhea, eosinophilia, and cholestatic jaundice.

D. Antidiarrheal Agents

1. *Imodium* (Loperamide; Taketomo et al., 2015)

   a. *Action.* Acts directly on the intestinal muscles through the opioid receptor to inhibit peristalsis and transit time. The drug reduces stool volume, causes decreased fluid and electrolyte losses, and demonstrates antisecretory activity.

   b. *Uses.* Used for treatment of acute diarrhea (FDA approved in children ≥2 years) although manufacturer recommends avoiding use in children younger than 2 years as acute enteritis often necessitates treatment of fluid and electrolyte imbalances; for chronic diarrhea associated with inflammatory bowel disease and intestinal failure, and to decrease volume of ileostomy output.

   c. *Dosage.* Acute diarrhea: In children 2 to 5 years weighing 13 to less than 21 kg, a dose of 1 mg after each subsequent loose stool, with dose repeated for each subsequent stool for a maximum of 3 mg/d; children 6 to 8 years weighing 21 to 27 kg, administer 2 mg for first loose stool, with 1 mg/dose repeated for each subsequent stool for a maximum of 4 mg/d; children 9 to 11 years weighing 27.1 to 43 kg, administer 2 mg for first loose stool, with 1 mg/dose repeated for each subsequent stool for a maximum of 6 mg/d; children older than 12 years, 4 mg for first loose stool, with 2 mg/dose repeated for each subsequent stool for a maximum of 8 mg/d. For chronic diarrhea related to intestinal failure or other noninfectious causes, larger doses are generally needed. Dosing initial 1 to 1.5 mg/kg/d in four divided doses with final dose range up to 0.5 mg/kg BID (twice a day).

   d. *Side effects* include dizziness, abdominal cramping, and constipation.

2. *Clonidine* (Catapres; Fragkos, Zárate-Lopez, & Frangos, 2016; Taketomo et al., 2015)

   a. *Action.* Stimulates α_2-adrenoreceptors in the brainstem resulting in decreased sympathetic outflow.

   b. *Uses.* Use to decrease GI losses in children with stomas related to the constipating side effect of the medication. Other more established uses include treatment of hypertension and use for withdrawal prophylaxis.

   c. *Dosage.* For GI use, patches have been used in dosing of 0.1 to 0.3 mg/24 hr with patches changed weekly.

   d. *Side effects* include hypotension, cardiac arrhythmia, agitation, constipation, diarrhea, and abnormal hepatic function tests.

E. Other Agents

1. *Lactulose* (Cephulac; Taketomo et al., 2015)

   a. *Action.* Hyperosmotic laxative; ammonia detoxicant.

   b. *Uses.* Used to prevent and treat portal-systemic encephalopathy. This treatment is controversial because the benefit of this therapy can be diminished relative to potential fluid and electrolyte disturbances.

   c. *Dosage.* For infants, administer 2.5 to 10 mL/d PO divided three or four times per day. In children, 40 to 90 mL/d PO divided three to four times per day. Adjust dosage to produce two to three stools per day.

d. *Side effects* include abdominal discomfort, diarrhea, nausea, and vomiting.

2. *Magnesium Hydroxide* (Milk of Magnesia; Taketomo et al., 2015)

a. *Action.* An antacid that can be used as a cathartic or laxative for constipation.

b. *Uses.* Used for bowel evacuation and treatment of hyperacidity.

c. *Dosage.* When used as a laxative in children ages 2 to 5 years, administer 5 to 15 mL/d PO or in divided doses. In children ages 6 to 12 years, administer 15 to 30 mL/d PO or in divided doses. As an antacid, administer 2.5 to 5 mL PO as needed.

d. *Side effects* include hypotension, diarrhea, respiratory depression, and hypermagnesemia.

3. *Polyethylene Glycol-Electrolyte Solution* (GoLY-TELY; Taketomo et al., 2015)

a. *Action.* Induces catharsis with strong electrolyte and osmotic effects.

b. *Uses.* Used as a bowel preparation for procedures and for treatment of constipation.

c. *Dosage.* For bowel preparation, 25 mL/kg/hr PO/NG until rectal effluent is clear.

d. *Side effects* include metabolic acidosis, potential for electrolyte disturbances, nausea, cramps, and abdominal distension.

4. *Polyethylene Glycol 3350* (MiraLax)

a. *Action.* An osmotic agent, causes water retention in the stool.

b. *Uses.* Used to treat occasional constipation.

c. *Dosage.* For infants, children, and adolescents, administer 0.2 to 0.8 mg/kg/d; maximum daily dose of 17 g/d.

d. *Side effects* include metabolic acidosis, potential for electrolyte disturbances, nausea, cramps, and abdominal distension.

F. Immunosuppressive Therapy

1. *Basic Principles.* Combination therapy is used to maximize therapeutic benefit of agents while minimizing associated toxicities, including infection and malignancy. Institution of specific protocols and organ-specific therapies exist with goals of therapy to maintain sufficient drug levels to prevent rejection. Combination protocols are used to increase drug efficacy and minimize drug toxicity.

2. *Tacrolimus* (Prograf; Taketomo et al., 2015)

a. *Action.* A calcineurin inhibitor that suppresses the synthesis of interleukin-2, the cytokine needed for lymphocyte activation.

b. *Dosage.* Administer 0.01 to 0.06 mg/kg daily via a continuous IV infusion or 0.10 to 0.3 mg/kg daily PO in divided doses twice a day. Dosing is variable depending on the organ transplanted and may be based on drug levels. Patients with renal or hepatic impairment should receive dosing from the lower end of the dosing ranges.

c. *Side effects.* With IV use, greater toxicity is observed with a high anaphylaxis risk, including arrhythmias, hypertension, nephrotoxicity, central nervous system (CNS) effects (insomnia, headache, tremor, seizure, paresthesia), hyperkalemia, hypomagnesemia, hyperglycemia, GI tract symptoms, alopecia, and lymphoproliferative disease (LPD).

3. *Cyclosporine* (Sandimmune; Taketomo et al., 2015)

a. *Action.* A calcineurin inhibitor that binds to the intracellular protein cyclophilin that inhibits T-cell proliferation through inhibition of interleukin-2 synthesis.

b. *Dosage.* Note that there are modified and nonmodified formulations of this medication. Nonmodified: administer 2 to 10 mg/kg daily via IV in divided doses every 8 to 24 hours for maintenance; postoperatively, administer 5 to 15 mg/kg daily PO divided every 12 to 24 hours; maintenance dosing is usually 3 to 10 mg/kg/d. Dosing is variable depending on the organ transplanted and may be based on drug levels. The PO dose is approximately three times the IV dose.

c. *Side effects* include hypertension, nephrotoxicity, CNS toxicity (headache, tremor, seizure, paresthesia), hypomagnesemia, GI tract symptoms, gum hyperplasia, hirsutism, and LPD.

4. *Corticosteroids.* Methylprednisolone (Solu-Medrol) and Prednisone (Taketomo et al., 2015)

a. *Action.* An anti-inflammatory agent that depresses the immune system by decreasing T-lymphocytes and monocyte activation.

b. *Dosage*

i. Methylprednisolone. Administer 0.5 to 1.7 mg/kg daily via IV in divided doses every 6 to 12 hours.

ii. Prednisone. Administer 0.05 to 2 mg/kg daily PO in divided doses one to four times daily.

c. *Side effects* include glucose intolerance, hyperglycemia, possible suppression of the hypothalamic–pituitary–axis, peptic ulcers, weight gain, hypertension, hyperlipidemia, sodium and water retention, osteoporosis, infection, abnormal hair growth and thinning, and increased risk of bruising and acne.

5. *Mycophenolate Mofetil* (Cellcept; Taketomo et al., 2015)

a. *Action.* An antimetabolite that inhibits T- and B-cell proliferation by inhibiting the inosine monophosphate dehydrogenase pathway, preventing lymphocyte proliferation.

b. *Dosage.* Administer 600 mg/m^2/dose twice daily PO; maximum daily dose of 2,000 mg/d.

c. *Side effects* include hypertension, headache, rash, nausea, vomiting, dyspepsia, cough, leukopenia, neutropenia, thrombocytopenia, increased malignancy risk, and anemia. Females within child-bearing years must receive counseling on pregnancy risk and have a pregnancy test prior to starting therapy, 2 weeks after starting therapy, and at follow-up visits.

6. *Azathioprine* (Imuran; Taketomo et al., 2015)

a. *Action.* Azathioprine is an antimetabolite that inhibits DNA synthesis.

b. *Dosage.* Initial dose is 3 to 5 mg/kg daily administered either PO or IV. Maintenance is 1 to 3 mg/kg per day taken once daily.

c. *Side effects* include bone marrow suppression (anemia, leukopenia), hepatotoxicity, pancreatitis, nausea and vomiting, increased malignancy risk, and mucosal ulceration.

NUTRITIONAL CONCEPTS

A. Nutrition Assessment

1. *Pediatric Critical Care Best Practices*

a. Thirty-one percent of pediatric intensive care unit (PICU) patients in an international point prevalence survey of 31 PICUs were determined to be malnourished (Mehta et al., 2012).

i. Malnourished patients included both underweight and overweight children. There is greater morbidity and mortality in the underweight child as compared to the overweight child.

b. Within 48 hours of admission, children in the PICU should undergo a detailed nutrition assessment, including a detailed dietary history, identification of changes in anthropometry, functional status, and nutrition-focused physical exam (Mehta et al., 2017).

2. *Anthropometrics*

a. An accurate weight (kg), length (cm), and body mass index should be documented at admission. Serial weight measurement is recommended as weight loss is the best single physical exam indicator of malnutrition risk.

b. A head circumference should be obtained in children younger than 3 years old (Mehta et al., 2017).

c. The z-scores for body mass index should be used to screen for extreme values (weight for length <2 years) or weight for age (if an accurate height is not available; Mehta et al., 2017).

3. *Assessment of Energy Needs* (kcal/kg/d)

a. Energy requirements are highly individual and vary widely (Verger, 2014).

i. Energy needs are dynamic, changing from a hypermetabolic to hypometabolic state through the trajectory of the PICU stay, largely related to changes in energy consumption and limited energy reserves.

b. The Society of Critical Care Medicine and A.S.P.E.N. recommend assessment of measured energy expenditure (MEE) by indirect calorimetry (IC; Mehta et al., 2017).

c. If IC is not feasible, the Schofield or Food Agriculture Organization/World Health Organization (WHO)/United Nations University equations may be used without the addition of stress factors.

d. Often, the requirement is determined by reference standards based on age for healthy children (Table 7.3), which should not be used for critically ill children.

B. Macronutrient, Micronutrient, and Fluid Requirements

1. *Carbohydrate, protein, and fat are the macronutrients.*

a. Recommended caloric distribution varies and for carbohydrates is 40% to 70%, protein is 7% to 21%, and for fat is 30% to 55%.

TABLE 7.3   Daily Estimated Energy Needs for Healthy Infants and Children

Age	kcal/kg/d
Up to 6 months	90–110
6–12 months	80–100
12–36 months	75–90
4–6 years	65–75
7–10 years	55–75
11–18 years	40–55

i.   A minimum protein intake of 1.5 mg/kg/d is recommended (Mehta et al., 2017).

ii. For obese patients, this guideline should be based on ideal body weight (Mehta et al., 2017).

b. Diets high in carbohydrates can increase carbon dioxide product and hamper ventilator weaning.

2. Micronutrients include vitamins, minerals, and electrolytes.

3. Fluid requirements vary as a function of age, weight, and clinical condition.

a. Calculation of maintenance fluids is used as a starting requirement for most children.

i.   First 10 kg (1–10 kg): 100 mL/kg

ii. Next 10 kg (11–20 kg): 50 mL/kg

iii. Over 20 kg (>20 kg): 20 to 25 mL/kg

iv. For a 10-kg child, the fluid requirement is a 1,000 mL a day, or 40 mL/hr.

C. Enteral Nutrition

1. Enteral route is preferred and should be used if at all possible and determined within 24 to 48 hours of admission (Mehta et al., 2017).

a. Promotes intestinal mucosal structure and gut absorptive and barrier functions (e.g., villi).

b. Is associated with fewer infectious and metabolic complications.

2. Estimated energy needs are greater for enteral feeds as all parenteral nutrition (PN) calories are directly absorbed. Most infants require 100 to 120 kcal/kg/d.

3. *Formula Selection*

a. Breast milk (BM) is the preferred source of nutrition for infants, nursing mothers should be provided with a breast pump if their infant is on NPO (nothing by mouth) status or cannot breastfeed. Selection of the appropriate formula is based on the patient's age and disease process (e.g., less protein may be needed in children with liver or renal disease). Premature infants require specialty formulas that are higher in calories per ounce and have additional vitamins and minerals.

4. Formulas have varying caloric density kcal/ounce.

a. Infants require 19 to 20 kcal/ounce, may increase to 24 kcal/ounce, 27 kcal/ounce, or 30 kcal/ounce for fluid restriction or to promote weight gain.

b. Children older than 12 months require 30 kcal/ounce formula.

c. For children younger than 12 months with poor weight gain, consider 45 kcal/ounce.

5. Enteral feeds can be administered orally, through an orogastric (OG)/NG tube, gastrostomy tube, or postpylorically through a gastrojejunostomy or jejunostomy tube.

6. Enteral nutrition is needed if the child has delayed gastric motility, intestinal dysmotility, or inability to tolerate gastric feeds or is at high risk for aspiration.

D. Parenteral Nutrition

1. An IV mixture of macronutrients (carbohydrates [dextrose or glucose], protein, and fat), and micronutrients (electrolytes, minerals, vitamins, and trace elements) for children that are unable to absorb nutrients through the GI tract.

a. Dextrose provides 3.4 kcal/g and constitutes 60% to 70% of the total PN caloric composition.

b. Protein can be administered as trophamine (recommended for infants younger than 1 year and for children with liver failure), or as clinisol or travasol (for children older than 1 year of age). Protein provides 4 kcal/g and should constitute up to 14% to 20% of the total PN caloric composition.

c. Fat emulsions (intralipid) may be administered as a separate solution to provide a major source of calories (20% solution provides 2 kcal/mL) and should constitute 30% to 50% of the total PN caloric intake. Providing 0.5 g/kg/d prevents essential fatty acid deficiency states.

d. Electrolytes, vitamins, minerals, and trace elements are added to these solutions to meet the child's known nutritional requirements.

2. PN can be administered through a peripheral or central line.

a. Formulations with a dextrose concentration greater than 12.5% should be administered centrally.

3. Common additives to the PN formulation include heparin, if central access is being used, and Ranitidine, if GI prophylaxis is indicated.

4. PN formulations can be commercial standard solutions or compounded individualized admixtures.

5. With PN, caloric needs are decreased by 10% to 15%, as compared to the enteral route.

6. PN "goals" are generally not achieved for 5 days, as macronutrients should gradually be advanced.

a. Possible alternatives to prescribing PN are to augment the child's nutrition by using dextrose 10% in water (D10W) and intralipids.

7. The Society of Critical Care Medicine and A.S.P.E.N. recommend not starting PN within the first 24 hours of PICU admission (Mehta et al., 2017). When PN should be initiated is not known and should be individualized and started within the first week of admission if unable to receive enteral nutrition (EN) or for severely malnourished patients or those at risk for nutritional deterioration (Mehta et al., 2017).

8. Complications of PN administration include bacteremia if central line is present, catheter-associated central line infection (central line-associated bloodstream infection [CLABSI]), metabolic derangement, and cholestatic jaundice.

NURSING MANAGEMENT OF TUBES AND DRAINS

A. NG Tube

1. An NG tube can be used for gastric decompression, feeds, fluids administration, and medication administration or for lavage in case of poisonings or GI hemorrhage.

2. The child's size and indication for NG placement will determine the size and type of tube that should be inserted.

a. Generally, smaller bore nonvented tubes are used for feeding.

b. Tubes used for decompression should not be used for feeds or medication administration as the necessary decompression ports may be too distal in the esophagus to safety administer feeds or medication. Do not tie off or obstruct the vent to prevent the backflow of gastric contents as this will block the vent and negate the function of the sump port.

3. See Table 7.4 for suggested steps for placing an NG tube.

4. Abdominal radiography is the most reliable method of confirming placement of an enteral tube; however, its use to verify enteral tube placement is not widespread in clinical practice due to the necessary radiation exposure (Lyman et al., 2016; Taylor, 2013). Evidence suggests that pH testing of GI secretions is the most accurate nonradiographic means of determining placement of an NG tube, although results are not 100% reliable (Gilbertson, Rogers, & Ukoumunne, 2011). Gastric aspirate has a pH of 5 or less and is usually grassy green or clear and colorless, with off-white to tan shreds of mucus (Irving et al., 2014; Taylor, 2013).

5. Nursing care involves adequately securing the tube to prevent inadvertent dislodgement, verifying position prior to use (if placement is in question radiologic verification is needed), flushing the tube after instilling medications or formula; if the tube is to be placed to suction, low intermittent suction should be used to minimize trauma to the gastric mucosa, recording input and output

TABLE 7.4 Nasogastric Tube Placement

1. Elevate the child's head of bed as tolerated.
2. To determine the length for nasal placement, measure from the child's nare, to the tip of the earlobe to midway between the xiphoid process and the umbilicus. For oral placement, the measurement should be started at the mouth.
3. Mark the correct length with an indelible marker or place a piece of tape around the tube.
4. Lubricate the end of the tube with water-soluble lubricant.
5. Insert the tube into the mouth or a patent nare and gently advance the tube. Encourage the child to swallow while inserting the tube.
6. Verify the tube placement by checking gastric pH or obtaining radiologic confirmation if placement is in question.
7. Secure the tube to the child's face.

Sources: Ellett, M. L. C., Cohen, M. D., Perkins, S. M., Croffie, J. M. B., Lane, K. A., & Austin, J. K. (2012). Comparing methods of determining insertion length for placing gastric tubes in children 1 month to 17 years of age. *Journal for Specialists in Pediatric Nursing, 17*(1), 19–32. doi:10.1111/j.1744-6155.2011.00302.x; Ellett, M. L. C., Cohen, M. D., Perkins, S. M., Smith, C. E., Lane, K. A., & Austin, J. K. (2011). Predicting the insertion length for gastric tube placement in neonates. *Journal of Obstetric, Gynecologic, and Neonatal Nursing, 40*(4), 412–421. doi:10.1111/j.1552-6909.2011.01255.x

every 4 hours, and performing oral care every 4 hours.

B. Gastrostomy Tube

1. A gastrostomy tube is used for fluid, feeds, and medication administration for children unable to tolerate oral intake. Only liquid medications should be administered through the gastrostomy tube. The tube may also be placed to gravity to allow for gastric decompression, although may not be as effective as decompression from an NG tube.

2. Gastrostomy tubes can be inserted via endoscope or percutaneous endoscopic gastrostomy (PEG) technique or surgically using an open or laparoscopic technique.

3. There are several types of tubes available, including low-profile skin-level devices (balloon and mushroom types) and balloon-ended tubes. The devices have a French size that indicates the diameter and a stem length, which is measured in centimeters.

4. Nursing care includes preventing inadvertent dislodgement (e.g., cover the tube with clothing, flex-net, bandage wrap, and disconnect tube extension sets when not in use), rotating the tube on a daily basis, and flushing the tube after instilling formula or medications to maintain patency. The tube site should be cleaned with soap and water. Care considerations for a newly placed gastrostomy tube (GT) include placing the tube to gravity in the immediate postoperative periods, "racking" or venting the tube to ensure the child can tolerate his or her own gastric secretions, and finally initiating feeds. If there is inadvertent dislodgement of the tube, it should be replaced within 3 to 4 hours with a GT study after replacement

to confirm the tube is intragastric. If the child has undergone a Nissen fundoplication at the same time as GT placement, tube feeds should be vented with a Farrell bag to allow the wrap to heal (the fundus of the stomach is wrapped and sutured around the distal esophagus and LES to prevent reflux) and allow for gastric decompression as needed.

5. All devices with balloons will require periodic replacement as the balloons will break down. If the tube falls out and was in place for less than 4 months, notify a practitioner from the service that placed the tube as a GT study may be ordered to verify correct position.

C. Nasojejunal Tube

1. A nasojejunal (NJ) tube (also referred to as a *postpyloric* or *postpyloric tube*) can be used for continuous feed, fluids, or medication administration for children at risk for aspiration or who do not tolerate gastric feeds. Feeds should be administered at a continuous rate as a bolus feed into the intestine may result in dumping, causing increased stool output and feeding intolerance.

2. The size of the tube is based on the size of the child. NJ tubes have either a guide wire or tungsten-weighted tip to facilitate placement.

3. The approximate length of the tube to be inserted is determined by measuring from the exit port of the tube from the child's nare to ear lobe, then from the ear lobe to the midway point between the xiphoid and umbilicus (Ellett et al., 2011, 2012).

4. At some organizations, prokinetic agents are administered to aid in successful passage of the postpyloric tube. The child should be placed right side lying as tolerated so the pylorus is in the lowest position, which will aid in placement. If this is not tolerated, the child should be placed supine with the head of bed elevated. Once gastric placement is achieved, the tube should be passed through the pylorus, instilling air or water, and advance until resistance is met.

5. Tube placement should be confirmed with an abdominal x-ray.

6. Nursing care involves adequately securing the tube to prevent inadvertent dislodgement, and may be secured with a bridling device, flushing the tube after instilling medications or formula, and performing oral care every 4 hours.

D. Surgical Drains

1. Surgical drains may be placed in or near the surgical wound to prevent the buildup of fluid and maintained until the amounts taper. Drains may be maintained to allow for the evaluation of the type of drainage after resuming a regular diet (e.g., Jackson-Pratt® drain positioned by a biliary anastomosis for bile).

2. There are two types of surgical drains, active drains (*closed* or *closed suction* drains) that use negative pressure to remove fluid, and passive drains (*open*) that depend on the high pressure in the wound and gravity to drain the surgical site (Durai & Ng, 2010). Active drains, such as a Jackson-Pratt or Hemovac drains, have an expandable chamber that creates suction to remove fluid from the wound. In order for the drain to work, the suction bulb must be depressed and emptied at a scheduled interval or when full in order for suction to be maintained. A passive drain, such as a Penrose drain, relies on gravity to remove fluid from the wound and is usually sutured in place.

3. Document the intake and output every 4 hours. Notify the provider of a significant increase or decrease in the amount or character of the drainage. The drain should be secured to prevent inadvertent dislodgement. The surrounding skin should be assessed for irritation or breakdown.

NURSING MANAGEMENT OF WOUND AND STOMA CARE

A. Wound Care

1. Abdominal wound care is variable and can be as simple as assessment for a wound infection (e.g., redness, warmth, pain, edema, foul-smelling drainage, or wound separation) to complex dressing changes involving negative pressure therapy. For complex wound care, consultation with a wound ostomy continence (WOC) nurse is appropriate.

2. Open-wound care should employ moist wound strategies. Wet to dry dressings will provide for gentle wound debridement and allow for wound granulation. Hydrocolloid and hydrofiber dressings (e.g., Aquacel) will allow for wicking of wound drainage, promoting an environment for wound healing.

3. Wounds with excessive drainage should have frequent changes with absorptive dressings that will aid in wound healing (e.g., Mepilex, thick foam).

B. Ostomy Care

1. An ostomy is a stoma that is surgically created from either the small intestine (ileostomy) or large intestine (colostomy) with the purpose of diverting waste outside the body. An ostomy appliance is placed to allow for the collection of stool.

2. *Stoma Assessment.* The bowel is highly vascularized and a stoma should be pink and moist. There are no nerves in a stoma. If a stoma becomes pale or dusky that should be reported to the provider as perfusion to that intestinal segment may be impaired. Stoma output varies related to what segment of the bowel is used for stoma creation; the more proximal the bowel the more acidic and liquid the output will appear. The more distal in the colon the stoma is placed, the thicker and more formed the stool, which will be thickest in the descending colon.

3. The ostomy appliance should be changed every 3 days or sooner if it leaks. The wafer should not be in place for longer than 3 days unless the patient is in the immediate postop period and output is minimal. A warm wet washcloth can be used to remove the old pouch. The skin should be pushed down versus pulling off the wafer as this is generally less painful. Clean the skin with water and allow the skin to dry. The new wafer can be cut according to the pattern. If there is not a pattern, placing a paper towel on top of the stoma will give an approximate measure of the size (dark and wet area on the paper towel can be used as a pattern) and the size to cut on the wafer for the stoma opening. After removing the paper on the wafer, place the wafer on the skin surrounding the stoma. Hold the wafer in place for 5 minutes to allow the plastic to melt and best adhere to the skin. Apply the bag to the appliance if not a one piece or already attached.

4. Nursing care includes emptying the bag when it is one-third full to extend the wafer adhering for a longer time to the skin. Pouches that become filled with air should be relieved to prevent wafer dislodgement. Measure and document the stoma effluence every 4 hours. Placing two to three cotton balls in the bag if the output is liquid will help absorb the effluence and prolong adherence of the appliance. If available, a WOC nurse should be consulted to optimize stoma care and educate the child and parents.

GASTROESOPHAGEAL REFLUX DISEASE

A. Definition and Etiology

1. GER is the involuntary movement of gastric contents from the stomach to the esophagus with or without regurgitation or vomiting. In the majority of infants, GER resolves by 1 year of age. GERD occurs with persistent GER that results in complications and impacts the child's quality of life.

2. *Etiology*

    a. At-risk children include those with prematurity, congenital esophageal abnormalities, congenital diaphragmatic hernia, neurologic impairment, cystic fibrosis, history of lung transplant, respiratory disorders, obesity, and family history of GERD.

B. Pathophysiology

1. Normally, the LES rests when there is a peristaltic wave and this relaxation is transient.

2. The LES rests (5–30 seconds) are of longer duration when the pressure in the esophagus is the same as the stomach (Barnhart, 2016) and is the physiological cause of GER.

C. Clinical Presentation

1. *History*

    a. Evaluate symptoms and what alleviates or aggravates them, dietary history, and comorbidities.

    b. GERD varies with age. Symptoms can range from persistent vomiting to intermittent spitting to apparent life-altering events with a significant decline at 1 year of age.

2. *Physical Examination*

    a. No specific examination findings are diagnostic of GER/GERD

    i. Review anthropometric measurements and growth charts.

    ii. Spitting and nonbloody and nonbilious vomiting are the most common symptom in infants. Other symptoms include feeding refusal, poor weight gain, respiratory symptoms, arching, choking, and coughing (Papachrisanthou & Davis, 2015).

    iii. In children, the most common symptoms are vomiting, heartburn, abdominal pain, and anorexia (Papachrisanthou & Davis, 2016).

3. *Diagnostic Tests*

    a. There is no single diagnostic test confirmatory of GER/GERD.

    b. According to the joint recommendations from the North American Society for Pediatric Gastroenterology, Hepatology and Nutrition and the European Society for Pediatric Gastroenterology, Hepatology and Nutrition (Vandenplas et al., 2009):

    i. Esophageal pH monitoring. This is a valid quantitative test of acid exposure; however, severity does not correlate with symptoms or complications.

    ii. Combined multiluminal impedance and pH monitoring. Detects acid and nonacid reflux episodes and is superior to pH monitoring for determining the relationship between the symptoms and disease.

    iii. Motility studies. Esophageal manometry studies may be abnormal but lack sensitivity and specificity for GERD diagnosis confirmation.

    iv. Endoscopy and biopsy. Endoscopically visible breaks in esophageal mucosa are the most reliable to diagnose reflux esophagitis and, although it is not diagnostic of GERD, it may be helpful for the diagnosis of other disorders.

    v. Upper GI. Not recommended for GERD diagnosis, may be helpful in determining alternate diagnoses.

    vi. Empiric trial of aid suppression. For the older child, a 4-week trial of a PPI is used for symptom improvement; however, this is not recommended in infants and younger children. Improvement in the child's heartburn does not confirm the GERD diagnosis as clinical improvement may be related to spontaneous improvement or placebo effect.

4. *Clinical Course*

   a. Persistent GER symptoms that progress to GERD with complications, including esophagitis and respiratory complications are expected.

D. Patient Care Management

   1. *Preventive Care or "Lifestyle Changes"*

     a. *Infants*

       i. Elevate head of bed to 30 degrees, minimize overfeeding, and consider a 1- to 2-week trial of hypoallergenic formula (Garth, 2016).

     b. *Children*

       i. Elevate head of bed, encourage left side-lying positioning, weight reduction if indicated; there is no evidence to support dietary modification (e.g., minimize caffeine, fatty or spicy foods, carbonation, eat small frequent meals; Garth 2016; Vandenplas et al., 2009).

   2. *Direct Care*

     a. *Pharmacology*

       i. Administer a PPI (up to 8 weeks)—not FDA approved in infants younger than 1 year.

       ii. Administer a histamine-2 receptor antagonist—generally first-line treatment.

       iii. Prokinetic agent—The adverse side effects outweigh potential benefit for GERD treatment and these agents are not recommended.

     b. *Surgical intervention*

       i. Indications for surgery include dependence on long-term medication therapy, nonadherence to medical therapy, repeated episodes of aspiration or related pneumonia episodes, and an apparent life-threatening event.

       ii. Nissen fundoplication may be performed open or laparoscopically and is a 360-degree circumferential wrap of the fundus of the stomach around the intra-abdominal esophagus.

   3. The child may be unable to "burp" or vomit, which can lead to gastric distension and, in rare cases, gastric rupture. The child may require placement of an NG tube or, if a gastrostomy tube is present, it is placed to gravity drainage. Feeds, if administered through an enteric tube, should be administered continuously and vented (with a Farrell bag or syringe) during the immediate postoperative period.

E. Outcomes

Symptoms that begin after 3 years of age are less likely to resolve without intervention.

ACUTE ABDOMINAL TRAUMA

Acute abdominal trauma is more often blunt versus penetrating, which is considered blunt abdominal trauma. The organs most commonly injured are the spleen and liver.

A. Definition and Etiology

Anatomic differences in children compared with adults include a body size that allows greater distribution of injury, a larger body surface area that allows for greater heat loss, abdominal organs that are more anterior with less SC fat protection, and a smaller blood volume resulting in hypovolemia with relatively smaller volume losses.

B. Pathophysiology

   1. *Blunt* injuries are caused by compression of solid or hollow viscous organs against the spine; rapid acceleration and deceleration with subsequent tearing of structures; or increased abdominal pressure resulting in contusion, laceration, or rupture of organs with subsequent hemorrhage. Solid organs are injured more often than hollow organs, and the most commonly injured organ is the spleen. Blunt trauma can result in lethal injury without visible signs of trauma.

   2. *Penetrating* injuries are most often caused by gunshot or stab wounds. The most common injury is to the hollow viscera. The onset of peritonitis may be immediate. Wounds that penetrate the abdomen usually require surgical exploration.

C. Clinical Presentation

   1. *History.* History is given by a parent or emergency responder report. If age appropriate, speak with the child and attempt to get a history. As with all trauma, if the history does not explain the injuries, providers should be suspicious of child maltreatment.

   2. *Physical Examination*

     a. Significant injuries to the head and extremities may overshadow abdominal injuries.

     b. Signs of injury are often subtle and include rebound tenderness, pain, rigidity, pallor, grunting respirations, hypotension, failure to respond to fluid resuscitation, and increasing abdominal girth. Acute abdominal distention occurs even with minor trauma, especially in infants and often in children as a result of crying and swallowing air. Distention may lead to vomiting and aspiration.

c. Signs of retroperitoneal bleeding include Cullen's sign (ecchymosis around the umbilicus) and Turner's sign (ecchymosis over the flank).

3. *Diagnostic Tests*

a. Abdominal x-rays, supine and lateral, are useful for determining intraperitoneal free air, ground-glass appearance (suggests intraperitoneal blood or urine), associated lower rib fractures (indicates severe force), and signs of an ileus.

b. Ultrasound (US), or FAST (focused abdominal sonography for trauma), is a rapid diagnostic tool used to identify intraperitoneal fluid in the hemodynamically unstable child with blunt trauma. However, FAST is poor at identifying organ-specific injury and therefore does not replace the abdominal CT as a tool for definitive diagnosis of abdominal injury. The sensitivity of the FAST exam is highly variable; however, use of FAST scans has reduced the number of CT scans in some institutions (Notrica, 2015).

c. Abdominal CT scan is the standard of care for evaluation of the peritoneal cavity and retroperitoneum in the hemodynamically stable child. The use of IV contrast is recommended to evaluate organ perfusion, bowel integrity, and the presence of intraperitoneal fluid (Ellison et al., 2015).

d. Diagnostic peritoneal lavage (DPL) is a technique that is rarely performed with the advent of newer imaging techniques (e.g., FAST exam) and involves the insertion of a catheter into the peritoneal cavity. Aspiration of blood is a positive tap. If no blood is obtained, then 10 mL/kg of normal saline (NS) or Ringer's lactate solution (RL) is infused through the catheter and the effluent is drained by gravity. Cell count and chemistries are obtained. White cell counts greater than 500 cells/mL, red cells counts greater than 100,000 cells/mL, amylase greater than 175 mg/dL, and aspirating stool or blood is a positive tap. A tap positive for blood indicates hemoperitoneum but provides no information on the bleeding source.

e. Complete blood count (CBC) and coagulation studies may help to evaluate bleeding.

f. The utility of other laboratory tests in the diagnosis of intra-abdominal injury is controversial. Elevated AST and ALT suggest liver injury (see Table 7.1). Elevated amylase and lipase suggest pancreatic injury.

g. Urinalysis should be obtained to evaluate for the presence of blood, which indicates kidney or bladder injury.

D. Patient Care Management

1. *Preventive Care.* Safety measures include appropriate child-restraint devices in automobiles and wearing appropriate protective gear when participating in contact sports.

2. *Direct Care*

a. Early management of airway, breathing, and circulation (ABC) has the most direct impact on survival. The critically ill child may require intubation and mechanical ventilation for stabilization of the airway and breathing. Circulatory stabilization requires the placement of large-bore IV lines and fluid resuscitation. Inadequate airway and fluid resuscitation are the leading causes of preventable death. Central venous pressure (CVP) and arterial blood pressure (BP) lines are placed to allow close monitoring of the child's intravascular volume and BP.

b. Current management of blunt abdominal trauma is based on the child's hemodynamic status (e.g., hemoglobin [Hgb] >7 mg/dL) as compared to injury severity grading scales. The mainstay of treatment remains nonoperative management for blunt solid abdominal organ injury (McVay, Kokoska, Jackson, & Smith, 2008).

c. Insertion of an NG or OG tube allows for gastric decompression, minimizes aspiration risk, and maximizes respiratory effort.

d. Serial laboratory studies are necessary for evaluation of injury, especially following the hematocrit, which is imperative to assess for ongoing bleeding. For blunt injuries for which serial values are being monitored, phlebotomy may be discontinued after two to three stable values (McVay et al., 2008).

e. Most solid-organ abdominal injuries are managed nonoperatively. The blood volume of a child is approximately 80 mL/kg. Fluid resuscitation guidelines include administering up to 40 mL/kg of saline or RL solution. If the child remains hemodynamically unstable, a blood transfusion should then be given. Indications for surgical exploration include massive fluid resuscitation

(>40 mL/kg of blood transfusions or more than 50% of blood volume), penetrating trauma, signs of peritonitis, radiographic evidence of pneumoperitoneum, and certain blunt injuries (e.g., diaphragmatic injury or bladder rupture).

3. *Organ-Specific Care*

a. The *spleen* is the most commonly injured abdominal organ in blunt abdominal trauma.

   i. Signs and symptoms include left upper quadrant (LUQ) tenderness, bruising, or abrasion, positive Kehr's sign (LUQ pain radiating to the left shoulder), signs of decreased perfusion (pallor, tachycardia, delayed capillary refill, and hypotension), and nausea and vomiting. Other signs may include Cullen's or Turner's sign.

   ii. Diagnostic studies. Abdominal x-ray examinations are rarely helpful but may demonstrate an elevated left hemidiaphragm or a medially displaced lateral stomach border suggesting splenic laceration. The hematocrit may be decreased related to bleeding, or leukocytosis may be noted. Definitive diagnosis is made by abdominal CT scan with contrast.

   iii. Classification is based on location and extent of injury (Table 7.5).

   iv. Management. The standard of care is nonoperative treatment in hemodynamically stable patients. See Table 7.6 for current activity restrictions, hospital length of stay, and imaging recommendations. Patients are NPO until stable. Surgery may include a *splenectomy* or *splenorrhaphy*. In most instances, suturing the injury or splenorrhaphy results in salvage of the spleen. The ultimate goal is preservation of the immune function of the spleen. Massive splenic injury requires a splenectomy. Postoperative care includes monitoring for potential complications such as atelectasis, bleeding, ileus, pain, and infection.

TABLE 7.5   Splenic Injury Scale

Grade	Injury Description
I	
Hematoma	Subcapsular, nonexpanding, <10% of surface area
Laceration	Capsular tear, nonbleeding, <1 cm of parenchymal depth
II	
Hematoma	Subcapsular, nonexpanding, 10%–50% of surface area, intraparenchymal, nonexpanding, <5 cm in diameter
Laceration	Capsular tear, 1–3 cm of parenchymal depth that does not involve a trabecular vessel
III	
Hematoma	Subcapsular, >50% of surface area or expanding, ruptured subcapsular or parenchymal hematoma, intraparenchymal hematoma, >5 cm or expanding
Laceration	>3 cm of parenchymal depth or involving trabecular vessels
IV	
Hematoma	Ruptured intraparenchymal hematoma with active bleeding
Laceration	Laceration involving segmental or hilar vessel producing major devascularization (>25% of spleen)
V	
Laceration	Completely shattered spleen
Vascular	Hilar vascular injury that devascularizes spleen

Source: Adapted from Lynch, J. M., Meza, M. P., Newman, B., Gardner, M. J., & Albanese, C. T. (1997). Computed tomography grade of splenic injury is predictive of the time required for radiographic healing. *Journal of Pediatric Surgery, 32*, 1093–1096. doi:10.1016/S0022-3468(97)90406-1

TABLE 7.6 Proposed Guidelines for Resource Use in Children With Isolated Spleen or Liver Injury

	CT Grade			
	I	II	III	IV
ICU (day)	None	None	None	1
Hospital stay	2	3	4	5
Predischarge imaging	None	None	None	None
Postdischarge imaging	None	None	None	None
Activity restriction (week)[a]	3	4	5	6

[a]Return to full-contact, competitive sports (i.e., football, wrestling, hockey, lacrosse, mountain climbing) should be at the discretion of the individual pediatric trauma surgeon. The proposed guidelines for return to unrestricted activity include "normal" age-appropriate activities.

Source: From McVay, M. R., Kokoska, E. R., Jackson, R. J., & Smith, S. D. (2008). Throwing out the "grade" book: Management of isolated spleen and liver injury based on hemodynamic status. *Journal of Pediatric Surgery*, 43(6), 1072–1076. doi:10.1016/j.jpedsurg.2008.02.031

v. Complications include rebleeding or splenic laceration 3 to 5 days after the initial injury. Splenectomized children are at risk for overwhelming postsplenectomy infection (OSI). *Streptococcus pneumoniae* is the most common causative agent. Vaccination against encapsulated bacteria, including *S. pneumoniae, Haemophilus influenzae* type b, and *Neisseria meningitides,* is recommended after splenectomy. Daily penicillin prophylaxis is recommended in children younger than 5 years and for 2 years following splenectomy and longer if there are other immunosuppression factors or a history of OSI (Buzelé, Barbier, Sauvanet, & Fantin, 2016). Parents should be taught signs and symptoms of infection and when to seek medical attention. Children who sustain an isolated splenic injury are restricted from contact sports and strenuous physical activity for a period consisting of the grade of injury plus 2 weeks.

b. The *liver* is second only to the spleen as a major source of hemorrhage and is the most common source of lethal hemorrhage. Bleeding stops spontaneously with most injuries.

  i. Signs and symptoms include right upper quadrant (RUQ) tenderness, ecchymosis, abrasion, enlarging abdominal girth, signs of

shock, and associated injuries such as lower rib fractures, pelvic fracture, or head injury.

  ii. Diagnostic studies. Definitive diagnosis is made with abdominal CT scan with contrast. Elevated transaminases are highly suggestive of liver injury, especially AST greater than 200 IU/L and ALT greater than 100 IU/L (Puranik, Hayes, Long, & Mata, 2002). A rapidly falling hematocrit suggests severe liver injury. See Table 7.6 for suggested radiologic monitoring to assess healing or continued bleeding based on the grade of injury.

  iii. Classification. Injuries are graded according to increasing severity (Table 7.7).

  iv. Management is similar to the treatment of splenic injury and involves supportive care with a nonoperative approach (see Table 7.6). Nonoperative management requires close monitoring of vital signs and physical examinations. Fever, leukocytosis, and abdominal tenderness remote from the liver injury may indicate an occult injury. Serial hematocrits, coagulation studies, chemistries, and transaminase levels should be monitored for significant liver dysfunction and monitored until stable. Close monitoring for ongoing bleeding is necessary, and patients should remain on strict bed rest until they are stable. Surgery is indicated for the hemodynamically unstable child, signs of peritonitis, or transfusion requirements exceeding 50% of the estimated blood volume during the first 24 hours (Garcia & Brown, 2003). Children with isolated hepatic injury are restricted from contact sports and strenuous physical activity for a period consisting of the grade of injury plus 2 weeks.

  v. Complications of operative management include delayed bleeding, abscess formation, abdominal compartment syndrome, biliary obstruction, and biloma.

c. The *pancreas* is located deep in the upper abdomen and is infrequently injured unless a significant sustained force compresses it against the spine. The classic injury is compression by bicycle handlebars in which the child flips over the bike and is impaled in the epigastrium by the handlebars. Other mechanisms include motor vehicle collisions and child maltreatment.

  i. Signs and symptoms include diffuse abdominal tenderness, deep epigastric pain radiating to the back, and bilious vomiting. Pain may diminish within the first 2 hours of injury and worsen with the

TABLE 7.7   Liver Injury Scale

Grade[a]	Injury Description	ICD-9	AIS-90
I			
Hematoma	Subcapsular, <10% of surface area	864.01	2
		864.11	
Laceration	Capsular tear, <1 cm parenchymal depth	864.02	2
		864.12	
II			
Hematoma	Subcapsular, 10%–50% of surface area; intraparenchymal, <10 cm in diameter	864.01	2
		864.11	
Laceration	1–3 cm parenchymal depth, <10 cm in length	864.03	2
		864.13	
III			
Hematoma	Subcapsular, >50% of surface area or expanding; ruptured subcapsular or parenchymal hematoma		3
	Intraparenchymal hematoma >10 cm or expanding		
Laceration	>3 cm parenchymal depth	864.04	3
		864.14	
IV			
Laceration	Parenchymal destruction involving 25%–75% of hepatic lobe or 1-3 Couinaud's segments within a single lobe	864.04	4
		864.14	
V			
Laceration	Parenchymal destruction involving >75% of hepatic lobe or >3 Couinaud's segment within a single lobe		5
Vascular	Juxtahepatic venous injuries; i.e., retrohepatic vena cava/central major hepatic veins		5
VI			
Vascular	Hepatic avulsion		6

AIS, Abbreviated Injury Scale; ICD, International Classification of Diseases.

[a]Advance one grade for multiple injuries, up to grade III.

Source: From Moore, E. E., Cogbill, T. H., Jurkovich, G. J., Shackford, S. R., Malangoni, M. A., & Champion, H. R. (1995). Organ injury scaling: Spleen and liver (1994 revision). *Journal of Trauma and Acute Care Surgery, 38*(3), 323–324. Retrieved from https://journals.lww.com/jtrauma/Fulltext/1995/03000/Organ_Injury_Scaling__Spleen_and_Liver__1994.1.aspx

release of enzymes over the next 6 to 8 hours (Intravia & DeBeradino, 2013).

ii.   Diagnostic studies

1) Amylase is elevated (reference range 0–88 IU/L). The extent of amylase increase alone does not correlate with the severity of injury and may be a nonspecific finding occurring with blunt injury in the absence of pancreatic injury.

2) Lipase (reference range, 20–180 IU/L). Elevation of amylase to greater than 200 IU/L and lipase greater than 1,800 IU/L correlates with significant pancreatic injury (Nadler, Gardner, Schall, Lynch, & Ford, 1999).

3) Diagnosis is usually made by abdominal CT scan with IV contrast.

4) US is useful for diagnosis of pseudocyst.

5) Magnetic resonance cholangiopancreatography (MRCP) or endoscopic retrograde cholangiopancreatography (ERCP) may be necessary to visualize ductal disruption or posttraumatic stricture.

6) Classification: Injury is graded based on the extent of parenchymal injury and the degree of disruption of the duct (Table 7.8).

TABLE 7.8 Pancreatic Injury Severity Scale

Class	Injury Description
I	Contusion or laceration without duct injury
II	Ductal transection or parenchymal injury with probable duct injury
III	Proximal transection or parenchymal injury with probable duct injury
IV	Combined pancreatic and duodenal injury

Source: Adapted from Jobst, M. A., Canty, T. G., & Lynch, F. P. (1999). Management of pancreatic injury in pediatric blunt abdominal trauma. *Journal of Pediatric Surgery, 34*(5), 818–823.

7) Management is nonoperative if there is no ductal disruption; although operative intervention with ductal disruption is controversial (Englum, Gulack, Rice, Scarborough, & Adibe, 2016). Supportive care interventions include NPO, NG tube for gastric decompression, IV fluids, and pain management. Parenteral nutrition should be considered if NPO longer than 3 days. Children are monitored for signs of infection. If a pancreatic pseudocyst (a loculated collection of pancreatic juices) develops, patients require 6 to 8 weeks of bowel rest with PN. Surgery is usually indicated for the treatment of distal transection of the pancreas. Surgery involves drainage, partial resection, or repair of lacerated ducts.

8) Complications include the development of pancreatic fistula or pseudocyst formation. Large cysts that have not resolved after 4 to 6 weeks require drainage. Surgical drainage, percutaneous by interventional radiology, and endoscopic drainage may be performed. Because the pancreas is stimulated with oral intake, feeding tolerance must be evaluated before pulling surgical drains.

d. *Stomach*

i. Signs and symptoms of injury include abrasion or contusion in the upper abdomen and bloody gastric drainage. A rigid abdomen with severe pain suggests perforation. Perforation leads to signs and symptoms of peritonitis within hours of injury.

ii. Diagnostic studies. Abdominal x-ray detects free air or abnormal NG tube position.

iii. Management includes surgical repair.

e. *Small and large intestine.* Small bowel injuries are the third most common site of abdominal organ injury in blunt trauma (Wise, Mudd, & Wilson, 2002). Common mechanisms include the lap-belt syndrome and abuse. The colon and rectum are rarely injured in children, and injuries to these organs usually occur in the presence of maltreatment.

i. Signs and symptoms include bloody gastric drainage, absent bowel sounds, tympanic sounds on percussion, midabdominal ecchymosis, seat-belt sign, and pain that increases as peritonitis develops. Signs and symptoms of peritonitis include severe abdominal pain, tenderness, guarding, distension or rigidity, redness, absent bowel sounds, fever, leukocytosis, and respiratory distress. Evaluation of a rectal injury requires rectal examination and is often done with the patient under anesthesia.

ii. Diagnostic studies. Abdominal x-rays with supine and lateral decubitus views may reveal air–fluid levels, dilated loops of bowel, bowel-wall thickening, or a chance fracture (lumbar spine fracture). CT scan with IV contrast may have greater sensitivity and specificity.

iii. Management requires surgical repair and generally involves segmental resection with primary anastomosis and possible ostomy placement. Supportive care includes frequent monitoring, NG decompression, replacement of excessive gastric output, stress ulcer prophylaxis, antibiotic therapy, fluid and electrolyte management, PN, and pain management.

iv. Complications. Delayed perforation, stricture formation, adhesions, and short bowel syndrome may occur.

E. Outcomes

See specific organ for complications.

ACUTE GI TRACT HEMORRHAGE

A. Definition and Etiology

1. Acute bleeding from the GI tract is usually classified as either upper or lower tract bleeding.

2. Etiology is based on age. Tables 7.9 and 7.10 outline the causes of upper and lower GI bleeding.

B. Pathophysiology

The child presenting with sudden massive blood loss is at risk for hemodynamic instability. The first priority is

TABLE 7.9   Causes of Upper GI Bleeding in Infants and Children

Neonates	Infants–Adolescents
Swallowed maternal blood, esophagitis	Esophagitis
Gastritis	Gastritis
Gastroduodenal ulcer	Gastroduodenal ulcer
Coagulopathy associated with infection, liver failure	Esophageal varices
Vascular anomaly	Gastrointestinal duplication
Hematologic (vitamin K deficiency)	Mallory–Weiss tear Vascular anomaly Coagulopathy Caustic ingestion

GI, gastrointestinal.

TABLE 7.10   Causes of Lower GI Bleeding in Infants and Children

Age	Causes
Neonates	Milk protein allergy Necrotizing enterocolitis Hirschsprung's enterocolitis Midgut volvulus Hematologic (vitamin K deficiency) Coagulopathy
Infant	Milk protein allergy Anal fissure Intussusception Infectious enterocolitis Meckel's diverticulum Vascular anomaly
Child	Anal fissure Juvenile polyps Infectious enterocolitis Inflammatory bowel disease Henoch–Schonlein purpura Hemolytic-uremic syndrome Vascular anomaly
Adolescent	Anal fissure Infectious enterocolitis Inflammatory bowel disease Vasculitis Hemorrhoids NSAID enteropathy

GI, gastrointestinal; NSAID, nonsteroidal anti-inflammatory drug.

Sources: Adapted from Lirio, R. A. (2016). Management of upper gastrointestinal bleeding in children: Variceal and nonvariceal. *Gastrointestinal Endoscopy Clinics of North America, 26*(1), 63–73. doi:10.1016/j.giec.2015.09.003; Sahn, B., & Bitton, S. (2016). Lower gastrointestinal bleeding in children. *Gastrointestinal Endoscopy Clinics of North America, 26*(1), 75–98. doi:10.1016/j.giec.2015.08.007

to determine the extent of the blood loss and establish whether perfusion is compromised. Greater than 15% circulating blood volume (CBV) loss results in stimulation of autonomic cardiovascular responses to maintain BP and perfusion. Greater than 20% CBV loss results in decreased systolic BP and metabolic acidosis. Rapid fluid resuscitation is required, or cardiovascular collapse and death may occur. *Upper GI bleeding* is defined as bleeding that originates proximal to the ligament of Treitz. Lower GI bleed occurs distally to ligament of Treitz.

C. Clinical Presentation

1. *History*

   a. Presentation of GI bleeding is shown in Table 7.11.

   b. Comorbidities (liver disease), medications (e.g., steroids, nonsteroidal anti-inflammatory drugs [NSAIDs]), and possible exposures should be assessed.

2. *Physical Examination*

   a. The location of bleeding can be identified by the color and source of the bleeding. Hematemesis is the result of acute blood loss from the upper GI tract and presents as coffee grounds emesis or frank blood. Hematochezia is bright- or dark-red blood per rectum. Melena is caused by the digestion of blood in the GI tract and presents as black, tarry stools and indicates an upper GI source of bleeding. Occult bleeding is the result of chronic blood loss.

   b. Signs and symptoms of hypovolemic shock occur with acute bleeding and include tachycardia, weak peripheral pulses, pallor and mottled color, cool skin, and oliguria. BP may be normal despite significant blood loss; hypotension is a late sign of shock.

3. *Diagnostic Tests*

   a. Laboratory studies. CBC needed to evaluate for anemia and thrombocytopenia; prothrombin time (PT) and partial thromboplastin time (PTT) to evaluate for coagulopathies; serum fibrinogen and fibrin split products to evaluate for disseminated intravascular coagulation (DIC); type and crossmatch for potential blood transfusion; guaiac test to evaluate for blood in stool or gastric fluid; chemistries, ammonia, and liver function tests (LFTs) to screen for liver dysfunction; and arterial blood gas (ABG) is measured to monitor for metabolic acidosis. If bloody diarrhea is present, send for stool culture and fecal leukocytes. A CBC, urinalysis, blood urea nitrogen (BUN), and creatinine

TABLE 7.11 Presentation of GI Tract Bleeding

Presentation	Definitions
Acute bleeding	
Hematemesis	Bloody vomitus; either fresh, bright-red blood or dark, digested blood with "coffee ground" appearance
Melena	Black, sticky, tarry, foul-smelling stools caused by digestion of blood in the GI tract (seen in both upper GI and lower GI tract bleeding)
Hematochezia	Fresh, bright-red blood passed from the rectum
Chronic bleeding	
Occult	Trace amounts of blood in normal-appearing stools or gastric secretions; detectable only with a guaiac test

GI, gastrointestinal.

Source: Modified from Huether, S. E., McCance, K. L., & Tarmina, M. S. (1994). Alterations of digestive function. In K. L. McCance & S. E. Huether (Eds.), *Pathophysiology: The biological basis for diseases in adults and children* (2nd ed.). St Louis, MO: Mosby-Year Book.

should be obtained in patients with suspected hemolytic-uremic syndrome.

b. Abdominal x-ray examination involves a supine and lateral decubitus view to evaluate for bowel gas pattern suggesting bowel obstruction, air–fluid levels, or pneumoperitoneum. Bowel-wall thickening suggests colitis.

c. Endoscopy provides direct visualization of the GI tract to determine injury, structural defects, or source of bleeding. An upper endoscopy is the preferred diagnostic procedure to evaluate bleeding of the upper GI tract and for therapeutic treatment (injection, cautery and mechanical therapy for nonvariceal bleeding, and variceal ligation or banding for variceal bleeding; Lirio, 2016). Colonoscopy is performed for lower GI bleeding.

d. Radionuclide studies are indicated for midintestinal bleeding and are effective tests for locating subacute or intermittent bleeding. Two types are used: technetium-labeled sulfur colloid (more sensitive) and technetium-pertechnetate-labeled red blood cells (RBCs). Demonstration of IV Tc-99m pertechnetate uptake by ectopic gastric mucosa in a Meckel's scan is helpful in diagnosing Meckel's diverticulum.

4. *Clinical Course*

a. Course is variable depending on the source and etiology. Upper GI variceal bleeding can result in sudden, massive blood loss and hypovolemic shock.

D. Patient Care Management

1. *Preventive Care*

a. Assess for signs of respiratory distress and hemodynamic instability.

2. *Direct Care*

a. Secure two large-bore IVs for fluid resuscitation as needed. Administer fluid (20 mL/kg of NS or RL) or blood transfusion (20 mL/kg or more as indicated) until peripheral circulation is adequate. After central line and arterial line placement, continuously monitor CVP and BP for response to fluid resuscitation and the need for continued therapy. The initial hematocrit may be misleading; if so, serial measurements are needed.

b. Place an NG tube and administer room temperature saline lavage until bleeding stops.

c. Administer H_2-histamine receptor antagonists, PPIs, and sucralfate to minimize bleeding and prevent rebleeding.

d. Endoscopic modalities, including injection, cautery, and mechanical therapy, may be used for nonvariceal and variceal ligation or banding for variceal bleeding (Lirio, 2016).

3. *Supportive Care*

a. Continuously monitor vital signs.

b. Monitor PT, PTT, and fibrinogen for coagulopathies. Administer vitamin K (AquaMEPHYTON), platelets, or fresh frozen plasma (FFP) as necessary.

c. Monitor electrolytes, BUN, and creatinine for potential renal dysfunction. Monitor urine output via a urinary catheter.

d. Monitor serum ionized calcium following transfusion for potential hypocalcemia.

e. Monitor for signs of further bleeding, including poor perfusion, abdominal pain, increased abdominal girth, decreased bowel sounds, hematemesis, and hematochezia.

f. Assess for signs and symptoms of abdominal perforation, including fever, severe or persistent abdominal pain, and abdominal rigidity.

4. *Esophageal Varices*

a. Acute treatment involves the administration of vasopressin (Pitressin), or octreotide (Sandostatin; see "Pharmacology" section earlier in this chapter). Insertion of a Sengstaken–Blakemore tube may be performed if endoscopy is not available. The tube has three separate lumens for gastric suction, inflation of gastric balloon, and inflation of esophageal balloon. Balloons must be deflated every 12 to 24 hours. Ensure patency of the gastric suction lumen by irrigating frequently. Frequent serious complications, including perforation or erosion of the esophagus or stomach (from hyperinflation or prolonged inflation of the balloons), limit its usefulness.

b. Endoscopic variceal ligation or banding is the treatment of choice.

c. Surgery is considered if other therapies are ineffective. Shunting procedures divert blood flow from the liver and allow decompression of the portal system with portal hypertension. Specific entities that may require surgery include Meckel's diverticulum, duplication cyst, midgut volvulus, NEC, and intussusception (if radiologic enema reduction not effective), and a refractory bleeding ulcer.

E. Outcomes

Complications include rebleeding, shock, sepsis, and DIC.

GI TRACT ABNORMALITIES

GI tract abnormalities are often detected in the prenatal period. Congenital anomalies are summarized in Table 7.12.

ACUTE SURGICAL ABDOMEN

A. Definition and Etiology

Acute surgical abdomen refers to the sudden onset of abdominal pain and tenderness that warrants evaluation for surgical intervention that is usually caused by a bowel infarction, obstruction, or perforation. Causes in neonates include NEC, intussusception, and midgut volvulus. Causes in children and adolescents include appendicitis (a perforated appendix is a common cause of peritonitis), Meckel's diverticulum, inflammatory bowel disease, omental torsion, ovarian torsion, intussusception (not reduced radiologically), incarcerated inguinal hernia, and trauma. Intraluminal bowel obstructions in children can be caused by foreign bodies, bezoars, with extramural causes from bowel adhesions, hernias, and internal volvulus.

B. Pathophysiology

1. Peritoneal inflammation (peritonitis) occurs as a result of injury or contamination. Primary peritonitis occurs with no obvious cause of contamination, but infection is indirectly introduced into the peritoneal cavity from the bloodstream or lymphatics. Secondary peritonitis occurs as a result of direct GI tract injury, such as with trauma. The inflammatory response causes exudation of fluid into the peritoneal cavity. Hypovolemia may occur as fluid shifts into the peritoneal cavity.

2. Upper GI tract perforations result in leakage of hydrochloric acid, digestive enzymes, or bile causing chemical peritonitis.

3. Lower GI tract perforation results in the leakage of fecal material, which releases aerobic and anaerobic bacteria into the peritoneum. Endotoxins may be released and cause bacterial peritonitis and sepsis.

4. Injury to the peritoneum causes decreased bowel motility and usually results in an ileus.

5. Obstruction can be complete, partial, or intermittent. Bowel proximal to the obstruction becomes distended due to a collection of air and GI tract contents. Distal bowel collapses from a lack of intraluminal content; therefore, proximal obstructions create more bowel collapse. With a distal obstruction, there is greater bowel distension and resultant abdominal distension.

C. Clinical Presentation

1. *History.* Variable depending on the location of the obstruction, the type of obstruction, and whether the obstruction is complete or partial. The onset, progression, location, and presence of other symptoms should be evaluated (e.g., stooling pattern, pain, NG output [bilious output indicative of an obstruction]). Presentation can be acute with signs of peritonitis (e.g., volvulus, traumatic visceral perforation, postsurgical bowel obstruction) or subtle and chronic with incomplete or recurring bouts of obstruction (e.g., intussusception).

TABLE 7.12 Congenital Gastrointestinal Abnormalities

Diagnosis	Etiology and Risk Factors	Pathophysiology	Signs and Symptoms	Nursing Diagnoses	Patient Care Management	Complications
Omphalocele	Cause unknown; may be caused during the second stage of rotation of the midgut with incomplete return of the bowel into the abdomen at 10–11 weeks gestation	Herniation of abdominal organs (intestine and liver) out of the abdomen. Usually covered by a peritoneal sac with the umbilical arteries and veins inserting into the apex of the defect. Associated anomalies include cardiac defects, neurologic abnormalities, genitourinary abnormalities, skeletal abnormalities, chromosomal abnormalities, malrotation of the intestine, Beckwith–Wiedemann syndrome	Size of the defect is variable. Dehydration, hypothermia, hypoglycemia, and respiratory distress (dependent on lesion size)	Potential for alteration in breathing patterns: ineffective r/t abdominal hernia. Potential for fluid volume deficit: actual r/t increased insensible water loss and third spacing. Potential for alteration in nutrition: actual r/t NPO status. Impairment of skin integrity: actual r/t abdominal hernia. Alteration in comfort r/t postoperative pain	1. Stabilize the airway 2. Cover exposed abdominal hernia with warm, moist dressing; cover dressing with plastic. Defect may be covered with bowel bag 3. Maintain NPO status 4. Place OG/NG tube 5. Maintain neutral thermal environment 6. Monitor I & Os 7. Monitor electrolyte status 8. Provide IV hydration (may require 1.5–2 times maintenance fluids) 9. Evaluation for associated anomalies: cardiac echo, renal ultrasound, chromosomal analysis 10. Repair of defect: primary surgical closure, staged silo closing, or secondary epithelization of defect 11. Postoperative care a. PN with enteral feeds when ileus resolved b. Management of fluid and electrolyte status c. Monitor for infection d. Pain management	Intestinal obstruction, Respiratory distress, Sepsis, Wound infection, Feeding intolerance, GERD, Sac rupture, Vascular compromise of abdominal contents and lower extremities once the defect is reduced

(continued)

TABLE 7.12 Congenital Gastrointestinal Abnormalities (*continued*)

Diagnosis	Etiology and Risk Factors	Pathophysiology	Signs and Symptoms	Nursing Diagnoses	Patient Care Management	Complications

Gastroschisis	Cause unknown; 50% of infants are born prematurely	Evisceration of abdominal contents, usually lateral and to the right of the umbilicus, may be the small and large intestine; no protective membranes
		
		Associated anomalies include intestinal stricture and atresia
			Size of defect usually smaller than an omphalocele
			
			Intestine may be edematous and inflamed due to exposure to amniotic fluid
			
			Bowel exposure precursor to prolonged ileus and motility
				Potential for alteration in breathing patterns: ineffective r/t abdominal hernia
				
				Potential for fluid volume deficit: actual r/t increased insensible water losses and third spacing
				
				Alteration in nutritional status: actual r/t NPO status and postop ileus
				
				Impairment of skin integrity: actual r/t abdominal hernia
				
				Alteration in comfort: r/t surgical procedure
					1. Cover exposed abdominal hernia with warm, moist dressing; cover dressing with plastic
					Defect may be covered by a bowel bag
					2. Maintain NPO status
					3. Place OG/NG tube
					4. Maintain neutral thermal environment
					5. Monitor I & Os
					6. Monitor electrolyte status
					7. Provide IV hydration
					8. Repair of defect: primary closure or silo staged reduction with surgical repair of the abdominal wall after the herniated bowel has been returned to the abdominal cavity
					9. Postoperative care
					  a. PN
					  b. Manage fluid and electrolyte status
					  c. Monitor for infection
					  d. Encourage pulmonary toilet
					  e. Pain management
						Intestinal obstruction
						Respiratory distress
						Sepsis
						Wound infection
						Feeding intolerance (GERD)
						Partial/complete bowel infarction with resultant SGS

Malrotation with volvulus	Abnormal rotation and fixation of the intestine; most commonly occurs in infancy (80% in the first month of life); however, may occur at any age	Complication of malrotation. The intestine returns from the umbilical cord about week 10 of gestation, undergoes a counterclockwise rotation about the axis of the superior mesenteric artery, followed by fixation to the posterior abdominal wall; abnormal twisting causes vascular obstruction with development of midgut necrosis, unless immediate diagnosis and surgery occur	Bilious vomiting. Melena or currant-jelly stools. Abdominal distension. X-ray can reveal variable findings: normal gas pattern, duodenal obstruction, multiple dilated bowel loops. An upper GI with small bowel follow-through evaluates the position of the ligament of Treitz, duodenal obstruction, and proximal jejunum in the right abdomen	Alteration in nutrition: actual r/t NPO status. Alteration in comfort: actual r/t pain associated with vascular compromise and associated postoperative pain	1. Maintain NPO status 2. Provide IV hydration 3. Prepare child for emergency surgery 4. Postsurgical care a. PN b. Manage fluid and electrolyte status c. Monitor for infection d. Encourage pulmonary toilet e. Pain management	Sepsis. Bowel infarction with resultant SGS
Intestinal atresia	Etiology thought to be related to absence of recanalization or vascular injury to the intestine at 8 weeks gestation. Obliteration of the intestinal lumen due to occlusion or total absence	Lack of patency of a bowel segment	Proximal obstruction: Bilious vomiting, duodenal (double bubble on AXR). Distal obstruction: abdominal distension, vomiting	Alteration in nutritional status: actual r/t NPO status. Alteration in comfort r/t associated postoperative pain	1. Maintain NPO status 2. Provide IV hydration 3. Prepare for palliative/corrective surgery 4. Postoperative care a. PN b. Manage fluid and electrolyte status c. Monitor for signs and symptoms of infection d. Encourage pulmonary toilet e. Pain management	Intestinal perforation. Ileus

(continued)

TABLE 7.12   Congenital Gastrointestinal Abnormalities *(continued)*

Diagnosis	Etiology and Risk Factors	Pathophysiology	Signs and Symptoms	Nursing Diagnoses	Patient Care Management	Complications
Intussusception	Frequently preceded by gastroenteritis, lead point intussusception is caused by a specific anatomic instigator (e.g., polyp, enlarged lymph node, tumor); most commonly occurs in children 5–12 months of age	One segment of the intestine invaginates into another (usually the ileum into the cecum); the entrapped bowel initially develops venous obstruction with eventual arterial obstruction and gangrene	Recurrent and severe paroxysmal abdominal pain Bloody stool Signs of bowel obstruction: Bilious vomiting, abdominal distension, RUQ may have sausage-shaped mass	Alteration in nutrition: actual r/t NPO status Alteration in comfort: pain associated with lesion	1. Provide IV fluids 2. Maintain NPO status 3. Nonsurgical repair with contrast enema 4. Surgical reduction, if radiologic intervention unsuccessful 5. Postsurgical care a. Provide IV hydration b. Monitor for infection c. Encourage pulmonary toilet d. Pain management	Intestinal perforation Intestinal infarction Shock
TEF	History of maternal polyhydramnios Abnormal separation of the esophagus in relation to the trachea Associated with VACTERL anomalies	Five types of the anomaly can occur: Type A: Isolated EA Type B: EA with proximal TEF Type C: EA with distal TEF (most common type) Type D: EA with proximal and distal TEF Type E: Isolated TEF (referred to as an H-type)	Dependent on type of anomaly Dysphagia Inability to pass OG/NG tube Choking/cyanosis with feeding Recurrent pneumonia	Potential for ineffective airway clearance r/t dysphagia Potential for fluid volume deficit r/t continuous suctioning of oral/gastric secretions Alteration in nutritional status: actual r/t feeding difficulties, NPO status	1. Maintain NPO status 2. Provide IV hydration 3. Keep the HOB elevated 4. Suction upper airway to clear oral secretions 5. Evaluate for other anomalies 6. Surgical repair/palliation of defect 7. Postoperative care a. Management of fluid and electrolyte status b. Monitor for infection c. Encourage pulmonary toilet d. Pain management	Respiratory distress Aspiration Esophageal stricture Anastomotic leak

Diaphragmatic hernia	Failure of diaphragm closure or return of the intestine prior to diaphragmatic closure around 10 weeks of gestation	Herniation of the abdominal organs into the thoracic cavity Herniation of the intestine into the thorax with resultant lung hypoplasia (usually left; right may be affected if there is displacement of the mediastinum)	Respiratory distress Heart tones shifted to the right Scaphoid abdomen	Alteration in breathing patterns: ineffective r/t pulmonary hypoplasia Alteration in nutritional status: actual r/t NPO status	1. Maintain NPO status 2. Place NG tube for gastric decompression 3. Place right-side down to augment pulmonary perfusion 4. Pulmonary management: mechanical ventilation; oscillatory ventilation; ECMO may be indicated 5. Prepare for emergent surgical repair	Respiratory failure Pneumothorax Sepsis

Hirschsprung's disease	Failure of innervation of GI tract around 5–12 weeks of gestation	Peristalsis in lower GI tract ceases; stool cannot be passed	Newborn: Fails to pass meconium within 24–48 hours after birth
			Signs of intestinal obstruction: Bilious vomiting, abdominal distension
			Child: Constipation, ribbonlike stool, abdominal distension, visible peristalsis; may develop enterocolitis
				Potential for fluid volume deficit r/t NPO status, vomiting
				Alteration in nutritional status: Actual r/t feeding difficulties, NPO status
				Impairment of skin integrity: Actual r/t colostomy
				Alteration in comfort r/t postoperative pain
					Neonate
					1. Maintain NPO status
					2. Provide IV hydration
					3. Pass NG tube if vomiting
					4. Prepare for rectal biopsy and possible surgical correction vs. colostomy
					5. Postoperative care
					  a. Manage fluid and electrolyte status
					  b. Monitor for infection
					  c. Wound care, colostomy usually present
					  d. Encourage pulmonary toilet
					  e. Pain management
						Obstruction
						Malnutrition
						Enterocolitis

AXR, abdominal x-ray; EA, esophageal atresia; ECMO, extracorporeal membrane oxygenation; GERD, gastroesophageal reflux disease; GI, gastrointestinal; HOB, head of bed; I & O, input and output; NG, nasogastric; NPO, nothing by mouth; OG, orogastric; PN, parenteral nutrition; r/t, related to; RUQ, right upper quadrant; SGS, short gut syndrome; TEF, tracheoesophageal fistula; VACTERL, vertebral defects, anal atresia, cardiac defects, tracheoesophageal fistula, renal anomalies, and limb abnormalities.

2. *Physical Examination*

a. Obstruction results in abdominal distention, tenderness, bilious vomiting, possible fever, and absent or hyperactive bowel sounds. With a proximal obstruction, the abdomen may be scaphoid and with a distal obstruction, there is abdominal distension.

b. Perforation causes fever, pain, and possibly signs of respiratory distress, including tachypnea, retractions, flaring, grunting, and acidosis.

c. Signs of third spacing include increased abdominal girth and hypovolemia (tachycardia, decreased peripheral perfusion, decreased urine output, and hypotension [late sign]).

d. Symptoms of peritonitis include fever, nausea, marked abdominal distention or rigidity, erythema over the abdomen, absent or hypoactive bowel sounds, diffuse abdominal pain, guarding of the abdomen, diarrhea, and rebound tenderness.

3. *Diagnostic Tests*

a. Abdominal x-ray examination may reveal a paucity of gas, dilated loops of bowel, or air–fluid levels with a bowel obstruction and is usually the first radiologic study done. A lateral view reveals the presence of free air with bowel perforation.

b. Abdominal US or MRI are often done to evaluate for appendicitis as nonionizing radiation is employed. A recent systematic review reported MRI had comparable sensitivity (92%–100%) and specificity (89%–100%) for the diagnosis of appendicitis as compared to CT scan (Ogunmefun, Hardy, & Boynes, 2016).

c. Abdominal CT scan with IV and PO contrast is used to evaluate suspected abscess or mass.

d. Air enema is often done instead of a contrast enema and is a diagnostic and therapeutic treatment for intussusception. Typically, air enema results in successful reduction of the obstructed bowel with reported success rates of 50% to 80% (Makin & Davenport, 2016). Generally, water-soluble contrast is used if attempting reduction.

e. Upper GI series is the gold standard for making the diagnosis of a midgut volvulus, although this abnormality is often appreciated from an abdominal CT scan.

4. *Clinical Course*

a. Varies depending on the surgical pathology. Generally, symptoms are progressive. A child with significant intra-abdominal pathology may eventually develop mental status changes and become somnolent.

D. **Patient Care Management**

1. *Direct Care*

a. Provide frequent vital-sign monitoring with assessment for respiratory distress. Elevate the head of the bed 30 to 45 degrees to enhance respiratory effort.

b. Place an NG tube for gastric decompression and drainage and maintain low intermittent suction if a complete or proximal obstruction is suspected.

c. Monitor intake and output, as oliguria commonly requires fluid boluses. Placement of a urinary catheter may be indicated.

d. Surgical intervention may be indicated for persistent abdominal pain, evidence of localized peritonitis (erythema over a portion of the abdomen), and the presence of free air on abdominal x-ray examination.

e. Analgesia as needed for pain. Typically, an IV opioid is administered either as an intermittent bolus or a continuous infusion with or without a patient-controlled analgesia unit. Opioids will slow bowel motility and often the pain regimen includes IV Ofirmev (acetaminophen) or IV NSAIDs when the child is NPO.

f. Administer broad-spectrum antibiotics with peritonitis.

2. *Supportive Care*

a. Perform pulmonary toilet to prevent atelectasis.

b. Frequent ambulation should be encouraged.

c. Deep vein thrombosis prophylaxis with use of sequential compression device and SC heparin or lovenox (enoxaparin) administration for at-risk children.

E. **Outcomes**

Complications include sepsis, perforation, need for bowel resection, adhesions with resultant obstruction, and abscess formation.

NECROTIZING ENTEROCOLITIS

A. **Definition and Etiology**

1. NEC is a multifactorial disease of the bowel with the greatest incidence in the premature neonate.

2. NEC is usually a disease of the neonate and is characterized by widespread inflammation of the gut; however, older children can have presentations with classic findings, including pneumatosis intestinalis. NEC is seen primarily in premature infants (90%) and is related to dysbiosis or altered bacterial colonization of the intestinal flora (Gupta & Paria, 2016). In near-term and term infants, hypoxic or ischemic insults are dominant risk factors.

3. Risk factors for the premature infant include receiving enteral feeds (greater incidence with commercial formulas as compared to BM) and presence of intrauterine growth retardation.

B. Pathophysiology

Despite research efforts, the pathophysiology of NEC is yet to be determined. Current thought is the disease occurs because of the dysbiosis, which leads to an unbalanced proinflammatory response that leads to mucosal disruption and eventual bowel necrosis in infants being enterally fed. Although spontaneous intestinal perforation is often termed NEC; researchers postulate an alternate pathophysiology, as there is minimal gut inflammation (Gupta & Paria, 2016).

C. Clinical Presentation

1. *History.* Can have an abrupt onset with fulminant presentation rapidly progressing to death. In its milder forms, NEC has many of the same signs and symptoms of sepsis (e.g., feeding intolerance, increased gastric residual volumes, bloody stools).

2. *Physical Examination.* See Table 7.13 for modified Bell's criteria, which are routinely used to diagnosis and stage the disease.

3. *Diagnostic Tests*

a. Abdominal x-ray examination with supine and lateral views may reveal pneumatosis intestinalis, dilated loops of small bowel, and pneumoperitoneum if perforation has occurred.

b. Abdominal US is becoming increasingly important in determining when surgical intervention may be indicated and is more sensitive in detecting portal venous gas and intra-abdominal free fluid (Gupta & Paria, 2016).

4. *Clinical Course*

a. Initially, symptoms of NEC are nonspecific and progress per Bell's criteria as outlined in Table 7.13. The classic triad is abdominal distention, bilious vomiting, and blood in the stools.

b. Signs of progressive NEC include discoloration of the abdominal wall, respiratory distress, hypotension, leukopenia, thrombocytopenia, and a WBC count reflecting a shift to the left.

D. Patient Care Management

1. *Preventive Care.* Preventive care focuses on preventing prematurity; there is and some evidence that there is a lower incidence in neonates who are prescribed probiotics and fed BM versus commercial formulas.

2. *Direct Care*

a. Infants are kept NPO with an NG tube to low intermittent suction for gastric decompression. Fluids and electrolytes are monitored, and PN is provided. When perforation has occurred, broad-spectrum antibiotic therapy is prescribed with a cephalosporin and aminoglycoside.

b. Respiratory and cardiac status are closely monitored with frequent monitoring of vital signs and serial abdominal girth measurements.

c. Guaiac stool testing is used to detect occult bleeding. Serial platelet counts and serial abdominal x-ray examinations are used to monitor progression.

d. Surgery is indicated if signs of perforation, peritonitis, or clinical deterioration are evident despite medical management.

3. *Outcomes*

a. Complications include being rendered short-gut with intestinal failure.

b. Mortality is 30% and for neonates requiring surgery, the mortality is as high as 45% (Hull et al., 2014).

HYPERBILIRUBINEMIA

A. Definition and Etiology

1. Hyperbilirubinemia is an elevation in the level of total serum bilirubin (TSB); it results from an imbalance between bilirubin production and excretion.

2. Bilirubin is the byproduct of the heme portion of the breakdown of the hemoglobin molecule.

3. Hyperbilirubinemia is an elevated level of serum bilirubin. Indirect prehepatic-unconjugated bilirubin elevations may be physiologic rather than

TABLE 7.13   Staging Criteria for Necrotizing Enterocolitis

Stage 1A (Suspect) a. Systemic manifestations: Temperature instability, lethargy, apnea, bradycardia b. GI tract manifestations: Poor feeding, increasing gastric residual volumes, emesis (may be bilious or have positive results for occult blood), mild abdominal distention, occult blood in stool c. Radiologic findings: Normal or intestinal dilation
Stage 1B (Suspect) a. Systemic manifestations: Temperature instability, lethargy, apnea, bradycardia b. GI tract manifestations: Poor feeding, increasing gastric residual volumes, emesis (may be bilious or have positive results for occult blood), mild abdominal distention, occult blood in stool, hematochezia c. Radiologic findings: Normal or intestinal dilation
Stage 2A (Definite—Mildly Ill) a. 1B signs and symptoms b. Marked abdominal distention and decreased bowel sounds c. Abdominal radiographs show significant intestinal distention with ileus, pneumatosis intestinalis
Stage 2A (Definite—Moderately Ill) a. 1B signs and symptoms plus thrombocytopenia and metabolic acidosis b. Marked abdominal distention and tenderness c. Abdominal radiographs with possible ascites and portal venous gas
Stage 3A (Advanced—Bowel Intact) a. Same signs and symptoms as in stage 2 plus deterioration in vital signs, increased apnea, shock, disseminated intravascular coagulation b. Same as 2A and evidence of peritonitis
Stage 3A (Advanced—Bowel Perforated) a. Same signs and symptoms as in stage 3A—bowel intact b. Same signs and symptoms as in stage 3A—bowel intact c. Abdominal radiographs show pneumoperitoneum

GI, gastrointestinal.

Sources: Modified from Bell, M. J., Ternberg, J. L., Feigin, R. D. Keating, J. P., Marshall, R., Barton, L., & Brotherton, T. (1978). Neonatal necrotizing enterocolitis: Therapeutic decisions based upon clinical staging. *Annals of Surgery,* 187(1), 1–7. Retrieved from https://www.ncbi.nlm.nih.gov/pmc/articles/PMC1396409; Gupta, A., & Paria, A. (2016). Etiology and medical management of NEC. *Early Human Development, 97,* 17–23. doi:10.1016/j.earlhumdev.2016.03.008

pathologic. Direct posthepatic-conjugated bilirubin elevations are always pathologic. The terms *direct* and *indirect* are used interchangeably with conjugated and unconjugated hyperbilirubinemia. Direct hyperbilirubinemia includes conjugated and delta bilirubin measurements.

4. Premature neonates; infants with traumatic births and increased hemolysis; breastfed infants; infants of East Asian, Native American, and Greek descent; ABO incompatibilities; Rh isoimmunization; glucose-6-phosphate dehydrogenase deficiency; pyruvate kinase deficiency; and infants of diabetic mothers are at higher risk for developing neonatal or physiologic jaundice or hyperbilirubinemia (Watson, 2009).

B. Pathophysiology

1. Fat-soluble bilirubin binds to albumin as indirect (prehepatic-unconjugated) bilirubin for transport to the liver. In the liver, fat-soluble bilirubin is detached from albumin and conjugated with glucuronic acid, rendering the bilirubin water soluble. Increases in indirect bilirubin result when the liver is not able to conjugate the bilirubin with impaired synthetic function.

2. Direct (posthepatic-conjugated) bilirubin is excreted into the hepatic ducts and eventually into the intestine. Impaired excretion of direct bilirubin into the bile ducts leads to increased levels of conjugated bilirubin as increased amounts are reabsorbed into the blood.

3. Impaired synthetic function and obstruction increase total bilirubin.

4. Three types of jaundice (prehepatic, hepatocellular, cholestatic) can occur. Prehepatic jaundice is usually caused by hemolysis. The total bilirubin is increased with the majority of the bilirubin in the indirect form. Hepatocellular jaundice results from liver dysfunction characterized by hepatic inflammation (infection, hepatitis, drug induced). The total bilirubin is increased. Cholestatic jaundice results from failure of biliary excretion. An increase in direct bilirubin is present.

5. Physiologic jaundice is a transient hyperbilirubinemia that is frequently observed in otherwise completely healthy newborns. Bilirubin values peak at day 3 of life and usually normalize by 2 weeks of age.

C. Clinical Presentation

1. *History.* Indirect hyperbilirubinemia is most common in premature infants in the neonatal period, with serum bilirubin levels peaking at 48 to 96 hours of life. If direct hyperbilirubinemia is present, the infant or child should be evaluated for other signs of liver disease.

2. *Physical Exam. Jaundice* is an accumulation of yellow pigment in the skin and other tissues and is evident when total bilirubin is greater than 3 mg/dL. *Kernicterus* is the presence of yellow pigment in the basal ganglia of the brain and is a complication of severe unconjugated hyperbilirubinemia. Bilirubin can enter the brain if it is not bound to albumin (unconjugated) or if there has been damage to the blood–brain barrier. Signs of kernicterus include a sluggish Moro reflex, opisthotonus, hypotonia, vomiting, high-pitched cry, seizures, and paresis of gaze (sun-setting sign). Dark-colored urine and pale-colored stool may occur in conjugated hyperbilirubinemia.

3. *Diagnostic Tests.* Indirect, direct, and total bilirubin levels are elevated. See Table 7.1 for reference ranges.

D. Patient Care Management

1. Management of indirect hyperbilirubinemia includes phototherapy by bilirubin lights or bilirubin blankets and is based on the infant's age and TSB (American Academy of Pediatrics Subcommittee on Hyperbilirubinemia [AAP], 2004). As much skin surface as possible should be exposed. Cover eyes to protect from light and provide eye care every 4 hours. Fluid requirements are increased up to 20% because of increased insensible water losses. With excessive hyperbilirubinemia, exchange transfusion and pharmacologic interventions (i.e., phenobarbital administration) may be indicated.

2. Management of direct hyperbilirubinemia depends on the etiology (see "Liver Failure" section)

E. Outcomes

Indirect hyperbilirubinemia can result in kernicterus or brain damage.

PANCREATITIS

A. Definition and Etiology

1. Pancreatitis is a diagnosis that is increasingly occurring in children and is classified as acute, acute recurrent, and chronic, which is characterized by ongoing inflammation of the pancreas.

2. Types of pancreatitis as defined by the International Study Group of Pediatric Pancreatitis (Morinville et al., 2012): acute, acute recurrent, and chronic.

  a. Acute pancreatitis (AP) requires two of the following:

    i. Abdominal pain compatible with AP

    ii. Serum amylase and/or lipase three or more times the upper limit of normal

    iii. Imaging with findings of AP

  b. Acute recurrent pancreatitis (ARP) is defined as two or more episodes of AP with interval return to baseline of at least a month with pain resolved and normalized amylase and lipase.

  c. Chronic pancreatitis (CP) requires

    i. Typical abdominal pain with imaging findings

    ii. Exocrine insufficiency with imaging findings

    iii. Endocrine insufficiency plus abdominal pain

3. Causes are diverse and include biliary (e.g., gallstones or cholelithiasis associated with hemolytic disorders, including spherocytosis, beta-thalassemia, and sickle cell disease), anatomic (e.g., blunt abdominal trauma, such as bicycle handlebar injuries, motor vehicle crashes), medications (e.g., L-asparaginase, valproic acid, Prednisone), metabolic (e.g., diabetic ketoacidosis, hypertriglyceridemia, hypercalcemia), and genetic abnormalities (e.g., serine protease-inhibitor [SPINK1 N345], protease inhibitor [PRSS1 R122H], cystic fibrosis transmembrane conductance regulator

[CFTR DeltaF508, 5T]; Kramer & Jeffery, 2014; Poddar, Yachha, Mathias, & Choudhuri, 2015).

B. Pathophysiology

1. Injury to the acinar cells leads to the release of proteases and other enzymes (e.g., elastase, lipase) with resultant autodigestion.

2. The inflammatory cascade causes edema and local inflammation and triggers inflammatory mediators and trypsin to be released, causing abdominal pain.

3. Release of inflammatory mediators leads to systemic inflammatory response syndrome (SIRS) with the potential for renal and pulmonary sequelae with resultant dehydration and the potential for thrombosis.

4. AP involves a single episode; with recurrent episodes or CP, morphologic changes in the pancreas begin to interfere with exocrine and endocrine functions, resulting in CP.

C. Clinical Presentation

1. *History.* Classic symptoms of pancreatitis in children are abdominal pain that is typically most intense in the epigastrium, nausea, vomiting, and anorexia.

2. *Physical Examination.* Symptom severity varies from mild abdominal pain to signs and symptoms of severe shock and end-organ failure. Although more common in adults, back and flank pain are also common as the organ is retroperitoneal. Moving and eating intensify the pain. A bluish discoloration around the umbilicus (Cullen's sign) or in the flanks (Turner's sign), signify hemorrhagic pancreatitis.

3. *Diagnostic Tests*

    a. Laboratory tests

        i. Amylase and lipase are enzymes derived from pancreatic acinar cells and will be elevated; lipase has a longer half-life and may remain elevated, whereas amylase levels typically peak approximately 48 hours after the onset of pancreatitis and may normalize with delayed presentations (Abu-El-Haija, Lin, & Palermo, 2014).

        ii. Other labs that may be evaluated include calcium, triglyceride levels, CBC, liver transaminases, bilirubin level, and BUN.

    b. Radiologic findings (see Table 7.2)

        i. Abdominal US recommended as initial imaging as it can confirm the diagnosis and assist with identifying contributing abnormalities.

        ii. Abdominal CT scan is the second most common imaging method as it can diagnose and identify etiologies and visualize masses, necrosis, and hemorrhage (Abu-El-Haija et al., 2014).

        iii. Use of MRCP is controversial for an initial episode of AP. MRCP can detect intrahepatic and pancreatic duct abnormalities (Abu-El-Haija et al., 2014).

4. *Clinical Course.* Varies based on the type of pancreatitis.

D. Patient Care Management

1. *Preventive Care.* Alleviate the cause of the pancreatitis.

2. *Direct Care for AP*

    a. Hydration with aggressive IV fluid administration is indicated with the initiation of one and a half to two times maintenance dose with D5.9NS (Szabo, Fei, Cruz, & Abu-El-Haija, 2015).

    b. Nutrition management has changed from maintaining NPO status to early EN. Begin with a clear diet at admission and advance to a regular diet if tolerated within 6 hours (Szabo et al., 2015). The goal of early EN is to maintain the gut barrier and prevent bacterial translocation (Szabo et al., 2015). PN should be prescribed for children who do not tolerate EN.

    c. Pain management is usually accomplished with the use of opioids and nonsteroidal anti-inflammatory agents (e.g., Toradol [ketorolac], and IV Ofirmev [acetaminophen]). The use of morphine and other opiate derivatives is theoretically less desirable in patients with pancreatitis, because these medications increase spasm of the sphincter of Oddi and may cause additional pain, although there is no current evidence to support this.

    d. IV antibiotics should be administered when pancreatic necrosis is present.

    e. Surgical intervention is indicated with a cholecystectomy for gallstone pancreatitis; for CP, the modified Puestow procedure is most commonly performed.

3. *Supportive Care.* Prevent thrombotic events with deep vein thrombosis prophylaxis.

E. Outcomes

1. Complications include pseudocyst formation and endocrine dysfunction (e.g., hyperglycemia).

2. Approximately 10% of children will develop CP after experiencing AP; the presence of a peripancreatic necrosis at initial presentation is an independent predictor of CP (Hao, Guo, Luo, & Guo, 2016).

3. Median hospital stay is a week and most children have complete recovery.

GALLBLADDER DISEASE

A. Definition and Etiology

1. Gallbladder disease, or cholecystitis, is inflammation of the gallbladder, which is most commonly caused by gallstones.

2. Gallbladder disease in children is increasing due to improved diagnostic modalities (US) and the obesity epidemic (Svensson & Makin, 2012).

3. Cholecystitis is inflammation of the gallbladder, which most commonly caused by gallstones. There are two types of disease: acalculous or calculous, depending on the presence of cholelithiasis.

4. There is a known spectrum of gallbladder disease, which ranges from biliary colic/dyskinesia, cholelithiasis, acute acalculous cholecystitis, choledocolithiasis to cholangitis.

5. Etiologies for acalculous disease are most commonly associated with sepsis or a severe infection. Calculous from nonhemolytic cholelithiasis—formation of gallstones in the absence of a hemolytic disease, including obesity, PN administration, history of an ileal resection (e.g., NEC), volvulus, cystic fibrosis, medications (e.g., Ceftriaxone and Furosemide), and pregnancy. Calculous from hemolytic cholelithiasis—bile in these patients has an increased amount of unconjugated bilirubin, leading to the formation of gallbladder sludge and thus the increased risk for cholelithiasis, which can occur with sickle cell disease, thalassemia, spherocytosis, and Gilbert syndrome.

B. Pathophysiology

1. The gallbladder is stimulated to contract due to hormones (cholecystokinin and motilin) that are released when fats are present in the duodenum. Gallbladder contraction propels bile down the common bile duct, through the sphincter of Oddi, and into the duodenum (Mouat, 2012).

2. Regardless of the etiology, there is stasis within the gallbladder.

3. With gallstone presence there is sludge formation and inflammation, which may lead to obstruction and further inflammation (Mouat, 2012).

4. Bile stasis and bacterial overgrowth lead to the release of lysolecithin (phospholipid) and other proinflammatory agents that exacerbate the inflammatory response (Mouat, 2012).

5. The pain is attributed to the increased pressure within the gallbladder.

C. Clinical Presentation

1. *History*

   a. *Acalculous.* Episodic RUQ pain occurs.

   b. *Calculous.* With cholelithiasis—there can be "silent stones" that are recognized incidentally on imaging; these children can be asymptomatic.

2. *Physical Examination*

   a. *Acalculous.* Fever, vomiting, and RUQ pain, and positive Murphy's sign (pain on deep inspiration when the inflamed gallbladder is palpated).

   b. *Calculous.* Range of presentation from children having fever, RUQ/abdominal pain, positive Murphy's sign, and vomiting.

3. *Diagnostic Tests*

   a. Laboratory evaluation

     i. There may be elevated liver transaminases, bilirubin level, and white blood cell count.

   b. Radiologic evaluation

     i. US will reveal a thickened gallbladder that contains debris; gallstones may or may not be present.

     ii. ERCP can be done to evaluate the pancreas and common bile duct with possible stone removal if present.

     iii. MRCP can be done with no radiation exposure to define and evaluate the biliary structures; however, this is strictly diagnostic and there can be no intervention.

4. *Clinical Course.* Variable depending on the etiology.

D. Patient Care Management

1. *Acalculous*

a. Offer supportive care and administer antimicrobials for self-limiting cases.

b. Cholecystectomy needed for progressive gallbladder distension or clinical deterioration.

2. *Calculous*

a. ERCP may be indicated if a stone is present with common bile duct dilation prior to a cholecystectomy. A surgeon may delay performing a cholecystectomy to allow for resolution of the inflammation, which will be evident with the resolution of fever, pain, and normalization of lab values.

b. Cholecystectomy
  i. Gallbladder removal either by an open or laparoscopic technique.

E. Outcomes

Complications include a bile leak and pancreatitis.

GI INFECTION

A. Definition and Etiology

1. GI infections include a multitude of acute diarrheal infections including viral, bacterial, and parasitic infection with organisms including *Clostridium difficile* and *vancomycin-resistant enterococcus.*

2. Acute diarrhea is a sudden change in the frequency and consistency of stools.

3. The most common etiology of diarrhea is viral. There has been a sustained decrease in the incidence of Rotavirus since the addition of Rotavirus vaccines to the recommended immunization schedule in 2006.

4. *C. difficile* is an anaerobic, spore-forming, toxin-forming, gram-positive bacillus bacteria that is being diagnosed with increasing frequency and is associated with antibiotic usage. *Vancomycin-resistant enterococcus* is increasingly being diagnosed in children and is associated with *C. difficile*

infection, the use of immunosuppressive therapies and significant antibiotic exposure.

B. Pathophysiology

1. Acute diarrhea alters the GI tract and can lead to dehydration. Dehydrated patients are deficient in both fluids and electrolytes and are at risk for acute kidney injury.

2. *C. difficile* is a gram-positive organism and is part of the normal GI bacterial flora. When risk factors exist, *C. difficile* will replicate and lead to colonization. Once colonization of the colon occurs, the bacteria begin to release two distinct toxins. Toxin A is an enterotoxin that disrupts colonic mucosal adherence to the basement membrane and causes damage to the intestinal villi. Toxin B is a cytotoxin that induces apoptosis, which leads to neutrophilic infiltration and inflammation of the colon.

C. Clinical Presentation

1. *History.* Infection is often hospital acquired and is associated with antibiotic usage.

2. *Physical Examination.* All children with diarrhea and dehydration will have a history of inadequate fluid intake and excessive fluid loss. The child may be febrile and usually is irritable, experiences abdominal pain and looks ill; there may or may not be associated vomiting. Signs of dehydration include sunken eyes, dry mucous membranes, and a sunken fontanelle in infants. The child will be tachycardic, and signs of compensated or hypovolemic shock may be present.

3. *Diagnostic Tests*

a. If there is blood or mucous in the stool, stool studies should be obtained. The stool should be sent to identify presence of white blood cells, bacterial culture, and *C. difficile* toxin (in children older than 1 year) and ova and parasites. Stool testing for children younger than 1 year is not recommended due to the high carriage rate (American Academy of Pediatrics Committee on Infectious Diseases, 2013).

b. Initial blood work typically includes evaluation of a serum chemistry panel and a CBC. Once the serum sodium concentration is determined, the estimate of the severity of dehydration (based initially on clinical examination alone) is modified as needed. Often these children have a metabolic acidosis, which may be evident from the low carbon dioxide level and an elevated BUN from the dehydration on the chemistry panel.

4. *Clinical Course.* Course is variable depending on the infecting organism and child's comorbidities.

D. Patient Care Management

1. *Preventive Care.* Good handwashing with soap and water and donning appropriate personal protective equipment are the keys to preventing the transmission of these infectious diseases.

2. *Direct Care*

a. Children with diarrhea from a bacterial cause require contact isolation until associated symptoms resolve and antibiotic therapy is complete. Contact isolation must be enforced with meticulous attention to handwashing because most of these organisms are contagious and are a frequent cause of nosocomial infection.

b. Obtain an accurate weight in kilograms as soon as possible after admission and on a daily basis during hospitalization. This weight measurement can be helpful in determining the severity of dehydration and evaluating the patient's response to therapy. Weight measurements are most reliable if the child is weighed on the same scale at the same time every day.

c. Take accurate intake and output measurements and notify the provider if the child's urine output is less than 0.5 to 1 mL/kg/hr.

d. Although the majority of acute diarrhea infections are caused by viral pathogens, antibiotics are administered for some bacteria or culture-proven parasitic infections.

    i. For positive *C. difficile* infection, the causative antibiotic is discontinued if possible, and a 7-day oral course of metronidazole (Flagyl) administered is provided. Oral vancomycin can also be administered to patients who cannot tolerate metronidazole or for any adolescent patients who are breastfeeding or pregnant.

3. For the child who is experiencing concomitant vomiting and diarrhea, ondansetron (Zofran) can help with symptom control. For children with mild dehydration, the medication can be administered as an oral disintegrating tablet. IV administration is recommended for children with moderate or severe dehydration (see "Pharmacology" section).

4. *Supportive Care*

a. Treatment becomes supportive as diarrhea resolves. Initially, when stools are frequent and watery, the child is NPO and maintenance fluid requirements are provided intravenously.

b. The irritated GI tract requires a period of rest, followed by the gradual resumption of oral feedings with oral electrolyte solutions. Once stool output has decreased and the child is no longer vomiting, clear liquids are offered and enteral feeding can be advanced slowly as tolerated to an age-appropriate diet. If diarrhea resumes during diet advancement, the child should be placed back on a clear diet or the last tolerated intake.

E. Outcomes

Although these illnesses are self-limiting, they contribute to the morbidity of children cared for in the PICU.

HEPATIC FAILURE

Hepatic failure can occur as chronic, "decompensated" chronic, or acute-chronic liver failure and acute liver failure (ALF).

A. Acute Liver Failure

1. *Definition of ALF*

a. The Pediatric Acute Liver Failure (PALF) study group has refined the definition of ALF as a syndrome, not a disease, with the following criteria:

    i. Hepatic-based coagulopathy defined as a PT ≥15 seconds or INR ≥1.5 not correctable with vitamin K in the presence of hepatic encephalopathy

    ii. PT ≥20 seconds or INR ≥2 regardless of hepatic encephalopathy

    iii. Biochemical evidence of acute liver injury

    iv. No known evidence of chronic liver disease (Sundaram, Alonso, Narkewicz, Zhang, & Squires, 2011)

b. Other ALF definitions (Sundaram et al., 2011):

    i. Hyperacute liver failure is fulminant hepatic failure (FHF) with the time from jaundice to encephalopathy less than 7 days.

ii. ALF as FHF with the time from jaundice to encephalopathy between 7 and 28 days.

iii. Subacute liver failure as FHF from the time from jaundice to encephalopathy more than 28 days.

2. Liver disease is a significant problem, with 15,000 children hospitalized each year (American Liver Foundation, 2013), which is a statistic that has remained unchanged over the past 25 years.

3. *Etiology of ALF*

a. Hepatitis (inflammation of the liver) is the most frequently identified cause of hepatic failure. Hepatotropic viral infectious causes include the following:

  i. Hepatitis A virus (HAV)

  1) On average, the incubation period is 28 days.

  2) Serologic markers for HAV include hepatitis A antibodies of the immunoglobulin M (IgM) class (anti-HAV IgM), whose presence reflects active or recent HAV infection, and hepatitis A antibodies of the immunoglobulin G (IgG) class (anti-HAV IgG), whose presence reflects immunity.

  3) The Advisory Committee on Immunizations Practices recommend routine vaccination for children at age 2 years living in communities with high rates of hepatitis A (Alaska, Arizona, California, Idaho, Nevada, New Mexico, Oklahoma, Oregon, South Dakota, Utah, and Washington), for those who have planned travel to endemic areas, and day-care workers.

  4) Disease transmission is via the oral–fecal route. Food, water, and shellfish contaminated by the virus are the usual sources.

  ii. Hepatitis B virus (HBV)

  1) The incubation period is, on average, 80 days.

  2) Hepatitis B vaccine is part of the American Academy of Pediatrics recommended immunization schedule and has led to a decline in the incidence; need for booster unclear.

  3) Serologic markers of HBV include hepatitis B surface antigen (HbsAg), whose presence reflects acute or

chronic infection; hepatitis B e antigen (HbeAg), whose presence reflects active HBV infection with active viral replication and high infectivity; antibody to hepatitis B surface antigen (anti-HBs), whose presence reflects clinical recovery and immunity; and HBV quantification with polymerase chain reaction (PCR), which reflects a specific quantity of active HBV.

  4) Disease transmission occurs through the exchange of blood or body fluids. Neonates can acquire the virus via maternal transmission.

  5) Disease presentation varies and may consist of a prodrome, followed by insidious onset, with symptoms usually resolving within 1 to 3 months. Unfortunately, there is a cadre of patients that develop chronic disease. A small percentage of infected individuals develop FHF.

  iii. Hepatitis C virus (HCV)

  1) Incubation time is 2 to 26 weeks.

  2) Serologic markers for HCV include anti-HCV antibody, indicating exposure to HCV and PCR, whose presence reflects HCV infection.

  3) Perinatal transmission is now the most common mode of acquiring HCV in children (Lee & Jonas, 2015).

  4) No vaccine available.

  iv. Clinical presentation of hepatitis involves three stages:

  1) *Preicteric stage* has a duration of approximately 1 week. Signs and symptoms include fever, chills, anorexia, malaise, abdominal pain, nausea, vomiting, joint pain, hepatomegaly, and lymphadenopathy. HAV is characterized by nonspecific features of viral illness, including fever, headache, anorexia, and nausea. HBV is characterized by arthralgia, arthritis, transient skin rash, and later malaise, nausea, vomiting, and low-grade fever. Jaundice usually occurs 10 to 12 days after the onset of symptoms.

  2) *Icteric stage* has a duration of 2 to 6 weeks. Signs and symptoms include weakness, fatigue, pallor, jaundice, dark urine, pale-colored stool, and pruritus.

3) During the *posticteric stage,* there is resolution of the jaundice, darkening of the stools, and normalization of LFT values. Complete recovery occurs in most cases.

v. Other viral causes include herpes simplex virus, Epstein–Barr virus (EBV), adenovirus, parvovirus, varicella, and cytomegalovirus (which may be congenitally acquired). Infants are at risk if the mother is infected with a primary infection and active infection is present at birth.

b. Neonatal "giant cell" hepatitis is a histologically descriptive term. The disease is characterized by large cells with many nuclei. The cause is most likely related to an autoimmune process.

c. Drug-induced acute hepatic failure.

i. The *liver* is the most common site for drug metabolism. Children receiving drugs known to be hepatotoxic should have serial LFT monitoring while receiving therapy. The risk of developing FHF increases with continued use of the drug in the presence of developing hepatitis.

ii. The most common toxic drugs are acetaminophen (Tylenol), ecstasy (methyldioxymethamphetamine), anticonvulsants (phenytoin [Dilantin] and valproate [Depakene]), methotrexate, halothane, and isoniazid.

d. Wilson disease is an autosomal-recessive disorder that results in excessive accumulation of copper in the organs. The biochemical disorder of copper metabolism is a defect in the copper adenosine triphosphatase transporter, with decreased copper excretion, defective incorporation of copper into ceruplasmin, and copper accumulation (Carlson, Al-Mateen, & Brewer, 2004). Liver dysfunction manifestations are variable and the child may present with FHF. Medical therapy includes administration of *d*-penicillamine and dietary restrictions of copper. Liver transplantation is indicated in the presence of FHF or cirrhosis with decompensation.

4. *Pathophysiology*

a. Pathophysiology of ALF is presumed to be multifactorial. Portal-systemic shunting (caused by progressive liver destruction) allows blood flow from the intestine to be shunted around the liver, bypassing any remaining viable hepatocytes. The liver is unable to remove toxic metabolites normally formed by intestinal bacterial degradation of proteins, amino acids, and blood (e.g., ammonia). Altered blood–brain permeability is hypothesized to be related to toxin(s) of intestinal origin bypassing the portal filtration, resulting in a disruption of the blood–brain barrier.

b. Neurologic pathophysiology

i. Multiple proposed etiologies

1) Mechanism of the formation of cerebral edema is not known.

2) High ammonia levels play a central role; although level does not correlate with exam and seems to be related to the accumulation of other neurotoxic substances.

c. Renal pathophysiology

i. More than one type of renal failure may be present. Careful differentiation of the type of renal failure must be made before appropriate therapy can be initiated.

ii. *Prerenal azotemia* occurs when prerenal blood flow and renal perfusion are compromised. Treatment includes addressing the cause of decreased renal perfusion (i.e., fluid resuscitation).

iii. *Acute tubular necrosis* is related to parenchymal damage to the kidney associated with a chronic prerenal or postrenal condition (e.g., toxic chemical exposure or glomerulonephritis). It may occur with concomitant sepsis, hemorrhage, and ischemia.

iv. *Hepatorenal syndrome* (functional renal failure of liver disease) is likely to be related to an unidentified vasoconstrictive substance causing a decrease in renal perfusion resulting in oliguric renal failure in the presence of hepatic failure. Renal failure resolves with improvement of the hepatic dysfunction; however, the associated mortality is high.

d. Hematologic pathophysiology

i. *Coagulopathy* is related to an abnormal production of prothrombin and other clotting factors produced by the liver, signifying impaired hepatic synthetic function, and ineffective removal of activated clotting factors.

ii. *Hypersplenism* results from increased portal venous pressures delaying the blood flow through the splanchnic bed with resultant congestion and enlargement of the spleen. Splenic overactivity increases destruction of RBCs, platelets, and WBCs. The sequelae of splenomegaly includes anemia, platelet dysfunction (quantitative and qualitative), leukopenia, and DIC.

5. *Clinical Presentation*

a. History

b. Physical examination

6. *Signs and Symptoms*

a. Staging of hepatic encephalopathy

  i. Stage I. Normal level of consciousness, periods of lethargy and euphoria

  ii. Stage II. Disorientation, increased drowsiness, and agitation with mood swings

  iii. Stage III. Marked confusion, sleeping most of the time

  iv. Stage IV. Coma

b. Jaundice. Yellow discoloration of the skin, mucous membranes, and sclera is caused by excessive bilirubin levels.

c. Renal-failure symptoms depend on the type of renal failure the child is experiencing. Azotemia should be evaluated carefully in the presence of hepatic failure, as nitrogenous wastes cannot be metabolized appropriately. Increased serum creatinine levels and oliguria are present.

d. Coagulopathy is recognized by an elevated PT. A PT that is uncorrectable despite IV vitamin K (AquaMEPHYTON) administration reflects significant parenchymal disease. In addition, there will be platelet dysfunction. Other signs include bruising and bleeding from mucosal surfaces and the presence of petechiae.

B. Chronic Liver Failure

1. *Definition*

a. The difference between acute and chronic disease presentation relates to the rate of parenchymal (organ-specific tissue) injury. Fibrosis leads to cirrhosis with development of portal hypertension evident by the presence of hepatosplenomegaly, varices, and ascites.

b. Most children have a chronic presentation of hepatic failure versus an acute presentation.

2. *Etiology*

a. Nonalcoholic fatty liver disease

  i. Most common cause of chronic liver disease in children in Western countries.

  ii. Affects up to 10% of U.S. children (Corte et al., 2012).

  iii. Etiology

    1) Multifactorial

    2) Multihit

    3) Insulin resistance causes increased levels of fatty acids, which results in fatty infiltration or steatosis.

    4) Hit continues as the increased fatty acids cause apoptosis of the hepatocytes *or* a second hit from the gut and adipose tissue-derived endotoxin causes progression to nonalcoholic steatohepatitis (NASH).

3. *Diagnosis*

a. Liver biopsy for definitive diagnosis

b. Elevated ALT

  i. Not excessive (1–4 × reference range)

  ii. Does not correlate with the degree of steatosis or fibrosis.

c. Pediatric symptoms. Fatigue, hepatomegaly, obesity with central adiposity (waist circumference may correlate with disease severity), RUQ or epigastric pain, and acanthosis nigricans

d. Treatment

  i. Gradual weight loss and physical activity

  ii. Pharmacologic agents:

  • No evidence that any agents help

  • Vitamin E and metformin are the most common agents that have been prescribed

4. *Pathophysiology*

a. *Hepatosplenomegaly.* The liver becomes firm and enlarged with regeneration, and the liver and spleen become enlarged due to vascular engorgement.

b. *Varices.* With intrahepatic fibrosis, there is obstruction of blood flow with formation of collaterals in the esophagus and rectum. These veins are thin walled and prone to developing varicosities (i.e., rectal, esophageal) and GI tract bleeding.

c. *Ascites* is related to the accumulation of fluid in the abdomen related to altered plasma oncotic pressure (decreased albumin production) and increased portal venous pressure. Increased abdominal girth, everted umbilicus, bulging flanks, positive fluid wave, and respiratory distress are noted.

d. *Malnutrition* is evident because of inadequate bile salts and the child's inability to absorb fat-soluble vitamins (A, D, E, and K). Poor weight gain and deficiencies of vitamin A (causing atrophy of the epithelial tissue and night blindness when severe), vitamin D (causing rickets), vitamin E (causing muscle degeneration, megaloblastic anemia, hemolytic anemia, creatinuria, target cell anemia, spur cell anemia, and peripheral neuropathy), and vitamin K (causing hypoprothrombinemia resulting in coagulopathy) are noted. Adequate glucose is necessary to maintain normal blood glucose levels.

e. *Pruritus* is related to bile salt deposition on the epidermis related to defective biliary drainage causing an accumulation of pruritogens. Constant itching can be accompanied with skin breakdown and secondary infection.

f. *Asterixis.* "Liver flap" is a flapping tremor of the hand noted when both arms are raised with forearms fixed and the hands dorsiflexed.

g. *Rickets* are caused by an abnormal bone formation related to a deficiency of vitamin D, calcium, and phosphorus. Pathologic fractures and bone malformations result.

h. *Telangiectasis* (vascular spiders, spider angiomas, spider nevi) are skin lesions consisting of a central arteriole from which smaller vessels radiate. Spontaneous bleeding from lesions can occur.

i. *Xanthomas* are fatty nodules that develop in the SC skin layer due to disturbances in lipid metabolism.

5. *Signs and Symptoms of Chronic Liver Disease*

   a. Jaundice

      i. Seen with both acute and chronic liver failure

      ii. Accumulation of yellow pigment in the tissues

      iii. Cephalocaudal distribution:

        • Head and sclera = 5

        • Trunk = 10

        • Distal extremities = 15

6. *Diagnostic Tests*

   a. Comprehensive blood chemistries, hematology and coagulation studies, US, CT scan, liver biopsy, endoscopy, and LFTs (see Table 7.2) may be useful in the determination of pathology as described previously.

7. *Patient Care Management*

   a. Disease specific preventive care

b. Direct care

   i. Management of encephalopathy

      1) Monitor for signs of increased ICP or neurologic dysfunction. Placement of an ICP monitoring device may be contraindicated in the presence of coagulopathy. Provide intubation when appropriate for airway control and hyperventilation.

      2) Intervene to decrease serum ammonia with administration of neomycin to decrease GI tract ammonia formation and lactulose (Cephulac) to acidify colonic flora and promote ammonia elimination. Restrict dietary protein.

   ii. To manage hepatorenal syndrome, monitor fluid and electrolyte status and correct electrolyte imbalances. Dialysis may be indicated (hemodialysis or continuous venovenous hemofiltration).

   iii. Manage coagulopathy by administering blood products (FFP by bolus or continuous infusion, platelets, packed RBCs, and factor VII); IV vitamin K (AquaMEPHYTON) therapy may be required.

   iv. Management of portal hypertension

      1) *Variceal bleeding* is treated with pharmacologic agents (i.e., vasopressin [Pitressin], octreotide [Sandostatin], and propranolol [Inderal]), endoscopic band ligation of varices, the Sengstaken–Blakemore tube (see "Acute Treatment of Esophageal Varices" in "Acute GI Tract Hemorrhage" section), or surgical intervention with a portosystemic shunt, or any combination of these. The use of propranolol (Inderal) is controversial as side effects, including heart block, exacerbation of asthma and altered physiologic response to hypoglycemia, may be detrimental. Currently, endoscopic banding or ligation is the most common initial treatment for children with hemorrhagic complications of variceal bleeding (Lirio, 2016). However, these procedures do not treat the cause of portal hypertension and for many children portosystemic shunting is appropriate.

      2) The goal of portosystemic shunts is to redirect portal blood flow into the systemic venous circulation, decreasing the

portal venous pressure. Central shunts (portacaval shunt) are created by anastomosis of the portal vein to the inferior vena cava. Distal splenorenal shunts are created by anastomosis of the splenic vein to the left renal vein. Nonshunt surgical procedures, including the Sugiura procedure (devascularization of the upper and lower two thirds of greater and lesser curvature of the stomach and ligation of select gastric vessels), are not as successful as shunt procedures. Complications of shunting procedures include thrombosis of the anastomotic vessel, elevated ammonia levels, peptic ulcers, aggravated hepatic failure, and ascites.

3) Management of splenomegaly. A spleen guard is a custom-fitted plastic device to cover and protect the spleen. Children with spleen guards must avoid contact sports.

4) Management of ascites. Sodium restriction and diuretic therapy (IV furosemide [Lasix]), or hydrochlorothiazide and spironolactone (Aldactazide) can help to control fluids. Paracentesis may be used when respiratory compromise occurs. It may precipitate fluid shifts. Complications include infection and hemorrhage.

8. *Outcomes.* Complications of acute hepatic failure include encephalopathy; cerebral edema, which is a major cause of mortality for children with FHF; hepatorenal syndrome; and coagulopathies resulting in GI tract, cerebral, and pulmonary hemorrhage. Associated mortality for children is as high as 70% to 90%.

LIVER TRANSPLANTATION

A. Definition and Etiology

1. Liver transplantation is replacement of the liver that has failed with a segment or whole-cadaver liver or a segment of the liver from a living related or nonrelated donor.

2. Biliary atresia is the most common indication for pediatric liver transplantation. The incidence is one per 10,000 to 19,000 in Europe and North America (Verkade et al., 2016). Biliary atresia is a congenital defect of unknown cause that involves the absence or obstruction of the intrahepatic and extrahepatic

bile ducts. With the development of fibrosis, bile flow is obstructed. Progressive disease with resultant fibrosis and eventual cirrhosis occurs.

3. *Metabolic Diseases*

a. *Alpha-1 antitrypsin ($\alpha_1 AT$) deficiency* is transmitted via an autosomal-recessive trait. Only 5% to 20% of $\alpha_1 AT$-deficient children develop liver disease. The disorder involves a deficiency of $\alpha_1 AT$, which is a polymorphic glycoprotein synthesized by the liver. Liver dysfunction is usually evident as cholestasis during the neonatal period, and cirrhosis develops in later childhood. Children with $\alpha_1 AT$ deficiency are at increased risk for developing hepatocellular carcinoma.

b. *Tyrosinemia* is an autosomal-recessive trait that results in deficiency of fumarylacetoacetate hydrolase (FAH) activity. Children with tyrosinemia have an increased risk for developing hepatocellular carcinoma.

c. *Urea cycle disorders* are a group of diseases resulting from the lack of enzymes in the pathway that metabolizes proteins. They are associated with elevated levels of the metabolite byproduct, ammonia, for which liver transplantation is curative.

4. *Intrahepatic Cholestasis*

a. *Progressive familial intrahepatic cholestasis (PFIC)* is a group of autosomal-recessive inheritance disorders that constitute a group of three types of disorders (PFIC type 1, 2 [impaired bile salt secretion], and 3 [reduced biliary phospholipid secretion]) with varied clinical characteristics and familial patterns of occurrence (Srivastava, 2014). It is characterized by a paucity of bile duct development with the presence of cholestatic jaundice and pruritus. Children with PFIC type 2 have a high incidence of liver tumors and monitoring is recommended from infancy (Srivastava, 2014). Effective treatment includes nutritional support, surgical biliary diversion, and liver transplantation for many children (Srivastava, 2014).

b. *Alagille syndrome (arteriohepatic dysplasia)* is an autosomal-dominant trait (Alagille et al., 1987). The syndrome's characteristics include a broad forehead, indented chin, vertebral defects, pulmonary artery stenosis, and congenital heart disease. Cholestasis may resolve in infancy with recurrence later in childhood.

5. *Malignant Disease*

a. *Hepatoblastoma* usually occurs as a mass lesion composed of epithelial cells or a mixture of epithelial and mesenchymal components. Seventy-five percent of these cases occur before age 3 years. The abdomen may enlarge with the presence of an abdominal mass.

b. *Hepatocellular carcinoma* is a highly malignant tumor characterized by anaplastic hepatocytes. It has a peak incidence in infancy, with another peak between the ages of 10 and 15 years. Signs and symptoms include abdominal swelling with associated pain and discomfort, fever, nausea, vomiting, weight loss, lethargy, and jaundice.

B. Pathophysiology

Children with ALF and acute-on-chronic liver failure are often candidates for liver transplantation when end-stage liver disease occurs (see "Liver Failure" section).

C. Clinical Presentation

1. *Contraindications to Transplantation.* There are no absolute contraindications to liver transplantation. The presence of metastatic disease or sepsis is a relative contraindication.

2. *Pretransplant Considerations*

a. Pretransplant considerations involve a medical workup that includes a thorough history and examination, laboratory tests, assessment for evidence of portal hypertension, and assessment of portal vein patency. Family preparation and education are extensive and include education about the pretransplant process, the transplant operation, and care during the posttransplant period.

b. The pediatric end-stage liver disease (PELD) model and model for end-stage liver disease (MELD) are used to generate a score for candidates to determine liver allocation. Scores for children 11 years and younger are determined by the PELD model and the scores for children 12 years and older are calculated based on the MELD model. The child's PELD score is based on age, growth failure, bilirubin level, INR, albumin, and whether child is younger than 1 year old. The MELD score (which can range from 6 to 40) is based on bilirubin level, INR serum creatinine, and serum sodium (United Network for Organ Sharing [UNOS], 2017). Priority is given to patients who are status 1A (sudden and severe onset ALF and are expected to live hours to a few days) and 1B (very sick, chronically ill pediatric patients <18 years old), and children

with certain diseases (e.g., certain metabolic diseases, hepatoblastoma; UNOS, 2017).

D. Patient Care Management

1. Liver transplantation orthotopic and living-related procedures

a. *Orthotopic liver transplant (OLTx)* refers to the replacement of the diseased liver with the liver or liver segment from a cadaver. A living-related transplant is performed following the donation of part of the liver from a healthy donor. Increasingly, OLTx is being performed on children with shared donor grafts (e.g., split grafts).

b. The transplant procedure is divided into three phases: preanhepatic (recipient's hepatectomy), anhepatic (recipient liver has been excised and donor liver is implanted), and neohepatic (reperfusion of the new graft). There are vascular anastomoses (including the portal vein and hepatic artery) and a biliary reconstruction is done depending on the recipients' disease process and size of the native bile duct. Children with biliary atresia or those with small bile ducts require biliary reconstruction to a piece of the intestine.

c. This biliary anastomosis is generally performed via a roux limb and is created as either a hepaticojejunostomy or a choledochojejunostomy depending on which duct is attached to the jejunum. In children with a disease with a normal biliary system, biliary anastomosis can be completed as an anastomosis between the two bile ducts as a choledocholedocostomy.

2. *Postop Nursing Care*

a. Promote pulmonary toilet. After resolution of the existing coagulopathies, initiate chest physiotherapy. Evaluate diaphragm function with an US if the child fails extubation twice.

b. Treat hypertension with antihypertensives. The first-line drug in the immediate postoperative period is institution specific; sodium nitroprusside, sublingual nifedipine (Procardia), or hydralazine are drugs that may be used when necessary.

c. Monitor Jackson–Pratt drainage. Bloody drainage may indicate surgical bleeding. The presence of bile in a surgical drain could indicate a bile leak.

d. Avoid rapid correction of coagulopathies. Hematocrit is maintained at approximately 30%. Subclinical anticoagulation is used for vessel thrombosis prophylaxis and is initiated when the PT is less than 17 seconds. Aspirin decreases platelet aggregation. Dipyridamole (Persantine) is a platelet adhesion inhibitor. Dextran decreases blood viscosity and platelet adhesiveness. Heparin may be used as a prophylactic anticoagulant.

e. Other commonly used medications include immunosuppressive therapy (see "Pharmacology" section earlier in this chapter) and drugs for infection prophylaxis. Broad-spectrum IV antibiotics are given perioperatively. Co-trimoxazole (Bactrim) is prescribed indefinitely for *Pneumocystis carinii*, *nocardia*, and *toxoplasmosis* prophylaxis. Nystatin (Mycostatin) is an antifungal agent used for thrush prophylaxis.

E. Complications and Outcomes

1. *Rejection*

    a. Signs and symptoms may include fever, RUQ tenderness, light-colored stools, dark-colored urine; however, most rejection episodes are diagnosed with asymptomatic elevation of liver enzymes.

    b. Liver biopsy is used for definitive diagnosis. Before the biopsy, check platelet count and PT. If the child is being treated with anticoagulants, consideration should be given to holding anticoagulation prior to the biopsy. US marking is used when necessary (e.g., may be done in the presence of abnormal anatomic findings, as in the presence of a reduced-size graft following liver transplantation). Monitoring for complications of the biopsy includes frequent assessment of vital signs for the assessment of hemorrhage, chest x-ray examination to rule out pneumothorax, and serial hematocrit measurements.

    c. Treatment is augmentation of the child's immunosuppression.

2. *Infection* is the leading cause of morbidity and mortality following transplantation.

    a. *Bacterial infections* occur most often within the first 30 days. Common causes include preexisting disease conditions; central lines; surgical intervention; and posttransplantation factors, including transfusion requirements and dosing of immunosuppressive agents. Treatment is antibiotic therapy.

    b. *Viral infections* usually occur from 31 to 180 days following transplantation. Infections caused by opportunistic or immunomodulating viruses commonly occur in the first 6 months

following transplantation. Common organisms include cytomegalovirus and EBV. After the 6-month posttransplant period, community-acquired infections are common as for any child. Primary infections occur when the patient becomes infected with a virus with no previous exposure. Secondary infection involves the reactivation of a latent virus. Recovery from a secondary infection is usually easier than recovery from a primary infection. Treatment is antiviral therapy. Acyclovir (Zovirax) inhibits viral DNA synthesis of the herpesviruses. Ganciclovir (Cytovene) inhibits the CMV DNA polymerase. Side effects include impaired renal function, neutropenia, thrombocytopenia, confusion, and nausea.

3. *LPD and EBV Infection.* LPD is characterized by the development of continually proliferating B lymphocytes, presumably stimulated under the influence of EBV. LPD is diagnosed by tissue biopsy with histologic evidence and is necessary to guide treatment. Treatment involves reducing or discontinuing the child's immunosuppression, initiating antiviral therapy, use of monoclonal antibody therapy (e.g., Rituximab), or chemotherapy.

4. *Survival* is estimated to be at 80% at 1 year.

INTESTINAL FAILURE/SHORT GUT/ INTESTINE TRANSPLANTATION

A. Definition and Etiology

1. Intestinal failure/short gut is the loss of the absorptive function of the intestine, with resulting malabsorption and malnutrition necessitating PN support. Although the terms *intestinal failure* and *short gut syndrome* (SGS) are sometimes used interchangeably, children can have intestinal failure when they have dysfunctional intestine with normal bowel length.

2. Intestinal failure is inadequate GI function to maintain nutrition and hydration necessitating PN support because of malabsorption and malnutrition. SGS is the most common indication for intestine transplantation. Short gut can occur secondary to congenital and acquired disease processes.

    a. *Congenital conditions* include gastroschisis, malrotation with volvulus, intestinal atresias, and total colon Hirschsprung's disease requiring surgical resection (see Table 7.12).

b. *Acquired conditions* include NEC (see "Necrotizing Enterocolitis" section) and traumatic injuries.

3. Other indications include intestinal dysmotility (e.g., intestinal pseudoobstruction, aganglionosis) and enterocyte absorptive impairment (microvillus inclusion disease and tufting enteropathy), or disease-associated loss of absorption.

B. Pathophysiology

1. Each infant- or child-rendered short gut is unique as successful intestinal adaptation is dependent on the type and length of bowel segment present.

  a. At birth, the normal estimated bowel length is 250 ± 40 cm (Goulet, Ruemmele, Lacaille, & Colomb, 2004).

  b. Infants can experience acceptable intestinal adaptation with less than 15 cm of intestine if the ileocecal valve is intact, and with 30 to 45 cm of intestine if the ileocecal valve is absent or does not function (Fishbein & Matsumoto, 2006).

  c. Intestinal adaptation occurs by increasing existing bowel surface area and functional abilities over a period of weeks to many months and is dependent on the etiology of the SBS and the functional state of the remaining bowel.

  d. Intestinal adaptation is characterized by increasing intestinal mass, lengthening of villi, and improved absorption at the epithelial level.

  e. Successful adaptation is described as the ability to achieve normal growth, fluid balance, and electrolyte levels without PN.

2. There are a multitude of mechanisms that contribute to malabsorption, including acid hypersecretion, rapid intestinal transit, and loss of surface area and impaired residual bowel with bacterial overgrowth and bile acid wasting.

C. Clinical Presentation

1. *History.* Most children younger than the age of 1 year are rendered short gut from a congenital anomaly or NEC. History is variable as there are both congenital and acquired etiologies with various disease trajectories.

2. *Physical Examination.* Specific exam consideration includes careful monitoring of growth parameters, signs and symptoms of liver dysfunction (see "Liver Failure" section specifically findings with cholestasis), integrity of central venous access, and skin integrity of diapered patients as excess secretion of bile acids may result in a severe diaper rash.

3. *Diagnostic Tests*

  a. An upper GI series with small bowel follow through may be done to determine bowel length and evaluate bowel caliber, if bowel lengthening procedure is being considered.

  b. A breath hydrogen test can be performed to evaluate for bacterial overgrowth.

  c. Although endoscopy is not indicated for this reason, if done, a culture of duodenal fluid can be obtained to evaluate for bacterial overgrowth.

4. *Clinical Course*

  a. Trajectory is variable depending on etiology, remaining bowel, and retained function.

D. Patient Care Management

1. *Preventive Care.* Optimize the medical and surgical management of neonates with congenital disorders to promote intestinal adaptation and bowel salvage with the goal of optimizing the enteral diet, PN prescription, treatment of bacterial overgrowth, administration of antacids and antisecretory agents, and use of antidiarrheal (stool bulking) agents.

2. *Direct Care*

  a. Monitor stool and urine output.

    i. Stool output should be replaced for output greater than 40 mL/kg/d. Most common replacement fluid is RL 0.5 mL:mL or mL:mL.

  b. Use enteral and PN nutrition.

    i. Fluid requirements are upwards of 100 to 200 mL/kg/d.

    ii. Caloric requirements are 100 to 150 kcal/kg/d.

    iii. EN promotes adaptation and BM is preferred with an associated shorter duration of PN dependence. If maternal or banked BM is not available, elemental hydrolyzed formulas are preferred. Duocal or microlipids may be used as caloric supplements.

    iv. PN prescriptions should minimize intralipids (0.5 gm/kg/d adequate to prevent essential fatty acid deficiency) levocarnitine should be added, trace elements manipulated (limit copper and selenium; remove manganese and chromium), glucose infusion rate should be optimized and wean or cycle PN as feasible. Alternative lipid formulations are being used that minimize the inflammatory effect on the liver, minimizing and reversing cholestatic changes. Unfortunately, available products are expensive and not FDA approved (Omegaven and Smoflipid 20% [soya oil, medium-chain triglyceride, olive oil, and fish oil]).

c. Use oral and enteral rehydration solutions as needed and may augment IV fluids as stool replacement, which may be added to enteral feedings.

d. Treat bacterial overgrowth with the cycling of antibiotics to prevent resistance. Metronidazole (Flagyl), sulfamethoxazole (Bactrim), and rifaximin (Xifaxin) are commonly used.

e. Antacid therapy is prescribed to minimize acid hypersecretion.

f. Administer antisecretory and antidiarrheal/bulking medications as prescribed (e.g., Imodium [loperamide] or Catapres [clonidine]; see "Pharmacology" section). Clonidine is most commonly used for children to slow ostomy effluence. Products to slow gastric motility (pectin and Benefiber) may be prescribed.

g. Bowel-lengthening surgical procedures.

  i. Bowel-lengthening procedures are considered for dilated loops of bowel (>2 cm) or complications from the dilated bowel loops (e.g., bacteremia from bacterial intestinal translocation or intolerance of enteral feeding advances).

  ii. The Bianchi procedure is the oldest procedure and involves a longitudinal incision to create two tubes to lengthen the bowel that are reconnected to create a longer, narrower single-lumen intestinal segment. The Kimura procedure is an alternative procedure for children with SGS and inadequate mesentery who are not candidates for the Bianchi procedure. The serial transverse enteroplasty procedure augments bowel length and peristalsis by stapling dilated bowel in a zigzag fashion to achieve a greater mucosal absorptive surface area and decreased bowel diameter.

h. Intestinal transplantation is considered for children experiencing complications of PN, including liver failure, loss of greater than two or more venous access devices, recurrent central-line catheter infections, and recurrent severe dehydration. The ideal intestine donor has the same blood type, weighs within 10% of the recipient's body weight, and is of similar age as the recipient. All intestine recipients have a stoma to allow for bowel surveillance and access for endoscopy and biopsy. See Figure 7.3 for the common intestinal transplant procedures. Postop care for the intestine recipient is summarized in Table 7.14. Complications of intestine transplant procedures include rejection, infection, and posttransplant lymphoproliferative disease (PTLD). Signs and symptoms of intestinal graft rejection include a pale or dusky stoma, an increase or decrease in enteric output, abdominal pain, and guaiac-positive output. Postoperative endoscopic biopsies of the transplanted bowel are made through the child's stoma on a routine and as-needed basis. Rejection is usually diagnosed with endoscopy and biopsy the gold standard.

3. *Supportive Care.* Children with intestinal failure should be referred to an intestinal rehabilitation team, which is usually composed of a gastroenterologist with specific expertise, advanced practice nurse, nutritionist, surgeon, social worker, and speech therapist.

E. Outcomes

1. *PN-induced cholestasis* is a possible complication of intestinal failure in patients with resultant concomitant liver and intestinal failure. Cholestasis or a bilirubin level greater than 2 mg/dL occurs in 40% to 60% of children with intestinal failure (Sondheimer et al., 1998) and contributes to the greatest morbidity and mortality for these children.

  a. Measures to reduce the incidence of cholestasis

    i. PN manipulations with cycling, lipid minimization, and limiting and/or removing trace elements.

    ii. EN with the promotion of breastmilk as optimal.

    iii. Decrease central line infection rates with antibiotic and ethanol locks. Ethanol locks are incompatible with heparin and should be instilled for 2 to 4 hours.

    iv. Cycle enteral antibiotics to treat bowel bacterial overgrowth.

  b. Success for these children is defined by liberation from PN and normal growth and development.

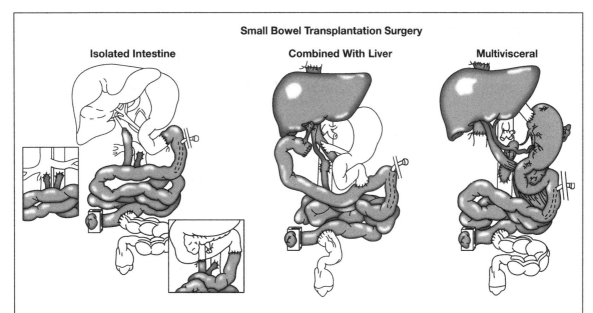

FIGURE 7.3   Common intestinal transplant procedures. The three basic intestinal transplant procedures (the graft is shaded). With the isolated intestine, the venous outflow may be to the recipient portal vein (center), to the inferior vena cava (left), or to the superior mesenteric vein (right).

Source: From Reyes, J. D. (2006). Intestinal transplantation. *Seminars in Pediatric Surgery, 15,* 228–234. doi:10.1053/j.sempedsurg.2006.03.010

TABLE 7.14   Nursing Care of the Intestine Transplant Recipient

Liver–intestine ABCs in the pediatric intensive care unit include airway, bowel integrity, and caloric or hydration requirements.
- Assess and support the child's ABC.
- Bowel integrity is initially assessed by physical appearance of the stoma (normal stoma appears pink and moist and an ostomy is created at the time of surgery and allows for frequent biopsies) and enteric output. An NG tube is placed for bowel decompression.
- Initial caloric requirements are met with PN.
- Enteral feedings are initiated as soon as possible after the transplant. The children generally have a gastrostomy tube or jejunostomy tube placed to allow for an initial slow rate of tube feedings.
- Hydration should be carefully assessed with quantitative assessment of input and output (urine, gastric, ostomy, stool output).
- Critical care goals are to support the patient to be hemodynamically stable and free of requirement for mechanical ventilation.
- Airway clearance and spontaneous ventilation may be ineffective as a result of the lengthy abdominal procedure and resultant anesthetic administration, visceral edema, and pain. With the resolution of postoperative coagulopathies, aggressive chest physiotherapy is initiated. Intestine recipients generally require mechanical ventilation longer than isolated liver recipients because intestine recipients typically are in poor health before the transplant and often have a precarious fluid balance.
- Optimize pain management.
- Additional challenges include open abdominal wounds and surgical reexploration for complications such as perforation or bleeding.

ABC, airway, breathing circulation; NG, nasogastric; PN, parenteral nutrition.

CASE STUDIES WITH QUESTIONS, ANSWERS, AND RATIONALES

Case Study 7.1: Blunt Abdominal Trauma: Bike and Belly Blues

Evan was out riding his bike. He fell with his handlebars "bumping into his chest bones." His mother brought him to the emergency department when he complained of significant abdominal pain 6 hours after his injury. He was diagnosed with a Grade 2 injury by CT scan.

1. What is the most commonly injured solid organ in children?
   A. The liver
   B. The spleen
   C. The pancreas
   D. The left kidney

2. A research study found that if a child is going to fail nonoperative management, this usually occurs within what time frame?
   A. 4 hours
   B. 8 hours
   C. 12 hours
   D. 16 hours

3. What is the anticipated time frame for his activity restriction?
   A. 2 weeks
   B. 3 weeks
   C. 4 weeks
   D. 6 weeks

Case Study 7.2: Acute Abdomen With Intra-Abdominal Pressure Monitoring

Madeline is a 10-year-old who has undergone surgery for a volvulus, which necessitated bowel resection. As she experienced significant third spacing with bowel edema, a three-way urinary catheter was inserted to allow for intra-abdominal pressure monitoring. Her pressure was noted to be trending upward.

1. What value is considered an elevated IAP in the critically ill child?
   A. >12 mmHg
   B. 4 mmHg
   C. 2 mmHg
   D. 10 mmHg

2. What value is considered to be indicative of abdominal compartment syndrome, warranting surgical intervention?
   A. 20 mmHg with oliguria
   B. 14 mmHg
   C. 10 mmHg
   D. 4 mmHg with oliguria

ANSWERS AND RATIONALES

Case Study 7.1

1. **B.** Most common mechanisms for injury are motor vehicle collision and falls; other common causes are bicycle injuries (handlebars) and maltreatment. Blunt trauma occurs in 80% of injuries versus 20% for penetrating injuries and is responsible for most abdominal injuries. The most commonly injured organs in the child with blunt abdominal injury is the spleen due to the lack of protection by the rib cage and the elasticity of the supportive ligaments. The liver is second to the spleen as a major source of hemorrhage and is the most common source of lethal hemorrhage. The pancreas is infrequently injured. The classic injury is compression by bicycle handlebars in which the child flips over the bike and is impaled in the epigastrium by the handlebars. The left kidney is not preferentially injured as compared to the right kidney.

2. **C.** A retrospective study found that children that were going to fail nonoperative management with a splenic injury had hemodynamic instability within 12 hours of hospital admission.

3. **C.** Nonoperative management is the mainstay of treatment for children with blunt abdominal injuries. Children who sustain an isolated spleen injury are restricted from contact sports and strenuous activity for a period consisting of the grade of the injury plus 2 weeks. Therefore a child with a grade 2 injury would be restricted from activity for 4 weeks.

Case Study 7.2

1. **A.** Elevated intra-abdominal pressure in a child is defined as greater than 12 mmHg. Normal IAP in a well child is 0 mmHg and in a child on positive pressure ventilation is 1 to 8 mmHg.

2. **A.** A child with a significant intra-abdominal pathologic condition may eventually develop mental status changes (generally a late and subtle sign). Intra-abdominal hypertension is defined as an intra-abdominal pressure (IAP) of 12 mmHg or more based on three standardized measurements obtained at least 4 to 6 hours apart (Kirkpatrick et al., 2013). Abdominal compartment syndrome is defined as an IAP >20mmHg and the onset of new or worsening organ failure directly attributed to elevated IAP.

REFERENCES

Abu-El-Haija, M., Lin, T. K., & Palermo, J. (2014). Update to the management of pediatric acute pancreatitis: Highlighting areas in need of research. *Journal of Pediatric Gastroenterology and Nutrition, 58*(6), 689–693. doi:10.1097/MPG.00000000000360

Alagille, D., Estrada, A., Hadchouel, M., Gautler, M., Odièvre, M., & Dommergues, J. P. (1987). Syndromic paucity of interlobular bile ducts (Alagille syndrome or arteriohepatic dysplasia): Review of 80 cases. *The Journal of Pediatrics, 110*(2), 195–200. doi:10.1016/S0022-3476(87)80153-1

American Academy of Pediatrics Committee on Infectious Diseases. (2013). *Clostridium difficile* infection in infants and children. *Pediatrics, 131*(1), 196–200. doi:10.1542/peds.2012-2992

American Academy of Pediatrics Subcommittee on Hyperbilirubinemia. (2004). Management of hyperbilirubinemia in the newborn infant 35 or more weeks of gestation. *Pediatrics, 114*(1), 297–316. doi:10.1542/peds.114.1.297

Barnhart, D. C. (2016). Gastroesophageal reflux disease in children. *Seminars in Pediatric Surgery, 25*(4), 212–218. doi:10.1053/j.sempedsurg.2016.05.009

Bell, M. J., Ternberg, J. L., Feigin, R. D., Keating, J. P., Marshall, R., Barton, L., & Brotherton, T. (1978). Neonatal necrotizing enterocolitis: Therapeutic decisions based upon clinical staging. *Annals of Surgery, 187*(1), 1–7. Retrieved from https://www.ncbi.nlm.nih.gov/pmc/articles/PMC1396409

Buzelé, R., Barbier, L., Sauvanet, A., & Fantin, B. (2016). Medical complications following splenectomy. *Journal of Visceral Surgery, 153*(4), 277–286. doi:10.1016/j.jviscsurg.2016.04.013

Carlson, M. D., Al-Mateen, M., & Brewer, G. J. (2004). Atypical childhood Wilson's disease. *Pediatric Neurology, 30*(1), 57–60. doi:10.1016/S0887-8994(03)00422-3

Corte, C. D., Alisi, A., Saccari, A., De Vito, R., Vania, A., & Nobili, V. (2012). Nonalcoholic fatty liver in children and adolescents: An overview. *Journal of Adolescent Health, 51*(4), 305–312. doi:10.1016/j.jadohealth.2012.01.010

Durai, R., & Ng, P. C. (2010). Surgical vacuum drains: Types, uses, and complications. *AORN Journal, 91*(2), 266–274. doi:10.1016/j.aorn.2009.09.024

Ellett, M. L. C., Cohen, M. D., Perkins, S. M., Croffie, J. M. B., Lane, K. A., & Austin, J. K. (2012). Comparing methods of determining insertion length for placing gastric tubes in children 1 month to 17 years of age. *Journal for Specialists in Pediatric Nursing, 17*(1), 19–32. doi:10.1111/j.1744-6155.2011.00302.x

Ellett, M. L. C., Cohen, M. D., Perkins, S. M., Smith, C. E., Lane, K. A., & Austin, J. K. (2011). Predicting the insertion length for gastric tube placement in neonates. *Journal of Obstetric, Gynecologic, and Neonatal Nursing, 40*(4), 412–421. doi:10.1111/j.1552-6909.2011.01255.x

Ellison, A. M., Quayle, K. S., Bonsu, B., Garcia, M., Blumberg, S., Rogers, A., . . . Holmes, J. F. (2015). Use of oral contrast for abdominal computed tomography in children with blunt torso trauma. *Annals of Emergency Medicine, 66*(2), 107–114. e4. doi:10.1016/j.annemergmed.2015.01.014

Englum, B. R., Gulack, B. C., Rice, H. E., Scarborough, J. E., & Adibe, O. O. (2016). Management of blunt pancreatic trauma in children: Review of the National Trauma Data Bank. *Journal of Pediatric Surgery, 51*(9), 1526–1531. doi:10.1016/j.jpedsurg.2016.05.003

Fishbein, T. M., & Matsumoto, C. S. (2006). Intestinal replacement therapy: Timing and indications for referral of patients to an intestinal rehabilitation and transplant program. *Gastroenterology, 130* (2 Suppl.), S147–S151. doi:10.1053/j.gastro.2005.12.004

Fragkos, K. C., Zárate-Lopez, N., & Frangos, C. C. (2016). What about clonidine for diarrhoea? A systematic review and meta-analysis of its effect in humans. *Therapeutic Advances in Gastroenterology, 9*(3), 282–301. doi:10.1177/1756283X15625586

Garcia, V. F., & Brown, R. L. (2003). Pediatric trauma: Beyond the brain. *Critical Care Clinics, 19*, 551–561.

Garth, E. (2016). Gastroesophageal reflux. In A. Kline-Tilford & C. Haut (Eds.). *Lippincott certification review: Pediatric acute care nurse practitioner* (pp. 407–410). Philadelphia, PA: Wolters Kluwer.

Gilbertson, H. R., Rogers, E. J., & Ukoumunne, O. C. (2011) Determination of a practical pH cutoff level for reliable confirmation of nasogastric tube placement. *Journal of Parenteral and Enteral Nutrition, 35*(4), 540–544. doi:10.1177/0148607110383285

Goulet, O., Ruemmele, F., Lacaille, F., & Colomb, V. (2004). Irreversible intestinal failure. *Journal of Pediatric Gastroenterology and Nutrition, 38*(3), 250–269. Retrieved from https://journals.lww.com/jpgn/Fulltext/2004/03000/Irreversible_Intestinal_Failure.6.aspx

Gupta, A., & Paria, A. (2016). Etiology and medical management of NEC. *Early Human Development, 97*, 17–23. doi:10.1016/j.earlhumdev.2016.03.008

Hao, F., Guo, H., Luo, Q., & Guo, C. (2016). Disease progression of acute pancreatitis in pediatric patients. *Journal of Surgical Research, 202*(2), 422–427. doi:10.1016/j.jss.2016.01.016

Huether, S. E., McCance, K. L., & Tarmina, M. S. (1994). Alterations of digestive function. In K. L. McCance & S. E Huether (Eds.), *Pathophysiology: The biological basis for diseases in adults and children* (2nd ed.). St Louis, MO Elsevier.

Hull, M. A., Fisher, J. G., Gutierrez, I. M., Jones, B. A., Kang, K. H., Kenny, M., . . . Jaksic, T. (2014). Mortality and management of surgical necrotizing enterocolitis in very low birth weight neonates: A prospective cohort study. *Journal of the American College of Surgeons, 218*(6), 1148–1155. doi:10.1016/j.jamcollsurg.2013.11.015

Intravia, J. M., & DeBerardino, T. M. (2013). Evaluation of blunt abdominal trauma. *Clinics in Sports Medicine, 32*(2), 211–218. doi:10.1016/j.csm.2012.12.001

Irving, S. Y., Lyman, B., Northington, L., Bartlett, J. A., Kemper, C., & Novel Project Work Group. (2014). Nasogastric tube placement and verification in children: Review of the current literature. *Critical Care Nurse, 34*(3) 67–78. doi:10.4037/ccn2014606

Jacob, S. W., & Francone, C. A. (1989). *Elements of anatomy and physiology* (2nd ed.). Philadelphia, PA: W. B. Saunders.

Jobst, M. A., Canty, T. G., & Lynch, F. P. (1999). Management of pancreatic injury in pediatric blunt abdominal trauma. *Journal of Pediatric Surgery, 34*(5), 818–823. doi:10.1016/S0022-3468(99)90379-2

Kenner, C., & Lott, J. W. (Eds.). (2014). *Comprehensive neonatal nursing* (5th ed.). New York, NY: Springer Publishing.

Kirkpatrick, A. W., Roberts, D. J., De Waele, J., Jaeschke, R., Malbrain, M. L., De Keulenaer, B., . . . Pediatric Guidelines Sub-Committee for the World Society of the Abdominal Compartment Syndrome. (2013). Intra-abdominal hypertension and the abdominal compartment syndrome: Updated consensus definitions and clinical practice guidelines from the World Society of the Abdominal Compartment Syndrome. *Intensive Care Medicine, 39*(7), 1190–1206. doi:10.1007/s00134-013-2906-z

Kramer, C., & Jeffery, J. (2014). Pancreatitis in children. *Critical Care Nurse, 34*(4), 43–53. doi:10.4037/ccn2014533

Lee, C. K., & Jonas, M. M. (2015). Hepatitis C: Issues in children. *Gastroenterology Clinics of North America, 44*, 901–909. doi:10.1016/j.gtc.2015.07.011

Lirio, R. A. (2016). Management of upper gastrointestinal bleeding in children: Variceal and nonvariceal. *Gastrointestinal Endoscopy Clinics of North America, 26*(1), 63–73. doi:10.1016/j.giec.2015.09.003

Little, C. M. (2014). Fetal development: Environmental influences and critical periods. In C. Kenner & J.W. Lott (Eds.), *Comprehensive neonatal nursing* (5th ed., pp. 1–27). New York, NY: Springer Publishing.

Lyman, B., Kemper, C., Northington, L., Yaworski, J., Wilder, K., Moore, C., . . . Irving, S. Y. (2016). Use of temporary enteral access devices in hospitalized neonatal and pediatric patients in the United States. *Journal of Parenteral and Enteral Nutrition, 40*(4), 574–480. doi:10.1177/0148607114567712

Lynch, J. M., Meza, M. P., Newman, B., Gardner, M. J., & Albanese, C. T. (1997). Computed tomography grade of splenic injury is predictive of the time required for radiographic healing. *Journal of Pediatric Surgery, 32*, 1093–1096. doi:10.1016/S0022-3468(97)90406-1

Makin, E., & Davenport, M. (2016). Evaluation of the acute abdomen. *Paediatrics and Child Health, 26*(6), 231–238. doi:10.1016/j.paed.2016.01.006

Martin, S. A. (1992). The ABCs of pediatric LFTs. *Pediatric Nursing, 18*(5), 445–449.

McVay, M. R., Kokoska, E. R., Jackson, R. J., & Smith, S. D. (2008). Throwing out the "grade" book: Management of isolated spleen and liver injury based on hemodynamic status. *Journal of Pediatric Surgery, 43*(6), 1072–1076. doi:10.1016/j.jpedsurg.2008.02.031

Mehta, N. M., Bechard, L. J., Cahill, N., Wang, M., Day, A., Duggan, C. P., & Heyland, D. K. (2012). Nutritional practices and their relationship to clinical outcomes in critically ill children—An international multicenter cohort study. *Critical Care Medicine, 40*(7), 2204–2211. doi:10.1097/CCM.0b013e31824e18a8

Mehta, N. M., Skillman, H. E., Irving, S. Y., Coss-Bu, J. A., Vermilyea, S., Farrington, E. A., . . . Braunschweig, C. (2017). Guidelines for the provision and assessment of nutrition support therapy in the pediatric critically ill patient: Society of Critical Care and American Society for Parenteral and Enteral Nutrition. *Journal of Parenteral and Enteral Nutrition, 41*(5), 706–742. doi:10.1177/0148607117711387

Moore, E. E., Cogbill, T. H., Jurkovich, G. J., Shackford, S. R., Malangoni, M. A., & Champion, H. R. (1995). Organ injury scaling: Spleen and liver (1994 revision). *Journal of Trauma and Acute Care Surgery, 38*(3), 323–324. Retrieved from https://journals.lww.com/jtrauma/Fulltext/1995/03000/Organ_Injury_Scaling__Spleen_and_Liver__1994.1.aspx

Morinville, V. D., Husain, S. Z., Bai, H., Barth, B., Alhosh, R., Durie, P. R., . . . Uc, A. (2012). Definitions of pediatric pancreatitis and survey of present clinical practices. *Journal of Pediatric Gastroenterology and Nutrition, 55*, 261–265. doi:10.1097/MPG.0b013e31824f1516

Mouat, L. (2012). Cholecystitis. In K. Reuter-Rice & B. N. Bolick (Eds.), *Pediatric acute care: A guide for interprofessional practice* (pp. 489–491). Sudbury, MA: Jones & Bartlett.

Nadler, E. P., Gardner, M., Schall, L. C., Lynch, J. M., & Ford, H. R. (1999). Management of blunt pancreatic injury in children. *Journal of Trauma and Acute Care Surgery, 47*, 1098–1103. Retrieved from https://journals.lww.com/jtrauma/Abstract/1999/12000/Management_of_Blunt_Pancreatic_Injury_in_Children.20.aspx

Notrica, D. M. (2015). Pediatric blunt trauma: Current management. *Current Opinion in Critical Care, 21*, 531–537. doi:10.1097/MCC.0000000000000249

Ogunmefun, G., Hardy, M., & Boynes, S. (2016). Is magnetic resonance imaging a viable alternative to ultrasound as the primary imaging modality in the diagnosis of paediatric appendicitis? A systematic review. *Radiography, 22*(3), 244–251. doi:10.1016/j.radi.2016.01.001

Papachrisanthou, M. M., & Davis, R. L. (2015). Clinical practice guidelines for the management of gastroesophageal reflux and gastroesophageal reflux disease: Birth to 1 year of age. *Journal of Pediatric Health Care, 29*(6), 558–564. doi:10.1016/j.pedhc.2015.07.009

Papachrisanthou, M. M., & Davis, R. L. (2016). Clinical practice guidelines for the management of gastroesophageal reflux and gastroesophageal reflux disease: 1 year to 18 years of age. *Journal of Pediatric Health Care, 30*(3), 289–294. doi:10.1016/j.pedhc.2015.08.004

Poddar, U., Yachha, S. K., Mathias, A., & Choudhuri, G. (2015). Genetic predisposition and its impact on natural history of idiopathic acute and acute recurrent pancreatitis in children. *Digestive and Liver Disease, 47*(8), 709–714. doi:10.1016/j.dld.2015.04.012

Puranik, S. R., Hayes, J. S., Long, J., & Mata, M. (2002). Liver enzymes as predictors of liver damage due to blunt abdominal trauma in children. *Southern Medical Journal, 95*, 203–206. Retrieved from https://sma.org/southern-medical-journal/article/liver-enzymes-as-predictors-of-liver-damage-due-to-blunt-abdominal-trauma-in-children-2

Reyes, J. D. (2006). Intestinal transplantation. *Seminars in Pediatric Surgery, 15*, 228–234. doi:10.1053/j.sempedsurg.2006.03.010

Sahn, B., & Bitton, S. (2016). Lower gastrointestinal bleeding in children. *Gastrointestinal Endoscopy Clinics of North America, 26*(1), 75–98. doi:10.1016/j.giec.2015.08.007

Simone, S. (2001). Gastrointestinal critical care problems. In M. A. Q. Curley & P. A. Moloney-Harmon (Eds.), *Critical care nursing* (2nd ed.). Philadelphia, PA: W. B. Saunders.

Slaughter, J. L., Stenger, M. R., Reagan, P. B., & Jadcherla, S. R. (2016). Neonatal histamine-2 receptor antagonist and proton pump inhibitor treatment at United States children's hospitals. *Journal of Pediatrics, 174*, 63–70. e3. doi:10.1016/j.jpeds.2016.03.059

Sondheimer, J. M., Asturias, E., & Cadnapaphornchai, M. (1998). Infection and cholestasis in neonates with intestinal resection and long-term parenteral nutrition. *Journal of Pediatric Gastroenterology and Nutrition, 27*(2), 131–137. Retrieved from https://journals.lww.com/jpgn/Fulltext/1998/08000/Infection_and_Cholestasis_in_Neonates_with.1.aspx

Srivastava, A. (2014). Progressive familial intrahepatic cholestasis. *Journal of Clinical and Experimental Hepatology, 4*(1), 25–36. doi:10.1016/j.jceh.2013.10.005

Stark, C. M., & Nylund, C. M. (2016). Side effects and complications of proton pump inhibitors: A pediatric perspective. *Journal of Pediatrics, 168*, 16–22. doi:10.1016/j.jpeds.2015.08.064

Sundaram, S. S., Alonso, E. M., Narkewicz, M. R., Zhang, S., & Squires, R. H. (2011). Characterization and outcomes of young infants with acute liver failure. *Journal of Pediatrics, 159*, 813–818 .e1. doi:10.1016/j.jpeds.2011.04.016

Svensson, J., & Makin, E. (2012). Gallstone disease in children. *Seminars in Pediatric Surgery, 21*, 255–265. doi:10.1053/j.sempedsurg.2012.05.008

Szabo, F. K., Fei, L., Cruz, L. A., & Abu-El-Haija, M. (2015). Early enteral nutrition and aggressive fluid resuscitation are associated with improved clinical outcomes in acute pancreatitis. *Journal of Pediatrics, 167,* 397–402. e1. doi:10.1016/j.jpeds.2015.05.030

Taketomo, C. K., Hodding, J. H., & Kraus, D. M. (2015). *Pediatric & neonatal dosage handbook* (22nd ed.). Hudson, OH: Lexicomp.

Taylor, S. J. (2013). Confirming nasogastric feeding tube position versus the need to feed. *Intensive and Critical Care Nursing, 29*(2), 59–69. doi:10.1016/j.iccn.2012.07.002

United Network for Organ Sharing. (2017). Questions and answers for transplant candidates about liver allocation. Retrieved from https://www.unos.org/wp-content/uploads/unos/Liver_patient.pdf

Vandenplas, Y., Rudolph, C. D., Di Lorenzo, C., Hassall, E., Liptak, G., Mazur, L., . . . Wenzl, T. G. (2009). Pediatric gastroesophageal reflux clinical practice guidelines: Joint recommendations of the North American Society for Pediatric Gastroenterology, Hepatology, and Nutrition (NASPGHAN) and the European Society for Pediatric Gastroenterology, Hepatology, and Nutrition (ESPGHAN). *Journal of Pediatric Gastroenterology and Nutrition, 49,* 498–547. Retrieved from https://dev-journals2013.lww.com/jpgn/Fulltext/2009/10000/Pediatric_Gastroesophageal_Reflux_Clinical.22.aspx

Verger, J. (2014). Nutrition in the pediatric population in the intensive care unit. *Critical Care Nursing Clinics of North America, 26,* 199–215. doi:10.1016/j.ccell.2014.02.005

Verkade, H. J., Bezerra, J. A., Davenport, M., Schreiber, R. A., Mieli-Vergani, G., Hulscher, J. B., . . . Petersen, C. (2016). Biliary atresia and other cholestatic childhood diseases: Advances and future challenges. *Journal of Hepatology, 65*(3), 631–642. doi:10.1016/j.jhep.2016.04.032

Watson, R. L. (2009). Hyperbilirubinemia. *Critical Care Nursing Clinics of North America, 21*(1), 97–120. doi:10.1016/j.ccell.2008.11.001

Wise, B. V., Mudd, S. S., & Wilson M. E. (2002). Management of blunt abdominal trauma in children. *Journal of Trauma Nursing, 9*(1), 6–14. Retrieved from https://journals.lww.com/journaloftraumanursing/Abstract/2002/09010/Management_of_Blunt_Abdominal_Trauma_in_Children.2.aspx

8

HEMATOLOGY AND IMMUNOLOGY SYSTEMS

Jessica L. Spruit

DEVELOPMENTAL ANATOMY AND PHYSIOLOGY

A. Hematopoiesis

1. Hematopoiesis is the process by which blood cells are formed.

2. Anatomic sites of hematopoiesis vary with age.

a. During embryonic and fetal life, the yolk sac, liver, spleen, thymus, lymph nodes, and bone marrow are all involved (Fernández & de Alarcón, 2013; Sieff, Daley, & Zon, 2015).

b. At birth, hematopoiesis takes place in the bone marrow, called *red marrow*, of all bones.

c. After birth, the red (blood-forming) marrow is gradually replaced by yellow (fatty) marrow. By adulthood, red marrow exists only in the pelvis, vertebrae, cranium, and sternum.

3. Mature blood cells arise through a developmental process called *differentiation*.

a. Pluripotent hematopoietic stem cells give rise to many differentiated blood cells and also replenish themselves.

b. Pluripotent hematopoietic stem cells differentiate into *committed stem cells*. These cells are committed to develop and differentiate into a certain cell type (i.e., red blood cells [RBCs], platelets, white blood cells [WBCs]).

c. The process of development and differentiation is guided and stimulated by a variety of important growth factors and cytokines: erythropoietin (EPO; stimulates red cells), thrombopoetin (platelets), and granulocyte colony-stimulating factor (G-CSF) stimulates white cells.

4. Five types of cells arise from the stem cell. Each of these cells end with "-blast," which refers to a nucleated precursor cell (Porth, 2015).

a. Proerythroblasts form the mature erythrocyte (RBCs).

b. Megakaryoblasts form the mature thrombocytes (platelets).

c. Myeloblasts form the mature neutrophils, eosinophils, and basophils (each a type of WBC).

d. Monoblasts form the mature monocytes (a type of WBC).

e. Lymphoblasts form the mature lymphocytes (a type of WBC; Fernández & de Alarcón, 2013; Figure 8.1).

5. Development of the pluripotential stem cell into a mature hematopoietic cell (RBC, WBC, or platelet) occurs in approximately 1 to 2 weeks.

6. Alterations in the development of blood cell lines include aplasia, in which the bone marrow completely fails to develop stem cells, and hypoplasia, in which the bone marrow develops an abnormally low number of stem cells.

B. Immune System

1. Functionally and anatomically, there is overlap with the hematopoietic system and hematopoiesis.

2. *Lymphocytes* are a type of WBC whose role is to provide protection to the organ via development of various types of immunity. There are two main types of lymphocytes: B cells (involved with humoral immunity (HI), the production of antibodies), and T cells (involved with cellular immunity; Pai & Reinherz, 2015).

3. The *primary lymphocytic tissue organs* describe the key sites of development of lymphocytes. B lymphocytes develop in the bone marrow. T lymphocytes develop in the thymus, which is located in the anterior mediastinum, behind the sternum (Pai & Reinherz, 2015).

4. *Secondary lymphoid tissue or organs* are sites for storage, division, and activation of lymphocytes.

a. The spleen is important for HI and for cellular immunity as well. It is also rich in macrophages (phagocytic cells) and serves as a normal site for destruction of old or damaged red cells.

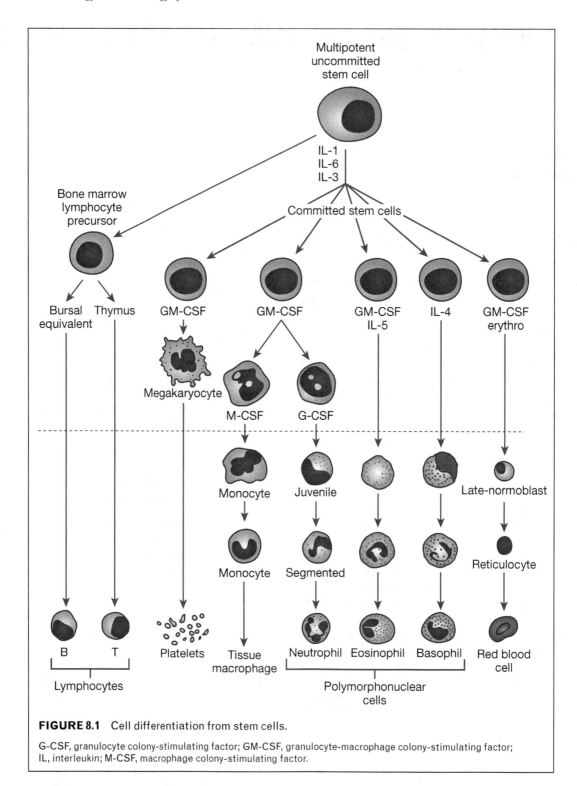

FIGURE 8.1 Cell differentiation from stem cells.

G-CSF, granulocyte colony-stimulating factor; GM-CSF, granulocyte-macrophage colony-stimulating factor;
IL, interleukin; M-CSF, macrophage colony-stimulating factor.

b. Lymphatic channels transport fluid from the interstitium around the cells in the body, through lymph nodes, and eventually empty into a large lymphatic vessel called the *thoracic duct*.

c. Lymph nodes are bean-shaped structures located along the length of the lymphatic vessels. Lymph nodes are distributed throughout the body and clustered in groups, both superficial and deep.

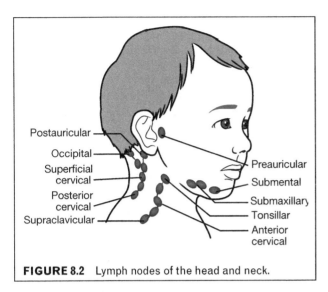

FIGURE 8.2 Lymph nodes of the head and neck.

Lymph nodes function as filters and are important sites of lymphocyte activation and differentiation. Lymph nodes of the head and neck are illustrated in Figure 8.2. Epitrochlear and inguinal lymph nodes should also be assessed.

d. Mucosa-associated lymph tissues (MALT) are dispersed throughout the body and line mucosal surfaces (i.e., the gastrointestinal [GI] tract, lungs, skin). They are located within or close to sites of potential invasion by bacteria or foreign substances.

e. The liver is rich in a particular type of macrophage called *Kupffer's cells*. These have filtering functions similar to the spleen although they are less effective.

C. Committed Hematologic Lines

1. *RBCs, or erythrocytes*, develop from erythroid precursor cells under the influence of EPO.

a. *Reticulocytes* represent the stage of maturation that occurs just before the erythrocyte matures. Reticulocytes are normally present in small numbers in the peripheral blood and are increased during states of erythroid stimulation. They quickly (in 24–48 hours) mature into RBCs.

b. *Mature RBCs* have a life span of 120 days. Their main function is to pick up oxygen as they move through the pulmonary capillaries and deliver that oxygen to the tissues.

c. *Hemoglobin* is a large, complex, iron-containing protein that fills RBCs and is responsible for the RBCs' oxygen-carrying abilities.

　i.　Normal adult hemoglobin is called *Hgb A*.

　ii.　Hemoglobin F (fetal Hgb) is present in large concentrations in the fetus, but it

rapidly declines after birth and is present in only minimal amounts in children and adults.

d. Normal RBC production requires adequate amounts of iron, folic acid, and vitamin B_{12}.

e. Anemia represents a decreased number of red cells or hemoglobin, with a resultant decrease in oxygen-carrying capacity. Anemia can result from decreased production of red cells, increased destruction of RBCs, or blood loss. Anemia is measured as a decrease in hematocrit and hemoglobin; it is usually defined as two standard deviations below the mean for the normal population (Brugnara, Oski, & Nathan, 2015).

f. The RBCs carry a variety of important *surface antigens* that are important in transfusion medicine. The most important antigens are A and B. The presence or absence of these determine one's blood group. Other antigen groups are also important; the Rh system is of considerable significance in pediatrics, where maternal sensitization to the D antigen can lead to hemolytic disease of the newborn.

2. *Leukocytes (WBCs)* are a heterogeneous group of cells that serve in a variety of ways to protect the organism. Phagocytosis, humoral and cellular immunity, and mediators of the inflammatory response are all important components of host defense. Granulocytes (neutrophils), lymphocytes (discussed separately), monocytes, eosinophils, and basophils are the different types of WBCs.

a. *Neutrophils* account for the largest component of total circulating WBCs, approximately 55% (age related). Neutrophils are the most active in phagocytosis (Moriber, 2014).

　i.　Neutrophils originate and mature in the bone marrow and can be found in blood vessel walls, intravascular spaces, tissues, and bone marrow.

　ii.　The mature form of the neutrophil is *polymorphonucleated (PMNs or "poly")*. PMNs normally constitute the majority of the circulating neutrophils and are phagocytic and active in inflammation and tissue damage. PMNs are the first WBCs to respond to infection and the most numerous WBCs at the site of infection.

　iii.　The immature form of the neutrophil has an unsegmented-appearing nucleus and is referred to as a *band*. The immature form lacks complete phagocytic ability and normally constitutes less than 10% of the circulating neutrophils.

iv. *Neutrophilia* is an increased number of circulating neutrophils, often accompanied by an increase in the number of immature *neutrophils* (bands). Neutrophilia is associated with infections; situations that increase cardiac output (stress response associated with surgery, hemorrhage, or emotional distress such as intense crying); or increased release of epinephrine, adrenocorticotropic hormone (ACTH), or adrenal corticosteroids. Neutrophilia is also sometimes seen following administration of granulocyte colony-stimulating factor (G-CSF).

v. *Neutropenia* refers to a decreased number of circulating neutrophils with the understanding that normal values are based on age, race, and other factors (Dinauer, Newburger, & Borregaard, 2015); it is often associated with malignant conditions and marrow hypoplasia or aplasia.

vi. WBCs mature in the bone marrow for approximately 10 days. WBCs then are released into the circulation, circulate in the blood for 4 to 8 hours, and then circulate another 4 to 5 days in the tissues. The life span of WBCs is shortened in the presence of an infection (Porth, 2015).

b. *Eosinophils* normally account for 2% to 5% of the circulating WBCs and have weak phagocytic activity (Porth, 2015). Eosinophils may have a role in "turning off" the immune response because the eosinophil is the last to arrive at the site of infection. Cytoplasmic granules contain chemical substances that destroy parasitic worms and act on immune complexes involved in allergic responses.

i. *Eosinophilia* refers to an increased number of eosinophils that is greater than normally present. The eosinophil count may rise as high as 50% of the circulating WBCs with parasitic infection and less often with allergic conditions.

ii. *Eosinopenia* refers to a decreased number of eosinophils; this decrease is not clinically significant and is rarely recognized clinically, as it requires an absolute eosinophil count. There are at least two known mechanisms that produce eosinopenia: primary elevation of adrenal corticosteroids or epinephrine and acute inflammation or stress causing release of adrenal corticoids and/or epinephrine (Dinauer et al., 2015).

iii. From the bone marrow, eosinophils are released into the circulation and migrate to tissues. Unlike other granulocytes, eosinophils may recirculate back and forth between the circulation and the tissues.

c. *Basophils* represent the smallest proportion of granulocytes, accounting for fewer than 1% of circulating WBCs. Cytoplasmic granules contain chemical substances (e.g., histamine, heparin, and probably serotonin) that are released and participate in inflammation and allergic responses.

i. Production and life span of the basophil are not thoroughly understood.

ii. *Basophilia* is an increased number of circulating basophils, often associated with allergic responses, infections, and chronic inflammatory diseases (Dinauer et al., 2015).

iii. *Basophilopenia* is a decreased number of circulating basophils, and may occur in thyrotoxicosis and after treatment with thyroid hormones (Dinauer et al., 2015).

d. *Mononuclear phagocytes (monocytes and macrophages)* normally constitute 3% to 8% of circulating WBCs. Produced in the bone marrow and spending only a brief time in the circulation, most monocytes migrate into the tissues and differentiate into macrophages (Porth, 2015).

i. *Monocytosis,* an increase in the number of circulating monocytes, is observed in patients with bacterial, protozoan, parasitic, or rickettsial infections. It is also a hallmark finding in juvenile myelomonocytic leukemia and may be observed in other oncologic disorders (Dinauer et al., 2015).

ii. *Monocytopenia* is a decrease in the number of circulating monocytes. It may be observed after glucocorticoid administration and infections with endotoxemia. In addition, monocytopenia is described as a primary feature of MonoMAC syndrome, which predisposes patients to infections and certain malignancies (Dinauer et al., 2015).

iii. *Macrophages* are not quantified in the serum and have a long life span; some live for years. Macrophages commonly reside in a specific tissue, although a small percentage may wander. Examples of fixed macrophages include alveolar macrophage, Kupffer's cells in the liver, microglial cells of the brain, and spleenic macrophages. Macrophages play a primary role in *nonspecific* defenses through the ability to phagocytose. They are capable of phagocytosing larger and greater numbers of particles than the neutrophil or the monocyte. Macrophages also play a primary role in *specific* defense through processing and presentation of the antigen to the helper T cell (Dinauer et al., 2015).

3. *Lymphocytes* (lymphoid lineage) are the primary immune cells associated with humoral and cell-mediated immunity (CMI), although a small portion of lymphocytes (natural killer [NK] cells) are nonspecific in nature.

    a. *Lymphocytes* account for 10% to 40% of the circulating WBCs. They are produced in the bone marrow and then migrate to other parts of the body to differentiate and mature into several distinct subsets.

        i. Cells that migrate to the thymus differentiate into T lymphocytes (T cells) and mediate CMI.

        ii. Cells that migrate to the bursa equivalent in the human (thought to be the bone marrow) differentiate into B lymphocytes (B cells) and mediate HI (involving antibody production).

        iii. NK cells constitute a subset of lymphocytes that is nonspecific in nature, and attack infectious microbes and tumor cells (Tortora & Derrickson, 2014).

    b. *Lymphocytosis*, an increase in the number of circulating lymphocytes, is often noted in patients with viral infections (such as infectious mononucleosis or infectious hepatitis) or lymphocytic leukemia or lymphoma.

    c. *Lymphopenia*, a decrease in the number of circulating lymphocytes, is often noted in patients with congenital immunodeficiency, AIDS, uremia, or following administration of corticosteroids or ACTH.

    d. *T lymphocytes, or T cells*, normally constitute 65% to 85% of all lymphocytes. T cells mediate CMI, which confers a component of specific, acquired immunity and protects from infections with intracellular organisms, such as viruses, fungi, protozoa, and helminthic parasites. T cells are involved in the elimination of mutated or tumor cells and the immune response triggered during tissue graft or organ transplantation.

        i. Subsets of T lymphocytes have been identified through the identification of specialized molecules of the cell membrane surfaces, referred to as *clusters of differentiation (CD)*.

        ii. Helper T cells (CD4) send chemical signals (via lymphokines) to the cytotoxic T cells, macrophages, and NK cells. They have an important role in the activation of B cells.

        iii. Suppressor T cells (CD8) send a signal to inhibit actions of B cells, helper T cells, and killer T cells.

        iv. Cytotoxic or killer T cells (CD8) eliminate targets *directly* by chemical destruction and play a role in the rejection of tissue transplantation.

    e. *B lymphocytes, or B cells*, normally constitute up to 35% of circulating lymphocytes. B cells mediate HI through transformation into a plasma cell, which then secretes immunoglobulin (Ig). HI confers a component of specific, acquired immunity and protects the host from bacterial infection and viral invasion.

    f. *NK cells* normally constitute 5% to 10% of the total lymphocyte count. NK cells have neither B- nor T-cell markers and are referred to by many other names (e.g., non-B cells, non-T cells, null cells). The target for the NK cell is the tumor cell or microbe-infected cell. The NK cells' cytotoxic abilities are nonspecific in nature because they can destroy the target without prior sensitization (Tortora & Derrickson, 2014).

    g. *Memory cells* have CD according to the various distinct cell types (helper, suppressor, or cytotoxic T or B cell). They are programed to recognize the original invading microorganism on subsequent invasions. Memory cells initiate a secondary response and may result in elimination before any signs or symptoms of infection are seen.

4. *Platelets (Thrombocytes)*. Megakaryoblasts mature into megakaryocytes.

    a. Megakaryocytes break into pieces (budding) forming *platelets*, which are released into the bloodstream. Granulocyte-macrophage colony-stimulating factor (GM-CSF), stem cell factor, and interleukin-3 (IL-3) have been shown to stimulate the growth of megakaryocytes but are ineffective clinically. Thrombopoietin receptor agonists have recently been approved for certain indications in children and may also be helpful.

    b. Two thirds of mature platelets circulate in the bloodstream, and one third are stored in the spleen but are released if needed to maintain hemostasis. The life span of platelets produced in vivo is 7 to 10 days; transfused platelets have a shorter life span, usually 3 to 4 days. Thrombocytes usually are removed by the spleen or incorporated into a clot.

    c. Thrombocytes are minute round or oval discs. Platelet performance depends on the quantity of platelets (platelet count: 150,000–400,000 cells/mm^3) and the quality of function. *Adhesiveness* is stickiness, the ability to attach to blood vessel walls and surfaces. *Aggregation* is the process in which the first-arriving platelets release substances that further recruit platelets so a platelet plug is formed.

d. Aggregation is increased with secretion of epinephrine and serotonin, substances found on the surface of platelets. Functions are decreased in the presence of antiprostaglandins such as aspirin (see "Hematologic and Immunologic Pharmacology" section, Platelet Suppressor Agents).

e. Newly produced platelets are more effective than those that have been in the circulation for a few days.

D. Plasma Factors

Plasma factors describe more than 40 substances or protein molecules in blood and tissues that are involved in the clotting cascade.

1. *Procoagulants*, also known as *plasma clotting factors*, promote coagulation. Clotting factors lead to the formation of a fibrin clot. They are referred to by Roman numerals and the name of the substance. Anticoagulants are produced in the liver except for factor VIII (formation site unknown). Vitamin K is required for the production of factors II, VII, IX, and X. Factors are circulated in inactive form until stimulated to initiate clotting (see "Plasma Factors" section). All factors act in concert in vivo to respond to tissue or blood cell injury. Consumption of the procoagulants results in their destruction.

2. *Anticoagulants Inhibit Coagulation*

a. Circulating anticoagulants are antithrombin III, protein C, and protein S. Antithrombin III inactivates thrombin and inhibits factor X. Protein C inactivates factors V and VIII, stimulates fibrinolysis, and elevates levels of tissue plasminogen activator (tPA). Protein activates protein C.

b. The fibrinolytic system's major component is *plasminogen*. Plasminogen is produced in the liver and circulated in the plasma. Concentrations increase in response to inflammatory states. Plasminogen is converted to plasmin, which has the ability to digest fibrinogen and fibrin. A by-product is D-dimer, an indicator of the breakdown of cross-linked fibrin. tPA further stimulates the conversion of plasminogen to plasmin. It is synthesized by endothelial cells of the vessels and is stimulated by tissue anoxia or damage to the endothelial lining of vessels. tPA will not activate plasminogen in the absence of fibrin.

c. The antithrombin system involves a plasma protein that inactivates thrombin, and active clotting factors not used in the clotting process.

3. *Coagulation* depends on a balance between the procoagulants and the anticoagulants. A balance is needed to maintain blood as a fluid when the vasculature is intact and uninjured. Anticoagulants usually predominate until a blood vessel or tissue is injured (Table 8.1).

TABLE 8.1 Nomenclature for Coagulation Factors

Factor	Synonym
I	Fibrinogen
II	Prothrombin
III	Tissue thromboplastin
IV	Calcium
V	Proaccelerin
VI	Not assigned
VII	Proconvertin
VIII	AHF
IX	Plasma thromboplastin component (Christmas factor)
X	Stuart factor (Stuart-Prower factor)
XI	PTA
XII	Hageman factor
XIII	FSF

AHF, antihemophilic factor; FSF, fibrin-stabilizing factor; PTA, plasma thromboplastin antecedent.

Note: The *antithrombin system* involves a plasma protein that inactivates thrombin and active clotting.

Source: Modified from Gordon, J. B., Bernstein, M. L., Rogers, M. C. (1992). Hematologic disorders in the pediatric intensive care unit. In M. Rogers (Ed.). *Textbook of pediatric intensive care* (2nd ed.). Baltimore, MD: Williams & Wilkins.

FUNCTIONS AND PHYSIOLOGIC MECHANISMS

A. Red Blood Cells

The *RBC function* is to transport oxygen from the lungs to the tissues. Oxygen-carrying capacity is determined by the amount of hemoglobin available, the amount of dissolved arterial oxygen, and cardiac output.

B. White Blood Cells

1. *Functions*

   a. *Defense.* WBCs protect the body's internal environment from "nonself" antigens or microorganism invasion by inactivating, destroying, or eliminating "nonself" antigens (Pai & Reinherz, 2015).

   b. A *DNA code* at the molecular level assists the immune system in discriminating "self" from "nonself" or "altered self." Nonself is composed of foreign or alien molecular structures and is referred to as *antigenic* or as an *antigen*. Antigens are identified by characteristic shapes on their cell surfaces, referred to as *epitopes*. Antigens may carry several epitopes on their cell surface, making them capable of stimulating several different T and B lymphocytes (Moriber, 2014).

   c. *Major histocompatibility complex (MHC)* molecules serve as the genetic blueprint and allow lymphocytes to ignore self-antigens expressed on tissues (Moriber, 2014). The MHC molecules specific to the human species are human leukocyte antigens (HLAs) and are located on chromosome 6. HLA antigens are located on the surfaces of most nucleated cells in the body as well as on platelets. HLA antigens are inherited according to Mendelian laws, with an individual's genotype determined by one paternal and one maternal haplotype. Close relatives share some of these antigens, whereas identical twins share all these antigens.

   d. *HLAs* of the MHC are divided into three classes (I, II, and III) based on function, types of cell antigens expressed on the cell membrane surfaces, and structure.

   i. *Class I* includes HLA-A, -B, and -C antigens and are found on all nucleated cell surfaces and platelets. Class I antigens serve as identification markers of self, assist in the elimination of cells infected with intracellular microorganisms and of mutated or malignant cells, and are involved in the rejection of tissue grafts. Class I antigens are the target antigens recognized by the cytotoxic T cells.

   ii. *Class II* includes HLA-DR, HLA-DQ, and HLA-DP in humans. Class II antigens serve as identification markers of exogenous antigens and assist in the elimination of extracellular microorganisms. Class II molecules are expressed on B cells, monocyte–macrophages, and dendritic cells. Expression may also be induced by inflammatory mediators and cytokines on T lymphocytes (Pai & Reinherz, 2015).

   iii. *Class III* plays an important role in the innate immune system and encodes many elements of the complement system (Moriber, 2014).

   e. *Homeostasis.* WBCs remove old or damaged debris from the circulation.

   f. *Surveillance.* WBCs recognize and guard against the development, growth, and dissemination of abnormal cells.

2. *Physiologic mechanisms* of WBCs are usually categorized by three lines of defense, each representing increasingly more complex and sophisticated means of protection and methods of elimination.

   a. The *first line of defense* involves the child's natural, innate barriers with unique physical, chemical, and mechanical capabilities. This provides a nonspecific or generic defense with immediate onset.

   i. Physical and mechanical barriers prevent or minimize entry and attachment of the antigen. These include the phenomenon of simple chemicals on the skin, which inhibit colonization and promote destruction of microorganisms, mucus traps in the respiratory and GI tract, hair and cilia traps, saliva, tears, and urine (dilution and washing away of antigens), defecation and vomiting (expulsion of invading organisms), and an intact GI lining (Moriber, 2014). Many factors associated with critical illnesses are thought to threaten the barrier role of the gut mucosa and increase the risk of translocation of gram-negative bacteria or endotoxins.

   ii. Chemical barriers deter attachment, survival, and replication of antigen. These include the acidic pH of the skin; lysozymes present in saliva, tears, and nasal secretions; gastric secretions; and unsaturated fatty acids in sweat and sebaceous glands.

b. The *second line of defense* involves the inflammatory response, phagocytosis, and complement activation. It is nonspecific or generic in nature with immediate onset once triggered, if the first line of defense is ineffective.

    i. The local *inflammatory response* is a sequential reaction to injury hallmarked by the release of numerous chemical mediators such as histamine, bradykinin (and other kinins), serotonin, and prostaglandins. The goals of inflammation include localization, dilution, and destruction of the offending antigen, maintenance of vascular integrity, minimization of tissue damage, and transportation of cells and substances to the area.

    ii. *Vascular response* is characterized by immediate vasoconstriction, which facilitates fibrin plug formation and WBC, RBC, and platelet margination. Vasodilation facilitates cell and cell products to move close to the area of injury. Capillary permeability assists in cell and cell-product movement from the vascular space into the tissues. Local increases in hydrostatic pressure and increased oncotic pressure of proteins in the interstitium leads to edema (Grossman, 2014d).

    iii. *Cellular response* involves margination or paving of the lining of cells along the capillary endothelium to prepare for movement from the intravascular space to the tissue. Margination is facilitated by the vascular response because fluid leakage into the interstitium results in an increased blood viscosity and a decreased blood flow. Following the leukocyte accumulation that occurs in margination, cytokines are released, causing the endothelial cells lining the vessels to express cell adhesion molecules. *Adhesion* allows the process of transmigration as the endothelial cells separate. *Transmigration* allows the leukocytes to move through the vessel wall and migrate into tissue spaces while influenced by chemotactic factors (Grossman, 2014d). *Chemotaxis* involves chemical signals to attract cells to the site of injury. Substances that serve as chemotactic chemicals include chemokines, protein fragments, and bacterial and cellular debris (Grossman, 2014d). The final phase of cellular response is *phagocytosis*, in which monocytes, neutrophils, and tissue macrophages engulf and degrade bacterial and cellular debris (Grossman, 2014d).

    iv. Other components of the inflammatory response, biochemical mediators, and plasma enzyme cascades facilitate the inflammatory response through diverse but complementary actions. Numerous biochemical mediators have been identified, such as prostaglandins, leukotrienes, endorphins, and histamine. The primary nonspecific plasma enzyme cascades include complement, coagulation (involved in the vascular response via hemostasis; see "Coagulation Factor" section, Coagulation Cascade), fibrinolysis (primary activity is the degradation of fibrin clot; see "Plasma Factors" section, Fibrinolytic System), and kallikrein or kinin (bradykinin; enhances inflammatory response by promoting vasodilation, increased capillary permeability, neutrophil chemotaxis, and other actions).

    v. Phagocytosis. Phagocytes include granulocytes (especially neutrophils) and monocytes or macrophages. The purpose of phagocytosis is to capture, engulf, and destroy the antigen. In addition, phagocytosis may eventually present the antigen to the helper T lymphocyte. The process of phagocytosis is complex and involves several mechanisms.

    1) Recognition of the antigen as nonself.

    2) Adherence or attachment of the phagocyte to the antigen or invader.

    3) Ingestion or engulfment is performed through the use of pseudopods. Eventually the antigen is taken into the phagocyte's cytoplasm, where it is enveloped in a sac (phagosome).

    4) Killing and degradation occur when the antigen-containing sac is subjected to lysozyme and the process known as the respiratory (oxidative) burst, containing hydrogen peroxide, superoxide anion, and hydrochlorite anion. Some microorganisms are ingested but not necessarily killed. For instance, the toxins from staphylococci may in turn kill the phagocyte. Others, such as tubercule bacilli, may multiply within the phagosome and eventually destroy the phagocyte.

    vi. The complement system works through innate and adaptive immunity to localize and destroy microorganisms. Complement proteins C1 to C9 normally circulate in the plasma in the inactive form, making up approximately 10% to 15% of plasma proteins.

Three independent pathways may lead to activation of the complement system in an innate response; these include the *classical*, *lectin*, and *alternative* pathways. The distinguishing features of these pathways are the proteins used in the early phases of activation. The reaction of each pathway is described in three phases: initiation or activation, amplification of inflammation, and membrane attack response.

1) In the activation phase, the alternative pathway is activated by microbial cell surfaces in the absence of antibodies. The classical pathway is part of the HI, activated by antibodies bound to antigens. The lectin pathway is activated with plasma lectin binds to mannose on microbes and activates the classical system (Moriber, 2014).

2) Activation of complement protein C3 is central to the inflammatory response. This leads to enzymatic cleavage into a larger C3b and smaller C3a fragment, which go on to attach to the microbe to initiate phagocytosis and to serve as a chemoattractant for neutrophils, respectively. C3b also works to cleave C5 into two fragments as part of an enzymatic response, leading to vasodilation, vascular permeability,

and late-step membrane attack responses (Moriber, 2014).

3) Late-step responses involve C3b as it binds to other complement proteins and stimulates additional responses through the influx of neutrophils and vascular phase of acute inflammation. Fluid and ions enter cells and cause lysis when complement C5b initiates C6, C7, C8, and C9 to form a membrane attack complex (MAC) protein.

c. The *third line of defense* involves specific, acquired immunity and is triggered if the first and second lines of defense are ineffective in eliminating or containing the antigen. The immune response is a highly complex sequence of events that is triggered by an antigen and integrally associated with other physiologic events, including but not limited to complement activation and the clotting and fibrocytic systems (Moriber, 2014). Hallmarks of the third line of defense include specificity, the ability of a lymphocyte to respond to a single antigen for which it was designed, and memory (i.e., the ability of a lymphocyte to recall prior exposure to an antigen and respond in an accelerated, potentiated manner). Specific acquired immunity may be obtained either passively or actively and naturally or artificially (Table 8.2).

TABLE 8.2   Acquired, Specific Immunity: Definition, Acquisition, and Characteristics

Types of Acquired, Specific Immunity	Definition and Acquisition	Characteristics
Passive Immunity		
Natural	Acquired through natural contact with *antibody* transplacentally or through colostrum and breast milk (e.g., IgG and IgA from mother to fetus or neonate)	No participation of the host; a transfer of preformed substances or sensitized cells from an immunized host to a nonimmunized host
Artificial	Acquired through the administration of *antibody* or antitoxin (e.g., gamma-globulin, tetanus)	Onset is immediate, but duration is temporary
Active Immunity		
Natural	Acquired through natural infection; the body is exposed to an *antigen* and mounts an immune response to that antigen (e.g., chickenpox)	Active participation of the host following exposure to an antigen either naturally (subclinical or clinical disease) or artificially through immunization
Artificial	Acquired through inoculation with a variant *antigen*, but usually not the entire antigen (e.g., immunization, attenuated virus)	Provides slow antigen-specific development of antibody, but provides permanent or long-lived immunity to that antigen

IgA, immunoglobulin A; IgG, immunoglobulin G.

Source: Adapted from Mudge-Grout, C. L. (1992). *Immunologic disorders.* St Louis, MO: Mosby-Year Book.

i. Specific acquired immunity occurs in phases. Recognition and processing of the antigen are the primary responsibilities of the macrophage, although the B lymphocyte may participate. Once identified as nonself, or foreign, the macrophage ingests the antigen and, through an enzyme-mediated reaction, begins "antigen processing." When "antigen processing" is complete, the macrophage reexpresses the processed antigen on its membrane surface in conjunction with HLA antigen. Antigen presentation to the B or T lymphocyte occurs (Moriber, 2014). Processing and presentation of the antigen trigger the immune response to facilitate elimination.

ii. Acquired immunity comprises two different, but closely interrelated, antigen-specific immune responses (Figure 8.3):

1) HI, which is mediated by B lymphocytes, results in the synthesis and secretion of immunoglobulins and *indirectly* eliminates or impedes the antigen. HI provides protection primarily from encapsulated pyogenic bacterial infections (Moriber, 2014).

2) CMI, which is mediated by T lymphocytes, *directly* eliminates the antigen. CMI protects from viral, bacterial, and parasitic infections; plays a role in rejection of foreign grafts; and participates in delayed hypersensitivity reactions (Porth, 2015).

iii. Humoral immunity. B lymphocytes can be activated without the help of the T lymphocyte, as in T-cell-independent antigen response, but most commonly are activated with the assistance of the T lymphocyte, as in the T-cell-dependent antigen response. B cells transform into plasma cells, which synthesize and secrete immunoglobulins and subsequently interact with the antigen for which it was made. Immunoglobulins (antibodies) are glycoproteins produced by plasma cells in response to an antigen (Moriber, 2014).

iv. There are five major classes of immunoglobulins: IgG, IgA, IgM, IgD, and IgE (Moriber, 2014; Table 8.3).

1) IgG makes up approximately 75% of total immunoglobulins and possesses antiviral, antitoxin, and antibacterial properties. This is the only type of IgG that crosses the placenta, and therefore, protects the newborn. IgG activates complement and binds to macrophages (Moriber, 2014).

2) IgA comprises approximately 15% of the immunoglobulin present; it is found in secretions and protects the mucous membranes.

3) IgM is prominent in early immune responses, responsible for activating complement, and forms natural antibodies such as ABO blood antigens. It makes up approximately 10% of immunoglobulins.

4) IgD is found on B lymphocytes and is necessary for the maturation of mature B cells.

5) IgE is involved in parasitic infections and allergic and hypersensitivity reactions.

v. Outcomes of antigen–antibody interaction include *neutralization* (antibody binds the antigen, causing the antigen to be ineffective or to promote removal by phagocytes), *agglutination* (antibody combines with the antigen to form clumps), *precipitation* (antibody combines with the antigen to make an insoluble lattice formation that precipitates), *opsonization* (antibody coats the antigen, enhancing phagocytosis), *complement* (antibodies activate complement, thus causing target cell lysis), and *antibody-dependent cytotoxicity* (antibody facilitates lysis of the antigen by another immune cell).

vi. Primary response. Antibody production occurs 2 to 10 days after the first exposure, and the response peaks in 1 to 3 weeks. Immunoglobulin M (IgM) is followed by an IgG response.

vii. Secondary, or memory phase, response is the response that occurs with exposure to a previously encountered antigen. Memory cells are responsible for the rapid (in 1–2 days), prolific, sustained response to the familiar antigen. Antibody response is primarily IgG at much higher titers for a shorter period compared with the primary response (Moriber, 2014).

viii. Cell-mediated immunity involves T-lymphocyte recognition and activation. T lymphocyte binds to the antigen *and* to a class I or class II protein on the surface of an antigen-presenting cell (usually the macrophage). Class I HLA antigens are required for cytotoxic T-lymphocyte activation. Class II HLA antigens are required for helper T-lymphocyte activation.

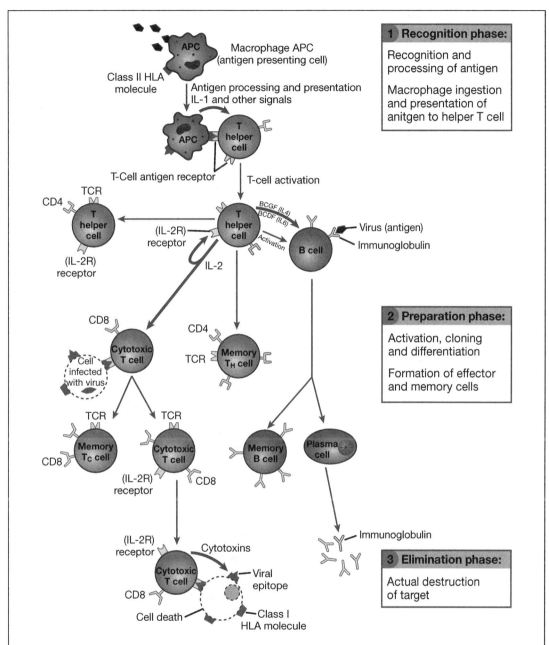

FIGURE 8.3 The specific immune response consists of three distinct phases: (1) the recognition phase, which involves the recognition and processing of antigens; (2) the preparation phase, which focuses on activation, cloning, and differentiation of cells; and (3) the elimination phase, in which the target in the cell is destroyed. Through the interdependence of B and T cells, both humoral and cell-mediated immunity are initiated.

CD4, cluster of differentiation 4; CD8, cluster of differentiation 8; CMI, cell-mediated immunity; HI, humoral (immunoglobulin) immunity. HLA, human leukocyte antigen; IL-1, interleukin-1; IL-2R, interleukin-2 receptor; TCR, T-cell receptor.

ix. Communication among all the cells participating in the immune response is facilitated through the secretion of *cytokines*. Cytokines are hormone-like substances that function to upregulate and downregulate immunologic, inflammatory, and reparative host responses. Cytokines secreted by lymphocytes are referred to as *lymphokines*. Cytokines secreted by monocytes or macrophages are referred to as *monokines*.

TABLE 8.3   Human Immunoglobulins

Ig	Percentage in Serum	Location	Activity and Function
IgG	75%	Most abundant intravascularly	Only immunoglobulin to cross placenta
		Also in extravascular spaces (e.g., lymph, colony-stimulating factor)	Primary antibody class
			Activates complement
			Takes 10–14 days after antigen stimulation to develop sufficient IgG titer in primary response; only 4 days in secondary response
			Appears 1 week after IgM and peaks in 1–3 weeks or longer after IgM peaks
			Promotes phagocytosis via opsonization
IgA	15%	Found in mucous membrane secretions	Two types: serum and secretory
		Intravascular	Primary defense against local invasion of body surfaces and orifices
IgM	10%	Intravascular only	Promotes phagocytosis
			Can activate complement
			Participates in blood transfusion reactions; makes antibodies for "nonself" ABO blood groups
			Made in utero and may indicate the presence of an intrauterine infection or ABO incompatibility
			First made in response to an antigen
			Predominant in a primary infection
			Peaks 1–2 weeks after infection
			Increases in chronic infections
IgE	0.1%	Found in serum bound to mast cells and basophils	Triggers release of histamine and other mediators from mast cells and basophils
			Involved in type I immediate hypersensitivity or anaphylactic reactions
			Defense against parasite infections
IgD	<1%	Found in serum located on surface of B cells	Function not yet defined
			May participate in B-cell differentiation
			Increases in chronic infection

Ig, immunoglobulin.

Sources: Data from Grady, C. (1988). Host defense mechanisms: An overview. *Seminars in Oncology Nursing, 4*(2), 92. doi:10.1016/0749-2081(88)90064-2; Mudge-Grout, C. L. (1992). *Immunologic disorders*. St Louis, MO: Mosby–Year Book; Selekman, J. (1991). Pediatric problems related to the immunologic system. In V. D. Feeg & R. E. Harbin (Eds.), *Pediatric nursing: Core curriculum and resource manual*. Pitman, NJ: Anthony Jannetti.

Cytokines are distinct from endocrine hormones in that they are produced by a number of cells rather than by a specialized gland, they do not usually present in the serum, and they act in a paracrine (locally near the producing cell) or autocrine (directly on the producing cell) fashion rather than on distant target cells. Selected cytokines are described in Table 8.4.

x. Developmental distinctions occur in the third line of defense. The infant's B cells are deficient in producing comparable adult levels

TABLE 8.4 Selected Cytokines: Source and Functions

Type	Source	Functions
IL		
IL-1 (endogenous pyrogen)	T cell, B cell, macrophage, endothelium, tissue cell	Enhances T-cell growth and function; stimulates macrophages; immunoaugmentation
IL-2 (T-cell growth factor)	T cells	Promotes T-cell and B-cell growth; activates T cell; enhances NK activity
IL-3 (multi-CSF)	T cells, mast cells	Stimulates growth of immature hematopoietic precursor cells (e.g., granulocytes, macrophages, RBCs, platelets, and mast cells)
BCGF (IL-4)	T cells	Enhances B-cell growth and function
BCDF (IL-6)	T cells	Enhances B-cell growth and function
INTERFERONS		
Interferon alfa	Lymphocytes, NK cells, macrophages, fibroblasts, epithelial cells	Enhances NK activity; provides antiviral protection; induces HLA-I expression; induces fever; generates cytotoxic T lymphocytes; induces macrophage killing of tumor cells
Interferon beta	Fibroblasts, macrophages, epithelial cells	Provides antiviral protection
Interferon gamma	T cells, NK cells	Activates macrophages; induces macrophage killing of microorganism and tumor cells; regulates action of certain cytokines; increases NK cell activity; increases expression of Fc receptor and HLA-I antigens
Tumor necrosis factor	Macrophages, T cells, and others	Enhances destruction of tumor cells
CSFs		
G-CSF	Monocytes, macrophages, endothelial cells, and fibroblasts	Stimulates growth and activation of neutrophils
M-CSF	Monocytes, macrophages, endothelial cells, and fibroblasts	Stimulates growth and activation of monocytes
GM-CSF	T cells, endothelial cells, and fibroblasts	Stimulates growth and activation of neutrophils, eosinophils, and macrophages

CSF, colony-stimulating factor; G-CSF, granulocyte colony-stimulating factor; GM-CSF, granulocyte–macrophage colony-stimulating factor; HLA, human leukocyte antigen; ; IL, interleukin; M-CSF, macrophage colony-stimulating factor; NK, natural killer; RBCs, red blood cells.

Sources: Data from Mudge-Grout, C. L. (1992). *Immunologic disorders.* St Louis, MO: Mosby–Year Book; Plaeger, S. F. (1996). Principal human cytokines. In E. R. Stiehm (Ed.), *Immunologic disorders in infants and children* (4th ed.). Philadelphia, PA: WB Saunders.

and subclasses of immunoglobulins. Serum immunoglobulin levels, the degree of synthesis at birth, and the age at which the levels are comparable to the adult are reflected in Table 8.5. The IgG level seems comparable between the newborn and the adult, but this level reflects the transplacental acquisition of maternal antibody during primarily the third trimester of gestation. The infant is lowest in immunoglobulin concentrations at about 4 to 5 months of age, when maternal IgG begins to decrease through natural catabolism and when infant synthesis of immunoglobulin is low. This period is referred to as physiologic hypogammaglobulinemia. During this time, the infant is most susceptible to infections caused by viruses, candida, and acute inflammatory bacteria (*Staphylococcus aureus, Streptococcus pyogenes, Streptococcus pneumoniae, Haemophilus influenzae* type B, and *Neisseria meningitidis*). This state can be prolonged to such an extent that the young child suffers from recurrent and severe infections.

C. Platelets

1. *Function.* The function of platelets is to maintain normal hemostasis and vascular integrity when a blood vessel wall is injured.

2. *Hemostasis* is a complex interaction among three responding systems (Grossman, 2014c).

a. Vascular constriction: Injury to a vessel wall leads to the release of chemical signals, such as endothelin 1, and constriction of the injured vessel within seconds. This smooth muscle contraction reduces blood flow to the area.

b. Formation of the platelet plug: Platelets rush to the area of injury where they are activated by cytokines and initiate the process of adhesion. The platelet surface changes, becoming "sticky" and attracting additional platelets (Figure 8.4).

c. Blood coagulation: Two coagulation pathways, the intrinsic and extrinsic pathways, lead to the activation of factor X, converting prothrombin to thrombin, and converting fibrinogen to fibrin threads.

3. *Physiologic conditions* influencing platelet response can be quantitative (increase or decrease in number) or qualitative (abnormal function).

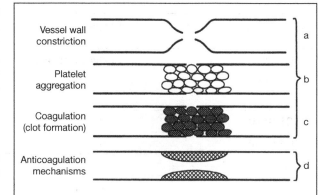

FIGURE 8.4 Hemostatic response of platelets. Major mechanisms involved in primary hemostasis (*a*) through (*c*). Injury results in vessel wall constriction, platelet aggregation, and clot formation. Anticoagulation mechanisms (*d*) reestablish blood flow by lysing the clot.

Source: From Harvey, M. (1986). *Study guide to core curriculum for critical care nursing* (p. 162). Philadelphia, PA: W. B. Saunders.

TABLE 8.5   Serum Immunoglobulins: Developmental Perspectives

Ig	Synthesis by Fetus (Gestation Week)	Percentage of Adult Levels at Birth	Age at Which Adult Levels are Achieved (Years)
IgM	10.5	10%	1–2
IgD	14	Small amount	1
IgG*	12	110%**	4–10
IgA	30	Small amount or none	6–15
IgE	10.5	Small amount	6–15

Ig, immunoglobulin.

*Crosses placenta; **Greater than or equal to maternal level.

Source: From Rosenthal, C. H. (1989). Immunosuppression in the pediatric critical care patient. *Critical Care Nursing Clinics North America, 1*(4), 779.

a. An increase in the number of circulating platelets (platelet count) usually occurs after acute blood loss to enhance hemostasis.

b. *Thrombocytopenia*, defined as a platelet count lower than 150,000/mm³, can result from decreased production, increased destruction, or increased trapping in the spleen (splenic sequestration). Causes of thrombocytopenia include medications (see "Therapeutic Modalities That Depress the Functions of the Hematologic and Immunologic Systems" section), renal or liver disease, cardiopulmonary bypass or hemodialysis, aplastic anemia, immune thrombocytopenic purpura (ITP), thrombotic thrombocytopenic purpura (TTP), heparin-induced thrombocytopenia (HIT), viral diseases, disseminated intravascular coagulation (DIC), radiation to the bones, and malignancies involving the bone marrow (displacement of normal stem cells with malignant cells). Thrombocytopenia may also result from congenital disorders, such as thrombocytopenic absent radii (TAR), congenital amegakaryocytic thrombocytopenia (CAMT), and Wiskott–Aldrich syndrome (WAS; Lambert & Poncz, 2015).

c. Platelet function can be impaired by medications (e.g., aspirin, nonsteroidal anti-inflammatory drugs [NSAIDs]; see "Therapeutic Modalities That Depress the Functions of the Hematologic and Immunologic Systems" section), renal disease, and inherited disorders such as Glanzmann thrombasthenia and platelet-type von Willebrand disease (Lambert & Poncz, 2015). Uremia causes reversible impairment of qualitative platelet function. Impaired platelet function results in bleeding in areas abundant in capillaries, such as the mucous membranes in the GI tract, the vagina, the bladder, and the nasopharynx, producing petechiae or ecchymosis or both.

d. Most platelet problems in critical care are due to thrombocytopenia rather than to decreased function of the platelets. Hemostasis begins to be affected when the platelet count is below 80,000 to 100,000/mm³, but bleeding is unlikely until the platelet count is less than 25,000/mm³. If the platelet count is less than 50,000/mm³, easy bruising may occur. If the platelet count is less than 10,000 to 20,000/mm³, spontaneous bleeding may occur, especially if the child is anemic or febrile. If the platelet count is 10,000/mm³, severe spontaneous or intracranial bleeding may occur.

e. Critically ill children may bleed as a result of sepsis, trauma, malignancy, toxins, and immunologic reactions. Correcting the underlying cause of the bleeding will often lead to resolution of bleeding. In addition, DIC, as described later in this chapter, is a frequent cause of excessive bleeding in the critically ill child (Lambert & Poncz, 2015).

D. Plasma Factors

1. *Procoagulants* contribute to the process of secondary hemostasis, which is represented by the formation of a fibrin clot and trapping of RBCs at the site of the initiating primary hemostatic plug.

2. *Enzymes and proteins* amplify initial activation of a soft clot to an appropriately sized, fully developed clot.

3. *Factors* play a role in initiating primary nonspecific plasma enzyme cascades.

4. *Coagulation cascade* starts within the bloodstream itself *(intrinsic)* or outside the bloodstream *(extrinsic)*. The process results in blood changing from a liquid to a gel state by the ultimate conversion of fibrinogen to insoluble fibrin polymers. Contraction of the fibrin network follows, causing the plug to retract, the walls of the damaged vessel to come together, and the injured vessel wall to seal shut.

a. The *intrinsic pathway* is activated when platelets contact collagen or damaged endothelium. Its function is screened by partial thromboplastin time (PTT).

b. The *extrinsic pathway* is activated when tissue factor is released from injured tissues, such as when tissues have been cut in surgery. Its function is screened by prothrombin time (PT).

c. The *common pathway* is the part of the coagulation cascade that is activated by the intrinsic or extrinsic pathway. The final step is a fibrin mesh within the platelet plug. Thrombin stimulates the platelets to further aggregate. Fibrin is an essential portion of a clot, soluble until polymerized by factor XIII, which converts it to a stable (insoluble) clot. The function of the common pathway is screened by both the PT and PTT.

5. *Anticoagulant mechanisms* function to maintain blood as a fluid to maintain vascular patency. The system must turn off the various coagulation pathways to reestablish blood flow through an injured vessel, maintain vascular patency, and modulate the balance between the clotting and lysing systems.

a. The *fibrinolytic system* involves the process of lysing a clot. Plasminogen is the precursor to the active part, which is plasmin. It is produced in the liver and circulated in the plasma.

The conversion to plasmin is increased in states such as inflammation and coagulation or in the presence of tPA. Plasmin lyses fibrin clots by digesting fibrin or fibrinogen. Plasmin splits fibrin into smaller elements called *fibrin split products (FSPs)* or *fibrin degredation products (FDPs)*. FSPs impair platelet aggregation, reduce prothrombin, and interfere with polymerization of fibrin.

b. The *antithrombin system* defends against excessive clotting and maintains blood as a fluid. The blood vessel wall has sites that allow thrombin to be inactivated by antithrombin III. Disorders of antithrombin mechanism include congenital thrombotic disorders (thrombophilia) and hepatic failure.

CLINICAL ASSESSMENT

A. History

1. *Chief complaint* is noted in the patient's or the primary caretaker's own words.

2. *History of Present Illness*

    a. Activity intolerance, fatigue, and weakness; shortness of breath and dyspnea; and "racing heart"

    b. Fever or chills, chronic or recurrent infection, lymphadenopathy, skin rash, and joint pain

    c. Petechiae, bruising, or abnormal bleeding (either prolonged after a minor injury or spontaneous)

3. *Patient Health History*

    a. Record immunizations and previous immunologic testing.

    b. The patient's diet and nutrition history is described, including recent weight gain or loss, dietary restrictions, food dislikes and intolerance, and routine dietary intake, including cultural adherence. All blood cell lines are dependent to some extent on adequate nutritional intake. In particular, iron, vitamin B_{12}, and folic acid are needed for RBC development.

    c. Allergies and hypersensitivities are noted, including allergies to inhalants (e.g., animal dander, pollens), contactants (e.g., fibers, chemicals, latex), injectables (e.g., drugs, blood transfusions), or ingestants (e.g., foods, food additives, drugs) and the symptoms accompanying the allergic or hypersensitivity reaction.

    d. Previous surgeries that may impair hematologic or immunologic status are noted, including organ or tissue transplantation, thymectomy, or splenectomy.

    e. Inquire about medical conditions that might impair hematologic or immunologic status. Abnormalities of RBCs are seen with anemia or malabsorption syndromes. Liver or spleen disorders (functional splenectomy), chronic or recurrent infections, mononucleosis, or problems with wound healing may impact WBC function or numbers. Platelets may be abnormal with prolonged or excessive bleeding or menorrhagia. Plasma factors may be implicated in hemarthrosis. Cancer, bone marrow abnormalities, congenital blood disorders, and immunodeficiency all can affect hematologic and immune status.

    f. General symptoms include fatigue, change in level of activity, weakness, headache, chills, fever, weight loss, failure to thrive, night sweats, poor wound healing, malaise, pain, prolonged or excessive bleeding, excessive bleeding related to dental extractions, and menorrhagia.

    g. See Table 8.6 for specific symptoms of concern.

    h. Psychosocial history should include recent stresses or life-changing events, response to stress, and coping methods.

4. Family history of RBC, WBC, platelet, and coagulation factor abnormalities is noted.

    a. *RBC abnormalities* include jaundice, anemia, and RBC dyscrasia, such as sickle cell anemia.

    b. *WBC abnormalities* include malignancies; frequent, recurrent, or chronic infections; congenital immunodeficiencies; acquired immunodeficiencies; and autoimmune disorders.

    c. *Platelet abnormalities* include any bleeding disorders or predisposition to bleeding or clotting.

    d. *Congenital bleeding disorders* include hemophilia, von Willebrand disease, and clotting disorders (thrombophilia).

    e. Any *symptoms of blood disorders* similar to the patient's symptoms are noted.

5. *Medication History*

    a. *Prescription agents* used to treat existing hematologic or immunologic conditions may include multivitamins, iron preparations (oral or parenteral), vitamin B_{12}, folic acid, or EPO for

TABLE 8.6 Symptoms of Concern

System	Symptoms of Concern
Neurologic	• Confusion, restlessness, syncope, irritability, impaired consciousness or somnolence • Deficits in sensory and/or motor function; altered cranial nerve function (cough, gag, swallow, blink)
Skin	• Prolonged bleeding, bruising easily, petechiae, jaundice, pallor, lesions, ulcers, decreased skin turgor, rhinitis, dermatitis, urticaria, eczema
Eyes	• Visual disturbances, retinal hemorrhages, pallor, erythema of conjunctivae
Nose and mouth	• Epistaxis, gingival bleeding, sore or ulcerated tongue, mucositis, candidiasis, vesicular crusting lesions
Lymph nodes	• Adenopathy (enlargement) or tenderness • Tachypnea, respiratory tract infection, respiratory distress, dyspnea, orthopnea, cough, hemoptysis, sputum, chest pain
Respiratory	• Bleeding from nose or endotracheal tube
Cardiovascular	• Hemodynamic instability • Oozing from venipuncture, intra-arterial, or intravenous sites • Pale skin and mucous membranes, vasculitis
GI	• Frank or occult bleeding in GI contents • Anorexia, altered bowel sounds, diarrhea, constipation, melena, vomiting, hematemesis, protuberant abdomen (not age-related), abdominal pain, masses, hepatosplenomegaly
GU	• Hematuria, menorrhagia, urinary tract infection
Mobility	• Ataxia, paresthesias • Altered level of activity • Muscle weakness • Pain in joints, back, shoulders, bones • Hemarthrosis

GI, gastrointestinal; GU, genitourinary.

RBC deficiencies. A wide variety of agents used to treat infection, autoimmune disorders, and malignancies affect WBC number and function and the ability of the body to mount an inflammatory response. Examples of such agents include antineoplastic agents, antibiotics, antivirals or antiretrovirals, antifungals, NSAIDs, and CSFs. Antiplatelet agents, such as aspirin, may compromise clotting functions. Anticoagulants affect plasma factors. Evaluate agents used to treat nonhematologic or immunologic conditions that adversely affect hemopoietic function (see "Therapeutic Modalities That Depress the Functions of the Hematologic and Immunologic Systems" section).

b. *Nonprescription* drugs include common agents such as aspirin, and also substances used as recreational drugs.

6. *Social–Cultural History*

a. Environmental exposures may include radiation, either inadvertent exposure or radiation therapies (total or localized), or inadvertent exposure to chemicals such as benzene, lead, and insecticides.

b. Discuss recent travel, especially outside the United States.

c. Determine whether the patient is sexually active (including nonconsensual sex). Evaluate sexual preference, safer sex practices, and multiple partners.

d. Determine tobacco and alcohol use. Alcohol consumption reduces the intake of essential nutrients and vitamins and may affect RBC production, platelet function, and clotting mechanisms.

e. Evaluate the use of complementary therapies and other interventions used by the patient and family.

B. Physical Examination of the Patient

1. *Inspection* (see Table 8.6)

2. *Auscultation*

a. Heart sounds, including gallop, rhythm, and pericardial rubs (may indicate an inflammatory process)

b. Lung sounds, including rales, rhonchi, and pleural rubs

3. *Palpation*

a. Palpate superficial lymph nodes for location, size, tenderness, fixation, and texture (see Figure 8.2). In pediatric patients between infancy and adolescence, palpable lymph nodes less than 3 mm are considered normal and those in the cervical and inguinal areas may be up to 1 cm in size. It is important to assess the texture, temperature, tenderness, and mobility of these nodes. If the nodes are discrete, easily mobile, and nontender, they may not always be of clinical significance. The increased incidence of infection in children means the frequency of inflammatory adenopathy is higher. Supraclavicular lymphadenopathy should be addressed with a high index of suspicion, as these nodes enlarge with Hodgkin's lymphoma (Jarvis, 2016).

b. Examine for sternal or rib tenderness, joint mobility and tenderness, and bone or abdominal tenderness.

c. Palpate liver and spleen for size and tenderness. Tenderness may be indicative of an inflammatory process or an enlarged organ with stretching of the capsule secondary to bleeding or malignancy. Assess for complications of portal hypertension (hepatomegaly or splenomegaly). Hepatosplenomegaly may also be noted in patients with numerous hematologic and oncologic disorders (e.g., hemolytic anemia, immunodeficiency disorders, and cancer).

INVASIVE AND NONINVASIVE DIAGNOSTIC STUDIES

A. Complete Blood Count (CBC)

1. *RBC Count*

a. Normal is approximately 4.5 to 6 × 10⁶ million/mm³ (varies with age; Table 8.7)

b. RBCs are *reduced* in anemia from any cause and will be relatively decreased in a patient experiencing fluid overload.

c. RBCs are *increased* in chronic hypoxemia, high altitude, and polycythemia.

2. *Hemoglobin (Hgb)* measures the oxygen-carrying capacity of the RBC and gives it the red color.

a. Normal (see Table 8.7)

b. Hgb × 3 is an approximation of the patient's hematocrit.

c. Hgb is reduced in anemia from any cause and relatively with fluid overload.

d. Hgb is increased in polycythemia and relatively with severe dehydration.

3. *Hematocrit (Hct)* compares the volume of RBCs with the volume of plasma; it is measured as percentage of total RBC volume.

a. Normal (see Table 8.7)

b. Hct is reduced in anemia from any cause and will be relatively decreased in a patient experiencing fluid overload.

c. Hct is increased in polycythemia and relatively with severe dehydration.

4. *Peripheral smear* enables a more exact evaluation of blood cell size, shape, and composition and is especially useful in evaluating anemia and confirmation of thrombocytopenia.

5. *Reticulocyte count* is the number of young RBCs. It indicates the proportion of immature RBCs in the circulation and is helpful in determining the cause of anemia in some children. The reticulocyte count measures the responsiveness and potential of the bone marrow to respond to bleeding or hemolysis.

a. Normal. 0.5% to 2% (may vary from one laboratory to another)

b. The reticulocyte count is reduced after a blood transfusion, in aplastic conditions, or in nutritional anemias.

c. The reticulocyte count is increased in hemolytic anemia, after blood loss, and with bone marrow recovery as a compensatory mechanism.

6. *Total WBC Count*

a. Normal WBC is approximately 5,000 to 10,000/mm³ (age specific; see Table 8.7).

b. Variations in the total WBC count include leukocytosis, an elevation in WBC count above normal range, and leukopenia, a reduction in WBC count below normal range.

TABLE 8.7   Hematologic Values During Infancy and Childhood

Age	Hemoglobin (g/dL)		Hematocrit (%)		Reticulocytes (%)	MCV (fl)	Leukocytes (WBC/mm³)		Neutrophils (%)		Lymphocytes (%)	Eosinophils (%)	Monocytes (%)
	Mean	Range	Mean	Range	Mean	Lowest	Mean	Range	Mean	Range	Mean*	Mean	Mean
Cord blood	16.8	13.7–20.1	55	45–65	5	110	18,000	(9,000–30,000)	61	(40–80)	31	2	6
2 weeks	16.5	13–20	50	42–66	1		12,000	(5,000–21,000)	40		63	3	9
3 months	12.0	9.5–14.5	36	31–41	1		12,000	(6,000–18,000)	30		48	2	5
6 months–6 years	12.0	10.5–14	37	33–42	1	70–74	10,000	(6,000–15,000)	45		48	2	5
7–12 years	13.0	11–16	38	34–40	1	76–80	8,000	(4,500–13,500)	55		38	2	5
Adult													
Female	14	12–16	42	37–47	1.6	80	7,500	(5,000–10,000)	55	(35–70)	35	3	7
Male	16	14–18	47	42–52		80							

fl, temtoliters; MCV, mean corpuscular volume; WBC, white blood cell.

*Relatively wide range.

Source: From Christensen, R. D., & Ohs, R. K. (1996). Development of the hematopoietic system. In R. E. Behrman, R. M. Kliegman, & A. M. Arvin (Eds.), *Nelson textbook of pediatrics* (15th ed.). Philadelphia, PA: W. B. Saunders.

c. Total WBC count reflects only those WBCs in the intravascular space (excluding the marginal pool). WBCs are also located in the following:

  i. Marginal pool. Cells are temporarily sequestered in small vessels or adhere to the walls of large blood vessels.

  ii. Tissues. Nearly twice as many neutrophils are found in the tissues as in the intravascular space.

  iii. Bone marrow. The bone marrow is the primary storage area for mature neutrophils.

7. *Differential WBC count* measures the five subcategories of circulating WBCs and is reported as a percentage of the total WBC count. It evaluates the bone marrow's ability to produce those particular cells (see Table 8.7) and indicates the type of cell that is excessively prominent. *Neutrophil shifts* are the number of "segs," or "bands" as reported in the differential WBC count, which may be interpreted in two ways:

a. As an indication of the cell's maturity, a "shift to the left" indicates predominantly immature neutrophils (bands), as seen in acute infection, tissue injury, or use of CSFs (Grossman, 2014b).

b. A "shift to the right" indicates an increased number of mature neutrophils, called "segs" because of their segmented nucleus, which can be observed in patients experiencing pernicious anemia (vitamin B_{12} deficiency), folate deficiency, stress, epinephrine, and corticosteroid therapy (Grossman, 2014b).

8. *Absolute cell counts* specifically quantifiy a particular cell line and may be derived for any cell line. Following is an example calculation of an absolute neutrophil count (ANC):

a. Obtain patient's total WBC count (i.e., WBC = 5 k/mm³).

b. Translate the total WBC count into an absolute number (*k* means 1,000 cells; therefore, 5 × 1,000 = 5,000 or an absolute WBC count of 5,000/mm³).

c. Obtain WBC differential and add the percentages of "polys" plus "bands" (polys = 60% plus bands = 10%; therefore, 60% + 10% = 70%).

d. Translate the percentage of "polys" plus "bands" into an absolute number by dividing by 100 (70% ÷ 100 = 0.7).

e. Multiply the absolute WBC count by the absolute "polys" plus "band" count (5,000 × 0.7 = 3,500; therefore, ANC = 3,500/mm³).

9. *Absolute neutrophil count*

a. Normal. 1,500 to 7,200/mm³ (may vary in infants and with race)

b. Interpretation:

  i. ANC less than 1,000. Moderate risk for infection

  ii. ANC less than 500. High risk for infection

10. *Absolute lymphocyte counts* were once thought to be comparable across ages. Although total lymphocyte count and subsets of lymphocytes are equivalent percentages of the WBC count in all ages, the young child's higher WBC count yields greater absolute numbers of lymphocytes and subsets of lymphocytes.

a. A lymphocyte count of less than 15% to 20% of the differential WBC count is considered abnormal.

b. Lymphocyte subset determinations are capable through monoclonal antibody technology. Quantifying lymphocyte subsets is useful in monitoring a patient's response to immunosuppressive therapy during the organ transplant process, an infectious process or an immune disorder, and the effect of medications on the patient's immune system.

  i. CD4 count (helper T lymphocyte). Cytomegalovirus (CMV) and Epstein–Barr virus (EBV) may result in a transient decrease in CD4 helper cells (Lexicomp, 2004).

  ii. CD8 count (suppressor or cytotoxic T lymphocyte). Viral illnesses may result in a marked increase in CD8 suppressor or cytotoxic cells (Lexicomp, 2004).

  iii. CD4:CD8 (helper-to-suppressor or cytotoxic) lymphocyte ratio. Normally there are more helper than suppressor or cytotoxic T lymphocytes. The normal ratio is greater than 1.0 (Lexicomp, 2004). Patients initially diagnosed with AIDS commonly demonstrate an elevation of CD8 suppressor or cytotoxic cells below 400 and a decrease of CD4 helper cells, resulting in a low CD4:CD8 ratio (Lexicomp, 2004).

B. Other Immune-Related Diagnostic Testing

1. *Erythrocyte sedimentation rate (ESR)* is a nonspecific indicator of acute inflammatory response. In many cases, the ESR is so nonspecific that it has little clinical utility as a single value, but following trends is helpful to assess the effectiveness of therapies. In the immunocompromised child, it may be one of the few objective measurements of response to therapy or relapse.

    a. ESR measures the amount of RBCs that settle in 1 hour. Normal values for the modified Westergren technique range from 4 to 20 mm/hr for a child, 0 to 15 mm/hr for adult males, and 1 to 20 mm/hr for adult females (Gilbert-Barness & Barness, 2010; Grossman, 2014b).

    b. Elevated rates occur in many conditions, including acute and chronic inflammatory conditions, including cytokine release syndrome, hypersensitivity conditions, vasculitis, and systemic lupus erythematosus (Grossman, 2014b).

    c. Decreased rates occur in sickle cell anemia, polycythemia, spherocytosis, and congestive heart failure (Gilbert-Barness & Barness, 2010).

2. *C-reactive protein (CRP)* is a nonspecific indicator of active inflammation.

    a. CRP, produced by the liver during periods of inflammation, enhances phagocytic activity of phagocytes, particularly of the neutrophil.

    b. CRP rises rapidly under an inflammatory stimulus, such as infection or injury. Levels are inappropriately low in systemic lupus erythematosus and scleroderma (Gilbert-Barness & Barness, 2010).

3. *Histocompatibility testing* identifies the HLA antigens, the child's genetic blueprint (Moriber, 2014).

    a. Histocompatibility testing is used for tissue typing for transplantation and forensics (Moriber, 2014).

    b. Two methods are used for histocompatibility testing: tissue typing and crossmatching.

        i. *Tissue typing* is the determination of an individual's HLA class I and II specificities. This is routinely performed for organ and tissue transplantation using complement-dependent cytotoxic assay.

        ii. *Crossmatching* is performed before solid organ transplantation to prevent (*or minimize*) risk of rejection after surgery.

        iii. Crossmatching detects the presence of antibodies in the recipient's serum that are directed against the HLA antigens of the potential donor. Various methods are used to complete HLA testing, with most patients awaiting transplantation undergoing initial crossmatching tests, including lymphocytes, T- or B-lymphocyte-enriched preparations, preformed antibodies, and auto-crossmatch.

    c. Molecular typing can be performed to define further DNA sequencing and assist in the selection of a more complete or precise match between the donor and recipient bone marrow cells.

4. *Complement assays* evaluate the primary complement components of the classic pathway and some of the components of the alternate pathway (Mudge-Grout, 1992). Total hemolytic complement 50 (C5H50) is used to test the integrity of the entire complement system because the entire cascade must be intact to reflect a normal level. The individual complement components (both from a total and functional perspective) also are measured (Gilbert-Barness & Barness, 2010).

5. *Total immunoglobulin level* and levels for the various classes and subclasses are measured. Normal immunoglobulin levels vary with age; therefore, it is imperative that age-adjusted values be used for all comparisons. Immunoglobulin levels can be diagnostic of congenital or primary immunodeficiencies (quantitative testing). If immunoglobulin levels are normal, in spite of suspected immunodeficiency, evaluation of the function and effectiveness of the immunoglobulin responding to an antigen may be indicated (qualitative testing).

6. *Coombs test, or direct antiglobulin test (DAT),* is used to diagnose autoimmune hemolytic anemia (AIHA) through detection of immunoglobulin or complement on the RBC surface (Chou & Schreiber, 2015). Agglutination or clumping occurs if the RBCs are coated with antibodies or complement. The greater the quantity of antibodies against the RBCs, the more clumping will occur. Any clumping is read as a positive result using a scale of 1 to 4+. Coombs test differentiates types of hemolytic anemia and detects immune antibodies (Gilbert-Barness & Barness, 2010).

    a. *Direct Coombs test* is an antiglobulin test that determines that serum antibodies (IgG) have attached to RBCs. It is used to detect newborn hemolytic disease, autoimmune processes in newborns and children, or hemolytic transfusion reactions. After transfusion, a positive result may indicate an antibody-mediated hemolytic reaction, but a negative result does not rule out such a condition because the transfused RBCs may have been completely destroyed in the recipient's bloodstream by the time the sample was drawn. A normal response is negative.

    b. *Indirect Coombs test* is a type of antibody screening that detects specific serum antibodies (IgG) to RBC antigens that are in the serum but not attached to the RBCs. It is used to detect IgG-positive antibodies in maternal blood and the newborn and is performed before RBC transfusions to detect any incompatibilities other than major ABO groups. A normal response is negative.

7. *Detection of antibody and antigens* is accomplished through a variety of in vitro techniques such as immunodiffusion, agglutination, enzyme-linked immunosorbent assay (ELISA), monoclonal antibodies, radioimmunoassay (RIA), and others.

  a. ELISA. See "AIDS" section.

  b. Monoclonal antibodies are laboratory-produced antibodies for a single "destiny" antigen that are used for prevention, diagnosis, and treatment of graft rejection and graft versus host disease (GVHD).

   i. Monoclonal antibodies can also be used to monitor subsets of T lymphocytes at the site of organ graft to assist in the diagnosis or monitoring of graft rejection.

   ii. Monoclonal antibodies are used on serum, urine, sputum, and stool samples (among others) to diagnose infections with microorganisms such as herpes simplex virus, streptococci, *Chlamydia*, and *Pneumocystis carinii*.

   iii. Monoclonal antibodies assist in the identification of cells and tissues (e.g., B- and T-lymphocyte differentiation, or HLA or blood typing) and are used in the diagnosis of various diseases (e.g., cancer, autoimmune disease).

   iv. Monoclonal antibodies to various tumor antigens or tumor products can be used in vitro to confirm the diagnosis of certain types of cancers. A radioactive tracer can be attached to monoclonal antibodies so that after the monoclonal antibodies are administered, a body scan may reveal where the cancer is located.

C. Coagulation

1. *Platelet Count*

  a. Normal. 150,000 to 400,000/mm³

  b. For hemostasis, 50,000/mm³ is usually adequate.

2. *Prothrombin Time (PT).* Assesses the extrinsic coagulation system by measuring factor VII and the common pathway or factors I (fibrinogen), II (prothrombin), V, and X.

  a. Normal. Control is usually 10 to 11 seconds (normal controls are established by the

individual laboratory; Branchford & Di Paola, 2015).

  b. Abnormal values are the result of factors less than 40% (Browarsky, 2010).

  c. PT is prolonged with oral anticoagulants, DIC, liver disease, long-term use of antibiotics, vitamin K deficiency, and phenytoin use.

  d. Prolonged PT in the absence of other abnormalities may indicate factor VII deficiency (Branchford & Di Paola, 2015).

3. *International Normalization Ratio (INR).* INR is the standardized method of expressing prolonged PT; this is helpful when monitoring Coumadin-type anticoagulants, as different thromboplastin preparations and different laboratories yielded diverse results (Branchford & Di Paola, 2015).

4. *Activated partial thromboplastin time (APTT)* assesses the factor I (fibrinogen), II (prothrombin), V, VIII, IX, X, XI, and XII. APTT measures the time needed for a fibrin clot to form. The blood specimen is first mixed with a phospholipid source and surface-activating agent. The specimen is incubated for approximately 2 to 5 minutes and then an activating agent (calcium chloride) is added (Branchford & Di Paola, 2015).

  a. Normal APTT is usually 26 to 35 seconds (normal controls are established by the individual laboratory) in children, and 30 to 54 seconds in term infants (Branchford & Di Paola, 2015).

  b. APTT is prolonged with heparin therapy, DIC, severe vitamin K deficiency, liver disease, hemophilia, and some von Willebrand disease.

  c. Any sample with heparin contamination falsely elevates the PTT, thrombin time (TT), and FSPs. Contamination of central venous catheters with heparin may be a common cause of prolonged PT in hospitalized infants and children (Branchford & Di Paola, 2015). Venipuncture is a more reliable method for obtaining accurate values, although ensuring adequate "waste" prior to obtaining the specimen may assist with this limitation.

5. *TT* reflects the time for thrombin to convert fibrinogen to fibrin.

  a. Normal. 10 to 15 seconds

  b. Results are normal in factor VIII deficiency.

  c. Results are prolonged when coagulation is inadequate due to decreased thrombin activity, DIC, antithrombin activity such as heparin therapy, insufficient or abnormal fibrinogen, or uremia.

6. *Fibrinogen*

   a.   Although normal values of fibrinogen range from 200 to 400 mg/dL, only 70 to 100 mg/dL is required for hemostasis to occur.

   b.   Decreased values reflect a risk of bleeding. Decreased values may be present in consumption disorders, such as DIC, and are also seen in hepatic dysfunction (Branchford & Di Paola, 2015).

   c.   Increased values may reflect a hypercoagulable state or inflammatory conditions secondary to activation of plasma enzyme cascades.

7. D-*dimer*. Measures the degradation of crosslinked fibrin; a specific test for DIC.

   a.   Normal. A D-dimer level of 0.5 µg/mL is normal; any positive test is considered significant (Gilbert-Barness & Barness, 2010)

   b.   Increased values are seen in DIC and inflammatory states.

8. *Specific factor assays* measure amounts of each of the various plasma proteins such as II, V, VII, VIII, IX, XI, and XII.

9. *Thromboelastography (TEG)* is a valuable study used to assess platelet function and the process of hemostasis, from clot formation to dissolution (Branchford & Di Paola, 2015).

10. *PFA-100* is a relatively new test, designed to simulate in vivo platelet adhesion and aggregation. This test may be useful in screening von Willebrand factor (vWF) levels, as it is inversely proportionate. Additional investigations are ongoing as PFA-100 accurately detects severe bleeding disorders that would likely have significant clinical symptoms adequate for diagnosis and is not currently sensitive or specific enough to screen for platelet disorders (Branchford & Di Paola, 2015).

11. *Platelet Function Tests*. The most common is platelet aggregometry, which may be influenced by medications and may require a "wash out" period of approximately 10 days to provide an accurate result (Branchford & Di Paola, 2015).

12. *Global clotting assays*, including TEG and thrombin generation assays (TGA) are gaining interest as a potential solution to the challenges of great phenotypic variability (Branchford & Di Paola, 2015).

   a.   TEG. Monitors the entire process of coagulation from clot formation to its dissolution, providing a continuous profile of overall rheology changes (Branchford & Di Paola, 2015).

   b.   TGA. Currently considered difficult to perform, although used extensively in research. Investigations of how to use TGA to monitor hemophilia treatment and anticoagulation therapy are underway (Branchford & Di Paola, 2015).

13. *Activated clotting time (ACT)* is a bedside assessment that measures the level of heparin anticoagulation for patients on an extracorporeal life support circuit. A common target that balances the risk of bleeding and risk of clotting is between 180 and 200 seconds (Maclaren, Conrad, & Dalton, 2016).

D. **Blood Typing**

1. *More than 300 different antigens* have been identified against human blood cells, each of which can cause antigen–antibody reactions.

2. *ABO* is one system for typing the antigens for individuals.

   a.   There are four blood groups (phenotypes). An individual inherits a specific type of blood; each type of blood has a specific antigen makeup with the antibodies described.

      i.   Group A. Natural anti-B antibodies are present in the plasma.

      ii.   Group B. Natural anti-A antibodies are present in the plasma.

      iii.   Group AB. No natural anti-A or anti-B antibodies are present in the plasma.

      iv.   Group O. Both natural anti-A and anti-B antibodies are present in the plasma.

   b.   ABO compatibility is essential for blood transfusion.

3. *Rh system* is a second important blood antigen grouping system involving several other antigens found on RBCs.

   a.   The most potent and easy to detect is the Rh D antigen. Absence of the D antigen is termed *Rh negative*. If the Rh D antigen is detected, the blood is termed *Rh positive*.

   b.   A person first must be exposed to Rh antigen before a significant reaction will occur. IgG antibodies can develop to the Rh antigens after sensitization by prior transfusion or pregnancy. A transfusion of Rh-positive blood to a sensitized Rh-negative person can provoke acute hemolysis.

   c.   Coombs test, or DAT, is used to determine the presence of IgG antibodies (Rh factor antibodies in an Rh-negative person).

4. *Cold-Reactive Autoantibodies.* IgM antibodies present in the plasma of some persons can cause RBCs to clump when (a) complement fixation occurs and (b) blood plasma temperature is below normal body temperature. Antibodies react to RBCs regardless of the blood type of donor blood and may lead to circulatory impairment and RBC hemolysis. Screening is done by indirect agglutination tests and actual measurement by the antiglobulin test. The reaction is often not significant clinically because optimal activation of these antibodies is at 4°C. Reduce potential for reactions by administering blood through a warming system.

5. *Warm-Reactive Autoantibodies.* IgG autoantibodies can cause a patient to react to his or her own RBCs as well as donor cells at 37°C. In cases of warm reactive AIHA, the DAT may reveal IgG plus complement, IgG only, or complement only. Although not fully understood, there seems to be an association between the IgG subtype (IgG_1, IgG_2, IgG_3, IgG_4) and the strength of the reaction and rate of RBC destruction (Chou & Schreiber, 2015).

E. Radiologic Examination

1. *Chest x-ray examination* is commonly valuable in detecting and tracking various inflammatory or malignant processes. However, just as other signs and symptoms of infection are masked during neutropenia, the chest x-ray examination may also be unreliable in revealing pneumonia in some immunocompromised children (Dinauer et al., 2015). Thoracic CT produces a much higher yield and is recommended in those neutropenic patients at risk for a complicated pulmonary infection. It has been observed in some neutropenic patients that once the neutrophil count begins to increase to a near-normal level, the chest x-ray results may worsen, revealing the existing pneumonia.

2. *Diagnostic imaging studies* of other areas of the body are indicated by the child's history and physical examination.

F. Biopsies

1. *Bone Marrow.* The bone marrow may be examined through a bone marrow aspirate (aspiration of fluid of the bone marrow) and biopsy (needle core biopsy) of the bone.

    a. *Purpose.* Biopsy provides a histologic and hematologic examination of cellular components of the blood.

    b. *Technique.* The patient is usually sedated, and the patient's respiratory status is closely monitored. The preferred site is the posterior, superior iliac crest. In the case of difficult procedures or if unable to place the patient in a prone position, it is possible to obtain aspiration and biopsy from the anterior iliac crest. If the patient is younger than 1 month of age, the preferred site is the tibia.

    c. A *contraindication* is respiratory compromise such that positioning the patient for the procedure would exacerbate the compromise.

    d. *Complications* include bleeding, pain, and infection at the site.

    e. *Transfusions* given just before a biopsy is done will not affect bone marrow results.

2. *Lymph Node Biopsy or Excision*

    a. *Purpose.* The purpose is to evaluate the architectural structure and histologic characteristics.

    b. *Techniques.* The patient is usually under general anesthesia. Areas other than the inguinal area are preferred for biopsy as they pose less risk for infection. Use the inguinal site only if other sites do not demonstrate enlargement.

    c. *Contraindication.* Bleeding and the inability to safely administer adequate analgesia are contraindications of biopsy.

    d. *Complications* include bleeding, pain, and infection at the site.

HEMATOLOGIC AND IMMUNOLOGIC PHARMACOLOGY

Numerous medications affect the hematologic and immunologic systems of the body. Mechanisms by which pharmacologic agents directly affect the hematologic and immunologic systems include those that increase production of cell lines (e.g., CSFs or growth factors) or that decrease production or increase destruction of cell lines or entire bone marrow production (e.g., chemotherapeutic agents). Side effects of pharmacologic agents on the hematologic and immunologic systems vary in intensity and range of cells affected (one cell line vs. the entire bone marrow function).

A. Therapeutic Modalities That Enhance the Functions of the Hematologic and Immunologic Systems

    1. *EPO*

        a. *Indications* include anemia of prematurity, chronic kidney disease, zidovudine-induced anemia, or anemia from bone marrow suppression following chemotherapy, medication administration, and bone marrow transplant (BMT). EPO is useful in other conditions for which transfusions are to be avoided, such as those not consenting to transfusions for religious reasons.

b. *Mechanisms of action.* EPO promotes RBC production by stimulating the division and differentiation of erythroid progenitor cells. EPO first releases reticulocytes into the bloodstream, which is followed by an increase in hemoglobin and hematocrit (Lexicomp, 2016).

c. *Side effects* are generally well tolerated.

   i. Irritation at the injection site may occur.

   ii. Self-limiting side effects include nausea, vomiting, and flu-like syndrome.

   iii. In adult patients who have had long-term hemodialysis therapy, hypertension, thrombosis, and seizures have been reported to be associated with EPO.

   iv. Black box warnings have been issued for erythropoiesis-stimulating agents related to increased risk of cardiovascular events, including myocardial infarction, stroke, venous thromboembolism, and mortality when the target hemoglobin levels exceed 11 g/dL. Increased risk for similar adverse cardiovascular events was reported in chronic kidney disease patients as well. In addition, breast, cervical, head and neck, lymphoid, and non–small-cell lung cancer patients were found to have shortened overall survival and/or increase tumor progression/recurrence risk when erythropoiesis-stimulating agents (ESAs) were administered to maintain hemoglobin >12 g/dL. A recommendation of using the lowest effective dose has been issued as a result of these warnings (Lexicomp, 2016).

2. *Myeloid Growth Factors.* Filgrastim (G-CSF), sargramostim (GM-CSF; see Table 8.4 and Figure 8.1)

   a. *Indications.* Myeloid growth factors are used to reduce the duration of neutropenia (and associated infection risk) associated with administration of chemotherapy, immunosuppressants, or bone marrow transplantation. These growth factors are also being used in patients with severe chronic neutropenia due to congenital neutropenia, cyclic neutropenia, or idiopathic neutropenia, in the treatment of neonatal neutropenia, and in AIDS patients receiving zidovudine (Lexicomp, 2016).

   b. *Mechanism of action.* Growth factors stimulate maturation of myeloid precursors.

      i. G-CSF effects are more selective than those of GM-CSF because G-CSF stimulates the production, maturation, and activation of neutrophils without affecting monocytes or eosinophils. G-CSF increases neutrophil migration and cytotoxicity (Lexicomp, 2016).

      ii. GM-CSF is multipotent or has the potential to stimulate the proliferation, differentiation, and functional activity of several cell lineages, including neutrophils, monocytes, eosinophils, and macrophages (Lexicomp, 2016).

   c. The most *common side effect is* a flu-like syndrome, including low-grade fever, bone pain, chills and rigor, myalgias, and headache. The severity of symptoms is variable and is influenced by the dose, route of administration, and schedule. Symptoms are reversible once the agent is discontinued, and recovery time is variable, ranging from days to several weeks. "First-dose effect" can occur with symptoms that include hypotension, tachycardia, flushing, and syncope. This is rare and limited to the first dose.

B. Therapeutic Modalities That Depress the Functions of the Hematologic and Immunologic Systems

1. *Marrow-suppressive agents* that are administered for another purpose but suppress RBC, WBC, and platelet production and activity.

   a. *Chemotherapeutic agents*

      i. Indications include cancer and immunologically mediated diseases such as rheumatoid arthritis or lupus nephritis.

      ii. Mechanisms of action. Chemotherapeutic agents interfere with the normal cycle of cell replication; they especially affect cells with short life spans or those in a constant state of reproduction such as blood cells, hair cells, and cells lining the GI tract.

      iii. Hematologic side effects involve failure of the bone marrow to develop the cell line. Such aplasia is dose dependent and usually reversible.

(Nurses administering chemotherapy and other biologic agents on a regular basis should receive training and maintain competency through the Association of Pediatric Hematology/Oncology Nurses [APHON] Chemotherapy and Biotherapy Provider Course.)

b. *Antibiotics, antivirals, and antiretrovirals*

i. Chloramphenicol (Chloromycetin). Classic example

1) *Indications* include infection by susceptible organisms, such as *Salmonella*, rickettsia, *H. influenzae*, or pathogens commonly found in patients with cystic fibrosis. Chloramphenicol crosses the blood–brain barrier and is particularly effective in central nervous system (CNS) infections caused by susceptible organisms. Newer cephalosporins, however, have largely replaced chloramphenicol for *H. influenzae* meningitis and its use is limited to situations where less toxic medications are either contraindicated or ineffective (Lexicomp, 2016).

2) Mechanism of action is through inhibition of bacterial protein synthesis. It is usually bacteriostatic but can be bacteriocidal against common meningeal pathogens *(H. influenzae, N. meningitidis, S. pneumoniae)*.

3) Hematologic side effects are both dose related and idiosyncratic (e.g., aplastic anemia). Reversible bone marrow suppression, which is primarily characterized by anemia (with or without thrombocytopenia and leukopenia), is believed to be *dose related*. It is more likely to occur in patients receiving large doses, prolonged therapy, or serum concentrations greater than or equal to 25 mcg/mL. It is more common than aplastic anemia and is reversible within 1 to 3 weeks after the drug is discontinued. Hemolysis has occurred in patients with glucose-6-phosphate dehydrogenase (G6PD) deficiency who receive chloramphenicol. *Bone marrow aplasia* is rare, *idiosyncratic*, and frequently fatal. It is not dose related and occurs weeks to months after the drug is discontinued. The mechanism of action is unknown.

ii. Trimethoprim–sulfamethoxazole (TMP–SMX, Bactrim)

1) Indications include pneumocystis pneumonia (PCP; caused by Pneumocystis jirovecii pneumonia [PJP]) prophylaxis and treatment.

2) Mechanisms of action. TMP–SMZ interrupts bacterial folic acid synthesis and growth as it inhibits dihydrofolic acid formation (Lexicomp, 2016). Most bacteria are more susceptible to the combination of agents than to either agent used alone. Individual agents at therapeutic levels are bacteriostatic, but the combination is usually bacteriocidal.

3) Side effects. Most common are rash (secondary to a hypersensitivity to the sulfonamide component), fever, nausea and vomiting, and neutropenia. Less common are thrombocytopenia, hepatitis, azotemia, bone marrow aplasia, and hemolytic anemia (secondary to hypersensitivity and G6PD deficiency). Discontinuation of medication is associated with complete resolution of neutropenia.

iii. Linezolid (Zyvox)

1) Indications include community- and hospital-acquired pneumonia, skin and soft-tissue infections, endocarditis, and infection by other drug-resistant organisms such as vancomycin-resistant *Enterococcus faecium* and methicillin-resistant *Staphylococcus aureus* (MRSA; Lexicomp, 2016).

2) Mechanisms of action. Bacterial protein synthesis is inhibited by preventing the formation of 70S initiation complex, which is necessary for bacterial translation. Linezolid is bacteriostatic against enterococci and staphylococci and bacteriocidal against most streptococci (Lexicomp, 2016).

3) Hematologic side effects include anemia, leukopenia, eosinophilia, neutropenia, and thrombocytopenia.

iv. Zidovudine (previously known as azidothymidine, AZT; see "AIDS" section) was the first licensed antiretroviral drug for HIV infection.

1) Mechanisms of action. Zidovudine, a thymidine analog, inhibits viral replication, interfering with viral RNA-dependent polymerase. Other dideoxynucleosides are commonly used in children (e.g., didanosine (or ddI), stavudine, lamivudine) and have less hematologic toxicity than zidovudine.

2) Hematologic side effects involve anemia, neutropenia, and thrombocytopenia.

v. Ganciclovir

1) Indications include prophylaxis and treatment of CMV in the immuno-compromised patient; ganciclovir also provides antiviral activity against herpes simplex virus 1 and 2 (Lexicomp, 2016).

2) Mechanisms of action. Ganciclovir is a derivative of acyclovir that belongs to a class of agents called *purine nucleosides*. This purine analog acts by incorporation into nucleic acids of DNA. This leads to abnormal transcription and translation and the loss of viral infectivity.

3) Hematologic side effects. May cause anemia, neutropenia (ANC <500/mm^3), and thrombocytopenia.

vi. Foscarnet (Foscavir)

1) An alternative to ganciclovir; indications include prophylaxis and treatment of CMV in the immunocom-promised patient. Foscarnet also provides antiviral activity against herpes simplex virus infections and acyclo-vir-resistant herpes zoster infections (Lexicomp, 2016).

2) Mechanisms of action. Foscarnet acts as a noncompetitive inhibitor of viral RNA and DNA polymerases. Foscarnet is a virostatic agent (Lexicomp, 2016).

3) Hematologic side effects. May cause abnormal WBC differential, abnormal platelet function, bone marrow sup-pression leading to anemia, granulocy-topenia, leukopenia, neutropenia, and thrombocytopenia (Lexicomp, 2016)

2. *Marrow-suppressive agents* given to suppress one or more type of WBCs (therapeutic immunosup-pression) that have dose-related effects leading to an increased risk of infection.

a. *Corticosteroids*

i. Indications include certain malignancies, treatment of acute or chronic GVHD, preven-tion and treatment of rejection of transplanted tissue, hypersensitivity reactions, and other inflammatory diseases. Corticosteroids do not reduce hemolysis in transfusion reactions, but they ameliorate drug-induced hemolysis. In ITP, corticosteroids are thought to act by inhibiting the phagocytosis of antibody-as-sociated coated platelets, thus increasing the platelet life span.

ii. Mechanisms of action. Corticosteroids alleviate temporary lymphocytopenia and reduce the migration of neutrophils and monocytes to sites of inflammation. Other actions include decreasing the number of cells available to participate in the inflamma-tory response; stabilizing the vascular beds by decreasing capillary permeability, thus inhibiting the movement of cells from the vascular space to the tissues; and reducing the functional capabilities of immunologi-cally active cells. Corticosteroids increase the neutrophil count secondary to mature neu-trophil release from the bone marrow and decrease movement of the neutrophils from the blood to the tissues.

iii. Side effects are significant, especially with long-term use, and include hypergly-cemia, hypertension, sodium and water retention, depression and sleep disturbances, increased risk of infection (especially viral and opportunistic infection), acne, delayed wound healing, and osteopenia.

b. *Cyclosporine A*

i. Indications include the prevention and treatment of GVHD; prevention of rejection of transplanted tissue, stem cells, or bone marrow; and treatment of other conditions such as severe aplastic anemia, nephrotic syndrome with focal glomerulosclerosis, and rheumatoid arthritis (Lexicomp, 2016).

ii. Mechanisms of action. Cyclosporine A (CSA) depresses the body's natural response to "nonself," antigenic tissue. CSA binds to cyclophilin intracellularly, forming an active, protein–drug complex. CSA inhibits the pro-duction and activation of the cytotoxic T lymphocytes secondary to calcineurin inhi-bition. Once T cells are activated, however, CSA cannot suppress T-cell proliferation. Thus, CSA works well at preventing but not treating rejection of transplanted tissues. CSA inhibits macrophage release but has little effect on function of B lymphocytes or T suppressor cells and antibody production.

iii. Administration. CSA is given intrave-nously or orally. Utilization of cyclosporine microemulsion (Neoral) has greatly reduced the absorptive variability previously asso-ciated with Sandimmune (Nevins, 2000). Continuous IV infusion is less toxic than bolus infusions and is often given in combi-nation with steroids.

iv. Side effects include nephrotoxicity, hypertension, hepatotoxicity, neurologic disturbances (seizures and posterior reversible leukoencephalopathy syndrome [PRES]), hyperglycemia, gynecomastia, hirsutism, and gingival hypertrophy.

c. *Tacrolimus*

i. Indications. Tacrolimus (Prograf) is a potent immunosuppressant used for the prevention and treatment of organ rejection in kidney, heart, and liver transplants. The frequency of use in the prevention and treatment of GVHD is increasing, although this remains an off-label indication (Lexicomp, 2016).

ii. Mechanism of action. Tacrolimus is a calcineurin inhibitor that suppresses the first phase of T-cell activation by blocking the production of calcineurin and IL-2 production.

iii. *Side effects* include nephrotoxicity, neurotoxicity (tremor, seizure, PRES), GI disturbances, hypertension, hyperglycemia, hypomagnesemia, nephrotoxicity, and infectious complications. Posttransplant lymphoproliferative disorder (PTLD) is the most severe complication associated with tacrolimus. It is believed that PTLD occurs as the result of active Epstein–Barr virus replication.

d. *Sirolimus (Rapamune)*

i. Indications. Used in combination with corticosteroids or a calcineurin inhibitor to prevent or treat transplanted organ rejection, to prevent acute GVHD in allogeneic stem cell transplantation, to treat refractory acute or chronic GVHD, and is therapeutic in vascular anomalies (Lexicomp, 2016).

ii. Mechanism of action. The mechanism of action for sirolimus differs from that of tacrolimus and cyclosporine. A mechanistic target or rapamycin (mTOR) inhibitor, sirolimus suppresses the second phase of T-cell activation.

iii. Side effects are often dose related, and include increased serum creatinine, hypertension, hypertriglyceridemia, increased lactate dehydrogenase (LDH), infection, and impaired wound healing (Lexicomp, 2016).

e. *Mycophenolate mofetil (MMF, Cellcept)*

i. Indications include prevention of rejection of transplanted tissues, treatment of chronic GVHD, uveitis, and refractory immune thrombocytopenia (Lexicomp, 2016). MMF is almost always used in conjunction

with other immunosuppressive therapies such as corticosteroids and calcineurin inhibitors.

ii. Mechanism of action. MMF is hydrolyzed to form mycophenolic acid (MPA). MPA causes a depletion of certain amino acids within the purine biosynthesis pathway, resulting in a cytostatic effect on T and B lymphocytes (Lexicomp, 2016).

iii. Side effects occur as the result of GI dysfunction (diarrhea, dyspepsia, anorexia, ulcers, pancreatitis), bone marrow suppression (leukopenia, neutropenia, anemia, thrombocytopenia), nephrotoxicity, and increased risk of infection.

f. *Azathioprine (Azasan, Imuran)*

i. Indications include prevention of kidney transplant rejection in adults and in the treatment of autoimmune diseases, including systemic lupus erythematosus, juvenile idiopathic arthritis, and inflammatory bowel disease (Lexicomp, 2016).

ii. Mechanisms of action. Azathioprine is a purine synthesis inhibitor. It blocks RNA and DNA synthesis, thus preventing cytotoxic T-cell proliferation and antibody production. It inhibits promyelocyte proliferation within the bone marrow.

iii. Side effects include bone marrow suppression, GI tract disturbances (nausea, vomiting, diarrhea), malaise, hepatotoxicity, increased risk of other cancers, and thrombocytopenia.

iv. Special considerations. Serious drug interactions can occur with allopurinol (Zyloprim), which inhibits the metabolism of azathioprine, causing increased serum levels of these active metabolites (mercaptopurinol), leading to increased toxicity. Therefore, a reduced dose of azathioprine is required if a patient is receiving both of these medications.

g. *Lymphocyte immune globulin preparations*

i. Production. Purified polyclonal immune globulins are derived from animal sources (commonly equine or rabbit), which are injected with human thymus or lymphoid cells. Antibodies are formed against these cells and accumulate in the animal's serum. The antibodies are extracted from the animal's serum, followed by purification to yield the immune globulin.

ii. Indications include prevention or treatment of acute rejection of transplanted tissue, prevention and treatment of GVHD following bone marrow transplantation, and aplastic anemia.

iii. Mechanisms of action. A purified, concentrated, and sterile gamma-globulin (IgG) reduces the number of circulating lymphocytes, making them susceptible to phagocytosis by macrophages.

iv. Preparations.

1) Antithymocyte globulin (ATGAM), also known as *lymphocyte immune globulin*, is produced from the serum of horses immunized with human thymus lymphocytes. It reduces the number of circulating, thymus-dependent lymphocytes.

2) Antithymocyte globulin (Thymoglobulin) is derived from the serum of rabbits.

v. Side effects of ATGAM and Thymoglobulin are similar and include fever, chills, anemia, thrombocytopenia, skin reactions (rash, pruritus, urticaria), and serum sickness-like symptoms (dyspnea; arthralgia; chest, back, and flank pain; diarrhea; nausea and vomiting).

vi. Infusions should be administered over a period of time determined to be safe by the pharmacy. If the patient experiences fever, chills, or other mild symptoms during the infusion, the rate may be slowed to improve tolerance (Lexicomp, 2016).

vii. Anaphylaxis is uncommon but may occur anytime during therapy. Observe the child continuously for possible allergic reactions throughout the infusion. Preinfusion treatment with an antipyretic, antihistamine, or steroid is highly recommended. Perform an intradermal skin test before administration to rule out serious allergic reactions before the administration of ATGAM. The patient may require ATGAM desensitization if the patient has positive results from a skin test. A test dose is not administered before the initiation of thymoglobulin; however, it is necessary to premedicate with an antipyretic, antihistamine, and steroid. Given the risk for serious reaction, immediate access to epinephrine and other emergency equipment is recommended (Lexicomp, 2016).

viii. Other effects may include reactivation of CMV, herpes simplex virus, or EBV or antigen- or antibody-induced glomerulonephritis.

3. *Monoclonal Antibodies.* Several types of monoclonal antibody are available for the treatment of hematologic, oncologic, and immunologic disorders. These include rituximab, infliximab, alemtuzumab, and eculizumab (Solaris, complement inhibitor).

a. *Rituximab* (Rituxan, anti-CD20)

i. Indications. Used to treat CD20-positive diseases, such as non-Hodgkin's lymphoma (NHL), chronic lymphocytic leukemia, and systemic autoimmune diseases such as AIHA. In addition, Rituxan has been used in chronic GVHD, PTLD, and chronic ITP (Garzon & Mitchell, 2015; Lexicomp, 2016).

ii. Mechanism of action. CD20 regulates cell cycle initiation; rituximab binds to the antigen on the surface of CD20 cells and activates complement-dependent B-cell cytotoxicity (Lexicomp, 2016).

iii. Side effects. Fever, fatigue, chills, gastric disturbances, anemia, lymphopenia, leukopenia, neutropenia, thrombocytopenia, increased risk of infection, and infusion-related reactions such as angioedema, bronchospasm, fever, headache, changes in blood pressure, pruritus, rash, and urticaria (Lexicomp, 2016).

b. *Infliximab* (Remicade, tumor necrosis factor blocking agent)

i. Indications. Used to treat Crohn's disease, ulcerative colitis, and severe rheumatoid arthritis (Food and Drug Administration [FDA] approved for adults at this time); Lexicomp, 2016).

ii. Mechanism of action. Binds to tumor necrosis factor alpha and interferes with its activity, including induction of proinflammatory cytokines, enhancement of leukocyte migration, activation of neutrophils and eosinophils, and induction of acute-phase reactants (Lexicomp, 2016).

iii. Side effects. May cause fatigue, chills, gastric disturbances, anemia, leukopenia, thrombocytopenia, increased risk of infection, and infusion-related reactions. Premedication for infusion-related reactions with acetaminophen and diphenhydramine may be considered. Patients with a history of severe reaction may also require corticosteroid premedication (Lexicomp, 2016).

c. *Alemtuzumab* (Campath, anti-CD52)

    i. Indications. Current labeled indications include treatment of B-cell chronic lymphocytic leukemia and relapsing multiple sclerosis; however, off-label uses include administration as part of a stem cell transplant conditioning regimen, induction therapy for renal transplant, and treatment of steroid refractory acute GVHD.

    ii. Mechanism of action. CD52 is a nonmodulating antigen on the surface of B and T lymphocytes, that also affects monocytes, macrophages, NK cells, and certain granulocytes. Antigen-dependent lysis of malignant cells occurs after binding with CD52 (Lexicomp, 2016).

    iii. Side effects. May cause headache, fatigue, insomnia, skin rash, urticaria, gastric disturbances, anemia, lymphocytopenia, and increased risk of infection. Due to the increased risk of infection, prophylactic antimicrobials should be administered. In addition, antiemetics may prevent or reduce symptoms such as nausea and vomiting (Lexicomp, 2016).

d. *Eculizumab* (Solaris, complement inhibitor)

    i. Indications. Current labeled indications include treatment of atypical hemolytic–uremic syndrome (a.0) and paroxysmal nocturnal hemoglobinuria (PNH; Lexicomp, 2016).

    ii. Mechanism of action. The MAC is blocked, which results in stabilization of hemoglobin and reduced need for transfusions of packed red blood cells (PRBCs). Eculizumab binds to complement protein C5, preventing cleavage to C5a and C5b fragments, thus inhibiting formation of terminal complexes (Lexicomp, 2016).

    iii. Side effects. May cause hypertension, peripheral edema, headache, skin rash, pruritus, gastric disturbances, renal insufficiency, fever, increased risk for infection, and infusion-related reactions. Due to the increased risk of infection, patients must receive the meningococcal vaccine at least 2 weeks prior to the initiation of treatment and education about serious signs/symptoms of infection should be provided. In addition, due to the risk of infusion-related reactions, patients should be monitored for 1 hour after completion of the infusion (Lexicomp, 2016).

4. *Platelet-Suppressive Agents.* Given for another purpose that results in the suppression of platelet activity.

    a. *Aspirin* (ASA)

        i. Indications include the need for antipyretic, anti-inflammatory, analgesic, or antiplatelet effects.

        ii. Mechanisms of action. ASA inhibits platelet aggregation by inhibiting thromboxane A_2 for the life of an exposed platelet (7–10 days). Effects do not disappear with drug clearance. ASA also inhibits prostacyclin.

        iii. Hematologic side effects include the prolongation of bleeding time to one to three times normal. If aspirin is given to those with liver disease or to those receiving anticoagulant therapy, the effects are amplified.

    b. *NSAIDs* (e.g., Ibuprofen, Naproxen)

        i. Indications include the need for anti-inflammatory, analgesic, and antipyretic actions.

        ii. Mechanism of action involves a decrease in function of platelets, which is reversible on the affected platelet when the NSAID is eliminated from the blood.

        iii. Hematologic side effects include prolonged bleeding time.

5. *Agents Affecting Plasma Clotting Factors*

    a. *Heparin* is an anticoagulant made from porcine intestinal mucosa or bovine lung.

        i. Indications include prophylaxis and treatment of deep-vein thrombosis, pulmonary embolism, and other thromboembolic disorders. Also, heparin is used as an anticoagulant during extracorporeal procedures, hemodialysis or hemofiltration, cardiac catheterization, or for hemodynamic monitoring. Heparin may also be used for selected causes of DIC, such as acute promyelocytic leukemia (APL), and to maintain patency of vascular access devices.

        ii. Mechanisms of action. Heparin inhibits clot formation but has no effect on formed clots. It dramatically accelerates the body's own anticoagulant mechanism, particularly that provided by antithrombin III (enhances the inactivation of thrombin II, inhibits X). Heparin promotes the destruction of factor X and has a direct inhibitory effect on factors IX, X, and thrombin. It also prevents conversion of fibrinogen to fibrin (Lexicomp, 2016).

iii.   Administration. For acute thrombosis, continuous IV infusion is preferred. Titrate to maintain the PTT or APTT one and a half to two times normal (Lexicomp, 2016). After acute anticoagulation is achieved, initiate concomitant oral therapy with warfarin (Coumadin) or an alternative oral anticoagulant.

iv.   Side effects are reversed with protamine sulfate, which binds heparin to a complex that lacks anticoagulant activity. Bleeding occurs, especially with children who have deficiencies of coagulation factors, such as hemophilia, or those with liver disease, platelet dysfunction syndromes (such as with aspirin therapy), peptic ulcer disease, and severe hypertension. HIT is a potential side effect. See "Heparin-Induced Thrombocytopenia" section for more information.

b.   *Warfarin* (Coumadin) is an anticoagulant.

i.   Indications include prophylaxis thromboembolic disorders, chronic anticoagulant therapy, such as long-term oral treatment of deep venous thrombosis and prevention of intracardiac clot formations associated with decreased wall motion, such as chronic atrial fibrillation.

ii.   Mechanisms of action. Warfarin inhibits the liver's activation of factor VII, followed by depression of factors II, IX, and X. It also increases plasma antithrombin III levels. Effectiveness is dependent on absorption from the GI tract, vitamin K status of the patient, and rate of hepatic metabolism of warfarin.

iii.   Administration. The oral route is used and dose is titrated to achieve an INR that is increased two to 3.5 times. Frequent, routine monitoring is required.

iv.   Side effects. Minor to life-threatening GI tract bleeding may occur. Side effects are reversed with vitamin K. Many drug interactions are possible, resulting in excessive anticoagulation; therefore, the nurse should consult with the pharmacist about any possible drug interactions before administration of warfarin.

c.   *Apixaban (Eliquis)* is an anticoagulant. At this time, safety and efficacy have not been established in patients younger than 18 years of age.

i.   Indications include reduction in risk of stroke and embolism in atrial fibrillation, thromboprophylaxis in acute medical illness, and treatment or secondary prevention of deep venous thrombosis and/or pulmonary embolism (Lexicomp, 2016).

ii.   Mechanisms of action. Apixaban is a direct activated factor Xa inhibitor.

iii.   Administration. The oral route is administered twice daily without regard to food. Apixaban may be preferable in some cases, as routine monitoring is not required while on this medication (Lexicomp, 2016).

iv.   Side effects. Sensitivity reactions, bleeding, risk of thrombosis if discontinued prematurely (Lexicomp, 2016).

d.   *Fibrinolytic agents* are drugs that dissolve clots (thrombus).

i.   Indications include great vein, atrial, arterial, and renal vein thromboses; occlusion of grafts; superior vena cava syndrome; and obstruction of vascular access devices such as central lines.

ii.   Mechanisms of action. Fibrinolytic agents promote conversion of plasminogen into plasmin and induce systemic fibrinolysis. Plasmin is a proteolytic enzyme that degrades proteins.

iii.   Specific agents

1) Streptokinase, a biologic product of certain strains of streptococci, is antigenic in nature. Repeat exposures to this drug increase the risk of anaphylaxis and are not recommended.

2) Urokinase, initially isolated from urine and fetal kidney cells, is produced using recombinant DNA technology and is not antigenic. This enzyme directly activates plasminogen. It has a lower incidence of allergic reactions than streptokinase, but availability varies.

3) Alteplase (tPA) activates plasminogen in the presence of fibrin. It binds to fibrin in the clot and converts entrapped plasminogen to plasmin. Concurrent heparin or antiplatelet therapy is sometimes given. It has the advantage of relatively selectively activating only the plasminogen bound to fibrin.

iv.   Monitor fibrinogen levels, fibrinogen degradation products, PT, PTT, CBC; look for evidence of bleeding such as hematuria and gingival bleeding.

v. Side effects. There is an increased risk of bleeding in children who have had major surgery within the preceding 10 days, a biopsy, or a history of active bleeding, especially from the GI tract. As with heparin, risks of bleeding must be weighed against the risks of the thrombosis. Effects can be reversed with the administration of fresh frozen plasma (FFP).

BLOOD COMPONENT THERAPY

A. Blood Products

Blood products commonly used for critically ill pediatric patients, indications, dosages, and nursing implications are outlined in Table 8.8.

B. Special Donor Designation and Crossmatching Issues

1. Knowledge regarding special donor requirements of individual patients is vital. Document the number of products available for immediate transfusion and when to send blood for type and cross.

2. Donor-directed (designated) blood is the donation of blood by family or friends for a specific patient.

   a. This is not possible for emergent needs.

   b. This has not offered a safety advantage over volunteer donors. There is a potential for clerical errors resulting from the additional steps in the donation process as well as from inaccurate history disclosure.

   c. Directed donation from parents to neonates is not recommended due to maternal alloantibodies and maternal antibodies in the infant's circulation.

   d. Directed donation from family members is not recommended for any patient who is a candidate for bone marrow transplantation.

3. HLA-matched platelets are needed when a patient has developed antibodies to antigens on platelets (e.g., multiple transfusions). This minimizes the chance of reaction to donor platelets so that the patient achieves an adequate rise in platelet count.

4. Patients who require lifelong transfusions (e.g., sickle cell disease patients) may develop multiple alloantibodies to donor blood antigens, which make crossmatching difficult.

5. O-negative unmatched blood may be given to patients with an urgent, life-threatening need for RBCs.

C. Modification of Blood Products

The goal of modification before transfusion is to minimize the risks of transfusions for patients with special needs.

1. *Leukodepletion* is used for patients who have experienced febrile transfusion reactions to decrease frequency of recurrent febrile nonhemolytic transfusion reactions, reduce incidence of HLA alloimmunication, and reduce risk of transfusion-transmitted CMV (American Association of Blood Banks [AABB], 2017).

   a. Leukodepletion does not prevent transfusion-associated graft versus host disease (TA-GVHD; AABB, 2013).

   b. Apheresis granulocytes should not be administered through a leukocyte reduction filter (AABB, 2017).

2. *Irradiation*

   a. This process destroys the leukocytes' ability to engraft in the immunosuppressed patient at risk for TA-GVHD (AABB, 2013).

   b. Irradiation is indicated for patients who are susceptible to TA-GVHD, including recipients of products from a blood relative, patients who are receiving hematopoietic stem cell transplantation, select immunocompromised patients, and transplant candidates whose donor has been selected for HLA compatibility (AABB, 2013).

   c. Irradiated blood products pose no danger to healthcare personnel (AABB, 2013).

3. *Filtration at the Bedside*

   a. To remove clots and aggregates, 150 to 260 micron filters are used.

   b. Each filtered set can be used for up to 4 units and should hang no longer than 4 hours.

   c. WBC filters may be used if indicated and if leukofiltration is not accomplished before storage at the blood bank.

D. Administration of Blood Products

Recent literature has suggested a general hemoglobin threshold of 7 g/dL for PRBC transfusion in acute a critically ill children, with some exceptions based on cardiac pathophysiology and other specific conditions (Chegondi, Sasaki, Raszynski, & Totapally, 2016; Lacroix, Tucci, & Du Pont-Thibodeau, 2015).

1. A *blood warmer* is indicated for transfusions of more than 1 unit of blood every 10 minutes, exchange transfusions in neonates, hypothermic

TABLE 8.8 Blood Products Commonly Used in the PICU

Blood Product	Indication	Dosage	1) Must be ABO Compatible 2) Compatibility Tested	Expected Response/ Estimated Change	Rate of Administration	Available Modifications	Special Considerations
Whole blood 500 mL/U	Symptomatic deficit of oxygen-carrying capacity plus hypovolemic shock Massive blood loss Exchange transfusions	20 mL/kg initially, followed by volume necessary to stabilize child's condition	1) Yes (must be ABO identical; Rh positive may receive Rh negative) 2) Yes	6 mL/kg increases Hgb by 1 g/dL	As fast as tolerated	Warmed Irradiated Leukocyte-depleted CMV negative, frozen, deglycerolyzed	Rarely used, usually for massive acute blood loss Platelets, WBCs, and clotting factors within stored whole blood are not functional
PRBCs 200–350 mL/U	Anemia/ symptomatic deficit of oxygen-carrying capacity ± hypovolemia	10–20 mL/kg	1) Yes 2) Yes	3 mL/kg increases Hgb by 1 g/dL 10 mL/kg increases Hct by 10%	2–4 hr	Washed Warmed Irradiated Leukocyte-depleted CMV negative, frozen, deglycerolyzed	Multiple transfusions may result in dilution of coagulation factors Wait 4–6 hours after transfusion to check hematocrit
Platelets 50–75 mL/U (random donor); 200–300 mL for pheresed units*	Thrombocytopenia (usually platelet count <10,000–20,000 or <50,000 with active bleeding) Abnormal platelet function	1–2 units/10 kg	1) Yes (preferred) 2) No	1 U/10 kg increases platelet count by approximately 50,000 mm³	As fast as tolerated, but usually not faster than 1 mL/kg/min	Irradiated Leukocyte-depleted CMV negative Volume-reduced Single donor HLA matched	Premedicate with acetaminophen or diphenhydramine for prevention of reaction Do not use microaggregate filters High risk of alloimmunizations with repeated transfusion Transfusion not indicated in platelet-destruction conditions, except in emergency

(continued)

TABLE 8.8 Blood Products Commonly Used in the PICU (*continued*)

Blood Product	Indication	Dosage	1) Must be ABO Compatible 2) Compatibility Tested	Expected Response/ Estimated Change	Rate of Administration	Available Modifications	Special Considerations
Fresh frozen plasma 200–250 mL/U	Deficit of plasma coagulation factors (prolonged PT, PTT) Provides plasma for volume expansion plus all coagulation factors Provides low levels of factor V and VIII	Clotting deficiency: 10–15 mL/kg Acute hemorrhage: 15–30 mL/kg	1) Yes 2) No		Depends on patient tolerance; not faster than 1 mL/kg/min, not slower than 4 hours	Irradiated	Should not be used for hypovolemia/ hypoproteinemia unless coagulation values are prolonged Must be used within 6 hours of thawing
Cryoprecipitate 10–40 mL/bag	Hemophilia A, only in special situations with directed donors Hypofibrinogenemia Factor XIII deficiency von Willebrand disease	1 unit per 5 kg DIC 1–2 bags/10 kg Additional doses at 8- to 12-hour intervals based on factor VIII levels and clinical status of patient	1) No 2) No		As fast as tolerated; usually not faster than 1 mL/kg/min	Irradiated	Must be used within 4 hours of thawing for pooled units; 6 hours for single unit Transmission of infections such as HIV and hepatitis B and C can occur Large doses in patient with normal fibrinogen may lead to hyperfibrinogenemia leading to acute thrombosis and DIC
Factor VIII Concentrate[†]	Hemophilia A	As described in "Hemophilia" section, based on goal factor recovery	1) No 2) No		Rate of administration per manufacturer	Stable with refrigeration weeks to months Most patients receive recombinant factor to decrease risk of virus transmission	Patient may develop antibodies to factor VIII resulting in less effectiveness of product

				1 U/kg factor will increase level about 1%–2%	Rate of administration per manufacturer	Most patients receive recombinant factor to decrease risk of virus transmission	Patient may develop antibodies to factor IX resulting in decreased effectiveness of product
Factor IX Concentrate†	Hemophilia B	As described in hemophilia section, based on goal factor recovery	1) No 2) No	1 U/kg factor will increase level about 1%–2%	Rate of administration per manufacturer	Most patients receive recombinant factor to decrease risk of virus transmission	Patient may develop antibodies to factor IX resulting in decreased effectiveness of product
Albumin 5% and 25%	Hypovolemia Hypoproteinemia 25% severe burns	5%: 10–20 mL/kg 25%: 0.5–1 g/kg depending on indication	1) No 2) No		5%: as fast as tolerated 25%: slower than 5%, as tolerated	NA	No infectious risk Risk of circulatory overload secondary to increased osmotic pressure, especially with 25% albumin Use within 6 hr of entering container
IVIG pools of plasma (>1,000) donors 90%–95% is IgG	Antibody deficiency disorders: congenital and acquired, including high-risk, LBW infants; patients posttransplant	(Dose varies per manufacturer)	1) No 2) No		Per individual manufacturing preparation; infuse slowly over 15–30 minutes and then gradually increase to max rate as tolerated		Reactions occur in 10%–15% of IVIG infusions, usually mild, not anaphylactic

CMV, cytomegalovirus; DIC, disseminated intravascular coagulation; HLA, human leukocyte antigen; IVIG, Intravenous immune serum globulin; LBW, low birth weight; PICU, pediatric intensive care unit; PRBCs, packed red blood cells; PT, prothrombin time; PTT, partial thromboplastin time.

*May give low volume; †Dose is dependent on manufacturer and patient weight.

patients, and those who have cold agglutinin disease.

    a. Warming prevents severe hypothermia, dysrhythmias, and cardiac arrest.

    b. Devices should be temperature controlled and heated through an inline system only.

    c. RBCs heated above 37°C may hemolyze.

2. *Mechanical pumps* (e.g., volumetric or syringe pumps) may be used to administer RBCs at a specific rate with minimal hemolysis. Pumps should be tested and validated for use with blood components (AABB, 2013).

3. *Reduced-volume blood products* (i.e., platelets) may be available from the blood bank and used for infants and children who need small-volume infusions or those who require a longer duration of infusion (AABB, 2013).

    a. RBC volumes may be ordered in small aliquots. Several aliquots may be prepared from a single donor unit, thus limiting donor exposure and risks.

    b. Small aliquots in specific amounts may be provided by the blood bank, occasionally in a syringe.

E. Complications

Primary prevention includes meticulous verification of the patient's identification and specific unit crossmatching. Table 8.9 summarizes reactions, signs and symptoms, and treatments for transfusion reactions. Early detection of reactions includes staying with the patient and administering the initial part of the transfusion slowly prior to increasing it to a more rapid rate (AABB, 2013).

    1. *Hemolytic Reaction*

    a. Most serious reaction occurs when the patient has antibodies to an antigen on the transfused RBCs (e.g., ABO incompatibility from mismatched blood).

    b. Reactions may be immediate (fever, hematuria, chills, dyspnea, chest/back pain), or delayed (2–14 days) after transfusion with anemia, unexplained fever, and decreased hemoglobin/hematocrit.

    c. Hemolytic reactions often result in a positive DAT (AABB, 2013).

    d. Acute reactions require supportive care, including correction of coagulopathy when present, maintenance of blood pressure, and careful attention to ensure adequate urine

TABLE 8.9 Transfusion Reactions to Blood or Blood Products

Reaction	Cause	Signs and Symptoms	Treatment
Anaphylaxis (occurs with infusion of only a few milliliters of product)	• Most often caused by antigen–antibody complexes involving antibodies to IgA • IgA deficiency	• Bronchospasm • Cough • Respiratory distress • Hypotension* • Urticaria • Vomiting	• Discontinue transfusion • Keep vein open with 0.9% sodium chloride, or NS (use completely new tubing set) • Notify physician • Administer epinephrine, steroids • Respiratory support • Deglycerolized (washed) red cells in future transfusions
Acute hemolytic transfusion reaction	• Transfusion of ABO-incompatible blood resulting in hemolysis of red cells	• Fever, chills* • Hypotension* • Hemoglobinemia • Hemoglobinuria • Lumbar pain (classic sign) • Shock • Dyspnea • Diaphoresis • Anxiety (impending sense of doom) • Chest pain • Restlessness • DIC	• Stop transfusion • Keep vein open with NS (completely new tubing set) • Notify physician • Treat shock and/or respiratory distress • Osmotic diuresis to prevent acute tubular necrosis • Treat DIC

(continued)

TABLE 8.9 Transfusion Reactions to Blood or Blood Products *(continued)*

Reaction	Cause	Signs and Symptoms	Treatment
Nonhemolytic	• Recipients reacting to poorly defined transfused antigens or recipient's antibodies reacting to transfused leukocytes and/or plasma proteins	• Fever (mild to severe)* • Chills • Headaches • Palpitations • Hives • Local erythema • Itching	• Stop transfusion • Keep vein open with NS (completely new tubing set) • Notify physician • Relieve symptoms (antipyretics, antihistamines) • If reaction mild, such as urticaria and/or slight fever and chills, may consider continuing transfusion after antihistamine; may also consider premedication and/or leukocyte-depleted products for future transfusions
TACO	• Transfused volume exceeds capacity of circulatory system, resulting in circulatory overload and pulmonary edema	• Respiratory distress • Hypoxia • Rales on auscultation • Hypertension	• Close monitoring of fluid status is warranted • Small volume transfusions may be indicated to reduce the risk of TACO secondary to large volume transfusions • Immediate interventions for pulmonary edema may include diuretics and colloid infusions
TRALI	• Immune response associated with granulocyte activation/degranulation and alveolar capillary membrane injury in response to a variety of factors, including WBC antibodies and accumulation of proinflammatory molecules in stored blood products	• Onset within 6 hours of transfusion • Acute onset of hypoxemia • Noncardiogenic pulmonary edema	• Aggressive respiratory support (often including mechanical ventilation) • Immediate notification of blood bank

DIC, disseminated intravascular coagulation; IgA, immunoglobulin A; NS, normal saline; TACO, transfusion-associated circulatory overload; TRALI, transfusion-related acute lung injury; WBC, white blood cell.

*Consider bacterial contamination of product.

output. Delayed reactions usually require no treatment (AABB, 2013).

2. *Febrile Nonhemolytic Reaction*

a. In a febrile nonhemolytic reaction, the temperature increases by greater than or equal to 1°C as a result of an immune response to infused WBCs or the action of cytokines.

b. Discontinue transfusion if patient's temperature rises 1°C or more above baseline.

c. The incidence of febrile nonhemolytic reactions decreases with the use of leukocyte-reduced blood products (AABB, 2013).

d. Antipyretics may be administered for symptom relief (AABB, 2013).

3. *Allergic Reaction*

a. If the reaction is mild (local erythema, pruritis), transfusion is temporarily stopped, antihistamine is given, and infusion may be restarted if symptoms are resolving. Patient is pretreated with antihistamine before subsequent transfusions.

b. Anaphylactic reactions with more severe symptoms of bronchospasm and hypotension are rare. Reaction typically occurs after a few milliliters of blood product is transfused, often in patients who are IgA or haptoglobin deficient. Interventions include discontinuing the product as well as administering epinephrine, fluids, and corticosteroids (AABB, 2013).

c. Washed cellular products may be helpful in preventing or reducing the severity of such reactions (AABB, 2013).

4. *Alloimmunization*

a. Risk is related to the immunizing substances that exist in blood components, forming antibodies against antigens on the surface of donor cells. Primary immunization presents days to weeks after the immunization takes place and is often without symptoms. However, these antibodies will destroy future transfused cells that possess targeted antigens upon their subsequent transfusion.

b. Alloimmunized patients who receive platelet transfusions receive no therapeutic effect. Single-donor or HLA-matched platelets may offset this problem.

c. Patients who are alloimmunized against red cell antigens may hemolyze donor cells.

d. Leukocyte-depleted blood components reduce risk of alloimmunization.

5. *Transfusion-associated circulatory overload (TACO)* occurs when transfusion volume exceeds circulatory system capacity.

a. Blood bank can divide red cells (aliquots) and provide "volume-reduced" platelets for volume-sensitive patients.

b. Volumes and rates of transfusion should be based on patient's size, fluid status, and clinical state.

c. Treatment of pulmonary edema should be treated immediately, often with diuretics and supportive care, and administration of colloid products should be reduced (AABB, 2013).

6. *Transfusion-related acute lung injury (TRALI)* is a serious immunologic complication posttransfusion, characterized by acute onset of hypoxemia and non-cardiogenic pulmonary edema without other identifiable causes (AABB, 2013).

a. Onset is within 6 hours of a blood component transfusion, and recognition of symptoms and potential correlation to a previous transfusion should prompt immediate notification of blood-bank services to complete necessary evaluations (AABB, 2013).

b. The cause may be WBC antibodies from sensitized donors, prior transfusion or transplantation, or stores of proinflammatory molecules in the blood product (AABB, 2013).

c. Treatment includes aggressive interventions to support the respiratory system, often including mechanical ventilation.

d. One of the leading causes of transfusion-related mortality (El Kenz & Van der Linden, 2014)

7. *Citrate Toxicity*

a. CPDA (citrate–phosphate–dextrose–adenine) is still used in some blood centers to preserve blood. Citrate anticoagulant causes depression of ionized calcium (AABB, 2013).

b. Patients who receive very rapid transfusions or multiple transfusions over a short period and patients with existing hepatic or renal dysfunction and those with circulatory collapse preventing adequate hepatic blood flow are at risk (AABB, 2013).

c. Complications of citrate toxicity include the metabolic derangement of hypocalcemia (ionized). Ventricular arrhythmias may occur if large volumes of citrated blood products are delivered rapidly through a central venous catheter (AABB, 2013).

d. Monitoring should include ionized calcium and electrocardiograms, as serum calcium is not necessarily reflective of ionized versus complexed hypocalcemia (AABB, 2013).

8. *Transmission of infectious diseases* is greatest with paid donors, multiple transfusions, and pooled plasma fractions. Mandatory screening of donor blood for hepatitis (B and C), HIV, human T-cell lymphotrophic virus (anti-HTLV-I/II), West Nile Virus, and CMV before it is transfused decreases the risk.

9. *Bacterial transmission* remains a risk of blood component transfusions. It is more likely for products that require thawing in a water bath or those stored at room temperature, such as platelets.

a. Contamination is confirmed by prompt Gram staining of the residual blood in the blood bag. Also, culturing the blood bag and filter may provide further evidence of the specific organism.

b. Clinical symptoms are noted in Table 8.9. Management includes immediate discontinuation of the transfusion, obtaining blood cultures, and initiation of broad-spectrum antibiotics plus supportive treatment.

c. Bacterial sepsis may result from infected blood products, and will often present as high fever, chills, hypotension, and hemodynamic instability during or shortly after a blood product transfusion. Such reactions may require vasopressors and other interventions to maintain vital organ function in the pediatric intensive care unit (PICU; AABB, 2013).

10. *Coagulopathy* can occur during massive transfusion (replacement of more than one blood volume).

a. The patient's body cannot replace more than a small fraction of coagulation factors and platelets, and stored blood has lost activity for platelet and coagulation factors.

b. It is recommended that for every 3 units of RBCs administered, the child also receives 1 unit of FFP and 1 unit of platelets. Coagulation studies may be done to determine specific component requirements.

11. *TA-GVHD* occurs when T lymphocytes present in donated blood react against recipient's tissues. It occurs most often in severely immunocompromised patients or after bone marrow transplantation. TA-GVHD has also been reported in patients who were being treated with purine analogues such as fludarabine. Although leukocyte reduction is not adequate in the removal of T lymphocytes, this can be prevented by irradiation of donor blood (AABB, 2013).

12. *Metabolic complications* are associated with massive transfusion or when a patient has severe liver or kidney disease. Hypothermia and hypocalcemia can occur and are addressed in Chapter 5. An additional metabolic abnormality may be hyper- or hypokalemia.

13. *Iron overload* occurs with chronic infusions over an extended period (years) in patients with severe chronic anemia (e.g., sickle cell anemia). It is due to the quantity of iron administered by transfusion being greater than that which is excreted. Overload results in deposits of iron in the cells of the myocardial, endocrine, and liver cells, leading to organ damage. It is managed by giving an iron-chelating agent or phlebotomy.

SYSTEM DYSFUNCTIONS

Anemia

A. Definition and Etiology

Anemia is defined as a reduction in red cell mass or blood hemoglobin concentration or a combination of the two.

B. Pathophysiology

Pediatric anemia most frequently occurs as the result of a decrease in RBC production, an increase in RBC destruction, a combination of the two, or blood loss. Decreased production may be due to ineffective erythropoiesis or absolute failure of erythropoiesis. Aplastic anemia is associated with pancytopenia (decreased RBCs, platelets, and WBCs) and hypocellular bone marrow without dysplasia or fibrosis (Hartung, Olson, & Bessler, 2013).

C. Clinical Presentation

The most significant problems seen in PICU patients with anemia include decreased oxygen carrying capacity, altered tissue perfusion, and altered fluid volume. Nursing assessment and management are targeted at these three key problems.

1. *History.* Signs and symptoms of anemia vary with the rapidity of its onset and with the underlying cause. If anemia develops rapidly, signs and symptoms may be more pronounced. If anemia develops more slowly, compensatory mechanisms such as expanding plasma volume decrease the cardiovascular symptoms. The patient may have only slight dyspnea on exertion despite significant anemia. Young children will self-regulate dyspnea by decreasing their activity level. Patients may report a history of fatigue, cold intolerance, dizziness, dyspnea, and decreased physical activity tolerance (Brugnara et al., 2015).

2. *Physical Examination*

a. Clinical signs and symptoms include tachycardia, tachypnea, diminished level of consciousness, lightheadedness, postural hypotension, and pallor of skin and mucous membranes.

b. Jaundiced skin and icteric sclera may be indicative of a hemolytic process.

3. *Diagnostic Tests*

    a. Laboratory data. Hemoglobin less than two standard deviations below the mean for the normal population is considered consistent with anemia (Brugnara et al., 2015).

    b. Additional tests, including a complete blood cell count, reticulocyte count, and evaluation of a peripheral blood smear, will aid in the evaluation of anemia, potentially identifying other cell lines involved (Brugnara et al., 2015).

    c. Evaluation for G6PD, hemoglobin electrophoresis, and iron studies should also be performed (Brugnara et al., 2015).

    d. Studies to evaluate for intravascular hemolysis, such as LDH, will also assist in evaluation for hemolytic anemia (Brugnara et al., 2015).

D. Patient Care Management

    1. *Preventive Care*

        a. Prevent iatrogenic anemia caused by large quantities of blood required for diagnostic procedures.

        b. Use smaller blood collection tubes; modern blood chemistry analyzers can perform a number of tests on a few drops of serum.

        c. Monitor and document cumulative total volume of blood drawn.

        d. Use diagnostic techniques to obtain capillary blood for testing whenever practical.

    2. *Direct Care*

        a. Administer blood products as ordered.

        b. Improve oxygenation. Reduce fear and anxiety to minimize oxygen demand. Assist in activities to reduce physiologic oxygen demand. Administer supplemental oxygen as ordered (only effective if adequate hemoglobin is present to carry the oxygen). Use semi-Fowler's position for optimal ventilation–perfusion match.

        c. Administer EPO in selected situations to promote endogenous RBC production.

    3. *Supportive Care*

        a. Decreased gas exchange occurs related to decreased red cell mass or decreased hemoglobin production.

WBC Hypoactivity

A. Definition and Etiology

WBC hypoactivity may be the result of decreased numbers of WBCs or subtypes of WBCs, or a consequence of dysfunction within WBCs.

B. Pathophysiology

Various conditions may cause WBC hypoactivity, including deficiencies, pharmacologic therapies, and the presence of malignancy.

C. Clinical Presentation

    1. *History*

        a. In some cases, WBC deficiency will be diagnosed at birth on a newborn screening evaluation.

        b. In others, patients may present with a history of multiple or atypical infections.

    2. *Physical Examination*

        a. Local signs and symptoms of inflammation include erythema, edema, warmth, pain, and decreased function of an affected area. Also note the presence and characteristics of exudate (serous vs. suppurative).

        b. Systemic clinical signs and symptoms of infection include body temperature below 36°C or above 38°C, tachycardia, tachypnea, altered mental status (e.g., confusion, irritability), diaphoresis, rigors or chills, and generalized symptoms such as change in activity level, fatigue, or malaise.

    3. *Diagnostic Tests*

        a. Alterations in WBC count. Leukocytosis, leukopenia, increased number of bands

        b. Positive blood or body fluid cultures

        c. Significant findings in site-specific diagnostic tests (e.g., pneumonia demonstrated on a chest radiograph)

D. Patient Care Management

    1. *Preventive Care*

        a. Institute good handwashing and universal precautions for all individuals who may have contact with the patient. Use proper technique for initiating and maintaining all intravascular lines and during all invasive procedures. Promote optimal fluid and nutritional intake.

b. Ensure a clean environment and restrict the patient's contact with individuals who may have infectious processes. Use a health screening tool for siblings wishing to visit the patient. Prevent the spread of infectious processes through the use of appropriate isolation procedures.

c. Critically ill children have a higher risk of developing impaired skin integrity secondary to inadequate nutrition, decreased oxygenation/ perfusion, immobility, immunosuppression, and use of medical technology and invasive procedures. The goal of nursing care is to promote skin integrity.

d. Assess and monitor skin integrity, body orifices, IV sites, and pressure areas for evidence of inflammation, infection, or skin breakdown.

2. *Direct Care*

a. Nurses caring for hematology/oncology patients on a regular basis should familiarize themselves with the clinical practice guidelines from the professional organization dedicated to the nursing care of these patients, the APHON.

b. Assess for and differentiate between inflammation and infection, which are not synonymous terms. Although all infections occur in the presence of inflammation, not all inflammation indicates infection. Infection is the pathologic process caused by the invasion of normally sterile tissue, fluid, or body cavity by pathogenic or potentially pathogenic microorganisms (Levy et al., 2003). Special attention must be paid to patients in whom the cardinal signs of the local inflammatory response may be diminished or absent (e.g., immunocompromised patients, patients receiving medications suppressing the inflammatory response, newborns with a delayed or limited ability to localize infection). In these patients, the most reliable signs of the local inflammatory response are often pain, fever, and other subtle changes in the vital signs.

c. Assess and monitor specific sites for infectious processes.

    i. Pulmonary or lower respiratory tract infection. Note tachypnea, any change in level of consciousness, feeding, behavior or activity level, presence of cough, signs of respiratory distress, and abnormal breath sounds.

    ii. Bacteremia, both primary and catheter related. Note systemic signs and symptoms of infection.

d. Assess for and differentiate between systemic infection and a systemic inflammatory response syndrome. SIRS is the acute development of two or more of the following (American College of Chest Physicians/Society of Critical Care Medicine, 1992):

    i. Fever (>38°C) or hypothermia (<36°C)

    ii. Tachycardia (outside age-appropriate range)

    iii. Tachypnea (outside age-appropriate range)

    iv. Alteration in WBC count, either leukocytosis (WBC >12,000/mm^3; use age-appropriate range [see Table 8.6]), leukopenia (WBC < 4,000/mm^3), or greater than 10% bands

    v. It is important to note that there has been debate about the sensitivity and specificity of SIRS criteria. Adult criteria is evolving and the pediatric nurse is encouraged to stay informed as these guidelines and recommendations evolve.

e. Administer prescribed antimicrobial agents and monitor response. Dilute medication per formulary guidelines to diminish venous irritation and ensure complete administration by following antibiotic with an adequate flush. Establish a schedule to maximize pharmacologic effects and minimize late administration. Assess for superinfections that may occur with long-term antibiotic use. Accurately obtain labs to assess kinetic levels of antimicrobials as ordered.

f. Administer granulocytes or biologic response modifiers as ordered.

g. Institute measures to decrease the patient's risk of infection with endogenous organisms. Assist in personal hygiene measures (oral care, etc.) as indicated. In collaboration with the physician, explore the possibility of using the patient's GI tract for feeding to minimize the risk of bacterial translocation.

3. *Supportive Care*

a. Administer supportive care per PICU guidelines paying careful attention to organ function and frequent assessment to identify dysfunction promptly.

b. Support the family of a critically ill child with explanations of care, education, and opportunities for involvement in family-centered care as appropriate.

4. *Collaborative Diagnoses and Comorbidities*

a. Patients are at risk for infection resulting from unintentional stressors (e.g., immunodeficiency, malnutrition, iatrogenic interventions such as placement of multiple invasive devices, immobility, or environmental pathogens) or intentional stressors (e.g., bone marrow suppression in preparation for transplantation or therapeutic regimens, including chemotherapy or radiation).

  i. Differentiate between hyperthermia and fever:

    1) Hyperthermia occurs when body temperature exceeds the set point secondary to cytokine activity. This response is often secondary to microorganisms and substances called *pyrogens*. Noninfectious processes can also cause fever, such as malignancy and pulmonary emboli (Porth, 2015).

    2) Hyperpyrexia, or fever, is an elevation in set point such that the body temperature is regulated at a higher level and typically occurs as the result of an infectious process.

  ii. Clinical signs and symptoms of fever include elevated temperature of 38° to 41°C. Young infants and immunocompromised patients may respond with hypothermia in the presence of infection. Other symptoms include tachycardia; tachypnea; altered mentation, confusion, or irritability; warm, dry skin with flushed cheeks; and diaphoresis.

  iii. Positive implications of increased temperature include enhanced activity of cells of the immune system and a nonconducive environment for the growth and activity of invading microorganisms (antigens). Negative implications of increased temperature include increased metabolic demand, increased insensible water loss and potential dehydration, discomfort, and fatigue.

  iv. Interventions

    1) Monitor and document fever pattern. In collaboration with the physician or advanced practice provider, determine the cause of fever. Fever may be the only sign of infection in the immunocompromised patient, and the patient is presumed to have an infection until proven otherwise.

    2) Monitor for dehydration. Estimate insensible water losses. In collaboration with the physician or advanced practice provider, evaluate the need for adjustment of fluid requirements.

    3) Identification of the source of infection is a primary concern in a febrile patient. Indwelling catheters should be sampled for culture. If possible, two peripheral blood samples should be obtained from separate venipuncture sites. Other cultures that may be obtained include sputum, tracheal, routine urinalysis and culture, and a stool examination and culture (especially if diarrhea is present).

    4) In collaboration with the physician or advanced practice provider, consider the administration of antipyretics (only after the fever is evaluated) and broad-spectrum antibiotic therapy (until the specific cause of the infection is determined). Keep in mind that some antipyretics, such as ibuprofen, may affect the platelets in such a way that they are contraindicated in the thrombocytopenic patient.

    5) Institute measures to decrease the temperature when the patient is febrile. Remove excess clothing or bed linens. Apply cool moist compresses, especially to the forehead and axilla. Use a cooling blanket but discontinue use if shivering ensues. Prevent chills or shivering because the associated peripheral vasoconstriction may actually further increase body temperature and decrease heat loss (Porth, 2015).

    6) Institute measures to increase comfort when the patient is febrile. Change wet bed linens in the presence of diaphoresis or with the use of a cooling blanket. Cool the patient's room if possible. Provide rest periods.

    7) If possible, discontinue medications that may cause fever as an adverse reaction.

b. Patients are at risk for altered integrity of mucous membranes resulting from oral infection or the side effects of chemotherapy or radiation.

   i. Assessment

   1) This is a common, dose-limiting toxicity caused by chemotherapy, radiation, and neutropenia.

   2) Clinical signs and symptoms are variable and range from reddened areas to deep ulcerations. Other manifestations include pain; dysphagia; thick oral secretions; the presence of white patches; cracked, dry lips; scalloping of the tongue edges; and drooling. The risk of infection increases greatly with impaired tissue integrity within the oral cavity. The fungal infection candidiasis (moniliasis or thrush) is identified by microscopic examination of scrapings (Porth, 2015). Appropriate antifungals, such as nystatin mouth rinse, may be indicated.

   ii. Implications of altered oral mucous membranes include impaired integrity and increased risk of infection, inadequate nutritional intake or absorption, pain, and difficulty swallowing or speaking (if not intubated).

   iii. Interventions. Assess and monitor the condition of the oral mucosa. Institute measures to prevent inflammation (mucositis) or to prevent further injury to existing inflammation. Avoid exposure to chemical or physical irritants, and provide adequate fluid intake. Provide oral hygiene measures at least three times a day. Provide treatment based on assessment findings, and institute measures to increase comfort. If the patient is able to tolerate PO intake, encourage bland, soft foods that are not especially dry for pain control and effective swallowing.

WBC Hyperactivity

Hypersensitivity Reactions

A. Definition and Etiology

Hypersensitivity reactions are classified according to the source of the antigen that stimulates the immune response (Table 8.10). Type I immediate hypersensitivity reaction or anaphylaxis results in hyperactivity of the surveillance function of the immune system.

B. Pathophysiology

The pathophysiology of the four types of hypersensitivity reactions are described in Table 8.10.

C. Clinical Presentation

1. *History.* Clinical signs and symptoms typically occur within minutes of exposure to the antigen and are the result of the action of inflammatory mediators on surrounding tissues and blood vessels (Porth, 2015).

2. *Physical Examination*

   a. Increased capillary permeability can lead to profound hypotension, circulatory collapse, and facial edema.

   b. Constriction of smooth muscle can result in wheezing, crackles, and progressive difficulty in breathing and stridor.

   c. An influx of eosinophils can produce erythema and pruritus.

3. *Diagnostic Tests.* Although a hypersensitivity reaction may prompt testing for allergies and sensitivities, diagnostic confirmation is not required at the time of an actual reaction and should not be performed as it may delay critical interventions.

D. Patient Care Management

1. Diagnosis and management of anaphylaxis are based on clinical manifestations.

2. Maintain oxygenation and ventilation. Administer supplemental oxygen as needed. Intubation and mechanical ventilation may be necessary. In the presence of tracheal or laryngeal edema, intubation may be difficult and there is a possibility that the patient may require an emergency tracheotomy. Epinephrine 1:1,000 is administered for treatment of bronchoconstriction, per pediatric advanced life support (PALS) protocol.

3. Support circulation with fluid administration and epinephrine administration to counteract vasodilation. Other vasoactive medications (e.g., dopamine, norepinephrine) may be required.

4. *Administer Prescribed Medications.* Antihistamines serve as antagonists to most of the effects of histamine. Bronchodilators relax bronchial smooth muscle. Corticosteroids are anti-inflammatory agents that serve to enhance the effects of bronchodilators.

5. Identify the antigen and avoid future exposures.

TABLE 8.10 Hypersensitivity Reactions

Type	Description	Example
Type I (anaphylactic reaction)	Triggered in response to an exposure to an environmental antigen Mediated by IgE antibodies that bind to specific receptors on the surface of mast cells and basophils Results in the release of a host of mediators to produce a classic anaphylactic response	Anaphylaxis Asthma Allergic rhinitis, hay fever
Type II (tissue-specific hypersensitivity)	Triggered by the presence of an antigen found only on a cell or tissue Mediated by antibody (usually IgM, but also IgG) through two different mechanisms (complement and Fc receptors on phagocytes) Results in the destruction of the antibody-coated cell with consequences dependent on the cell that is destroyed (e.g., RBC, WBC, or platelet)	ABO incompatibility Rh incompatibility Drug-induced thrombocytopenia
Type III (immune complex reaction)	Triggered by the formation of antigen–antibody complexes that activate the complement cascade Immune complexes are formed in the circulation and are later deposited in blood vessels or healthy tissue; multiple forms of the response exist depending on the type and location of the antigen Results in local edema and neutrophil attraction and thus degradative lysosomal enzymes resulting in tissue injury	Serum sickness Glomerulonephritis
Type IV (delayed hypersensitivity)	Triggered by the recognition of an antigen Mediated by activated T lymphocytes and release of lymphokines, which then stimulate the macrophage to phagocytize foreign invaders and some normal tissue Results in a delayed onset; does not have an antibody component; this response is strictly a cellular reaction	Contact sensitivities such as poison ivy and dermatitis Tuberculin reactions Graft rejection

Ig, immunoglobulin; RBC, red blood cell; WBC, white blood cell.

Autoimmune Disease

A. Definition and Etiology

Autoimmune disease is the hyperactivity of the homeostasis function of the immune system.

B. Pathophysiology

1. The homeostasis function of the immune system removes old and damaged "self" components from the body.

2. The immune system mistakenly identifies itself as "nonself" and begins to form antibodies (autoantibodies) against its own healthy cells (autoantigens). This results in the development of immune complexes that are deposited in tissues (e.g., skin, joints, kidneys) and in tissue damage.

C. Examples of autoimmune diseases of childhood include systemic lupus erythematosis and juvenile-onset diabetes mellitus.

PLATELETS AND PLASMA FACTORS

Bleeding Disorders

A. Definition and Etiology

Bleeding disorders may be the result of inadequate platelet production, excess platelet destruction, abnormal function, impairment of the coagulation stage of hemostasis, or disordered vessel integrity (Grossman, 2014c).

B. Pathophysiology

1. Bone marrow dysfunction, as in the case of severe aplastic anemia, causes inadequate platelet production.

2. Platelet destruction is the result of an immune process, such as the platelet antibodies responsible for ITP, or a nonimmune process such as mechanical destruction by prosthetic valves or excess consumption in processes such as acute DIC or TTP.

3. Defects in von Willebrand factor or other inherited diseases, such as hemophilia A and B, are responsible for disordered bleeding.

4. Bleeding may be the result of medications that predispose a patient to bleeding, such as heparin, NSAIDs, and aspirin (Grossman, 2014c).

C. Clinical Presentation

1. *History*

Patients and caregivers may report a history of excessive bruising or bleeding. Reports of blood in the stool, emesis, urine, or during routine activities, such as flossing or brushing teeth, should alert the healthcare provider to a potential bleeding disorder. In addition, the history may reveal prolonged bleeding after minor injuries.

2. *Physical Examination*

a. Assessment should include vital signs (tachycardia and hypotension), fluid and electrolyte status (decreased urine output, emesis, diarrhea), characteristics of fluid losses (assess for gross or occult blood), perfusion status, capillary refill, mental status, and urine output.

b. Use urine and stool tests to detect the presence of blood.

3. *Diagnostic Tests*

a. Coagulation studies, including the PT, PTT, and fibrinogen, should be assessed.

b. Additional studies to evaluate factors VIII and V may also be indicated, as well as an evaluation of natural anticoagulants, including protein C, protein S, and antithrombin III.

c. TEG and TGA, as described previously in this chapter, may also be useful as a global clotting assays (Branchford & Di Paola, 2015).

D. Patient Care Management

1. *Preventive Care*

a. Identify which patients are at increased risk for bleeding.

b. Avoid intramuscular and subcutaneous injections; if necessary, apply pressure for 10 minutes. If intravascular access is needed, peripheral IV access rather than central access poses less risk for trauma and bleeding to the patient.

c. Provide a safe environment, such as padding the side rails and other firm surfaces, especially if the child is combative or at risk for seizure activity.

d. Do not administer aspirin or NSAIDs because of their effects on platelets. Parents should be taught to read nonprescription medication labels to avoid giving the child aspirin.

e. Prevent intracranial bleeding related to increased intracranial pressure. Teach the patient to avoid the Valsalva maneuver and to cough, sneeze, and blow nose gently.

f. Administer stool softeners.

g. Provide mouth care with foam swabs and a mild saline or bicarbonate and peroxide solution. Do not floss if thrombocytopenia is present.

h. Administer vitamin K (normally obtained from diet and enteric bacterial synthesis) when indicated. Vitamin K is needed for factors II, VII, IX, and X to be effective. Deficiencies are seen with malnutrition, obstructive biliary disease, liver disease, and with use of certain broad-spectrum antibiotics. Vitamin K can be administered orally if absorption is not impaired, subcutaneously, intramuscularly, and intravenously. Anaphylactoid reactions are rare but are seen more often with the IV route (Pipe & Goldenberg, 2015).

2. *Direct Care*

a. Volume replacement. Administer crystalloids or colloids or both, blood products, and vasoactive infusions as ordered.

b. Control of bleeding. Apply direct pressure or cold compresses, and elevate the extremity. Application of topical hemostatic agents may also be necessary.

3. *Collaborative Diagnoses and Comorbidities.* Hypovolemia related to bleeding

RBC DISORDERS

Sickle Cell Disease

A. Definition and Etiology

1. Sickle cell disease (SCD) is the general term used to describe a group of genetic disorders that are characterized by mutations in the hemoglobin gene. These mutations lead to sickling of the RBCs in response to deoxygenation.

2. SCD is a serious, chronic, autosomal-recessive, hemolytic disease. The most common forms are hemoglobin SS disease (HbSS), hemoglobin SC disease (HbSC), hemoglobin S-beta thalassemia (HbSβthal), and other rare variants. Clinical manifestations will vary in type and severity among each of these phenotypes.

3. SCD occurs almost exclusively in individuals of African descent and typically manifests at approximately 1 year of age when most of the fetal hemoglobin (HbF) has been replaced with HbSS or HbSC (Heeney & Ware, 2015)

B. Pathophysiology

1. When the oxygen saturations fall, RBCs with HbSS (an abnormal form of hemoglobin associated with SCD) become crescent or sickle shaped. These sickled RBCs become trapped in small vessels, leading to erythrostasis and occlusion of the microvasculature. Hypoxemia, acidosis, hypothermia or hyperthermia, and dehydration lead to further sickling and increased viscosity of the blood.

2. Masses of sickled RBCs occlude blood vessels, leading to thrombosis, ischemia, and infarction. Specific organs involved will present with signs of hypoperfusion, vascular occlusion, and tissue ischemia. The body recognizes and hemolyzes the abnormal RBC structure. Sickled RBCs may return to normal shape when the blood is more oxygenated (such as in the pulmonary vein). However, after repeated occasions, a portion of RBCs released into free circulation will be more sensitive to mechanical trauma, even normal trauma experienced during circulation, or they will not return to their nonsickled shape even when the blood is well oxygenated.

C. Clinical Presentation

1. *History*

a. Nearly all states (44 per the 2015 publication by the National Institutes of Health [NIH]) provide screening for SCD as part of the newborn screen, which will assist in diagnosis prior to requirement of a blood transfusion or development of clinical manifestations.

b. High-risk infants, identified as those of African, Mediterranean, Middle Eastern, Indian, Caribbean, and South and Central American ancestry, should be screened if they are born in states that have not standardized a hemoglobinopathy initial screening test (NIH National Heart, Lung, and Blood Institute, 2015).

2. *Physical Examination*

a. Clinical manifestations occur secondary to the anemia and organ dysfunction caused by vascular occlusion. Specific symptoms include painful episodes, including aching bones, especially hands and feet in infants; sudden severe abdominal pain; chest pain; and splenomegaly in young children. Older children and adolescents

with SCD may report pain in the lumbosacral spine, knee, shoulder, elbow, and femur.

b. The spleen is nonfunctional in children with HbSS disease, even if the spleen is enlarged.

c. SCD is not associated with bleeding.

d. Impaired growth and development, failure to thrive, and increased tendency to develop serious infections are results of decreased splenic function (Table 8.11).

3. *Diagnostic Tests*

a. Peripheral blood smear will show sickled erythrocytes. If only the sickle cell trait is present, the smear will be normal.

b. Hemoglobin electrophoresis indicates the precise type of hemoglobinopathy as it differentiates between types of hemoglobin and reports the percentage of blood composition of each.

c. CBC reflects hemolytic anemia with reduced hemoglobin, hematocrit, and RBC count because the spleen has destroyed sickled cells. Platelets and reticulocyte count may be elevated as a compensatory response to anemia.

d. Bilirubin may be elevated because of the hemolysis of the sickled cells.

e. Radiologic findings

i. Bone x-rays may show no abnormality in the face of severe bone pain.

ii. Chest x-rays may show cardiomegaly and pulmonary infiltrate with acute chest syndrome (ACS).

iii. Transcranial Doppler screen (TCD) measures the blood velocity in the circle of Willis. Identification of intracranial arterial vasculopathy and thus, higher risk of stroke, is possible via this method. Interventions for primary and secondary stroke prevention based on this assessment have proven effective (Heeney & Ware, 2015).

iv. CT scan and MRI/magnetic resonance angiography (MRA) should be performed after stabilization if a cerebrovascular accident (CVA) is suspected.

D. Patient Care Management

1. *Pain Management*: *Supportive Interventions*

a. Prevent pain by rapid recognition and management of dehydration, hypoxemia, and acidosis to prevent sickling.

TABLE 8.11 Clinical Manifestation of Sickle Cell Anemia*

Manifestation	Comments
Anemia	Chronic, onset 3–4 months of age; may require folate therapy; hematocrit usually 18%–26%
Aplastic crisis	Parvovirus infection, reticulocytopenia; acute and reversible; may need transfusion
Sequestration crisis	Massive splenomegaly (may involve liver), shock; treat with transfusion
Hemolytic crisis	May be associated with G6PD deficiency
Dactylitis	Hand–foot swelling in early infancy
Painful crisis	Microvascular painful vaso-occlusive infarcts of muscle, bone, bone marrow, lung, intestines
Cerebrovascular accidents	Large- and small-vessel occlusion → thrombosis/bleeding (stroke); requires chronic transfusion
Acute chest syndrome	Infection, atelectasis, infarction, fat emboli, severe hypoxemia, infiltrate, dyspnea, absent breath sounds
Chronic lung disease	Pulmonary fibrosis, restrictive lung disease, cor pulmonale
Priapism	Causes eventual impotence; treated with transfusion, oxygen, or corpora cavernosa-to-spongiosa shunt
Ocular	Retinopathy
Gallbladder disease	Bilirubin stones; cholecystitis
Renal	Hematuria, papillary necrosis, renal-concentrating defect; nephropathy
Cardiomyopathy	Heart failure (fibrosis)
Skeletal	Osteonecrosis (avascular) of femoral or humeral head
Leg ulceration	Seen in older patients
Infections	Functional asplenia, defects in properdin system; pneumococcal bacteremia, meningitis, and arthritis; deafness from meningitis in 35%; *Salmonella* and *Staphylococcus aureus* osteomyelitis; severe *Mycoplasma* pneumonia
Growth failure, delayed puberty	May respond to nutritional supplements
Psychologic problems	Narcotic addiction (rare), dependence unusual; chronic illness, chronic pain

G6PD, glucose-6-phosphate dehydrogenase.

*Clinical manifestations with sickle cell trait are unusual but include renal papillary necrosis (hematuria), sudden death on intraocular hyphema extension, and sickling in unpressurized airplanes.

Source: From Scott, J. P. (2000). Hematology. In R. E. Behrman & R. M. Kliegman (Eds.), *Nelson's essentials of pediatrics* (4th ed.). Philadelphia, PA: W. B. Saunders.

b. Obtain a history of past and present pain management.

c. Conduct frequent, ongoing pain assessments using the appropriate pain scale for age, developmental level, and clinical condition.

d. Use analgesics and anti-inflammatory agents as indicated and ordered. Monitor effectiveness in decreasing pain. Patient-controlled analgesia is an effective method to use to achieve adequate pain control.

e. Use nonpharmacologic pain management techniques as indicated (e.g., heat, massage, distraction, guided imagery).

f. In selected clinical situations (e.g., severe ACS) RBC transfusion or exchange transfusion is given to decrease the percentage of

HbSS-containing RBCs. Goal is usually a hematocrit of 25% to 30% with less than 30% HbS. Avoid raising the hematocrit to more than 35% because this will increase the viscosity of the blood and promote increased sickling.

2. *Bed rest* minimizes oxygen demand and consumption.

3. *Hydroxyurea.* Hydroxyurea enhances the production of HbF, thereby decreasing the ability of the RBCs with HbSS to sickle. Indications for hydroxyurea therapy are limited to severe complications such as frequent pain episodes, acute chest, severe symptomatic anemia, or other severe vaso-occlusive events. Frequency monitoring for toxicities is required for patients receiving hydroxyurea therapy. In addition, guidance regarding contraception methods is necessary for males and females, as hydroxyurea is a teratogen (NIH, 2015).

4. *Bone marrow or stem cell transplant* is the only current therapy that may provide a cure for SCD. Results of matched sibling donor (MSD) bone marrow transplantation are promising, with reports of greater than 90% survival and approximately 85% survival without SCD. Research regarding the use of alternative donors, such as umbilical cord blood (UCB), matched unrelated donors (MUDs), and haploidentical donors, is ongoing (NIH, 2015).

5. *Gene therapy* may offer a future cure for SCD. Gene transfer to correct the molecular defect in the hemoglobin is under investigation as a future treatment.

6. *Transfusion therapy* may include episodic or chronic transfusions of RBCs (Heeney & Ware, 2015).

   a. Simple transfusions are useful in the treatment of symptomatic anemia, severe or progressive ACS, splenic sequestration, stroke, and priapism.

   b. Exchange transfusions withdraw blood (manually or through erythrocytapheresis) and then transfuse nonsickle cell blood. The goal of this therapy is to reduce the HbS concentration to less than 30%.

   c. Episodic transfusions may be simple or exchange transfusions; these are useful in the treatment of an acute event. Goal hemoglobin will not exceed 10 to 11 g/dL.

   d. Chronic transfusions are indicated for severe cases in which the risk of morbidity from sickle cell outweighs the risk of chronic transfusion therapy (allosensitization, infection, iron overload).

Chronic transfusions are usually performed every 4 weeks and may involve simple or exchange transfusions to maintain HbS less than 30%.

   e. Transfusions may also be indicated to achieve a preoperative Hgb greater than 10 g/dL prior to surgical procedures (Heeney & Ware, 2015).

7. *Collaborative Diagnoses and Comorbidities.* Patients are at risk for impaired gas exchange, activity intolerance, and pain.

8. *Goals and Desired Patient Outcomes: Prevention of Complications*

   a. Promote early diagnosis through newborn screening.

   b. Encourage follow-up in a comprehensive sickle cell clinic.

     i. Educate the family regarding the importance of mandatory prophylactic penicillin starting at 2 months of age. Discontinuation of penicillin prophylaxis is controversial.

     ii. Teach parents that fever (temperature >38.5°C) or other signs of infection, such as lethargy, irritability, poor oral intake, chills, or vomiting, must be promptly evaluated to determine the source of the fever and the need for treatment (NIH, 2015).

     iii. Teach parents to palpate the spleen for possible enlargement.

   c. Prevent crises through prevention of dehydration, hypoxemia, and acidosis.

   d. Prevent infection with all recommended childhood vaccines. Children with SCD require additional immunizations, including four doses of the seven-valent pneumococcal-conjugated vaccine (Prevnar) followed by two additional doses of the 23-valent pneumococcal polysaccharide vaccine (Pneumovax) starting at 24 months old. Children with SCD can begin to receive annual influenza vaccines after 6 months of age (NIH, 2015).

E. Complications of SCD

1. *Infections* are a major cause of morbidity and mortality for children with SCD. The most common cause of death in children with SCD is *S. pneumoniae* sepsis.

   a. Compromised function of the spleen leads to an increased susceptibility to encapsulated bacteria. There is an increased risk of *S. pneumoniae* (pneumococcus) and *H. influenzae* type b infections. Any clinical pneumonia decreases the effectiveness of oxygenation, thereby increasing sickling of RBCs.

b. Prevention. Prophylactic penicillin should be initiated upon diagnosis of SCD. Penicillin VK is administered twice daily though 5 years of age; the dose is age dependent (NIH, 2015).

c. Assess for infections requiring immediate attention and admission to the hospital; fever greater than 38.5°C is considered an emergency. Note significant pain, fever, and chills. Patients with SCD typically have a slightly elevated WBC count; but with infection, the WBC count further increases to greater than 30,000/mm³. Chest radiographic examination demonstrates significant pulmonary infiltrates if infection involves the pulmonary system.

d. Management. Obtain blood cultures and immediately begin empiric antibiotics, including coverage for pneumococcus and *H. influenzae*. Urine and throat cultures may also be required, as are urinalysis and chest x-ray if symptomatic. Toxic-appearing children with a concern for meningitis require evaluation with a lumbar puncture (NIH, 2015).

2. *Splenic sequestration crisis* is a life-threatening complication. Acute pooling of blood in the splenic sinuses results in a rapid decrease in Hgb. This results in acute splenic enlargement, significant anemia with 2 g/dL of greater fall in hemoglobin, and, if severe, can progress rapidly to hypovolemic shock and death. First cases of splenic sequestration are typically seen in children between the ages of 3 months and 5 years (NIH, 2015).

a. Assessment. Clinically, acute weakness, pallor, abdominal distention and pain, tachycardia, tachypnea, dyspnea, splenomegaly, and left upper quadrant pain are noted. Laboratory results demonstrate a rapid fall in hemoglobin and hematocrit (Heeney & Ware, 2015; NIH, 2015).

b. Management. Immediate management is focused on the restoration of circulating volume and oxygen-carrying capacity. This is accomplished by emergent RBC transfusion. Cardiovascular status is the primary concern in this complication and, with restoration of intravascular volume and cardiovascular function, improvement in splenic sequestration will take place. It is important that RBC transfusions do not increase the hemoglobin to the patient's baseline, as trapped RBCs will be released from the spleen with recovery. Emergent splenectomy is not indicated (Heeney & Ware, 2015; NIH, 2015).

c. Recurrence of splenic sequestration is common, often within 2 to 3 months. Management strategies following splenic sequestration may include continued observation, chronic transfusion therapy, or splenectomy. The goal of transfusion therapy is to maintain the HbS level at less than 30%. Following a splenectomy or if the spleen fibroses, the child will need preventive strategies for infection as described previously. Adults are not susceptible to these crises because their spleens are atrophied (called *autosplenectomy*) because of repeated infarctions (Heeney & Ware, 2015; NIH, 2015).

3. *Aplastic crisis* is a transient episode of failure of RBC production that can be life threatening. It is usually associated with human parvovirus B19, leading to transient suppression of erythropoiesis.

a. Assessment. Clinical manifestations of severe anemia including fever, anorexia, lethargy, tachypnea, tachycardia, nausea, vomiting, abdominal pain, and headache are noted (not splenomegaly). Laboratory results show a rapid decrease in hemoglobin, low reticulocyte count (<1%) in peripheral blood, and low RBC precursors in the bone marrow aspirate. A concurrent episode of ACS may be seen.

b. Management. Transfuse with RBCs slowly to alleviate signs or symptoms of inadequate tissue oxygenation; repeated transfusions may be indicated. Protective isolation may be used. All caretakers must adhere to isolation guidelines.

4. *Acute Chest Syndrome*

a. ACS is defined as respiratory symptoms associated with a pulmonary infiltrate on chest radiograph. In children, ACS is often associated with infection. In adults, ACS is usually seen after a severe, bony, painful crisis. Contributing causes include infection, sickling of RBCs in pulmonary vasculature, hypoventilation secondary to pain, hypoventilation secondary to opioid analgesics, asthma or reactive airway disease, and bone marrow/fat embolism. The major concern is that a vicious cycle of pulmonary vaso-occlusion, poor oxygenation of blood, increased RBC sickling, and more vaso-occlusion will ensue. Vascular occlusion of branches of the pulmonary artery leads to infarction of the lung. The syndrome may be self-limited, particularly when it involves a small area of pulmonary parenchyma, but it can rapidly progress and become massive and fatal. A chronic pattern seen in this syndrome leads to chronic scarring of the lung as seen on x-ray examination. Repeated episodes lead to restrictions of vital capacity, pulmonary hypertension, and cor pulmonale.

b. Assessment. Clinical course is variable, ranging from mild symptoms to a rapidly progressing and fatal respiratory failure.

   i.   Clinical appearance. Patient will have fever accompanied by chest pain, cough, nasal flaring, accessory muscle use, wheezing, dyspnea, tachycardia, and tachypnea.

   ii.   X-ray. Pulmonary infiltrate may not be prominent, especially if the patient is dehydrated; it may progress to a complete "white-out."

   iii.   Laboratory results. Blood and sputum cultures may be positive for organisms.

   iv.   Arterial blood gases. Variable degrees of hypoxia may be seen.

c. Management. The patient should be admitted to the hospital and monitored closely due to the high risk of morbidity and mortality.

   i.   Presence of pneumonia must be ruled out. However, it is usually very difficult to distinguish between pulmonary infarction and pneumonia, and the processes are likely to coexist. In younger patients, pneumonia is more likely to be the cause of symptoms. In older patients, pulmonary infarction is the more common cause.

   ii.   Initiate broad-spectrum antibiotics for *S. pneumoniae, H. influenzae,* and *Mycoplasma pneumoniae* immediately if new pulmonary infiltrates are seen on radiographic examination.

   iii.   Administer supplemental oxygen to hypoxic patients. Bronchodilators may be effective in patients with obstructive disease and incentive spirometry should be encouraged. Adequate analgesia therapy is necessary for patients experiencing hypoventilation secondary to chest pain. Noninvasive ventilation with continuous positive airway pressure (CPAP) or bilevel positive airway pressure (BiPap) may be indicated for patients with inadequate respiratory effort. Those with respiratory failure will require mechanical ventilation (Heeney & Ware, 2015).

   iv.   Simple or exchange transfusion may be indicated if poor respiratory function is seen (NIH, 2015).

5. *Vaso-occlusive crisis (pain crisis)* is one of the most debilitating problems for SCD patients. It can occur in any organ system and is characterized by obstruction of small arterioles by sickled RBCs, resulting in ischemia of tissues, organ dysfunction, and pain. Onset is unpredictable with varied frequency, intensity, duration, and severity. Precipitating factors include infection, fever, dehydration, trauma, or exposure to cold. Uncomplicated acute pain is self-limited and often lasts hours to a few days. For some patients, pain episodes may last weeks. Chronic pain can be psychologically and physically debilitating and can last 3 to 6 months or more (NIH, 2015).

a. Assessment. Diagnosis is by history, not by laboratory test or radiographic examination. Clinical appearance demonstrates severe deep pain at any site, commonly musculoskeletal, in extremities, back, chest, or abdomen. Chest radiographic examination is used if chest pain is present to rule out ACS. During infancy the syndrome is characterized by a dactylitis, or "hand–foot" syndrome, with soft-tissue swelling, heat, and pain of the dorsum of the hands, feet, fingers, and toes.

b. Management

   i.   Management of vaso-occlusive disease requires disruption of the cycle of hypoxemia and sickling by providing adequate hydration, oxygenation, antibiotic therapy if infection is suspected, and rapid pain assessment and control (NIH, 2015).

   ii.   Initially rule out other causes of pain, such as osteomyelitis, bone infarction, and other causes for chest or abdominal pain.

   iii.   Hydration. Administer IV fluids at one to 1.5 times the maintenance rate. Potassium chloride may be added pending serum potassium values; additional adjustments may be made as needed based on evaluation of serum chemistries (NIH, 2015). A recent Cochrane review stated that there is no recommended type of fluid replacement for sickle cell crisis and that more research is needed to indicate whether hypotonic saline is of benefit (Okomo & Meremikwu, 2015).

iv. Administer supplemental oxygen if the patient is hypoxic.

v. If fever is higher than 38.5°C, blood cultures should be obtained and empiric IV antibiotics initiated.

vi. Relief of acute, severe pain begins with opioid therapy, often via parenteral morphine or an alternative. Opiates may be delivered via patient-controlled analgesia. Careful monitoring for side effects, including sedation and respiratory depression, is necessary (NIH, 2015).

vii. Chronic pain relief may be achieved through sustained-release or long-half-life opioids. Clinicians should anticipate physical dependency and tolerance (both physiologic responses), and should not confuse these with addiction (psychologic dependence; NIH, 2015).

viii. Oral pain medications may be used to treat children with mild to moderate pain and may include NSAIDs or acetaminophen. In addition, an intravenous NSAID, ketorolac, may be utilized (NIH, 2015).

ix. Adjuvant therapies may include anxiolytics, anticonvulsants, antidepressants, and clonidine (NIH, 2015).

6. *Cerebrovascular accident (CVA)* is an acute infarction in the brain, most commonly related to intracranial arterial stenosis or obstruction, which can result in stroke. Other complications, such as ACS, infection, aplastic crisis, and dehydration, may also cause an acute infarct in patients with a chronic vasculopathy. The incidence of CNS events in children in the first 20 years of life is approximately 0.7% (Heeney & Ware, 2015).

a. Assessment. Clinical appearance demonstrates hemiparesis, headache, dizziness, lethargy, aphasia, focal seizures, gait and visual disturbances, or alteration in mentation or alertness.

b. Radiologic studies. Initial stabilization should be performed prior to radiographic evaluation. Noncontrast CT of the brain is the initial study, and may be followed by MRI with diffusion-weighted imaging (DWI) and fluid-attenuated inversion recovery (FLAIR). MRI results may be normal initially because several days of evolution are necessary to detect an edematous infarcted area. Arteriogram is not commonly used, but when it is performed, administration of hyperosmolar contrast requires preparation with hydration and transfusion to lower HbS to less than 30% before the scan is done. Contrast material may increase sickling. Low-ionic strength contrast medium is preferable (Heeney & Ware, 2015).

c. Management. The goal is to prevent progression of the CVA. Emergent management includes initiation of IV hydration and simple transfusion with a goal Hgb of more than 10 g/dL or an exchange transfusion. Use strategies to maintain normal intracranial pressure. Administer anticonvulsants if seizures occur. Patients are at risk for recurrence of CVA. Therefore, a chronic RBC transfusion program may be initiated to maintain HbSS levels at less than 30%. Patients may require iron chelation therapy to treat iron overload.

7. *Bone marrow necrosis and fat embolism* are caused by microinfarctions of bone or marrow. Secondary embolization of fat or marrow particles leads to pulmonary infarction or fat globules in the coronary, cerebral, and renal microvasculature, resulting in renal, neurologic, or respiratory failure, which is frequently fatal.

a. Assessment. Clinically, severe bone pain, fever, neurologic abnormalities, or respiratory distress are noted. Lipid or fat may be present in sputum specimens.

b. Management includes administration of supplemental oxygen, simple or exchange transfusion, and ventilatory support as needed.

8. *Multi-organ system failure (MOSF)* is an unusual clinical condition for patients with SCD resulting from several of the aforementioned complications. Episodes of pain complicated by the acute failure of at least two of three organs (lung, liver, or kidney) may result in a severe, life-threatening complication of pain episodes in patients with otherwise mild SCD. MOSF is associated with an unusually severe vaso-occlusive crisis for the child and a high baseline hemoglobin level, which may or may not be associated with an infection. The cause is undefined but is assumed to be from the diffuse microvascular occlusion and tissue ischemia simultaneously in multiple organs and the sequestration and destruction of RBCs, leading to further tissue ischemia from the decreased oxygen-carrying capacity.

a. Assessment. Clinically, the child has fever, a rapid fall in hemoglobin and platelet count, nonfocal encephalopathy (confusion, lethargy), and rhabdomyolysis. Laboratory results show hypoxia and elevation of liver enzymes, bilirubin, PT, and creatinine. Radiographic findings include pulmonary infiltrates.

b. Management. Transfusion, if aggressive and prompt, may reverse the syndrome. Exchange transfusion may be necessary for young children. Provide hydration and IV analgesia.

9. *Priapism,* a painful, involuntary erection of the penis, occurs as sickled cells are trapped in the penis. Although it may resolve spontaneously and require only analgesics, management may involve hydration, exchange transfusion (if condition does not resolve in 4–6 hours), and surgery to aspirate the stagnant blood and administer local vasodilators (NIH, 2015).

WBC DISORDERS: IMMUNODEFICIENCY DISEASES

Despite the type of stressor (e.g., congenital, acquired, intentional, and unintentional), the final common pathway or outcome of immunodeficiency or immunosuppression is impaired immune function or immunocompromise. Immunodeficiency is a permanent state of impaired immune function that is usually genetic or congenital in nature, but may be acquired Immunosuppression is a state of impaired immune function that can be intentional or unintentional and is usually temporary.

Congenital Immunodeficiency Diseases

A. Disorders are characterized by an inadequate number or inadequate function of one or more of the components of the immune system resulting from a genetic or congenital condition. Disorders are divided by involvement of B lymphocytes, T lymphocytes, phagocytes, complement, or a combination of these components.

B. *Humoral or B-lymphocyte disorders* are characterized by B-cell dysfunction and diminished immunoglobulin production. This deficiency predisposes children to recurrent infections by *S. pneumoniae, H. influenzae, Staphylococcus aureus,* and other gram-negative bacteria (Moriber, 2014).

1. These are a diverse group of immunodeficiencies that may manifest as a deficiency in all classes of immunoglobulins (panhypogammaglobulinemia), as a deficiency in only one class of immunoglobulin (hypogammaglobulinemia), or as a combination of deficiencies in some classes with overproduction of immunoglobulin in another class.

2. IgA deficiency is the most common primary immunodeficiency and results in increased incidence of early, recurrent infections, allergies, and autoimmune conditions. Another example of a B-lymphocyte disorder includes X-linked agammaglobulinemia and combined variable immunodeficiency (CVID).

3. B-lymphocyte deficiencies are frequently interrelated with T-lymphocyte dysfunction (see "Combined B- and T-lymphocyte Disorders").

4. Etiology and pattern of infections include enteroviruses and bacterial infections as described earlier. Humoral deficiency does not predispose the patient to fungal infections (Moriber, 2014).

C. *T-lymphocyte disorders* are characterized by an inadequate number or function of T lymphocytes. These patients have a limited ability to produce mature T lymphocytes, resulting in the inability to assist in the activation of the immune response.

1. T-lymphocyte disorders are associated with the survival and replication of intracellular organisms inside host immune cells. T cells also play a role in the control of malignancies and coordination of overall immune response. These diverse functions result in many different immunologic responses (Moriber, 2014).

2. Examples of T-lymphocyte disorders include DiGeorge syndrome and X-linked immunodeficiency with hyper-IgM.

3. Etiology and pattern of infections most often include herpes viruses, fungi, and bacteria, including *Salmonella typhi* and mycobacteria. Opportunistic infection with organisms, such as *Candida albicans* and *Aspergillus fumigatus,* pose a risk to these patients (Moriber, 2014).

D. *Phagocyte dysfunction disorders* are disorders resulting from diverse extrinsic or intrinsic factors.

1. *Extrinsic factors*

i. Deficiency in opsonization related to decrease in either antibody or complement

ii. Suppression of neutrophils or altered chemotaxis of neutrophils related to deficiency or alteration in complement

iii. Decreased circulating lymphokines

iv. Medications with immunosuppressive effect on phagocyte function or number

2. *Intrinsic factors.* Defects in the metabolic pathway of phagocytes.

3. Examples of primary disorders of phagocytosis include chronic granulomatous disease (CGD) and leukocyte adhesion deficiency (LAD). Secondary disorders of phagocytosis may be drug induced (corticosteroids or immunosuppressive therapy) or related to diabetes mellitus (Moriber, 2014).

4. Etiology and pattern of infection demonstrate an increased incidence of staphylococcal infections. Patients with phagocytic disorders are considered at risk for infection with gram-negative bacterial and fungal infections despite a "normal" WBC count. Fungal infections, including *C. albicans and Nocardia,* are also associated with disorders of phagocytosis (Moriber, 2014).

5. Patients with inadequate numbers of phagocytes are referred to as *neutropenic* (total WBC number is decreased) or *granulocytopenic* (number of PMNs and bands decrease). These are clinical states rather than immunodeficiency disorders.

E. *Complement disorders* are characterized by the absence of an inhibitor or a deficiency in one or more of the specific complement components.

1. Deficiencies for each of the key components of complement have been described; however, an increase in the susceptibility to infection is commonly noted for deficiencies in C1q, C3, and C4 (Moriber, 2014).

2. Examples of complement disorders include hereditary deficiency of complement proteins and acquired disorders that consume complement disorders (Moriber, 2014).

3. Etiology and pattern of infection include an increased risk of encapsulated bacterial infection, especially *S. pneumoniae.* In addition, patients may develop autoimmune disease such as vasculitis and systemic lupus erythematosus (Moriber, 2014).

F. *Combined B- and T-lymphocyte disorders* involve the humoral and CMI responses and result in a wide variety of immunodeficiencies.

1. Combined immunodeficiencies are caused by mutations in multiple genes and lead to immunodeficiency through their influence on lymphocyte response, cytokines, or MHC antigens (Moriber, 2014).

2. This is the most severe of all the immunodeficiencies because the patient is unable to form antibody (B lymphocyte), orchestrate the immune response (T lymphocyte), and destroy virally infected cells and cells infected with intracellular microorganisms (T lymphocyte).

3. Examples of combined immunodeficiencies include severe combined immunodeficiency disorders (SCIDs), Wiskott–Aldrich syndrome, ataxia-telangiectasia, and combined immunodeficiency syndrome. Combined immunodeficiency may also result from exposure to radiation, cytotoxic pharmacologic agents, and immune suppression (Moriber, 2014).

4. Etiology and pattern of infection include infection from all types of microorganisms (bacterial, fungal, viral, and protozoal). Infections are often severe and recurrent.

Severe Combined Immunodeficiency

A. *Pathophysiology.*

SCID has been linked to 13 mutations; almost half of those mutations are X-linked defects in the common gamma chain. In the other approximately 55% of patients, mutations are inherited in an autosomal recessive pattern (Moriber, 2014). The most common form of X-linked SCID is caused by a mutation in the IL2RG gene. This leads to defective T-lymphocyte differentiation and production. One of the most common forms of autosomal recessive SCID is adenosine deaminase (ADA) deficiency. This leads to accumulation of toxic purine metabolism, causing destruction of T cells and organ damage (Moriber, 2014).

B. *Clinical Presentation*

1. *History*

a. SCID is initially characterized by an unusual frequency of common infections, chronic diarrhea, and failure to thrive (Bonilla & Notarangelo, 2015).

b. Symptoms of SCID may be delayed by weeks to months because of the protection of maternal antibodies (Bonilla & Notarangelo, 2015).

2. *Physical Examination.* Infections are characteristic in terms of severity, recurrence (persistent in nature), type of organism, and location (common sites include the respiratory tract, mucous membranes, liver, GI tract, and blood). Oral candidiasis is resistant to therapy. Chronic diarrhea responds poorly to alterations in diet and may become life-threatening.

C. *Diagnostic Tests*

1. Peripheral blood lymphocyte phenotype will reveal the presence or absence of lymphocyte subsets (T, B, and NK cells).

2. Erythrocyte and leukocyte enzymes, such as ADA and nucleoside phosphorylase, are assessed to determine the cause of SCID. ADA is not detectable in ADA-deficiency SCID and will be normal in X-linked SCID.

3. Chest x-ray examination demonstrates a small or absent thymus.

D. Patient Care Management

1. *Preventive Care.* Pretransplant management includes isolation to prevent infection and meticulous skin and mucosal hygienic care. Patients must be monitored closely for indications of infection (fever may be the only sign). Antibiotics, antivirals, and antifungal agents are administered as appropriate. All RBC transfusions must be irradiated to prevent transfusion-related GVHD.

2. *Direct Care*

a. Stem cell transplantation is considered to be the first-line therapy for the treatment of SCID.

b. Immune reconstitution involves palliative enhancement of immune function. Intravenous immune serum globulin (IVIG) administration is used in severely ill children: 100 to 400 mg/kg via IV every 1 to 4 weeks.

c. Enzyme-replacement therapy involves injections of polyethylene glycol-conjugated bovine ADA each week. Although this option is often well tolerated and effective in improving immune function, immune reconstitution remains incomplete with this method (Bonilla & Notarangelo, 2015).

d. Gene therapy has yielded encouraging results to date, especially for patients who do not have an adequate HLA-matched donor for hematopoietic stem cell transplantation (Bonilla & Notarangelo, 2015).

3. *Supportive Care*

a. Infection can progress to sepsis, septic shock, and death (see discussion in Chapter 9) on septic shock.

b. Failure to thrive and malnutrition may require the use of parenteral nutrition.

c. The following increase the risk of these patients developing GVHD:

  i. Immunocompetent lymphocytes are transfused from the mother to the fetus or infant during gestation or delivery.

  ii. Nonirradiated blood products are administered.

d. Administration of live vaccines may result in an active infection; therefore, early identification and careful selection of which vaccines are administered is essential.

4. *Collaborative Diagnoses and Comorbidities*

a. Altered protection related to primary immunodeficiency

b. Potential for infection related to primary immunodeficiency, effects of prescribed medications, and malnutrition

c. Potential for hyperthermia due to infectious processes

d. Potential for impaired gas exchange related to pulmonary infections (e.g., PCP, other opportunistic infections)

e. Potential for fluid–volume deficit due to infectious processes, chronic and unresponsive diarrhea, and fever

f. Potential for altered nutrition that does not satisfy body requirements, related to frequent or chronic infectious processes, and chronic and unresponsive diarrhea

g. Potential altered growth and development related to prolonged or repeated illness or hospitalization

5. *Goals and Desired Patient Outcomes*

a. Augment or improve the child's immune system.

b. Protect from acquisition of infection (avoid live virus immunizations).

c. Detect, identify, and eradicate infections or neoplastic disease.

Acquired Immune Deficiency Syndrome

A. Definition and Etiology

HIV infection is the presence of the HIV, which causes a wide spectrum of disease and a varied clinical course.

1. AIDS is the portion of the HIV disease that represents the most advanced stage of the clinical spectrum and is considered a chronic illness today (U.S. Department of Health and Human Services [HHS], n.d.-a; Grossman, 2014a).

2. The incubation, or latency stage, is the period from HIV infection to clinical manifestations of the disease; shorter incubation periods in children with perinatally acquired HIV have been noted than for children or adults with other modes of transmission.

3. Incidence. The number of pediatric HIV infections has decreased since the implementation of maternal antiretroviral therapy during pregnancy.

   a. Estimated AIDS diagnoses (adjusted) in 2014 (Centers for Disease Control and Prevention [CDC], 2015):

   • Children younger than 13 years of age: 159 cases

   • Adolescents 13 to 14 years: 33 cases

   • Adolescents between 15 and 19 years: 1,664 cases

   • Young adults 20 to 24 years: 7,144 cases

   • In 2014, adolescents and young adults between 13 and 24 years of age accounted for more than 20% of new HIV diagnoses (CDC, 2015).

4. Mode of transmission. Children are most commonly infected by HIV through one of the following means:

   a. Transmission from mother to infant is the most common method of HIV contraction in children, accounting for approximately 90% of cases. This transmission may occur in utero, during the birthing process, or through ingestion of breast milk (Grossman, 2014a).

   b. General recommendations for an HIV-infected pregnant woman to take the same regimen as a nonpregnant adult have been made, noting that consideration of adverse effects on the woman, fetus, or infant and an assessment of benefits and risks must be included (HHS, n.d.-b). Currently, this includes zidovudine and additional antiretroviral therapies as indicated and evaluated as safe (Grossman, 2014a).

   c. Exposure to infected blood or blood products or sexual contact with an infected individual is a much less common method of infection in children and adolescents. Since blood screening was

initiated in 1985, transmission via blood products is no longer considered a transmission risk (Grossman, 2014a).

5. The classification of stages for HIV infection was revised in 2014 to create a single definition. Five stages (0, 1, 2, 3, or unknown) are used for surveillance staging of disease. Stages 1, 2, and 3 are based on an age-appropriate peripheral CD4+ T-lymphocyte count. Certain opportunistic infections are diagnostic of stage 3 disease regardless of the CD4 T-lymphocyte count, unless criteria for stage 0 are met (Selik et al., 2014).

B. Pathophysiology

1. HIV, a ribonucleic acid (RNA) retrovirus, causes AIDS. When a retrovirus infects a cell, the viral RNA is transcribed backward ("retro-") into the host DNA. The virus then uses the host cell's enzymes to direct the synthesis of new viral RNA and proteins to assemble new virus particles. The HIV interrupts normal cellular activity and function and ultimately causes the host cell to die, thereby releasing new virus into the circulation and infection of more host cells.

2. The principal, but not exclusive, target of the HIV is the CD4+ helper T lymphocyte, which orchestrates both CMI and HI. HIV causes the number and function of the helper T lymphocytes to decline, creating a decline in immune function and response and an imbalance in the ratio of helper T lymphocytes to suppressor or cytotoxic T lymphocytes (CD4–CD8). As the number of CD4 (helper T lymphocytes) declines, the patient becomes increasingly immunocompromised and at risk for opportunistic infection or malignancy. (Grossman, 2014a).

C. Clinical Presentation

1. *History*

   a. Initially, patients may be asymptomatic or develop viral symptoms similar to EBV or mononucleosis illness (Sterling & Chaisson, 2015).

   b. Patients may report symptoms including fever, fatigue, rash, headache, arthralgia, myalgia, night sweats, or GI disturbances with acute HIV infection (Grossman, 2014a).

   c. The most common presentations of children with HIV include failure to thrive, CNS abnormalities, and developmental delays (Grossman,

2014a). An additional complaint may include recurrent bacterial infections.

d. Infants born with HIV often weigh less and have shorter lengths (Grossman, 2014a).

2. *Physical Examination.* Physical examination may reveal oral candidiasis, chronic diarrhea, lymphadenopathy, hepatosplenomegaly, failure to thrive, eczematous rash, neurologic abnormalities (e.g., microcephaly, encephalopathy, dementia, developmental delay, loss of attained milestones), fever, and salivary gland (parotid) enlargement.

D. Diagnostic Tests

1. Virology assays, preferably HIV RNA and HIV DNA nucleic acid tests (NATs), must be used for the diagnosis of children younger than 18 months with a history of perinatal HIV exposure. HIV antibody tests should not be used in this population, as the sensitivity and specificity of this test in the first months of life is less than that of the virologic tests. (HHS, n.d.-b)

2. The timing of testing is dependent on risk factors such as exposure and risk for perinatal transmission.

3. Virologic diagnostic testing for infants with perinatal exposure is recommended at 14 to 21 days of life, 1 to 2 months of life (2–4 weeks after completion of antiretroviral prophylaxis), and 4 to 6 months. (HHS, n.d.-b)

4. Positive tests during the assessments described previously should be validated with an additional virologic test on a second specimen as soon as possible.

5. Definite negative testing is established when nonbreastfed infants test negative twice (initially at 1 month of age and a second at ≥4 months of age or two negative tests obtained at ≥6 months of age). (HHS, n.d.-b)

6. Children who are not exposed during the perinatal period or those exposed older than 24 months of age should be tested using HIV antibody tests. If infection is suspected, additional confirmation with NAT may be necessary to diagnose HIV.

7. HIV culture is not routinely used as part of diagnostic testing.

8. Monitoring of HIV infection involves assessment of the absolute CD4 lymphocyte count and plasma HIV RNA (viral load) upon diagnosis. In children who are not immediately started on antiretroviral

therapy, these levels should be monitored every 3 to 4 weeks. (HHS, n.d.-b)

9. Drug resistance testing, preferably with genotypic resistance testing, is recommended prior to therapy initiation for all treatment-naïve patients.

10. In children who do receive antiretroviral therapy, testing of the absolute CD4 lymphocyte count and viral load is recommended approximately 2 to 4 weeks after initiation of therapy to assess response and adherence. Routine assessment every 3 to 4 months for the first 2 years of therapy is also recommended.

11. After 2 to 3 years of demonstrated adherence, adequate CD4 counts, and stable clinical status, the frequency of CD4 count assessment can be decreased to every 6 to 12 months.

12. CBC may reveal anemia and thrombocytopenia.

13. Routine monitoring of CBC with differential, serum chemistries, and other diagnostic tests may be indicated by the type of antiretroviral therapy used or clinical status.

14. Lymph node biopsies often reveal marked follicular hyperplasia with an abundance of B cells.

E. Clinical Course

Clinical course and manifestations are very different from those manifested in adult patients. The course of the disease is more accelerated, with most children symptomatic before 2 years compared with 8 to 10 years for adults. The pattern of disease also varies with the age of the patient, with children experiencing a higher incidence of bacterial infections compared with adult patients, neurodevelopmental alterations (including developmental delay), failure to thrive, and different types of cancers rather than Kaposi sarcoma (e.g., lymphoma; Weinberg, 2000).

F. Patient Care Management

1. *Preventive Care*

a. HIV is present in many body fluids, including blood. Universal blood and body fluid precautions should be used for all patients, including those children who are HIV infected. Use gloves when handling any body secretions including blood, stool, vomitus, or nasogastric (NG) drainage or performing invasive procedures. Use barrier precautions or protective wear (gown and protective eyewear) to prevent skin and mucous membrane contamination. Hands should be washed following glove removal.

b. Parenteral exposure to infected blood by accidental needlestick injury is the overwhelming cause of HIV in healthcare workers (Havens & Committee on Pediatric AIDS, 2003). There is a decreased risk with the use of needleless systems, placement of needles and other "sharps" in puncture-resistant containers for disposal, and avoidance of recapping, bending, or removing needles from disposable syringes (Havens & Committee on Pediatric AIDS, 2003). It is important to report all exposures to an employee's occupational health department to be counseled on the risk of acquiring HIV and other blood-borne illnesses. In addition, postexposure prophylaxis (PEP) for HIV may be offered to the healthcare worker.

2. *Direct Care*

a. Suppress or inhibit viral replication and prevent the development or progression of immunodeficiency.

b. Combination therapy is warranted in the treatment of HIV due to its various effects on the stages of replication. The classes of current antiretroviral medications include the following (Grossman, 2014a):

i. Reverse transcriptase inhibitors. Inhibit replication of HIV by acting on the enzyme reverse transcriptase

ii. Protease inhibitors. Inhibition is achieved through binding to the protease enzyme, preventing cleavage into individual proteins

iii. Fusion/entry inhibitors. These stop the entrance and fusion of HIV with the CD4+ cell, blocking the insertion of HIV genetic information

iv. Integrase inhibitors. Prevent the HIV genome from integrating into the host's genome by blocking the integration step of the viral cycle

v. Multidrug combination products

c. Therapies are continuously investigated and developed. For the most up-to-date information, refer to aidsinfo.nih.gov/drugs.

d. Management of children with HIV/AIDS in the ICU varies with the reason for their admission. One common threat to children with HIV is respiratory failure secondary to PCP.

i. PCP is a major cause of early mortality in children with HIV, often occurring in the phases of disease with the peak age of onset between 3 and 6 months (Grossman, 2014a).

ii. PCP is considered a fungus based on DNA analysis, but also has biologic features of a protozoa. Transmission is likely airborne in nature (Mofenson et al., 2009).

iii. The greatest risk factor for PCP infection in HIV-infected patients is severe compromise, or a marked decrease in CD4 count and percentage.

iv. Signs and symptoms include fever, tachypnea, dyspnea, cough, respiratory distress, and hypoxia. Additional symptoms may include decreased oral intake, diarrhea, and weight loss. Auscultation may reveal bilateral basilar rales.

v. Chest x-ray may be unremarkable or may reveal perihilar infiltrates early in the disease course. Later in the disease course, diffuse parenchymal infiltrates with "ground-glass" appearance may be appreciated (Mofenson et al., 2009).

vi. Four clinical findings have been identified as independently associated with PCP in children with pneumonia: age younger than 6 months, tachypnea greater than 59 breaths per minute, arterial hemoglobin saturation less than or equal to 92%, and lack of emesis.

vii. Diagnostic findings. Definitive diagnosis is made when clinical symptoms are accompanied by evidence of the organism. Samples to accomplish this include sputum analysis, NG aspirates, washings via bronchoalveolar lavage, and open-lung biopsy (Mofenson et al., 2009).

viii. Prophylaxis for infants should be initiated within 4 to 6 weeks of age. Children should receive prophylaxis based on current recommendations that consider age and CD4 counts (Mofenson et al., 2009). The preferred medication for chemoprophylaxis is TMP–SMX; it is generally well tolerated, effective, affordable, and has a broad spectrum of antimicrobial activity. Current dosage recommendations are TMP dose 150 mg/m^2/d divided in two equal doses on 3 consecutive days each week (Mofenson et al., 2009). Alternative medication regimens may include Dapsone, Atovaquone, or aerosolized pentamidine (Mofenson et al., 2009). Prophylaxis may be discontinued when CD4 counts reach certain age-dependent levels (Mofenson et al., 2009).

ix. Treatment. Definitive treatment is aimed at eradicating the organism. First-line therapy is TMP–SMX dosed according to age and weight. Alternatives have been identified for adults with limited data in children, including intravenous pentamidine, atovaquone, dapsone/TMP, and clindamycin (Mofenson et al., 2009).

x. Use of a short course of steroids may prevent or suppress the inflammatory response and reduce pulmonary edema secondary to PCP when initiated within 72 hours of diagnosis in moderate to severe PCP (Mofenson et al., 2009).

xi. Supportive treatment is provided. Most patients require oxygen administration. Mechanical ventilation is indicated with respiratory failure if PaO_2 cannot be maintained at 60 mmHg or greater with inspired O_2 fraction of 50% or greater.

3. *Collaborative Diagnoses and Comorbidities*

a. Potential for infection related to the HIV/AIDS disease process, immunodeficiency, effects of prescribed medications, and malnutrition

b. Potential for impaired gas exchange related to pulmonary infections (e.g., PCP, other opportunistic infections)

c. Potential for fluid volume deficit as a result of chronic diarrhea and fever

d. Potential for altered nutrition that does not satisfy body requirements, related to the HIV/AIDS disease process, nausea, vomiting, diarrhea, and effects of prescribed medications

e. Potential neurologic status changes related to HIV/AIDS disease process

f. Potential altered parenting related to chronicity of diagnosis and critical illness

g. Potential for ineffective coping (parent, child, sibling) related to the chronicity of the disease, repeated hospitalizations, critical illness, death of a family member, or anxiety and fear of infection or stigma

h. Potential for transmission of the disease related to high-risk-taking behavior and lack of knowledge regarding mode of transmission

4. *Goals and Desired Patient Outcomes*

a. Suppress retroviral replication.

b. Augment or improve the child's immune system.

c. Detect, identify, and eradicate infections or neoplastic disease.

d. Educate the patient and family about viral transmission and ways to reduce exposures.

e. Counsel adolescents and young adults about high-risk behaviors and the dangers of viral transmission.

G. Impact of HIV on Other Organ Systems

1. *Respiratory System.* In addition to PCP, there is a risk for tuberculosis, bacterial sinusitis, bronchitis, otitis, and pneumonia secondary to *S. pneumoniae* and *Haemophilus. Pseudomonas aeruginosa* and *Staphylococcus* infections often occur more frequently in HIV-infected individuals (HHS Panel on Opportunistic Infections in HIV-Infected Adults and Adolescents, n.d.).

2. *Cardiovascular System.* Left ventricular dysfunction and cardiomyopathy are seen frequently by ECG, but are generally not clinically significant. These may be related to the occurrence of congestive heart failure and arrhythmias (Weinberg, 2000).

3. *CNS.* CNS complications in pediatric HIV are common. It is estimated that progressive encephalopathy occurs in about 20% to 40% of children with HIV infection (Weinberg, 2000). Cerebral atrophy and bilateral calcification of the basal ganglia and frontal white matter are commonly seen by neuroimaging (Weinberg, 2000).

4. Malignancies may also be increased in individuals with HIV (Grossman, 2014a).

5. *Recurrent Bacterial Infections.* Children with HIV are at risk for recurrent, invasive bacterial infections with organisms that include *S. pneumoniae, H. influenzae, and Salmonella* spp. (HHS Panel on Opportunistic Infections in HIV-Infected Adults and Adolescents, n.d.).

Secondary Immunodeficiency

A. A large percentage of children admitted to the ICU are immunocompromised as a result of an acquired defect in immune function.

B. Secondary immunodeficiency is caused by a variety of stressors, including, but not limited to anesthesia, tissue injury (e.g., surgery, trauma, thermal injuries), medications (see "Hematologic and Immunologic Monitoring" section), malignancy, and malnutrition (acute and chronic).

C. Although the pathophysiology of the defects in immune function differs slightly with each of the aforementioned stressors, the implications of these are the same as found in the "WBC Hypoactivity" section.

COAGULOPATHIES AND PLATELET DISORDERS

Disseminated Intravascular Coagulation

A. Definition and Etiology

1. DIC is a serious bleeding disorder resulting from activation of the coagulation sequence with a subsequent decrease in clotting factors and platelets, leading to uncontrolled bleeding (Grossman, 2014c).

2. DIC is not a primary disease or primary bleeding disorder. DIC is always a result of another disease or condition. It is often associated with shock, infections, hemolytic processes (such as transfusion of mismatched blood), and severe tissue damage (such as extensive burns or trauma, rejection of transplants, and postoperative damage, especially after extracorporeal circulation). Possible additional causes are neoplastic disorders (especially APL), septic shock, severe hypovolemic shock, and heat stroke (Grossman, 2014c; Wilson, 2015).

B. Pathophysiology

Coagulation mechanisms are abnormally stimulated.

1. *Clotting Component.* Widespread and rapid formation of fibrin thrombi in the microcirculation results in the consumption of certain clotting factors and platelets. The presence of fibrin thrombi in the microcirculation (microclots) leads to ischemic tissue injury. If significant microinfarction occurs, organ function is impaired, leading to brain, kidney, liver, or lung injury (Grossman, 2014c; Wilson, 2015).

2. *Hemorrhagic Component.* As the clots are lysed and clotting factors, fibrinogen, and platelets are consumed, blood loses its ability to clot (consumptive coagulopathy). A stable clot, therefore, cannot be formed at injury sites, thus predisposing to hemorrhage. Clotting factors and platelets cannot be made by the body as fast as they are used (Grossman, 2014c; Wilson, 2015).

C. Clinical Presentation

1. *History.* Two categories of symptoms occur; however, many patients may have laboratory evidence of DIC without clinical signs.

2. *Physical Examination*

a. *Clotting.* Symptoms include spontaneous, easy, or disproportionately severe bruising; intramuscular hematoma (spontaneous or trauma related); cool, mottled skin; pallor; and circulatory failure. Thrombosis of peripheral or central veins leads to absent popliteal, posterior tibial, or pedal pulses; cyanosis of fingers, toes, earlobes, or tip of the nose; and tissue necrosis and gangrene.

b. Bleeding in a patient with no previous bleeding history or out of proportion to the degree of thrombocytopenia is noted as a range from prolonged oozing from venipuncture sites and bleeding around intranasal, endotracheal, and urethral catheters to profuse hemorrhage from all orifices. Subtle to occult bleeding occurs. Systemic signs include the following:

  i. Skin. Petechiae, ecchymosis, purpura, and hematoma

  ii. Head. Gingival bleeding and epistaxis

  iii. Genitourinary. Hematuria

  iv. GI tract. Hematemesis and melena

  v. Neurologic. Headache and altered level of consciousness

  vi. Cardiovascular. Symptoms of shock

3. Diagnostic tests from invasive and noninvasive diagnostic studies. No single laboratory test confirms the diagnosis of DIC.

a. Platelet count is decreased in approximately 50% of patients, likely secondary to consumption (Wilson, 2015).

b. Coagulation tests (Wilson, 2015)

  i. PT is prolonged in approximately 50% to 60% of patients.

  ii. PTT is prolonged in approximately 50% to 60% of patients.

  iii. Fibrinogen level is decreased.

  iv. Fibrinogen degradation products (FDPs) and D-dimer are elevated.

v. Protein C, S, and antithrombin are markedly decreased.

vi. The most sensitive tests include prothrombin fragment 1.2 and thrombin–antithrombin (TAT) complexes, as they are markers of endogenous thrombin generation.

vii. A diagnostic scoring system for DIC that was proposed by the International Society on Thrombosis and Hemostasis is widely used in ICUs. This system assigns a score based on the assessment of platelet count, elevation of fibrin-related markers, prolonged PT, and fibrinogen levels. A score of 5 or more is considered compatible with overt DIC. The sensitivity and specificity of this system are estimated at greater than 90%; however, it can only be applied in children who have an identified underlying cause of DIC.

D. Patient Care Management

1. *Preventive Care.* Early detection and prompt management can prevent complications and death. Primary disorders associated with DIC must be treated.

2. *Direct Care*

a. Treatment of the underlying cause is essential in the treatment of DIC (Wilson, 2015).

b. If the symptoms of thrombosis or bleeding are mild, no specific therapy is needed. Begin specific treatments only when significant bleeding or organ dysfunction related to DIC occurs.

c. Administer blood products to replace coagulation factors in patients who are symptomatic; do not treat based on laboratory values alone. Provide platelet transfusions to maintain a goal level of $50,000/mm^3$. FFP provides clotting factors; large volumes may be required to correct coagulopathies. Cryoprecipitate provides needed fibrinogen and factor VIII. Use in addition to FFP or whole blood as needed. Goal fibrinogen concentrations should be greater than 1.5 g/L. Goal PT values are less than double the normal range (Wilson, 2015). Fresh whole blood is used if bleeding is profuse to supply all clotting factors and platelets. This will also serve as a volume expander and will increase the oxygen-carrying capacity by increasing the hemoglobin.

d. Supportive strategies to control bleeding with recombinant factor VIIa have been reported to be of benefit, but data is limited and reports are often anecdotal. Potential complications, including thrombotic adverse events, necessitate randomized controlled trials prior to this intervention becoming a recommendation (Wilson, 2015).

e. Heparin by continuous infusion has not yet been proven to be beneficial in controlled clinical trials. It may be reasonable to administer therapeutic doses in patients with chronic DIC, overt thromboembolism, and conditions of excessive fibrin deposition such as purpura fulminans (Wilson, 2015).

f. Provide normal perfusion by fluid replacement.

g. Improvement is reflected by increased fibrinogen concentrations and platelet count. Any increase in fibrinogen or platelet count is an encouraging indication that the consumption process has been interrupted and bleeding will be under control.

3. Complications are related to end-organ hypoxic or ischemic changes. Multifocal neurologic defects are due to multiple small brain infarcts. Thrombosis of blood vessels supplying the kidney cortex may result in renal failure. Pulmonary embolism and adult respiratory distress syndrome (ARDS) may occur. Acute ulceration and GI bleeding, intraabdominal bleeding, intrahepatic hemorrhage, and mesenteric thrombosis may occur.

4. *Collaborative Diagnoses and Comorbidities*

a. There is a potential for bleeding and hemorrhage.

i. Maintain mucous membrane and skin integrity.

ii. Monitor internal bleeding and control overt bleeding.

b. Patients are at risk for impaired cardiac output due to blood loss.

c. There is a potential for impaired gas exchange related to blood loss.

i. Maintain hemoglobin above 10 g/dL.

ii. Treat hypoxemia.

5. *Goals and Desired Patient Outcomes*

a. Correct the primary problem.

b. Perfuse vital organs until primary problem and DIC are controlled.

Immune Thrombocytopenic Purpura

A. Definition and Etiology

1. ITP occurs in about one in 10,000 children annually; it is the most common autoimmune disorder affecting a blood element (Wilson, 2015).

2. Two forms of ITP exist: acute and chronic. Acute ITP is usually self-limited and involves children younger than 10 years of age. It is often preceded by a viral infection or vaccination. Chronic ITP is persistent thrombocytopenia with a platelet count of less than 150,000 for greater than 6 months. Chronic ITP is associated with age older than 10 years, female gender, and insidious onset (Wilson, 2015).

3. Spontaneous recovery occurs with a normal platelet count within 4 to 8 weeks of diagnosis in approximately 50% of patients. Approximately two thirds of patients with ITP will recover their platelet count within 3 months of diagnosis. In patients with thrombocytopenia longer than 6 months, approximately one third will recover spontaneously (Wilson, 2015).

4. The peak age of diagnosis is 2 to 6 years old (Wilson, 2015).

B. Pathophysiology

1. The decreased platelet count is immune mediated, and *purpura* means bruises caused by bleeding into the skin.

2. The body develops antibodies against its own platelets. These antibodies coat the surface of the platelets and cause the immune system to see the platelet as "foreign" or "nonself" and destroy it. Antibodies directed against specific platelet antigens lead to platelet destruction. Bleeding may occur when platelets are less than 50,000/mm^3. The spleen is the site of antibody production and of destruction of sensitized platelets. Bone marrow produces platelets as rapidly as possible, but the platelets are quickly destroyed (in a few hours). Increased sequestration of platelets in the spleen further limits the availability of platelets to the circulation.

3. Exact cause is often not known; other possible causes of the thrombocytopenia must be ruled out, such as a toxin or drug exposure. Viral illnesses precede the onset of symptoms in most cases in children.

C. Clinical Presentation

1. *History.* The history of the child indicates previous good health; some report a recent viral illness. Seasonal fluctuation, with cases occurring more frequently in the spring, has been noted (Wilson, 2015).

2. *Physical Examination*

a. Patients present most commonly with petechiae and ecchymosis. Less common sites of bleeding include epistaxis, oral mucosa bleeding, hematuria, hematochezia, and melena. Adolescent females may experience menorrhagia (Wilson, 2015).

b. Symptoms, such as malaise, bone pain, and adenopathy, should alert the clinician to consider other diagnoses, such as leukemia (Wilson, 2015).

3. *Diagnostic Tests*

a. It is essential to exclude other causes of accelerated platelet destruction or decreased production of platelets by the bone marrow. Rule out leukemia, meningococcal meningitis, sepsis, systemic lupus erythematosus, and DIC.

b. CBC. Platelet count is decreased, approximately 80% of children will have counts below 20,000/μL.

c. PT and PTT are usually normal.

d. Bone marrow aspirate may be indicated depending on the type of therapy being considered (Wilson, 2015).

e. Differentiation from hemolytic–uremic syndrome (HUS)

i. HUS is a triad of hemolytic anemia, thrombocytopenia, and renal failure, all of which involve diffuse endothelial cell damage, activation of platelets, and widespread involvement of multiple organ systems.

ii. HUS is similar to ITP in that HUS is usually associated with infection or viral illness and that many children have bruising and petechiae from severe thrombocytopenia.

iii. HUS is different from ITP in that HUS is associated with oliguria or anuria with elevated blood urea nitrogen (BUN) and with neurologic symptoms such as seizures or coma.

iv. The average course of illness for HUS is 4 to 6 weeks.

4. *Complications.* Intracranial bleeding is the most serious complication, occurring in fewer than 1% of patients with ITP.

D. Patient Care Management

1. Acute ITP is usually self-limited with most pediatric patients recovering without treatment. Life-threatening bleeding occurs only rarely.

2. The American Society of Hematology has produced guidelines that recommend treatment with IVIG or a glucocorticoid in patients who have platelet counts less than 20,000/μL plus significant mucosal bleeding, or those with platelet counts less than 10,000/μL with minor purpura (Wilson, 2015).

3. Glucocorticoids are thought to be effective for ITP due to their inhibition of phagocytosis and antibody synthesis. They have also demonstrated improved platelet production and increased microvascular endothelial stability. Traditional regimens have used doses of 2 mg/kg/d of prednisone for a duration of 21 days. Side effects, including weight gain, fluid retention, cushingoid facial features, hyperglycemia, hypertension, emotional lability, growth retardation, avascular necrosis, and osteoporosis, should be considered (Wilson, 2015).

4. IVIG therapy has been shown to cause a rapid increase in platelet counts secondary to the inhibition of phagocytic activity. Total doses of 2 g/kg divided over 2 to 5 days have been used traditionally. The response seen often lasts only 2 to 4 weeks. Side effects, including nausea, headache, light-headedness, fever, and aseptic meningitis, should be considered (Wilson, 2015).

5. Splenectomy may be used in chronic ITP with high risk for hemorrhage. Due to the risk of sepsis, however, this treatment option is often delayed until at least 5 years of age (Wilson, 2015).

6. Immunosuppressive agents, including monoclonal antibodies (rituximab or alemtuzumab), have been anecdotally reported as effective. Other immunosuppressive agents, such as azathioprine, cyclophosphamide, tacrolimus, MMF, and vinca alkaloids, have been reported as effective for refractory or chronic ITP to varying extents (Wilson, 2015).

7. $Rh_o(D)$ is used for the treatment of chronic ITP in nonsplenectomized $Rh_o(D)$ antigen-positive patients. This is an alternative therapy for patients who are not eligible for splenectomy or other therapies (Wilson, 2015).

8. *Collaborative Diagnoses and Comorbidities*

   a. Potential for impaired skin and mucous membrane integrity

   b. Potential for hemorrhage

9. *Goals and Desired Patient Outcomes*

   a. Individualization of the treatment plan.

   b. Protection from sources of trauma. Parents should be taught to make the environment as safe as possible (bumper pads on the crib, avoid toys with sharp or hard surfaces). Older children should not play contact sports; restrict bicycle use.

   c. Avoid other platelet-damaging drugs such as aspirin.

   d. Control bleeding.

   e. Maintain adequate platelet count.

10. Patients with ITP may present to the PICU for life-threatening hemorrhage (such as intracranial hemorrhage) and will likely receive multimodal therapy with all or a combination of IVIG, anti-D, high-dose glucocorticoids, and platelet transfusions. Additional therapies that have been used in this clinical scenario include recombinant factor VIIa and emergent splenectomy (Wilson, 2015).

Heparin-Induced Thrombocytopenia

A. Definition and Etiology

1. HIT has a median platelet count of approximately 50,000/μL after 5 to 10 days of heparin therapy initiation. A rapid-onset pattern can occur if a patient has been exposed to heparin in the recent past (i.e., less than 100 days), with symptoms occurring within the first 24 hours of reexposure (Wilson, 2015).

2. Approximately 1% to 5% of adults on heparin therapy develop HIT. The complication is seen less in children and is practically nonexistent in neonates (Wilson, 2015).

3. Risk for development of HIT increases with therapeutic drug dosing, bovine products, and unfractionated forms of heparin (Wilson, 2015).

B. Pathophysiology

An immune reaction against a complex of heparin and platelet factor 4 (PF4). PF4 is a normal element in platelet granules that binds to heparin. This binding of antibody produces immune complexes that activate platelets and lead to thrombosis (Grossman, 2014c).

C. Clinical Presentation

1. *History.* An unexplained drop in platelet count should raise the suspicion of HIT.

2. *Physical Examination.* Signs of clotting (increased bruising, thrombus formation) or bleeding appear if the platelet count is extremely low.

3. *Diagnostic Tests.* Laboratory confirmation of heparin-PF4 antibodies along with clinical findings can confirm the diagnosis (Wilson, 2015).

D. Patient Care Management

1. Immediate discontinuation of heparin is necessary when HIT is diagnosed. (Grossman, 2014c; Wilson, 2015).

2. Alternative anticoagulation methods are necessary to prevent thrombosis recurrence; this may include synthetic antithrombin argatroban and synthetic pentasaccharide fondaparinux (Wilson, 2015).

PLASMA CLOTTING FACTOR DISORDER

Hemophilia

A. Definition and Etiology

1. Hemophilia is a disorder of hemostasis of one or more clotting factors.

2. Sex-linked recessive traits occur almost exclusively in males; female carriers transmit the disease. Of the severe bleeding disorders, hemophilia A and B are the most common (DiPaola, Montgomery, Cox Gill, & Flood, 2015; Taylor, Valentino, & Osborn, 2012).

3. In hemophilia A, inheritance of an abnormal gene results in decreased or absent factor VIII production. Hemophilia B is caused by a defective factor IX gene and deficient factor IX.

4. Hemophilia affects approximately one in 5,000 males; it is estimated that 80% to 85% of affected individuals have hemophilia A (DiPaola et al., 2015).

B. Pathophysiology

1. *Types*

a. Hemophilia A. Deficient in factor VIII; also called *classic hemophilia.*

b. Hemophilia B. Deficient in factor IX; also called *Christmas disease.*

2. Factor X activation is dependent on factors VIII and IX. When factor VIII or IX are absent, the ability to generate thrombin and fibrin is seriously compromised (DiPaola et al., 2015).

3. Formation of a normal clot at sites of bleeding is prevented. The degree of bleeding is related to the degree of factor deficiency. Hemophiliacs are susceptible to persistent bleeding or severe hematoma formation following relatively minor trauma. Severe hemophilia, defined as less than 1% of normal factor levels, is more likely to be associated with spontaneous bleeding (Taylor et al., 2012).

C. Clinical Presentation

1. *History*

a. About 30% of affected individuals do not have a family history of the disease (Grossman, 2014c).

b. Bleeding during circumcision occurs in approximately 30% of male infants with hemophilia (DiPaola et al., 2015).

2. *Physical Examination*

a. Bleeding can occur anywhere in the body following trauma or normal activity or occurs spontaneously.

b. Specific signs and symptoms include the following:

   i. Slow, persistent, and prolonged bleeding from minor injuries and small cuts

   ii. Uncontrollable hemorrhage subsequent to dental extraction or irritation of the gums

   iii. Epistaxis, especially after a facial injury

   iv. Hematuria

   v. Ecchymosis and subcutaneous hematomas (petechiae are rare)

   vi. Neurologic manifestations from bleeding near peripheral nerve leading to compression of the nerves

   vii. Bleeding into joints (hemarthrosis), which may lead to severe joint deformity, especially knees, ankles, and elbows; this causes permanent crippling

3. *Diagnostic Tests*

a. Hemophilia A

   i. Factor VIII assay. Decreased levels and increased PTT

      1) Less than 1% of normal level represents severe hemophilia. Child is at risk for spontaneous and trauma-induced hemorrhage from infancy.

2) When children have 2% to 5% of the normal level of factor VIII, they will likely experience a moderate clinical course. In the case of trauma or surgery, however, supportive treatment will be necessary.

3) Patients who have greater than 5% of the normal level of factor VIII will likely have a mild clinical course. These patients do not often require supportive treatment.

ii. Factor VIII activity levels should be assessed.

iii. CBC. Normal results are seen, including platelet count.

b. Hemophilia B

i. Factor IX assay. Decreased levels

1) Less than 1% of normal level represents a severe bleeding tendency.

2) One percent to 3% of normal level represents a moderate degree of bleeding tendency.

3) Five percent to 25% of normal level represents a mild degree of bleeding tendency.

4) Greater than 25% of normal level represents significant bleeding only in cases of trauma or surgery.

ii. PT is normal and PTT is prolonged (usually at least 60 seconds in children with severe deficiencies).

iii. CBC results are normal, including platelet count.

c. Radiographic findings. Major joint destruction following repeated hemorrhages.

D. Patient Care Management

1. Immediate evaluation and interventions as indicated are essential to high-quality care of children with hemophilia.

2. Decisions regarding prophylaxis and treatment in the event of bleeding are based on information about the patient's history, including response to therapy and presence of inhibitors, and the characteristics of pharmacological interventions, including half-life and volume of distribution.

3. *Hemophilia A Management* (DiPaola et al., 2015)

a. Prophylactic regimens may be used prior to any bleeding episodes or early in the course of a potential bleed depending on the center where the child is being treated.

b. Adequate management of mild to moderate hemorrhage requires a factor VIII level of 30 to 50 U/dL.

c. Desmopressin acetate (DDAVP) may be adequate for treatment in mild to moderate bleeding episodes.

d. For severe, life-threatening bleeding or preparation for surgery, it is necessary to restore the clotting factor level to normal (100–150 U/dL) in the acute phase and maintain a level of at least 50 to 60 U/dL for 5 to 7 days, followed by a maintenance program that maintains the level at 30 U/dL for 5 to 7 additional days. In cases such as this, factor VIII can be administered every 12 hours or via continuous infusion.

e. Recombinant products are preferred over plasma-derived products. A formula has been identified to calculate the dose of factor VIII.

Dose of factor VIII (in units) = U/dL of rise in plasma factor VIII required × body weight in kilograms × 0.5.

f. Routine bleeding episodes often require one to two doses of replacement factor to achieve adequate hemostasis.

g. The half-life of factor VIII is approximately 10 to 12 hours.

4. *Hemophilia B Management* (DiPaola et al., 2015)

a. Goal levels of factor IX are approximately 25 to 30 U/dL.

b. Recombinant products are preferred over plasma-derived products. A formula has been identified to calculate the dose of factor VIII:

Dose of factor IX (in units) = U/dL of rise in plasma factor VIII required × body weight in kilograms.

c. When using recombinant factor IX, the dose should be increased by 1.2- to 1.5-fold to ensure adequate recovery of levels.

d. The half-life of factor IX is longer than factor VIII, lasting approximately 18 to 24 hours, and increasing the interval of time between doses.

5. *Collaborative Diagnoses and Comorbidities*

a. Potential for hemorrhage related to deficiency of factor VIII or IX

i. Provide immediate and often repeated administration of factor VIII or IX, depending on the diagnosis. Only recombinant factor products should be used. Occasionally patients will develop inhibitors or antibodies to their factors. Other activated factor products may be indicated.

ii. Local control of hemarthrosis includes elastic wraps and ice packs to the affected limb to reduce swelling, bleeding, and pain. Elevation of the extremity, restriction of normal activity for 48 hours to prevent rebleeding, and pain control are important.

b. Potential for impaired skin and mucous membrane integrity

i. Prevent injury. Venipunctures should be done only in antecubital, external jugular, or other superficial veins. Hold pressure for a minimum of 15 minutes and avoid intramuscular injections. Counseling should include the appropriate level of activity for the child, including contact sports.

ii. Avoid NSAIDs and aspirin.

iii. Provide education to caregivers.

iv. Provide genetic counseling.

v. Teach how to recognize a bleeding episode, which measures should be done first, and how to differentiate between episodes that can be controlled at home and those that require hospital care.

6. *Goals and Desired Patient Outcomes*

a. *Restore normal clotting activity.* For mild hemorrhages, supplemental factor administration is needed to achieve specific levels (for hemophilia A and hemophilia B as described previously) to control bleeding. For major bleeding, correction to 100% activity is recommended.

b. Minimize tissue and joint damage.

c. Preparation for the child in need of surgery is administration of 80% to 100% of normal factor level. Keep the level above 30% to 50% during the postoperative course.

E. Complications

1. Hematoma formation, which can be large, results in compression of vital structures. Hematomas may produce fever, leukocytosis, severe pain, and hyperbilirubinemia as a result of RBC degradation.

2. *Progressive Arthropathy.* Inflammatory and hypertrophic changes occur in the synovial tissue. Over time, this results in erosion of cartilage and bone.

3. Intracranial bleeding associated with trauma may be related to subdural, epidural, intracerebral, subarachnoid, or rarely intraspinal sites.

4. Inhibitor to factor VIII or IX may develop.

ONCOLOGIC EMERGENCIES

Tumor Lysis Syndrome

A. Definition and Etiology

1. Tumor lysis syndrome (TLS) is the most common pediatric oncology emergency, characterized by metabolic derangements secondary to the release of intracellular contents from tumor cells into the bloodstream. The classic triad includes the following:

a. Hyperuricemia (most common finding)

b. Hyperkalemia

c. Hyperphosphatemia

2. TLS is most commonly associated with cancers that have high tumor burden, such as NHL, Burkitt lymphoma, and acute lymphoblastic leukemia (ALL; Mullen & Gratias, 2015).

3. Predictors of TLS include the following:

a. Bulky disease on diagnosis

b. Adenopathy

c. Hepatosplenomegaly

d. Leukocytosis

e. Elevated LDH

f. Renal impairment

4. The onset of TLS may occur at the onset of therapy initiation, or may precede diagnosis as cells lyse prior to treatment (Coiffier, Altman, Pui, Younes, & Cairo, 2008; Mullen & Gratias, 2015).

B. Pathophysiology

1. Massive cell lysis occurs in the setting of rapid proliferation, large tumor burden, and high chemosensitivity of cells.

2. Lysis leads to the release of intracellular contents, including intracellular anions, cations, and other breakdown products (Mullen & Gratias, 2015).

C. Clinical Presentation

1. *History*

a. The highest incidence of TLS has been reported in patients with NHL and B-cell ALL. Children and adolescents with acute myeloid leukemia (AML), chronic lymphocytic leukemia, and Hodgkin's lymphoma are also at risk, although these diseases are less commonly associated with the development of TLS.

b. Newly diagnosed patients should be thoroughly evaluated for TLS at the time of presentation and during initiation of cytotoxic therapy.

c. Evaluation of hydration status and kidney function is also essential in preventing further complications associated with TLS (Coiffier et al., 2008; Madden, 2012; Mullen & Gratias, 2015).

2. *Physical Examination*

a. Patients with TLS may complain of lethargy, nausea, anorexia, and muscle cramps.

b. Signs of TLS include diarrhea, vomiting, edema, fluid overload, and tetany.

c. Additional clinical manifestations may include cardiac arrhythmias (related to hyperkalemia), oliguria or anuria, and altered level of consciousness.

3. *Diagnostic Tests*

a. Routine, frequent monitoring of serum electrolytes with special emphasis on potassium, phosphorus, calcium, LDH, uric acid, BUN, and creatinine should be performed. These assessments are often required at least every 6 to 8 hours for at-risk patients.

b. According to Hande–Garrow definition, laboratory TLS involves the following electrolyte abnormalities within 4 days of the initiation of therapy (Mullen & Gratias, 2015):

   i.   Twenty-five percent increase from pretreatment values of potassium, uric acid, phosphate, or urea nitrogen

   ii. Twenty-five percent decrease in hypocalcemia

c. According to Hande–Garrow definition, clinical TLS involves laboratory TLS as described previously and at least one of the following (Mullen & Gratias, 2015):

   i.   Serum creatinine greater than 2.5 mg/dL

   ii. Serum potassium greater than 6.0 mmol/L

   iii. Serum calcium less than 6.0 mg/dL

   iv. Development of life-threatening arrhythmia or death

d. An additional definition, Cairo–Bishop provides a definition and grading classification of TLS based on the presence of laboratory TLS and an assessment of the degree of abnormalities in creatinine, the presence and need for intervention of cardiac arrhythmias, and presence and extent of seizure activity. This system includes assessment of laboratory values and clinical status for a longer duration, from 3 days prior to therapy initiation to 7 days from initiation (Coiffier et al., 2008).

e. ECG may be indicated for patients with hyperkalemia due to the risk of cardiac arrhythmia.

f. EEG may be necessary for patients who experience seizure activity.

D. Patient Care Management

1. It is important to remember that certain factors, including preexisting kidney impairment and dehydration, may exacerbate the effects of excess metabolites (Coiffer et al., 2008; Mullen & Gratias, 2015).

2. *Aggressive hydration* (once renal failure or oliguria are ruled out) is the most important intervention for children, as this will promote urinary excretion of uric acid and phosphorus and improve glomerular filtration.

3. The recommended fluid is 5% dextrose and an age-appropriate sodium chloride solution at two times maintenance, or 125 mL/m²/hr. Of note, the addition of sodium bicarbonate is not routinely recommended but may be considered in certain patient circumstances. Potassium should not be added to any fluids, given the risk of hyperkalemia with TLS (Coiffier et al., 2008)

4. Ensure adequate hydration is achieved by monitoring for urine output of at least 100 mL/m²/hr and urine specific gravity less than or equal to 1.010 (Coiffier et al., 2008).

5. *Treatment of hyperkalemia* (potassium >5.0 or trend in the upward direction) may involve several strategies (Coiffier et al., 2008):

a. Continuous cardiorespiratory monitoring for at-risk patients is indicated even in the setting of a normal baseline ECG, as the continued destruction of tumor cells may lead to hyperkalemia at various times during diagnosis and the initiation of therapy.

b. Sodium polystyrene solfonate (1 g/kg/dose) is indicated for moderate hyperkalemia (≥6.0 mmol/L without symptoms).

c. Albuterol nebulization is needed for severe hyperkalemia (≥7.0 mmol/L and/or symptomatic).

d. A bolus dose of insulin (0.1 unit/kg) with concurrent dextrose administration (400 mg/kg of glucose, ratio of 1 unit of insulin for every 4 g of glucose) is administered for severe hyperkalemia (Committee on Drugs, 1998).

e. Loop and thiazide diuretics may be useful for a transient decrease in hyperkalemia.

f. Stabilization of the cardiac membrane with calcium gluconate should be performed in patients with life-threatening arrhythmias secondary to hyperkalemia. Unless the patient is symptomatic with certain arrhythmias, calcium infusions should not be administered due to the risk of calcium phosphate or calcium carbonate precipitation in the setting of hyperphosphatemia and alkalization. This approach to hyperkalemia is unique; in most critical care cases, calcium should be administered as a priority intervention to stabilize the cardiac membrane (Mirrakhimov, Voore, Khan, & Ali, 2015).

g. Dialysis may be used when TLS persists despite the interventions described.

6. Treatment of hyperphosphatemia (phosphorus ≥5.0 mg/dL) may involve several therapies (Coiffier et al., 2008):

a. Oral phosphate binders, such as aluminum hydroxide, for initial treatment

b. Severe cases with impaired renal function may require hemodialysis, peritoneal dialysis, or continuous venovenous hemofiltration.

7. Treatment of hyperuricemia (uric acid ≥ 8.0 mg/dL or 25% increase from baseline) may be achieved through one of two recommended pharmacologic strategies (Coiffier et al., 2008):

a. Allopurinol may be administered IV or PO to inhibit the production of uric acid. It is important to note that this does not degrade uric acid that is present at the time of initiation; therefore, this is preferable for prophylaxis in medium-risk patients.

b. Recombinant urate oxidase (rasburicase) may be administered IV and is recommended for children with TLS or those considered to be high risk as it directly breaks down uric acid.

Hyperleukocytosis

A. Definition and Etiology

1. Hyperleukocytosis is a WBC count greater than 100,000 cells/mm³.

2. It has been reported that hyperleukocytosis occurs in approximately 5% to 20% of children with leukemia, most frequently in infant and T-cell ALL.

3. This oncologic emergency increases the risk of leukostasis and related complications.

4. Clinical leukostasis, the sludging of circulating blasts in the microvasculature, occurs most often in children with AML (Henry & Sung, 2015; Mullen & Gratias, 2015; Newman, 2012).

B. Pathophysiology

1. Although not fully understood, increased blood viscosity seems to contribute to leukostasis in the microvasculature. An additional complicating feature is the large size and limited deformability of blasts (Henry & Sung, 2015; Mullen & Gratias, 2015).

2. Adhesion molecules and the potential of leukemic blasts to promote their own adhesion to the endothelial lining may also contribute to the development of leukostasis, although this is being investigated.

C. Clinical Presentation

1. *Physical Examination*

a. Patients may be asymptomatic with hyperleukocytosis; however, clinical symptoms of leukostasis may evolve rapidly (Newman, 2012).

b. Symptoms are dependent on the microvasculature involved and may include the following:

i. Lungs. Tachypnea, hypoxia, dyspnea, acute respiratory disease syndrome, respiratory failure

ii. Neurologic symptoms. Headache, tinnitus, dizziness, ataxia, mental status changes, seizures, stroke

iii. Renal failure

iv. Priapism

v. Cardiac failure

vi. Dactylitis

2. Diagnostic tests include a CBC significant for greater than 100,000 WBCs/mm³.

D. Patient Care Management

1. The most important intervention to prevent or reduce complications is to rapidly reduce the number of WBCs through appropriate cytotoxic therapy per the oncology team (Henry & Sung, 2015; Mullen & Gratias, 2015; Newman, 2012).

a. For CNS disease, cranial radiation therapy may be indicated.

b. Patients with ALL may benefit from low-dose prednisone therapy to reduce hyperleuko-cytosis.

c. Hydroxyurea has been reported as effective in decreasing WBC and blast counts.

2. Aggressive hydration is indicated to promote blood flow and dilution of the hyperleukocytosis.

3. As described previously, the addition of urate oxalate decreases the risk for TLS, potentially decreasing the number of patients with acute hyperleukocytic leukemias who develop leukostasis. In addition, patients should be monitored closely for TLS.

4. It is unclear whether leukapheresis and exchange transfusion are indicated for patients with ALL and AML; these therapies are discouraged in APL (Henry & Sung, 2015; Mullen & Gratias, 2015).

5. Transfusions of RBCs should be minimized until the WBC is reduced due to potential complications of increased blood viscosity.

Superior Mediastinal Syndrome

A. Definition and Etiology

1. Space-occupying lesions in the anterior mediastinum and related complications are a commonly encountered pediatric oncologic emergency.

2. Complications of anterior mediastinal masses include superior vena cava syndrome, compression of the heart or pulmonary vessels, and tracheal compression. The phrase *superior mediastinal syndrome (SMS)* describes the secondary compression of the great vessels and tracheobronchial tree by an anterior mediastinal mass (Mullen & Gratias, 2015).

3. The most common malignancies associated with anterior mediastinal masses include NHL, ALL, Hodgkin's lymphoma, and neuroblastoma.

B. Pathophysiology

1. The anterior mediastinum is an anatomic component outlined by the sternum, thoracic inlet, and anterior border of the heart. The presence of a space-occupying lesion in that area may cause compression of the heart and pulmonary vasculature, great vessel (superior vena cava syndrome), and tracheobronchial tree.

2. Superior vena cava syndrome is the restricted blood return to the right atrium and impaired venous drainage from the head, neck, and upper extremities.

3. Tracheobronchial compression may cause respiratory compromise; this is especially relevant in children who have smaller, relatively compressible airways (Henry & Sung, 2015; Newman, 2012).

C. Clinical Presentation

1. *History*

a. Patients may present with varying degrees of respiratory distress such as cough or wheeze, facial/neck/upper airway edema, or altered mental status.

b. Respiratory symptoms are often worse in the supine position due to the pressure of the anterior mediastinal mass on the rest of the chest structures.

c. More severe cases may present with shock related to cardiac compromise or respiratory failure.

2. *Physical Examination*

a. Evidence of *airway obstruction.* cough, hoarseness, orthopnea, anxiety, cyanosis

b. Evidence of *cardiovascular compromise.* Venous engorgement of the face, neck, and upper extremities; syncope; and altered mental status (Henry & Sung, 2015)

3. *Diagnostic Tests*

a. Chest x-ray may demonstrate the presence of a mass. This diagnostic method may be better tolerated due to the various positions it can be obtained in and the brief duration of time required.

b. Chest CT is a valuable diagnostic tool; however, if the patient is not stable, the duration of time in the supine position or anesthesia required may be prohibitive of this study (Mullen & Gratias, 2015).

c. Echocardiogram will evaluate for pericardial effusion and superior vena cava obstruction.

d. Biopsy and pathology review of the tumor to confirm the diagnosis is valuable; however, lifesaving cytotoxic therapy should not be delayed until a diagnosis is established in critically ill patients. Analysis of pleural fluid may be diagnostic in patients with pleural effusion (Mullen & Gratias, 2015).

e. Bone marrow aspirate and biopsy may be diagnostic.

D. Patient Care Management

1. Patients with SMS are at great anesthetic risk. When possible, spontaneous respiration should be maintained to maintain muscle, airway, and chest wall tone. In addition, spontaneous respiration maintains the negative pressure of the chest (Mullen & Gratias, 2015).

2. Neuromuscular blockade agents should be avoided (Mullen & Gratias, 2015).

3. When patients require anesthesia, all caregivers should be notified of the risk for a difficult airway and close monitoring should be provided. Consideration of the physiologic processes may be offered prior to intubation and initiation of anesthesia.

4. Some patients may benefit when placed in the prone position to reduce the pressure of an anterior mediastinal mass.

5. Empiric therapy may be indicated as a lifesaving intervention if a diagnosis cannot be established. This is often accomplished using radiation, steroids, and combination chemotherapy (Mullen & Gratias, 2015).

6. When a diagnosis is established, appropriate treatment should be initiated per the pediatric oncology team.

Spinal Cord Compression

A. Definition and Etiology

1. Spinal cord compression affects approximately 3% to 5% of pediatric patients with cancer, and is most often diagnosed at the time of presentation (Mullen & Gratias, 2015).

2. The diagnoses of neuroblastoma, soft-tissue sarcomas, Ewing sarcoma, and rhabdomyosarcoma account for approximately 50% of tumors causing spinal cord compression (Mullen & Gratias, 2015).

B. Pathophysiology

Most tumors that cause spinal cord compression are extradural.

C. Clinical Presentation

1. *History.* Most patients who present with spinal cord compression will report *back pain*. It is important to investigate the description of pain, including duration, onset, relieving factors, and type of pain experienced.

2. *Physical Examination. Neurologic disturbances* may vary depending on the extent of compression.

Symptoms may include ataxia, gait disturbance, incontinence, decreased strength, reflexes, or sensory.

3. *Diagnostic Tests*

a. Spinal radiograph may reveal the presence of a compressive spinal region, often describing a paraspinal soft-tissue mass. Additional descriptions may include widening of interpeduncular distances, enlargement of the neural foramina, and lytic or sclerotic changes to adjacent bone.

b. MRI is the preferred method of evaluation if the radiograph is normal but concern for compression persists. It is also useful in detecting spinal cord compression, and can assist in the categorization of extradural, intradural–extramedullary, or intramedullary involvement (Henry & Sung, 2015).

D. Patient Care Management

1. The primary goal is immediate relief of compression as prevention of further neurologic loss of function and restoration of lost function are ideal outcomes of initial interventions. This may require multimodal therapy and should also strive to obtain tissue via biopsy to accurately diagnose the underlying condition.

2. Therapeutic interventions include the following:

a. Rapidly administer dexamethasone in the setting of high suspicion and neurologic dysfunction.

b. Oral steroids may be administered if no neurologic symptoms are present (Henry & Sung, 2015).

c. Perform surgical decompression via laminectomy.

d. Chemotherapy may reduce tumor burden and corresponding spinal cord compression. Most of the research in this modality has been in the setting of neuroblastoma or Ewing sarcoma (Mullen & Gratias, 2015).

e. Radiotherapy is effective against most pediatric tumors causing this complication. It is important to consider the side effects of radiotherapy, including stunted growth of the spinal column, scoliosis, and risk of secondary malignancies. The young child may also require anesthesia for the successful administration of radiotherapy over several doses (Henry & Sung, 2015; Mullen & Gratias, 2015).

HEMATOPOIETIC STEM CELL (BLOOD OR BONE MARROW) TRANSPLANTATION

A. Definition and Explanation of Terms

1. Hematopoietic stem cell transplantation (HSCT) involves the transplantation of pluripotential hematopoietic stem cells capable of self-renewal and terminal differentiation, giving rise to an entirely new hematopoietic system for the patient. The terms bone marrow transplant (BMT) and HSCT can be used interchangeably.

2. There are two types of HSCT

a. *Autologous transplant* uses stem cells from the patient's own marrow or peripheral blood. Stem cells are collected through an apheresis procedure in which the patient receives G-CSF (often during recovery from previous chemotherapy) to increase the level of CD34+ cells in peripheral circulation or a bone marrow harvest when marrow is aspirated (most often from the posterior superior iliac crests bilaterally) repeatedly. The stem cells are then processed and frozen to preserve viability of the cells. After high doses of chemotherapy and radiation to remove cancer cells from the patient's body, the stem cells are thawed and reinfused into the patient as a hematopoietic "rescue" from the marrow ablation secondary to high doses of chemotherapy.

b. *Allogeneic transplant* is the transplantation of cells from a nonself donor. This type of transplant is performed to correct congenital or acquired defects in marrow production, immune function, or a combination of the two. There are many sources of allogeneic stem cells:

   i. Bone marrow is obtained through a surgical procedure called a *bone marrow harvest*. The patient undergoes general anesthesia and marrow is extracted from the bilateral superior iliac crests. The volume aspirated from the patient is based on the donor weight and cell dose requested by the transplanting center.

   ii. Peripheral blood stem cells (PBSCs) are obtained through a peripheral blood apheresis procedure. Donors receive G-CSF therapy prior to the collection to increase the circulating CD34+ cells. The patient does not require sedation for this procedure but may experience side effects of G-CSF (as described previously in this chapter) or the anticoagulant from the pheresis circuit. In addition, if adequate IV access is not established

peripherally, placement of a temporary central catheter may be necessary.

   iii. Umbilical cord blood is donated at the time of delivery and cryopreserved for potential donation for HSCT transplantation.

3. Allogeneic donors may include the following:

a. *MSD.* This refers to a sibling who has demonstrated histocompatibility (perfectly matching [10/10] or near-perfect match [9/10] HLA antigens).

b. *Syngeneic transplant* uses stem cells taken from an identical twin that are reinfused into the ill twin. Usually there are few complications because of identical gene makeup. A less aggressive conditioning regimen is required because only removal of the tumor is needed, not ablation of the marrow to prevent graft rejection.

c. *Haploidentical family donor.* This often involves a parent or child of the recipient, a donor who is a half-match of measured HLA antigens. This type of transplant is of emerging interest due to the increased availability of suitable donors as a result of its use and improved technology and outcomes.

d. *MUD.* This refers to a volunteer donor from a bone marrow registry with histocompatibility (HLA antigens). In cases in which a perfect match is not available, a mismatched unrelated donor (MMUD) may also be identified (e.g., 7 out of 8 HLA match). At some centers, removal of the T lymphocytes from the marrow before reinfusing the marrow into the donor may minimize the incidence of GVHD.

e. *Umbilical cord blood* from an unrelated donor is administered.

4. *Indications.* HSCT is a primary therapy in the treatment of cancer, diseases that affect the immune and hematopoietic systems, and certain inherited diseases including (Diver, 2012; Haining, Duncan, El-haddad, & Lehmann, 2015):

a. *Malignancies*

   i. Autologous indications. Hodgkin's lymphoma, NHL, neuroblastoma, CNS tumors

   ii. Allogeneic indications. ALL (refractory, recurrent, high-risk diseases), AML (certain indications based on risk and response), chronic myelogenous leukemia (for patients refractory to tyrosine–kinase inhibitors), juvenile myelomonocytic leukemia (JMML), Hodgkin's lymphoma, NHL

b. Immunodeficiency disorders (allogeneic transplant). SCID, WAS, LAD

c. Hemoglobinopathies (allogeneic transplant) SCD, thalassemia, PNH

d. *Osteopetrosis*

e. Bone marrow failure syndromes (allogeneic transplant). Aplastic anemia, Fanconi anemia, dyskeratosis congenita, Diamond–Blackfan anemia

f. Lysosomal/perioxisomal diseases (allogeneic transplant). Mucopolysaccharoidosis (MPS 1: Hurler's syndrome), X-linked adrenoleukodystrophy (ALD), Krabbe disease, metachromatic leukodystrophy

g. Hemophagocytic lymphohistiocytosis (HLH)

5. Success of this treatment is related to the elimination of the underlying problem, prevention of rejection, prevention of GVHD, and appropriate control over the potential multi organ complications that occur in the weeks after transplant while waiting for the return of the transplanted bone marrow function.

B. Process of HSCT

1. *Evaluation.* HSCT candidates are evaluated for their underlying disease process and baseline organ function. Psychosocial evaluations are necessary to ensure that adequate support is mobilized to promote adherence with frequent monitoring, complex medication regimens, and continued follow-up for years posttransplant.

2. *Conditioning Regimens.* The conditioning, or preparative, regimen is used to prepare the patient for transplant. This requires eradication of malignancy for patients with cancer, administration of immunosuppression to prevent rejection, and therapy to induce marrow aplasia adequate for the underlying condition and type of transplant (Haining et al., 2015). This requires the use of chemotherapy, radiation therapy, and other immunosuppressive agents. There are varying degrees of preparative regimen intensity:

a. *Myeloablative regimen.* This strives to eliminate hematopoietic function of the marrow. Often indicated in malignancies for which eradication of disease remains a priority. Myeloablative regimens have traditionally used total body irradiation (TBI) or Busulfan; however, alternative regimens have also utilized agents, including cyclophosphamide, clofarabine, etoposide, fludarabine, and melphalan.

b. *Nonmyeloablative regimens.* Full myeloablation is not required in patients with impaired function at baseline or in those with immunodysfunction. To minimize toxicity in such situations, nonmeyloablative regimens have been designed and may include the same agents in lower doses or alternative pharmacologic agents.

3. *Infusion.* The donated stem cells are infused into the patient who has completed the conditioning regimen.

a. Marrow and PBSCs obtained from a donor are administered fresh whenever possible at a rate determined by the volume compared to recipient weight to prevent complications such as fluid overload. In addition to fluid overload, potential complications related to the transplant are similar to those described previously in this chapter.

b. Cryopreserved products, including autologous infusions and UCB, are administered rapidly, often within 30 minutes of thawing to preserve cellular viability. In addition to standard transfusion reactions, the recipient may experience side effects of the preservative in the product. When dimethyl sulfoxide (DMSO) is used as a preservative, it is important to ensure the daily dose administered is safe for the recipient's weight. It may be necessary to deliver the transplant over 2 days in such cases to prevent adverse events related to preservative toxicity.

c. One important concept unique to HSCT is the ability to administer ABO-incompatible blood products, as HSCT evaluates histocompatibility using HLA antigens. In the case of ABO-incompatible infusions, premedication and monitoring should be performed per institution protocols.

4. Engraftment is defined by an absolute neutrophil count of greater than 500 for 3 consecutive days.

a. The timing of engraftment is dependent on the type of HSCT and source of stem cells. Autologous products generally engraft before allogeneic transplants. Regarding stem cell source, PBSCs are the first to engraft, followed by marrow, and finally UCB. In order to be considered successful, engraftement must take place within 28 days for PBSCs and marrow, and 42 days for UCB products.

b. RBC and platelets recover after neutrophils. Engraftment of platelets is declared when the patient maintains minimum counts greater than 7 days posttransfusion.

c. Normal WBC count may return in a few weeks; however, effective function of the WBCs may take up to 1 year.

d. If the transplanted stem cells are of a different RBC type, close collaboration with the blood bank is needed to administer the appropriate products.

C. Posttransplant Management

1. Reconstitution of a near-normal immunologic status takes place progressively over a period that may last several months to more than 1 year following the SCT. The process is longer for allogeneic recipients than autologous recipients.

2. *Immunosuppression.* To prevent GVHD, patients are given immunosuppressive drugs (tacrolimus, mycophenolate mofetil, cyclosporine).

3. Supportive care is needed to manage electrolyte imbalances and nutritional deficits, deficient blood components, and infections.

a. Enteral nutrition, total parenteral nutrition, and fluid replacements may be needed.

b. RBC and platelet transfusions are administered to maintain patient-specific minimum values, which are determined by the underlying disease and comorbidities (e.g., patients with a history of surgical resection of CNS mass or active bleeding may require higher platelet thresholds). If an invasive procedure is planned, then the platelet count should be in the 50,000 to $100,000/mm^3$ range. Clotting factors should be replaced with appropriate blood products, such as FFP when the PT or PTT is prolonged, if the fibrinogen level is decreased, or if there is active bleeding.

c. G-CSF may be indicated in the posttransplant period to support engraftment. G-CSF should be avoided in certain malignancies.

d. Prophylactic antimicrobials often consist of antifungals, antivirals, and antibiotics. In the setting of fever, broad-spectrum, empiric antibiotics should be initiate immediately. Upon identification of organisms, antimicrobial therapy may be adjusted. Patients may remain on antibiotics until engraftment is achieved. Many prophylactic therapies will continue through the first 100 to 365 days of transplant, depending on the level of immunosuppression, presence of comorbidities, and other clinical factors.

e. Pain related to severe mucositis usually is effectively managed through the use of continuous narcotic infusions, often in the form of PCA.

f. Antiemetic therapies are required during administration of the conditioning regimen and often in the posttransplant period. Many children require multimodal therapy.

D. Acute Complications

1. *Infection* is the leading cause of morbidity and mortality in the posttransplantation patient.

a. For weeks after the transplant, these neutropenic and immunosuppressed patients are highly susceptible to bacterial, viral, and fungal infections despite aggressive antibiotic and antifungal therapy and protective environments. A routine strategy for prevention of infection is high-efficiency particle air (HEPA) filtered air and positive pressure rooms to decrease risk of fungal infections. Other requirements include strict handwashing techniques, meticulous central venous catheter care, prophylactic antibiotics, antivirals and antifungals, and daily mouth care. CMV-negative blood products are used if both the donor and recipient of the marrow are CMV-negative. Leukocyte-reduced blood products may also be used to decrease the risk of transfusion-related CMV infection (Haining et al., 2015).

b. Identification of the *signs and symptoms* of infection must be immediately followed by prompt and aggressive treatment to avoid septic shock and death. Signs and symptoms may be obscured in neutropenic patients. Therefore, all fevers are regarded as infectious in nature until proven otherwise (Henry & Sung, 2015).

c. Management includes antibiotics, antifungals, and antiviral agents.

2. *Hepatic Dysfunction.* Veno-occlusive disease (VOD) is usually observed approximately 10 to 20 days after chemotherapy (Haining et al., 2015).

a. *Definition and etiology.* VOD is a clinical syndrome characterized by hepatomegaly, right upper quadrant tenderness, hyperbilirubinemia, and fluid retention. It may occur after an allogeneic or autologous transplant. Some risk factors have been identified, including Busulfan-based chemotherapy regimens, prior intensive chemotherapy, use of TPN for more than 30 days, preexisting iron overload, and unrelated donor transplantation (Haining et al., 2015).

b. *Pathophysiology.* VOD is a complex process caused by damage to the endothelial cells and hepatocytes. Following this initial event, subendothelial edema occurs along with microthromboses, fibrin deposition, and expression of factor VIII and vWF within the venular walls, leading to decreased or obstructed blood flow. Later in the process, collagen deposits within the ventral lumens and contributes to the obliteration of lumens and hepatocyte necrosis. In severe cases, portal flow is reversed and hepatorenal syndrome may lead to MOSF (Haining et al., 2015; Richardson et al., 2013).

c. *Clinical presentation*

i. Physical examination. Patients may have fluid retention, tender hepatomegaly, hyperbilirubinemia, and pulmonary infiltrates or edema. Renal insufficiency may result from VOD thought to be related to portal hypertension (Haining et al., 2015).

ii. Diagnostic tests. Two criteria have been developed to diagnose VOD: (Richardson et al., 2013)

1) *Seattle criteria* require at least two of the following clinical features within the first 30 days of transplant: jaundice, painful hepatomegaly or ascites, and unexplained weight gain.

2) *Baltimore criteria* require a serum bilirubin greater than or equal to 2.0 mg/dL and at least two of the following: hepatomegaly, ascites, greater than or equal to 5% weight gain.

3) *Liver ultrasound with Doppler flow* may also be helpful in assessing the flow of blood through the portal vein. Early in the disease course, the ultrasound findings may be normal; therefore, repeated, daily imaging may be warranted (Haining et al., 2015).

4) *Evaluation of other causes* is necessary to distinguish VOD from processes such as sepsis, acute GVHD, medication hepatotoxicity, or portal vein thrombosis.

5) *Liver biopsy* is considered the gold standard for diagnosis; however, this procedure is difficult and the risks may be prohibitive in the setting of immunosuppression, coagulopathy, and clinical instability (Haining et al., 2015).

d. *Patient care management* (Haining et al., 2015; Richardson et al., 2013)

i. Supportive care continues to be the mainstay of treatment, including aggressive fluid management, maintenance of intravascular volume, adequate oxygen support, and transfusion support as indicated. Fluid management may require renal replacement therapy (Chima, Abulebda, & Jodele, 2013)

ii. Mild to moderate VOD may be self-limited. Severe or refractory VOD is associated with poor outcomes.

iii. Ursodeoxycholic acid has been used as a prophylactic strategy, although efficacy is unclear.

iv. Defibrotide, a polydeoxyribonucleotide, has been used prophylactically and as treatment for VOD with success reported in clinical trials, likely due to its antithrombotic and thrombolytic activity.

v. Other possible treatment may include high-dose corticosteroids (Chima et al., 2013).

3. *GI Tract Dysfunction*

a. *Definition and etiology.* Many HSCT patients suffer from a breakdown in the integrity of the mucosal defense system. This complication is increased in myeloablative regimens and in specific agents associated with greater toxicity.

b. *Pathophysiology.* GI dysfunction is caused by direct toxicity of chemotherapy and radiation, which provides a portal of entry for infection from the denuding of the epithelial lining of the entire GI tract mucosa.

c. *Clinical presentation*

i. Physical examination. Signs and symptoms include mucositis (inflammation of all mucous membranes, which is quite painful); nausea, vomiting, and diarrhea (hypovolemia and significant electrolyte imbalances); and hemorrhage from a site in the GI tract. It is important to note that patient may complain of pain, dysphagia, and anorexia secondary to mucositis even if the physical examination of their oral cavity is unremarkable.

ii. Diagnostic tests. Upper and lower GI scope procedures with biopsy may be used to evaluate the origin of mucositis (tissue biopsies may be sent for pathologic review for GVHD or infectious etiology) if the course does not improve upon engraftment and hematologic recovery, as expected.

d. *Patient care management*

i. Mucositis. Often peaks 10 to 14 days posttransplant, as the WBC count remains extremely low. The severity of swelling and pain is variable. Use appropriate antibiotics, meticulous oral hygiene, and aggressive pain control. In the absence of other complicating factors, such as infection or GVHD, inflammation will heal with neutrophil engraftment.

ii. Nausea and vomiting. Aggressive use of antiemetics, especially in combinations individualized to patient response, is indicated.

iii. Diarrhea. Maintain fluid and electrolyte balance, evaluate infection to ensure additional therapies are not warranted, provide symptomatic relief, and protect the skin in the rectal area from severe excoriation and breakdown.

iv. Hemorrhage. Maintain hemodynamic stability and find and treat the source; angiography and surgery may or may not be performed, depending on the determination of the risks compared with the benefits.

4. *Renal Dysfunction*

a. Renal dysfunction is a frequently seen complication and is caused by toxicities of chemotherapy, antibiotics, antifungals, and other pharmacologic agents and is aggravated by any prerenal problems, such as decreased renal perfusion from hypovolemia or obstructive uropathy secondary to clots and hematuria noted in BK viruria.

b. Up to 50% of HSCT recipients will have evidence of an acute kidney injury and 5% to 20% may develop chronic kidney disease (Chima et al., 2013).

c. Diagnosis, signs and symptoms, and laboratory results are detailed in the renal system (see Chapter 5).

d. Specific differences regarding renal dysfunction in the HSCT patient include the following:

i. Hyperkalemia may or may not occur.

ii. Hypokalemia frequently occurs, often requiring IV potassium replacement. In patients receiving CSA or amphotericin B, potassium continues to be wasted in the urine unless the patient becomes anuric.

iii. Increased BUN is difficult to interpret, as it is influenced by processes other than decreased glomerular filtration rate. Steroids and the presence of blood in the GI tract can significantly increase BUN without any alteration in renal function.

e. Hemofiltration or dialysis is occasionally required to correct life-threatening electrolyte imbalances, eliminate waste products, and restore fluid balance.

5. Pulmonary complications may have acute or late onset and lead to higher mortality in HSCT when compared to patients who do not develop these complications. Pulmonary complications posttransplant involve a broad spectrum of processes, as briefly described in the following section, and may follow autologous or allogeneic transplantation (Haining et al., 2015).

a. *Definition and etiology.* Acute lung injury is a common indication for admission of the HSCT to the ICU. Risk factors for pulmonary complications include preexisting lung dysfunction related to previous chemotherapy, infection, previous surgical procedures involving the lung, use of radiotherapy, and presence of GVHD (Haining et al., 2015). Pulmonary complications posttransplant involve a broad spectrum of processes, as briefly described in the following section, and may follow autologous or allogeneic transplantation (Chima et al., 2013; Haining et al., 2015).

i. *Idiopathic pneumonia syndrome (IPS)* is an acute complication that may be fatal. Patients have evidence of respiratory compromise including hypoxia and radiographic imaging will demonstrate a diffuse infiltrate unrelated to fluid overload, infection, renal failure, or cardiac dysfunction (Haining et al., 2015).

ii. *Diffuse alveolar hemorrhage (DAH)* is an acute complication that often presents in the first 1 to 3 months posttransplant with cough, shortness of breath, and hypoxemia. Although frank hemoptysis is rare, diagnosis is made based on increasingly bloody bronchoalveolar fluids. Radiographic imaging will reveal diffuse infiltrates, typically noted centrally (Haining et al., 2015).

iii. *Bronchiolitis obliterans syndrome (BOS)* is an obstructive syndrome that leads to obliteration of the small airways. Chest radiograph will demonstrate hyperinflation secondary to the obstruction and CT will demonstrate ground-glass appearance and bronchiectasis.

iv. *Bronchiolitis obliterans organizing pneumonia (BOOP)*, or *cryptogenic organizing pneumonia (COP)*, is a late complication that indicates the presence of granulation tissue within the alveolar ducts and alveoli. The onset may be as slow as 2 years posttransplant. Chest CT will demonstrate patchy airspace disease and a ground-glass appearance.

b. *Pathophysiology.* The processes involved are dependent on the type of pulmonary complication. The pulmonary parenchyma is injured in interstitial pneumonitis and ARDS. Periengraftment respiratory distress syndrome and DAH involve the pulmonary vascular endothelium. BOOP and BOS involve the airway epithelium (Chima et al., 2013; Haining et al., 2015).

c. *Clinical presentation* (Chima et al., 2013; Haining et al., 2015)

   i.   Physical examination. Signs and symptoms vary depending on the underlying process and site of tissue injury, but may include fever, cough, dyspnea, hypoxemia, hemoptysis, tachypnea, and reduced forced vital capacity (FVC) and forced expiratory volume in the first second of exhalation (FEV$_1$).

   ii.   Diagnostic tests. See Chapter 2 for more information on pulmonary diagnostic tests.

   1) Chest radiograph is easy to obtain and provides valuable diagnostic information early in the setting of respiratory compromise.

   2) Chest CT will provide more specific information when it can be performed safely.

   3) Echocardiogram is useful in the diagnosis of pulmonary hypertension.

   4) Bronchoalveolar lavage (BAL) is useful in the identification and diagnosis of infectious organisms and evaluation of aspirates.

   5) Open lung biopsy may be indicated for focal processes.

   6) Pulmonary function tests will assist in the identification of restrictive and obstructive lung disease.

d. *Patient care management* (Chima et al., 2013; Haining et al., 2015)

   i.   Treatment is dependent on the underlying pathophysiology and also involves supportive care in the form of broad-spectrum antimicrobial coverage, assessment of fluid status, supplemental oxygen therapy, and mechanical ventilation (invasive and noninvasive) as indicated.

   ii.   Initial treatment for many noninfectious complications may include *systemic* corticosteroids. This pharmacologic intervention has been effective in conditions with inflammatory or immune processes, such as DAH, BOOP, and IPS. Of note, BOS has not responded as well to corticosteroids as BOOP.

   iii.   *Azithromycin* has been reported to be a useful adjunct in some patients with BOS.

   iv.   Additional immunosuppressive agents, including tumor necrosis factor (TNF)-α blockers (etanercept), have also been used. Specific pharmacologic interventions based on the underlying physiologic processes are being evaluated to improve the management of posttransplant pulmonary complications.

6. *Cardiac Complications*

   a. *Definition and etiology.* Cardiac complications are caused by cancer therapy, especially anthracyclines, cyclophosphamide, or radiation to the chest administered as as part of the conditioning regimen or given before SCT.

   b. *Pathophysiology.* Heart failure often leads to pulmonary edema. This results from a loss of myocardial fibrils, mitochondrial changes, and cellular degeneration; chronic changes, such as fibrosis, are common. Cardiac complications may occur early in the post-SCT period.

   c. *Clinical presentation*

   i.   Physical examination. Signs and symptoms include weight gain, peripheral edema, tachycardia, dyspnea on exertion, orthopnea, rales, and rhonchi.

   ii.   Diagnostic tests. Echocardiogram is used to measure shortening or ejection fractions.

   d. *Patient care management.* Patients may continue to deteriorate, as chronic and cumulative damage is usually irreversible. Treatment is limited to supportive measures, including precise fluid management, judicious use of diuretics and inotropic agents, use of pharmacologic agents to promote effective contractility, maintaining comfort, and decreasing myocardial oxygen consumption and stress.

7. Hemorrhagic cystitis causes significant morbidity for the SCT patient.

   a. *Definition and etiology.* Cystitis is caused by bladder toxicity from chemotherapy, most often associated with cyclophosphamide.

   b. *Pathophysiology.* A metabolite produces ulceration of the bladder mucosal tissue. Small vessels in the underlying tissue hemorrhage into the bladder. Viruses of the bladder mucosa, specifically BK virus, may also cause hematuria.

   c. *Clinical presentation*

      i.   Physical examination. Signs and symptoms include red-tinged urine with clots, dysuria or frequency of urination, and symptoms of urethral obstruction from clots such as pain. This can lead to postrenal failure if not corrected.

      ii. Diagnostic tests

         1) Urinalysis will detect the presence of hematuria and other products in the urine.

         2) Bladder ultrasound indicates the presence of clots or thickened bladder wall.

         3) Infectious studies to evaluate for viral and bacterial organisms are also helpful in diagnosis.

   d. *Patient care management*

      1) Mild cases respond to aggressive hydration with resolution in 1 to 2 days.

      2) Severe cases may require continuous bladder irrigation with a three-way Foley catheter or administration of anti-infectives intravesicularly.

      3) Platelets are used to maintain platelet counts at higher than 20,000/mm^3 for a child who is not bleeding or higher than 50,000/mm^3 for a child who is bleeding.

      4) Cystoscopy is used to cauterize the bleeding ulcerative areas; it is usually not a long-term solution because of the diffuse widespread area affected.

8. *Acute GVHD*

   a. *Definition and etiology.* Acute GVHD represents a rejection interaction between recipient tissues and donor T lymphocytes. It predominantly involves the skin, GI tract, and the liver. It is rare for GVHD to occur in syngeneic or autologous transplants. There is increased risk with partially matched allogenic transplants. GVHD is reported almost exclusively in the allogeneic transplant setting, although there are rare reports of GVHD in autologous transplantation. GVHD is a significant cause of morbidity and mortality in allogeneic transplants.

   b. *Pathophysiology.* Acute GVHD results from histocompatibility differences between the donor cells (graft) and the recipient (host). The effector mechanisms and release of inflammatory mediators that result from T cells leads to tissue damage. This tissue damage is exacerbated by preexisting compromise of the tissues (related to the conditioning regimen or other immunologic events). Further damage then results from release of cytokines in response to immune events and inflammation (Haining et al., 2015).

   c. *Clinical presentation*

      i.   Physical examination. Signs and symptoms are not always immediately recognized because symptoms may mimic other problems such as infection, VOD, hepatitis, and toxic effects of chemotherapy. Organ-specific manifestations include the following:

         1) Skin GVHD. Onset of a maculopapular skin rash initially involving the palms and soles and later progressing centrally may cause intense pruritus and progress to bullous lesions and ulceration. Skin GVHD occurs at or near the time of WBC engraftment. The stage of skin GVHD is assigned according to the percentage of body surface involved. Desquamation and bullae indicate stage 4 disease.

         2) Gastrointestinal GVHD. Nausea; vomiting; abdominal cramping; anorexia; paralytic ileus; green and watery, and heme-negative diarrhea. Later, heme-positive diarrhea occurs as more of the intestinal mucosa begins to slough. Hypoalbuminemia is noted. The stage of GI GVHD is based on the volume of diarrhea output daily, either in mL/kg or mL/m^2 in children. A daily average of output calculated over 3 days is generally used to assign a stage. The presence of severe pain and ileus indicates stage 4 disease.

         3) Liver GVHD. Right upper quadrant pain, hepatomegaly, jaundice, ascites (rare), elevated liver enzymes, and bilirubin occur. The stage of liver GVHD is based on the total bilirubin level.

         4) The degree of organ system involvement is graded from I to IV, based on

a combination of three organ-specific stages. Higher grade indicates more severe disease.

ii. Diagnostic tests. Diagnosis is made by biopsy of the skin or rectal or liver tissue. If biopsy is not possible or the patient is not stable, clinical diagnosis is adequate to initiate therapy.

d. *Patient care management*

i. Prophylaxis. Morbidity and mortality are lessened by prevention rather than treatment of established GVHD. Interventions include selection of histocompatible donors, immunosuppressive therapy as described previously in this chapter, and removal of T cells from the donor marrow before transplantation (associated with a risk of engraftment failure). Irradiation of all blood products before transfusion results in the inactivation of T lymphocytes, whereas adequate platelet and RBC function is maintained.

ii. Treatment of acute GVHD includes corticosteroids (first line), topical or system-specific therapies, and other forms of immunosuppression as described previously in this chapter. Various combinations are warranted depending on the organ systems involved and other factors such as presence of infection underlying indication for transplantation; investigations of such therapies are ongoing. There is no standard for second-line therapy. Complications, including death, of infections remain a significant threat to the long-term survival of immunocompromised patients with GVHD.

iii. Assess early clinical manifestations of GVHD. Distinguish GVHD from other complications such as antibiotic or chemotherapy reactions, irritated bowel, infections, and radiation toxicity.

iv. Appropriate skin care will provide comfort and reduce the risk of infection. Low air-loss beds decrease discomfort of pressure points and may facilitate exudate absorption. In addition to topical immunosuppressants, gentle moisturizes are recommended. Provide pain-control measures for the pain associated with skin desquamation.

v. Provide measures to resolve the GI tract effects of GVHD. Watch for hypovolemia and shock through strict monitoring of intake and output, daily weights, and assessment of electrolytes. The patient may need to be

NPO to provide gut rest and reduce further gut activation of the GVHD. Clean the perineal area and soothe irritated skin. Assess for rectal lesions. Assessment should evaluate for the presence of GI tract bleeding.

vi. Careful attention to pharmacologic agents that may compromise organ function in the setting of GVHD is warranted to prevent further complications.

vii. Increased infection prophylaxis may be required for patients with acute GVHD and increased levels of immunosuppression. An example of this is the need to increase antifungal prophylaxis in the setting of high-dose steroids to provide prophylaxis for *Aspergillus*. In addition, a high index of suspicion should be exercised with evidence of infection, as patients may not mount an adequate response and display classic symptoms. Risk of rapid deterioration and mortality secondary to infection is high in such patients.

9. *Chronic GVHD*

a. *Definiton and etiology.* Chronic GVHD typically occurs beyond 100 days; however, it is increasingly defined by the presentation rather than the time frame it presents. Chronic GVHD is disabling and potentially life-threatening. Risk factors include HLA-mismatched transplants, older patient or donor age, use of female donors for male recipients, and is associated with higher morbidity and mortality in patients who have progressive disease after acute GVHD.

b. *Pathophysiology.* Although not completely understood, it seems that donor T-cells recognize minor histocompatibility antigens or lose peripheral T-cell tolerance. Chronic GVHD manifests similar to autoimmune disorders (Haining et al., 2015).

c. *Clinical presentation*

i. Physical examination. Signs and symptoms vary by the organ system involved, often resemble autoimmune systemic collagen vascular diseases, and may include the following:

1) Skin. Lichen planus, hypo/hyperpigmentation, erythema, dryness, scleradermatous changes that may limit range of motion (Haining et al., 2015)

2) Ocular. Dry eyes, photophobia

3) Oral. Dry mouth, leukoplakia, depapillation or scalloping of the tongue, lichen planus-like lesions

4) Liver. Obstructive jaundice, bridging necrosis, cirrhosis

5) GI system. Anorexia, malabsorption, weight loss, diarrhea, nausea, vomiting

6) Musculoskeletal system. Myositis and tendonitis lead to progressive joint involvement and limited range of motion

7) Pulmonary. Obstructive lung disease progressive to bronchiolitis obliterans

8) Immune system. Persistent immunodeficiency with profound depression of B and T-cell function

9) Staging is based on the degree of organ involvement and characterizes limited disease as that involving localized area of the skin or hepatic dysfunction; extensive disease indicates generalized skin involvement of limited manifestations in addition to other system involvement; work to clarify the grading and staging of chronic GVHD is ongoing

ii. Diagnostic tests. Chronic GVHD diagnosis can be made based on clinical manifestations. Biopsy of involved tissues will also confirm the diagnosis.

d. *Patient care management* requires the support of many specialists as part of an interprofessional team. Corticosteroids are the first-line therapy. As with acute GVHD, no standard regimen has been developed for steroid-refractory cases. Additional therapeutic options that have been evaluated include extracorporeal photopheresis, immunosuppression through the use of monoclonal antibodies (such as rituximab), mycophenolic acid, rapamycin, and pentostatin. Efforts to improve the treatment of chronic GVHD and reduce toxicities, morbidity, and mortality are ongoing (Haining et al., 2015).

i. The pathophysiology and treatment of chronic GVHD causes significant immune dysfunction and increases the risk of serious infection and death as well as organ toxicity. Infection prophylaxis is indicated based on the degree of immunosuppression and diligent monitoring should evaluate for evidence of infection.

ii. Patients with immune dysfunction related to their GVHD may have reduced IgG2 and IgG4, decreased mucosal IgA, and functional asplenia. This predisposes them to infection with encapsulated organisms, viral reactivation (such as varicella-zoster and herpes simplex), PCP, and chronic infections (such as sinusitis, bronchitis, and conjunctivitis; Haining et al., 2015). Prophylaxis for PJP as described earlier is indicated. Penicillin VK as prophylaxis for encapsulated organisms in the setting of functional asplenia may also be indicated in patients with chronic GVHD (Haining et al., 2015).

CASE STUDIES WITH QUESTIONS, ANSWERS, AND RATIONALES

Case Study 8.1

Eleven-year-old Ethan was admitted to the PICU for metabolic derangements consistent with tumor lysis syndrome secondary to newly diagnosed cancer.

1. Which of the following diagnoses is most likely for Ethan?

A. Neuroblastoma

B. Hodgkin's lymphoma

C. Burkitt lymphoma (non-Hodgkin's lymphoma [NHL])

D. Chronic myelogenous leukemia

2. As you review Ethan's labs, you would expect all of the following EXCEPT:

A. Hyperuricemia

B. Hyperkalemia

C. Hyperphosphatemia

D. Hypermagnesemia

3. You know that which of the following interventions would be indicated for Ethan?

A. Pharmacologic agents for hyperuricemia, such as rasburicase

B. Initiation of continuous cardiorespiratory monitoring

C. Administration of aggressive hydration via intravenous fluids and close monitoring of urine output

D. B and C only

E. All of the above

4. An ECG obtained on Ethan for hyperkalemia of 7.2 mmol/L reveals peaked T-waves. The most important, immediate intervention is

A. Nebulized albuterol

B. IV administration of calcium gluconate

C. A bolus of insulin and dextrose 25% infusion

D. Oral allopurinol

Case Study 8.2

Seventeen-year-old Latoya was diagnosed with severe aplastic anemia and is currently awaiting the HLA typing of her siblings to determine whether or not she will proceed with MSD HSCT. During this time, she is receiving supportive care and requires a transfusion of PRBCs today. During the transfusion, she becomes febrile to 39.2°C and reports new-onset headache. She does not have any evidence of respiratory distress or hemodynamic instability, but you note chills and a couple of mild urticarial lesions.

1. You suspect that Latoya is experiencing which of the following transfusion reactions?
   A. Nonhemolytic reaction
   B. Anaphylaxis
   C. Acute hemolytic reaction
   D. Transfusion associated circulatory overload

2. Your immediate intervention for Latoya is
   A. Obtain blood to send to the blood bank for laboratory evaluation
   B. Stop the transfusion and administer 0.9 NaCl to maintain patency of the IV
   C. Administer intramuscular epinephrine
   D. Slow the rate of infusion while administering an antipyretic and antihistamine

Answers and Rationales

Case Study 8.1

1. **C.** Malignancies with bulky disease and high growth rates are at the highest risk for TLS. TLS in solid tumors, such as neuroblastoma and Hodgkin's lymphoma, is rare. Although acute lymphoblastic leukemia (ALL) may be associated with TLS, the risk of chronic myeloid leukemia (CML) causing TLS is less.

2. **D.** The breakdown of tumor cells leads to the release of intracellular contents into the circulating blood stream, causing hyperuricemia, hyperkalemia, and hyperphosphatemia. Hypocalcemia may also be observed. Derangements of magnesium are not associated with TLS.

3. **E.** All of the interventions listed earlier would be appropriate for a patient, such as Ethan, who is admitted to the PICU with TLS. Rasburicase breaks down uric acid that accumulates during cell lysis. Cardiorespiratory monitoring should be observed continuously, as continued breakdown of tumor cells secondary to spontaneous lysis or initiation of therapy may lead to hyperkalemia. Aggressive hydration promotes urinary flow, leading to excretion of uric acid and phosphorus. Patients should be monitored to ensure their cardiac and kidney functions tolerate the aggressive hydration.

4. **B.** Administration of calcium gluconate is reserved for symptomatic patients with severe hyperkalemia only. Calcium gluconate is utilized to stabilize the cardiac membrane and would be the most critical, immediate intervention for Ethan. Nebulized albuterol and insulin/dextrose would all be effective in reducing the hyperkalemia in Ethan; however, they will take time to act and will not address the emergency of potentially fatal cardiac arrhythmia. Administration of sodium polystyrene sulphonate and sodium bicarbonate may also be effective in reducing the serum potassium. Oral allopurinol is effective in decreasing the production of uric acid during tumor cell lysis.

Case Study 8.2

1. **A.** The description of fever, chills, urticaria, and headache are consistent with a nonhemolytic transfusion reaction. If Latoya was experiencing anaphylaxis, you would expect to see respiratory distress in the form of bronchospasm, cough, or difficulty breathing. In addition, patients may experience involvement of their skin (urticaria), hemodynamic instability (hypotension), and GI disturbances (vomiting). Acute hemolytic reactions produce fever, chills, the classic sign of lumbar pain, shock, dyspnea, anxiety, chest pain, and restlessness as a response to hemolysis secondary to ABO incompatibility. TACO may present as respiratory distress secondary to fluid overload and pulmonary edema.

2. **B.** The most important intervention is to stop the transfusion that is causing the described reaction. It may be necessary to send specimens to the blood bank for evaluation, but immediate stabilization of the patient is a priority. Intramuscular epinephrine is indicated in anaphylaxis. Although it may be possible to complete the infusion after administration of an antipyretic and antihistamine, the transfusion should be stopped until those medications can be administered and symptoms subside.

REFERENCES

American Association of Blood Banks, American Red Cross, America's Blood Centers, & Armed Services Blood Program. (2017). Circular of information for the use of human blood and blood components. Retrieved from https://www.aabb.org/tm/coi/Documents/coi1017.pdf

American College of Chest Physicians/Society of Critical Care Medicine Consensus Conference: Definitions for Sepsis and Organ Failure and Guidelines for the Use of Innovative Therapies in Sepsis. (1992). *Critical Care Medicine, 20*(6), 864–874. Retrieved from https://journals.lww.com/ccmjournal/Abstract/1992/06000/American_College_of_Chest_Physicians_Society_of.25.aspx

Bonilla, F. A., & Notarangelo, L. D. (2015). Primary immunodeficiency diseases. In S. H. Orkin, D. E. Fisher, D. Ginsburg, A. T. Look, S. E. Lux, & D. G. Nathan (Eds.), *Nathan and Oski's hematology and oncology of infancy and childhood* (8th ed.). Philadelphia, PA: Elsevier Saunders.

Branchford, B., & Di Paola, J. (2015). Approach to the child with a suspected bleeding disorder. In S. H. Orkin, D. E. Fisher, D. Ginsburg, A. T. Look, S. E. Lux, & D. G. Nathan (Eds.), *Nathan and Oski's hematology and oncology of infancy and childhood* (8th ed.). Philadelphia, PA: Elsevier Saunders.

Browarsky, I. L. (2010). Coagulation disorders. In E. Gilbert-Barness & L. A. Barness (Eds.), *Clinical use of pediatric diagnostic tests* (2nd ed.). Amsterdam, the Netherlands: IOS Press.

Brugnara, C., Oski, F. A., & Nathan, D. G. (2015). Diagnostic approach to the anemic patient. In S. H. Orkin, D. E. Fisher, D. Ginsburg, A. T. Look, S. E. Lux, & D. G. Nathan (Eds.), *Nathan and Oski's hematology and oncology of infancy and childhood* (8th ed.). Philadelphia, PA: Elsevier Saunders.

Centers for Disease Control and Prevention. (2015). HIV surveillance report, 2014 (Vol. 26). Retrieved from http://www.cdc.gov/hiv/library/reports/surveillance

Chegondi, M., Sasaki, J., Raszynski, A., & Totapally, B. R. (2016). Hemoglobin threshold for blood transfusion in a pediatric intensive care unit. *Transfusion Medicine Hemotherapeutics, 43*(4), 297–301. doi:10.1159/000446253

Chima, R. S., Abulebda, K., & Jodele, S. (2013). Advances in critical care of the pediatric hematopoietic stem cell transplant patient. *Pediatric Clinics of North America, 60*, 689–707. doi:10.1016/j.pcl.2013.02.007

Chou, S. T., & Schreiber, A. D. (2015). Autoimmune hemolytic anemia. In S. H. Orkin, D. E. Fisher, D. Ginsburg, A. T. Look, S. E. Lux, & D. G. Nathan (Eds.), *Nathan and Oski's hematology and oncology of infancy and childhood* (8th ed.). Philadelphia, PA: Elsevier Saunders.

Christensen, R. D., Ohs, R. K. (1996). Development of the hematopoietic system. In R. E. Behrman, R. M. Kliegman, & A. M. Arvin (Eds.), *Nelson textbook of pediatrics* (15th ed.). Philadelphia, PA: W. B. Saunders.

Coiffier, B., Altman, A., Pui, C.-H., Younes, A., & Cairo, M. S. (2008). Guidelines for the management of pediatric and adult tumor lysis syndrome: An evidence-based review. *Journal of Clinical Oncology, 26*(16), 2767–2778. doi:10.1200/JCO.2007.15.0177

Committee on Drugs. (1998). Drugs for pediatric emergencies. *Pediatrics, 101*(1), 433–443. doi:10.1542/peds.101.1.e13

Dinauer, M. C., Newburger, P. E., & Borregaard, N. (2015). Phagocyte system and disorders of granulopoiesis and granulocyte function. In S. H. Orkin, D. E. Fisher, D. Ginsburg, A. T. Look, S. E. Lux, & D. G. Nathan (Eds.), *Nathan and Oski's hematology and oncology of infancy and childhood* (8th ed.). Philadelphia, PA: Elsevier Saunders.

DiPaola, J., Montgomery, R. R., Cox Gill, J., & Flood, V. (2015). Hemophilia and von Willebrand disease. In S. H. Orkin, D. E. Fisher, D. Ginsburg, A. T. Look, S. E. Lux, & D. G. Nathan (Eds.), *Nathan and Oski's hematology and oncology of infancy and childhood* (8th ed.). Philadelphia, PA: Elsevier Saunders.

Diver, J. L. (2012). Bone marrow transplant and graft-versus-host disease. In K. Reuter-Rice & B. Bolick (Eds.), *Pediatric acute care: A guide for interprofessional practice.* Burlington, MA: Jones & Bartlett.

El Kenz, H., & Van der Linden, P. (2014). Transfusion-related acute lung injury. *European Journal of Anesthesiology, 31*, 345–350. doi:10.1097/EJA.0000000000000015

Fernández, K. S., & de Alarcón, P. A. (2013). Development of the hematopoietic system and disorders of hematopoiesis that present during infancy and early childhood. *Pediatric Clinics of North America, 60*(6), 1273–1289. doi:10.1016/j.pcl.2013.08.002

Garzon, A. M., & Mitchell, W. B. (2015). Use of thrombopoietin receptor agonists in childhood immune thrombocytopenia. *Frontiers in Pediatrics, 3*, 70. doi:10.3389/fped.2015.00070

Gilbert-Barness, E., & Barness, L. A. (2010). *Clinical use of pediatric diagnostic tests* (2nd ed.). Amsterdam, the Netherlands: IOS Press.

Gordon, J. B., Bernstein, M. L., Rogers, M. C. (1992). Hematologic disorders in the pediatric intensive care unit. In M. Rogers (Ed.). *Textbook of pediatric intensive care* (2nd ed.). Baltimore, MD: Williams & Wilkins.

Grady, C. (1988). Host defense mechanisms: An overview. *Seminars in Oncology Nursing, 4*(2), 86–94. doi:10.1016/0749-2081(88)90064-2

Grossman, S. (2014a). Acquired immunodeficiency syndrome. In S. C. Grossman & C. M. Porth (Eds.), *Porth's pathophysiology: Concepts of altered health states* (9th ed., pp. 361–380). Philadelphia, PA: Wolters Kluwer/Lippincott Williams & Wilkins.

Grossman, S. (2014b). Blood cells and the hematopoietic system. In S. C. Grossman & C. M. Porth (Eds.), *Porth's pathophysiology: Concepts of altered health states* (9th ed., pp. 638–647). Philadelphia, PA: Wolters Kluwer/Lippincott Williams & Wilkins.

Grossman, S. (2014c). Disorders of hemostasis. In S. C. Grossman & C. M. Porth (Eds.), *Porth's pathophysiology: Concepts of altered health states* (9th ed.). Philadelphia, PA: Wolters Kluwer/Lippincott Williams & Wilkins.

Grossman, S. (2014d). Inflammation, tissue repair, and wound healing. In S. C. Grossman & C. M. Porth (Eds.), *Porth's pathophysiology: Concepts of altered health states* (9th ed., pp. 306–328). Philadelphia, PA: Wolters Kluwer/Lippincott Williams & Wilkins.

Haining, W. N., Duncan, C. N., El-haddad, A., & Lehmann, L. (2015). Principles of bone marrow and stem cell transplantation. In S. H. Orkin, D. E. Fisher, D. Ginsburg, A. T. Look, S. E. Lux, & D. G. Nathan (Eds.), *Nathan and Oski's hematology and oncology of infancy and childhood* (8th ed.). Philadelphia, PA: Elsevier Saunders.

Hartung, H. D., Olson, T. S., & Bessler, M. (2013). Acquired aplastic anemia in children. *Pediatric Clinics of North America, 60*(6), 1311–1336. doi:10.1016/j.pcl.2013.08.011

Harvey, M. (1986). *Study guide to core curriculum for critical care nursing* (p. 162). Philadelphia, PA: W. B. Saunders.

Haven, P. L., & Committee on Pediatric AIDS. (2003). Postexposure prophylaxis in children and adolescents for nonoccupational exposure to human immunodeficiency virus. *Pediatrics, 111*(6), 1475–1489.

Heeney, M. M., & Ware, R. E. (2015). Sickle cell disease. In S. H. Orkin, D. E. Fisher, D. Ginsburg, A. T. Look, S. E. Lux, & D. G. Nathan (Eds.). *Nathan and Oski's hematology and oncology of infancy and childhood* (8th ed.). Philadelphia, PA: Elsevier Saunders.

Henry, M., & Sung, L. (2015). Supportive care in pediatric oncology: Oncologic emergencies and management of fever and neutropenia. *Pediatric Clinics of North America, 62*, 27–46. doi:10.1016/j.pcl.2014.09.016

Jarvis, C. (2016). *Physical examination and health assessment.* (7th ed.). St. Louis, MO: Elsevier.

Lacroix, J., Tucci, M., & Du Pont-Thibodeau, G. (2015). Red blood cell transfusion decision making in critically ill children. *Current Opinion in Pediatrics*, 27(3), 286–291. doi:10.1097/MOP.0000000000000221

Lambert, M. P., & Poncz, M. (2015). Inherited platelet disorders. In S. H. Orkin, D. E. Fisher, D. Ginsburg, A. T. Look, S. E. Lux, & D. G. Nathan (Eds.), *Nathan and Oski's hematology and oncology of infancy and childhood* (8th ed.). Philadelphia, PA: Elsevier Saunders.

Levy, M. M., Fink, M. P., Marshall, J. C., Abraham, E., Angus, D., Cook, D., . . . Ramsay, G. (2003). 2011 SCCM/ESICM/ACCP/ATS/SIS International Sepsis Definitions Conference. *Intensive Care Medicine*, 29(4), 530–538. doi:10.1007/s00134-003-1662-x

Lexicomp Online Laboratory Values. (2004). Retrieved from http://www.cronline.com/crlsql/servlet/cronline

Lexicomp Online. (2016). Retrieved from http://online.lexi.com/lco/action/home

Maclaren, G., Conrad, S. A., & Dalton, H. J. (2016). Extracorporeal life support. In D. G. Nichols & D. H. Shaffner (Eds.), *Rogers' textbook of pediatric intensive care* (5th ed., pp. 581–599). Philadelphia, PA: Wolters Kluwer.

Madden, J. R. (2012). Tumor lysis syndrome. In K. Reuter-Rice & B. Bolick (Eds.), *Pediatric acute care: A guide for interprofessional practice*. Burlington, MA: Jones & Bartlett.

Mirrakhimov, A. E., Voore, P., Khan, M., & Ali, A. M. (2015). Tumor lysis syndrome: A clinical review. *World Journal of Critical Care Medicine*, 4(2), 130–138. doi:10.5492/wjccm.v4.i2.130

Mofenson, L. M., Brady, M. T., Danner, S. P., Dominguez, K. L., Hazra, R., Handelsman, E., . . . Van Dyke, R. (2009). Guidelines for the prevention and treatment of opportunistic infections among HIV-exposed and HIV-infected children. *Morbidity and Mortality Weekly Report*, 58, 1–166. Retrieved from https://www.cdc.gov/mmwr/preview/mmwrhtml/rr5811a1.htm

Moriber, N. A. (2014). Innate and adaptive immunity. In S. C. Grossman & C. M. Porth (Eds.), *Porth's pathophysiology: Concepts of altered health states* (9th ed., pp. 276–305). Philadelphia, PA: Wolters Kluwer/Lippincott Williams & Wilkins.

Mudge-Grout, C. L. (1992). *Immunologic disorders*. St Louis, MO: Mosby-Year Book.

Mullen, E. A., & Gratias, E. (2015). Oncologic emergencies. In S. H. Orkin, D. E. Fisher, D. Ginsburg, A. T. Look, S. E. Lux, & D. G. Nathan (Eds.), *Nathan and Oski's hematology and oncology of infancy and childhood* (8th ed.). Philadelphia, PA: Elsevier Saunders.

National Institutes of Health National Heart, Lung, and Blood Institute. (2015). The management of sickle cell disease. Retrieved from https://www.nhlbi.nih.gov/files/docs/guidelines/sc_mngt.pdf

Nevins, T. E. (2000). Overview of new immunosuppressive therapies. *Current Opinion in Pediatrics*, 12(2), 146–150. Retrieved from https://journals.lww.com/co-pediatrics/Abstract/2000/04000/Overview_of_new_immunosuppressive_therapies.11.aspx

Newman, A. R. (2012). Leukemia and lymphoma. In K. Reuter-Rice & B. Bolick (Eds.), *Pediatric acute care: A guide for interprofessional practice*. Burlington, MA: Jones & Bartlett.

Okomo, U., & Meremikwu, M. (2015). Fluid replacement therapy for acute episodes of pain in people with sickle cell: A review. *Cochrane Database of Systematic Reviews*, 2015(3), CD005406. doi: 10.1002/14651958.CD005406.pub4

Pai, S. Y., & Reinherz, E. L. (2015). Immune response. In S. H. Orkin, D. E. Fisher, D. Ginsburg, A. T. Look, S. E. Lux, & D. G. Nathan (Eds.), *Nathan and Oski's hematology and oncology of infancy and childhood* (8th ed.). Philadelphia, PA: Elsevier Saunders.

Pipe, S., & Goldenberg, N. (2015). Acquired disorders of hemostasis. In S. H. Orkin, D. E. Fisher, D. Ginsburg, A. T. Look, S. E. Lux, & D. G. Nathan (Eds.), *Nathan and Oski's hematology and oncology of infancy and childhood* (8th ed.). Philadelphia, PA: Elsevier Saunders.

Plaeger, S. F. (1996). Principal human cytokines. In E. R. Stiehm (Ed.), *Immunologic disorders in infants and children* (4th ed.). Philadelphia, PA: WB Saunders.

Porth, C. M. (2015). *Essentials of Pathophysiology* (4th ed., p. 241–296). Philadelphia, PA: Lippincott Williams & Wilkins.

Richardson, P. G., Ho, V. T., Cutler, C., Glotzbecker, B., Antin, J. H., & Soiffer, R. (2013). Hepatic veno-occlusive disease after hematopoietic stem cell transplantation: Novel insights to pathogenesis, current status of treatment, and future directions. *Biology of Blood and Marrow Transplant*, 19(1 Suppl.), S88–S90. doi: doi:10.1016/j.bbmt.2012.10.023

Rosenthal, C. H. (1989). Immunosuppression in the pediatric critical care patient. *Critical Care Nursing Clinics North America*, 1(4), 779.

Scott, J. P. (2000). Hematology. In R. E. Behrman & R. M. Kliegman (Eds.), *Nelson's essentials of pediatrics* (4th ed., pp. 00–00). Philadelphia, PA: W. B. Saunders.

Selekman, J. (1991). Pediatric problems related to the immunologic system. In V. D. Feeg & R. E. Harbin (Eds.), *Pediatric nursing: Core curriculum and resource manual*. Pitman, NJ: Anthony Jannetti.

Selik, R. M., Mokotoff, E. D., Branson, B., Owen, S. M., Whitmore, S., & Hall, H. I. (2014). Revised surveillance case definition for HIV infection—United States, 2014. *Morbidity and Mortality Weekly Report*, 63, 1–10. Retrieved from https://www.cdc.gov/mmwr/preview/mmwrhtml/rr6303a1.htm?s_cid=rr6303a1_w

Sieff, C. A., Daley, G. Q., & Zon, L. I. (2015). Anatomy and physiology of hematopoiesis. In S. H. Orkin, D. E. Fisher, D. Ginsburg, A. T. Look, S. E. Lux, & D. G. Nathan (Eds.), *Nathan and Oski's hematology and oncology of infancy and childhood* (8th ed.). Philadelphia, PA: Elsevier Saunders.

Slota, M. C. (Ed.). (2006). *Core curriculum for pediatric critical care nursing* (2nd ed.). St.Louis, MO: Elsevier.

Sterling, T. R., & Chaisson, R. E. (2015). General clinical manifestations of human immunodeficiency virus infection (including acute retroviral syndrome and oral, cutaneous, renal, ocular, metabolic, and cardiac diseases). In J. E. Bennett, R. Dolin., & M. J. Blaser (Eds.), *Mandell, Douglas, and Bennett's principles and practice of infectious diseases* (8th ed., pp. 1541–1557). Philadelphia, PA: Elsevier Saunders.

Taylor, A., Valentino, L., & Osborn, K. (2012). Hemophilia. In K. Reuter-Rice & B. Bolick (Eds.), *Pediatric acute care: A guide for interprofessional practice*. Burlington, MA: Jones & Bartlett.

Tortora, G. J., & Derrickson, B. (2014). *Principles of anatomy and physiology* (14th ed., pp. 661–687). Hoboken, NJ: Wiley.

U.S.Department of Health and Human Services. (n.d.-a). AIDSinfo. Retrieved from https://aidsinfo.nih.gov

U.S.Department of Health and Human Services Panel on Antiretroviral Therapy and Medical Management of Children Infected with HIV. (n.d.-b). Guidelines for the use of antiretroviral agents in pediatric HIV infection. Retrieved from http://aidsinfo.nih.gov/contentfiles/lvguidelines/pediatricguidelines.pdf

U.S.Department of Health and Human Services. Panel on Opportunistic Infections in HIV-Infected Adults and Adolescents. (n.d.). Guidelines for prevention and treatment of opportunistic infections in HIV-infected adults and adolescents: Recommendations from the Centers for Disease Control and Prevention, the National Institutes of Health, and the HIV Medicine Association of the Infectious Diseases Society of America. Retrieved from https://aidsinfo.nih.gov/contentfiles/lvguidelines/adult_oi.pdf

U.S. Department of Health and Human Services Panel on Treatment of Pregnant Women with HIV Infection and Prevention of Perinatal Transmission. (n.d.). Recommendations for the use of antiretroviral drugs in pregnant women with HIV infection and interventions to reduce perinatal HIV transmission in the United States. Retrieved from http://aidsinfo .nih.gov/contentfiles/lvguidelines/PerinatalGL.pdf

Weinberg, G. (2000). Antiretroviral therapy of human immunodeficiency virus infection. In G. L. Mandell, J. E. Douglas, & R. Bennett (Ed.), *Principles and practices of infectious diseases* (5th ed.). New York, NY: Churchill Livingstone.

Wilson, D. B. (2015). Acquired platelet defects. In S. H. Orkin, D. E. Fisher, D. Ginsburg, A. T. Look, S. E. Lux, & D. G. Nathan (Eds.), *Nathan and Oski's hematology and oncology of infancy and childhood* (8th ed.). Philadelphia, PA: Elsevier Saunders.

9

MULTISYSTEM ISSUES

SECTION I. MULTIPLE TRAUMA

Frances Blayney and Colleene Young

Critically injured children and their families require the expertise of a multiprofessional team consisting of pediatric nurses, intensivists, and other healthcare professionals to provide optimal trauma care. Children are different from adults and they exhibit unique physiological response to polytrauma/multiple trauma compared to adults (Table 9.1). This section on multiple trauma covers knowledge of developmental considerations, mechanisms of injury, specific injuries, treatment of injuries, and prevention strategies to assist the pediatric intensive care unit (PICU) nurse in the provision of safe, effective, quality care for the injured child and family. Pediatric trauma patients may suffer severe disabilities as a result of their injuries, which may require long-term care and pose a financial burden on society.

Children are unique and require special resources. Trauma centers or healthcare systems need to be able to provide care according to their needs and develop plans to ensure those needs are met and specialized care is provided. Such care is optimally provided at pediatric hospitals that are dedicated to children and have demonstrated expertise and commitment in caring for pediatric trauma patients. It is vital that the trauma team and trauma surgeon be properly trained and specifically credentialed by the hospital to provide pediatric trauma care (American College of Surgeons [ACS], 2014). Healthcare professionals must advocate for the needs of the injured pediatric patient within the community by establishing close working relationships with other hospitals. There are different levels of pediatric trauma centers based on annual admissions with Level I centers admitting at minimum more than 200 injured children under the age of 15 each year and Level II centers admitting more than 100 injured children younger than the age of 15 each year. All Level I and II pediatric trauma centers must have systems in place to screen and identify for child maltreatment and nonaccidental trauma (NAT). Pediatric patients sustaining major trauma must be fully evaluated by the trauma team (with specialists in pediatric surgery, anesthesiology, neurosurgery, orthopedic

surgery, emergency medicine, radiology, and rehabilitation) and be able to respond when needed to deliver the appropriate care as expeditiously as possible to limit the extent of the injury.

Minimum criteria for activation of pediatric trauma teams include (ACS, 2014):

- Hypotension by age criteria

- Gunshot wounds (GSWs) to the neck, chest, abdomen, or extremities proximal to the elbow or knee

- Glasgow Coma Score (GCS) of less than 9 or deteriorating by 2, with a mechanism due to the trauma

- Patients transferred from other hospitals requiring blood transfusions to maintain vital signs

- Intubated patients transferred from the scene, patients in respiratory compromise or requiring an emergent airway, or intubated patients with respiratory compromise transferred from another hospital

- Per emergency department physician's discretion

There must be collaboration among all critical care providers and the trauma service caring for a pediatric trauma patient. All Level I and II pediatric trauma centers need to have surgeons certified or eligible for certification by the American Board of Surgery. All Level I and II pediatric trauma centers must submit data to the National Trauma Data Bank (NTDB) and all data should be benchmarked with national pediatric trauma data from such registries as the NTDB or Pediatric Trauma Quality Improvement Program (TQIP). In addition, pediatric trauma surgeons and other healthcare providers should have structured education specific to care for pediatric trauma patients. The education available includes, but is not limited to, Pediatric Advanced Life Support (PALS) from the American Heart Association (AHA); courses such as Pediatric Care After Resuscitation (PCAR) from TCAR Education Programs; Emergency

TABLE 9.1 Comparison of Adult and Pediatric Physiologic Response to Polytrauma

Factor	Adults	Children
Timing of organ failure	48–72 hours after injury	Immediately after injury
Organ failure sequence	Sequential	Simultaneous
Acute lung injury	High risk	Low risk
Systemic inflammatory response	Robust	Dampened
Local inflammatory response	Dampened	Robust
Death due to pelvic fracture	High risk	Low risk
Morbidity	Associated with pelvic fracture	Associated with organ injuries
Neurologic injury	Low recovery rate	High recovery rate

Source: From Pandya, N. K., Upasani, V. V., & Kulkarni, V. A. (2013). The pediatric polytrauma patient: Current concepts. *Journal of the American Academy of Orthopaedic Surgeons, 21*(3), 170–179. doi:10.5435/JAAOS-21-03-170

Nursing Pediatric Course (ENPC) and Trauma Nursing Core Course (TNCC) from Emergency Nurses Association; courses from the American Academy of Pediatrics (AAP), the American College of Emergency Physicians, and the Advanced Trauma Life Support (ATLS) from the ACS. Pediatric trauma mortality is significantly improved in pediatric trauma centers or adult centers with pediatric trauma certification, compared to just Level I or II adult trauma centers (Daley, 2015).

EPIDEMIOLOGY AND INCIDENCE

A. Epidemiology

1. For all children aged 1 to 19 years, accidental injury (unintentional injury) is the leading cause of death, with motor vehicle traffic-related deaths the number one cause in that category. Other fatal childhood injuries, in order, are suffocation, firearms, and drowning/submersion (Nance, 2015). The data also indicate that firearm incidents occur 38 to 81 times more frequently than suffocation and drowning/submersion incidents, respectively. According to the Centers for Disease Control and Prevention's (CDC) National Vital Statistics System, in 2014 suicide became the second leading cause of death in the 10 to 14 and the 15 to 24 age groups. Homicide is the third leading cause of death in the 1 to 4 and 15 to 24 age groups (CDC & National Center for Injury Prevention and Control, 2014).

2. In the Traffic Safety Facts annual report for 2015 from the National Highway Traffic Safety Administration (2017), fatal crashes increased by 7.2% in 2015 compared with 2014, which is the largest increase in one year since 1965 to 1966. Although the percentage of alcohol-impaired driving fatalities declined over the past two decades, the rate increased in 2015. Several factors influence childhood injuries:

a. Age and stage of development
b. Gender
c. Behavior
d. Environment

3. Developmental milestones also correlate with the mechanism of pediatric injuries.

B. Age and Stage of Development, Gender

Children's abilities to react and respond to others, to coordinate, anticipate, and judge the consequences of their actions are factors that change predictably as children's physical, communicative, social, and intellectual abilities develop. The mechanism and outcomes of injury varies by age. There are very interesting statistics in the Pediatric Annual Report 2015 regarding gender. For example, females showed a higher incident rate than males in falls and motor vehicle accidents (MVAs), but lower fatality rates. Females had a higher incident of hot object/substance injuries than males and a higher fatality rate for this injury type. With firearms as the mechanism of injury, males had a fourfold incident rate, yet females had a higher firearms fatality rate (Nance, 2015).

C. Mechanisms of Injury

Falls are the leading cause of nonfatal injury and are most common from infancy through age 14. Children tend to fall from objects, balconies, windows, and trees. Falls occur most often in homes, followed by schoolyards and playgrounds. The next major mechanism of injury is MVAs, followed by pedestrian injury (i.e., when children are struck by motor vehicles; Table 9.2). Most pediatric injuries occur as a result of blunt trauma with penetrating trauma accounting for only a small portion. Head injuries are the most severe type of blunt trauma and are responsible for the most deaths (Nance, 2015).

D. Environment

1. Although they constitute a smaller percentage of injuries than does blunt force, penetrating injuries in children have increased in recent years, attributable in large part to the proliferation of handguns, increased gang violence, drug use, and the trafficking of drugs. Rgardless of age, poverty is the major factor influencing the rate of penetrating injury (Schecter, Betts, Schecter, & Victorino, 2012).

2. In 2014, state and local child protective services received approximately 3.2 million referrals for child abuse or neglect, of which 702,000 children were determined to be victims and resulted in 1,580 pediatric deaths. Most of the deaths were children younger than 3 years of age, with the highest rates of child abuse occurring in children younger than age 1 (U.S.

Department of Health & Human Services [HHS], 2016). As demonstrated in earlier reports, neglect comprised the greatest percentage of maltreatment incidents at 75%. Physical abuse was second at 17%. Important to note is that children may have suffered multiple types of maltreatment at the same time or repeatedly, but it was counted as one type.

3. Child maltreatment resulting from blunt trauma to the head or from shaking is the leading cause of head injury among infants and young children. Boys have a higher incidence of child fatalities from maltreatment than girls (2.48 per 100,000 population of male children compared to 1.82 per 100,000 population of female children). Child sexual abuse is four times higher among females than among males with one in five girls suffering from child sexual abuse (National Center for Victims of Crime, n.d.). The victimization rate of children younger than 1 year has had the largest increase in all age groups for the past 5 years (HHS, Administration for Children & Families [ACF], Administration on Children, Youth and Families, & Children's Bureau, 2016).

4. For every child who dies of an injury caused by abuse, 40 others are hospitalized and 1,120 are treated in emergency departments. An estimated 50,000 children acquire permanent disabilities each year from abuse. The American Society for Positive Care of Children, State of America's Children 2014 report, states that child abuse and neglect costs the U.S. $80 billion each year.

TABLE 9.2   Leading Causes of Injury

Age	Rank	<1	1–4	5–9	10–14	15–19
Mechanism	1 Highest	Firearms	Firearms	Firearms	Firearms	Firearms
	2	MV Transport	MV Transport	MV Transport	MV Transport	MV Transport
	3	Cut/Pierce	Transport Other	Transport Other	Transport Other	Cut/Pierce
	4	Struck by, Against	Struck by, Against	Cut/Pierce	Cut/Pierce	Transport Other
	5	Fall	Cut/Pierce	Struck by, Against	Struck by, Against	Fall

Source: Adapted from "Case Fatality by Selected Mechanism of Injury and Age." Committee on Trauma, American College of Surgeons. NTDB Annual/Pediatric Report 2015. Chicago, IL. The content reproduced from the NTDB remains the full and exclusive copyrighted property of the American College of Surgeons. The American College of Surgeons is not responsible for any claims arising from works based on the original data, text, tables, or figures. Nance, M. L. (Ed.) (2015). *National Trauma Data Bank 2015: Pediatric annual report.* Retrieved from https://www .facs.org/~/media/files/quality%20programs/trauma/ntdb/ntdb%20pediatric%20annual%20report%202015%20final.ashx

5. As has been shown, the statistics on unintentional injury leading to death, injuries, and disability in the pediatric population are alarming and push us to find solutions and educate our communities.

INJURY PREVENTION AND FAMILY EDUCATION

In all age groups, prevention is paramount to safety and health. When children are admitted to the ICU, nurses are primary advocates for preventive care and guidance. Using knowledge of child development as a foundation, safety education and anticipatory guidance for both parents and children can be incorporated

into many nursing interventions and parent teaching (Table 9.3). Although it is difficult to approach the subject of prevention in a critical setting, the opportunity to teach families about how to prevent recurring injuries should not be lost.

MECHANISMS OF INJURY

Mechanism of injury can be described as the effect of energy on human tissue. Several mechanisms of injury are responsible for pediatric trauma, including kinetic, thermal, electrical, chemical, and radiant energy. It follows that specific injuries are classified according to the responsible mechanism. Other mechanisms

TABLE 9.3 Developmental Risk Factors and Education

Developmental Risk Factors	Mechanisms/Types of Injury	Prevention Strategies and Parent Teaching
Infant		
Learns to roll, sit, crawl, and walk	Falls (most frequent) • Walker related • Rolling from high surfaces • Fall from adults' arms	Use safety straps in • High chair • Stroller • Changing table • Swing • Infant seat Keep doors closed to stairs and laundry chutes Do not open windows more than 4 inches
Cries to communicate until language develops	Homicide	Promote parenting skills and coping interventions • Support networks • Health promotion (balanced diet, adequate sleep)
Depends on others for needs and safety	Drowning Burns/scalding MVAs	Never leave child unattended in • Bathtub, pool, water sources • Walker Test temperature of water before bathing Use safety locks/gates on stairs, doors, and windows Use ACT mnemonic: *A*void heat stroke by never leaving child in car; *C*reate a reminder in back seat; *T*ake action—call 911 if you see a baby left in a car Restrain infant in an approved rear-facing infant seat in rear seat
Explores through touch, taste, feelings, and motion	Suffocation Choking Aspiration Poisoning Burns/scalding	Avoid drinking hot liquids, cooking, smoking while holding infant Test temperature of food before feeding and water before bathing Use flame-retardant nightwear Crib should not have moveable side rails; lower mattress when infant can sit Keep crib free of toys, blankets; crib should only have a firm mattress covered with a tight-fitting crib sheet

(continued)

TABLE 9.3   Developmental Risk Factors and Education *(continued)*

Developmental Risk Factors	Mechanisms/Types of Injury	Prevention Strategies and Parent Teaching
		Crib corner posts should not stick up more than 1/16 of an inch Keep small objects, inappropriate toys, and household items out of reach Avoid latex balloons Position infant on back for sleep
Toddler		
Explores his or her body and the world	Fall from greater heights than infants • Windows • Porches • Playground equipment Riding toys	Use safety locks/gates on stairs, doors, and windows Lower mattress when infant can sit Supervise playground activity Keep doors closed and use child protective devices on doorknobs Have child wear a helmet
Desires increased independence	Choking	Cut food into small pieces Avoid foods such as peanuts, hard candy, and popcorn Remind toddlers not to run with food/toys in their mouths
Lacks concept of danger Lacks comprehension of cause–effect	Heat injuries, burns/scalds Chemical burn injuries Drowning	Avoid drinking hot liquids, cooking, or smoking while holding child Test temperature of food before feeding and water before bathing Use flame-retardant nightwear. Never leave child unattended in bathtub, pool, water sources Avoid latex balloons Use electrical outlet covers Keep appliances and cords out of reach Avoid tablecloths Help child avoid dangerous situations by teaching and reinforcing associated risks Restrain toddler in an approved car seat in rear seat
Preschool Age		
Desires increased independence Learns skills by imitating others Develops increased motor skills Lacks well-developed sense of direction Lacks well-developed peripheral vision Experiences the world through egocentrism, imagination, and fantasy	Bike vs. pedestrian accidents Falls	Provide safe riding toys Avoid permitting child to ride on inappropriate equipment such as tractor, lawn mower, ATV Teach street safety by informing child of stop/look/listen and the buddy system when crossing the street Teach helmet safety Use safety locks/gates on stairs, doors, and windows Supervise playground activity Keep doors closed and use child protective devices on doorknobs Use electrical outlet covers Keep appliances and cords out of reach Help children avoid dangerous situations by teaching and reinforcing associated risks
General age-specific safety	Burns (fire related burns are most common; overall rare in this age)	Keep pot handles turned inward or toward back of stove Keep matches and lighters out of reach Teach child to stop, drop, and roll Use three-point restraints or approved car seat in motor vehicle

(continued)

TABLE 9.3   Developmental Risk Factors and Education *(continued)*

Developmental Risk Factors	Mechanisms/Types of Injury	Prevention Strategies and Parent Teaching
School Age		
Well-developed motor skills **May lack the cognitive skills to analyze and judge situations accurately** **Increasingly advanced motor skills** **Learning to ride bicycle**	MVAs Falls • Balconies • Windows • Playground equipment • Trees Head injuries	Avoid riding inappropriate equipment/toys such as lawn mower or ATV Teach street safety by looking both ways, holding hands, and not crossing the street alone Teach helmet safety Supervise playground activity Teach swimming skills and water safety
Increasing independence **Developing relationship with peers** **General age-specific safety**	Burns (fire-related burns are most common; overall are rare in this age)	Help children avoid dangerous situations and remind them of potential dangers Keep pot handles turned inward Keep matches and lighters out of reach Teach child to stop, drop, and roll Use three-point restraints in rear seat of motor vehicle.
Adolescent		
Increased activity in sports **Able to drive motor vehicles**	MVAs Spinal cord injuries, head injuries, and long-bone fractures	Use three-point restraints in motor vehicle Encourage adolescents not to use drugs and alcohol and never before driving a motor vehicle or getting into a car with someone who has Encourage use of helmets with motorcycles, bicycles, skateboards, and sports activities
Desires increased independence	Drowning Firearm injuries Homicide/suicide	Validate peer pressure while helping adolescent live within the limits set by his or her parents Teach swimming skills and water/boat safety
Developing relationship with peers **Participates in risk-taking behavior and succumbs easily to peer pressure** **Believes injury will not happen to him or her; judgment may not be well defined**		Teach firearm safety • Treat firearms with respect • Do not play with firearms • Treat all firearms as if they are loaded • Use gun locks if gun is in home and store ammunition in a separate place from firearm
All Age Groups		
General safety		Teach parents and children that restraint devices are the most effective safety devices in preventing serious injury and death in MVAs (American College of Surgeons, 2003) Use age-appropriate restraint device and position while in motor vehicle Teach child to treat driveways and parking lots the same as streets Firearm safety • Keep firearms in areas secure from children • Utilize gun locks if firearms are in home and store ammunition in a separate place from firearm • Reinforce gun safety and not to play with guns

(continued)

TABLE 9.3   Developmental Risk Factors and Education *(continued)*

Developmental Risk Factors	Mechanisms/Types of Injury	Prevention Strategies and Parent Teaching
		Teach swimming skills and water safety Restrict exposure/teach safety related to environmental elements such as sun/cold Encourage use of helmet and protective gear for bike riding and appropriate sports
Maintain a safe environment		Increase knowledge related to age-appropriate toys/activities and playground equipment Have smoke detectors/fire ladders and fire extinguishers in home Practice fire and emergency evacuation plans at home at least every 6 months
Safety around animals	Animal bites	Introduce infants to pets slowly and cautiously Teach children pet safety Teach not to tease animals Teach not to approach unfamiliar animals Teach injury prevention as part of a healthy lifestyle Healthcare professionals should help increase parents' awareness of the community programs that can help them with injury prevention and the challenges they may face in keeping their children safe

ATV, all-terrain vehicle; MVAs, motor vehicle accidents.

include water submersion, cold exposure, asphyxia, and intentional injury (see "Child Maltreatment" section).

A. Kinetic Energy

Kinetic energy is the energy of motion. The equation for kinetic energy is KE = mass × velocity^2/2. This means, for example, in a frontal collision, an increase in 40% of speed produces almost a 100% increase in force (Criddle, 2013; Hodnick, 2012). Kinetic energy is the force that is responsible for most traumatic injuries. Kinetic forces cause blunt, crush, shear, acceleration–deceleration, and penetrating injuries.

1. *Blunt-Force Trauma.* Most pediatric injuries are due to blunt-force trauma, which results in injuries to the solid and hollow organs as well as to the long bones. It also produces crushing, shearing, or tearing of tissue both externally and internally. Some examples of blunt-force trauma are falls, MVAs, seat belt injuries, and pedestrian versus motor vehicle. Children who are hit by moving vehicles will often have multiple injuries. The patterns of injuries that occur when a child is struck by a vehicle depend primarily on

two factors: the size of the child and type of vehicle involved.

2. *Crush Injury.* A crush injury occurs when compressive strain (energy) is concentrated in one body area. Crush injuries include animal bites, being caught in machinery or equipment (e.g., finger caught in a car door).

a. Patients who experience crush injuries from extreme forces (e.g., high-speed MVAs, earthquakes) are at particular risk for the development of rhabdomyolysis and myoglobinuria. Volume depletion from fluid sequestration in damaged tissues and poor fluid intake can lead to acute kidney injury (AKI).

b. Myoglobinuria is usually associated with rhabdomyolysis or muscle destruction. The cellular release of myoglobin is often accompanied by an increase in creatinine kinase (CK). When excreted into the urine, myoglobin can precipitate tubular obstruction and AKI. Myoglobinuria causes little or no morbidity or mortality except when it is associated with the secondary complications of rhabdomyolysis, including hyperkalemia, hypocalcemia, acidosis, and AKI. In patients experiencing myoglobinuria, physical examination reveals generalized muscle weakness (often with painful muscle groups), trauma, or areas of ischemic pressure necrosis where the patient has lain for extended periods. Expect any patient with extensive trauma to have some degree of myoglobinuria (Devarajan, 2015).

i. Animal bites can lead to a localized infection, cellulitis, and, in some instances, to surgical intervention. Bites vary from a small puncture wound or laceration to crushing of major arteries, veins, and nerves. Children are most likely to be involved in animal bites from cats, dogs, ferrets, and other small animals. Most bites occur at home by the family dog (Ginsburg & Hunstad, 2016).

ii. Dog bites may result in a child being admitted to the ICU, depending on the location and severity of the bite. Dog bites are associated with a lower incidence of infection than human bites. However, cat bites or scratches have a higher risk for infection (>50%; Babovic, Cayci, & Carlsen, 2014; Ginsburg & Hunstad, 2016). Bites to the airway region may be severe and require mechanical ventilation and surgery. Underlying injuries, such as fractures, may also be present. Potential complications include infection (most common) and rabies (most serious).

iii. Parental concerns are often focused on cosmetic implications for the future and on bleeding. The discrepancy between the potential complications and common parental concerns presents teaching opportunities for critical care nurses.

iv. Wound care should include irrigation under pressure and cleansing of the site with benzalkonium chloride to kill rabies. A wound culture should be obtained. The nurse should anticipate radiographic studies and administration of tetanus toxoid and antibiotics (Ginsburg & Hunstad, 2016).

v. Providing education to the family regarding prevention strategies for the future is crucial. Education should include information about how to approach dogs and other animals, when to avoid approaching them, as well as available community resources for dog-bite education (AAP, 2015).

3. *Shear Injury.* Shear injury occurs when forces are applied in opposite directions (as when the brain moves within the cranium). When a shear injury is present in the absence of a significant trauma history and in combination with retinal hemorrhages, inflicted trauma, such as shaken baby syndrome (SBS), must be ruled out (see "Child Maltreatment" section).

4. *Acceleration–Deceleration Injury.* Acceleration–deceleration injuries occur when a body stops suddenly and the internal organs keep moving inside the body, for example, in a high-speed MVA. The internal organs and vessels (e.g., spinal cord, hepatic artery and vein, descending thoracic aorta) rupture or tear. This type of injury can occur in a high-speed MVA when the child is thrust against the seat belt. This also applies to the brain moving within the cranial vault. This injury is historically referred to as "coup contra coup." The brain hits an object when the forward thrust is stopped and hits the back of the skull when the backward motion is stopped.

5. *Penetrating Injury*

a. Penetrating injuries occur from firearms (the most deadly), knives, or other sharp objects.

b. The severity of knife wounds is related to the anatomic area inflicted with the knife, the length of the blade, and the angle of penetration. An exit wound may or may not be present and the blade may be impaled. Objects and toys can become missiles that can penetrate a child's body. A young child running with a toy in his or her mouth who subsequently falls can sustain a penetrating injury to the oropharynx. Damage to the internal organs results from kinetic force along the path of the penetrating object (Hodnick, 2012).

c. Firearm injuries are one of the leading causes of injury deaths in the United States. The case fatality rate for children is 15.4% compared to suffocation at 27.7% and drowning/submersion at 14.6% (Nance, 2015). Injuries from low-velocity weapons are generally less destructive than from high-velocity weapons (e.g., semiautomatic weapons) because velocity plays a more important part in the kinetic energy equation (see previous discussion on kinetic energy). Injuries from firearms are related to the type of weapon, size, caliber of bullet, muzzle velocity of the projectile, number of bullets that penetrate the body, bullet trajectory, and the distance from which the firearm was discharged. Dense organs, such as the liver and muscles, or fluid-filled organs, such as the heart or gastrointestinal (GI) system, sustain greater damage than less dense organs, such as the air-filled lungs. The damage to body tissues from a bullet or missile is related to three processes: tearing and crushing of the tissues, cavitation, and shock waves. Cavitation is the development of a cavity along the track of the projectile as the projectile comes into contact with the relatively liquid human body. The "temporary" cavity closes as the energy dissipates, but there may be enough tissue injury from the projectile that a permanent cavity is created along the central core of the projectile tract. As the energy of the projectile increases, the size of the temporary cavity increases, causing considerable damage. This is one of the reasons that high-velocity, high-energy weapons cause so much damage. Another reason is the shock waves generated by high-velocity, high-energy weapons. In the human body, shock waves refer to a rapid change in temperature, pressure, or density secondary to the projectile (Hodnick, 2012).

6. *GSW Characteristics.* GSWs to the head are less common than are GSW to the extremities and are understandably more fatal. The bullet may course through multiple routes once it is in the body. It may ricochet off bone, resulting in bony fragments. Moreover, the bullet itself may fragment. Fragments of any type will increase the size and severity of the wound. A bullet may tumble or somersault within the body, causing increased damage and greater wound severity. Penetrating forces produce entrance and often exit wounds. This is important to keep in mind when performing a primary survey.

7. *Bullet Wounding Mechanisms.* Tearing and crushing of tissues occurs when the missile initially strikes. Yaw is the deviation of a bullet from a straight path. If the bullet strikes the body at an angle, the angle of yaw is increased and more damage occurs (Hodnick, 2012). Temporary cavitation occurs as a result of the bullet losing energy to the surrounding tissues as it enters the body. This cavity can exceed the size of the bullet and it is achieved within milliseconds of penetration. Cavitation is defined by bullet velocity. It is produced from the effects of combustion (muzzle blast) and is commonly seen with shotgun wounds. Internal explosion of gas and powder results in burns to the surrounding tissue.

8. *Risk for Injury.* Bone, brain, liver, spleen, and fluid-filled organs (e.g., heart, GI tract) can be damaged severely by the formation of a temporary cavity because of the greater amount of energy imparted to this dense and relatively inelastic tissue. Lower density, elastic tissues (e.g., the lung) are less affected by cavitation because less energy is transferred to the tissue. Nursing implications and treatment for GSW patients and basic principles (airway, breathing,

circulation [ABCs]) of trauma apply to victims of GSW.

9. The primary survey should also include rapid assessment for the location of entry and exit wounds. The nurse should be aware that GSW to the neck could cause significant airway complications (e.g., hematoma, direct injury to the larynx). Anticipation of endotracheal intubation or emergent cricothyrotomy for GSW to the neck is prudent.

a. It is understandable that if multiple body regions are affected, this will increase the likelihood of death. Most children who arrive at trauma centers alive but subsequently die of nonintracranial fatal firearm injuries, die quickly as the result of major vascular and thoracic injuries (Hodnick, 2012).

b. "Damage control" for abdominal injuries is intended for severe hemorrhage uncontrolled with aggressive fluid and blood product administration. The cascade of physiologic derangements that often accompany severe hemorrhage refractory to fluid administration plays a large part in patient demise. The cascade includes a triad of acidosis, hypothermia, and coagulopathy. Damage control entails initial laparotomy with control of hemorrhage and contamination followed by an ICU course of aggressive resuscitation aimed at restoring metabolic homeostasis. After this, definitive repair of injuries and abdominal closure 12 to 48 hours after the initial laparotomy are recommended (Hughes, Burd, & Teach, 2014).

c. Following the primary survey, intravascular access should be established and fluids administered (20 mL/kg). Accurate, precise description of the wound and surrounding landmarks should follow. If the GSW is to the child's head, the nurse should anticipate CT scan, surgical debridement, and antibiotic therapy postoperatively if complications of infection develop. GSW to the abdomen can result in immediate peritonitis (e.g., major vascular injuries, hollow organ injuries).

d. Several wound outcome measures should be assessed throughout the child's ICU course, including the incision color, the surrounding tissue (degree, color, and pain intensity), and progression of exudate (type, color, and amount). The nurse should also asses the type of closure materials present: sutures (most common), staples, tissue adhesive, adhesive tapes, and laser tissue bonding (Al-Mubarak & Al-Haddab, 2013).

e. Vigilant pulmonary, neurologic, and peripheral vascular assessment is necessary to detect complications such as bullet embolization. If bullet embolization is suspected or confirmed, anticipate surgical debridement and anastomosis of the involved injured major vessels. Wounds that are close to major vessels warrant astute observation for hematoma formation. GSW to bones are treated as compound fractures that require surgical exploration and debridement.

f. It is advisable to start teaching the family as close to the ICU admission as possible. Teaching should include prevention and signs and symptoms of posttraumatic stress disorder (PTSD).

B. Exposure Injuries

1. *Thermal Injury.* Thermal injury occurs when the rate of heat absorption is greater than the rate of heat dissipation and results in scalds and flame burns (see "Section IV. Burns" later in the chapter).

2. *Electrical Injury.* When electricity—either through current or lightning—comes into contact with the body, its electrical energy is converted to heat. The heat causes injury. Most electrical injuries are due to low-voltage alternating current in the home setting (see "Section IV. Burns").

3. *Chemical Injury.* When a chemical is applied to the body, it causes injury by either producing heat or denaturing protein (see "Section II. Toxicology" and "Section IV. Burns"). An example of chemical injury is an abusive parent who pours bleach on a child's skin.

4. *Radiant Burns.* Exposure to the sun or to nuclear or therapeutic radiation can cause radiant burns (see "Section IV. Burns").

5. *Heat and Cold Exposure Injuries*

a. Environmental exposure during extreme cold results in hypothermia and frostbite. Hypothermia begins when a child's temperature is 35°C. Children are at risk for hypothermia because of their large body surface area (BSA)-to-mass ratio and because they have less subcutaneous fat for heat production. Blood loss, alcohol use, and the injuries themselves may be hypothermia-related conditions.

b. Frostbite may accompany hypothermia and multiple trauma injuries and occurs when ice crystallizes in the body's extracellular and intracellular fluid. Frostbite usually affects the areas most exposed (e.g., fingers, hands, feet, toes, ears, nose; Zonnoor, 2017). The severity of frostbite and resultant tissue injury depends on the absolute temperature and the duration of exposure. The wind-chill factor will also greatly affect the severity of frostbite. A review of the literature has shown novel, eccentric causes of frostbite, such as inhalant abuse (Koehler, 2014), recreational use of nitrous oxide and toluene (Koehler, 2014; Van Amsterdam, Nabben, & Van den Brink, 2015). Frostbite from these causes is related to the coldness of pressurized gas. Although a number of frostbite classifications exist, the grades for the severity of frostbite injury presented by Cauchy, Chetaille, Marchand, and Marsigny (2001) are useful in that they are descriptive and also predictive of the extent of injury and probable outcome. The grades are assigned after rewarming.

i. Grade 1. Absence of initial lesion; no blisters. On day 2: no need for bone scanning; prognosis: no amputation, no sequelae.

ii. Grade 2. Initial lesion on distal phalanx; clear blisters. On day 2: bone scan shows hypofixation of radiotracer uptake area; prognosis: tissue amputation; fingernail sequelae.

iii. Grade 3. Initial lesion on intermediary and proximal phalanx; hemorrhagic blisters on digit. On day 2: bone scan shows absence of radiotracer uptake on digit; functional sequelae.

iv. Grade 4. Initial lesion on carpal/tarsal; hemorrhagic blisters over carpal/tarsal region. Day 2: bone scan shows absence of radiotracer uptake area on the carpal/tarsal region; prognosis: bone amputation of limb with possible systemic involvement, sepsis, functional sequelae (Cauchy et al., 2001).

c. The goal of frostbite treatment is to save as much tissue as possible to regain maximal function and to prevent complications. The focus of frostbite treatment is rapid rewarming when it is permanent (as refreezing causes more tissue injury), pain control, reperfusion, infection prevention, safe manipulation of the affected region, prevention of future reperfusion, and manipulation of body part. Combination therapy (pharmacologic and nonpharmacologic interventions) can be useful (see Chapter 1).

d. Wash wounds with mild soap and water if they appear clean. Consider chlorhexidine gluconate if wounds appear or are suspected of being soiled. If a dressing is required, use a nonadherent dressing to provide a pain-free, nonocclusive barrier. Anticipate administering prophylactic antibiotics and tetanus toxoid. The draining or aspiration of clear blisters is controversial and should be a multidiscipline decision. Hemorrhagic blisters should not be drained. This type of blister implies a deeper injury and should be left intact to prevent infection and desiccation (Zonnoor, 2017).

e. Rapid rewarming in circulating water is the definitive treatment for frostbite. The circulating water allows for a constant temperature of 37°C to 39°C to be applied to the affected areas. The temperature of the water should be closely monitored to avoid slow rewarming or overheating. Antiseptic solutions, such as povidone–iodine or chlorhexidine, may be helpful when added to the bath. Thawing of the injured area can take from 20 to 40 minutes for superficial injuries and up to an hour for deep injuries. "The most common error in this stage of treatment is premature termination of the rewarming process because of reperfusion pain" (Zonnoor, 2017). Avoid applying dry heat as the loss of temperature sensitivity in the injured area may lead to burns. Prevent mechanical friction by avoiding tissue-to-tissue contact and touching the extremity to the sides during a rewarming bath. Elevate and splint the affected extremity and apply sterile nonadherent dressings. Local wound care should be followed diligently with frequent assessment for signs of infection. Daily hydrotherapy is recommended for 30 to 40 minutes at 40°C (Zonnoor, 2017).

f. Prolonged environmental exposure to heat may result in heat-related illnesses spanning from heat cramps, heat exhaustion/heat syncope to heat stroke. Of these, heat stroke is a true medical emergency. It is crucial to detect and treat the less dangerous heat-related illnesses before they progress to heat exhaustion and finally heat stroke. Children are at risk for heat-related emergencies because they acclimate more slowly to exercise in the heat compared with adults (exertional heat stroke; Laskowski-Jones, 2010). Other predisposing risk factors for heat stroke that may be considered unique for the pediatric population include, but are not limited to, dehydration, fatigue, sleep deprivation, fever, muscular exertion, history of seizures, sunburn, and the use of certain drugs (e.g., alcohol, amphetamines, cocaine; Bakar & Schleien, 2016). Heat illness is caused by the body's inability to manage heat. Heat exhaustion and heat stroke occur when the body's thermoregulatory mechanisms are no longer able to maintain a body temperature around 37°C/98.6°F. Factors that may contribute are high temperature, high humidity, and physical exertion in high temperatures making evaporative cooling less effective. Children and the elderly have physiologic limitations, especially if combined with chronic illness (Glazer, 2005).

g. Heat exhaustion is a milder illness than heat stroke. Exercise-related heat exhaustion may occur as exercising muscles create 10 to 20 times more heat than muscles at rest. Core body temperatures with heat exhaustion are between 37°C/98.6°F and 40°C/104°F. Symptoms include nausea, vomiting, dizziness, fatigue, weakness, and headache. Treatment consists of vigorous rehydration with intravenous (IV) fluids if mental status or GI problems preclude oral intake. Children experiencing heat exhaustion should be moved to a cooler environment and measures to cool the body (e.g., ice packs to the neck or axilla, cool towels, fanning) should be used (Glazer, 2005; Laskowski-Jones, 2010).

h. Heat stroke is an acute medical emergency caused by an extreme buildup in body heat with core body temperatures usually between 40°C/104°F and 44°C/111.2°F (Bakar & Schleien, 2016). It is life threatening with a mortality rate of around 10% despite good medical management. Shock, circulatory abnormalities, disseminated intravascular coagulation (DIC), rhabdomyolysis, arrhythmias, and seizures are prominent features. Treatment involves immediate transport to an emergency medical facility. Rapid reversal of hyperthermia is the main goal, starting before transport utilizing whatever means available (most likely evaporative cooling). After arrival at a medical facility, rapid cooling may be accomplished by immersion cooling and internal cooling procedures such as gastric, bladder, and rectal cold-water lavage. More extreme rapid cooling methods include peritoneal and/or thoracic lavage and cardiopulmonary bypass (Bakar & Schleien, 2016; Glazer, 2005). The pediatric patient with heat stroke will require close management of circulation, hydration, and intensive multisystem monitoring and support.

C. Drowning, Submersion, and Anoxic Injury

1. Drowning is a common and highly preventable cause of death in childhood. Children aged 1 to 4 years have the highest rate of morbidity and mortality from drowning; about one in five people who die from drowning are children aged 14 and younger (CDC, 2017). The definition of *drowning* is a process resulting in primary respiratory impairment from submersion or immersion in a liquid medium (ILCOR Advisory Statement on Drowning, 2003). The child may survive the event or not. Drowning is a type of asphyxial injury. Other examples of asphyxial injuries include inhalation, traumatic asphyxia, apnea, strangulation, suffocation, foreign-body aspiration, and adolescents playing the "choking game" or committing suicide by hanging (Byard, Austin, & Van den Heuvel, 2011; Toblin, Paulozzi, Gilchrist, & Russell, 2008). The "choking game" is either self-strangulation or strangulation by another person using his or her hands or a noose to achieve a state of euphoria, which is brief and attributed to cerebral hypoxia (Toblin et al., 2008).

2. The three most important risk factors that contribute to drowning and near drowning are the following:

   a. Inability to swim or the overestimation of swimming capabilities

   b. Risk-taking behavior

   c. Inadequate adult supervision. Sites where childhood drownings occur may be distinguished as domestic (e.g., bathtubs, buckets), artificial pools (e.g., swimming pools, hot tubs), natural freshwater (e.g., ponds, pits), and salt water (Semple-Hess & Campwala, 2014). Most drownings occur in June, July, and August in backyard pools (Laskowski-Jones, 2010).

3. *Pathophysiology*

   a. The actual process of drowning occurs when the victim's airway is beneath the surface of the water. Voluntary breath holding occurs, which may only last for 20 seconds to maximum of around 60 seconds, at which time small amounts of water are aspirated into the airways. The presence of water in the airways triggers coughing and laryngospasm. The victim is unable to breathe, which leads to hypoxia, hypercarbia, and acidosis. The hypoxia to the brain leads to loss of consciousness (LOC) and apnea. The laryngospasm stops and the victim may aspirate larger volumes of water. The sustained hypoxia leads to cardiac deterioration and multiple organ failure (Semple-Hess & Campwala, 2014).

   b. Cardiac pathophysiologic changes associated with submersion injury are the consequence

of the hypoxia and acidosis. Hypothermia may play a role depending on the temperature of the water. Dysrhythmias associated with cardiac dysfunction due to drowning generally progress from tachycardia to bradycardia to pulseless electrical activity (PEA) to asystole (Semple-Hess & Campwala, 2014). Pulmonary pathophysiologic changes are related primarily to intrapulmonary shunting from a variety of factors: bronchospasm, impaired gas exchange due to aspiration of fluids into the lungs, washout of surfactant, alveolar injury, and atelectasis (Semple-Hess & Campwala, 2014). Research has now shown that there are no clinical differences in pulmonary injury whether fresh water or salt water is aspirated. The type of fluid aspirated should also be kept in mind. Dirty stagnant water may breed infectious injury and chemical aspiration from gastric contents or cleaning solutions may lead to chemical pneumonitis (Semple-Hess & Campwala, 2014). In addition, submersion injury victims intubated and on mechanical ventilation will be at increased risk for ventilator-associated pneumonia (VAP).

4. *Hypothermia* Hypothermia is often associated with submersion injuries and the severity of the hypothermia is dependent on the temperature of the water. It has been hypothesized that cold water is protective as it elicits the "dive reflex" and causes hypothermia. Both the diving reflex and the hypothermia provide protection of vital organ function by decreasing metabolic demand and reducing the damaging effects of hypoxia (Quan, Mack, & Schiff, 2014). The mammalian "dive reflex" is elicited by the face coming in contact with cold water and consists of breath holding, intense peripheral vasoconstriction with bradycardia, decreased cardiac output, and increased mean arterial pressure (MAP). However, physiologic studies have found the diving reflex to be transient and ultimately not a protection or a predictor of survival in drowning victims (Quan et al., 2014, 2016).

5. *Recovery and Outcome*

   a. In a recent study performed by Quan et al. (2016), the strongest outcome predictor was submersion duration. They found that less than 5-minute submersion durations were associated with favorable outcomes. The worst outcomes were at submersion durations longer than 25 minutes. A longer than 25-minute submersion duration was statistically found to be invariably fatal. Their conclusion is that submersion duration greater than 10 minutes has a very low likelihood of a good outcome (Quan et al., 2016). There is no question regarding the critical role of bystander CPR in the survival of the drowning victim. Immediate CPR, as soon as it is possible and safe, will help to restore oxygenation and ventilation (AHA, 2015; Venema, Groothoff, & Bierens, 2010).

b. Prediction of functional neurologic outcome versus death or severe disability becomes more reliable with time as the child is treated and recovery or response to therapy is observed. Neurologic examination within the first 24 to 72 hours of therapy (combined with other imaging and testing procedures) is the best indicator of neurologic outcome (Ibsen & Koch, 2002). Magnetic resonance spectroscopy rather than CT scan may be useful in the early evaluation of hypoxic–ischemic injury (Ibsen & Koch, 2002). Early EEG is complicated by the use of sedatives, analgesics, and muscle relaxants consistent with resuscitation and initial treatment. A flat or severely attenuated EEG or burst suppression record is often a poor prognostic indicator, but it is most likely reflective of the initial insult and resuscitation. Similar findings that persist in the absence of such medications are more predictive of a poor neurologic prognosis (Isben & Koch, 2002).

6. *Treatment in the ICU*

a. An important focus of treatment for a drowning victim is core rewarming. Passive and active rewarming procedures are used based on the degree of hypothermia. Passive methods would involve removing all wet garments and covering the victim with warm blankets. Active rewarming includes external and internal measures. External measures are the use of hot packs, heating lamps, or forced-air external warmers. Internal active rewarming would include warming IV fluids, warm humidified oxygen (either through face mask or endotracheal tube [ETT]), warm saline lavage of stomach, peritoneum, rectal, and even mediastinal spaces. Most aggressive and most efficient would be the use of extracorporeal circulation (ECC) or extracorporeal membrane oxygenation (ECMO) rewarming technique (Biagas & Aponte-Patel, 2016).

b. The goal of mechanical ventilation after hypoxic-ischemic injury is to optimize ventilation and oxygenation and to maintain normocarbia (Hazinski, 2013).

c. Fluid resuscitation and inotropic agents may be required to restore adequate tissue perfusion as a result of impaired myocardial contractility, persistent hypoxemia, hypothermia, acidosis, suboptimal intravascular volume, and electrolyte abnormalities (Caglar & Quan, 2016). Long-term morbidity and mortality after near drowning are due to hypoxic–ischemic brain injury. However, reduction of increased intracranial pressure (ICP) has not been proved an effective cerebroprotective strategy in drowning victims (Biagas & Aponte-Patel, 2016; Caglar & Quan, 2016).

HISTORY

A. Trauma Resuscitation

Trauma resuscitation begins immediately after the injury, with first aid initiated by family or bystanders, and continues with the prehospital care providers and emergency department staff. The initial assessment and treatment must be organized and methodical to decrease trauma-related morbidity and mortality.

B. Injury History

1. The history surrounding the injury is obtained from family, bystanders, prehospital providers, and the patient (if possible). Pertinent historical information is obtained and relates to three important areas: mechanism of injury, patient history, and the plausibility of the mechanism of injury and patient history. The critical care nurse plays a pivotal role in assimilating details specific to the mechanism of injury and the presenting injury and complications. The following serves as a guide for the nurse and lists basic information that should be obtained relative to each mechanism of injury.

a. *Motor vehicle occupant.* Scene fatalities, use of restraining devices (e.g., car seat, three-point restraints, booster seat, lap belt), front or backseat passenger, ejection from the vehicle, site of impact (e.g., side, rear end, head on), motor vehicle speed, object of collision (e.g., oncoming vehicle, stationary vehicle, or object), passenger compartment intrusion, entrapment

b. *Pedestrian versus motor vehicle crash.* Speed of the vehicle, travel of the patient after the impact, being run over by or pinned under the vehicle, the type of surface on which the patient landed, the point of impact on the patient's body

c. *Bicycle versus motor vehicle crash.* Speed of the bicycle, speed of the vehicle (if moving), use of a bicycle helmet

d. *Fall.* The height from which the patient fell, the number of steps, the surface onto which the patient landed, and the area of body that hit the ground first

e. *Penetrating injury.* The type of weapon used, number of bullets fired, caliber of bullets, firing range, number, and location of stab wounds

2. The following questions related to the injury history help elicit valuable information to anticipate ICU course and outcome.

a. *Airway.* Did the child have a choking or vomiting episode? Was assistance needed to maintain the child's airway?

b. *Breathing.* Did the child stop breathing or have difficulty breathing? If so, for how long did this occur? Was rescue breathing initiated?

c. *Circulation.* Was blood lost? About how much? Was cardiopulmonary resuscitation (CPR) initiated? How long was it in progress?

d. *Disability.* Did the child sustain an LOC? If so, for how long? Was the child easily arousable? Does the child have antegrade (loss of memory after the injury) or retrograde (loss of memory before the injury) amnesia? Does the child recognize family members and familiar objects? Was the child able to wiggle his or her fingers and toes? Did the child appear flaccid? Did the child appear frightened, apprehensive, or anxious?

e. *Other.* Was any first aid administered? Were any splints or bandages applied? Did the child get up and walk around after the injury or was the child found in the same position as immediately following the injury?

3. Additional information may integrate the mechanisms of injury with the patient's social history. Family and developmental history may be elicited from the following questions:

a. *Developmental plausibility.* Is the mechanism of injury consistent with the injuries seen and the history related to these injuries? Does the mechanism of injury match the patient's history? That is, if the mechanism of injury in an infant was a fall from a couch (approximately 1 foot high) onto a carpeted floor and the infant is in

cardiopulmonary arrest, intentional injury must be suspected (see "Child Maltreatment" section).

b. *Credibility of witnesses.* Are family members or bystanders changing their stories to match the child's injuries? Are witnesses reluctant to divulge information? For example, the mechanism of injury in a 13-year-old child is a GSW to the chest from a drive-by shooting. It is a warm evening; all the neighbors are outside, and yet no one sees the car or driver. Such witnesses may be afraid to come forward for fear of gang retaliation.

c. *Patient's overall appearance.* How does the child appear overall? Does the child appear well nourished and clean? Is the child's appearance developmentally appropriate? Does the child appear to be the correct size and weight for his or her age? Does the child have any bruises, scars, or other signs of child maltreatment? How is the parent–child relationship? Does the parent or caregiver comfort or scold the child for the injury? Does the parent label the child as "clumsy" or "accident prone"? Does the child go willingly to strangers or shrink from human touch? (see "Child Maltreatment" section).

C. Patient Health History

1. Parents may have been involved in the injury and may be receiving treatment elsewhere (e.g., for an MVA). Family members called to the hospital might not be able to provide information about the patient's health history. Parents or legal guardians must be notified when an injury occurs; however, emergency treatment is not withheld until parental consent is obtained.

2. The critical care nurse can use the acronym SAMPLE to guide the assessment of the basic past health history (AAP & AHA, 2016, p. 38):

a. Signs/symptoms

b. Allergies to medications, food, latex, and so on

c. Medications the patient regularly receives (both over-the-counter and prescription); last dose and time of recent medications

d. Past medical history or illness as well as special needs (e.g., hearing impairment, use of special devices)

e. Last meal eaten

f. Events or environment that led to the injury (obtained in injury history)

INITIAL ASSESSMENT

The initial assessment of the multiply injured child includes the primary and secondary assessments. Children have unique anatomic and physiologic features that make them different from adults. These features should be taken into consideration when conducting the primary and secondary assessments.

A. Primary Assessment

1. In the primary assessment, life-threatening injuries are detected and treated. Life-threatening injuries include airway obstruction; open, tension, and bilateral hemopneumothoraces; traumatic arrest; flail chest; cardiac tamponade; and hemorrhagic shock.

2. Life-saving interventions are initiated simultaneously with the detection of these injuries and include airway stabilization and restoration of breathing and circulation.

3. *Airway and Cervical Spine Assessment*

  a. Pediatric developmental considerations (Table 9.4; see "Respiratory System" and "Neurological System" within the table)

  b. Assessment and interventions

   i. The airway is assessed for patency. The presence of loose teeth, vomit, and blood is determined and cleared if possible and safe to do so. Cervical spine injury is assessed very carefully and prehospital protocols have been developed to guide emergency medical services (EMS) in recognizing clinical evidence for a cervical spine injury or a high suspicion of injury. The automatic use of cervical spine immobilization with rigid cervical collars and straight backboard for any or all trauma patients has been a topic of much debate in the research. Studies have shown that cervical immobilization is not effective and can have harmful effects when improperly applied (Bledsoe & Carrison, 2015; E. Kim et al., 2013; Morrissey, Kusel, & Sporer, 2014; Sundstrøm, Asbjørnsen, Habiba, Sunde, & Wester, 2014). If cervical spine injury is clinically assessed or a high suspicion remains, recommendations are to secure the child to the backboard and stabilize the neck to prevent movement. Various cervical stabilization techniques are used, including leaving the infant in the car seat and the use of properly fitting collars either rigid or soft and placing on a firm/rigid backboard. Proper alignment is a challenge for the young infant and child trauma patients due to their large occiput causing flexion of the cervical spine, which can cause airway compromise or aggravation of an existing spinal cord injury. The guideline is to assess the infant or child's occiput in relation to the board and pad the upper back to align the external auditory meatus to the shoulders (M. Crowley, 2014).

   ii. Signs and symptoms of spinal cord injury are quickly ascertained, such as numbness, tingling, and inability to wiggle the toes and fingers. If initiated, full spinal immobilization is maintained throughout the initial treatment until discontinued by a physician.

TABLE 9.4 Pediatric Developmental Considerations

Anatomy and Physiology	Significance	Age Anatomy Matures
RESPIRATORY SYSTEM		
Oxygen consumption higher compared with adults Lower FRC	Hypoxemia occurs more rapidly when distressed Shorter safe apnea time Results in ↑ respiratory rates Smaller intrapulmonary oxygen stores	Increases with age
Small length and diameter of airways	Predisposition to obstruction, infection, and atelectasis	Resolves with age and growth
Shorter trachea	Predisposition to inadvertent extubation Unintentional head movement may displace ETT	Resolves with age

(continued)

TABLE 9.4 Pediatric Developmental Considerations *(continued)*

Anatomy and Physiology	Significance	Age Anatomy Matures
Large head with prominent occiput, short neck, weak shoulder girdle Cartilages of infant's larynx and trachea are soft	Predisposition to upper airway obstruction by position alone Makes visualization of cords difficult on laryngoscopy Easily compressed by hyperextension or hyperflexion of the neck—obstructing airway	2–6 years
Narrow nasal bridge; obligate nose breathers	Predisposition to nasal obstruction by foreign body, trauma, secretions, edema, or surgery	3–6 months
Large tongue Large, floppy, U-shaped epiglottis	↑ Likelihood of airway occlusion ↑ Sensitivity to edema, trauma, and infection ↑ End expiratory pressure during respiratory failure	Up to 10 years 2 years
Weaker hyoepiglottic ligament (at base of vallecula attaches the epiglottis to base of the tongue)	Curved blades aimed at the vallecula to lift epiglottis from the airway may not work in infants and young children	
Cricoid cartilage most narrow aspect of trachea causing funnel shape	↑ Susceptibility to trauma, edema, and infection 1 mm of edema ↑ resistance to airflow by factor of 16[a], which ↑ work of breathing in infants and young children Foreign bodies may become lodged below the cords May provide an effective seal around ETT (uncuffed)	Varies with age and growth Generally <10 years About 6–8 years
Diaphragm is primary muscle of respiration Diaphragm sits horizontally in infants	Generates large negative pressure in thorax ↑ In abdominal contents can compromise diaphragmatic movement (bleeding in trauma; swallowing air when crying) Contraction of diaphragm draws lower ribs inward ↓ Efficiency of diaphragmatic effort in breathing	4–5 years Varies with age and growth
Immature development of intercostal and abdominal muscles	These muscles cannot be relied upon for respiratory effort, they fatigue more easily and predispose infants and young children to atelectasis and respiratory failure Infant compensates by ↑ respiratory rate	Transition from abdominal to costal breathing at 2–3 years, completed by 7 years
Right and left mainstem bronchi at 55 degree angles	Intubation of either mainstem bronchi equally possible High risk of bilateral aspiration	1–2 years
Immature alveolar system causing ↓ number of alveoli and ↓ surface area for gas exchange	↓ Diffusion ↑ Shunting	8 years

(continued)

TABLE 9.4   Pediatric Developmental Considerations *(continued)*

Anatomy and Physiology	Significance	Age Anatomy Matures
Chest wall in younger children is cartilaginous Thin chest wall	Blunt and penetrating energy forces easily transmit to underlying lung and cardiac tissue Breath sounds easily transmitted allowing false assumption that breath sounds are equal	About 10 years
Ribs: flexible, attach horizontally instead of bucket-handle attachment in mature rib cage Soft, thin, more compliant chest wall	Limits ability to ↑ tidal volume with chest excursion Less effective at protecting upper abdominal structures and lungs	About 10 years
Infant's upper airway very reactive	Makes ETT intubation difficult Stimulation of hypopharynx may cause vigorous gagging and laryngeal spasm	
Faster respiratory rate and smaller tidal volumes	Greater insensible pulmonary fluid loss If trauma in closed space ↑ RR may lead to ↑ uptake of smoke and toxic gases More prone to fatigue and respiratory failure	
Cardiovascular System		
Low cardiac stroke volume High cardiac rate	↑ Rate doubles cardiac output (twice that of an adult) to meet needs for ↑ metabolic rate Little/limited ability to ↑ their stroke volume	After 6–8 years
Higher oxygen requirement and faster metabolic rate	Requires higher cardiac output per kilogram of body weight	Varies with age and growth
Circulating blood volume small (80 mL/kg) but larger mL/kg basis than adults Children may have a blood loss of up to 25%–30% before BP changes	Small amounts of blood loss can ↓ circulating volume and ↓ perfusion Hypotension is a late sign of circulatory compromise Assessment of perfusion parameters is best indication of worsening perfusion	
Cardiac output rate dependent in infants and young children	Tachycardia is initial response to hypovolemia and ↓ oxygen delivery Tachycardia may be first and only sign of impending shock	
Proportionately, larger volume of blood in the head	Rapid onset of cerebral edema and ↑ ICP	2–6 years
Immature adrenergic receptors	Limited response to sympathetic innervation in stress due to trauma, blood loss, surgery	About 2 years
Parasympathetic nervous system more mature at birth	↑ Sensitivity to vagal stimulation causing bradycardia	About 1 year

(continued)

TABLE 9.4 Pediatric Developmental Considerations *(continued)*

Anatomy and Physiology	Significance	Age Anatomy Matures
Greater BSA in proportion to their body weight Higher extracellular-to-intracellular fluid volume ratio	Requires proportionally more fluid during resuscitation Will require maintenance fluid	
Neurological System		
Large head-to-body ratio Weak neck muscles Spinal facet joints horizontally oriented Lax ligaments	With falls or ejection or struck then flown—the head will land or hit first Predisposes children to head trauma More head and neck movement in children—maximal movement at C1–C3 in young children; maximal movement at C5–C6[b] in older children Predisposes children to neck trauma; younger children have more high-level cervical injuries, fewer fractures, more dislocations, more spinal cord injuries[c]	Up to 6–8 years Young child <12 years Older child >12 years
Skull is soft and compliant	Less protection for brain tissue; more susceptible to injury	Bone growth in childhood Complete ossification by early 20s
Fontanelles open	Open fontanelles and sutures may allow for ↑ICP delaying herniation but hiding signs of tissue injury	Anterior fontanelle closes at 12–18 months
Sutures not fused (children <2 years)	Predisposes to diastatic fractures	
Nerve myelination not complete at birth	Unmyelinated brain tissue is particularly vulnerable to injury, especially shearing forces	Visible growth up to 2 years, maturation in adolescence, adult
Physical and psychological age-related milestones	Important to know whether milestones have been reached as initial neuro assessment is performed	
Exposure		
Immature thermostatic control Less adaptive behavioral reaction to cold stress[b] Large body surface to body mass (BSA to weight) Decreased subcutaneous fat Inability to shunt blood away from skin when cold	↓Ability to adjust to temperature changes More prone to hypothermia (which can slow resuscitative measures) and frostbite Susceptible to convective and conductive heat loss ↓Ability to maintain temperature; T ↓36.5°C causing ↑metabolic rate, ↑oxygen consumption and metabolic acidosis	6 months to 1 year Develops with maturation
Nonshivering thermogenesis	Brown fat broken down to provide warmth; ↑oxygen consumption and leads to decompensation	After 6 months
Thinner skin Inefficient sweating Higher metabolic rate Unable to care for themselves or to control their environment	Susceptible to significant burn injuries from exposure to less heat compared to adults Easily internally bruised Higher incidence of heatstroke—most severe form of heat-related illnesses	

(continued)

TABLE 9.4 Pediatric Developmental Considerations *(continued)*

Anatomy and Physiology	Significance	Age Anatomy Matures
Abdomen		
Round protuberant abdomen Immature abdominal muscles Rib cage higher and pelvis small[d]	Little protection for underlying solid and hollow abdominal organs Solid organs in abdomen proportionately larger Abdominal organs prone to injury Trauma forces readily commuted to internal organs without bruising	
Sigmoid colon and ascending colon not completely attached to peritoneal cavity	More prone to deceleration injuries[e]	
Glucose		
Children more prone to hypoglycemia	Monitor blood glucose frequently in burns or trauma	
Coagulopathy		
Early trauma induced coagulopathy[f] Local activation of the coagulation system after trauma	Most commonly encountered complication of trauma Independent predictor of mortality	
Eustachian Tube		
Eustachian tube is short and horizontal	More prone to infection	Begins slanting downward between 6 and 8 years
Behavior/Ability to Cooperate		
Infants and young children are scared and anxious	Performing a physical exam on infants and young children is challenging due to their anxiety and fear Important to approach with calmness, confidence, and compassion	

BP, blood pressure; BSA, body surface area; ETT, endotracheal tube; FRC, functional residual capacity; ICP, increased intracranial pressure; RR, respiratory rate.

Sources: Adapted, modified, and updated from Crowley, C. M., & Morrow, A. I. (1980). A comprehensive approach to the child in respiratory failure. *Critical Care Nursing Quarterly, 3*(1), 27–44.

[a]Kline-Tilford, A. M., Sorce, L. R., Levin, D. L., & Anas, N. G. (2013). Pulmonary disorders in nursing. In M. F. Hazinski (Ed.), *Nursing care of the critically ill child* (3rd ed., pp. 483–561). St. Louis, MO: Elsevier.

[b]Hardcastle, N., Benzon, H. A., & Vavilala, M. S. (2014). Update on the 2012 guidelines for the management of pediatric traumatic brain injury—Information for the anesthesiologist. *Pediatric Anesthesia, 24*(7), 703–710.

[c]Sundstrøm, T., Asbjørnsen, H., Habiba, S., Sunde, G. A., & Wester, K. (2014). Prehospital use of cervical collars in trauma patients: A critical review. *Journal of Neurotrauma, 31*(6), 531–540.

[d]Emergency Nurses Association. (2013). *ENPC provider manual* (4th ed.). Des Plaines, IL: Author.

[e]Zonnoor, B. (2017). Frostbite. In D. M. Elston (Ed.), *Medscape*. Retrieved from https://emedicine.medscape.com/article/926249-overview

[f]MacLeod, J. B., Winkler, A. M., McCoy, C. C., Hillyer, C. D., & Shaz, B. H. (2014). Early trauma induced coagulopathy (ETIC): Prevalence across the injury spectrum. *Injury, 45*(5), 910–915.

4. *Respiratory Assessment*

a. Developmental considerations (Table 9.4; see "Respiratory System" section within the table)

b. Assessment and interventions

i. Respirations are assessed by observation and inspection. The qualities of respirations are determined by assessing the presence of breath sounds high in the axillae and anterior chest. Unequal bilateral breath sounds may indicate a pneumothorax on the diminished side. Signs of respiratory distress include retractions of the intercostal muscles, nasal flaring, grunting (in infants), adventitious breath sounds, diminished, or absent breath sounds. Rescue breathing with 100% oxygen via bag-valve mask (BVM) is initiated in the apneic or bradypneic child.

ii. The chest is exposed and inspected for any surface trauma, penetrating wounds, paradoxical movements, and flail segments. The rib cage is gently palpated for tenderness, crepitus, and flail segments. The sternum is palpated for tenderness as well.

5. *Circulatory Assessment*

a. Developmental considerations (Table 9.4; see "Cardiovascular System" section within the table)

b. Assessment and interventions

i. Circulation is assessed by auscultation of heart sounds for their rate, rhythm, and quality. If the pulse is absent or if peripheral pulses or blood pressure (BP) are nonpalpable in the presence of an electrical rhythm (PEA), chest compressions are immediately initiated. Muffled heart tones, distended neck veins (if visible), and shock may indicate cardiac tamponade, which may necessitate pericardiocentesis or open pericardiotomy. Major external hemorrhage is controlled by applying direct pressure.

ii. Peripheral circulation is assessed by palpating the radial or brachial pulse, measuring capillary refill time (should be ≤2 seconds), assessing skin color (pink), and temperature (warm). Deviations in peripheral circulation may indicate decreased blood flow to the periphery, which can result in decreased oxygen and substrate delivery to the tissues.

6. *Neurologic Assessment*

a. Developmental considerations (Table 9.4; see "Neurologic System" section within the table)

b. Assessment and interventions

i. A brief neurologic evaluation establishes the patient's LOC and pupillary size and reactivity. Responsiveness may be more difficult to evaluate in the preverbal child. Alterations in developmentally expected behaviors (e.g., lack of stranger anxiety in an 8-month-old infant, decreased muscle tone in a 2-month-old infant or inability to focus and follow objects in a 6-month-old infant), may indicate changes in neurologic functioning. Changes in the child's LOC may indicate decreased oxygenation (pulmonary exchange) or perfusion (hypovolemia), not necessarily brain injury.

ii. Throughout the primary assessment, the nurse talks to the child to determine his or her LOC and to provide emotional support. The AVPU method of evaluation determines the child's response to stimulation (Emergency Nurses Association, 2013):

- *A*wake
- Responsive to *v*erbal stimuli
- Responsive to *p*ainful stimuli
- *U*nresponsive

iii. The infant should respond by looking around and being wary of strangers. The verbal child should be able to state his or her name and perhaps other information. The child who changes from awake to sleepy to disoriented should be watched closely. The Pediatric Glasgow Coma Score (PGCS) should be obtained to record the best eye, motor, and verbal responses (see "Clinical Assessment of Neurologic Function" in Chapter 4 for information on the GCS).

7. *Exposure*

a. Developmental considerations (Table 9.4; see "Exposure" section within the table)

b. Assessment and interventions. The child is completely undressed to allow inspection of all injuries. Overhead warming lights and warm ambient temperature should help maintain body temperature within a normal range. Warm blankets should be applied to respect modesty, prevent convective heat loss, and promote comfort.

B. Secondary Assessment

A complete head-to-toe assessment is conducted to detect and treat all non–life-threatening injuries.

1. The head is examined for depressions, lacerations, hematomas, and impaled objects. The anterior and posterior fontanelles in infants are palpated. A tense and bulging fontanelle may indicate increased ICP. The scalp is palpated for lacerations and observed for dirt, glass, and other debris.

2. The face is inspected for deformities, lacerations, foreign bodies, and impaled objects. The orbits, facial bones, and mandible are palpated for pain and crepitus. Asymmetric facial movement is observed, which may indicate facial nerve paralysis. Classic LeFort (facial) fractures, although rare in children, should be suspected in any blunt force or penetrating facial trauma. Malocclusion is indicative of a fractured mandible. An example of a combined traumatic finding to the head or face would be a child with a self-inflicted GSW to the mandible who has a palate impaled with a tongue piercing.

3. The eyes are assessed for pupillary reactivity, symmetry, and extraocular movements. Blood in the anterior chamber of the eye (hyphemia) should be reported immediately because this finding indicates a serious injury. Foreign bodies should be noted, and penetrating objects should be stabilized in place with gauze and tape. A ruptured globe is possible if the eye is swollen shut and bruised and a penetrating or direct blunt force was applied during the injury. The presence of tearing should be noted as well. Visual acuity may be easily assessed by asking the young child to point to an object or by having an older child verbalize his or her ability to see. The presence of contact lenses should be ascertained, and the contact lenses removed. Periorbital bruising or "raccoon's sign" is indicative of a basilar skull fracture. Scleral hemorrhage may be observed if compression forces were applied at the time of injury.

4. The ears are examined for cerebrospinal fluid or bloody drainage. Such drainage can be collected onto a gauze pad; however, the ear is never packed with gauze. Hematotympanum should be noted. Ecchymosis over the mastoid process or "Battle's sign" is indicative of a basilar skull fracture. When ecchymosis over the mastoid process is noted, the skull fracture is more than 12 hours old. Ear lacerations should be covered with gauze soaked in normal saline (NS) until definitive repair is scheduled.

5. The nose is examined for cerebrospinal fluid or bloody drainage, deformities, lacerations, or bruising. Drainage can be collected onto a gauze pad, but the nares are not packed with gauze.

6. The oral cavity, including the tongue, mucous membranes, and teeth, is examined for injury. Displaced permanent teeth can be placed in milk or NS and dated. Debris should not be removed from the tooth because this material aids in reimplantation. Dental apparatus, such as braces, may have been damaged during the injury and should be assessed by a pediatric dentist or orthodontist.

7. The neck examination involves opening the front piece of the cervical collar for inspection of the anterior neck. The neck is assessed for lacerations, swelling, deformities, jugular vein distention, and impaled objects. The neck is palpated for pain, tenderness, and subcutaneous emphysema. Tracheal positioning is noted. Normal position is midline. The larynx is palpated for integrity. A fractured larynx is easier to palpate than visualize. The awake child's voice is assessed for hoarseness or changes. A hoarse or "gravelly" voice may also indicate tracheal trauma and the possible need for airway intervention. After the neck is assessed, the collar is secured.

8. The chest is reinspected for symmetry, flail segments, open wounds, and impaled objects. The anterior chest is examined for cutaneous lesions that might indicate underlying pulmonary or cardiac injury. The chest is auscultated for the presence of normal and adventitious breath sounds. The anterior rib cage and both clavicles are palpated for pain and tenderness. Pain with inspiration should be noted. The heart sounds are auscultated and should be clear and distinct. The point of maximal impulse (PMI) should be noted.

9. The abdomen is observed for distention, bruising, penetrating wounds, and impaled objects. Bowel sounds should be auscultated. The abdomen is then palpated for pain, rigidity, and tenderness. The lower abdomen is palpated for bladder tenderness and distention.

10. The pelvis is palpated for tenderness and intactness. Any pain or displacement on palpation is indicative of a pelvic fracture. Femoral pulses are assessed for equality and strength. The bladder is palpated for distention. The genitalia, urinary meatus, perineum, and rectum are inspected for signs of trauma, bleeding, and impaled objects. Blood at the urinary meatus may indicate a urethral tear. The prostate gland is difficult to palpate in the preadolescent boy. A flaccid rectal sphincter is indicative of spinal cord injury. The rectal examination may be deferred in cases of severe rectal trauma when an examination under anesthesia (EUA) or surgical intervention is needed or when a foreign body is lodged in the rectal vault. Priapism may be noted. Anal examinations specific to abuse are difficult to interpret due to a number of variables: (a) the size of the object introduced, (b) the presence of force, (c) use of lubricants, (d) degree of cooperation from the victim, (e) the number of episodes of penetration, (f) the time since the last contact (Herrmann, Banaschak, Csorba, Navratil, & Dettmeyer, 2014).

11. The extremities are inspected for any deformities, open wounds or fractures, contusions, and impaled objects. Each extremity is palpated for pain and peripheral pulses are assessed for equality and amplitude. Skin color and temperature are reassessed as well as is capillary refill time. The responses given when asking the child to wiggle his or her toes and fingers and asking whether he or she can feel the nurse touching the toes and fingers indicate neurovascular and neuromotor integrity. Hand grasps and foot flexion and extension determine strength and motor nerve functioning.

12. The back examination involves carefully log rolling the child to inspect the back. To log roll the child, one person is assigned to keep the child's head midline and to execute the move. Additional staff members are needed to roll the child onto his or her side at the surgeon's command. Another person examines the back for any deformities, lacerations, hematomas, impaled objects, or abrasions on the posterior surface and flank. Each vertebra is palpated for stability and the presence of pain. After this examination, the surgeon gives the command to roll the child to the supine position, maintaining in-line cervical stabilization the entire time. The child's motor and neurovascular statuses are assessed immediately before and after the log rolling to assess the presence of spinal cord injury.

13. Vital signs and pulse oximetry readings are measured continuously and recorded every 5 minutes until the child is stable and then every 15 minutes for the first hour of treatment. Temperature is measured frequently to evaluate the effectiveness of warming measures and to detect and treat hypothermia. The child's vital signs should be compared with age-appropriate norms for heart rate, respiratory rate, and BP. Immediately after the injury, however, the child's physiologic requirements may not fall within age-appropriate ranges. Therefore, these parameters should serve as a guide only.

C. Trauma Scoring

1. After the primary and secondary assessments are completed in the field or emergency department (ED), a trauma score (TS) and a PGCS score are assigned. TS determinations are integral to the appropriate triage to pediatric trauma centers. TS systems are intended to be simple and based on rapidly obtainable clinical findings. TSs utilized are easy to calculate as well as sensitive enough to include pediatric patients who require a higher level of expertise and care (Brazelton & Gosain, 2016).

2. Validated triage scoring systems for pediatric trauma include the PGCS, TS, Revised Trauma Score (RTS), and the Pediatric Trauma Score (PTS). The PTS, utilized at many pediatric emergency departments, assesses six parameters important in the outcome of pediatric trauma: size, airway, blood pressure, central nervous system (CNS), fractures, and wounds (Denke, 2013). This scoring system has been validated as a reliable predictor of injury severity as well as an indicator for triage to an appropriate pediatric trauma center. The TS assesses respiratory rate and effort, BP, and capillary refill. It also includes the GCS score. The RTS comprises the GCS score (see Chapter 4), BP, and respiratory rate. Ideally, TSs are calculated during three phases: in the prehospital setting, on arrival to the ED, and 1 hour later.

INITIAL TREATMENT

A. Airway and Cervical Spine

1. In the unconscious child, the airway initially is opened and maintained using the jaw-thrust maneuver. This maneuver is the safest technique for opening the airway in the child with a suspected cervical spine injury (AAP & AHA, 2016). The head-tilt/chin-lift method is not used in pediatric trauma patients because this method may convert a cervical spine fracture without neurologic injury into a cervical spine fracture with neurologic injury. Because the child's oral cavity is relatively small, the upper airway is easily obstructed by the lax oropharyngeal musculature in the unconscious child.

2. Foreign material (e.g., teeth, vomit, or blood), is cleared from the oral cavity with a tonsillar tip (Yankauer) suction tube. Stimulation of an intact gag reflex must be avoided as gagging, vomiting, and aspiration may result. Blind finger sweeps are not recommended for foreign-body removal in infants and young children because foreign material may be displaced distally and injury to the friable oral mucosa may result.

3. An oropharyngeal airway may be placed in unconscious children to maintain airway patency. Oral airway size must be appropriate because an artificial airway that is too small may push the tongue backward. One that is too large may damage the delicate, soft intraoral tissues causing bleeding and swelling and further complicating airway management. The oropharyngeal airway is measured from the corner of the mouth to the angle of the jaw (AAP & AHA, 2016). This type of airway is inserted directly using a tongue blade to pull the tongue forward. This airway is not rotated 90 degrees as in the adult because damage may occur to the oral tissues. Furthermore, the tongue may be displaced posteriorly into the pharynx, causing an airway obstruction.

4. Nasopharyngeal airways are not recommended in pediatric trauma patients. In the child with a head injury, a basilar or cribriform plate fracture may be present. During insertion of a nasopharyngeal airway, entry into the cranial vault may occur.

5. These basic airway maneuvers are acceptable for short-term airway control. Endotracheal intubation is preferred for extended periods. The equipment is prepared and cardiorespiratory and pulse oximetry monitors are used. The child's vital signs are closely monitored for cardiac dysrhythmias, lower oxygen saturation, or bradycardia. During endotracheal intubation, neutral cervical spine alignment is maintained by the surgeon or another skilled practitioner to avoid hyperextension. Endotracheal intubation is best accomplished by rapid sequence technique by a skilled practitioner.

6. A combination of medications is often used during rapid sequence intubation to prevent increased ICP and to produce adequate states of sedation, analgesia, and paralysis (Stewart, Bhananker, & Ramaiah, 2014). Succinylcholine and rocuronium both have a short onset of action. Succinylcholine is used when a fast-acting and short duration paralytic agent is required. For example, in head trauma patients for whom the neurological exam is essential or in a trauma patient who has recently eaten and has a full stomach. Due to its nondepolarizing effects, succinylcholine must be used cautiously in trauma patients with long-bone fractures as fasciculation may occur and in patients with known or suspected hyperkalemia. Routine use of atropine as a premedication for intubation in nonneonates is controversial, especially if used to prevent dysrhythmias. There are also no studies that validate the use of a minimum dose of atropine (AAP & AHA, 2016). The sedatives, anesthetic, and neuromuscular blocking agents (NMBA) used are based on the condition and stability of the patient and the treating physician's discretion. For a normotensive patient, midazolam, etomidate, propofol, or thiopental may be used. Propofol has been reported to have a high potential for morbidity when used as an infusion in children, causing the "propofol infusion syndrome" (PIS; Loh & Nair, 2013). Etomidate is a short-acting sedative-hypnotic that is commonly used in rapid sequence intubation. Etomidate is known to blunt the normal stress-induced increase in adrenal cortisol production. It is for this reason that the cautious use of etomidate in septic or debilitated patients is warranted (see Chapter 2).

7. An uncuffed ETT is used in children 8 years of age and younger because the cricoid cartilage serves as an effective seal. The orotracheal route is preferred. The ETT is secured with tape and benzoin or with commercially prepared devices. An orogastric tube may be inserted after intubation to decompress the stomach. The gastric tube is measured from the corner of the mouth, over the ear to the xiphoid process, and marked with tape. Once the tube is properly placed, it is secured with tape. A chest radiograph is taken to confirm the ETT placement and depth, as well as the presence of the orogastric tube in the stomach. Indicators of correct airway placement include symmetric chest movement, equal bilateral breath sounds auscultated in all fields and absent over stomach, end-tidal carbon dioxide ($EtCO_2$) detection and condensation in the ETT. Endotracheal suctioning may be required if copious secretions or oral trauma are present.

8. The most common complication of endotracheal intubation is inadvertent intubation of the right mainstem bronchus or dislodgment of the ETT into the right mainstem bronchus if the patient is positioned for procedures or transported within the facility. When this situation arises, chest expansion may not be equal and breath sounds are absent or diminished in the left side of the chest. Pulse oximetry readings may be low and ventilation may be difficult. Prompt recognition of this complication is essential. It is corrected by withdrawing the ETT until equal breath sounds and equal chest movement are observed. Documentation of ETT placement measurement at the nose or lip is valuable.

9. In children in whom airway patency and control are not possible because of extensive craniofacial injuries, an emergency tracheostomy or cricothyrotomy may be required.

10. Spinal precautions are maintained during emergency treatment. Spinal precautions include the application of a rigid cervical collar, cervical immobilization device (CID) and an immobilization board. If the child vomits, the child is log rolled as a unit with the equipment remaining intact after which suctioning is performed. Anteroposterior, lateral, oblique, and odontoid cervical spine radiographs from C1 through T1 may be obtained to determine the presence of spinal fractures. When obtaining the lateral views, the child's arms are pulled downward by a surgeon or a nurse to allow for radiographic visualization of T1. The radiographs are assessed for vertebral symmetry, alignment, and spacing. If the child does not have radiographic evidence of bony spinal abnormalities and the child has normal neurologic findings and no pain on palpation, the spinal immobilization devices may be removed. Normal neurologic findings include absence of pain with full range of cervical motion. This is often difficult to assess in the presence of distracting injuries or head trauma. An MRI may be needed to evaluate the spine further.

B. Breathing

1. High-flow oxygen through a nonrebreather face mask at a flow rate of 10 to 15 L/min is administered. The face mask fits properly if it is snug and covers the nose and mouth. If the child will not tolerate a face mask and oxygen saturation levels are maintained at 98% to 99%, the oxygen can be administered in a blow-by fashion.

2. If apnea or shallow breathing occurs, ineffective respirations are present. In such cases, artificial ventilation is initiated with a BVM and 100% high-flow oxygen. If breathing is spontaneous, but effective respirations are not achieved, endotracheal intubation is performed. The chest should rise and fall symmetrically when the bag is squeezed. If the chest does not rise, the face mask and head should be carefully repositioned while maintaining spinal precautions. The BVM device should have a bag capacity of at least 450 mL, be self-refilling, and come in pediatric and adult sizes. The pop-off valve should be occluded to allow for the need for higher ventilation pressures.

3. A pulse oximeter detects the percentage of oxygen saturation in the blood and is a useful adjunct for determining adequacy of oxygenation.

4. Mechanical ventilation is initiated once proper endotracheal placement and adequate ventilation are achieved. The initial settings include an age-appropriate rate, 100% oxygen and a low positive end-expiratory pressure (PEEP). The ventilator settings are adjusted according to the child's response to treatment.

5. Life-threatening thoracic injuries include tension hemothoraces, pneumothoraces, and pericardial tamponade. All these conditions are rare but must be anticipated. Pneumothoraces are initially treated with rapid needle decompression followed by chest tube placement. Pericardial tamponade is treated with a pericardiocentesis or a pericardial window in the operating room.

C. Circulation

1. Cardiorespiratory and blood pressure monitors are employed immediately after the child's arrival at the hospital. The appropriate cuff size should be two thirds the size of the child's upper arm or thigh.

2. IV cannulation with the largest catheter diameter possible is attempted in the upper, preferably uninjured extremity. Intraosseous (IO) access should be considered if IV access cannot be achieved in a reasonable amount of time. If IO access is unsuccessful, central venous cannulation or cut down should be attempted by an experienced physician or surgeon in the antecubital space or via the saphenous system. During IV cannulation, blood is obtained and sent for the following tests, depending on the location of injury. In suspected abdominal trauma, the following are assessed: hemoglobin, hematocrit, and platelet count; electrolytes and glucose; blood urea nitrogen (BUN) and creatinine; amylase, lipase, aspartate aminotransferase (AST), and alanine aminotransferase (ALT). Creatinine phosphokinase (CPK) is assessed for a child with suspected cardiac trauma. Type and crossmatch or type and screen are required if operative management is anticipated or blood will be administered. Blood toxicology screening is done for patients with suspected drug or alcohol use. The IV crystalloid fluid of choice is lactated Ringers (LR) solution, which is administered at a maintenance rate in the absence of hypovolemic shock. The fluid is warmed if rapid infusion is administered. A stopcock can be connected to the tubing if fluid boluses are anticipated. Overhydrating is avoided in children with significant head injury to prevent cerebral edema.

3. In the tachycardic or hypotensive child, a 20 mL/kg fluid bolus of crystalloid is administered. If no improvement in heart rate or blood pressure is observed, a second bolus is administered. More than two boluses of fluid may be required. If no response is apparent, a 10-mL/kg bolus of warm, O-negative blood may be administered rapidly.

4. External hemorrhaging is controlled with direct pressure to the wound. Elevation of a bleeding extremity in conjunction with direct pressure may help to slow the bleeding process. Tourniquet and hemostat applications are controversial and are not used.

5. The application of a pneumatic antishock garment (PASG) has limited value in the pediatric population. Its use in children is generally limited to inflation of a leg compartment for splinting of a femur fracture.

6. Traumatic arrest (empty heart syndrome) is treated with CPR and rapid infusion of warmed crystalloid and blood products. Thoracotomy and open cardiac massage are rarely performed for blunt trauma and are usually a last-chance effort to resuscitate the child. Prognosis is poor.

D. Disability and Neurologic Checks

1. Frequent neurologic checks are performed to observe for changes in LOC, motor, and sensory function. The PGCS score is helpful to document serial neurologic assessments. Changes in the child's LOC may indicate hypovolemia or increased ICP. Vomiting and irritability are early signs of increased ICP. In infants, a bulging fontanelle or an increased head circumference is a late sign of increased ICP.

2. Normoventilation with 100% oxygen is initiated in the child with a severe head injury to keep the $PaCO_2$ between 35 and 45 mmHg. Hyperventilation is initiated to achieve a $PaCO_2$ of approximately 30 mmHg if signs of a lesion (e.g., epidural) or rapid decompensation are present. A $PaCO_2$ less than 28 mmHg may contribute to brain ischemia.

3. Procedures and treatments are explained to the child at a level he or she can understand. Words of praise and comfort go far to help reassure the frightened, injured child.

E. Exposure

1. Passive and active warming measures are initiated to prevent conductive and convective heat loss. Passive warming measures include warm blankets and increased ambient room temperature. Active warming measures include the administration of normothermic IV fluids and blood products to help with core warming.

2. Temperature measurements are obtained via the oral, rectal, or tympanic routes. Temperature probes on ETTs, esophageal probes, or urinary bladder thermistors are other options for temperature measurement.

F. Gastrointestinal and Genitourinary Systems

1. An orogastric or nasogastric tube (NGT; if no facial or cranial injury suspected) should be inserted to prevent gastric distention, vomiting, and aspiration. Initial drainage can be tested for the presence of blood. Gastric contrast can be administered through the gastric tube before CT testing.

2. In the absence of trauma or blood at the urinary meatus or suspected urethral trauma, an indwelling bladder catheter may be inserted and connected to a urinary drainage bag. If urethral trauma is suspected, a retrograde urethrogram must be performed before insertion of an indwelling bladder catheter. When drug or alcohol use is suspected, urinalysis and toxicology and blood toxicology screen are indicated. In postmenarchal females, urinary chorionic gonadotropin (UCG) testing should be done to rule out pregnancy.

3. A stool smear should be tested for occult blood.

G. Musculoskeletal System

1. All long-bone fractures are immobilized. The child's neurovascular status is assessed immediately before and after splinting to ensure that an injury has not occurred or been aggravated. Open fractures, lacerations, or wounds require careful evaluation and cleaning.

2. Amputated body parts are wrapped in dry or moistened gauze, sealed in a plastic bag, and then placed in an ice-water bath. At no time should the amputated part touch the ice directly, as tissue necrosis may occur. Subspecialists (e.g., plastic surgery, reimplantation specialists) will determine whether reattachment is possible after evaluating the child's amputated parts. Whether the child and family view the amputated part or injured limb is decided on an individual case basis. Younger children may become frightened of the wound, whereas older children may be curious, and their imagined injury may be worse than the reality (see Chapter 1). Tetanus prophylaxis, antibiotics, and analgesic administration are necessary.

SECONDARY INTERVENTIONS

A. Diagnostic Testing

1. During any intrahospital transport, an experienced nurse and physician should always accompany the child and be prepared to intervene should the child have any changes or he or she deteriorates. Appropriately sized resuscitation equipment consisting of an Ambu bag, mask, oral airway, oxygen tank, and intubation equipment (e.g., appropriate-sized ETT, blade, handle, and stylet) if needed. If the patient is already intubated, confirm that the ETT is secure prior to transport. The child should be monitored with at least the minimum of ECG, oximetry, and blood pressure capabilities. Additional considerations for safe transport are to have suction available and medications for sedation and/or intubation.

2. Chest radiographs are obtained to determine the placement of ETTs, gastric tubes, and chest tubes. They can be done at the bedside in the trauma room, and technology today allows immediate interpretation of the radiographs at the bedside. These films also confirm the presence of pneumothoraces or hemopneumothoraces, rib and clavicle fractures, and diaphragm integrity. Abdominal radiographs confirm the placement of gastric tubes and bladder catheters; stomach and intestine intactness can be observed as well. Free air is noted, and the pelvis is examined for fracture. Radiographs of the spine and extremities remain the standard diagnostic test for rapid evaluation screening for injuries to those areas. Skeletal radiographs are obtained according to the suspected injury and skeletal survey should be performed when there is a suspicion of NAT. If the child needs to be transported to the radiology department for additional radiographs, the nurse should remain with the patient to monitor his or her condition and explain procedures to help alleviate any anxiety the child may have or to administer sedation or pain medications if needed.

3. CT scanning is undertaken in children with significant head, face, chest, or hemodynamically stable abdominal trauma. CT scanning is the diagnostic modality of choice for blunt abdominal trauma. The use of oral contrast or IV contrast can improve the diagnostic capabilities of the CT scan. Contrast can be used in stable patients who are able to tolerate the time it takes to administer it. However, CT scans should not be delayed in more urgent cases. Angiography may be obtained for suspected severe vessel injury from blunt or penetrating trauma.

4. Diagnostic peritoneal lavage (DPL) use is decreasing with the emergence of focused assessment by sonography in trauma FAST). It is useful in detecting intra-abdominal blood (Bacade & Bowlling 2016). A FAST study can be done quickly at the bedside, is noninvasive, and can be repeated as serial diagnostic exams. Some of its limitations are inexperience of the operator and the fact that the FAST exam is insufficient in excluding injuries or in grading the injuries to solid organs. DPL has its limitations as it does not identify which organ may be injured or the grade

of the injury. There is also risk of perforation of the bowel with clinicians less experienced in performing DPL in the pediatric patient. Therefore, DPL is rarely performed to diagnose hemorrhage or visceral perforation in the pediatric population. CT scanning is still the procedure of choice to identify intra-abdominal injuries. DPL or FAST may be indicated when a CT scanner is unavailable, or when CT scan findings are normal but a hollow viscus injury is suspected (Simone, 2003).

5. Echocardiography (echo) can be useful in evaluating thoracic injuries because it can reveal functional or anatomic cardiovascular injuries or injuries adjacent to cardiovascular structures. An electrocardiogram may show rhythm disturbances, premature beats, or S–T segment changes, which may occur as a result of blunt-force trauma to the chest and can result in cardiac contusions.

B. Pain Assessment

1. There are many factors that can affect pain assessment in the pediatric patient. These can include developmental stage of the child, anxiety, past experiences, family perceptions, and medications, as well as the child's past experiences with medications. Pain can involve physical, social, and emotional factors. Pain can also be subjective and multidimensional (Joestlein, 2015). AAP states, "suffering occurs when the pain leads the person to feel out of control, when the pain is overwhelming, when the source of pain is unknown, when the meaning of pain is perceived to be dire, and when the pain is chronic" (AAP and American Pain Society, 2001, p. 793).

2. Inadequate pain management can have long- and short-term effects. This can lead to increased length of stay (LOS), as well as slower recovery and healing. It can cause emotional trauma and may cause analgesia to be less effective in future procedures (Joestlein, 2015). Fear and anxiety as well as separation from the parent(s) can increase the child's perception or experience of pain. The parent(s) or family member's beliefs or attitudes can alter or influence the child's perception of pain or the child's ability to admit whether he or she is experiencing pain. Some of these beliefs or attitudes include the parent's fear that their child could become addicted to pain medications, overdose, or experience negative side effects. It is imperative for the nurse to educate the patient and the family regarding pain management, which may lead to a better understanding of the rationale behind the use of pain medication, thus allowing for better pain control with less emotional or psychological trauma or fear of pain. The nurse needs to be able to identify both emotional and physical components of pain and know how to distinguish between the two.

3. The American Society of Pain Management Nursing (ASPMN) recommends using a modified Hierarchy of Pain Assessment Technique, which consists of self-reporting pain (if applicable) or reporting by proxy such as a parent or family member. It also should include looking for and identifying potential causes of pain, and observing patient behaviors while assessing pain (Herr, Coyne, McCaffery, Manworren, & Merkel, 2011). Self-reporting remains the recommended method to assess pain intensity and is used primarily for older children and adolescents. It is the most accurate measurement tool for pain assessment. Most self-reporting tools measure the sensory component of pain, not the behavioral component. However, factors, such as developmental age, behavioral conditions (e.g., autism), intubation, sedation, and/or chemically paralyzed patients, can limit the child's ability to convey whether he or she is experiencing pain. The nurse should document why the patient is unable to self-report pain, which pain assessment tool is being utilized, what the plan is for managing pain, as well as the patient's response to pain management interventions.

4. The Faces, Legs, Activity, Cry, and Consolability (FLACC) scale can be used with children as young as infants. There is also a modified version of the FLACC scale for cognitively impaired children. The FLACC scale lends itself well to children who have an artificial airway, who have significant cognitive delay, and who are unable to self-report pain because of conditions associated with multiple trauma (e.g., multiple surgical procedures; Willis, Merkel, Voepel-Lewis, & Malviyas, 2003). The acronym FLACC denotes the following assessment categories: face (expression, muscle movement), legs (position, movement), activity (body position, movement), cry (degree, quality), and consolability (degree, effective interventions; Merkel, Voepel-Lewis, Shayevitz, & Malviya, 1997).

5. The Behavioral Pain Assessment Scale is a valid, reliable, and clinically useful tool (Manworren & Hynan, 2003). Behavioral assessment tools are typically used in preverbal children, but can be used in the school-age child as well. It includes observing and assessing defined behaviors (e.g., crying, grimacing, or posturing), which may be associated with pain.

6. Pain rating scores, which may be numeric usually (i.e., on a scale of 1–10) or picture based, are commonly used for school-aged children to adolescents, but may be applicable for the younger child, especially the picture-based scale. Most of these pain assessment tools measure the intensity of the pain, but not the location of the pain or quality of the pain. Also, children may sleep or be withdrawn as a way to control pain. So it cannot be assumed that a sleeping child does not have pain.

7. Newborns experiencing trauma present unique challenges. The following are general principles for the prevention and management of newborn pain. Pain in newborns may be of a diagnostic (e.g., arterial puncture), therapeutic (e.g., chest tube insertion), or surgical nature. If a procedure is painful for adults, it should be considered painful in newborns. Newborns may experience a greater sensitivity to pain and are more susceptible to the long-term effects of painful stimulation (Anand, 2001). Hyperalgesia may be a problem for babies who have experienced previous tissue injury, postoperative pain, localized infection, or inflammation (Anand, 2001). Adequate pain management may be associated with decreased clinical complications and even decreased mortality. Sedatives do not relieve pain and may mask the newborn's pain response (Anand, 2001).

8. A combination of environmental, behavioral, and pharmacological interventions can prevent, reduce, and sometimes even eliminate newborn pain (Anand, 2001). An example would be the use of a sucrose pacifier and swaddling (behavioral and environmental management) together with fentanyl citrate (pharmacologic management) for a chest tube insertion procedure.

C. Emotional Support

1. The injured child experiences many painful and frightening events before, during, and after the injury. Children have fears of parental separation, pain, disfigurement, and mutilation. Nurses need to provide comfort and emotional support to the child and family during this time of crisis. There are several resources available to the critical care nurse to provide this support such as social work, support groups, and spiritual care. There has been a great deal of research and study dedicated to PTSD recently and its symptoms, which will be discussed later in this chapter.

2. The assignment of a primary nurse to the patient helps the child focus on one person and provide consistency for the child and family. Speaking in a calm, reassuring voice may help the child to relax or to be less fearful and allow trust to develop with the child.

For example, consider the child who receives spinal immobilization, standing at the child's side near chest level allows the child to see the nurse without attempting to move his or her head sideways; standing over the child's head may be frightening and intimidating. Holding the child's hand, stroking the child's hair, and talking calmly and confidently can help the child to gain trust.

3. Explanations for procedures should be age appropriate for the child and also given to the parents so that they can comprehend what is being done. This may involve the use of interpreters, child life specialists, and social workers to provide support. The truth should be told about any pain or discomfort that may occur as well as the healthcare team's interventions to prevent or limit any pain or discomfort the child may endure. Coping measures for painful procedures include deep breathing, guided imagery, counting, singing, or other activities that allow for distraction (e.g., such as videos, music). Allowing the child to wiggle a hand or foot gives the child some sense of control. Child life specialists can be of special assistance in identifying and implementing helpful coping skills that the child or parent(s) can apply to get through potentially scary and painful procedures. Use of pet therapy is now widely accepted to calm and distract children when it is deemed appropriate for the pet to be present at the bedside.

4. Parents or family members should be permitted to see the child as soon as possible. The nurse should explain to the family what they will see, hear, and smell upon entering the child's room as well as orienting the family that they may hear many different sounds or alarms. To alleviate fears that may be associated with the various alarms frequently heard within an ICU setting, the nurse should ensure family members that skilled staff are specially trained and knowledgeable in regard to what each alarm represents and that their child will be continually monitored to alert staff to any vital changes. Having child life specialists available to prepare siblings of a critically injured pediatric patient, especially prior to their first visit, on what they may experience or feel is helpful to prevent or limit the effects of a potentially traumatic experience. This is especially helpful if the sibling(s) was involved or witnessed the injuries incurred by the patient. Child life specialist and/or social work may be of assistance to family members in their decision making to allow siblings to visit, depending upon the severity of the injuries suffered. Sibling's age and developmental status may also be taken into account. Explain the current plans for the child's treatment to the family in language that they can comprehend. Encourage them to ask questions and allow them to be present and/or participate in medical rounds. The family is encouraged to touch and talk to the child and participate in his or her care whenever it is appropriate or safe to do so (e.g., changing a diaper, bathing, or turning the patient). However, the family should be educated on the effects of overstimulation of the patient and when physical or verbal interaction is appropriate or may be harmful. The family may welcome having a social worker, religious counselor, or other support person present. Parental presence during resuscitation is not only advocated, but encouraged. Family presence during their child's CPR provides the family with an awareness that every effort is being made to care and support their child. It also allows them to be with the child in the event the resuscitation efforts are not successful (Gilmer, 2016).

5. PTSD is becoming more recognized and studied in the pediatric population, especially in children who are victims of trauma, child maltreatment (which is also referred to as NAT), or who have experienced inadequate pain management. It is estimated that one in six children and/or parent(s) will develop PTSD after a traumatic event, which can lead to poorer physical and functional recovery (Kassam-Adams, Marsac, Hildenbrand, & Winston, 2013). PTSD symptoms that go unrecognized may inhibit full recovery, lead to inadequate coping skills, and an increased use of healthcare services. The Medical Trauma Working Group of the National Child Traumatic Stress Network defined pediatric medical stress as "a set of psychological responses of children and their families to pain, injury, serious illness, medical procedures, and invasive or frightening treatment experiences" (para. 1). Injuries that can cause PTSD include various forms of violence, burns, animal bites, accidents, and NAT. Persistent PTSD symptoms can impair daily functioning. The healthcare team should optimize pain management, minimize traumatic procedures and encourage the child and parent(s) or family members to verbalize their fears, and provide reassurance and realistic hope. Parent(s) have a key role in the child's recovery; however, the parent(s) may also experience PTSD. Their responses can affect how the child copes with the event or situation. This can lead to the parent's inability to assist the child in coping with the traumatic event.

6. Seeking professional social support has shown to decrease PTSD symptoms after traumatic events, injuries, or experiences. Professional social support may include the services of a child life specialist and social worker as well as pet therapy, music therapy, art therapy, imagery, and psychological support. Social withdrawal is associated with an increased risk

TABLE 9.5   Posttraumatic Stress Disorder Syndrome Risk Factors and Symptoms

Risk Factors For PTSD	Symptoms Indicating PTSD
Peritrauma subjective life threat: child believes he or she could have died or injury was life threatening Peritrauma fear: psychological reactions of PTSD, depression, or anxiety Little or no past trauma support from parents, friends, or teachers Past trauma experience with poor family functioning Posttrauma coping strategies (e.g., withdrawal, distraction, or suppression of thoughts)	Invasion or intrusion of distressing memories, dreams with trauma reminders Avoids thoughts, feelings, people, activities that remind the individual of the traumatic event Dissociated feelings of reality or altered sense of oneself or surroundings Changes in mood or cognition Persistent negative expectations of self, others, or of the world Negative emotions and feelings of detachment Changes in arousal that include hypervigilance, sleep disturbance, exaggerated startle response, and/or difficulty concentrating

PTSD, posttraumatic stress disorder.

of PTSD. Follow-up therapy should include identifying the child's coping mechanism as well as the child's interpretation of the injury or event to identify issues that could prevent the child's recovery. The natural psychological process for recovery includes thinking about the event balanced with distracting oneself or avoiding distressing reminders. Recovery may also be facilitated by reexperiencing and avoiding the distressing event or experience in doses so that the child does not get overwhelmed and allows him or her to process the event or experience (Table 9.5). PTSD symptoms may continue with the use of avoidance coping, blaming others, and other maladaptive behaviors such as suppression of the event.

SPECIFIC INJURIES

Critical care nurses need to have a strong understanding of the body's organ systems. This should include physiologic as well as anatomic organ system understanding as many trauma patients may have sustained injuries to more than one organ system, presenting as a multitrauma patient. The critical care nurse must be able to prioritize those injuries or complications, which may be life-threatening and intervene quickly, whereas other injuries that are non–life-threatening can be treated once the patient has been stabilized. Many times these complications may be masked in the multitrauma patient. The pediatric patient can decompensate quickly if the injuries or complications are not treated in a timely manner. For the purpose of discussion, specific body system injuries are briefly addressed in this section with the understanding that these injuries will not be isolated in the multiple trauma patient (Figure 9.1).

A. Head Injuries

1. According to the CDC, head injuries are the leading cause of injury-related deaths in children and adolescents. In 2015, the CDC reported an estimated 2.5 million ED visits, 280,000 hospitalizations, and 50,000 deaths among all age groups with an increase seen in those younger than 1 to 4 years and 15 to 24 years. Of those deaths, the most common mechanism of injury was due

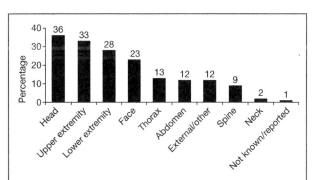

FIGURE 9.1   Incidents of trauma based on body region.

Source: Adapted from "Incidents and Case Fatality Rate by AIS Body Region." Committee on Trauma, American College of Surgeons. NTDB Annual/Pediatric Report 2015. Chicago, IL. The content reproduced from the NTDB remains the full and exclusive copyrighted property of the American College of Surgeons. The American College of Surgeons is not responsible for any claims arising from works based on the original data, text, tables, or figures.

Source: Nance, M. L. (Ed.). (2015). *National Trauma Data Bank 2015: Pediatric annual report*. Retrieved from https://www.facs.org/~/media/files/quality%20programs/trauma/ntdb/ntdb%20pediatric%20annual%20report%202015%20final.ashx

to MVA. The medical system spends over $1 billion annually on pediatric traumatic brain injury (TBI; Schaller, Lakhani, Hsu, 2015). Other common causes of TBI in pediatrics include NAT, falls, auto versus pedestrian collisions, assault, violence, and sports. The majority of these injuries are due to blunt-force trauma. Children have proportionately larger heads with weaker cervical ligaments and muscles, leading to an increased incidence(s) of head trauma as well as an increase in severity of injuries. There is also a proportionately larger volume of blood in the pediatric head, which can cause a rapid onset of cerebral edema and increased ICP. Children's (<2 years of age) skulls tend to be softer and the cranial suture lines are not completely fused, which can predispose them to diastatic fractures or separation of the bones at the suture line. The thin pliable skull provides less protection for the brain, making children more vulnerable to shearing from linear and rotational forces. Traumatic injuries to the head may impact the skull, neural tissue, and/or the cerebral vasculature. Head trauma can be either from primary or secondary causes. Primary TBI is a direct result of an injury when it occurs. Secondary TBI occurs as a result of the initial injury that can lead to cerebral edema, hypoxic–anoxic brain injury, bony fragments impinging on the brain, and/or delayed vascular injuries. Care of the TBI patient is aimed at preventing or controlling secondary injuries. TBI is divided into mild (GCS 13–15), moderate (GCS 9–12), and severe (GCS ≤8). CT scans can be performed quickly to assess for hemorrhages, hematomas, midline shifts, skull fractures, excess cerebrospinal fluid (CSF), edema, or herniation. MRI scans can be performed if the patient is stable, due in part to the length of time required to complete the scan. MRI can be useful to assess for extra-axial hemorrhage and ischemia.

2. Mild head trauma, such as a concussion, occurs when injury to the head arises from blunt trauma or acceleration/deceleration forces. One or more of the following conditions must be present for a diagnosis of mild TBI:

   a. Temporary confusion, disorientation, or impaired consciousness

   b. Loss of memory during the time immediately before, during, or after the injury

   c. A period of unconsciousness lasting no longer than 30 minutes; the patient may also present with seizures that occur right after the injury or later postinjury, irritability, lethargy, vomiting, headaches, dizziness, fatigue, poor concentration, and/or behavior disturbances

3. Moderate head injuries can be considered contusions or bleeds. Contusion injuries cause a more prolonged compromise of cerebral function than concussions. They are most often due to coup-contre coup type injuries (brain mass hitting the sides of the skull) from the rapid acceleration/deceleration as experienced in MVA whiplash-type injuries. The patient may have an LOC or decreased LOC, focal neurologic abnormalities, or coma.

4. Types of bleeds in the brain include subdural, subarachnoid, epidural, and intraparenchymal hemorrhage. Surgical evacuation of head bleeds or hematomas may be considered in patients with midline shifts, mental status changes, or focal neurologic defects.

   a. A subdural hemorrhage is the accumulation of blood between the dura and the arachnoid space and is the most common type of bleed in children. They can be classified as acute, subacute, or chronic and are venous in nature. A child who presents with an acute subdural hemorrhage will have immediate alterations in cerebral functioning. A child who has a subacute subdural hemorrhage may develop signs and symptoms of decreasing LOC that can occur over a 2-week period. Children with a chronic subdural hemorrhage may not be diagnosed until months after the injury occurred, when they manifest signs of personality, behavioral or cognitive changes, or develop an onset of seizures. A subdural hemorrhage conforms to the brain on CT scan.

   b. A subarachnoid hemorrhage occurs when blood is between the arachnoid space and the meningeal layers. A common cause of this type of bleed occurs with violent shaking as in "SBS" in NAT. A lumbar puncture (LP) can confirm this type of bleed, but should not be performed until subdural or epidural bleeds have been ruled out and the patient is not at risk for increased ICP.

   c. Epidural hemorrhage occurs when blood accumulates between the skull and dura. It is most commonly associated with a middle meningeal tear. The child can have rapid deterioration of his or her mental status if not treated, which can lead to coma and/or death. An epidural hemorrhage is often associated with a skull fracture causing a laceration of the artery. Epidural hemorrhages tend to appear more convex or lenticular in shape on the CT scan.

   d. Intraparenchymal hemorrhage is blood that accumulates in the brain tissue. A large hemorrhage may require surgical evacuation to limit the risk of herniation. This can be caused by rapid acceleration/deceleration injuries such as those experienced in an MVA. Although some bleeds may be iatrogenic and not caused by external trauma, trauma remains the most common cause of head bleeds in the pediatric patient.

5. Children with mild to moderate head injuries usually will require hospitalization if they have any neurologic deficits, seizures, nausea or vomiting, severe headache, fever, prolonged change in LOC, skull fracture, ataxia, blurred vision, unequal pupils, confusion, slurred speech, fluid leak from the ears or nose, abnormal patterns or changes in breathing, altered LOC, or suspected child maltreatment. Assessment of children with mild to moderate head injuries should include serial neurologic evaluations with measurement of the LOC, pupillary response, motor and sensory response, and vital signs. This may also include serial scans to assess for increase or change in any head bleed or if the child's condition changes or worsens. Changes in the child's LOC may indicate increasing ICP, which requires prompt intervention and notification of neurosurgery to prevent subsequent deterioration and possible brainstem herniation.

6. Severe head injuries may cause diffuse cerebral swelling and edema. Diffuse axonal injuries are considered severe TBI. They are usually the result of shearing injuries to the axons of the white mater being torn, which also can occur due to twisting or rotational forces and can be caused by the rapid acceleration/deceleration. They can also be seen in children who experience NAT from violent shaking and/or slamming of the head against a solid object with increased force. There is disruption of the cortex and the lower brainstem. These patients may present or lapse into a coma state. Signs of a severe head injury include a decreased LOC, posturing, combative behavior, and other abnormal neurologic findings. Children with severe head injuries most likely will require airway and ventilatory control, especially if the GCS is less than eight.

7. The goal of any child with a TBI is to control and prevent hypotension and hypoxemia, which can lead to secondary injuries. The metabolic demands (e.g., oxygen consumption) increase significantly in a child with TBI. A child with TBI should be kept normothermic and measures taken to prevent fevers. Although seizure prophylaxis is not usually indicated, if the child develops seizures, they must be treated immediately. Nutritional support should be implemented as soon as possible.

TABLE 9.6   Goals of TBI Management

Adequate oxygenation and normocapnia
SBP and MAP monitored to avoid hypotension
Normothermia <38°C
Avoid hyponatremia, which may cause cerebral edema
Normalize electrolytes and prevent hyperglycemia
Closely monitor urine output for risk of DI or SIADH and treat immediately
Monitor serum osmolality
Closely monitor labs as TBI patients are at risk for anemia and coagulopathy (recommend maintaining a goal Hgb >7 dL)

DI, diabetes insipidus; Hgb, hemoglobin; MAP, mean arterial pressure; SBP, systolic blood pressure; SIADH, syndrome of inappropriate antidiuretic hormone; TBI, traumatic brain injury.

8. The ACS (2015) trauma quality-improvement program recommends the following best practices in management of TBI (Table 9.6).

 a. ICP monitoring may be recommended or indicated if the GCS is less than 8 and there is evidence of an injury on the CT scan. The gold standard for measuring ICP is an external ventriculostomy drain (EVD) connected to a catheter placed in the ventricle that allows for monitoring the pressure in the cranium and permits for drainage of CSF to decrease elevated ICP. An elevated ICP can be caused by edema (either cellular or extracellular), cerebral venous outflow obstruction, hyperemia (loss of autoregulation or vasodilation), a mass effect (e.g., increase in hemorrhage), and disturbances in CSF circulation. Elevated ICP is a reliable predictor of poor neurologic function as well as decreased cerebral perfusion pressure (CPP). Although brain hypoxia can still occur even with normal ICP and CPP.

 b. The ACS recommends a three-tier approach to manage TBI.

  i. Tier 1 includes keeping the head of bed elevated greater than 30 degrees and head midline to improve venous outflow, provide short-acting sedation and analgesia (e.g., fentanyl, Propofol, or versed) for intubated patients, an EVD for intermittent CSF drainage, frequent and ongoing neuro exams, and consideration of repeated CT scans to help guide treatment. If the ICP remains greater than 20 to 25 mmHg, progress to Tier 2.

  ii. Tier 2 management includes intermittent hyperosmolar therapy (i.e., mannitol 0.25–1 gm/kg) as needed for increased ICP. With the use of mannitol, serum sodium and osmolality levels should be monitored every 6 hours because it is an osmotic diuretic and should be used cautiously, especially in hypotensive patients. Mannitol should not be given if serum osmolality levels are greater than 320 to 360 mOsmol/L as it can lead to dehydration, which can cause further swelling in the brain. Hypertonic saline or 3% saline may also be considered and is usually given every 6 hours over 30 to 60 minutes preferably in a central venous line, with the dosage of 6.5 to 10 mL/kg or as a continuous infusion of 0.1 to 1 mL/kg in order to maintain an ICP less than 20 mmHg. Three percent saline increases plasma osmolality and creates an osmolar gradient to decrease fluid in the cranial space. Serum sodium should be monitored frequently (e.g., every 6 hours) as it can cause hypernatremia. The goal is to maintain a CPP greater than 50 mmHg, which is calculated by subtracting the ICP from the MAP (MAP – ICP = CPP). Additional goals are to prevent hypoxia, PaO_2 less than 60 mmHg, and maintain the $PaCO_2$ at 30 to 35 mmHg. Hyperventilation may be used in an acute elevated ICP crisis. However, $PaCO_2$ less than 30 mmHg can cause vasoconstriction from alkalosis, which can lead to decreased cerebral blood flow (CBF). These patients should be intubated and may require neuromuscular blockade (NMB) to better control their respiratory function. Perform hourly neuro checks or more frequently if necessary and repeat CT scans if neurologic changes are evident. If the ICP continues to remain greater than 20 to 25 mmHg despite Tier 2 interventions, then Tier 3 interventions may be indicated.

iii. Tier 3 may require surgical intervention known as a *decompressive craniectomy*. NMB may continue to be indicated as long as the patient is adequately sedated. Use of a barbiturate or propofol coma may be indicated for patients with malignant or uncontrolled intracranial hypertension. Use of these agents can cause severe hypotension so BP must be closely monitored as hypotension can lead to decreased CPP and CBF. Continuous EEG can be utilized to identify burst suppression.

c. Hypotension with or without hypoxia causes significant mortality rates in children compared with rates in adults. Use of inotropic support may be needed to keep MAP elevated to thereby maintain an adequate CPP. A CPP less than 40 mmHg is consistently associated with increased mortality (Parrillo, 2003). However, children recover more frequently and with less disability than similarly injured adults, which suggests that TBI in children may preserve cerebral oxygenation and perfusion better than TBI in adults (Daley, 2015).

9. *Concussion*

a. There has been an increased focus of study in the area of concussion and postconcussion syndrome. As of 2014, all 50 states have passed concussion legislation to promote safety in youth sports and require that athletes be medically cleared after concussion to return to sports by a qualified medical professional. The Zachary Lystedt Law passed in Washington in 2009 requires student athletes be removed from competition when a head injury is suspected. Dr. Ivet Hartonian of the American Academy of Neurology defines concussion as "biomechanically induced clinical syndrome related to alterations in brain function that can affect memory and orientation" (Hartonian et al., 2013). The injury can be to the head, face, neck, or even a blow elsewhere to the body with force transmitted to the head. Concussions are more a functional injury rather than a structural injury. An estimated 300,000 to 1 million sports-related TBIs occur annually in the United States (Yue et al., 2016). Postconcussion symptoms include headache, fatigue, dizziness, as well as neurocognitive and neuropsychotic deficits such as difficulty concentrating, forgetfulness, and depression. Other symptoms can be sleep disturbances as well as continued or recurrent headaches. The athlete may have slow reaction times and balance impairments. If these symptoms persist, it can lead to absences from school, risk for second impact syndrome, and possibly chronic traumatic encephalopathy (CTE), which can have long-term implications for disability and even death (Yue et al., 2016). CTE is a progressive neurodegenerative disorder with symptoms that include irritability, impulsivity, attention difficulties, memory impairments, depression, and gait disturbances (Rose, Weber, Collen, & Heyer, 2015; Table 9.7).

TABLE 9.7   Potential for School Accommodations for Postconcussion or Concussion Syndrome

Workload overall	Excuse of school absences Shortened school days Provide for rest breaks during class or between classes Extend assignment(s) deadline(s) Postpone examinations (particularly standardized tests)
Physical exertion	Provide extra time to travel between classes Excuse participation in physical education classes and/or sports Minimize flights of stairs and limit weight of backpack
Poor concentration, slowed mentation	Provide additional time for test taking and homework assignments Have student sit closer to teacher(s)/instructor(s) Provide class notes Allow tests to be taken in separate, quite room
Sensitivity to light and noise	Provide quiet room for lunch/breaks Minimize band, choir, or shop classes Allow ear plugs (outside of classrooms) Allow for a hat and/or sunglasses Sit in area of classroom with dimmer lighting Minimize time on computer screens
Visual disturbances	Minimize reading or allow breaks while reading (may need assistance with reading) Provide a note-taker or scribe Minimize use of computer screens

Source: Adapted from Rose, S. C., Weber, K. D., Collen, J. B., & Heyer, G. L. (2015). The diagnosis and management of concussion in children and adolescents. *Pediatric Neurology, 53*(2), 108–118.

b. CT scans and MRI scans are not required as the scan will usually appear normal. Adolescents may have a higher risk for prolonged symptoms and headaches compared to younger children. Girls report more symptoms, may perform worse on neurocognitive and reaction time testing, and take longer to recover than boys (Blume, 2015).

c. Concussion exam should consist of evaluating mental status, cranial nerve coordination, vision exam, balance testing, physical exam, history and mechanism of injury, and a funduscopic exam to rule out papilledema or other signs of increased ICP. There are multiple assessment tools to evaluate the effects of concussions such as the Sports Concussion Assessment Tool 3 (SCAT3), which was developed by the Concussion in Sport Group (McCrory et al., 2013). Management includes education for the child and family regarding symptoms and expected recovery, possible lifestyle changes, importance of adequate rest, proper nutrition, sleeping habits, and adequate hydration (Blume, 2015). Nonsteroidal anti-inflammatory drugs (NSAIDs) should be

avoided in the first 24 to 48 hours due to their risk for bleeding, but acetaminophen can be taken safely. Prescription drugs, such as opioids, should be avoided because they can have a negative effect on arousal and cognition.

10. Skull fractures are described by type: linear, depressed, compound, basilar, ping-pong, and growing. Seventy five percent of pediatric skull fractures are linear. Depressed skull fractures can cause disruption of the skull's integrity and impinge on the brain itself. A compound skull fracture requires a tremendous amount of force. A child with a compound skull fracture should exact a high suspicion for NAT. Basilar skull fractures occur at the base of the skull and usually will have CSF leaking from the nose or ears, have the appearance of "raccoon eyes" and/or hemotympanum. The child may also have "Battle's sign," which is ecchymosis behind the ears. A child with a basilar skull fracture may also have an injury to the cochlear, ocular, and facial nerves. These fractures are considered open fractures and there is a risk of infection or meningitis. Any child with a suspicion of a basilar skull fracture should not have an

NGT inserted due to the risk of it being directed into the brain as a result of the open fracture. A child with a depressed or basilar skull fracture may present with altered LOC, focal neuro findings, LOC greater than 1-minute, multiple episodes of emesis, or a bulging fontanel in children younger than 2 years of age whose fontanel has not completely closed.

B. Maxillofacial Injuries

1. Unique features of pediatric facial trauma are related to the underdevelopment and continued growth of the pediatric facial skeleton. The child's midface and lower facial growth are much slower than the upper facial growth. Also, the child's midfacial growth occurs in a vertical and anterior direction. Because the cranium makes up a larger proportion of the craniofacial skeleton in younger children, they will likely experience more frontal-orbital injuries (Boyette, 2014). Brain growth will continue to expand in the cranium and is about 85% of the adult size around age 5 and the eye orbit rapidly grows to about 90% of the adult size during this time period. There is gradual pneumatization of the paranasal sinuses, which grow at different rates; this variation is thought to be the reason for a decreased frequency of facial fractures in children due to their bones being more solid. Nasal growth usually reaches adult-sized width within about 1 year, but the length of the nose does not grow until the teen years. The child also has more or larger buccal fat pads that help to disperse the force of a blow to the midface region. This makes the facial skeleton more stable and less susceptible to fractures. Unerrupted teeth in the maxilla and mandible help to contribute to more dense and stable bone thereby requiring increased force to cause a fracture in this area in the younger child (Boyette, 2014). Diagnosis of facial fractures in pediatrics is often challenging and may be missed on imaging. Assault and MVAs are the most common causes of pediatric facial trauma. According to the NTDB (2015), the mandible was the bone most often fractured (32.7%) in the facial skeleton, followed by the nasal bone (30.2%), and maxilla/zygoma (28.6%). Pediatric facial fractures tend to indicate a high-energy trauma and often are associated with trauma to other organ systems. Up to 55% of pediatric facial trauma patients have concomitant injuries and infants and toddlers have a significantly higher incidence of severe intracranial injuries, usually related to NAT. Maxillofacial injuries include trauma to the dentition, mandible, and midface and should be suspected in children who sustain blunt or penetrating forces to the face. The face is assessed for bruising, lacerations, open wounds, and impaled objects; for symmetry; and intactness of cranial nerves.

The nose is palpated for tenderness, observed for bruising, and the nares examined for bleeding or blood clots. The face is palpated for "step-offs," tenderness, and pain. The maxilla is palpated for continuity and loose or missing teeth are noted, as is the presence of orthodontic appliances. The exam should also include pupil reaction and size, visual acuity, presence of diplopia, and extraocular movement. The physical exam should be done as gently as possible as the pediatric patient may not cooperate. Anteroposterior, open mouth, panorex radiographs, and CT scanning may be obtained in the stable child to determine the extent and location of facial injuries. CT scan remains the gold standard for identifying facial fractures.

2. *Mandibular Fractures.* A mandibular fracture may be suspected if the child is unable to open and close his or her mouth or if a malocclusion is present. In girls, usually younger than 12 years, the most frequent area for mandibular fractures is the condyle and is commonly associated with falls, whereas in boys aged 13 to 18 years, the most common area is the ankle and is usually related to assault or contact sports. Challenges to mandibular fracture management are related to unerrupted teeth, temporomandibular joint dysfunction, and facial growth disturbances. Most fractures can be treated with conservative measures, such as a soft diet, especially if it is a nondisplaced fracture, which does not affect dental occlusion. Displaced fractures of the condyle should have a closed reduction and in the case of severe comminuted or multiple fractures, open reduction is indicated. Internal fixation similar to that of adults can be used in the older child if they have reached skeletal and dental maturity. In the younger child with developing dentition, screws may be required to avoid unerrupted teeth. A single mini-plate fixation is generally used for stabilization. Children may have concerns about their inability to talk. Speech therapy can be helpful to teach the child alternate methods for communication. The older child and adolescent may have concerns about his or her appearance and should be reassured that any bruising and/or edema will subside over time. Careful attention is given to airway management and oral hygiene as well as antibiotics if there is a risk for infection.

3. Dental injuries occur from direct-force trauma to the face. In very young children, only the temporary (primary) teeth may be involved; however, if the injury displaces or avulses the temporary dentition, the underlying follicles (the location of the developing permanent teeth) may be involved. The most serious damage to teeth occurs in the permanent teeth that have a partially developed root (Council on Clinical Affairs, 2011).

4. *Orbital Fractures.* Ophthalmology should be consulted for all orbital fractures. Orbital roof fractures are the most common type of orbit fracture in children under 10 years of age because the "crumple zone" of the frontal sinus is not fully developed. With an increased ratio of the cranial vault to the facial skeleton, fracture of the frontal bone and superior orbital rim and roof are more common in children under 5 years old. Orbital roof fractures rarely require surgical intervention, except when there is muscle entrapment, which limits extraocular eye movement or exophthalmos and is usually caused by a depressed fracture. The child may have pain with eye movement, nausea, vomiting, and bradycardia. Muscle entrapment should be repaired as quickly as possible as children begin to heal rapidly and it can result in fibrosis and shortening of the muscle within a few days. The child may experience diplopia that can last for several months or may become permanent. If globe rupture is suspected, the eye should be covered with a protective device and an immediate ophthalmology exam performed. Ocular trauma can affect the external socket, the eyeball, or both. A challenge in management of ocular trauma is scar tissue development, which can inhibit regenerative capabilities. The conjunctiva, lens, and eyelid can regenerate, but the optic nerve and retina cannot.

5. Midfacial fractures are classified using the LeFort categories. A LeFort I fracture is a transverse fracture across the maxilla above the alveolar process and horizontal plate of the palatine and palatal process of the maxilla and involves the nose and anterior teeth. The LeFort II fracture is a pyramidal fracture that involves the orbital floors, lamina papyracea of the ethmoid bone, and separation of the frontal nasal suture. A LeFort III fracture involves craniofacial disarticulation in which the facial bones are separated from the cranial buttress systems and involves the orbits. The LeFort fractures tend to be the most life-threatening of the facial fractures and can cause profuse bleeding, loss of oral cavity structural integrity, and malocclusion of teeth (Engman-Lazear, 2015). LeFort fractures are treated with internal fixation.

6. Nasal fractures occur in the bony pyramid, cartilaginous nasal vault, the septum, or all three. "Open book" fractures are seen only in children and are usually caused by a direct frontal blow to the nose. It can cause blood to develop and spread apart the nasal bones centrally. A septal hematoma needs urgent surgical evacuation to prevent cartilage necrosis and saddle-nose deformity. Treatment may be immediate or delayed, depending on the child's condition. Treatment is a closed reduction under general anesthesia for the younger child and local anesthetic with IV sedation may be adequate in older children.

C. Spinal Cord Injuries

1. *Spinal Cord Injuries Without Radiographic Abnormalities (SCIWORA)*

a. Spinal cord injuries occur less frequently than injury to other body systems, but can have a lifelong impact on the child and the family. When these injuries do occur, outcomes may be permanent and can be devastating. Children have proportionately larger heads, and a higher center of gravity. Their neck muscles are not as well developed and flexion and extension injuries can be common. This laxity of the juvenile spine allows for spinal cord injuries to occur without bony abnormalities. Thus it is also referred to as *SCIWORA.* Compression and contusion injuries are more common than transection of the spinal cord. Children experience a higher incidence of compression injuries and fewer fractures compared to adults. The younger child experiences injuries that are higher in the cervical spine compared to older children due in part to the immature musculature, ligaments, and larger, proportionately heavier head. The most common mechanisms of spinal injuries in pediatrics are caused by MVAs, followed by falls, sports-related activities, violence, or assault. Neck injuries may also involve damage to ligaments, vasculature, and the airway may be compromised.

b. There are three horizontal zones for classification of neck injuries. Zone 1 is from the sternal notch to the cricoid cartilage. Zone 2 is from the cricoid cartilage to the angle of the mandible. Zone 3 is from the angle of the mandible to the base of the skull (Daley, 2015). C2 fractures also known as *hangman's fracture* is the most lethal fracture of the spine and causes loss of respiratory drive requiring immediate intubation while maintaining cervical spine stability. It is usually caused by hyperextension of the spine and cord disruption. Another cause of this type of fracture can be from improperly positioned seat belts in which the child slides down during a collision and is strangled by the seatbelt during the rapid acceleration–deceleration events. C3 to C7 fractures are commonly due to ligamentous injuries. Thoracic spine injuries generally are due to compression injuries and commonly are the result of falls. Fractures in the thoracolumbar area are usually due to burst injuries.

c. Cord syndromes may be caused by edema to the spinal cord or compression and can be proximal or distal to the injury. Anterior cord syndrome is usually caused by hyperflexion of the neck and can cause complete motor paralysis below the level of the injury, causing the patient to feel pain, but not light touch. There is a loss of corticospinal and spinothalamic pathways with preservation of posterior column function. Central cord syndrome is usually due to compression injuries and can cause muscle weakness or paralysis, affecting the upper extremities more than the lower extremities as a result of injuries to the centrally located fibers affecting upper motor limb and spinothalamic function. Brown–Sequard syndrome (half-cord syndrome) occurs when half the cord is injured causing paralysis and proprioception loss on the same side of the cord damage, causing loss of pain and temperature sensation on the opposite side of the cord injury, often resulting from penetrating spinal cord injuries and damage to the ascending spinothalamic fibers and motor pathways. These cord syndromes may or may not be reversible depending on the extent of the injury and degree of edema to the spine.

d. SCIWORA was introduced by Prang and Wilheger and defined as "clinical symptoms of traumatic myelopathy with no radiologic or computed tomographic features of spinal fracture or instability" (Pang & Wilberger, 1982/2012, p. 115). The pediatric spine is not completely calcified and allows stretching of the cord beyond its limits or severs the roots without any radiologic evidence. In SCIWORA, the child's vertebral column can stretch up to 2 inches, whereas the cord itself may only stretch about a quarter of an inch without causing cord disruption. Therefore, the vertebral column is stretched within its normal limits, but beyond the limits of the spinal cord, thus causing the cord to be compromised and causing neurologic symptoms, but with a normal cervical spine x-ray and CT scan (Engman-Lazear, 2015). This is almost exclusively a pediatric diagnosis. It is more common in the younger child and occurs more frequently within the cervical spine, predominately between levels C1 and C4. The thoracic spine is the next most frequently injured area of the spine, with lumbar injuries being less common in children. Thoracic spine injury is most frequently associated with high-energy causes, such as MVAs, and is generally seen in conjunction with other injuries, especially head injuries. The child may present with neurologic and/or motor deficits, but x-rays and CT scan usually appear normal with no abnormalities. There can be a delayed onset of symptoms, including paresthesia of the legs and hands, generalized weakness, and a burning sensation down the spine associated with neck movement. This delay can occur up to 4 days postinjury. The neurological deficit is generally more severe in the upper extremities than the lower extremities. The child may complain of muscle spasms and demonstrate limited neck mobility. SCIWORA injuries are classified into four types: Type I have no detectable abnormalities, type IIA have extraneural abnormalities, type IIB have intraneural abnormalities, and type IIC has both intraneural and extraneural abnormalities (Boese & Lechler, 2013). MRI scan is used to identify soft-tissue injuries of the intraneural and extraneural spinal structures and is helpful in determining the prognosis of the injury, but not necessarily the stability of the spine. It is important to understand that once a SCIWORA injury is diagnosed, the child is at increased risk for recurrence of this injury. Recurrent injuries are typically more severe than initial injuries and some patients with SCIWORA may not fully recover and have permanent disability. Patients with SCIWORA may be placed in external braces, such as a stiff cervical collar for several months, to prevent further injury; these injuries are treated conservatively.

2. *Management of Spinal Injuries*

a. If complete spinal immobilization is necessary, it should be maintained until it is clinically determined that a spinal cord injury is not present. Children with high spinal cord injuries must receive airway control and mechanical ventilation, whereas children with lower cervical injuries are closely observed for worsening of their respiratory status. Children with high spinal cord lesions may require more IV fluid than children with lower spinal cord lesions because spinal shock causes peripheral vasodilatation (warm shock) and relative hypovolemia. Therefore, at a minimum, normal maintenance infusion rates are required. Infusion of vasopressors, such as dopamine or phenylephrine (Neo-Synephrine) may also be indicated. High-dose methylprednisolone (30 mg/kg) is administered early in the treatment regimen (generally within 6–8 hours of the injury) to be effective and is then continued as an infusion for 24 to 48 hours. Prophylactic gut protection must be given to prevent GI bleeds. Patients may be at risk for hyperglycemia so monitoring of glucose levels is important. The child in spinal immobilization should be log rolled and skin assessed for breakdown and/or pressure areas. The nurse needs to evaluate bilateral extremity strength or weakness, movement and sensory intactness. Lateral, anteroposterior, and odontoid radiographs of the cervical spine should be obtained, along with anteroposterior and lateral views of the thoracic and lumbar spine if indicated. Flexion–extension radiographs to determine stability of the bony canal are not performed until it is determined that spinal cord injury is not present. Such flexion–extension tests may be performed in SCIWORA injury once additional diagnostic testing is completed. Serial neurologic assessments are performed to determine whether the injury is worsening. Children with spinal injuries or fractures may require use of a cervical collar for immobilization and to maintain alignment. Surgical intervention and use of halo traction or vest for stabilization may also be utilized. Education for the family and child is important to prevent skin breakdown and prevent infection at the pin sites. There may be an emotional impact to the child associated with such injuries that needs to be addressed. Child life specialists can be helpful in providing support and coping mechanisms.

b. The unconscious, multiply injured child should remain in complete spinal immobilization until he or she is awake and able to complete a neurologic examination (Figure 9.2). Additional diagnostic tests, such as MRI or somatosensory-evoked potentials (SSEPs), may be indicated to determine the presence of or extent of a spinal cord injury. An MRI may also be effective in evaluating possible spinal cord injuries in the obtunded, unconscious, or intubated patient (Frank, Lim, Flynn, & Dormans, 2002).

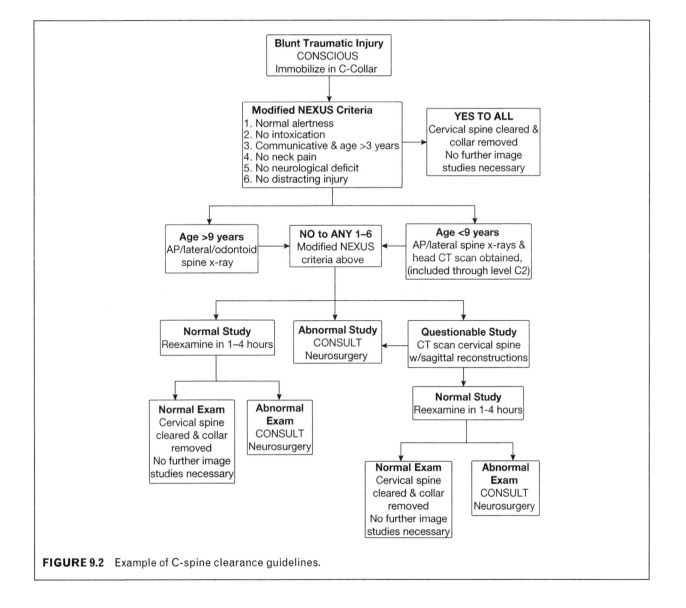

FIGURE 9.2 Example of C-spine clearance guidelines.

D. Thoracic Injuries

1. Thoracic injuries are the second leading cause of death in children after brain or neurologic trauma. The child's thoracic cavity is very pliable with greater cartilage content and incomplete ossification of the rib cage, which lends itself to more mediastinal mobility. Thus, rib fractures are less common in pediatrics than adults and most thoracic injuries can be managed nonoperatively unless there is significant hemorrhage involved. Rib fractures are usually the result of a tremendous amount of force. Fractures of the first two ribs may cause brachial plexus or subclavian artery injuries. Fractures of ribs 9 to 12 can be associated with liver or splenic injuries.

2. Pulmonary contusions and pneumothorax are the most common thoracic injuries in children and can occur without rib fractures being present. They are most often caused due to blunt-force trauma. The child may have shortness of breath (SOB), tenderness over the area, bruising, dyspnea, rales, hypoxia, and possibly hemoptysis. The child may not present until 12 to 24 hours after the injury has occurred. Management of pulmonary contusions depends on the severity of the injury and the symptoms. They may only require oxygen therapy, but in severe cases intubation and ventilatory support (which is rare) may be required. Pulmonary contusions can cause inflammation leading to edema, atelectasis, and consolidation. Most contusions will resolve in 7 to 10 days and are managed medically with supportive therapy. The goal of management is to prevent respiratory failure so adequate oxygenation and pain control are key, along with aggressive pulmonary toilet. *Pneumothorax* refers to an accumulation of air in the pleural space and can lead to a collapsed lung. The patient may have a sudden onset of SOB with chest pain, causing the child to take shallow and/or rapid respirations. There are decreased or absent breath sounds over the affected area and it is hyperresonant to percussion. The definitive diagnosis is made by chest x-ray (CXR). Some pneumothoraces can be treated with oxygen therapy and resolve, whereas others may require a needle decompression or a chest tube placed until the lung reexpands. Tension pneumothorax can cause air to compress the lung and, as the pressure expands, the injured lung is deviated to the unaffected side. This can lead to tracheal deviation. If not treated quickly, the patient can develop cardiorespiratory compromise, which can result in cardiopulmonary arrest. A needle thoracostomy should be performed emergently until a chest tube can be placed.

3. Hemothorax is due to vascular injuries in the thoracic cavity resulting in blood accumulating in the pleural space. This can be caused by blunt force or penetrating injuries. Massive hemorrhaging can lead to a tension hemothorax, causing cardiopulmonary compromise, which leads to cardiopulmonary arrest. The child may present with signs of hypovolemic shock, anemia, SOB, and tachypnea. A blood loss of 20 mL/kg is equal to 20% to 25% of the child's total blood volume and may need multiple blood transfusions to adequately resuscitate.

4. Pericardial tamponade is most commonly associated with penetrating injuries, whereas cardiac contusions are usually associated with blunt trauma. Both types of injuries can lead to a pericardial tamponade. With pericardial tamponade injuries, blood fills the pericardial sac restricting the heart's ability to contract and can lead to cardiac arrest. This can occur very rapidly as the child's pericardial sac is small and as little as 25 to 50 mL of blood can result in a tamponade. Pericardial tamponade occurs more often in adolescents than in younger children. The child may present with a weak, thready, and rapid pulse. He or she may show signs of shock, have pulsus paradoxus, narrow pulse pressure, distended neck veins, and muffled or distant heart tones. These are late signs and require emergent attention. Treatment includes a pericardiocentesis or, in severe cases, an open surgical exploration. Cardiac contusions are generally treated medically with supportive therapy. The child may have dysrhythmias, elevated cardiac enzymes, and possibly cardiac dyskinesis.

5. Diaphragm injuries may be caused by a tear oftentimes resulting from blunt-force trauma (e.g., MVA). Increased abdominal pressure can be transmitted to the diaphragm, causing it to tear. It usually affects the left side more often than the right side. Abdominal contents can migrate into the thoracic cavity, causing respiratory distress by compressing the lungs. Bowel sounds may be auscultated in the chest cavity and, if an NGT is placed, it is seen in the chest on x-ray. Surgical repair is indicated.

6. Tracheobronchial injuries may occur after blunt-force trauma to the chest and usually within 1 inch of the carina. It is equally distributed between both the left and right main bronchus. The child may present with significant dyspnea, hemoptysis, pneumothorax, hemothorax, pneumomediastinum, crepitus, or hemorrhage. The patient will probably require intubation and ventilatory support. Large tears generally require surgical repair, whereas small tears can heal on their own. A child who has fractures from ribs 1 to 5 and has a persistent pneumothorax with dyspnea, should raise a high suspicion of a tracheobronchial injury.

7. Common thoracic injuries and their symptoms and treatments are outlined (Table 9.8).

TABLE 9.8 Thoracic Injuries

Condition	Clinical Manifestations	Treatment
Rib fractures	Pain Crepitus Bruising	Medicate for pain; splinting
Closed pneumothorax	Dyspnea Tachypnea Decreased or absent breath sounds on the affected side Pain Dullness with percussion	Needle thoracostomy; insertion of chest tube
Open pneumothorax	Sucking noise on inspiration Bubbling noise on expiration Dyspnea Tachypnea	Application of an occlusive dressing, taped on three sides
Tension pneumothorax	Dyspnea Jugular vein distention Decreased or absent breath sounds on the affected side Tracheal deviation away from the affected side Decreased or absent chest wall movement Hyperresonance with percussion Possible mediastinal shift away from the affected side	Needle thoracostomy; insertion of a chest tube
Hemothorax	Dyspnea Tachypnea Tachycardia Pallor Restlessness Hypotension Dullness with percussion Decreased or absent breath sounds	Insertion of a chest tube Fluid resuscitation
Pulmonary contusion	Dyspnea	Oxygenation Ventilation
Cardiac contusion	Tachycardia Dysrhythmias Chest pain	Oxygenation Fluid administration Cardiac monitoring
Tracheobronchial rupture	Crepitus Subcutaneous emphysema Pneumomediastinum Pneumopericardium	Intubation Ventilation
Pericardial tamponade	Beck's triad (muffled heart tones, decreased arterial pressure, elevated venous pressure) Agitation Decreased peripheral perfusion Pulsus paradoxus Jugular vein distention	Ventilation Pericardiocentesis Fluid resuscitation Cardiac monitoring Thoracotomy

E. Abdominal Injuries

1. Abdominal trauma in pediatrics presents with different injuries than abdominal trauma in adults. The solid organs (liver, spleen, kidneys) are proportionately larger in children and are more prone to injury. The child's abdomen begins at the nipple line and the abdomen is more thin walled and lacks the musculature to protect the organs, thus making them more susceptible to rupture. The diaphragm is also more horizontal and does not provide much protection for the liver or spleen. Organs in the abdominal cavity are not well protected by fat pads and are more suspended making them more prone to shearing injuries with acceleration/deceleration forces. The abdominal organs are more frequently torn or lacerated from the pedicle. Abdominal injuries in children may be harder to diagnose as the vital signs in children do not change as early compared to adults and signs of peritoneal injury or irritation can be masked, altered, or delayed.

2. The most common cause of abdominal injuries in pediatrics is blunt-force trauma usually due to MVAs and then secondarily caused by pedestrian injuries (e.g., auto versus pedestrian). In children younger than age 3 years, the cause most often is NAT due to the child being kicked or punched in the abdomen causing compression of the organs. In school-age children, another common mechanism of injury is improper seat belt positioning or bike injuries in which the child hits the handlebars. Handlebar injuries are also common in the older child. The most frequent organ injured is the spleen followed by the liver, kidney, and then the GI tract. The majority of blunt abdominal injuries in pediatrics are stable and treated with nonoperative management (NOM). It is considered the standard of care with a 90% to 95% success rate, which was pioneered in pediatrics (Daley, 2015; Schnitzler et al., 2016). Only about 5% of NOM treatments fail in the pediatric patient and generally will occur within the first 12 hours postinjury most often due to shock, peritonitis, hemorrhage, pancreatic injury, hollow viscus injury, or ruptured diaphragm. If surgical exploration is indicated, it is usually due to shock from hemorrhage, peritonitis, pneumoperitoneum, free air in the abdomen, thickened bowel loops, or mesenteric inflammation present on imaging studies. The most common surgical procedure is an exploratory laparotomy. Laparoscopy exam can be performed in the hemodynamically stable patient and results in fewer adhesions, less pain, decreased coagulopathy, decreased postoperative ileus, and a decreased incidence of bowel obstructions compared to laparotomy procedures (Sharp & Holcomb, 2013). Mortality with blunt abdominal injuries is higher in pediatrics because many times they may have concurrent chest, head, and skeletal injuries. Penetrating trauma is not as common in pediatrics, but the highest incidence occurs in the adolescent age group and is most often associated with assault or violence. Penetrating abdominal injuries may or may not require surgical intervention. X-ray studies, ultrasound (US), and FAST are the first diagnostic tools utilized with suspected abdominal trauma as well as CT scan if the patient is stable. US technology has been improved with the development of contrast-enhanced ultrasonography (CEUS). The pediatric patient with abdominal trauma may present with signs and symptoms of shock, including hypotension, decreased perfusion, capillary refill, cool extremities, and decreased LOC. Treatment includes hemodynamic stability with fluid and/or blood product resuscitation. Attention needs to be given to prevent hypothermia as this can result in vasoconstriction, acidosis, and abnormal coagulopathy. Fluids given rapidly should be warmed. The patient may or may not have abdominal bruising present. A child with a "lap belt sign" from an MVA should elicit a high suspicion for spleen, liver, stomach, or bowel injuries due to the forceful retraction of the seat belt compressing the abdomen against the spine.

3. *General Signs and Symptoms of Abdominal Trauma*

a. *Spleen Injuries.* Splenic injuries are the most common abdominal injury in pediatrics and are graded on a scale of I to V depending on the severity of the trauma to the spleen with grade V laceration usually requiring a splenectomy. The splenic injuries grading scale is as follows (advance one grade for multiple injuries up to grade III):

- Grade I: Hematoma, subcapsular <10% surface area; laceration, capsular tear <1 cm parenchymal depth

- Grade II: Hematoma, subcapsular 10% to 50% surface area, intraparenchymal <5 cm in diameter; laceration, capsular tear of 1 to 3 cm parenchymal depth that does not involve trabecular vessel

- Grade III: Hematoma, subcapsular >50% surface area or expanding, ruptured subcapsular or parenchymal hematoma, intraparenchymal hematoma >5 cm or expanding; laceration, parenchymal depth >3 cm or involving trabecular vessels

- Grade IV: Laceration, involving segmental or hilar vessels producing major devascularization >25% of spleen

- Grade V: Laceration, spleen completely shattered; vascular injury, hilar vascular injury with devascularizes spleen (Moore, Cogbill, Malangoni, Jurkovich, & Champion, 1996)

The spleen is a highly vascularized organ and therefore the risk of bleeding is of great concern with splenic injuries. The chief complaints are usually upper abdominal pain in the left quadrant, left shoulder pain referred to as *Kehr's sign*, and may sometimes complain of chest pain. NOM is most often preferred and splenectomies are usually done as a last resort and performed based on the inability to control bleeding. The child's spleen can stop bleeding spontaneously; however, the child should be monitored in the ICU for up to 48 hours. The risks of having a splenectomy can result in the patient's decreased ability to fight infections, increased coagulopathies, abscess, and pneumonia. Serial laboratory studies should be obtained—specifically, hemoglobin and hematocrit (H/H) to monitor for bleeding. The patient should remain on bed rest up to 3 to 5 days depending on the severity of the injury and strict intake and output (I/O) should be monitored. The patient may be at risk for hypovolemic shock due to bleeding. In addition, a type and screen should be sent upon admission as well as coagulation studies. The patient will have physical activity restrictions for up to 4 to 8 weeks postinjury.

b. *Hepatic Injuries.* The liver is the second most injured solid organ in pediatric abdominal trauma and is most often caused by blunt trauma. The right lobe is more often injured due to its location and size. Liver injuries can result in serious blood loss because it is highly vascularized. Most common causes are MVAs, falls, auto versus pedestrian, and NAT. Liver injuries are also graded I to V depending on the severity of the injury. The following is the heptic injuries grading scale (advance one grade for multiple injuries up to grade III):

- Grade I: Hematoma, subcapsular <10% surface area; laceration, capsular tear <1 cm parenchymal depth

- Grade II: Hematoma, subcapsular 10%–50% surface area, intraparenchymal <10 cm in length; laceration, capsular tear 1–3 cm parenchymal depth, <10 cm in length

- Grade III: Hematoma, subcapsular >50% surface area of ruptured subcapsular or parenchymal hematoma, intraparenchymal hematoma >10 cm or expanding; laceration, parenchymal depth >3 cm

- Grade IV: Laceration, parenchymal disruption involving 25% to 75% hepatic lobe or one to three Couinaud's segments

- Grade V: Laceration, parenchymal disruption involving 75% of hepatic lobe or >3 Couinaud's segments within a single lobe; vascular injury, juxthepatic venous injuries (i.e., retrohepatic vena cava/central major hepatic veins)

- Grade V: Vascular injury, hepatic avulsion (Moore et al., 1996)

Most patients with hepatic injuries require NOM of their injuries with a success rate of 85% to 90%. The higher the grade of injury, the more difficult it is to hemodynamically stabilize the patient. Some patients with hepatic injuries may be treated with angiographic embolization to control bleeding. However, if this method is ineffective or the patient is hemodynamically unstable, surgical exploration may be required. In extreme cases, a hepatic lobectomy is performed to control the bleeding. If a patient requires 25 to 40 mL/kg/d or more of blood transfusions, this is also an indication for surgical exploration. Hepatic injuries have the highest mortality rate in pediatric abdominal trauma. The child may present with symptoms of right upper quadrant pain and tenderness, abdominal distention, increased abdominal girth, and signs of hypovolemic shock. Treatment of hepatic injuries requires close monitoring of vital signs (VS); strict I/O; serial laboratory studies (including H/H); coagulopathy studies, liver function tests (LFT), and serial abdominal girths (measured in the same location). Patients with hepatic injuries are at risk for developing atelectasis, pneumonia, abscess, hemobilia, and coagulopathy abnormalities.

c. *Kidney Injuries.* The kidney is the third most common solid organ injured in pediatric abdominal trauma. Kidney injuries are also graded I to V based on severity of injury and are mostly treated with NOM. The kidney injuries graded scale is as follows (advance one grade for multiple injuries up to grade III):

- Grade I: Contusion, microscopic or gross hematuria, urologic studies normal; hematoma, subcapsular, nonexpanding without parenchymal laceration

- Grade II: Hematoma, nonexpanding perirenal hematoma confirmed to renal retroperitoneum; laceration, parenchymal depth <1 cm of renal cortex without urinary extravagation

- Grade III: Laceration, parenchymal depth <1 cm or renal cortex without collecting system rupture or urinary extravagation

- Grade IV: Laceration, parenchymal laceration extending through renal cortex, medulla, and collecting system; vascular injury, main renal artery or vein injury with contained hemorrhage

- Grade V: Laceration, completely shattered kidney; vascular injury, avulsion of renal hilum, which devascularizes kidney (Moore et al., 1996)

Right kidney injuries may occur with hepatic injuries and left kidney injuries are more associated with splenic injuries due to their locations. The pediatric patient generally has less perirenal fat, smaller abdominal muscles, and less ossified ribs, which puts the child at greater risk for renal injuries and provides less protection compared to adults. However, most renal injuries tend to be low grade (I–II). Most kidney injuries in children are a result of blunt trauma, whereas penetrating injuries to the kidney are more often seen in adolescent males as a result of assault. The child may present with bruising over the umbilicus and flank area known as *Grey–Turner's sign*, hematuria, pain, and dyspnea. CEUS may be used to identify or grade kidney injuries but each kidney must be assessed individually because uptake of the contrast can be different depending on the extent of the injury to each kidney. Treatment is usually conservative with careful monitoring of VS, I/O, and urine output (especially changes in amount and color) so a Foley catheter should be placed and serial laboratory studies (H/H and electrolytes) performed. The patient should remain on bed rest for at least 24 hours or longer with higher grade injuries. In rare cases, a nephrectomy may be necessary if the damage is extensive or the bleeding cannot be controlled.

d. *Pancreas Injuries.* Pancreatic injuries are not common in pediatrics due to the pancreas's location in the retroperitoneal space of the abdominal cavity (Arslan et al., 2014). Most often it is related to blunt trauma and occurs more in the older child and adolescents such as compression injury of the abdomen against the handlebars in bike accidents. Pancreatic injuries can be difficult to diagnose because the patient may not exhibit abnormal findings. It is most often diagnosed by history of the mechanism of injury and revealed on CT scan. The amylase level may or may not be elevated, but an elevated amylase does not always indicate pancreatic injury. Pancreas injuries are also graded I to V (Table 9.9) based on severity of injury. NOM is recommended along with bed rest and placement of an NGT. Laboratory studies should include amylase, lipase, and serial glucose levels. In severe cases of pancreatic laceration, partial resection may be indicated; however, this is very rare.

e. *Stomach and Intestinal Injuries.* The stomach and intestines are considered hollow viscus organs. Injuries to the stomach and intestines are less common and the majority are due to blunt forces (e.g., MVAs, falls) and penetrating causes, especially in the adolescent age group as a result of assault. In the younger child, the cause is most often NAT. Another common cause of hollow viscus organ injuries is damage done by seat belt restraint in an MVA as a result of the rapid acceleration/deceleration and the tightening of the seat belt against the abdomen compressing against the spine and causing a rupture. This can cause bowel contents to leak out into the peritoneal space, which can lead to peritonitis. The child may present with abdominal bruising, pain, tenderness, abdominal distention, vomiting, and fluid in the peritoneal space on CT scan. The child may also have decreased urine output, and exhibit signs of shock and poor perfusion, especially to the lower extremities. Treatment requires hemodynamic stabilization, fluid resuscitation, surgical exploration and repair, and possible bowel resection of the injured area. Management includes close monitoring of VS, I/O, serial abdominal girths, perfusion assessment with close attention to the lower extremities, observing for signs of infection, antibiotic therapy, and pain control. Patients can be at risk for developing an ileus, abscess, and/or abdominal compartment syndrome (ACS).

f. *Bladder Injuries.* The bladder is considered an abdominal viscus organ in the younger child and is less protected when full. A full bladder can rupture between a car seat belt and the child's vertebral column as a result of a deceleration injury (Morey, et al. (2014, amended 2017), 2004). The bladder neck, especially in girls, is less protected. Boys are more vulnerable to urethral injuries as a result of the length and position of the urethra. The tissues of prepubescent girls are

TABLE 9.9   Pancreatic Injuries

Pancreatic Injury Scale		
Grade[a]	Injury Type	Injury Description
I	Hematoma Laceration	Minor contusion without duct injury Superficial laceration without duct injury
II	Hematoma Laceration	Major contusion without duct injury or tissue loss Major laceration without duct injury or tissue loss
III	Laceration	Distal transection or parenchymal injury with duct injury
IV	Laceration	Proximal[b] transection or parenchymal injury involving ampulla
V	Laceration	Massive disruption of pancreatic head

[a]Advance one grade for multiple injuries up to grade III.

[b]Proximal pancreas is to the patient's right of the superior mesenteric vein.

Source: Adapted from Moore, E. E., Cogbill, T. H., Malangoni, M., Jurkovich, G. J., & Champion, H. R. (1996). Scaling system for organ specific injuries. Retrieved from http://www.aast.org/Library/TraumaTools/InjuryScoringScales.aspx

smaller and considerably more rigid than those of the adolescent or adult, thus increasing the risk of tearing with either blunt or penetrating trauma. Prepubescent girls also have a thin vesicovaginal septal wall.

   i. Ureteral elasticity and torso mobility allow for ureteral injuries to occur. In younger children, bladder rupture usually occurs more intraperitoneally and in adolescents is more extraperitoneal because the anatomical location varies between the two age groups. Rupture is often due to bone spicule in a pelvic fracture. The child may present with hematuria, complaints of suprapubic pain, and the inability to void.

   ii. A CT cystography is performed for diagnosis. Intraperitoneal rupture requires surgical repair, whereas extraperitoneal rupture usually does not. Injuries to the female genitalia occur from falls, straddle injuries, sexual abuse, or assault. These injuries are not easily observed in the ED and they may require EUA in the operating

room. Testicular trauma results from straddle-type injuries. Most testicular injuries occur in adolescents who are struck in the scrotum while playing sports or during an altercation. Testicular fractures can be diagnosed with US and then can be repaired. Direct forces are the most common causes of penile injuries (e.g., zipper injuries, toilet seat trauma).

g. *Penetrating Trauma.* Penetrating trauma has a higher likelihood of surgical management and may be done in stages in order to stabilize the patient. The first surgery may be done to control the bleeding and/or prevent further leakage of contaminated fluid as damage control. A reoperation may then be planned within the next 24 to 48 hours to perform the definitive repair when the patient may be more stable. This is done so the patient does not undergo a lengthy, possible life-threatening operation and will have less bowel edema. The abdomen may be kept open with a sterile occlusive dressing and closed at a later time. Management will include monitoring of VS; strict I/O; perfusion assessment; and assessing for signs of infection, ACS, and hypovolemia.

h. *ACS.* This can be as a result of complications from abdominal trauma or injuries. It is caused by increased pressure in the abdominal cavity, often caused by edema and fluid. It can cause decreased perfusion to the lower extremities and distal organs, as well as decreased cardiac output due to decreased venous return to the heart. If left untreated, it can lead to cardiorespiratory compromise and death. Early symptoms include decreased urine output, prolonged capillary refill to the lower extremities with weak pulses, and decreased perfusion as represented by a coolness to touch. Normal intra-abdominal pressure (IAP) is 0 to 5 mmHg. IAP greater than 10 mmHg is considered intra-abdominal hypertension (IAH). IAP of 10 mmHg to 15 mmHg may be associated with organ damage and sustained IAP greater than 20 mmHg to 25 mmHg is consistent with ACS. The patient may become oliguric with an IAP greater than 20 mmHg. If paracentesis is not effective at removing fluid or the edema continues, a decompressive laparotomy may be performed in order to preserve perfusion distally. The abdomen is left open with a sterile occlusive mesh dressing or a wound vacuum-type system (to keep the skin dry from fluids that may ooze from the open wound) until the IAP decreases or abdominal perfusion pressures (APP) remain above 50 mmHg. To calculate the APP, subtract the MAP from the IAP (MAP–IAP = APP). IAP can be measured by instilling fluid into the Foley catheter to measure bladder pressure, which is considered the gold standard for measuring IAP. Nursing care includes serial monitoring of IAP every 2 to 6 hours, strict I/O, VS, neurological assessments, circulatory checks, and laboratory studies such as LFTs, electrolytes, BUN, creatinine, lactate, and hematology labs as well.

F. Musculoskeletal Injuries

1. Musculoskeletal injuries commonly occur in children and include open and closed fractures, dislocations, nerve injuries, tendon injuries, and amputations. Growing bones are porous and more vascular, whereas the periosteum is strong and thick. These features lead to partial fracturing of the bone (e.g., greenstick fracture), rather than complete fractures. Although the thicker periosteum allows quicker fracture healing, it may impede fracture reduction (Daley, 2015; Ross & Juarez, 2016). Fracture healing occurs in three stages:

   a. Stage I. Inflammatory stage, during which a hematoma collects inside and outside of the bone.

   b. Stage II. Reparative phase during which cartilage formed from the hematoma is replaced by bone through endochondral ossification.

   c. Stage III. Remodeling phase is the process during which bone is renewed through formation and resorption of bone.

2. The same mechanism is at work as in the growth process of bones, which allows for more rapid healing of fractures in children (Ross & Juarez, 2016). The ligaments are strong, allowing for higher occurrence of fractures versus ligament injuries. Children have an epiphyseal growth plate (physis) located at the articulating ends of the bones between the epiphysis and metaphysis. The physis is responsible for longitudinal bone growth, and injury to the growth plate may result in growth disturbance or arrest. Growth generally is completed in boys by 16 years of age and in girls by 14 years of age. Fractures occurring near or at the physeal plate can be the most serious, as fractures in this area can cause premature growth cessation or deformities, so follow-up is imperative (Engman-Lazear, 2015). Obesity plays a large factor in children with musculoskeletal trauma, especially fractures with a higher incidence than nonobese children. Obese children tend to be more sedentary, have more weight to support on impact, poorer balance, and may not have enough

bone mineral density to support their increased weight. Childhood obesity has become a worldwide problem with an estimate of over 43 million children obese or overweight in 2010, including 32% of children and adolescents in the United States (Lazar-Antman & Leet, 2012). Lower calcium and milk uptake and an increase in carbonated-beverage consumption has been shown to increase risk for fractures.

3. Musculoskeletal trauma is suspected in the child with tenderness at the point of injury; soft-tissue swelling or discoloration; limitations in range of motion (ROM); loss of function; altered sensory perception; and changes in pulse, temperature, or capillary refill distal to the injury (Liebman, 2000). Musculoskeletal trauma is rarely life threatening, so the priorities of airway, breathing, and circulation are addressed before treating any fractures. Neurovascular status is assessed before and after any intervention, such as splinting, swathing, or dressing. Elevation of the injured extremity may be needed to decrease swelling and ongoing assessment is needed to prevent or identify compartment syndrome, which may occur. A child in pain can interfere with an accurate assessment of an orthopedic fracture so pain-control measures should be implemented and continued as needed. A pneumonic device useful when treating an orthopedic injury is known as the "5 Ps to orthopedic fractures": Pain, pallor, pulselessness, paresthesia, paralysis. The nonaffected side or extremity should be assessed first before assessing the affected side or extremity, by starting distal to the injury and then working the way back toward the injury. Starting at the injury site can cause pain and anxiety, thus hampering a true assessment. Tetanus prophylaxis may be recommended if unsure of the immunization status of the child. Radiographs include the joint above and below the injury with comparative views (radiographs of the injured and uninjured extremities).

4. Most fractures are simple and nondisplaced, requiring only the application of a cast. A schematic representation of fractures is found in Figure 9.3. The casted extremity is assessed for swelling of the toes or fingers, odor from the cast, changes in skin color and temperature. If the child complains of sharp pain or numbness, compartment syndrome should be suspected. Fracture stabilization is important to protect soft tissues, reduce pain, and facilitate rehabilitation. Treatment should be aimed at preventing prolonged casting or bed rest and to promote mobility as soon as possible (Pandya, Upasani, & Kulkarni, 2013).

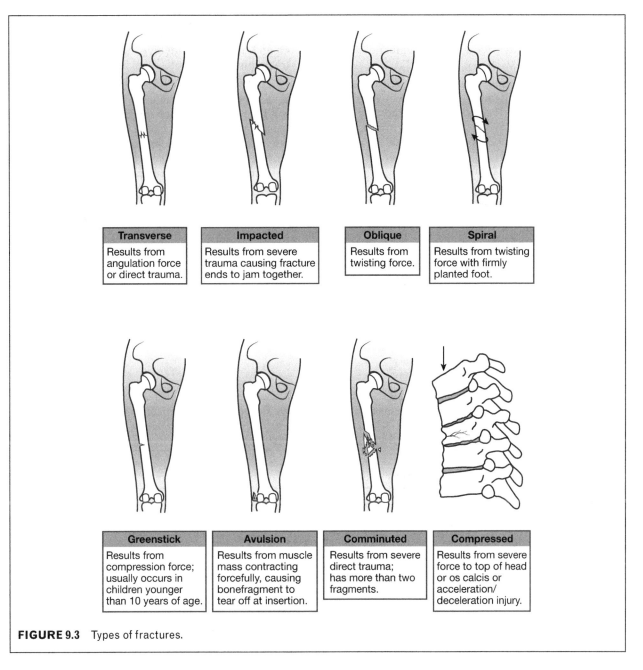

Transverse	Impacted	Oblique	Spiral
Results from angulation force or direct trauma.	Results from severe trauma causing fracture ends to jam together.	Results from twisting force.	Results from twisting force with firmly planted foot.

Greenstick	Avulsion	Comminuted	Compressed
Results from compression force; usually occurs in children younger than 10 years of age.	Results from muscle mass contracting forcefully, causing bonefragment to tear off at insertion.	Results from severe direct trauma; has more than two fragments.	Results from severe force to top of head or os calcis or acceleration/ deceleration injury.

FIGURE 9.3   Types of fractures.

5. Nondisplaced fractures may be too edematous to allow casting. In such cases, a splint is applied, and the cast can be applied later when the swelling has resolved. Displaced fractures may require a closed reduction in which the orthopedic specialist and nurse apply manual traction–countertraction to realign the fractured bone. Sedation is administered using IV analgesics and sedatives (e.g., midazolam, fentanyl, propofol, or ketamine). Once the fracture is reduced, the medications can be stopped, the cast applied, and postreduction radiographs obtained. If the closed reduction was not successful, an open reduction and internal fixation is required.

6. Open fractures are divided into three types.

    a. Type I open fractures are less than 1 cm long, are usually a clean puncture with little soft-tissue involvement, and can be treated with casting, provided a window is cut into the cast to allow for wound visualization and dressing changes.

b. Type II open fractures have a laceration greater than 1 cm with slight or moderate crushing and no extensive soft-tissue damage.

c. Type III injuries have extensive damage to soft tissues, muscle, skin, and neurovascular structures; contamination is present (Engman-Lazear, 2015). IV antibiotics are administered and wound may be irrigated. Debridement is continued every 24 to 48 hours until the wound is clean. Type II and III injuries may be treated with external fixation (Table 9.10).

7. Physeal fractures are described using the Salter–Harris classification and are outlined in Figure 9.4. Open fractures that involve the growth plate may be treated with smooth K-wires in addition to external fixation (Sahu & Ranjan, 2016).

8. Elbow fractures occur in children, with supracondylar fractures involving the distal humerus the most common. Injury to the brachial artery is most often associated with supracondylar and intercondylar fractures. If a brachial artery injury is suspected, an arteriogram must be performed, followed by

TABLE 9.10 Classification of Open Fractures

Type	Description
Type I	Wound <1 cm long Usually moderately clean puncture through which a spike of bone has pierced the skin Little soft-tissue damage No sign of crushing injury Fracture usually is simple, transverse, or short oblique with little comminution
Type II	Laceration is >1 cm long No extensive soft-tissue damage, flap, or avulsion Slight or moderate crushing injury Moderate comminution of fracture Moderate contamination
Type III	Extensive damage to soft tissues, including muscles, skin, and neurovascular structures High degree of contamination Great deal of comminution and instability as a result of high-velocity trauma
Type IIIA	Soft-tissue coverage of bone is adequate despite extensive laceration, flaps, or high-energy trauma Includes segmental or severely comminuted fractures from high-energy trauma regardless of size of wound
Type IIIB	Extensive injury to or loss of soft tissue, with periosteal stripping and exposure of bone Massive contamination Severe comminution from high-velocity trauma After irrigation and debridement, a segment of bone is exposed Local or free flap is needed for coverage
Type IIIC	Any open fracture associated with arterial injury that must be repaired, regardless of degree of soft-tissue injury

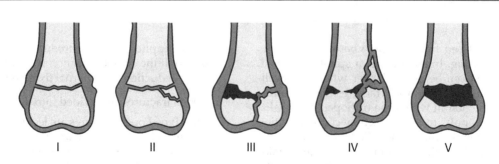

FIGURE 9.4   Salter–Harris fractures.

emergent surgical repair of the vessel. If not assessed rapidly and treated properly, complications can result. Extremity compartment syndrome can develop in less than 12 to 24 hours and will be discussed later in this chapter. A complete neurovascular assessment is performed along with Doppler examination of the arterial blood supply. Operative management for a closed reduction is undertaken. Skeletal or skin traction can be implemented, closed reduction and percutaneous pinning are options as well (Sahu & Ranjan, 2016). Careful ongoing evaluation of the child's neurovascular status is imperative. Use of physical therapy and occupational therapy can help the child and family cope with learning to use the nondominant arm if the dominant arm is injured. Elbow dislocations are uncommon. However, when they do occur it is usually due to an avulsed medial epicondyle trapped in the elbow joint and is most often associated with throwing actions. This is known as *Little Leaguer's elbow*. MRI will show edema around the bone and soft tissue. The child will have pain and tenderness over the medial condyle. If the medial condyle is displaced more than 3 mm on x-ray, surgical reduction and pinning may be indicated (Rosendahl & Strouse, 2016).

9. Shoulder injuries occur more in the adolescent age group oftentimes from contact sports or due to overuse related to throwing actions. "Little Leaguer's shoulder" will show a stress injury of the proximal humerus. X-rays show a widening and irregularity of the proximal humerus. Treatment is to stop the activity causing the injury, which will lead to resolution of the problem. Shoulder dislocation is the most common type of dislocation in pediatrics and is associated with skeletal immaturity. Traction may be used to reduce these dislocations; however, there is a risk for nerve and vessel entrapment (Rosendahl & Strouse, 2016).

10. Clavicle and forearm fractures are the most common fractures in children. Cast immobilization for forearm fractures is usually 4 to 6 weeks. Routine care for the cast and assessment for swelling and perfusion should be taught to the child and family.

11. Wrist and hand injuries usually are "Salter" type fractures involving the physis or as a plastic fracture of the distal radial metaphysis. "Gymnast's wrist" injury is a stress injury of the distal radial physis and on x-ray shows it widened and irregular. There is adjacent metaphyseal sclerosis and bone marrow edema is usually present on both sides of the physis (Rosendahl & Strouse, 2016). Continued gymnastic activity may lead to premature physeal fusion, causing radial shortening and predisposition to carpal impingement

and triangular fibrocartilage complex injury (Rosendahl & Strouse, 2016).

12. Knee, tibia, and fibula injuries are most often due to sports such as football, skiing, snowboarding, wrestling, basketball, and cheerleading. Meniscus and ligament (cruciate and collateral) injuries can occur, but generally not until skeletal maturity, making these injuries more common in the adolescent age group. The open physes are weaker than ligaments in the knee. Fractures of the tibia or fibula are common in the younger child. In the adolescent these fractures usually result from falls and pedestrian versus a motor vehicle. Treatment may include surgical repair and immobilization. Use of crutches is recommended to limit weight bearing and for bone growth and resolution (Rosendahl & Strouse, 2016). Twisting knee injuries and lower extremity injuries are more often associated with skiing, whereas upper extremity injuries are more associated with snowboarding.

13. Femoral fractures are common and require a tremendous amount of force, with about 70% occurring in the midshaft area, oftentimes caused by an MVA or pedestrian versus motor vehicle (Engman-Lazear, 2015). Femur fractures account for the most common major orthopedic injury in children. Femoral fractures peak in the toddler age group usually after a fall and in the adolescent age group commonly after a high-energy trauma (Daniels, Kane, Eberson, & Born, 2012). The injured thigh will be swollen, firm, appear shortened, may be bruised, and there is a risk for significant hemorrhage. The child is unable to move the leg and complains of pain. An anteroposterior radiograph should be obtained. Treatment varies according to the child's age, weight, the level of the fracture and pattern, and preference of the surgeon or institution. Ideally, the treatment should provide adequate stabilization, maximize comfort, allow for early mobilization, minimize caregiver needs, and limit scarring and complications (Narayanan & Phillips, 2012). Other factors that may influence which type of treatment is used include magnitude of displacement, extent of comminution, soft-tissue injuries, whether it is an open fracture, and the presence of other significant injuries. Femur fracture in pediatrics can be treated in a variety of ways, which include spica casts, skin traction, skeletal traction, internal fixation, bridge plating, external fixation, and flexible or rigid intramedullary (IM) nailing. Spica casts are oftentimes an option for children younger than 10 years and/or 30 kg or less. Advantages to spica casts include no scarring and less risk for infection, minimal hospitalization, and an alternative method for repair can easily be done if healing is not effective. Disadvantages include less comfort; increased responsibility for the caregiver; and may be associated with a more frequent loss of reduction, malunion, and shortening (Narayanan & Phillips, 2012). Spica casting is contraindicated in children if the shortening is 2 to 3 cm and if there are multiple injuries (Sahu & Ranjan, 2016). In cases of shortening, skeletal or skin traction is indicated until early callus formation is observed on radiographs. Skin traction has less morbidity than skeletal traction but is limited to about 5 to 10 pounds of traction across the fractured extremity, thereby reducing its effectiveness in restoring axial alignment. Skin traction risks include skin blistering, sloughing, and breakdown. Skeletal traction is effective in the initial management of pediatric femoral fractures. Physeal growth arrest is a serious complication following proximal or distal femoral traction (Daniels et al., 2012). Imprecise pin placement can cause varus or valgus alignment of the fracture. When skeletal traction is used, pin care is performed on a routine schedule to avoid infection. Signs of pin infection include tenting of the insertion site, redness, and drainage. Risks associated with traction or casting include malunion, osteomyelitis, skin breakdown, excessive shortening, and rotational deformities (Sahu & Ranjan, 2016).

a. External fixation, IM fixation, and plating are options for stabilizing femur fractures. External fixation has the capability to stabilize adjacent joints, to prevent excessive soft-tissue movement and contractures, and can be used until the patient is stable enough to undergo definitive fracture management (Mooney, 2012). External fixation has a higher risk of complications that include refracture (at pin-sites or fracture), pin-site infections, delayed union, and scars. Complications of external fixation include delayed union, pin infections, knee stiffness, and refracture after fixator removal. Due to these complications, external fixation generally is used in patients with open fractures, length-unstable fractures, or associated soft-tissue injury (Mooney, 2012).

b. IM nailing is the most popular management option for length-stable femoral shaft fractures in school-age children and adolescents. Flexible IM nails (titanium, elastic, stainless steel) are commonly used for femoral fracture fixation in school-age children and rigid trochanteric IM nails are used for adolescents.

c. Plating provides relative fracture stability without disruption of the soft-tissue envelope at the fracture site (Li & Hedequist, 2012). Stainless steel nails provide improved fixation in children with unstable diaphyseal femur fractures.

Internal fixation may require supplementary casting and may be useful in older children who are in less danger of growth plate injury (Sahu & Ranjan, 2016). Compression plating provides good control of bone fragments, a high rate of union, low risk for infection, ease of mobilization, and low risk for functionally important limb-length discrepancy (Sahu & Ranjan, 2016).

d. Pain and inflammation near a major joint may signal impending ectopic bone formation (Sahu & Ranjan, 2016). Physical therapy, pharmacologic management, and additional surgery may be required and subsequently affect recovery. Complications of IM nails and plating include infection, nail protrusion/migration, osteonecrosis, femoral deformities, and revision surgeries (Li & Hedequist, 2012; Narayanan & Phillips, 2012). Osteonecrosis may develop as a result of direct trauma to the vessel at the time of injury, kinking of the vessels with displacement, tamponade effect by intracapsular hematoma, or injury during treatment (Spence et al., 2016). Treatment strategies should be individualized and should include the parent and child in the decision making. With plating fixation, patients can begin hip and knee ROM activities post-operatively. Weight bearing with crutches is allowed until x-rays show callus formation, usually at 6 to 8 weeks postop and then advanced as tolerated. Patients then can resume normal activity. At about 6 months after the repair, the plate can be removed. Plate removal requires more surgery and the long scar may have cosmetic disadvantages (Sahu & Ranjan, 2016). After removal, weight bearing is encouraged as tolerated and activity is restricted for about 6 weeks to prevent fracture through the screw holes (Li & Hedequist, 2012).

14. Pelvic fractures can be life-threatening fractures secondary to compression forces that cause displacement of the pelvis ring, causing injuries to surrounding organs and vasculature. Pelvic fractures are defined as fractures of the bones of the pelvis or a separation of one of the two immobile joints in the pelvis, sacroiliac joint, or symphysis pubis. About 80% of pelvic fractures have multiple fracture sites and are associated with abdominal or GU trauma. Pelvic fractures are usually found in polytrauma patients and are due to high-energy mechanism impact (Miele et al., 2016). Patients with pelvic fractures are at risk for hemorrhage from multiple sources, including osseous, vascular, and visceral structures. Displaced pelvic fractures can injure paravaginal, superior gluteal, and internal iliac arteries, which can compromise the viability of the lower extremity. There is a higher proportion of iliac wing and pubic

ring fracture in younger children, and adolescents have a higher proportion of acetabular fractures and sacroiliac diastasis (Pandya et al., 2013). An anterior–lateral x-ray may confirm fractures. Visceral injuries associated with pelvic fracture may be very serious and may involve urologic and neurologic injuries. Specific neurologic injury may include the lumbosacral plexus when sacroiliac disruptions or sacral fractures are incurred. Initial assessment includes manipulation of the pelvis to assess for stability. If unstable, no further manipulation should be done as it may cause further hemorrhage. Hemodynamically unstable patients with an unstable pelvis should have a pelvic binder applied, in order to reduce blood loss and pelvic volume until stabilization of the pelvis can be performed. Emergent angiography and embolization may be needed with signs and symptoms of hemorrhaging and hemodynamic instability. Aggressive replacement of fluid and blood is vital to preventing neurovascular complications to the extremities. Nursing care involves neurocirculatory checks, serial laboratory studies, monitoring of VS, strict I/O, and routine postop care. Children with pelvic fractures require bed rest and attention must be given to prevent skin breakdown and pressure sores, as well as ensuring pulmonary toilet to prevent atelectasis. Unstable pelvic fractures may require the application of an external fixation device or, in rare cases, internal fixation may be required. Again, the psychological effects of immobility must be addressed and options for movement must be given (Sahu & Ranjan, 2016).

G. Nerve Injury

Nerve injury is suspected in any crushing trauma. Open wounds near the anatomic location for peripheral nerves should be an indication of nerve involvement (Sahu & Ranjan, 2016). Sensory loss is difficult to ascertain in young children; however, two tests can be administered to determine nerve damage. The first test is to observe for a lack of sweating in the affected area using an iodine starch test or a ninhydrin print test. The second test is the wrinkle test, in which the extremity is placed in warm water. If the skin wrinkles, the nerve is intact. Nerve injuries are graded from I to V, with grades I to II having the best chances for full recovery. Peripheral nerve injuries tend to heal better in children than in adults. It is believed that the child's brain plasticity assists in nerve regeneration. Children seem to need less formal sensory reeducation following peripheral nerve repair than adults, which may be due to their natural curiosity. The shorter distances required by axons to regenerate before reaching their end organ may also enhance nerve recovery. Moreover, the shorter distances peripheral pain impulses need to travel to reach the cerebral cortex may make up for injury or the degree of nerve myelination.

H. Amputated Digits

1. Amputated digits or extremities are classified as complete or incomplete. Traumatic amputations are rare, but do occur and the child should be taken to a facility with microsurgical capabilities for reimplantation, ideally, a pediatric level-I trauma center or an adult level-I trauma center with pediatric-trained specialists. Traumatic amputations are serious injuries and can result in prolonged hospitalizations and disability. Prior to reimplantation, the child must be stabilized and blood loss controlled. The amputated part needs to be assessed for viability of reimplantation. The stump needs to be gently cleaned and debrided with pressure applied to help control the bleeding. The debridement should occur within 6 hours of the amputation to preserve soft tissue and prevent infections. The stump should be elevated to limit or reduce swelling. X-rays of the stump and amputated part need to be taken to help identify the extent of the injury and landmarks for reattachment. The amputated part needs to be properly handled to prevent further tissue destruction. It should be properly cleaned and wrapped in moist gauze, then placed in a plastic bag or container. The container should be placed in a cooler on ice. The amputated part should not be placed directly on the ice as it can get too cold and at risk of developing frostbite which would make it not be suitable for reimplantation. The goal is to save as much of the physis as possible to allow bone growth in the developing child. Pediatric traumatic amputations tend to be more extensive and occur more often than in adults.

2. Specific management of the child with a traumatic amputation includes the following (Khan, Javed, Rao, Corner, & Rosenfield, 2016):

   a. Initial assessment, resuscitation, homeostasis, and necessary transfusions

      i. Wound management and stump protection (including cleaning and debridement)

      ii. Limb splinting in partial amputations

      iii. Antibiotics and tetanus prophylaxis

      iv. Appropriate transport of the amputated limb

      v. Appropriate imaging of the stump and amputated part

3. After reimplantation, the attached body area is assessed for bleeding and neurovascular integrity. The amputated area is carefully wrapped in sterile dressings, and care should be taken to shield the young child's view from the injury. The success of the reimplantation is related to the child's health condition and the viability of the tissues. If the reimplantation is not viable, the child may require prosthesis and subsequent rehabilitation. Unique pain challenges accompany amputation injuries. The psychological impact of traumatic amputations may include depression and PTSD in both the child and the family. Use of counseling, psychological support, social work, chaplain services, and a child life specialist should be implemented early to deal with these issues. Support groups of other families that have experienced similar injuries can help the child and family deal with this potentially life-changing event. Also, the family and child will require rehabilitation services (e.g., physical therapy, occupational therapy). Some complications related to traumatic amputations include soft-tissue injuries, anastomosis, painful neuromas, phantom limb pain, pressure ulcers, osseous overgrowth (which can cause skin perforations), and improper prosthetic fittings. Amputations occur from knives, bicycle spokes, and crushing injuries from lawn mowers, farm equipment, motor vehicles, and powerboats.

4. Neurovascular assessments include postoperative assessments of arterial and venous circulation. A sign of arterial occlusion is a pale, cool extremity with poor turgor. A sign of venous occlusion is a cyanotic, cool extremity with tense turgor. The extremity should be elevated unless there are signs of arterial compromise. The patient's room should be warmed or the reimplanted part warmed with devices that blow warm air without applying pressure in order to avoid vessel constriction. Brisk bleeding should be noted, and the physician notified immediately with any changes in perfusion, pulses, and color. Postoperative care includes wound care and dressing changes. The wound may require further debridement and the patient should be started on antibiotics to prevent infections. In some instances, medicinal leeches may be utilized to promote blood flow to the reimplanted area.

I. Tendon Injuries

Tendon injuries also occur with crush or open injuries, usually in the forearm and hand. The child may not be able to move or wiggle the fingers, or refuse to do so because of pain and discomfort. Operative management is necessary to repair tendons. Following tendon repair, the area is assessed for function and neurovascular status. Passive-flexion exercises are performed with the parents or therapist. Physical and occupational therapy are keys to an optimal recovery. Nerve and tendon injuries occur from crushing forces (e.g., lawn mowers or farm equipment).

DANGEROUS COMPLICATIONS OF MULTITRAUMA

Dangerous complications of multitrauma include, but are not limited to rhabdomyolysis, compartment syndrome, fat embolism syndrome (FES; Fort, 2003), and venous thromboembolism (VTE).

A. Rhabdomyolysis

1. Rhabdomyolysis is the disintegration of muscle tissue. Injured myocytes cause a massive influx of calcium ions, sodium ions, and fluid into the cytoplasm. Myoglobin, potassium, phosphate, and lactate are released into the intracellular fluid space, which can result in hypocalcemia, hyperkalemia, and acidosis (Baird & Cooper, 2016). Uric acid levels may also be elevated.

2. Several predisposing trauma-related conditions are associated with rhabdomyolysis and include crush injuries, electrical shock, severe burns, extended immobility, snake venom, substance abuse (i.e., alcohol, barbiturates, cocaine, street drug "ecstasy"), tetanus, and reperfusion to damaged cells (as in fasciotomy for compartment syndrome).

3. A classic sign associated with rhabdomyolysis is dark, reddish-brown urine. Laboratory findings reveal that serum CK, equals or exceeds a level 5 times that of normal. Myoglobin is present in the urine. Urine dipstick shows the urine to be heme positive without the presence of red blood cells (RBCs). Acute renal insufficiency (elevated BUN and creatinine) is a consequence of severe myoglobinuria wherein the globulin precipitates and blocks the urinary tubules. Myoglobin excretion is facilitated by alkalinization of the urine and increased urine flow.

4. Symptoms associated with rhabdomyolysis include muscle pain, weakness, decreased urine output, and cramping. Sinus tachycardia, nausea, vomiting, and fever are other symptoms. Neurologic symptoms of agitation and confusion may be evident. Renal manifestations of rhabdomyolysis may include decreased urine output, potential renal failure, and electrolyte abnormalities. Finally, a patient with this complication may have DIC.

5. *Nursing Implications and Treatment.* The nurse caring for a patient with rhabdomyolysis should prepare to normalize electrolyte values, administer IV crystalloids and, if hyperkalemia is present, treat with sodium bicarbonate, insulin, and glucose. Administering phosphate-binding antacids and diuretics is part of the therapy. Strict I/O is required and urine output should be at least 1 mL/kg/hr to ensure adequate flushing of the kidneys to prevent obstruction in the tubules due to cell breakdown.

B. Compartment Syndrome

1. Compartment syndrome occurs when pressure in the myofascial compartment exceeds capillary perfusion pressure so that blood flow decreases to the tissues. Occurrence is rare in children. Compartment syndrome is more often seen in the lower extremities compared to the upper extremities. If left untreated, it can cause myonecrosis, contractures, infection, neurologic dysfunction, and long-term disability. A high suspicion for compartment syndrome with recognition and intervention is critical to prevent morbidity and permanent disability. Infection is usually due to an inflammation response, resulting in endothelial injury and vascular permeability. Therefore, acute compartment syndrome is a surgical emergency. There is also concern for reperfusion injury. Late diagnosis can compromise circulation leading to tissue ischemia, cellular anoxia, and eventually tissue death, leading to amputation of the affected limb, or even death of the patient. Children, however, are more resilient than adults and tend to have better outcomes and recovery (Broom et al., 2016).

2. Trauma-related conditions associated with compartment syndrome include hemorrhage, edema, extravasation, extreme muscle inactivity, external forces (i.e., cast, eschar, and tight dressings), IV infiltration, burns, infection, vascular problems, crush injuries, fractures, falls, and snake bites.

3. Signs and symptoms of compartment syndrome can be subtle and include swelling, tenseness, tenderness along with paresthesia, hypoesthesia, or anesthesia of the affected limb. The extremity may be cool to touch and pale with prolonged capillary refill. Complete neuropathy may occur. Other indications of compartment syndrome include warm, shiny skin; loss of pulse (late sign); and pain, especially with movement or if pain is not relieved by analgesia or has increased analgesia requirements. The most common symptom, however, is swelling and pain. The child is usually not able to be consoled. The pain may also be nonspecific and compartment firmness is unreliable.

4. Children who are able to communicate may be able to describe "loss of two-point discrimination." This is the inability to distinguish between one or two stimuli (ends of a paperclip) touching the affected extremity. Diagnosis can be difficult in infants and toddlers younger than 3 years of age, uncooperative patients, patients with altered level of consciousness, and those patients with inconsistent clinical findings.

5. *Nursing Implications and Treatment.* Nurses have the following responsibilities when treating a patient with compartment syndrome:

    a. Keep the affected extremity at the heart level.

    b. Perform serial neurovascular examinations at least hourly.

    c. Anticipate fasciotomy.

    d. Monitor for the development of rhabdomyolysis.

6. Use of a noninvasive regional saturation (NIRS) monitor can be helpful in measuring tissue oxygenation to the affected area to help diagnose compartment syndrome. However, there are limitations due to skin pigmentation and subcutaneous fat (Broom et al., 2016). A fasciotomy may be indicated if intracompartmental pressures are greater than 30 mmHg, intracompartmental pressures are 15 mmHg to 25 mmHg with signs and symptoms present, or intracompartmental pressures of 25 mmHg without signs and the diastolic blood pressure minus the intracompartmental pressure is less than 30 mmHg (Wallin, Nguyen, Russell, & Lee, 2016). Usually, there are favorable outcomes if the fasciotomy is performed within 48 to 72 hours postinjury. A sterile occlusive dressing or wet-to-dry dressing wrapped in Kerlix changed every 8 to 12 hours is applied; and the skin is closed after the swelling has subsided and the extremity has adequate perfusion. Care must be taken to prevent infection and to assess for bleeding.

C. Fat Embolism Syndrome

1. FES is rare and oftentimes associated with long-bone fractures or after orthopedic surgery. It can be challenging to diagnose due to its nonspecific and respiratory distress symptoms being the most common in 90% of the cases. Many times it encompasses a triad of pulmonary, neurologic, and skin symptomatology (Newbigin et al., 2016). The triad of symptoms includes hypoxia, confusion, and petechial rash. However, this triad may not be present in all patients. FES diagnosis requires the presence of one major and four minor criteria (Table 9.11). Two theories described for FES is the mechanical theory in which fat globules enter the venous channels at the fracture site and embolization of these fat particles cause direct obstruction of pulmonary capillaries. The biochemical theory postulates the fat

TABLE 9.11   Fat Embolism Syndrome Criteria[a]

Major Criteria	Minor Criteria
Hypoxia (<60 mmHg O$_2$) Confusion Petechial rash	Pyrexia (>39°C) Tachycardia (>120 bpm) Retinal changes (petechiae) Anuria or oliguria Anemia (Hgb ↓ 20%) Thrombocytopenia ↓ 50%) Elevated ESR (>71 mm/hr) Fat macroglobulinemia

ESR, erythrocyte sedimentation rate; Hgb, hemoglobin.

[a]FES = one major + four minor criteria.

Source: Adapted from Newbigin, K., Souza, C. A., Torres, C., Marchiori, E., Gupta, A., Inacio, J., … Peña, E. (2016). Fat embolism syndrome: State-of-the-art review focused on pulmonary imaging findings. *Respiratory Medicine, 113*, 93–100.

emboli in the capillaries release free fatty acids and glycerol initiating an inflammatory cascade causing localized endothelial injury, permeability edema, and hemorrhage. FES may manifest within 12 hours postinjury or surgery with symptoms peaking within 48 to 72 hours. The petechial rash occurs over the anterior torso, axillary regions, and conjunctiva, but typically does not appear until 3 to 5 days after the onset of symptoms (Newbigin et al., 2016). Risk factors include high-velocity trauma, surgical delay of more than 10 hours to fix the fracture, fixation of multiple fractures during the same procedure, and contusion of the lung (Newbigin et al., 2016). FES should be considered whenever alveolar–arterial oxygen gradients deteriorate in conjunction with loss of pulmonary compliance and CNS deterioration. As ventilation becomes compromised secondary to decreases in pulmonary compliance, PaCO$_2$ levels increase. Hemodynamics deteriorate while pulmonary arterial pressures are increased, often accompanied by decrease in cardiac index. CXR may show bilateral diffuse or patchy ill-defined opacities and findings are generally nonspecific and are limited in the diagnosis of FES. CT scan is the imaging modality of choice. CT scan may show a patchy ground-glass opacity type picture and a smooth interlobular septal thickening. Cerebral manifestations of FES include confusion to encephalopathy. The patient may also have headaches, seizures, or become comatose. MRI is the imagining of choice for suspected cerebral fat embolus and generally shows multiple small scattered nonconfluent hyperintense lesions that involve both the gray and white matter. These lesions can appear within 4 hours after the onset of symptoms.

2. *Nursing Implications and Treatment.* There is no specific treatment for FES and treatment is generally supportive. Patients who develop FES usually have very good outcomes and symptoms are self-resolving. Patients with pulmonary involvement tend to have complete resolution within 2 weeks but there are some reported cases with chronic sequelae, which is rare. Cerebral FES patients' symptoms gradually resolve within a few weeks to a few months (Newbigin et al., 2016). Corticosteroid and heparin have been suggested as treatments for FES, but their use is controversial and has not shown to decrease morbidity or mortality (Newbigin et al., 2016).When caring for a patient at risk for the development of FES, the nurse should move the fractured extremity as little and as carefully as possible before fixation. Arterial blood gases (ABG), hemoglobin, hematocrit, and platelets should be monitored. Respiratory and neurologic status should be assessed for signs and symptoms of hypoxemia.

D. Venous Thromboembolism

1. Risk for the development of VTE is related to severe trauma, major vascular injury, central venous catheter placement, obesity, infection, immobilization, and lower extremity procedures such as osteotomies and long-bone fixation (Murphy, Naqvi, Miller, Feldman, & Shore, 2015). VTE occurs more commonly in adolescents and polytrauma patients with femur/femoral neck injuries, tibia, ankle, pelvic, and acetabulum injuries (Murphy et al., 2015). Patients with spinal cord injuries or spinal fractures are at high risk for VTE following trauma due to decreased mobility and oftentimes are restricted to bed rest. Diagnosis can be made via Doppler studies, angiography studies, or venogram. Thrombectomies may be performed in severe cases, but its use is still controversial. The patient may develop collateral vessels to provide circulation to the distal areas from the embolus.

2. *Nursing Implications for the Prevention of VTE.* Consider applying a sequential compression device (SCD) if the patient is at risk and unable to ambulate or perform leg and foot ROM exercises (Cummings & Byrum, 2001). The nurse should avoid applying SCDs when local leg conditions exist that would be compromised by the sleeves (e.g., dermatitis, vein ligation, skin graft, incisions). Ischemic vascular disease, massive edema of legs, pulmonary edema from congestive heart failure (CHF), extreme deformity or contracture of leg, and suspected preexisting VTE are additional contraindications for the use of SCD. The immobile or bed-rest patient should be turned frequently and interventions taken to prevent skin breakdown or pressure ulcers. The patient may also be placed on antifibrinolytic therapy such as low-molecular-weight heparin (LMWH), warfarin, aspirin, or heparin infusion. If the patient is placed on this therapy, there is an increased risk for bleeding and therefore precautions to prevent bleeding need to be implemented; such as prophylactic medications to prevent GI bleeds, monitoring of labs (e.g., anti-Xa levels, coagulopathy studies, H/H). Also, if the child is discharged home on antifibrinolytic therapy, education needs to be given to the patient and family to avoid contact sports or activities that could cause bleeding and notify their healthcare professional should they experience bleeding. The nurse should assess pedal and posterior tibial pulses every 1 to 2 hours for patients at risk, assess quality of pulses, capillary refill time, presence of cyanotic nail beds, cooler skin temperature, numbness, and/or tingling. Teach the child and family to report pain and cramping in the lower legs immediately and the child's family should be taught to avoid massaging the lower legs if they begin to hurt.

E. Vascular Injuries

1. Vascular injuries can occur most often with orthopedic injuries associated with long-bone fractures or supracondylar fractures. Trauma to a child's major artery can cause ischemia, growth retardation, compartment syndrome, Volkmann's contraction, and long-term disability.

2. Signs and symptoms include pulsatile bleeding, increase hematoma, weak or absent pulses, cold limb, bruit or thrill, decreased perfusion, and swelling. CT angiography (CTA) is the preferred method for diagnosis, but Doppler studies or arteriography can be used to diagnose. The clinician needs to differentiate between a thrombosis or spasm of the vessel. A spasm usually lasts less than 3 hours and absent pulses lasting longer than 6 hours could indicate a thrombosis present (Daley, 2015).

3. Treatment requires early intervention and most patients will likely undergo surgical repair. It is important to replace blood loss before surgical exploration. Mortality is associated generally with poor surgical access, mechanism of injury (such as shearing of the vessel), delay in diagnosis and treatment, or other concurrent injuries such as head trauma. Diagnosis can be difficult in pediatrics because of physiologic compensation masking signs of blood loss and other injuries. Nursing care includes monitoring of VS, assessing for bleeding, and perfusion.

CHILD MALTREATMENT

A. Definition

1. Child maltreatment also referred to as *NAT*, includes child abuse, neglect, and endangerment. It can include physical, emotional, psychological, and sexual abuse. NAT or child maltreatment occurs across all age groups, sexes, cultures, and socioeconomic groups. However, there is a higher incidence associated with poverty, substance abuse, and single-parent homes; one third of the victims are younger than the age of 3 months (Daley, 2015). Other risk factors include a special-needs child, parent with a history of abuse as a child, a nonbiological male in the house, domestic violence, and community violence. According to the HHS ACF, there were an estimated 3.6 million reports of possible abuse or neglect involving 6.6 million children in 2014 to child protective services. From that number, 1,580 children died from NAT or neglect. However, the number of children who are victims of abuse or neglect is thought to be higher because many cases are not recognized or reported (Crichton et al., 2016). Currently, there is no validated screening tool for NAT/neglect in the United States. Children's hospitals recognize child abuse with high-risk injuries twice as often as nonchildren's hospitals and abusive fractures seven times more often (Lindberg, Beaty, Juarez-Colunga, Wood, & Runyan, 2015). Missed diagnosis can lead to repeat abuse or escalation of injuries; and repeat victims of NAT are at a greater risk for morbidity and mortality. Victims of recurrent NAT have a higher mortality rate (25%) compared to mortality rates for victims of initial NAT (10%). The highest group of fatal NAT occurs in children younger than 3 years of age (Escobar et al., 2016).

2. The Child Abuse Prevention and Treatment Act (CAPTA) defines the terms *child abuse* and *neglect* as: "any recent act or failure to act on the part of a parent or caregiver which results in death, serious physical or emotional harm, sexual abuse or exploitation, or an act or failure to act which presents imminent risk or serious harm" (HHS, ACF, Administration on Youth and Families, Children's Bureau, 2010, p. 6). CAPTA identifies four major types of maltreatment: physical abuse, neglect, sexual abuse, and emotional or psychological abuse (Figure 9.5).

B. Etiology and Incidence

1. Numerous parental and child factors place a family at risk for child maltreatment (Table 9.12).

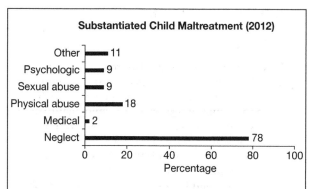

FIGURE 9.5 Substantiated child maltreatment.

Source: Adapted from Jackson, A. M., Kissoon, N., & Greene, C. (2015). Aspects of abuse: Recognizing and responding to child maltreatment. *Current Problems in Pediatric and Adolescent Health Care, 45*(3), 58–70. doi:10.1016/j.cppeds.2015.02.001

NAT victims had more severe head injuries, hollow viscus injuries, pancreatic injuries, and a higher injury severity score than children who were not victims of NAT. NAT victims were also more likely to die from their injuries compared to children who were not victims of NAT (Carter & Moulton, 2016). Children younger than 2 suffered more head trauma, older children suffered more abdominal and skeletal injuries, whereas adolescents are more prone to experience sexual abuse (Daley, 2015; Figure 9.6).

2. Reporting suspected child maltreatment or neglect by nurses and healthcare professionals is mandated by law. The person reporting does not need to have actual evidence or have witnessed the event. Nurses should report their suspicions to their local child protective services or child-abuse hotline.

TABLE 9.12   Common Indicators of Child Maltreatment

Family Behaviors
Inappropriate parent–child interaction Extremes of reactions to hospital staff (e.g., hostile, unconcerned) Unrealistic expectations of the child Parental denial of any knowledge of how injury occurred Attribution of blame to sibling for injury Inappropriate response to severity of injury by parent, such as underreacting or overreacting to child's condition
Child Behaviors
Extremes of behaviors (e.g., withdrawn, acting out) Lack of opposition to painful procedures Developmental delays Inappropriate sexual behavior Somatic complaints (e.g., chronic headaches, sleep disorders, enuresis) Suicidal behavior and threats Drug or alcohol abuse
Historical Findings
Story inconsistent with physical findings or developmental level Delays in seeking medical treatment Direct disclosure Repeat visits to the emergency department
Physical Findings
Multiple injuries in various stages of healing Injury type and location inconsistent with child's developmental level Characteristic pattern reflective of object used to cause injury (e.g., belt marks) Signs of poor overall care Genital bleeding or discharge in prepubescent children
Radiographic Findings
Multiple fractures Cortical metaphyseal fragmentation Traumatic involucrum Skull fractures Suture separation

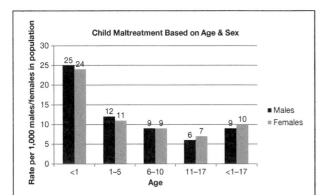

FIGURE 9.6 Child maltreatment based on age and gender.

Source: Adapted from U.S. Department of Health & Human Services, Administration for Children & Families Administration on Youth and Families, Children's Bureau. (2016). *Child maltreatment 2014*. Retrieved from http://www.acf.hhs.gov/programs/cb/research-data-technology/statistics-research/child-maltreatment

Most hospitals have social workers available to contact the appropriate services. Healthcare workers who "willfully" fail to report suspicious or known child abuse or neglect may face consequences of violating the law. Most states have a "good faith" law protecting the healthcare worker as long as the report is accurate and in good faith (Ross & Juarez, 2016). In suspected child abuse or neglect, social work can be helpful with child protective services in instituting visitor restrictions if there is a risk the parent or caregiver may attempt to leave the hospital with the child.

C. History of the Injury

1. Child physical abuse is suspected based on the physical findings and the history surrounding the injury. Physical abuse is the infliction of physical injury to a child. The history in relation to the injury is what differentiates intentional from unintentional harm.

2. The history of the injury should be obtained and well documented. Characteristics of the history that are consistent with child abuse include the following:

a. History is inconsistent with the injury.

b. Caregiver denies any knowledge of how the injury occurred.

c. Caregiver is reluctant to divulge information or changes the story.

d. Child is developmentally incapable of the injury.

e. There is a delay in seeking treatment.

f. Child has prior hospitalizations or injuries.

g. Caregiver's response is inappropriate to the level of injury.

h. Caregiver may not make eye contact.

i. History of previous placement in foster care or with a child protective agency.

3. All communication is documented using the child's and the caregiver's own words (Baird & Cooper, 2016; Daley, 2015).

D. Physical Abuse

1. *Cutaneous injuries* (e.g., bruises, bite marks, burns) occur from excessive force applied to the child from a caregiver and constitute one specific manifestation of physical abuse injury.

2. *Bruises*

a. Any bruises must be evaluated in light of the plausibility of the injury event as stated by the caregiver, the child's health history, the child's level of development, the presence of other injuries, and laboratory data. Patterns of bruising should be noted that could indicate an object used as well as location of the bruise. In toddlers and older children who are mobile, it is not uncommon to have bruises. However, nonmobile children and infants with bruises should raise a high suspicion for NAT.

b. Bruises commonly occur in young children as they run and play. Normally, bruises are small, few, and found on the extensor surfaces, such as the shins, elbows, chin, and knees. Bruises indicative of physical abuse are found on the face, head, and areas protected by clothing. Periorbital hematomas are especially suspicious for maltreatment. Bruises found on the chest, abdomen, thighs, buttocks, and back are also suspicious for physical abuse. These bruises are usually in various stages of healing and are numerous.

c. In infants, bruises may be seen near the mouth, lips, and frenulum resulting from physical forces when the caregiver repeatedly attempts to force-feed a bottle. Bruises or rope burns may be found around the neck, wrists, or ankles and indicate that the child was restrained. Blistering and abrasions may be present, which may indicate the child's struggle against the restraints. In infants and young children, paired oval bruises or pinch marks may be found on the cheeks, arms, earlobes, and other areas. To hide the marks, school-age children who have repeatedly been subjected to beatings and bruising prefer to wear long-sleeved and long-legged clothing, even in warm weather.

3. *Bite Marks*

   a. Bite marks are another cutaneous manifestation that is highly indicative of child abuse. Adult bite marks are differentiated from child bite marks by measuring the maxillary intercanine distance. A distance greater than 3 cm indicates an adult bite. Bites should be examined for size, shape, and be measured. As with all suspicious physical injuries, documentation with pictures should be added to the chart with description of size, shape, and location (Ginsburg & Hunstad, 2016).

4. *Burns*

   a. Burns may be thermal such as scalding of skin, contact with hot surfaces or flames, cigarette burns or lighters, chemical burns (e.g., inhaling or drinking caustic substances either forced or accessible without appropriate safe storage), and electrical burns (e.g., frayed electrical cords, wires, or unprotected electrical outlets). An unintentional scald burn can occur if the young child pulls a crock pot or pot of hot liquid onto himself or herself. The intensity of the burn would be greatest about the head, with the depth of burn tapering off as it reaches the chest. An intentional scald injury has a circumscribed area of injury that is full thickness and depicts the patterned configuration of a heating object (e.g., steam irons, curling irons, car cigarette lighters). Usually, no splash pattern is seen with intentional burns (Millward, Morgan, & Kelly, 2003). Abusive burns occur more on the extremities, buttocks, and/or perineum.

5. *Internal Organ Injuries*

   a. As with cutaneous lesions, the history of an internal organ injury is important to ascertain. Internal organ injuries occur from blunt forces applied to the children as they are struck, kicked, punched, beaten, thrown, or stabbed by caregiver(s). The manifestations of internal organ injuries are the same in both unintentional and intentional trauma. Liver lacerations, splenic rupture, pulmonary and cardiac contusions, as well as brain injuries can occur as a result of child maltreatment. Blunt abdominal trauma (most common type of inflicted abdominal trauma in children) is usually the result of a child being punched or kicked in the abdomen.

Intra-abdominal hemorrhage may result with few external signs. Visceral injuries rarely produce immediate specific signs or symptoms that lead to prompt identification. Inflicted abdominal injury should be suspected when there are the following:

   i. Clear signs of abdominal trauma

   ii. Unexplained shock

   iii. Unexplained cardiac arrest

   iv. Unconsciousness with suspected inflicted head injury

   v. Unexplained unconsciousness

   b. Severe internal injuries might not be immediately detected because of the caregiver's failure to give an accurate history of trauma and also because little or no external evidence of abdominal trauma may be seen at the time of examination. Children who sustain child maltreatment tend to be younger and preverbal and thus unable to verbalize how the injury occurred. These children are usually brought in for treatment because of worsening signs of injury such as abdominal distention, vomiting, or other vague parental history or complaints (Carter & Moulton, 2016).

   i. Emergent situations are those involving children brought to the hospital for treatment who have unstable VS, severe dehydration, malnutrition with possible progression to shock or other life-threatening injuries. When rib fractures are present, a significant force was applied to the chest (usually squeezing), and maltreatment must be suspected and investigated. Intracranial hemorrhage and abdominal injuries are associated with 20% of children with rib fractures (Lindberg et al., 2015). Treatment for inflicted abdominal and chest trauma is the same as for unintentional injury.

6. *Long-Bone Fractures*

   a. Maltreated children sustain long-bone fractures as their extremities are twisted and pulled by caregivers or from being thrown or beaten. Fracture patterns are consistent with the applied blunt forces and include spiral fracture of long bones (from intentional twisting), rib, skull, nose, or facial fractures; and femur fractures in children younger than 1 year of age. Fractures to the sternum, spinous processes, scapulae, and humeral fractures are seen in children younger than 3 years and are a result of blunt force. The young child is brought for treatment because of an inability to use an arm or to bear weight on a leg. The injured extremity appears deformed, painful, and swollen similar to unintentional musculoskeletal trauma. The AAP and College of Radiology recommend mandatory skeletal surveys in any child for whom there is suspicion of NAT. Children's bones tend to be more porous, less dense, and have lower bending strength, which allows them to bend more easily thus making them harder to break than in adults. Their periosteum is thicker, stronger, and less easily torn thereby preventing fractures or dislodgements. Fractures in children tend to require a great amount of force. Bone also forms more easily in children compared to adults and is more vascular so fractures may show varying states of healing (Ross & Juarez, 2016; Table 9.13).

7. *Head Trauma*

a. Head trauma from child abuse is the most common cause of child abuse-related deaths, but can also result in brain damage, psychological dysfunction, and physical impairments. Head trauma occurs from blunt forces (impact, shaking), penetrating forces (bullet), and lack of oxygenation (asphyxia). Impact injuries occur when the child is struck by a caregiver's hand or object or the child is thrown against an unyielding surface. Resulting injuries include brain insults,

skull fractures, facial fractures, possible eye and ear injuries. Penetrating injuries occur from bullets, knives, or other objects projected at the child, causing direct injuries to the brain, head, and face. Asphyxia from gagging or choking to stop the child's crying can lead to ischemia and brain damage (Millward et al., 2003).

b. Probably the most well-known form of child abuse is shaken baby syndrome. This syndrome occurs in children younger than 2 years. Violent shaking leads to the formation of a subdural hematoma, metaphyseal chip fractures, and retinal hemorrhages. The infant or toddler may have an avulsion fracture of the spinous process, fracture of the pars or pedicles, or compression of multiple vertebral bodies from severe shaking or battering (usually in the cervical spine area; C. Kim et al., 2016). The shaken baby may display lethargy; poor sucking ability; irritability; rhythmic eye opening and deviation; decerebrate or decorticate posturing; seizures; alterations in muscle tone; and decreased responsiveness to voice, touch, or pain. The child presents for treatment either seizing in cardiac arrest or with a history of a seizure. The definitive finding in shaken baby syndrome is the presence of retinal hemorrhages. Therefore, careful ocular examinations are imperative in any young child with a vague history who has seizures or suffered cardiac arrest. Many times the infant with retinal

TABLE 9.13   Radiologic Skeletal Injury Specificity

Specificity	Location	Mechanism
High	Classic metaphyseal lesion (corner fracture, bucket, or handle fracture) Rib fractures at any location (especially posterior, axillary, multiple, or bilateral) Scapular fractures (blade, acromial process) Spinous process fractures Sternal fractures Multiple fractures (especially bilateral)	Torsional force or traction injury Shaken baby syndrome and direct impact Direct force, severe twisting, or shaking Hyperflexion, hyperextension Direct force
Moderate	Fractures at different ages Epiphyseal separation Vertebral body fractures and subluxations Digital fractures Complex skull fractures Subperiosteal new bone formation	Compression, hyperextension, or hyperflexion Squeezing, forced hyperextension, trampling Direct impact
Low (Common)	Clavicular fractures Long-bone fractures Linear skull fractures	Sudden traction on the arm Gripping and twisting, direct impact Direct impact

Source: Adapted from Ross, A. H., & Juarez, C. A. (2016). Skeletal and radiological manifestations of child abuse: Implications for study in past populations. *Clinical Anatomy, 29*, 844–853. doi:10.1002/ca.22683

hemorrhages may end up blind as the retina cannot regenerate (Engman-Lazear, 2015).

8. Diagnostic tests for child maltreatment are summarized (Table 9.14).

9. Treatment is initiated based on the extent of the injuries with the most life-threatening injuries treated first. Surface bruises are photographed, measured, and their location documentated; then the photographs are placed in the child's medical record. Child protective services is contacted, usually by a social worker. The caregiver or parent is informed of the suspicion of child maltreatment (NAT), his or her reaction may range from relief to anger. It is best to have this information given to the family by the physician with a nurse or social worker in attendance. Child protective services will interview each parent/caregiver separately. If deemed abuse is suspected or confirmed, the home should be inspected and the removal of any

other children in the home may occur. Local police will be notified and will also interview the family members separately. The hospital's security officers may need to be nearby in the event the family reacts violently. Abused children may be placed in foster care and legal action may be taken against the family.

10. In the ICU, abused children may die of their injuries and be subject to coroner's review. Usually when this happens, any tubes may need to be left in the child until the coroner approves the removal or the child's body is transported to the coroner's office. Because the nurse is in the position to support both the child and family, it may be very difficult to support perpetrators suspected of inflicting the life-threatening injuries. Furthermore, if the child dies of the injuries, homicide charges may be filed. Nurses who care for such children may need support from other resources within the hospital such as employee assistance, social work, and/

TABLE 9.14 Diagnostic Tests Indicated in Child Maltreatment

Complete Blood Count	Comments/Rationale
Hematocrit, hemoglobin Coagulation studies Prothrombin time, partial thromboplastin time, platelets	Rules out shock, anemia Rules out organic cause of bruising or bleeding Elevated levels may be the first indicator of abdominal injury Elevated levels are indicative of extensive soft-tissue and muscle injury
Serum	
Amylase Creatine phosphokinase Syphilis serology Human chorionic gonadotropin Toxicology screen	Rules out sexually transmitted disease; suspect sexual abuse in all ages Rules out pregnancy; all postmenarcheal girls with a history suggesting sexual abuse Rules out forced or voluntary ingestions and chemical abuse Rules out renal trauma, dehydration, ingestions, sexual abuse
Urine	
Red blood cells, specific gravity, toxicology screen, culture, pregnancy test, test for sperm	Culture for gonorrhea, *Chlamydia*, and other sexually transmitted diseases is especially important with suspected sexual abuse Microscopic examination for sperm; may be omitted if >72 hours since abuse incident or if child has bathed
Cultures	
Wounds, throat, vaginal, rectal	
Vaginal Secretions	
Vaginal wet preparation Saline and potassium hydroxide with whiff test	*Trichomonas*, yeast, or *Gardnerella* infections
Radiologic Studies	
Skeletal x-ray film: Skull, ribs, extremities Bone scans Ultrasound, CT scan, MRI	Rules out fractures; common findings are multiple fractures Detects remote injuries and extremely recent injuries Important in detecting subtle intracranial and internal abdominal injuries

or chaplain services. Oftentimes, debriefing after such an emotionally draining and psychological experience can be helpful to acknowledge and recognize the commitment of the healthcare team.

E. Sexual Abuse

1. Sexual abuse is often defined as the involvement of children or adolescents in sexual activities they do not understand, to which they cannot give informed consent or that violate sexual taboos (Finkel & DeJong, 2001). CAPTA defines sexual abuse as "employment, use, persuasion, inducement, enticement, or coercion of any child to engage in or assist any other person to engage in any sexually explicit conduct or simulation of such conduct for the purpose of producing visual depiction of such conduct; or the rape and in cases of caregiver or interfamilial relationships, statutory rape, molestation, prostitution, or other form of sexual exploitation of children or incest with children" (CAPTA, 2010, p. 6). Sexual abuse comprises one or some combination of the following activities: fondling a child's genitals, intercourse, incest, rape, sodomy, exhibitionism, exploitation, digital or object penetration of the rectum or vagina, sexual touching, vaginal penile or rectal penile penetration, pornography, and prostitution. Similar to physical abuse, sexual abuse involves a host of family, child, and societal factors. Incest, for example, is allowed to continue in families that do not protect their children or that fail to have appropriate caregivers available. Children may be groomed by a perpetrator for increasing sexual involvement over a period of time. The relationship is kept secret and involves threats of harm or special favors. This may be confusing to the child because the activity may "feel good." Children do not know or understand the precise physical act of intercourse. The child feels guilty and betrayed as he or she continues in the relationship. If the child does come forward, the child's story may be discounted, allowing the abuse to continue.

2. Sexual abuse happens to both genders, to children of all ages, and to children in every socioeconomic strata. Poverty, drug abuse, alcoholism, unhappy family life, and living in a family without one or both natural parents may make the child vulnerable to this abuse. Sexual abuse not only is inflicted by adult caregivers, but also occurs by siblings, as well as adult authority figures (e.g., teachers or coaches) and sometimes through peer pressure. With the immergence of websites, social networks, and electronic devices, there has been an increase in deviant behavior leading to sexual abuse and, at times, leading to death or suicide of the victim.

3. Sexual assault (rape) occurs in children and adolescents and is the forcible act of intercourse. Young children who are victims of sexual abuse tend to act out sexually with their peers, siblings, and adults. They exhibit precocity in sexual remarks or questions that demonstrate their increased awareness of sexual behavior, and frequent and compulsive masturbation may occur (Millward et al., 2003). These children become obsessed with cleanliness to remove blood or secretions and to avoid "feeling dirty." They have a preoccupation with genital references and may even draw them (a finding that is uncommon in children without sexual abuse). Adolescents may become runaways, develop suicidal thoughts, or engage in prostitution (Millward et al., 2003).

4. *Assessment and Treatment.* The child with suspected sexual abuse may be brought in for treatment by a caregiver. The caregiver may state that abuse is known, or that the child has a vaginal or penile discharge or dysuria. Herpetic lesions to the mouth may be another complaint for treatment. Sexual abuse should be suspected in pregnant, young adolescents (10–14 years of age), especially if the pregnancy is concealed, or with vaginal or penile discharge, foreign bodies, sexually transmitted diseases, or rectal or vaginal pain (Millward et al., 2003).

5. The sexually abused or assaulted child must undergo a physical examination and interview. Experienced professionals in the care of these children must conduct these examinations to avoid contamination of evidence and to allow the child to tell the story only once. The physical examination may be deferred in the child with sexual abuse if the last episode occurred more than 72 hours before presentation (Millward et al., 2003). If the sexual abuse or assault occurred within 72 hours, the physical examination should be initiated.

6. The physical examination may be done with a parent or caregiver present, provided that person is not the perpetrator. A nurse or rape crisis counselor assumes the role of support person while another nurse assists with obtaining and labeling the specimens. The child can be placed on an adult's lap in the frog-leg position or assume a knee-chest position on the examination table. The left lateral decubitus position allows for examination of the rectum. If at any point the child does not cooperate with the examination and becomes upset and fearful, the examination is stopped. An EUA is then performed. The child is never restrained or forced to comply with the examination. Secondary abuse is caused by a physical examination that is so overzealous that it assumes a rape-like quality in the mind of the child

(Fleisher & Ludwig, 2000). The external genitalia are examined, and cultures for syphilis, gonorrhea, and chlamydia are obtained. Any lacerations, bruising, and bleeding are noted. A Wood's lamp is also used to observe for semen; a wet prep for sperm or semen detection is also obtained. In the adolescent female victim, a bi-manual pelvic examination is indicated. In young females, a pediatric ear speculum may be used to visualize the cervix and cultures obtained. The rectal area is examined for bruising, bleeding, or tearing and cultures obtained. In the male child, similar cultures of the meatus and rectum are obtained, and both areas are observed for bruising, lacerations, or tearing.

7. All evidence is obtained carefully and is secured in an assault kit that is usually provided by the local law enforcement agency. Such kits have prelabeled envelopes for specimen collection. Aside from the cultures, other specimens include a saliva sample, pubic hairs, a comb used to comb the hairs, fingernail scrapings, and blood specimens for venereal disease research laboratory (VDRL) test, HIV, hepatitis B, and human chorionic gonadotropin (HCG). Postmenarchal females are usually given the option to take a high dose of oral contraceptives to prevent pregnancy. Pharyngeal cultures are also obtained. The specimens are then sealed, and the collecting nurse's name written on the outside of the collection box. The box is then hand delivered to the hospital police for safe keeping. Everyone must sign for the box, or it is handed directly to the law enforcement agent, who signs for the box. This chain of evidence avoids potential mishandling or tampering, either of which may jeopardize the legal process. The child's clothes are also obtained and placed in paper bags and given to law enforcement. Follow-up is completed through the hospital, rape crisis center, or regular healthcare professional.

8. The examining professional carefully documents all the physical findings. The nurse documents the chain of evidence and the child's reaction to the examination. The sexually abused or assaulted child is interviewed by a trained professional. The parent(s) or caregiver and child are interviewed separately. The child is not asked any leading questions and is simply asked to talk about what happened. The child may use puppets or dolls to demonstrate what occurred. Using paper and crayons for drawing allows the nonverbal or preverbal child to depict the situation. The child is told that he or she did the right thing by coming forward with the story and that the child did not do anything wrong (Millward et al., 2003).

F. Neglect

1. Neglect is the most prevalent type of child maltreatment. Child neglect is a failure to provide for a child's basic needs. Child neglect can be physical, educational, emotional, a lack of supervision, and includes withholding medical treatment. It can be willful disregard for the child or the caregiver lacks the ability or resources to provide these needs. It can include nutritional neglect such as failure to thrive or lack of adequate nutrition. Obesity has been identified by the HHS as well as the CDC as an epidemic in the United States and is also considered a form of neglect. It is important to track growth measurements, head circumference, and body mass index. Other factors that may be associated with neglect include parental substance abuse, low self-esteem, social isolation, reliance on physical punishment for discipline, depression, and lack of knowledge regarding growth and development (Millward et al., 2003).

2. Neglected children may be brought for treatment by law enforcement authorities who respond to a complaint from a neighbor, teacher, or any concerned individual. Signs of neglect should be observed in children who are admitted for possible child maltreatment, ingestions, or drug overdoses (Table 9.15).

TABLE 9.15 Observed Forms of Neglect in Pediatric Medical Settings

Noncompliance of medical recommendations
Delay or failure to seek medical care
Inadequate nutrition, non–illness-related failure to thrive or unmanaged morbid obesity
Illicit drug exposure to newborns or pediatric ingestions
Injuries and ingestions resulting from inadequate protection from environmental hazards (e.g., guns, unrestrained in car)
Inadequate nurturance or affection
Inadequate clothing
Unmet educational needs

Source: Adapted from Jackson, A. M., Kissoon, N., & Greene, C. (2015). Aspects of abuse: Recognizing and responding to child maltreatment. *Current Problems in Pediatric and Adolescent Health Care, 45*(3), 58–70. doi:10.1016/j.cppeds.2015.02.001

G. Psychological Maltreatment (Emotional Abuse)

Emotional abuse usually occurs with other forms of maltreatment. Emotional or psychological abuse involves verbal abuse or mental injury. *Psychological abuse* is defined by the American Professional Society on the Abuse of Children as a "pattern of caregiver behavior or extreme incident(s) that convey to children that they are worthless, flawed, unloved, unwanted, endangered, or only of value meeting another's needs" (Jackson, Kissoon, & Greene, 2015, p. 66). Emotional abuse can be understood in terms of actions or lack thereof that could cause or have caused serious behavioral, cognitive, emotional, or mental disorders. In such instances, the caregiver or parent(s) do not provide a nurturing environment. The caregiver may berate, belittle, degrade, terrorize, isolate, and reject the children. Signs of emotional abuse include sleep and feeding disorders, hyperactivity, developmental delays, and excessively passive or aggressive behavior. These behaviors may be observed in children who are in the ICU for other reasons. Such behaviors should be brought to the attention of the physician and social worker so that investigations into the child's home life can be conducted.

H. Child Endangerment

Child endangerment can involve lack of or disregard for the child's safety that may or may not result in injury. It can include unrestrained or improperly restrained children in motor vehicles, hazardous or caustic substances not properly stored (allowing the child access to them), ingestion of medications, illicit drugs or alcohol, or inadequate supervision of the child. Another cause of child endangerment is associated with head injuries due to tipping over of televisions. The U.S. Consumer Product Safety Commission cited tip-over injuries from televisions as third on their list of the top five hidden household hazards and can cause skull fractures, head bleeds, concussions, and neck injuries due to improper securement of the television (Befeler, Daniels, Helms, Klimo, & Boop, 2014).

I. Munchausen Syndrome by Proxy

1. *Munchausen syndrome by proxy (MSBP;* also known more recently as factitious disorder imposed on another [FDIA or FDIoA]) is defined by the American Professional Society on the Abuse of Children as a form of child abuse, calling it "medical child abuse" (Ferrara et al., 2013; Gehlawat, Gehlawat, Singh, & Gupta, 2015). Asher first described the most extreme and dramatic form of factitious disorders called *Munchausen*

syndrome in 1951. Meadow, in 1977, described cases in which a parent or caregiver produced or feigned symptoms of nonexistent illnesses in their children so that the children had to undergo innumerable harmful examinations and treatments (Meadow, 1977). At this time the illness was called *MSBP* (Flaherty & MacMillan, 2013). The AAP defines this as "child abuse in the medical setting." It may include psychological, physical, medical neglect, and/or abuse. The caregiver receives attention as a result of the harm he or she has done to the child. It is intentional illness forced upon the child causing the child to undergo unnecessary tests and treatments resulting in harm, pain, and sometimes death of the child. The perpetrator is most often the mother or female caregiver who brings attention unto herself for having to care for a sick child. The caregiver will oftentimes fabricate emotional or behavioral conditions such as attention deficit disorders, hyperactivity, learning disabilities, psychosis, and dissociative disorders (Table 9.16). In addition, the caregiver may underreport signs and symptoms or exaggerate them. They may invent a history of illness or actually cause the signs and symptoms of an illness. The caregiver may sometimes coach the child on how to behave or to act sick, and, if the child is verbal, on what to say using medical terminology that may not be at the child's level of understanding (Flaherty & MacMillan, 2013). The majority of the children of MSBP are younger than 6 years of age and it occurs equally between males and females. MSBP is poorly understood and can be difficult to diagnose and treat. Many cases go undiagnosed. Approximately 75% of morbidity from fabricated child illness occurs while the child is hospitalized. Emphasis should be on the child as a victim undergoing unnecessary and harmful treatments instead of the caregiver's motivation or mental status. The perpetrator gains support of the healthcare team through skilled deceit, leading professionals to believe he or she is a devoted, loving parent or caregiver. The perpetrator "doctor shops" and "hospital jumps" so that tracking the child's true medical history is virtually impossible.

2. Caregiver risk factors include thriving on attention from physicians, insistence that the child cannot cope without the parent's attention, that the parent or caregiver has knowledge about healthcare or is involved in healthcare, is familiar with medical terminology or has a history of factitious, or somatoform, disorders. In addition, the

TABLE 9.16 Indicators for Possible Fabricated Illnesses in a Child

Diagnosis does not match objective findings
Signs or symptoms are bizarre
Parent, caregiver, or suspected offender does not express relief once child is improving or does not have confirmed diagnosis
Inconsistent history of symptoms from multiple observers
Parent's or caregiver's behavior does not match expressed distress or report of symptoms
Parent or caregiver insists on invasive, numerous, and/or painful procedures
Parent or caregiver insists on hospitalization
Signs and symptoms begin only in the presence of one parent or caregiver
Sibling has or had an unusual or unexplained illness or death
Sensitivity to multiple environmental substances or medicines
Failure of child's illness to respond to normal treatments or unusual intolerance to treatments
Parent or caregiver publicly solicits sympathy or donations or benefits for "rare" child's illness
Extensive, unusual illness history in the parent or caregiver; parent's or caregiver's family; or parent's or caregiver's history of somatization disorders

Source: Adapted from Flaherty, E. G., & MacMillan, H. L. (2013). Caregiver-fabricated illness in a child: A manifestation of child maltreatment. *Pediatrics, 132*(3), 590–597.

perpetrator may have felt unwanted as a child or is jealous of her or his own child; suffered a lack of maternal attention or love as a child; or feels acceptance and gets attention from the medical staff, which causes them to continue to harm their child (Table 9.16). Siblings may have complicated medical histories as well. There may be a history of unexplained sudden infant death syndrome (SIDS) of a sibling. More than one SIDS death is reason for a high index of suspicion. Questions the healthcare team should ask if a fabricated illness is suspected:

a. Are the signs and symptoms consistent with the illness or injury credible?

b. Was unnecessary or harmful treatment or medical care given to the child?

c. Who instigated the evaluations or treatment? Was it the caregiver or the healthcare team?

d. Was there intentional refusal to give medications, treatments, interventions, or were follow-up appointments missed that could help the child?

e. Countless methods of abuse may mark this disorder. Presentation is not typical and covers a broad range of symptoms. They include but are not limited to the following:

a. Falsifying signs and symptoms (e.g., apnea, cardiac arrest, GI bleeding, seizures, fever, rash, and CNS depression)

b. Poisoning (e.g., insulin, table salt, fingernail polish remover)

c. Contamination of blood, urine, or stool samples to feign a false result

d. Injection of urine, stool, saliva, or blood in IV access ports

e. Intentional suffocation

f. Blowing air in the gastric tube

g. Application of caustic substances to the skin

h. Withdrawal of blood from the IV line to cause anemia

i. Adding blood to the diaper to feign a GI bleed

j. Pouring chocolate milk (or similar substance) over the child and linen to resemble vomit

k. Excessive compassion toward the child when healthcare providers are present and ignoring the child when healthcare providers are not present (Flaherty & MacMillan, 2015; Jackson et al., 2015)

3. Documentation should describe details of the actual observation of the perpetrator's behavior, including interaction with the child, staff, physician, and family or significant others. Documentation should include not only what the nurse witnessed, but also what the caregiver reported to them, such as the child was apneic, crying, bleeding, seizing, or having emesis. Actual quotes should be documented not only gotten from the caregiver, but also what the child said. If the child is verbal, he or she should be questioned without the caregiver present regarding signs and symptoms, when they occurred, and where. Questions to ask if there is suspicion of a fabricated illness include family and

social history, including extended family and siblings. Documentation should also include the child's response to treatment.

CASE STUDIES WITH QUESTIONS, ANSWERS, AND RATIONALES

Multiple Trauma Case Studies

Case Study 9.1

Michael is a 5-year-old boy who suffered a traumatic amputation of his right arm. He was triaged at a pediatric Level I trauma center ED and emergently rushed to surgery. The multidisciplinary team included orthopedic surgeons, trauma surgeons, neurosurgeon, and plastic surgeons. After undergoing a 23-hour surgery for reimplantation of his right arm that was "ripped off" and disarticulated at the elbow, he required massive fluid resuscitation with crystalloids and blood products. He was admitted in critical condition to the PICU. Michael had suffered this injury after reaching into a commercial washing machine where his arm became entangled in the wet clothes, creating a tourniquet-like grasp onto his arm.

1. In the immediate postoperative period, what is the primary cause of shock in this patient?
   A. Cardiogenic shock
   B. Hypovolemic shock
   C. Neurogenic shock
   D. Septic shock

2. What are the neurovascular assessments required for patients who undergo reimplantation of a traumatic amputated limb?
   A. Pulses/capillary refill
   B. Color/temperature
   C. Sensation/movement
   D. All of the above

3. Due to Michael's prolonged surgery, aggressive fluid resuscitation and immobilization; he is at risk for which syndrome?
   A. Hepatic encephalopathy
   B. Diabetes insipidus (DI)
   C. Acute respiratory distress syndrome (ARDS)
   D. Nephrotic syndrome

Case Study 9.2

Molly was struck by a motor vehicle on the way to school and airlifted to a level I pediatric trauma center.

Her primary survey showed severely altered LOC, respiratory failure, hypovolemic shock, and distended abdomen. She was intubated, IV access obtained, fluid resuscitation (crystalloids and blood products were administered), radiologic studies were performed, and she was admitted to the PICU. Molly continued to be hypotensive in hypovolemic shock requiring 21 L of crystalloids and 15 L of blood products over a 12-hour period. CT scan results showed a grade V liver laceration. She underwent an emergent operative procedure at the bedside to control bleeding.

1. What type of surgical procedure was likely to have been performed?
   A. Portal vein ligation
   B. Hepatic lobectomy
   C. Damage control surgery
   D. None of the above

2. What are the complications of abdominal compartment syndrome?
   A. Oliguria
   B. Decreased cardiac output
   C. Bowel ischemia
   D. All of the above

3. Massive blood transfusions can lead to hypocalcemia?
   A. True
   B. False

Multiple Trauma Answers and Rationales

Case Study 9.1

1. **B.** Shock is most likely caused from massive blood loss from the traumatic amputation of his right arm.

2. **D.** Assessments should include perfusion parameters and nerve/motor function.

3. **C.** ARDS is a condition characterized by noncardiogenic pulmonary edema and is initiated by a variety of stimuli that trigger the release of systemic inflammatory mediators. Etiology includes among other factors, secondary or systemic injuries such as prolonged hypotension, trauma, sepsis, multiple blood transfusions and immobilization, and so forth.

Case Study 9.2

1. **C.** Damage control surgery is performed emergently to treat uncontrolled hemorrhage in an attempt to stabilize the patient. Definitive surgical

repair may be done in 24 to 48 hours later once the patient is stable.

2. D. All of the above. Abdominal compartment syndrome occurs from decreased perfusion to the abdominal organs and distal extremities caused by increased IAP associated with hemorrhaging and concomitant fluid resuscitation.

3. True. The anticoagulant added to banked blood is citrate which binds with calcium. With massive blood transfusions, it is important to monitor the patient's calcium as hypocalcemia can lead to more bleeding.

MULTIPLE TRAUMA REFERENCES

Al-Mubarak, L., & Al-Haddab, M. (2013). Cutaneous wound closure materials: An overview and update. *Journal of Cutaneous and Aesthetic Surgery, 6*(4), 174–188.

American Academy of Pediatrics. (2015). Animal bites—healthychildren.org. Retrieved from http://www.healthychildren.org/English/health-issues/conditions/from-insects-animals/Pages/Animal-Bites.aspx

American Academy of Pediatrics & American Heart Association. (2016). *Pediatric advanced life support (PALS) provider manual.* Dallas, TX: American Heart Association.

American Academy of Pediatrics and American Pain Society. (2001). The assessment and management of acute pain in infants, children, and adolescents. *Pediatrics, 108*(3), 793–797. doi:10.1542/peds.108.3.793

American College of Surgeons. (2003). Statement on safety belt laws and enforcement. Retrieved from https://www.facs.org/about-acs/statements/43-safety-belt

American College of Surgeons. (2014). Pediatric trauma care. In M. F. Rotondo, C. Cribari, & R. S. Smith (Eds.), *Resources for optimal care of the injured patient* (6th ed., pp. 65–75). Chicago, IL: Author. Retrieved from https://www.facs.org/~/media/files/quality%20programs/trauma/vrc%20resources/resources%20for%20optimal%20care.ashx

American College of Surgeons. (2015). ACS TQIP best practices in the management of traumatic brain injury. Retrieved from https://www.facs.org/~/media/files/quality%20programs/trauma/tqip/traumatic%20brain%20injury%20guidelines.ashx

American Heart Association. (2015). American Heart Association 2015 guidelines: Special circumstances of resuscitation. Retrieved from https://eccguidelines.heart.org/index.php/circulation/cpr-ecc-guidelines-2/part-10-special-circumstances-of-resuscitation

American Heart Association and International Committee on Resuscitation. (2015). CPR & ECC guidelines 2015: Cardiac arrest due to drowning. Retrieved from: https://eccguidelines.heart.org/index.php/circulation/cpr-eccguidelines-2/part-10-special-circumstances-of-resuscitation

Anand, K. J. (2001). Consensus statement for the prevention and management of pain in the newborn. *Archives of Pediatrics & Adolescent Medicine, 155*(2), 173.

Arslan, S., Güzel, M., Turan, C., Doganay, S., Dogan, A. B., & Aslan, A. (2014). Management and treatment of liver injury in children. *Turkish Journal of Trauma and Emergency Surgery, 20*(1), 45–50. doi:10.5505/tjtes.2014.58295

Babovic, N., Cayci, C., & Carlsen, B. T. (2014). Cat bite infections of the hand: Assessment of morbidity and predictors of severe infection. *Journal of Hand Surgery, 39*(2), 286–290.

Bacade, S. S., & Bowlling, R. H. (2016). Diagnostic imaging of the abdomen. In *Roger's textbook of pediatric intensive care* (pp. 1677–1704; 5th ed.).

Baird, J. S., & Cooper, A. (2016). Multiple trauma. In D. G. Nichols & D. H. Shaffner (Eds.), *Rogers' handbook of pediatric intensive care* (5th ed., pp. 404–427). Philadelphia, PA: Lippincott Williams & Wilkins.

Bakar, A. M., & Schleien, C. L. (2016). Thermoregulation. In D. G. Nichols & D. H. Shaffner (Eds.), *Rogers' handbook of pediatric intensive care* (5th ed., pp. 499–514). Philadelphia, PA: Lippincott Williams & Wilkins.

Befeler, A. R., Daniels, D. J., Helms, S. A., Klimo, P., & Boop, F. (2014). Head injuries following television-related accidents in the pediatric population. *Journal of Neurosurgery: Pediatrics, 14*(4), 414–417.

Biagas, K. V., & Aponte-Patel, L. (2016). Drowning. In D. G. Nichols & M. C. Rogers (Eds.), *Rogers' textbook of pediatric intensive care* (5th ed., pp. 428–435). Philadelphia, PA: Lippincott Williams & Wilkins.

Bledsoe, B., & Carrison, D. (2015). Why EMS should limit the use of rigid cervical collars. Retrieved from http://www.jems.com/articles/print/volume-40/issue-2/patient-care/why-ems-should-limit-use-rigid-cervical.html

Blume, H. K. (2015). Headaches after concussion in pediatrics: A review. *Current Pain and Headache Reports, 19*(9), 42.

Boese, C. K., & Lechler, P. (2013). Spinal cord injury without radiologic abnormalities in adults: A systematic review. *Journal of Trauma Acute Care Surgery, 75*(2), 320–330. doi:10.1097/TA.0b013e31829243c9

Boyette, J. R. (2014). Facial fractures in children. *Otolaryngologic Clinics of North America, 47*(5), 747–761.

Brazelton, T., & Gosain, A. (2016). Classification of trauma in children. Retrieved from http://www.uptodate.com

Broom, A., Schur, M. D., Arkader, A., Flynn, J., Gornitzky, A., & Choi, P. D. (2016). Compartment syndrome in infants and toddlers. *Journal of Children's Orthopaedics, 10*(5), 453–460.

Byard, R. W., Austin, A. E., & Van den Heuvel, C. (2011). Characteristics of asphyxial deaths in adolescence. *Journal of Forensic and Legal Medicine, 18*(3), 107–109.

Caglar, D., & Quan, L. (2016). Drowning and submersion injury. In R. M. Kliegman (Ed.), *Nelson textbook of pediatrics* (20th ed., pp. 561–568). St Louis, MO: Elsevier.

Carter, K. W., & Moulton, S. L. (2016). Pediatric abdominal injury patterns caused by "falls": A comparison between nonaccidental and accidental trauma. *Journal of Pediatric Surgery, 51*(2), 326–328.

Cauchy, E., Chetaille, E., Marchand, V., & Marsigny, B. (2001). Retrospective study of 70 cases of severe frostbite lesions: A proposed new classification scheme. *Wilderness and Environmental Medicine, 12*, 248–255.

Centers for Disease Control and Prevention. (2015). *Report to Congress on traumatic brain injury in the United States: Epidemiology and rehabilitation.* Atlanta, GA: National Center for Injury Prevention and Control, Division of Unintentional Injury Prevention.

Centers for Disease Control and Prevention. (2016). Natural disasters and severe weather. Retrieved from https://www.cdc.gov/disasters/extremeheat/index.html

Centers for Disease Control and Prevention. (2017). Leading causes of death reports, 1981–2016. Retrieved from https://www.cdc.gov/injury/wisqars/leading_causes_death.html

Centers for Disease Control and Prevention, National Center for Injury Prevention and Control, & Division of Unintentional Injury Prevention. (2012). National action plan for child injury prevention. Retrieved from http://www.cdc.gov/safechild/pdf/national_action_plan_for_child_injury_prevention.pdf

Children's Defense Fund. (2014). The state of America's children. Retrieved from www.americanspcc.org/wp-content/uploads/2014/03/2014-State-of-Americas-Children.pdf

Council on Clinical Affairs, American Academy of Pediatric Dentistry. (2011). Guideline on management of acute dental trauma. *Reference Manual, 34*(6), 230–238. Retrieved from www.aapd.org/media/policies_guidelines/g_trauma.pdf

Creel, J. (1988). Mechanism of injury due to motion. In J. E. Campbell (Ed.), *Basic trauma life support: Advanced prehospital care* (3rd ed., pp. 1–20). Englewood Cliffs, NJ: Prentice Hall.

Crichton, K. G., Cooper, J. N., Minneci, P. C., Groner, J. I., Thackeray, J. D., & Deans, K. J. (2016). A national survey on the use of screening tools to detect physical child abuse. *Pediatric Surgery International, 32*(8), 815–818.

Criddle, L. M., (2013). The Biomechanics of Trauma. *Pediatric care after resuscitation*. Product of TCAR Education Programs, The Laurel Group, Inc.

Crowley, M. (2014). Spinal cord and vertebral column trauma. In D. Gurney & Emergency Nurses Association (Eds.), *Trauma nursing core course (TNCC): Provider manual* (7th ed., pp. 173–192). Des Plaines, IL: Emergency Nurses Association.

Crowley, C. M., & Morrow, A. I. (1980). A comprehensive approach to the child in respiratory failure. *Critical Care Nursing Quarterly, 3*(1), 27–44.

Cummings, C. C., & Byrum, D. (2001). The beat goes on. *American Journal of Nursing, 101*(Suppl.), 9–12.

Daley, B. J. (2015, November 4). Considerations in pediatric trauma. Retrieved from http://www.emedicine.medscape.com/article/982711-overview In J. Geibel (Ed.), Medscape. Retrieved from https://emedicine.medscape.com/article/435031-overview

Daniels, A. H., Kane, P. M., Eberson, C. P., & Born, C. T. (2012). Temporizing management of pediatric femur fractures using J-splints. *Orthopedics, 35*(9), 773–776.

De Waele, J. J., Ejike, J. C., Leppäniemi, A., De Keulenaer, B. L., Delaet, I., Kirkpatrick, A. W., … Malbrain, M. L. (2015). Intra-abdominal hypertension and abdominal compartment syndrome in pancreatitis, paediatrics, and trauma. *Anestezjologia Intensywna Terapia, 47*(3), 219–227.

Denke N, (2013). Trauma. In _____ (Ed.), *Emergency Nursing Pediatric Course (ENPC) Provider Manual* (4th ed., pp. 261–293). Des Plaines, IL: Emergency Nursing Association

Devarajan, P. (2015). *Myoglobinuria*. Retrieved from http://www.emedicine.medscape.com/article/982711-overview

ENA. (2012–2013). *ENPC provider manual* (4th ed.). Des Plaines, IL: Emergency Nurses Association.

Engman-Lazear, S. (2015). *Course #92071: Care of the pediatric trauma patient*. Retrieved from http://www.netce.com/studypoints.php?courseid=1137

Escobar, M. A., Pflugeisen, B. M., Duralde, Y., Morris, C. J., Haferbecker, D., Amoroso, P. J., … Pohlson, E. C. (2016). Development of a systematic protocol to identify victims of non-accidental trauma. *Pediatric Surgery International, 32*(4), 377–386.

Etzel, K. A. (2006). Multiple trauma. In M. C. Slota & American Association of Critical-Care Nurses (Eds.), *Core curriculum for pediatric critical care nursing* (2nd ed., pp. 638–688). St Louis, MO: Elsevier Saunders.

Ferrara, P., Vitelli, O., Bottaro, G., Gatto, A., Liberatore, P., Binetti, P., & Stabile, A. (2013). Factitious disorders and Munchausen syndrome: The tip of the iceberg. *Journal of Child Health Care, 17*(4), 366–374.

Finkel M. A., DeJong A. R., (2001). Medical findings in child sexual abuse. Child Abuse Medical Diagnosis and Management, (2nd Edition, pp 207–286). Philadelphia: Lippincott, Williams and Wilkens.

Flaherty, E. G., & MacMillan, H. L. (2013). Caregiver-fabricated illness in a child: A manifestation of child maltreatment. *Pediatrics, 132*(3), 590–597.

Fort, C. W. (2003). How to combat 3 deadly trauma complications. *Nursing, 33*(5), 58–64.

Frank, J. B., Lim, C. K., Flynn, J. M., & Dormans, J. P. (2002). The efficacy of magnetic resonance imaging in pediatric cervical spine clearance. *Spine, 27*(11), 1176–1179.

Gehlawat, P., Gehlawat, V., Singh, P., & Gupta, R. (2015). Munchausen syndrome by proxy: An alarming face of child abuse. *Indian Journal of Psychological Medicine, 37*(1), 90.

Ginsburg, C. M., & Hunstad, D. A. (2016). Animal and human bites. In R. M. Kliegman (Ed.), *Nelson textbook of pediatrics* (20th ed., pp. 3447–3452). St Louis, MO: Elsevier.

Glazer, J. L. (2005). Management of heatstroke and heat exhaustion. *American Family Physician, 71*(11), 2133–2140.

Hardcastle, N., Benzon, H. A., & Vavilala, M. S. (2014). Update on the 2012 guidelines for the management of pediatric traumatic brain injury—Information for the anesthesiologist. *Pediatric Anesthesia, 24*(7), 703–710.

Hartonian, I., Babikian, T., Yudovin, S., Valino, H., Fischer, J., & Giza, C. (2013). Sport-related concussion in youth: Impact on behavioral functioning. *Neurology 80(7 Suppl.)*. Retrieved from http://n.neurology.org/content/80/7_Supplement/IN5-2.002

Hazinski, M. F. (Ed.). (2013). *Nursing care of the critically ill child* (3rd ed.). St. Louis, MO: Elsevier.

Herr, K., Coyne, P. J., McCaffery, M., Manworren, R., & Merkel, S. (2011). Pain assessment in the patient unable to self-report: Position statement with clinical practice recommendations. *Pain Management Nursing, 12*(4), 230–250. doi:10.1016/j.pmn.2011.10.002

Herrmann, B., Banaschak, S., Csorba, R., Navratil, F., & Dettmeyer, R. (2014). Physical examination in child sexual abuse: Approaches and current evidence. *Deutsches Ärzteblatt International, 111*(41), 692–703.

Hodnick, R. (2012). Penetrating trauma wounds challenge EMS providers. Retrieved from http://www.jems.com/articles/print/volume-37/issue-4/patient-care/penetrating-trauma-wounds-challenge-ems.html

Hughes, N. T., Burd, R. S., & Teach, S. J. (2014). Damage control resuscitation permissive hypotension and massive transfusion protocols. *Pediatric Emergency Care, 30*(9), 651–656.

Ibsen, L. M., & Koch, T. (2002). Submersion and asphyxial injury. *Critical Care Medicine, 30*(11), S402–S408.

ILCOR Advisory Statement on Drowning. (2003). Recommended guidelines for uniform reporting of data from drowning. Retrieved from http://circ.ahajournals.org/content/108/20/2565

Jackson, A. M., Kissoon, N., & Greene, C. (2015). Aspect of abuse: Recognizing and responding to child maltreatment. *Current Problems Pediatric Adolescent Healthcare, 45*(3), 58–70. doi:10.1016/j.cppeds.2015.02.001

Joestlein, L. (2015). Pain, pain, go away! Evidence-based review of developmentally appropriate pain assessment for children in postoperative setting. *Orthopaedic Nursing, 34*(5), 252–259. doi:10.1097/NOR.0000000000000175

Kassam-Adams, N., Marsac, M. L., Hildenbrand, A., & Winston, F. (2013). Posttraumatic stress following pediatric injury. *JAMA Pediatrics, 167*(12), 1158.

Khan, M. A., Javed, A. A., Rao, D. J., Corner, J. A., & Rosenfield, P. (2016). Pediatric traumatic limb amputation: The principles of management and optimal residual limb lengths. *World Journal of Plastic Surgery, 5*(1), 7–14.

Kim, C., Vassilyadi, M., Forbes, J. K., Moroz, N. W., Camacho, A., & Moroz, P. J. (2016). Traumatic spinal injuries in children at a single level 1 pediatric trauma centre: Report of a 23-year experience. *Canadian Journal of Surgery, 59*(3), 205–212. doi:10.1503/cjs.014515

Kim, E., Brown, K. M., Leonard, J. C., Jaffe, D. M., Olsen, C. S., & Kuppermann, N. (2013). Variability of prehospital spinal immobilization in children at risk for cervical spine injury. *Pediatric Emergency Care, 29*(4), 413–418. doi:10.1097/PEC.0b013e318289d743.

Kline-Tilford, A. M., Sorce, L. R., Levin, D. L., & Anas, N. G. (2013). Pulmonary disorders in nursing. In M. F. Hazinski (Ed.), *Nursing care of the critically ill child* (3rd ed., pp. 483–561). St. Louis, MO: Elsevier.

Koehler, M. M. (2014, May). Orofacial and digital frostbite caused by inhalant abuse. Retrieved from http://www.mdedge.com/cutis/article/82106/pediatrics/orofacial-and-digital-frostbite-caused-inhalant-abuse

Laskowski-Jones, L. (2010, June). Summer emergencies: Can you take the heat? *Nursing, 40*(6), 24–31. doi:10.1097/01.NURSE.0000376293.29982.ee

Lazar-Antman, M. A., & Leet, A. I. (2012). Effects of obesity on pediatric fracture care and management. *The Journal of Bone and Joint Surgery, 94*(9), 855–861.

Li, Y., & Hedequist, D. J. (2012). Submuscular plating of pediatric femur fracture. *Journal of the American Academy of Orthopaedic Surgeons, 20*(9), 596–603.

Liebman, M. A. (2000). Initial resuscitation of the pediatric trauma victim. In P. A. Moloney-Harmon & S. J. Czerwinski (Eds.), *The care of the pediatric trauma patient* (pp. 62–70). St Louis, MO: W. B. Saunders.

Lindberg, D. M., Beaty, B., Juarez-Colunga, E., Wood, J. N., & Runyan, D. K. (2015). Testing for abuse in children with sentinel injuries. *Pediatrics, 136*(5), 831–838.

Loh, N. W., & Nair, P. (2013). Propofol infusion syndrome. *Continuing Education in Anaesthesia Critical Care & Pain, 13*(6), 200–202.

MacLeod, J. B., Winkler, A. M., McCoy, C. C., Hillyer, C. D., & Shaz, B. H. (2014). Early trauma induced coagulopathy (ETIC): Prevalence across the injury spectrum. *Injury, 45*(5), 910–915.

Manworren, R. C. B., & Hynan, L. S. (2003). Clinical validation of FLACC: Preverbal patient pain scale. *Pediatric Nursing, 29*(2), 140–146.

Meadow, R. (1977). Munchausen syndrome by proxy, the hinterland of child abuse. *The Lancet, 310*(8033), 343–345. doi:10.1016/s0140-6736(77)91497-0

Merkel, S. I., Voepel-Lewis, T., Shayevitz, J. R., & Malviya, S. (1997). The FLACC: A behavioral scale for scoring postoperative pain in young children. *Pediatric Nursing, 23*(3), 293–297.

McCrory, P., Meeuwisse, W. H., Aubry M, Cantu, B., Dvořák, J., Echemendia, R. J., . . . Turner M. (2013). Consensus statement on concussion in sport: The 4th International Conference on Concussion in Sport held in Zurich, November 2012. *British Journal of Sports Medicine, 47*(5), 250–258. doi:10.1136/bjsports-2013-092313

Miele, V., Piccolo, C. L., Trinci, M., Galluzzo, M., Ianniello, S., & Brunese, L. (2016). Diagnostic imaging of blunt abdominal trauma in pediatric patients. *La Radiologia Medica, 121*(5), 409–430.

Millward, L. M., Morgan, A., & Kelly, M. P. (2003). *Prevention and reduction of accidental injury in children and older people: Evidence briefing*. London, UK: Health Development Agency.

Mooney, J. F. (2012). The use of "damage control orthopedics" techniques in children with segmental open femur fractures. *Journal of Pediatric Orthopaedics B, 21*(5), 400–403. doi:10.1097/BPB.0b013e32834fe897.

Moore, E. E., Cogbill, T. H., Malangoni, M., Jurkovich, G. J., & Champion, H. R, (1996). Scaling system for organ specific injuries. Retrieved from http://www.aast.org/Library/TraumaTools/InjuryScoringScales.aspx

Morey, A. F., Brandes, S., Dugi, D.D., Armstrong, J. H., Breyer, B. N., Broghammer, J. A.,... et al. (2014, amended 2017). *Urotrauma: AUA guideline*. American Urological Association Education and Research, Inc. Retrieved from https://www.auanet.org/guidelines/urotrauma-(2014-amended-2017)

Morina, N., Koerssen, R., & Pollet, T. V. (2016). Interventions for children and adolescents with posttraumatic stress disorder: A meta-analysis of comparative outcome studies. *Clinical Psychology Review, 47*, 41–54.

Morrissey, J. F., Kusel, E. R., & Sporer, K. A. (2014). Spinal motion restriction: An educational and implementation program to redefine prehospital spinal assessment and care. *Prehospital Emergency Care, 18*(3), 429–432. doi:10.3109/10903127.2013.869643

Murphy, R. F., Naqvi, M., Miller, P. E., Feldman, L., & Shore, B. J. (2015). Pediatric orthopaedic lower extremity trauma and venous thromboembolism. *Journal of Children's Orthopaedics, 9*(5), 381–384.

Nance, M. L. (Ed.). (2015). *National Trauma Data Bank 2015: Pediatric annual report*. Retrieved from https://www.facs.org/~/media/files/quality%20programs/trauma/ntdb/ntdb%20pediatric%20annual%20report%202015%20final.ashx

National Center for Victims of Crime. (n.d.). Child sexual abuse statistics. Retrieved from http://www.victimsofcrime.org/media/reporting-on-child-sexual-abuse/child-sexual-abuse-statistics

National Child Traumatic Stress Network. (2016). Medical trauma quote p. 1. Retrieved from https://www.nctsn.org/what-is-child-trauma/trauma-types/medical-trauma

National Highway Traffic Safety Administration. (2017). *Traffic safety facts: 2015 data*. Retrieved from https://www.nhtsa.gov/sites/nhtsa.dot.gov/files/documents/812409_tsf2015dataspeeding.pdf

Narayanan, U. G., & Phillips, J. H. (2012). Flexibility in fixation: An update on femur fractures in children. *Journal of Pediatric Orthopaedics, 32*(Suppl. 1), S32–S39.

Newbigin, K., Souza, C. A., Torres, C., Marchiori, E., Gupta, A., Inacio, J., … Peña, E. (2016). Fat embolism syndrome: State-of-the-art review focused on pulmonary imaging findings. *Respiratory Medicine, 113*, 93–100.

Pandya, N. K., Upasani, V. V., & Kulkarni, V. A. (2013). The pediatric polytrauma patient: Current concepts. *Journal of the American Academy of Orthopaedic Surgeons, 21*(3), 170–179. doi:10.5435/JAAOS-21-03-170

Pang, D., & Wilberger, J. E. (2012). Spinal cord injury without radiographic abnormalities in children. *Journal of Neurosurgery, 116*(6), 114–129. Original work published 1982. doi:10.3171/jns.1982.57.1.0114

Quan, L., Bierens, J. J., Lis, R., Rowhani-Rahbar, A., Morley, P., & Perkins, G. D. (2016). Predicting outcome of drowning at the scene: A systematic review and meta-analyses. *Resuscitation, 104*, 63–75.

Quan, L., Mack, C. D., & Schiff, M. A. (2014). Association of water temperature and submersion duration and drowning outcome. *Resuscitation, 85*(9), 790–794.

Rose, S. C., Weber, K. D., Collen, J. B., & Heyer, G. L. (2015). The diagnosis and management of concussion in children and adolescents. *Pediatric Neurology, 53*(2), 108–118.

Rosendahl, K., & Strouse, P. J. (2016). Sports injury of the pediatric musculoskeletal system. *La Radiologia Medicine, 121*(5), 431–441.

Ross, A. H., & Juarez, C. A. (2016). Skeletal and radiological manifestations of child abuse: Implications for study in past populations. *Clinical Anatomy, 29*, 844–853. doi:10.1002/ca.22683

Sahu, R. L., & Ranjan, R. (2016). Fracture union in percutaneous Kirschner -wire fixation in paediatric tibial shaft fractures. *Chinese Journal of Traumatology, 19*(6), 353–357. doi:10.1016/j.cjtee.2016.08.003

Schaller, A. L., Lakhani, S. A., & Hsu, B. S. (2015). Pediatric traumatic brain injury. *South Dakota Medicine, 68*(10), 457–461, 463.

Schecter, S. C., Betts, J., Schecter, W. P., & Victorino, G. P. (2012). Pediatric penetrating trauma: The epidemic continues. *Journal of Trauma and Acute Care Surgery, 73*(3), 721–725.

Schnitzler, E. J., Iölster, T., & Russo, R. D. (2016). The acute abdomen. In D. G. Nichols, & D. H. Shaffner (Eds.), *Roger's textbook of pediatric intensive care* (5th ed., pp. 7000–7001). Philadelphia, PA: Wolters Kluwer.

Semple-Hess, J., & Campwala, R. (2014). Pediatric submersion injuries: Emergency care and resuscitation. *Pediatric Emergency Medicine Practice, 11*(6), 1–21.

Sharp, N. E., & Holcomb, G. W. (2013). The role of minimally invasive surgery in pediatric trauma: a collective review. *Pediatric Surgery International, 29*(10), 1013–1018.

Simone, S., (2003). *Abdominal genitourinary injury.* In P. A. Moloney-Harmon & S. J. Czerwinski (Eds.), *The care of the pediatric trauma patient* (pp. 189–205). St Louis, MO: W. B. Saunders.

Spence, D., DiMauro, J., Miller, P. E., Glotzbecker, M. P., Hedequist, D. J., & Shore, B. J. (2016). Osteonecrosis after femoral neck fractures in children and adolescents. *Journal of Pediatric Orthopaedics, 36*(2), 111–116.

Stewart, J. C., Bhananker, S., & Ramaiah, R. (2014). Rapid-sequence intubation and cricoid pressure. *International Journal of Critical Illness and Injury Science, 4*(1), 42–49. doi:10.4103/2229-5151.128012

Sundstrøm, T., Asbjørnsen, H., Habiba, S., Sunde, G. A., & Wester, K. (2014). Prehospital use of cervical collars in trauma patients: A critical review. *Journal of Neurotrauma, 31*(6), 531–540.

Toblin, R. L., Paulozzi, L. J., Gilchrist, J., & Russell, P. J. (2008). Unintentional strangulation deaths from the "choking game" among youths aged 6–19 years—United States, 1995—2007. *Journal of Safety Research, 39*(4), 445–448.

U.S. Department of Health & Human Services, Administration for Children & Families, Administration on Youth & Families Children, Youth and Families, Children's Bureau. (2016). *Child maltreatment 2014.* Retrieved from https://www.acf.hhs.gov/sites/default/files/cb/cm2014.pdf

U.S. Department of Health & Human Services, Administration for Children & Families, Children's Bureau. (2016). Child abuse and neglect statistics. Retrieved from https://www.childwelfare.gov/topics/systemwide/statistics/can

Van Amsterdam, J., Nabben, T., & Van den Brink, W. (2015). Recreational nitrous oxide use: Prevalence and risks. *Regulatory Toxicology and Pharmacology, 73*(3), 790–796.

Venema, A. M., Groothoff, J. W., & Bierens, J. J. (2010). The role of bystanders during rescue and resuscitation of drowning victims. *Resuscitation, 81*(4), 434–439.

Wallin, K., Nguyen, H., Russell, L., & Lee, D. K. (2016). Acute traumatic compartment syndrome in pediatric foot: A systematic review and case report. *Journal of Foot and Ankle Surgery, 55*(4), 817–820.

Willis, M. H., Merkel, S. I., Voepel-Lewis, T., & Malviya, S. (2003). FLACC behavioral pain assessment scale: A comparison with the child's self-report. *Pediatric Nursing, 29*(3), 195–198.

Yue, J. K., Winkler, E. A., Burke, J. F., Chan, A. K., Dhall, S. S., Berger, M. S., … Tarapore, P. E. (2016). Pediatric sports-related traumatic brain injury in United States trauma centers. *Neurosurgical Focus, 40*(4), E3.

Zonnoor, B. (2017). Frostbite. In D. M. Elston (Ed.), *Medscape.* Retrieved from https://emedicine.medscape.com/article/926249-overview

SECTION II. TOXICOLOGY

Maureen A. Madden

Poisoning represents one of the most common medical emergencies encountered worldwide and is especially problematic for children, who constitute the population that is most vulnerable and at risk for unintentional and preventable poisonings. The scope of toxic substances involved in poisoning is very broad, requiring healthcare providers to have an extensive knowledge of signs and symptoms of poisoning, as well as specific therapeutic interventions and antidotes. The vast majority of children who ingest poisons suffer no harm. However, healthcare providers must recognize, assess, and manage those exposures that are most likely to cause serious injury, illness, or death and initiate appropriate management to minimize the physical injury that may occur. Those patients identified as most at risk are likely to require management in an ICU setting.

DEFINITIONS

A. Poisoning Versus Overdose

The term *poison* is often used to refer to nonpharmaceutical substances, and *overdose* is used for pharmaceuticals; however, any substance that enters the body and causes harm is a poison, and therefore the term *poisoning* is used in this section to describe the results of any exposure resulting in an adverse reaction such as injury, illness, or death.

B. Poison Exposure

Poison exposure means coming into some form of contact with a potentially harmful or toxic substance that can produce toxic effects. Such exposure can be through ingestion, inhalation, ocular or dermal contact, or parenteral injection.

C. Routes of Exposure

The manner in which a potentially toxic substance enters the body can influence the time of onset, intensity, and duration of toxic effects. Consistently, the most common route of exposure is ingestion. However, never overlook the importance of other routes of exposure, for example, inhalation and dermal routes for organophosphate insecticides; inhalation, nasal, ocular, and parenteral routes for drugs of abuse; ocular, dermal, oral, and inhalation for caustic chemicals; inhalation for gases, fumes, and vapors; and parenteral for envenomations. The effects of a poison exposure are determined by the degree of absorption of the substance into the bloodstream, the extent of metabolism to a less toxic or more toxic substance, distribution to target organs, and ultimate elimination from the body.

D. Acute Versus Chronic Exposure

Poisoning may be acute or chronic, but the overwhelming majority of human toxic exposures are acute with unintentional ingestions outnumbering intentional ingestions. Most poison exposures in children are the result of acute ingestion. Chronic overdoses, or an acute overdose of a drug also taken for a long period, are possible for children who require therapeutic drugs for medical conditions. Chronic exposures also occur for those abusing drugs, for victims of child abuse, and for victims of factitious disorder by proxy. Pharmacokinetics, toxic blood levels, and clinical manifestations of poisoning may differ between acute and chronic exposure to a drug. The cornerstone of treatment comprises a thorough evaluation of the poisoning exposure, careful assessment of the patient, and the application of supportive care as indicated. The most important aspect of managing a child with a potential poisoning exposure is meticulous attention to detail in both routine and intensive supportive care. When a toxic ingestion is suspected, initial management is always focused on stabilizing the patient's condition utilizing the priorities of resuscitation: airway, breathing, and circulation (ABCs); and securing rapid intravenous (IV) access before instituting additional management and therapeutic interventions.

ROLE OF THE POISON CENTER

A. The poison center is a valuable source of expert clinical toxicology information. There are 56 poison control centers operating in the United States, providing 24 hr/day, and 7 day/week assistance. The poison control centers are staffed by physician, pharmacists, nurses, and experts in toxicology and are able to:

    1. Provide expert advice about poisoning by drugs (legal, illegal, foreign, veterinary), household products, industrial chemicals, hazardous materials, environmental toxins, chemical warfare agents, drugs to treat exposure to biological warfare agents, snakes, spiders, plants, mushrooms, and pill identification.

2. Determine whether a constellation of symptoms could be caused by poisoning.

3. Locate sources for unusual antidotes (e.g., botulinum antitoxin, exotic snake antivenins), treatments, and laboratory studies.

4. Conduct clinical and epidemiologic research, providing education and information on new drugs and the most up-to-date treatment recommendations.

B. Each patient referred to the poison control center becomes an anonymous part of a national database, which collectively identifies actual and, in some cases, previously unsuspected hazards. These data are uploaded by your local poison center in real time to the American Association of Poison Control Centers National Poison Data System (NPDS), as part of syndromic surveillance for public health threats. Data also are used to reformulate or repackage products or to require removal of products from the market.

C. The Joint Commission on Accreditation of Healthcare Organizations requires that the poison center phone number be posted in every healthcare facility. All U.S. poison control centers share the same phone number, 1-800-222-1222, and calls are automatically routed to the local poison control center according to the initiating telephone exchange and area code.

EPIDEMIOLOGY AND ETIOLOGY

A. Epidemiology

1. The most comprehensive source of information about poison exposures in the United States is the "Annual Report of the American Association of Poison Control Centers' NPDS," published annually in the journal *Clinical Toxicology* and on the web at www.aapcc.org. It provides data for differentiation between common but relatively benign poison exposures and those with serious consequences.

2. In 2014, there were 2,165,142 human poison exposures reported to 56 poison centers in the United States. More than 91% of these exposures occurred in a residence. About 68% of the 2.2 million exposures reported to poison centers were treated at the exposure site, saving millions of dollars in medical expenses. A summary of the number of pediatric exposures and fatalities is found in Table 9.17 (Mowry, Spyker, Brooks, McMillan, & Schauben, 2015).

3. The most common poison exposures in children during 2014 are listed in Table 9.18. Table 9.19 lists those substances associated with the largest number of fatalities in all ages. This section focuses on the most dangerous poison exposures, rather than the most common.

B. Risk Factors

1. All ages are vulnerable to iatrogenic poisonings (e.g., incorrect drugs or routes of administration in a healthcare setting), environmental toxins (e.g., carbon monoxide, pesticides, contaminated water), inadvertent ingestion of substances improperly stored, and idiosyncratic reactions. Children of any age may be victims of child abuse or factitious disorder by proxy. The ingestion of a potentially poisonous substance typically represents a complex interaction of factors, including the child, substance, and environment. In addition, there are some age-related physiologic and behavioral factors that may predispose to, exacerbate, or mitigate poison exposures. Specifically, toddlers and adolescents demonstrate a bimodal high incidence of exposure to toxic substances.

TABLE 9.17   Number of Pediatric Poison Exposures, 2014

Age	Number of Exposures	Percentage of All Exposures	Number of Fatalities	Percentage of All Fatalities
Under 6	1,031,927	47.7	16	1.4
6–12	132,067	6.1	26	2.2
13–19	158,468	7.3	87	7.4

Source: Adapted from Mowry, J. B., Spyker, D. A., Brooks, D. E., McMillan, N., & Schauben, J. L. (2015). 2014 Annual Report of the American Association of Poison Control Centers' National Poison Data System (NPDS): 32nd annual report, *Clinical Toxicology, 53,* 962–1147. doi:10.3109/15563650.2015.1102927

TABLE 9.18   Most Common Poison Exposures, 2014

Younger Than Age 6 Years	All Ages
Cosmetics and personal care products	Analgesics
Household cleaning substances	Sedatives/hypnotics/antipsychotics
Analgesics	Unknown drug
Foreign bodies/toys/misc	Cardiovascular drugs
Topical preparations	Muscle relaxants
Vitamins	Antidepressants
Antihistamines	Antihistamines
Pesticides	Antimicrobials
GI preparations	Stimulants and street drugs
Plants	Anticonvulsants

GI, gastrointestinal.

Source: Adapted from Mowry, J. B., Spyker, D. A., Brooks, D. E., McMillan, N., & Schauben, J. L. (2015). 2014 Annual Report of the American Association of Poison Control Centers' National Poison Data System (NPDS): 32nd Annual Report, *Clinical Toxicology, 53*, 962–1147. doi:10.3109/15563650.2015.1102927

TABLE 9.19   The 10 Most Common Causes of Poison-Related Fatalities, All Ages, 2014

Miscellaneous sedative/hypnotics/antipsychotics
Miscellaneous cardiovascular drugs
Opioids
Miscellaneous stimulants and street drugs
Miscellaneous alcohols
Acetaminophen alone
Acetaminophen combinations
SSRIs
Miscellaneous fumes/gases/vapors
Miscellaneous antidepressants

SSRIs, selective serotonin reuptake inhibitors.

Source: Adapted from Mowry, J. B., Spyker, D. A., Brooks, D. E., McMillan, N., & Schauben, J. L. (2015). 2014 Annual Report of the American Association of Poison Control Centers' National Poison Data System (NPDS): 32nd annual report, *Clinical Toxicology, 53*, 962–1147. doi:10.3109/15563650.2015.1102927

2. The general concept of the "one-pill" rule states that a single adult therapeutic dose would not be expected to produce significant toxicity in a child. This is true for most agents but there are a small group of pharmaceutical agents and household products that can create life-threatening effects when ingested in very small quantities. A "sip or pill can kill," is a category of products with the potential to cause life-threatening toxicity or death in a child younger than 2 years of age, despite the ingestion of only one or two tablets or sips (Michael & Sztajnkrycer, 2004). Approximately 24 agents have the potential to be fatal to individuals with small body mass. Nine of the most commonly ingested agents in this category are calcium channel antagonists, camphor, clonidine and the imidazolines, cyclic antidepressants, opioids and opiates, diphenoxylate/atropine (Lomotil), salicylates, sulfonylureas, and toxic alcohols (methanol, ethylene glycol and isopropanol; Michael & Sztajnkrycer, 2004).

a. Infants are poisoned when parents misread or disregard medication labels, when potentially harmful substances are left within an infant's grasp, or when older siblings "feed" or "help with" infants. Immature GI tract flora predisposes infants to infant botulism from ingestion of honey and to methemoglobinemia from the ingestion of foods or well water high in nitrites. The infant's immature nervous system exacerbates the risk of poisoning by any CNS toxin. Rapid respiratory and metabolic rates increase the risk of carbon monoxide poisoning. Immature hepatic and renal systems may or may not increase the risk of poison exposures, depending on the specific mechanisms for metabolism and excretion. An infant's small body weight increases the potential for danger if an infant is envenomated by snakes or spiders.

b. Toddlers normal developmental characteristics increase the likelihood of ingestions in this age group. Toddlers are newly mobile, curious, and anxious to explore their environment through reaching, climbing, and tasting, yet too young to know what is dangerous and subsequently are poisoned when potentially poisonous substances are left within reach. There are three prominent reasons that typically put children at risk for toxic exposure: improper storage of substances in the home, children spending more time in other people's homes, and caregiver distraction. Other factors that put children at risk are a chaotic or stressful home environment; an unemployed or single-parent household; parental illness or disability; accessibility to toxic agents; lack of proper supervision; grandparent visiting or caretaking; and desire to imitate adult behavior, including taking of medicines (Calello & Henretig, 2014). Children are unable to distinguish medicines and household products from benign look-alikes such as candy and soft drinks. Physiologically, toddlers face the same risks as infants in terms of the nervous, hepatic, and renal systems; respiratory and metabolic rate; and body weight.

c. School-age children may not be able to read or may misinterpret label instructions on products and medicines, succumb to "dares" of classmates, and may not be able to predict the consequences of their actions. Because of wide variability in normal growth and development, it is difficult generally to predict the physiologic effects of many poison exposures in children.

d. Preteens and adolescents may misinterpret label instructions on products and medicines, succumb to "dares" of classmates, explore more widely outside the home and school environment, abuse drugs, or attempt suicide. The majority of ingestions in this age group occur in the home and

are intentional rather than accidental. Adolescent ingestions frequently involve multiple substances, are a result of either suicide attempts or substance abuse, and commonly a delay occurs between the ingestion and when medical attention is sought. Adolescents also have increased access to illicit and licit drugs and alcohol than younger children. Adolescents may be exposed to chemicals on the job. After about age 10, children metabolize acetaminophen as adults do (i.e., generate increased amounts of the hepatotoxic metabolite). As they near the upper end of the adolescent age range, physiologic responses approach, then equal, adult responses for all agents.

MANAGEMENT OF PATIENTS WITH POISON EXPOSURES

A. History

1. Most poisoning exposures in children younger than 6 years are unintentional and are not associated with malicious or suicidal intent. Poisonings in this age group usually involve one substance that is often nontoxic or minimally toxic. The amount ingested is usually small and children usually present for evaluation soon after ingestion. Usually the basic information is known: Children spill things, brag about taking medicine or "helping mommy," or act guilty about having done something "forbidden."

2. In the absence of history, a high index of suspicion is required to determine whether a poison exposure has occurred. Suspect a poison exposure when there is a sudden onset of illness; unexplained symptoms, findings, or laboratory values; an unusual complex of symptoms; exposure to a fire (carbon monoxide, cyanide); or psychiatric treatment in the child, a family member, or caretaker and therefore access to psychotropic drugs. In older children who are trauma victims, suspect drug or alcohol use as a precipitating factor. Also, previously undiagnosed medical conditions (e.g., glucose-6-phosphate dehydrogenase [G6PD] deficiency) may predispose to poisoning by some agents (naphthalene mothballs, dapsone), and the poison center can help identify such conditions.

3. To determine whether a poison exposure may have occurred, ask about medicines and products in the home; whether there have been visitors in the home or the child has visited elsewhere as an increasing number of exposures in children younger than 6 years of age involve ingestion of a grandparent's or elderly caretaker's medicine. These agents tend to be more toxic to children, often in sustained-release dosage forms. Ask whether herbal medicines, home remedies, or foreign preparations have been used or are available; or if the child has been breastfeeding. To assess environmental factors, ask whether anyone else is ill, for example, or whether there have been any home improvement projects or new appliances installed.

4. In addition to ascertaining the nature of any symptoms, history of an ingestion includes type and amount of ingestion if known; the possibility of multiple agents; the time of ingestion; time of presentation; any history of vomiting, choking, coughing, and/or alteration in mental status; and any interventions performed prior to presentation at the medical facility. This information can provide valuable clues in determining what the poison is or whether the available history is accurate.

B. Assessment

As previously stated, this section focuses on the most dangerous poison exposures; therefore, assessment and management consist of a thorough evaluation of the poisoning exposure, careful assessment of the patient, and the application of basic supportive care as indicated. When a toxic ingestion is suspected, initial assessment and management are always focused on first stabilizing the patient's condition utilizing the priorities of resuscitation, the ABCs, and securing rapid IV access. The poisoned patient often represents an acute-onset emergency with a broad range of multiorgan system pathophysiology. Any interventions related to the potentially urgent or emergent concerns of adequacy and stability of the respiratory system and circulatory system should supersede all other concerns and interventions.

In cases of poisoning, the letters D, E, and F can extend the initial stabilization mnemonic to include disability assessment, drugs, decontamination, ECG, and fever. These are important foci in the assessment and management of toxic exposures. The disability assessment includes a brief neurologic examination, including level of consciousness, pupillary size, and reactivity; drug therapy is the potential empiric use of items such as oxygen, dextrose, and naloxone. A point of care assessment of serum glucose is indicated for any patient who presents with altered mental status or lethargy as well as for any patient exposed to agents that might cause hypoglycemia. Hypoglycemia is one of the most easily detected and treatable effects secondary to toxic exposures.

1. Clinical assessment in cases of poison exposure is no different from physical assessment for any other medical emergency. Clinical syndromes, called *toxidromes*, comprise a constellation of signs and symptoms that suggest a specific class of poisoning as seen in Table 9.20. Toxidromes integrate initial vital signs, mental status changes, symptoms, clinical findings, and laboratory results to help identify the toxin and allowing initiation of appropriate treatment in a timely manner. The clinical examination needs to be focused on the central and autonomic nervous system, eye findings, changes in skin, oral and GI mucosa, and odors. These are the areas most likely affected in toxic syndromes. In the poisoned child, after appropriate stabilization, there may be a role for laboratory testing.

2. The need for laboratory assessment depends on whether the poison is known; if so, what the poison is; whether knowledge of test results will affect medical care, prognosis, or disposition of the patient; and, in some cases, whether there are medicolegal considerations. In addition, serum and/or urine toxicology screens may be necessary to rule out the possibility of exposure to additional unknown agents.

a. For many poisonings with *anticipated systemic effects*, baseline serum electrolytes; renal and hepatic functions; respiratory, cardiovascular, and hematologic parameters; and ABG analyses are necessary.

b. For some poisons, *quantitative measurement* in urine or serum determines whether treatment is needed. Examples include acetaminophen, aspirin, lead, ethylene glycol, and methanol.

c. In other cases, *laboratory studies* may confirm the presence of particular substances but do not alter patient care (e.g., tricyclic antidepressants [TCAs]).

d. At other times, *laboratory values* cannot be returned in time to influence patient care (e.g., cyanide).

e. In some cases, the *time* between exposure and collection of the laboratory specimen influences the interpretation of laboratory results (e.g., acetaminophen, aspirin, carbon monoxide) as the screening assay only reflects the presence or absence of drugs or metabolites at or above a threshold concentration at the time the specimen is collected. It does not exclude the presence of drug or metabolite, only that the substance was not present at the minimal threshold quantity.

TABLE 9.20   Table of Toxidromes

Toxidrome	Symptoms	Causative Agent
Sympathomimetic (stimulant)	Restlessness Excessive speech and motor activity Tremor Insomnia Tachycardia Hyperthermia Mydriasis Hallucinations	Amphetamines PCP Cocaine ADHD medications Cathinones Other stimulants
Sedative/hypnotic	Sedation Confusion Delirium Hallucinations Coma Paresthesia Diplopia Blurred vision Slurred speech Ataxia Nystagmus	Barbiturates Benzodiazepines
Opioid	Altered mental status Miosis Unresponsiveness Shallow respiration Bradypnea Bradycardia Hypotension Decreased bowel sounds Hypothermia	Narcotic agents Heroin Clonidine
Anticholinergic[a]	Fever Flushing Tachycardia Urinary retention Dry skin Blurred vision Mydriasis Decreased bowel sounds Ileus Myoclonus Psychosis Hallucinations Seizures Coma	Some mushrooms Cyclic antidepressants Antihistamines Atropinics Scopolamine Over-the-counter sleep preparations
Cholinergic[b]	Salivation Lacrimation Urination Defecation GI distress (diarrhea) Emesis Bradycardia	Organophosphates Insecticides Some mushrooms Black widow spider bites

ADHD, attention deficit hyperactivity disorder; GI, gastrointestinal; PCP, phencyclidine.

[a]Mnemonic: Hot as a hare, dry as a bone, red as a beet, mad as a hatter, blind as a bat.
[b]Mnemonic: SLUDGE.

f. When a poisoning is suspected but not known, a *comprehensive toxicology screen* may be helpful in identifying the agent. How "comprehensive" such a screen is varies from facility to facility; it is essential to know what was tested for before declaring such a screening result to be negative.

g. It is usual, and desirable, to "treat the patient, not the laboratory." When caring for a poisoned patient, the exact opposite is sometimes necessary to prevent devastating consequences. In some common, potentially fatal poisonings, *metabolites* are responsible for toxic effects, and ideally the patient would be treated before toxic metabolites are generated and while the patient is still asymptomatic. In cases of acetaminophen, ethylene glycol, and methanol poisoning, laboratory studies do guide therapy.

C. Interventions

As previously discussed, after ensuring basic stabilization, the use of specific interventions or therapies, including antidotes and enhanced elimination techniques, is limited to cases for which there is expectation that a defined benefit will outweigh the risk of the procedure. There are limited data and information to distinguish lethal concentrations of certain drugs and toxic substances in children and the newer or limited-use therapies have limited pediatric experience. Therefore, indications for the use of interventions in children may be different from those in adults and need to be carefully considered before implementing them.

1. *Prevention of Absorption.* Decontamination is the initial step as it will limit further absorption of the toxin. This may refer to removal from contaminated air, irrigation of exposed eyes and skin, or GI tract decontamination via adsorption or enhanced elimination techniques.

    a. *Ocular exposure* is treated by copious irrigation, at least 15 to 20 minutes for acidic substances and 30 minutes for alkaline substances, with subsequent reevaluation. One measure of the efficacy of irrigation is when a pH strip gently touched to the conjunctival cul-de-sac indicates a neutral pH. Ocular irrigation in children is difficult at best, and the optimal method to use is the one that can be initiated quickly and then maintained. Ocular irrigation in teens can be performed as in adults, with an irrigation device.

    b. *Dermal exposure* is also treated by copious irrigation for the times specified previously.

For older children, a shower is ideal. Ensure to protect staff from exposure to harmful substances with personal protective equipment, initiate irrigation, and remove and bag contaminated clothing.

    c. *GI tract decontamination* refers to the practice of functionally removing an ingested toxin from the GI tract in order to decrease its absorption. Historically, many approaches have been adopted, including gastric evacuation (forced emesis or gastric lavage), intragastric binding (most commonly by single or multidose activated charcoal), or enhancing transit of toxins to decrease total absorption time (whole-bowel irrigation [WBI] or cathartics). As clinical practice has evolved and understanding of the efficacy, risks, and benefits of decontamination have grown, many practices have fallen out of favor. No controlled clinical studies have demonstrated that "routine" GI decontamination reduces morbidity and mortality in poisoned patients. However, evidence suggests that decontamination may reduce the absorption of toxins in the GI tract and may be helpful in very select circumstances. The decision to perform GI decontamination is based upon the specific poison(s) ingested, the time from ingestion to presentation, presenting symptoms, and the predicted severity of poisoning. GI decontamination is most likely to benefit patients who present within 1 hour of a known ingestion of a toxic agent and symptoms have not yet begun. Once symptoms have begun it is typically too late to initiate this intervention (Green, Harris, & Singer, 2008). As such, there is no single preferred strategy for the management of gastric decontamination in pediatric poisonings. The decision to implement a gastric emptying technique is largely dependent upon clinical status and specific situations. Use of an individualized approach based on the timing of ingestion, type of substance, and the amount of the ingested substance in conjunction with the clinical status will dictate treatment choices.

    i. *Ipecac syrup* was once used to induce vomiting. The American Academy of Pediatrics no longer recommends the use of ipecac syrup to treat poisoning, even at home.

    ii. *Gastric lavage*, a form of gastric emptying, also known as *gastric irrigation*, is the process of cleaning out the contents of the stomach artificially. It is no longer considered the standard of care in pediatric patients as the associated potential risks typically outweigh the benefit and therefore is limited in use (Benson et al., 2013). It is sometimes used in patients with known life-threatening overdoses and it is only performed when a benefit is anticipated and one of the following conditions exist: the substance does not bind to activated charcoal, the opportunity to use activated charcoal is significantly delayed or missed, or the child presents within 1 hour of ingestion without significant CNS symptoms already present. Gastric emptying will have limited benefit if attempted more than 1 hour after ingestion because most toxins will have been absorbed or passed through the pylorus already, except for agents that slow gastric motility. The efficacy of gastric lavage is limited by the respective sizes of the child, the tube, and the ingestion, commonly in tablet form.

1) If gastric lavage is to be implemented, the procedure should be only done by individuals with expertise and understanding of the risks associated with the procedure. The procedure consists of first ensuring that the airway is secure and then obtaining the materials necessary for the gastric lavage, including warm NS for instillation. The largest possible orogastric tube should be used, usually a 16- to 32-gauge French. Instill 50 to 100 mL of warm NS at a time, and then allow it to remain in the stomach for a few minutes and drain by gravity. Repeat until lavage fluid is clear. Activated charcoal and a cathartic can be administered before the lavage tube is withdrawn if indicated by the specific suspected or known agent ingested.

2) Gastric lavage is contraindicated for ingestion of caustic substances and hydrocarbons due to the risk of mucosal burns and risk of aspiration of substances into the airway and pulmonary system.

iii. *WBI* can facilitate removal of select toxins from the GI tract in some patients, but there is no convincing evidence from clinical studies that it improves the outcome of poisoned patients. It can be considered for potentially toxic ingestions of sustained-release or enteric-coated drugs, particularly for those patients presenting greater than 2 hours after

drug ingestion when activated charcoal is considered to be less effective. WBI can also be considered for patients who have ingested substantial amounts of iron, lithium, or potassium as the morbidity is high and there is a lack of other potentially effective options for GI decontamination. WBI can be considered for removal of ingested packets of illicit drugs in "body packers." The concurrent administration of activated charcoal and WBI might decrease the effectiveness of the charcoal (Thanacoody et al., 2010).

1) The general procedure is the same as for bowel preparations. Secure the airway if necessary, and administer a polyethylene glycol–electrolyte solution until the rectal effluent is clear. The dose is 0.5 L/hr for young children and 1 to 2 L/hr for older children and adults. WBI is contraindicated in patients with bowel obstruction, perforation, or ileus, and in patients with hemodynamic instability or compromised unprotected airways.

iv. *Activated charcoal* is processed so that each molecule contains multiple binding sites. Activated charcoal adsorbs, or binds to, most clinically important drugs and poisons. This prevents absorption from the GI tract into the bloodstream. Activated charcoal does not adsorb metals (e.g., iron, lithium), caustic substances, ethanol, or many pesticides. When these substances are ingested, activated charcoal may still be indicated because of coingestants.

1) The usual dose of activated charcoal is 0.5 to 1 g/kg for young children, 25 to 50 g for older children, and 50 g per dose for adolescents and adults.

2) Activated charcoal should not be mixed with ice cream, syrups, or other items intended to improve palatability. The charcoal adsorbs many of these agents and would therefore be less effective.

3) Single doses of activated charcoal (SDAC) are indicated for the most serious poison exposures because it decreases the amount of toxic substance available for absorption into the bloodstream and should only be used for known serious poison exposures with early presentation, less than 1 hour

after ingestion, and before onset of symptoms, especially CNS symptoms (Juurlink, 2016). This intervention is often used in the prehospital or emergency room environments.

4) Multiple doses of activated charcoal (MDAC; every 2–6 hours) are recommended in the setting of life-threatening ingestions such as carbamazepine, dapsone, phenobarbital, salicylates, phenytoin, quinine, and theophylline, as it is useful in lowering toxic blood levels and shortening the course of poisoning of substances that undergo enterohepatic or enterogastric recirculation. Some drugs are partially metabolized in the liver, and then active drug is secreted into bile and deposited in the small bowel. Subsequent doses of activated charcoal adsorb the drug as this occurs. This is true regardless of the route of exposure. *Intestinal dialysis* takes advantage of concentration gradients. As drug is adsorbed to charcoal in the GI tract, previously absorbed, unmetabolized drug moves from receptor sites and intracellular spaces into the GI tract. As this occurs, it, too, is adsorbed by subsequent doses of activated charcoal. Aspirin ingestion is sometimes considered another indication for MDAC, due to the propensity of aspirin tablets to form bezoars, though evidence is lacking.

5) Cautions. To prevent a charcoal impaction, always check for active bowel sounds before administering a dose of charcoal. When MDAC are given, cathartics are occasionally administered no more than once, or occasionally twice, per day to prevent electrolyte imbalance and dehydration. Errors have occurred when charcoal suspension in sorbitol has been mistakenly administered instead of charcoal in an aqueous suspension. Charcoal is contraindicated with absent bowel sounds because it may indicate ileus or obstruction. Always reassess for bowel sounds before administering the next dose of charcoal.

v. Cathartics. Cathartics are no longer routinely recommended. If cathartics are used at all to treat a poisoning, sorbitol, and magnesium citrate are the most common.

1) *Sorbitol* may be combined with charcoal or administered afterward. It should be administered no more than once per day. The dose is 1 to 2 g/kg.

2) *Magnesium citrate* may be combined with charcoal or administered afterward. It should be administered no more than once per day with a dose of 4 mL/kg.

2. *Enhancement of Elimination.* The ability and possibility of enhancing elimination depend on a substance's volume of distribution and usual route of elimination.

a. *Ion trapping* is useful for some drugs that are more rapidly eliminated in an alkaline environment; examples include salicylates and phenobarbital. In these cases, administering sodium bicarbonate to alkalinize the urine enhances excretion. (Some drugs are more easily eliminated by acidifying the urine, but this is not recommended; precipitation of myoglobin and renal failure may occur.)

b. *Extracorporeal measures* to enhance elimination of toxins may be useful in certain dangerous poisonings by substances that can be retrieved from the vascular compartment. Depending on the child's age, hemodialysis can be used for salicylates, lithium, methanol, and ethylene glycol, among others; hemoperfusion may be used for theophylline; and exchange transfusion is sometimes used to treat "gray baby syndrome" induced by chloramphenicol.

c. *Lipid emulsion therapy (LET)* is increasingly being considered as a rescue antidote to treat lipophilic drug toxicities such as anesthetics, calcium channel blockers (CCBs), and TCAs. LET has a number of known complications, including lipemia interfering with laboratory testing, pancreatitis and associated symptoms of abdominal pain, nausea and/or vomiting, and ARDS. The limited data associated with use and the known complications of LET reserves its use for hemodynamically unstable patients in whom supportive efforts are not successful (Gosselin et al., 2015).

D. Administration of Antidotes

Few pharmacologic antidotes are available as seen in Table 9.21. Most poisonings are treated by

TABLE 9.21 Countermeasures for Selected Toxin Exposures

Toxin Exposure	Countermeasure
Acetaminophen (Tylenol/Paracetamol)	NAC
Anticholinergics	Physostigmine
Anticoagulants	Vitamin K_1, protamine
Benzodiazepines	Supportive care, flumazenil[a]
Botulism	Botulinum antitoxin, BIG
Beta-blockers	Glucagon
Calcium channel blockers	Calcium, glucagon
Cholinergic	Atropine Pralidoxime in organophosphate overdose
Carbon monoxide	Oxygen, hyperbaric oxygen
Cyanide	Amyl nitrate, sodium nitrate, sodium thiosulfate
Digoxin	Digoxin Fab antibodies (Digibind)
Iron	Deferoxamine
INH	Pyridoxine
Lead	British antilewisite, ethylenediaminetetraacetic acid, dimercaptosuccinic acid
Methemoglobinemia	Methylene blue
Opioids	Naloxone (Narcan)
Sulfonylureas (oral hypoglycemics)	Dextrose, octreotide
Toxic alcohols	Fomepizole, ethanol infusion, dialysis
Tricyclic antidepressants	Sodium bicarbonate

BIG, botulism immune globulin; INH, isoniazid; NAC, N-acetylcysteine.

[a]Flumazenil may precipitate seizures when used with patients who are chronic benzodiazepine users or in situations, including tricyclic antidepressant overdose.

Source: Adapted from Madden, M. A. (2015). Pediatric toxicology: Emerging trends. *Journal of Pediatric Intensive Care, 4*, 103–110.

decontamination followed by symptomatic and supportive care. If a specific antidote is indicated, it is described as part of the treatment for poisonings considered in the following sections.

E. Provision of Supportive Care

For all the substances discussed throughout this section, the premise is that initial stabilization techniques have been addressed and instituted when indicated. Provision of supportive care and symptom management from poisoning encompasses monitoring to ensure airway protection especially in the obtunded child, maintaining adequate oxygenation and ventilation, correction of any hypotension or hypertension, correction of acid–base or electrolyte disturbances, monitoring for dysrhythmias, rhabdomyolysis, and awareness of current medical problems and medications.

TABLE 9.22 Causes of Increasing or Recurring Symptoms and Drug Levels

Incomplete gastrointestinal decontamination: Virtually any solid dosage form
Drug concretion or bezoar. Examples: Aspirin, iron, meprobamate
Enterohepatic recirculation. Examples: Amitriptyline, digoxin, phencyclidine
Ingestion of anticholinergic drug, or drug with anticholinergic properties. Examples: Antihistamines, atropine, tricyclic antidepressants, glutethimide
Exposure to especially lipid-soluble substances. Examples: Some organophosphate insecticides, anesthetic agents, ethchlorvynol
Incorrect or incomplete history
Incorrect laboratory values
Reexposure in the hospital

Descriptions of individual toxins indicate whether one particular drug (e.g., antiarrhythmic, anticonvulsant, vasopressor) is preferred. Increasing or recurrent symptoms may be expected with some poisonings and occur unexpectedly in others. See Table 9.22 for possible reasons.

F. Prevention of Future Episodes

Circumstances contributing to iatrogenic poisonings must be considered. For young children, age- and development-specific poison-prevention teaching may be required. Suspicions of abuse require legal and social service involvement. Drug abuse prevention and treatment programs and psychiatric intervention may be required for older children and adolescents.

POISONINGS BY PHARMACEUTICAL AGENTS

A. Acetaminophen

Acetaminophen is contained within hundreds of prescription and nonprescription analgesics, both alone and in combination with other analgesics, including opioids; in combination with antihistamines in over-the-counter sleeping preparations; and in combination with decongestants, antihistamines, antitussives, expectorants, and analgesics in products to treat coughs, colds, and allergies. Most preparations are oral, but the drug also is available as rectal suppositories and an IV formulation.

1. Acetaminophen is rapidly absorbed from the GI tract, but food or coingestants may delay peak absorption until about 4 hours after ingestion.

2. Acetaminophen is metabolized in the liver. After about the age of 10 years, approximately 5% to 10% of the drug is metabolized by a hepatotoxic metabolite that is normally detoxified by the enzyme glutathione. In overdose, the body's glutathione stores are depleted, causing liver damage characteristic of acetaminophen overdose. In children younger than 10 years, a different metabolic pathway may be followed, presumably providing some degree of hepatic protection. This relative protection is not entirely reliable, and infants and young children can also die of hepatic injury after acute or chronic acetaminophen overdose. There is some renal metabolism of acetaminophen; therefore renal injury, although not as common as hepatic injury, is possible.

3. The toxic dose of acetaminophen is related to body weight (or ideal body weight in the case of markedly obese individuals); ingestions of unknown amounts or greater than 150 mg/kg require laboratory assessment of absorbed acetaminophen to predict toxicity.

4. Because the toxic effects of acetaminophen overdose are due to metabolites, symptoms of toxicity are delayed. Only rarely, after massive overdose, does a patient develop mental status changes, significant GI tract symptoms, and acidosis within hours after ingestion. Often there are no symptoms of overdose for 6 to 14 hours after ingestion. The earliest symptoms are nausea and vomiting. Within 24 to 48 hours after ingestion, hepatic enzymes elevate. The patient may experience increasing GI

tract symptoms and right upper quadrant pain, or the patient may feel relatively well. Within 72 to 96 hours after an untreated, severe overdose, hepatic encephalopathy with coagulopathies and hyperglycemia may ensue, followed rapidly by hepatic failure and death.

5. *Assessment*

a. History should include the specific name of the drug as there may be many formulations; the amount ingested; the time of ingestion; and whether ingestion was acute, chronic, or both; the type, onset, duration, or absence of symptoms; and whether there were coingestants.

b. Serum acetaminophen level should be obtained at least 4 hours after ingestion. Also baseline hepatic, renal, and hematologic studies, including prothrombin time (PT)/international normalized ratio (INR) as a measure of synthetic function of the liver, should be obtained if the level is toxic, if ingestion was large or chronic by history, or occurred more than 8 to 12 hours earlier.

6. Treatment of acetaminophen poisoning is straightforward and typically successful if the antidote administration of N-acetylcysteine (NAC), is initiated within 8 to 12 hours after ingestion, if indicated. A determination of need for intervention is made using the Rumack–Matthew nomogram. The nomogram is a sensitive risk-prediction tool and identifies patients at very low risk or very high risk of developing hepatotoxicity after acetaminophen overdose and stratify those who do or do not require administration of NAC. Patients with acetaminophen concentrations below the "possible" line for hepatotoxicity on the Rumack–Matthew nomogram may be discharged home after they are medically cleared. If the ingestion occurred with intent to do self-harm, a thorough psychosocial, psychological, and/or psychiatric evaluation is indicated before the patient can be discharged safely from the medical care facility. All patients above the nomogram line for possible hepatotoxicity should be treated with the specific antidote NAC, which serves as a glutathione precursor and substitute to prevent N-acetyl-p-benzoquinoneimine-induced (NAPQI) hepatocellular injury and decrease the risk of developing hepatotoxicity. The nomogram may be used most effectively after acute, single ingestions (where entire ingestion occurs within an 8-hour period), a known time of ingestion, immediate-release formulation, and in the absence of formulations or coingestants that alter absorption and bowel

motility (e.g., anticholinergics, opioids). Delayed treatment still has some utility. Indications for NAC include a toxic acetaminophen level in blood obtained 4 or more hours after ingestion and/or toxic ingestion by history or suspicion when laboratory results cannot be returned by 8 hours after ingestion. The entire course of therapy must be administered to every patient with an acute ingestion and a toxic acetaminophen level, even if the plasma acetaminophen level becomes negative. NAC is being used to treat effects of the toxic metabolite, not the parent compound.

a. Oral NAC

i. The loading dose is NAC 140 mg/kg administered orally (PO), followed by 70 mg/kg every 4 hours for 17 doses, for a total of 18 doses over 72 hours. Make a 3-to-1 dilution of the drug in juice or a beverage palatable to the patient. In an alert patient, offer the diluted drug over ice in a covered container.

ii. Administration of PO NAC is often complicated by vomiting induced by the poisoning and NAC itself. If a dose of NAC is vomited within 1 hour of administration, the dose must be repeated. If an antiemetic is required, use ondansetron or another antiemetic that does not require hepatic metabolism. If necessary for successful NAC administration, a duodenal tube may be placed with radiographic confirmation of placement.

b. IV NAC was approved by the U.S. Food and Drug Administration (FDA) in January 2004 under the brand name Acetadote and is now the recommended route for treatment by poison control. It is a 21-hour IV regimen consisting of three doses with a total dose of 300 mg/kg administered.

i. The loading dose is 150 mg/kg, administered over 60 minutes; second dose of 50 mg/kg (max dose 5 g) is infused over 4 hours. Finally, 100 mg/kg is infused over 16 hours (Taketomo, Hodding, & Kraus, 2015). Fluid and electrolyte imbalance is a concern for small children; call the poison center for additional dosing information. Poison control typically recommends the utilization of the IV formulation for increased tolerance and compliance.

c. Other treatment includes daily monitoring of hepatic enzymes and symptomatic and supportive care.

7. Special considerations include the need for a high index of suspicion. Acetaminophen poisoning is perfectly treatable if recognized early but potentially fatal if untreated. Those who recover and have no clinical or laboratory evidence of hepatic injury are not expected to experience sequelae. Those who develop liver failure from this poisoning may undergo successful liver transplantation.

B. Anesthetics for Topical Use

Anesthetics for topical use contain benzocaine, dibucaine, prilocaine, and lidocaine. They are found in prescription and nonprescription remedies, including teething lotions, first-aid creams, and drugs infiltrated into wounds before suturing. Children have died rapidly after the ingestion of dibucaine.

1. Children experience the rapid onset of dysrhythmias, seizures, and methemoglobinemia after ingestion or absorption of these drugs. As little as several milligrams is sufficient for toxic effects to occur.

2. Suspect methemoglobinemia in patients who are cyanotic and do not respond to oxygen. Methemoglobinemia is a disorder characterized by the presence of a higher than normal level of methemoglobin (metHb, i.e., ferric [Fe^{3+}] rather than ferrous [Fe^{2+}] hemoglobin) in the blood. Methemoglobin has a decreased ability to bind oxygen and results in an increased affinity of bound oxygen to the three other ferrous heme sites within the same hemoglobin unit. This leads to an overall reduced ability of the RBC to release oxygen to tissues, with the associated oxygen–hemoglobin dissociation curve shifted to the left. When methemoglobin concentration is elevated in RBCs, tissue hypoxia can occur due to the overall reduced ability of the RBC to release oxygen to tissues. Bedside pulse oximetry in the presence of methemoglobinemia may be misleading. The pulse oximeter only measures the relative absorbance of two wavelengths of light to differentiate oxyhemoglobin from deoxyhemoglobin. Methemoglobin increases absorption of light at both wavelengths and therefore offers optical interference to pulse oximetry by falsely absorbing light and generating false readings, plateauing at approximately 85%. Pulse oximetry measurements are often falsely high in those with high-level methemoglobinemia. The severity of the cyanosis does not correspond to the pulse oximetry reading: A patient may appear extremely cyanotic but still have a pulse oximetry reading in the high 80s. Newer pulse oximetry models have improved technology to differentiate methemoglobin.

3. Tentative diagnosis can be made by inspection of the blood. A drop of the patient's blood on a piece of filter paper appears brown next to a drop of "normal" blood. Laboratory confirmation reports a percentage of methemoglobin, the amount of normal hemoglobin that has been converted to methemoglobin and therefore cannot transport oxygen.

4. Specific treatment for methemoglobinemia is the IV administration of methylene blue. Treatment for other toxic manifestations is symptomatic and supportive.

C. Antidepressants

SSRIs have become more widely prescribed than TCAs and other cyclic antidepressants because there are fewer dangerous effects in overdose and fewer unpleasant side effects for patients. Poison center data support the widespread availability and lower toxicity of SSRIs compared with TCAs. In 2014, TCAs alone or formulated with other drugs accounted for 10,349 calls to poison centers and were associated with 46 fatalities and major life-threatening effects in 341 cases. The corresponding numbers for SSRIs were 31,169 exposures, with 99 fatalities and life-threatening effects in 118 cases.

1. TCAs include amitriptyline (Elavil), clomipramine (Anafranil), desipramine (Norpramin), doxepin (Sinequan), imipramine (Tofranil), nortriptyline (Pamelor), and others, both singly and in combination with other psychotropic agents. There are no approved therapeutic indications and no safe doses for these drugs in very young children, who may have access to drugs belonging to an older sibling or other family member. Imipramine is used in the treatment of nocturnal enuresis in older children. The TCAs may be used to treat depression in preteens and adolescents, although treatment with SSRIs is now more common. Evidence-based management guidelines for TCA poisoning are available from the American Association of Poison Control Centers (AAPCC).

    a. In general, these drugs are *rapidly absorbed* in the GI tract and undergo first-pass metabolism in the liver. Conjugates are then renally eliminated. Cyclic antidepressants are very lipophilic and highly protein bound, leading to large volumes of distribution. They have long elimination half-lives that often exceed 24 hours

(>31–46 hours for amitriptyline). In an overdose, altered pharmacokinetics may prolong elimination and increase toxic effects. Cyclic antidepressants have significant anticholinergic effects that can delay gastric emptying, particularly in large ingestions, with significant amounts of unabsorbed drug remaining in the GI tract. In addition, the acidosis that results from respiratory depression and hypotension reduces protein binding, resulting in higher serum levels of active free drug. Although the exact therapeutic mechanism of cyclic antidepressants is not known, it is most likely related to decreased central norepinephrine and serotonin reuptake, resulting in increased levels of these amines in the brain.

b. TCA's toxic effects are related to the following four pharmacologic effects: anticholinergic, direct alpha-adrenergic blockade, inhibition of norepinephrine and serotonin reuptake, and blockade of fast sodium channels in myocardial cells. The most serious adverse effects of cyclic antidepressant toxicity are due to CNS effects and cardiovascular instability. Depressed mental status is generally caused by the antihistamine and anticholinergic properties of cyclic antidepressants, whereas seizures are thought to be due to increased CNS levels of biogenic amines. Life-threatening cardiovascular complications are due to impaired conduction from fast sodium channel blockade. This alters depolarization, widens the QRS complex, and prolongs the PR and QT intervals. Impaired cardiac conduction may lead to heart block and unstable ventricular dysrhythmias or asystole. Cyclic antidepressants have also been shown to directly depress myocardial contractility. However, the profound hypotension seen in serious cyclic antidepressant poisoning is primarily due to vasodilatation from direct alpha-adrenergic blockade. Early hypertension may precede the significant hypotension characteristic of this poisoning.

c. The toxic dose cannot be predicted with certainty. Any amount is potentially dangerous for infants, toddlers, and young children. For adolescents and adults, the toxic amount is variable, with 10 to 20 mg/kg generally noted to cause significant toxicity. EMS transport, GI tract decontamination, and at least 6 hours of ED evaluation are required for all ingestions in young children and ingestions larger than a therapeutic dose in older children. A patient who develops any clinical signs of toxicity within the

6-hour observation period requires admission to a monitored bed until the patient has been asymptomatic for 24 hours.

d. The presentation of a tricyclic overdose is variable with cardiovascular and CNS symptoms predominating. A classic presentation of TCA overdose poisoning includes hypotension; metabolic acidosis; and numerous dysrhythmias, especially ventricular dysrhythmias and conduction delays and potentially the rapid onset of grand mal seizures and coma, perhaps within 30 minutes of ingestion. Common ECG findings are numerous, with sinus tachycardia being the most common, followed by prolonged PR and widening of QRS intervals with resultant ventricular arrhythmias.

e. When assessing the patient, strict attention to managing the ABCs is imperative. It is necessary to anticipate the potential need to secure the airway with intubation, if the patient is still conscious, as there may be a rapid change in mental status secondary to the CNS effects of the poisoning. The most useful laboratory study is ABG analysis. Symptomatic patients are likely to develop acidosis that is resistant to correction. Laboratory measurements of drug and metabolite levels correlate loosely with expected toxicity but are not necessary for patient care because they are not used to determine treatment.

f. Treatment includes implementing GI tract decontamination if the patient presents within 1 hour of ingestion and prior to onset of symptoms; maintaining serum pH between 7.45 and 7.55; cardiac monitoring; and treatment of hypotension, seizures, and dysrhythmias.

   i. Administer activated charcoal every 4 hours until the patient is asymptomatic; check for the presence of bowel sounds before each charcoal dose.

   ii. Sodium bicarbonate is the drug of choice to treat TCA poisoning. Life-threatening cardiovascular complications are due to impaired conduction from fast sodium channel blockade and the administration of sodium bicarbonate overcomes this blockade by the induction of alkalosis and resultant correction in acidosis, leading to decreased drug binding to sodium channels. This correction results in stabilization of the cardiac rhythm. Although hyperventilation is sometimes used to correct acidosis, sodium bicarbonate is preferred as it is much more effective.

iii. Lidocaine, magnesium sulfate, or overdrive pacing may be indicated for dysrhythmias unresponsive to a normalized pH. Recently, LET has been proposed as an effective antidote to treat cardiotoxicity from overdose of myocardium-poisoning lipophilic drugs, including CCBs, beta-blockers, digoxin, local anesthetics, cyclic antidepressants, antipsychotics, and atypical antidepressants. Although there are not enough data to support the routine use of IV LET as a rescue agent in all settings, treatment protocols have been developed regarding its use in specific clinical scenarios. Because the potential risks of administering high doses of LET should be considered only after advanced cardiac life support measures have been unsuccessful.

iv. Hypotension must be treated aggressively and may require invasive support if fluids, positioning, and norepinephrine are ineffective. The administration of hypertonic sodium chloride has been shown to be as effective as sodium bicarbonate in reversing QRS prolongation and hypotension.

v. Benzodiazepines, such as diazepam or lorazepam, may be used for the management of agitation or seizures. The pharmacologic effects of phenytoin may be elevated, increasing the pharmacologic effects and risk of toxicity so the use of phenytoin or fosphenytoin is to be avoided.

vi. Physostigmine is a short-acting cholinesterase inhibitor that has been described as causing asystole and seizures. There is no role for its use in the management of tricyclic toxicity.

g. Amoxapine is a cyclic antidepressant that causes few cardiovascular effects after overdose, but it is often associated with status epilepticus. An overdose of amoxapine requires aggressive seizure control, often including intubation and neuromuscular blockade.

2. Serotonin uptake inhibitors include citalopram (Celexa), fluoxetine (Prozac), fluvoxamine (Luvox), paroxetine (Paxil, Seroxat), sertraline (Zoloft, Lustral) and escitalopram (Lexapro, Cipralex).

a. Effects of single-drug overdoses tend to be mild, including drowsiness and GI effects. Citalopram especially is associated with a greater incidence of seizures and cardiac effects, including QTc prolongation. Early recognition is necessary to ensure appropriate resuscitative interventions and to limit exposure to other medications that may potentially exacerbate the serotonin syndrome and associated symptoms. Although most clinical symptoms are mild to moderate, patients have the potential to deteriorate quickly. In the syndrome's mildest stage, symptoms are often attributed to other causes, and in its most severe form, it can easily be mistaken for neuroleptic malignant syndrome. Severe serotonin toxicity is characterized by muscle rigidity, which can cause the body temperature to elevate rapidly to over 40°C. This hypertonicity can mask the classic and diagnostic signs of hyperreflexia and clonus. Patients may have unstable and labile vital signs with confusion or delirium and can experience tonic–clonic seizures. If the muscle rigidity and hyperthermia are not treated properly, patients can develop cellular damage and enzyme dysfunction leading to rhabdomyolysis, myoglobinuria, renal failure, metabolic acidosis, ARDS, and/or disseminated intravascular coagulation (Wang, Vashistha, Kaur, & Houchens, 2016).

b. *Serotonin syndrome* is a potentially life-threatening condition that can lead to multiorgan failure within hours if not recognized. It may occur idiosyncratically, after large overdoses, or especially with an overdose of more than one drug. It is caused by elevated serotonin levels in the central and peripheral nervous systems. The classic presentation is a triad of autonomic dysfunction, neuromuscular excitation, and altered mental status. Ascending neuromuscular effects may lead to respiratory compromise. Potential physical exam findings of autonomic dysfunction include diaphoresis, tachycardia, nausea and vomiting, and mydriasis. Other signs are hyperactive bowel sounds, diarrhea, and flushing. Clinical findings associated with neuromuscular excitation are myoclonus, hyperreflexia, hyperthermia, hypertonicity, and rigidity. Other signs are spontaneous or inducible clonus, ocular clonus, and tremor. Patients often present with confusion and agitation as well as anxiety, lethargy, and coma. The symptoms vary based on the severity of the serotonergic toxicity and may not present simultaneously (Wang et al., 2016).

c. There are several conditions that can alter the regulation of serotonin, including therapeutic doses, drug interactions, intentional or unintentional overdoses, and overlapping transitions between medications. The only drugs that have been reliably confirmed to precipitate serotonin syndrome are monoamine oxidase inhibitors (MAOIs), SSRIs, serotonin–norepinephrine reuptake inhibitors (SNRIs), and serotonin releasers. But there are other drugs that have been implicated with serotonin syndrome and are categorized into five different classes:

    i.   Drugs that decrease serotonin breakdown (e.g., MAOIs, linezolid, methylene blue, procarbazine)

    ii.   Drugs that decrease serotonin reuptake (e.g., SSRIs, SNRIs, TCA, opioids [meperidine, buprenorphine, tramadol, tapentadol], dextromethorphan, antiepileptics [carbamazepine, valproate], and antiemetics [ondansetron, granisetron, metoclopramide], and the herbal preparation St. John's wort)

    iii.   Drugs that increase serotonin precursors or agonists (e.g., tryptophan, lithium, fentanyl, and lysergic acid diethylamide [LSD])

    iv.   Drugs that increase serotonin release (e.g., fenfluramine, amphetamines, and methylenedioxymethamphetamine [MDMA; ecstasy])

    v.   Drugs that prevent breakdown of the agents listed earlier (e.g., erythromycin, ciprofloxacin, fluconazole, ritonavir, and grapefruit juice)

d. Treatment consists of two primary interventions: to discontinue the serotonergic agent and to provide supportive care. Treatment may include GI decontamination when appropriate. For severe serotonin toxicity, treatment should focus on management of the ABCs. The two primary life-threatening concerns are hyperthermia (temperature >40°C or 104°F) and muscle rigidity, which can lead to hypoventilation. Controlling hyperthermia and rigidity can prevent other severe complications such as rhabdomyolysis. Patients with severe serotonin toxicity should be sedated using benzodiazepines, neuromuscularly relaxed with a nondepolarizing medication, intubated, and supported with mechanical ventilation. This will reverse ventilatory hypertonia. Neuromuscular relaxation will also prevent the exacerbation of hyperthermia, which is due to muscle rigidity. Standard cooling measures should be used to manage hyperthermia.

Antipyretics have no role in the treatment of serotonin syndrome since the hyperthermia is not caused by a change in the hypothalamic temperature set point. Most patients demonstrate improvement within 24 hours of stopping the precipitating drug and implementing therapy.

    i.   Cyproheptadine is a serotonin and histamine antagonist with anticholinergic and sedative effects. Antiserotonin and antihistamine drugs appear to compete with serotonin and histamine, respectively, for receptor sites. The recommended initial dose of cyproheptadine is 12 mg, followed by 2 mg every 2 hours if symptoms continue. Maintenance dosing with 8 mg every 6 hours should be prescribed once stabilization is achieved. The total daily dose for adults should not exceed 0.5 mg/kg/d. Cyproheptadine is available only in oral form but can be crushed and administered via a nasogastric tube (Taketomo, Hodding, & Kraus, 2015).

e. Because patients are often prescribed more than one drug, those with a *history* of having overdosed on an SRI should be evaluated for coingestion of other drugs, especially other antidepressants.

D. Benzodiazepines

Benzodiazepines are used as adjuncts to anesthesia, as anticonvulsants, for muscle spasms, and for anxiety relief. Young children may have access to these drugs if they are being taken therapeutically by family members. They may also be abused or self-administered in suicide attempts. The combination of a benzodiazepine with ethanol or another CNS depressant significantly increases toxicity. In general, overdoses of these drugs can be successfully treated with respiratory support and sometimes the antidote flumazenil.

1. Commonly used benzodiazepines include alprazolam, clonazepam, oxazepam, lorazepam, diazepam, and chlordiazepoxide. Midazolam is used as an adjunct to anesthesia.

2. Benzodiazepines act by enhancing the effects of γ-aminobutyric acid (GABA), an inhibitory neurotransmitter in the brain. The many types of drugs within the class make it impossible to generalize about absorption and elimination. Some of those prescribed for therapeutic use in the outpatient setting (e.g., diazepam) have a long half-life; therefore, significant and prolonged respiratory depression should be anticipated in someone who abused the drug or took a large quantity.

3. Effects of overdose include respiratory and CNS depression, which may necessitate intubation and mechanical ventilatory support. In an uncomplicated overdose, there are no specific drug-related laboratory values of use. In a potential mixed overdose, determination of coingestants is important.

4. Flumazenil is the specific antidote. Flumazenil effectively reverses respiratory depression associated with benzodiazepine overdose, but there are contraindications. A test dose may be used to help determine whether respiratory depression is caused by a benzodiazepine overdose, although it should not be used to maintain wakefulness. Caution must be used to avoid precipitating withdrawal in a patient who is dependent on a benzodiazepine. Flumazenil should never be used if the patient has also overdosed on a TCA because an increased risk of seizures has been associated with this use. Likewise, flumazenil should not be used if the patient is known to have a seizure disorder.

5. Treatment includes primarily symptomatic and supportive care, including potential intubation. If the patient is habituated to the drug, withdrawal symptoms may occur. A protocol to prevent acute withdrawal and accomplish gradual withdrawal must be implemented.

E. Calcium-Channel Blockers

CCBs include amlodopine, diltiazem, nicardipine, nifedipine, verapamil, and others, in regular and sustained-release preparations. As indications for their use in cardiovascular disease and other conditions have increased, poison exposures and fatalities in children have also increased. No antidote or universally effective treatment exists. Aggressive GI tract decontamination may be necessary depending upon the clinical circumstances and vigorous supportive care are required.

1. CCBs are easily absorbed from the GI tract. Elimination rates vary but can be prolonged for days after an overdose.

2. Calcium is required for cellular contraction. These drugs, therapeutically and in overdose, slow the influx of calcium through calcium channels into

the intracellular space of cardiac nodal tissue, myocardial tissue, and vascular (especially arteriolar) tissue. The result is conduction delays, diminished cardiac output, and hypotension.

3. The toxic dose is variable but small. The ingestion of any amount (concept of "one sip or pill can kill") of any of these CCB agents should be considered potentially fatal in a child.

4. Physical assessment must be comprehensive. There are multiple mechanisms for hypotension (decreased cardiac output, diminished peripheral vascular resistance), hypoxia and apnea (bradydysrhythmias, heart block, decreased cardiac output), and metabolic acidosis (hypoperfusion, hypoxia). Also common are CNS depression, seizures, possibly hypoxic seizures, headache, flushing, and hyperglycemia (CCBs inhibit insulin release). Electrolyte monitoring, ABG analysis, ECG, and continuous assessment of respiratory and cardiovascular status are needed. Recognize that the patient may exhibit hypotension with relative preservation of mental status until cerebral perfusion is affected.

5. Treatment with GI decontamination may be considered because CCBs slow gastric motility and delay gastric emptying. Options include activated charcoal, gastric lavage, and consideration of WBI for ingestion of multiple tablets or sustained-release preparations. High-dose IV calcium chloride or calcium gluconate is indicated as theoretically it creates a concentration gradient large enough to partially overcome the channel blockade, driving calcium into the cells, although it is not usually effective. In a patient with stable electrolyte and acid–base status, calcium chloride is preferred because it contains a higher concentration of calcium. (Extravasation of calcium chloride can cause tissue necrosis, so placement and patency of peripheral IV lines must be checked before each administration by this route.) Insulin plus dextrose has been used to stabilize blood pressure in patients refractory to other treatments. The disruption of calcium homeostasis causes a negative chronotropic and inotropic effect and vasodilatation as well as impaired glucose metabolism. Glucagon may be used to increase the heart rate and conduction velocity, although it, too, is not always effective. Otherwise, treatment is symptomatic and supportive, including fluid resuscitation with crystalloid solutions. If volume expansion does not raise the blood pressure to the desired level, vasopressors (e.g., dopamine, epinephrine) can stimulate myocardial contractility and cause vasoconstriction supporting blood pressure and cardiac output. If refractory hypotension exists, various combinations of vasoactive infusions may be necessary. In the hypotensive and bradycardic patient, administer atropine.

6. Serum calcium levels must be monitored closely while treatment continues. In addition, other electrolytes must be serially monitored, including potassium, magnesium, and serum glucose levels. No absolute change in the quantity of the patient's calcium stores occurs, but there is a change in the distribution of calcium stores.

F. Chloroquine

Chloroquine is used to treat malaria and rarely for other medical conditions, such as rheumatoid arthritis. It is rapidly absorbed and has a narrow therapeutic margin. Exposures are unintentional in children, suicidal in adults, and a result of therapeutic error in all ages (i.e., taking the drug daily rather than weekly, as indicated). There is no antidote and no therapy has been proved to be effective for patients with severe chloroquine poisoning, which is usually fatal. Overdoses are infrequent, but apnea, hypotension, seizures, cardiorespiratory collapse, and death can occur within 30 to 60 minutes after ingestion.

1. The toxic dose of chloroquine overlaps the therapeutic dose. Chloroquine poisoning in children, although infrequent, is extremely dangerous because of the narrow margin between therapeutic and toxic doses. Children have died after ingestion of less than 300 mg.

2. If a patient survives to reach the ICU, treatment includes activated charcoal (and possibly a cathartic) if not already administered, and vigorous symptomatic and supportive respiratory, cardiac, and neurologic care. Epinephrine and diazepam are the drugs of choice for cardiac effects and seizures. Close monitoring of electrolytes is necessary. Patients are often hypokalemic.

G. Digitalis/Digoxin

Digoxin is a purified cardiac glycoside similar to digitoxin extracted from the foxglove plant. Digoxin overdoses in the pediatric population are usually acute, although chronic intoxication may occur. Children may have access to their own drugs or those of family members. Pediatric therapeutic doses must be carefully calculated and measured, and blood levels must be carefully monitored. Some plants contain cardiac glycosides with digitalis-like effects if ingested, including purple foxglove (*Digitalis purpurea*) and oleander (*Nerium oleander*). Poisoning by these plants is treated the same as digitalis poisoning.

1. Digitalis usually is absorbed rapidly and excreted renally.

2. The toxic effects of digitalis are exacerbations of therapeutic effects. Digitalis interferes with the Na^+–K^+–ATPase pump, found in smooth muscle and abundantly in cardiac tissue. Therapeutically, this maintains the correct proportions of intracellular and interstitial sodium, potassium, and calcium necessary for cellular contraction and nodal conduction. When the Na^+–K^+–ATPase pump is poisoned by toxic concentrations of digitalis, intracellular calcium levels rise, intracellular potassium is depleted, and serum potassium levels become markedly elevated. However, patients may present with hypokalemia when digitalis is administered chronically in conjunction with diuretics. Any and every dysrhythmia can result. Atrial dysrhythmias, bradycardia, and heart block are most common, along with ventricular irritability and hypotension.

3. A toxic dose can be estimated by history, but there is no substitute for laboratory evaluation of serum levels and careful evaluation of the patient. The therapeutic trough range is 0.5 to 2 ng/mL, but toxicity can occur within this range.

4. Clinical effects of acute overdose occur in the GI and cardiovascular systems: nausea, vomiting, hypotension, bradycardia, and dysrhythmias. In chronic overdose, visual changes are also described, especially yellow or green "halos" or "hazes." Laboratory evaluation of electrolytes, especially potassium, and renal function is needed, along with the serum digitalis level. Continuous ECG monitoring is essential.

5. Treatment of digitalis overdose includes prevention of absorption, intensive monitoring, administration of the antidote, and symptomatic and supportive care.

    a. GI tract decontamination may be indicated, particularly if there is a delay in obtaining the antidote digoxin immune Fab, with administration of MDAC to enhance clearance of digitoxin.

    b. Usual measures are indicated to treat bradycardia and other dysrhythmias, hypotension, and hyperkalemia.

    c. Administration of the antidote, digoxin immune Fab, quickly reverses severe hyperkalemia and life-threatening dysrhythmias. Care must be taken when administering the antidote in patients who are chronically treated with digoxin, as the reversal can lead to the occurrence of the underlying cardiac condition or arrhythmia. IV administration of 40 mg of digoxin immune Fab fragments (one vial) binds approximately 0.5 mg of digitalis. The poison center can help to make other dose determinations if the amount of ingested digitalis is not available. Patients with renal failure may need dialysis to remove the digoxin immune Fab complex.

d. If the antidote is not available, standard but aggressive treatment is needed to treat hyperkalemia (insulin, glucose, and sodium bicarbonate), support blood pressure, and treat dysrhythmias. Patients in renal failure require dialysis to remove digitalis.

e. Monitoring serum digoxin levels can be confusing after antidote administration, as some laboratory methods measure and report a concentration that includes both free digitalis and that bound to Fab. It is necessary to know whether reported digitalis levels are of free digitalis only. This is especially important for patients treated therapeutically with digitalis who must remain digitalized. Consultation with a cardiologist should occur for these patients.

H. Diphenoxylate and Atropine

Diphenoxylate–atropine combinations (e.g., Lomotil) are used to treat diarrhea in adults. There is no safe amount of this drug for young children. This is a category of products with the potential to cause life-threatening toxicity or death in a child younger than 2 years of age, despite the ingestion of only one or two tablets or sips. The combination of powerful opioid and anticholinergic effects is the reason for both its therapeutic usefulness in adults and its danger in young children.

1. The anticholinergic effects of atropine cause this drug to be retained in the GI tract for prolonged periods. The onset of opioid effects can be delayed for as long as 24 hours after ingestion.

2. Every child who ingests any amount of this drug must be monitored for 24 hours, ideally in an ICU setting, especially when symptomatic.

3. Treatment includes GI tract decontamination, symptomatic and supportive care, and careful monitoring for the onset of CNS and respiratory depression induced by diphenoxylate, the opioid component of this drug. Naloxone is effective for symptoms of opioid overdose.

I. Oral Hypoglycemic Agents

The mechanism of action of sulfonylureas or oral hypoglycemic agents, including glyburide and glipizide, results in increased insulin production, and can cause the delayed onset of significant hypoglycemia in children, even in single-tablet ingestions. Every young child who swallows even one of these pills requires GI tract decontamination when presenting early after ingestion and admission, with hourly serum glucose determinations, for 24 hours. If hypoglycemia occurs, treat with IV dextrose. Glucagon may be ineffective because small children have little stored glycogen. Octreotide, whose mechanism of action is theorized to suppress insulin release, may be administered to stabilize serum glucose in conjunction with dextrose infusion to prevent hypoglycemia.

J. Imidazoline Derivatives

Clonidine, like many other imidazoline derivatives, is usually thought of as a selective α_2-adrenergic agonist and is approved for use as a centrally acting antihypertensive, in addition to ocular and nasal vasoconstrictors as tetrahydrozoline, naphazoline, and oxymetazoline. All are α_2-agonists with mixed central and peripheral effects. A single tablet of clonidine, inadvertent application of even a used clonidine patch, or just several drops of the other drugs can cause the onset of coma, respiratory depression, and hypotension within 30 minutes of ingestion (or topical application for liquid vasoconstrictors and decongestants). GI tract decontamination is indicated for solid dosage forms with activated charcoal if the patient presents within 1 hour of ingestion and prior to symptoms. Symptomatic and supportive care is required for 24 to 36 hours, and a full recovery is expected.

K. Iron

Iron in the form of adult-strength supplements and prenatal vitamins with iron cause dangerous overdose in children younger than 6 years of age. Prescription-strength preparations may contain 60 to 65 mg of elemental iron per tablet, although some contain more than 100 mg of elemental iron. Fatalities in children from iron poisoning have declined because over-the-counter preparations now usually contain less than 30 mg of elemental iron per tablet. Overdoses of children's chewable multiple vitamins with iron may cause iron toxicity, but they have not been associated with iron-related fatalities in children. Iron supplements are sometimes used in suicide attempts by others, especially pregnant teenagers. The use of deferoxamine, a specific antidote, is important but may be limited in serious iron poisoning because of side effects, especially hypotension.

1. In overdose, iron causes significant corrosive injury to the GI tract. Absorption of iron is thus enhanced. Circulating free iron injures blood vessels and damages hepatocytes. As iron is metabolized, free hydrogen is released; in concert with other events, this produces metabolic acidosis.

2. Mild symptoms may occur with ingestion of more than 20 mg/kg of essential iron. Significant toxicity or death is possible with ingestions of more than 60 mg/kg; this amount of iron can be ingested by a 10-kg child who swallows just 10 typical prescription-strength adult preparations. The amount of essential iron in each iron salt varies; the potential risk is calculated by determining the iron salt and the amount of essential iron in each preparation, the number of pills missing, and the child's body weight. Actual risk is determined by serum iron levels and the presence or absence of symptoms.

3. The course of severe iron poisoning is typically described in five sequential phases, although individual patients may not always demonstrate each of the phases. There is no universal agreement as to number of phases or times assigned to those phases.

   a. Phase I usually occurs within the first 6 hours after ingestion, includes GI tract symptoms, possibly severe, consisting of hemorrhagic gastritis, vomiting, hematemesis, diarrhea, lethargy, and pallor. A patient is unlikely to develop significant systemic toxicity without first having GI symptoms. In severe cases, the GI losses of blood and fluid may be massive and lead to shock and coma.

   b. Phase II is a latent phase occurring about 6 to 12 hours after ingestion, during which the patient is asymptomatic or demonstrates an improvement in symptoms, especially when supportive care was initiated during phase I. The systemic insults described in phase I continue during this asymptomatic phase, and the patient abruptly enters phase III in serious ingestions. The only findings on examination may be lethargy, mild tachycardia, or tachypnea.

   c. Phase III occurs about 12 to about 24 hours after ingestion, involves a rapid onset of cardiovascular collapse and multisystem damage. Hypotension, marked metabolic acidosis, increasing lethargy and coma, seizures, pulmonary edema, hepatorenal failure with coagulopathies, shock, and hypoglycemia occur due to mitochondrial damage and hepatocellular injury.

   d. Phase IV occurs 2 to 3 days postingestion and is characterized by hepatic injury. Death may occur rapidly or after days or weeks of complications, including intestinal necrosis.

   e. Phase V occurs 2 to 6 weeks postingestion and is characterized by late scarring of the GI tract, which causes pyloric obstruction or hepatic cirrhosis. However, these complications are rare, even in severe cases.

4. Assessment of these patients includes careful evaluation of physical findings and laboratory results. Determine the nature of any symptoms and the time of onset compared with the time of ingestion.

   a. *Initial laboratory studies* include an ideal serum iron level, which is a peak level at 2 to 6 hours after ingestion, complete blood count (CBC), and electrolytes. Patients with more than mild GI tract symptoms also require ABG analysis and baseline hepatic and renal function studies. Typing and crossmatch are indicated if there is frank bleeding or guaiac-positive stools.

   b. *Iron tablets* (not pediatric chewable vitamins with iron) are radiopaque. An abdominal radiograph may permit counting of tablets in the child's GI tract, but a negative image cannot be used to rule out iron ingestion.

5. Treatment of the iron-poisoned child includes GI tract decontamination, chelation with deferoxamine, and symptomatic and supportive care.

   a. *GI tract decontamination* may include WBI. If an abdominal radiograph demonstrates iron pills in the intestinal tract, WBI is used until the appropriate number of pills is counted in the rectal effluent or until a repeat radiographic examination documents that the pills have been removed. Iron is not adsorbed to activated charcoal.

   b. *Chelation* is indicated if the serum iron level is greater than 350 mcg/dL in the presence of symptoms, or if the serum iron is greater than 500 mcg/dL. Deferoxamine is administered IV. The intramuscular route may be used only when severe symptoms are not present. The usual dose of deferoxamine is 15 mg/kg/hr. Higher doses are sometimes used but may be associated with hypotension. "Vin rosé-"colored urine, is a marker for elimination of deferoxamine-iron chelate, but this does not always appear and is not always reliable. Serum iron levels are more accurate.

   c. *Serum iron levels* must be repeated until it is certain that levels are dropping and that there is not a concretion, or clump, of iron tablets being slowly absorbed from the GI tract.

   d. *Symptomatic and supportive care* is required with aggressive measures to stop GI tract bleeding, correct hypovolemia and hypotension, and treat coagulopathies and other consequences of hepatic failure. After the acute phase passes, the patient will require follow-up with gastroenterology to monitor for GI obstruction secondary to strictures and scarring.

   e. *Iron poisoning* is associated with two special dangers. Parents and healthcare providers often think of iron as "just" a vitamin and are ignorant of the fact that quite small amounts of this essential element can cause fatalities in children. Second, the asymptomatic latent phase of iron poisoning fools parents and healthcare providers who misinterpret the absence of symptoms as absence of risk.

L. Isoniazid

Isoniazid (INH) is used to treat tuberculosis. Young children may have access to the drug, and it is used in suicide attempts by teenagers.

1. INH, given therapeutically or taken in overdose, depletes the body of pyridoxine (vitamin B_6). Pyridoxine is a cofactor in numerous enzymatic reactions, including those responsible for the generation of GABA. GABA is an inhibitory neurotransmitter in the CNS and the depletion leads to seizures.

2. An overdose of INH can precipitate depressed mental status or the onset of generalized tonic–clonic seizures, potentially within 30 minutes of ingestion as it is rapidly absorbed, and the subsequent development of severe acidosis.

3. The only effective treatment for INH-induced seizures is IV pyridoxine. If the dose of INH is known, the dose of pyridoxine is a milligram-per-milligram equivalent (70 mg/kg up to 5 g). If the dose is unknown, pyridoxine 5 g IV, should be administered (Taketomo et al., 2015). Benzodiazepine (lorazepam or diazepam) is an effective adjunct as it enhances the action of GABA, but it cannot assist with synthesis of GABA and is not a substitute for pyridoxine.

4. Once seizures are controlled, GI tract decontamination utilizing activated charcoal can be considered, but is likely to be ineffective due to time elapsed. Acidosis often corrects itself once seizures are controlled, but it is amenable to the usual therapies. Treatment otherwise is symptomatic and supportive.

M. Opioids

Opioids are found in a variety of prescription preparations and illicit or street drugs. Because the ICU nurse is familiar with the administration of opioid analgesics and antitussives, this section simply emphasizes a few points related to overdose.

1. The classic triad of symptoms (miosis, respiratory depression, and coma) may be masked by concomitant administration of other drugs. Abusers of stimulant drugs, such as cocaine and amphetamines, frequently use an opioid or other depressant simultaneously. Opioids may be abused inadvertently when drug dealers substitute them for or combine them with other drugs.

2. Young children can be markedly sensitive to some opioids. Dangerous situations may occur when parents each inadvertently administer a codeine-containing antitussive.

3. Some opioids are associated with clinically significant differences:

a. *Meperidine* (*Demerol*) use or abuse is not necessarily associated with pinpoint pupils. Also, normeperidine, the first metabolite of meperidine, is a CNS stimulant; chronic use or abuse is therefore associated with seizures.

b. *Propoxyphene* (*Darvon*) and *pentazocine* (*Talwin*) may require up to 10 mg of naloxone to reverse the respiratory depression they induce, much higher than the standard naloxone dose.

c. *Methadone* has a half-life of about 24 hours, much longer than other opioids, and requires sustained doses of naloxone by IV infusion to prevent respiratory depression until the methadone is eliminated.

4. Dermal patches and oral lozenges containing fentanyl, even if they were used and discarded, are a significant risk to children who access them, for example, by retrieving them from a trash can. Discarded fentanyl patches contain sufficient residual drug to seriously poison a child who chews, swallows, or applies one to the skin.

N. Salicylate Poisoning

Salicylate poisoning is most often due to aspirin. However, most fatal salicylate poisonings in children occur from ingestion of methyl salicylate (oil of wintergreen), a rapidly absorbed liquid, and from GI tract preparations containing bismuth subsalicylate. Older children and teenagers may take aspirin in suicide attempts. Although chronic salicylate poisoning may occur on therapeutic doses, such doses are rarely used in children.

1. Aspirin is rapidly absorbed. In therapeutic doses, it has a small volume of distribution and is bound to serum proteins. It undergoes hepatic metabolism and renal excretion. With chronic administration, receptors are saturated and free salicylate accumulates rapidly.

2. The actions of salicylate in overdose are complex and interdependent. Salicylates impair cellular respiration by uncoupling oxidative phosphorylation. Stimulation of the central respiratory drive causes primary respiratory alkalosis. A primary metabolic acidosis is independently caused by salicylates, eventually becoming the primary acid–base abnormality as mitochondria are affected. Interference with carbohydrate and lipid metabolism generates organic acids and ketone formation. Increased metabolic demands result in hypoglycemia, both in the serum and the CNS. Uncoupling of oxidative phosphorylation leads to hyperthermia. Direct CNS toxicity can cause tremor, agitation, seizures, and coma. Sequence and exact clinical effects depend on size, timing, and acuity of ingestion and the age and health of the patient. A careful evaluation of each patient's status and history is essential.

3. Acute toxicity generally correlates with ingested dose. Ingestions of greater than 150 mg/kg by history may be associated with mild toxicity, moderate toxicity ingestions up to 300 mg/kg, severe toxicity with doses of 300 to 500 mg/kg and greater than 500 mg/kg with fatality. Severe poisoning include high salicylate blood levels: 7.25 mmol/L (100 mg/dL) in acute ingestions or 40 mg/dL in chronic ingestions, significant neurotoxicity (agitation, coma, convulsions), kidney failure, pulmonary edema, or cardiovascular instability. Death is often a result of pulmonary edema leading to cardiovascular collapse. Optimally, plasma levels should be assessed 4 hours after ingestion and then every 2 hours after that to allow calculation of the maximum level, which can then be used as a guide to the degree of toxicity expected.

4. In the absence of history, suspect salicylate poisoning in a patient who presents with tachypnea, tachycardia, hyperthermia, diaphoresis, mental status changes, respiratory alkalosis, metabolic acidosis, or mixed acid–base abnormalities. If present, tinnitus is an important clue, as is frank or occult GI tract bleeding.

5. Treatment objectives include cardiopulmonary stabilization, prevention of absorption, correction of fluid deficits, correction of acid–base abnormalities, and enhancement of excretion and elimination. As with all significant overdoses, ABCs should be evaluated and stabilized as necessary. Dehydration and concomitant electrolyte abnormalities must be immediately corrected. Initial treatment includes GI decontamination, followed by MDAC administered every 4 hours with a cathartic once in 24 hours if salicylate levels continue to rise. Activated charcoal can limit further gut absorption by binding to the available salicylates. MDAC may enhance salicylate elimination and may shorten the serum half-life as well as assist in treating bezoars with ongoing absorption of salicylates, which should be suspected when salicylate levels continue to rise or fail to

decrease despite appropriate treatment. Hydration is essential but must be controlled to avoid precipitating pulmonary edema. Potassium supplementation is often needed. Renal excretion of salicylic acid depends on urinary pH. Alkalinization of blood and urine enhances urinary excretion. Ion trapping may occur, as aspirin is a weak acid and ionizes when exposed to a basic environment, such as alkaline urine, and is excreted more readily. The administration of sufficient amounts of sodium bicarbonate to correct acidosis and achieve a urine pH between 7.5 and 8 enhances renal excretion of salicylate. Hemodialysis can be used to enhance the removal of salicylate from the blood and is usually used in those who are severely poisoned. Otherwise, treatment must be aggressive, but primarily is symptomatic and supportive.

6. *Special Considerations*

a. Aspirin tablets may clump together in the stomach, forming concretions, or bezoars, that may be slowly absorbed over an extended period. If a large ingestion is suspected, it is essential to measure serial salicylate levels to avert the delayed onset of fatal effects as well as with ingestion of sustained-release forms of aspirin, which can result in the delayed onset of symptoms.

b. The time between ingestion and death from salicylate poisoning can often be measured in just hours, so a high index of suspicion and aggressive management are essential to prevent serious CNS effects and fatalities.

O. Sympathomimetics

Sympathomimetic drugs are represented by both legal and illegal agents in the pediatric age group: Cocaine is a legal, useful topical vasoconstrictor and a widely abused street drug; amphetamines are used as weight-control agents, to treat hyperactivity disorders, and as the street drug "speed"; legal decongestants and appetite suppressants are sold as "street speed" or amphetamine look-alikes. Ephedra, even if it is not available legally, can be obtained via the Internet. The use of designer and over-the-counter drugs has exploded, due to Internet and social media descriptions. Over-the-counter medications, particularly those containing dextromethorphan (known as *dex*), have become popular recreational drugs among adolescents in addition to the numerous emerging synthetic compounds and herbal agents. Children are poisoned by ingesting appetite suppressants or taking an overdose of cough, cold, or allergy preparations containing decongestants and by swallowing available street drugs. Adolescents are poisoned by taking overdoses of appetite suppressants, by abusing street drugs, or by attempting to avoid arrest by swallowing illicit drugs. Hallucinogenic amphetamines (MDMA, methylenedioxyamphetamine [MDA], Ecstasy, "Adam," "Eve") are abused as "party drugs" or "rave drugs." The intended use, route of administration, and duration of action of these drugs may differ, but the acute clinical effects are indistinguishable, and treatment of acute effects is essentially the same.

1. The toxic dose is variable and may be idiosyncratic. In street drugs, the actual amount of drug, as opposed to adulterants, is unknown.

2. Clinical effects are as expected for any sympathomimetic agent: tachycardia; hypertension; diaphoresis; mydriasis; agitation and tremulousness; and central vasoconstriction, including cardiac, cerebral, and visceral effects. In significant poisoning, ventricular dysrhythmias, seizures, hyperthermia, and coma may develop. The hallucinations sought by users of "party" or "rave" drugs are accompanied by other sympathomimetic effects, especially extreme hyperthermia.

3. Clinical assessment and laboratory evaluation are straightforward. As with all significant overdoses, ABCs should be evaluated and stabilized as necessary. When unknown agents are suspected, acetaminophen and salicylate levels should be obtained as they are common coingestants. ECG should be obtained to evaluate for conduction disorders, which are common with these category of agents. Dehydration and relative hypovolemia is common so fluid hydration status needs to be assessed and corrected. If the patient has severe agitation, serum electrolytes, renal function, and CK should be evaluated as rhabdomyolysis is a potential consequence. When possible, identification of the drug involved helps to predict the duration of effects: a few hours for cocaine unless complicated by cardiac, cerebral, or other events caused by vasoconstriction, hyperthermia, or seizures; 18 to 24 hours for amphetamines, with the same caveat; variable times are needed for the other drugs and are dependent to some extent on whether they are sustained-release preparations. Although radiographic examinations are not generally indicated in poisoning by sympathomimetic drugs, in the case of swallowed illegal drugs, they may help to visualize the number and location of the packets.

4. Treatment of these poisonings includes GI tract decontamination when indicated plus symptomatic and supportive care. A single dose of activated charcoal with a cathartic is indicated unless drug packets (e.g., vials, condoms, balloons, foil) have been swallowed. In these cases, WBI may be indicated until the packets pass. If agitation is present, it can be treated with the administration of benzodiazepines. Severe hyperthermia may result secondary to muscle rigidity and needs to be treated by minimizing muscle activity. If benzodiazepines do not adequately treat agitation and muscle rigidity, intubation with a nondepolarizing neuromuscular agent, to minimize hyperkalemia and rhabdomyolysis, may be required.

P. Synthetic and Herbal Products

The emergence of numerous synthetic compounds and herbal agents has led to significant rise in use of such agents among adolescents. These emerging substances are being used for recreational purposes without any knowledge of their potential harmful effects. These new substances have resulted in significant poisoning morbidity and mortality in the pediatric population, producing acute and chronic toxicity as well as numerous deaths. Spice, a synthetic cannabinoid, first marketed as an "herbal" product, and bath salts, synthetic cathinone stimulants that mimic cocaine-type effects, are the most well-known drug trends. Both types of products were marketed and sold in gas stations and over the Internet without any age restrictions in the United States before the Drug Enforcement Agency banned possession and sale of the chemicals that were utilized in the production of these agents. Yet a whole new line of synthetic and herbal products continues to emerge, marketed along the same pathways as spice and bath salts. The constantly changing names and product chemical contents create a challenging environment for healthcare professionals to understand the products being utilized. There are limited studies to track potency or side effects because of the nature of the constantly changing chemicals and ingredients. Many individuals are utilizing alternative or synthetic drugs under the false belief that they are legal substitutes for popular street drugs and are therefore safe. The manufacturers of these synthetic drugs change the chemical content, change the names, and mark the packaging as "not intended for human consumption" or "research chemical," which does not deter individuals from using them. These emerging drugs are also more readily available through legitimate sources such as convenience stores, gas station markets, gardening/plant stores, and via the Internet.

1. The toxic dose is variable and may be idiosyncratic. In street drugs, the actual amount of drug, as opposed to adulterants, is unknown.

2. Clinical effects are wide ranging as described in Table 9.23.

TABLE 9.23 Recreational Substances

Name	Street Name(s)	Clinical Presentation	Management/Treatment
Ethanol/ethyl alcohol	"Slimming" "Butt chug" "Boozy bears" (Drunk gummies; Rummy bears) "Eyeball shots" (Vodka eyeballing) Liquid hand sanitizer "Smoking alcohol" Snorting alcohol Alcohol-infused food substances	Acute ethanol intoxication can cause the following: CNS depression Mild vasodilatation leading to a modest decrease in blood pressure Flushed skin Urticaria Hypothermia Tachycardia Myocardial depression Variable pupillary response Respiratory depression Decreased pulmonary secretion clearance Decreased sensitivity to airway foreign body Diuresis Loss of behavior inhibitions Hypoglycemia Loss of fine motor control	Supportive care; correction of dehydration; correction of hypoglycemia
Synthetic cannabinoid receptor agonists	Spice, K2	Agitation, anxiety, paranoia, tachycardia, hypertension, muscle spasms, seizures, dystonia, diaphoresis, tremors, psychosis	Aggressive supportive care; benzodiazepines (lorazepam) for agitation and seizures; EEG if seizures are present or unexplained altered mental status; serial cardiac enzymes if chest pain present
Synthetic cathinone stimulants Mephedrone Methylone MDPV MDMA[a]	Bath salts, Ivory Wave, Vanilla Sky, Meow- Meow, Bliss, Molly, Ecstasy, E, Rolls, Beans	Agitation, insomnia, irritability, dizziness, depression, paranoia, delusions, seizures, panic attacks	Intravenous fluids and benzodiazepines; supportive care
Dextromethorphan	DXM, Skittles, Robo, Robotripping	*Nausea*, vomiting, nystagmus, dilated pupils, rash, ataxia, diaphoresis, fever, hypertension, bradypnea, urinary retention, diarrhea, tachycardia, hyperthermia, toxic psychosis, coma	Administer activated charcoal if presents in less than 1 hour after ingestion; naloxone may be administered for sedation and coma; evaluate for toxic effects of coingested drugs; supportive care
Salvia (*Salvia divinorum*)	Maria pastora, magic mint, diviner's sage, sally-D, sage of the seers	Subtle high to vivid psychedelic experience, including hallucinations, slurred speech, incoordination, psychomimetic experiences similar to psychosis, visual disturbances, dysphoria, mood swings, altered perception of self	Supportive care, symptoms short lived—up to 3 hours, administer benzodiazepines if combative

(continued)

TABLE 9.23 Recreational Substances *(continued)*

Name	Street Name(s)	Clinical Presentation	Management/Treatment
Energy drinks Caffeine and supplements	Red Bull Monster Rockstar 5-hr energy AMP	Contains caffeine and other energy-promoting substances (i.e., guarana) that result in CNS excitation, seizures, tachycardia, ventricular dysrhythmias; hypokalemia, hyperglycemia, vomiting, death	Benzodiazepines for agitation and seizures; dysrhythmias treated with beta-adrenergic blockers or lidocaine; correction of hypokalemia; concomitant ethanol intoxication is a real concern and requires supportive care and any other symptoms need to be addressed; ondansetron for vomiting; hemodialysis if indicated

CNS, central nervous system; MDMA, 3,4-methylenedioxymethamphetamine; MDPV, methylenedioxy-pyrovalerone.

[a]MDMA also commonly referred to as Ecstasy, Molly, E, X, Beans.

Source: Adapted from Madden, M. A. (2015). Pediatric toxicology: Emerging trends. *Journal of Pediatric Intensive Care, 4*, 103–110.

3. Clinical assessment and laboratory evaluation are straightforward. When possible, identification of the drug involved helps to predict the duration of effects.

4. Treatment of these poisonings includes GI tract decontamination when indicated and then aggressive symptomatic and supportive care.

POISONING BY NONPHARMACEUTICAL AGENTS

A. Carbon Monoxide

Carbon monoxide is a colorless, odorless, tasteless, nonirritating, and highly toxic gas. It is a major product of the incomplete combustion of carbon and carbon-containing compounds. The most common residential sources are house fires, exhaust from automobiles and gas-powered equipment, furnaces, space heaters, wood- and coal-burning stoves and fireplaces, gas ovens, and hot water heaters. Methylene chloride, found in paint strippers, is metabolized to carbon monoxide after ingestion, inhalation, or dermal absorption.

1. Carbon monoxide has an affinity for hemoglobin 200 times greater than that of oxygen. Besides displacing oxygen at hemoglobin receptor sites, it inhibits the release of oxygen from hemoglobin. Therefore inadequate amounts of oxygen are circulating, and that which is circulating is less available to tissues.

2. The effects of carbon monoxide poisoning are related to hypoxemia and the resultant direct tissue hypoxia; the greater the amount of carboxyhemoglobin, which is a stable complex of carbon monoxide that forms in RBCs when carbon monoxide is inhaled, the more severe the symptoms. Direct cellular toxicity also occurs. A carboxyhemoglobin level of about 10% may be associated with headache, nausea, and lethargy. As the carboxyhemoglobin level increases, GI tract and CNS symptoms increase. At a level of 50% the patient is unconscious, and victims of carbon monoxide exposure die at levels of about 70% or greater. Symptoms of chronic carbon monoxide exposure (e.g., due to malfunctioning furnaces or clogged chimneys) are often mistaken for a viral or flulike illness.

3. Evaluating victims of carbon monoxide poisoning requires close attention to symptoms experienced at any time since exposure, not just at the time of evaluation. Standard pulse oximetry, as with methemoblobin, cannot distinguish between carboxyhemoglobin and oxyhemoglobin. The carboxyhemoglobin level at the time of presentation may have declined markedly since the patient was exposed. Carboxyhemoglobin is measured via either arterial or venous blood, to assess lactate and acid–base status as measures of tissue hypoxia. Arterial blood is preferred for the diagnosis of carbon monoxide poisoning due to its precision in assessment of acidosis, especially lactic acidosis, which affects the assessment of the severity and management of carbon monoxide poisoning An ECG should be obtained to evaluate for myocardial ischemia. Cherry-red skin is a hallmark finding associated with carbon monoxide poisoning. After an acute exposure to carbon monoxide, those who have lost consciousness, even if they are now awake, and fetuses are at greatest risk.

4. The initial treatment for carbon monoxide poisoning is administration of 100% oxygen. Carbon monoxide elimination occurs primarily via the pulmonary circulation by competitive binding of hemoglobin to oxygen. The rate of elimination is related proportionally to the degree of oxygenation, atmospheric conditions, and minute ventilation. The half-life of carbon monoxide is approximately 300 minutes in an individual breathing room air. The application of high-flow oxygen via a nonrebreather mask can reduce the half-life to approximately 80 minutes. Hyperbaric oxygen, which has a pressure three times atmospheric pressure, reduces the half-life even further to approximately 20 to 30 minutes and is indicated for those who were or are unconscious, pregnant women, those who remain symptomatic after oxygen administration, those who have severe metabolic acidosis, concern for end-organ ischemia, and those with recurrent symptoms. Hyperbaric oxygen may improve tissue oxygenation by bypassing the normal transfer of oxygen via hemoglobin (Weaver, 2009).

5. Other treatment is primarily symptomatic and supportive.

6. *Special Considerations*

a. Children and household pets are at greatest risk for carbon monoxide poisoning because of their rapid respiratory and metabolic rates. When a family is poisoned by carbon monoxide, children are generally more seriously ill.

b. *Aggressive treatment* is required because long-term neuropsychiatric sequelae have been documented in adults with carbon monoxide exposure. Because of the difficulty or impossibility of conducting and interpreting such tests in children, long-term sequelae are postulated but not documented.

c. Consider carbon monoxide poisoning in any family or gathering in which a number of people become ill with GI and CNS complaints.

d. Unless the source of carbon monoxide is known (e.g., a suicide attempt with automobile exhaust, house fire) or remedied (e.g., repair of a faulty furnace), patients and their families must not return to a possibly contaminated environment.

e. Encourage the installation of carbon monoxide alarms in dwellings intended for human occupancy. Some individual states have mandated placement of carbon monoxide alarms in certain types of dwellings.

B. Caustic Substances

Caustic substances are strong acids or alkalis that cause chemical burns on the tissues that come in contact with the substance. Young children are injured by unintentional contact with household substances, especially with improper storage, whereas older children may ingest these substances in suicide attempts. Occasionally children are exposed when they attempt unsupervised experiments. Although the sources and mechanisms of injury are different, treatment and nursing care for both are essentially the same for both acids and alkalis. The single exception is hydrofluoric acid, which is considered separately.

Over the past 10 years, there has been an increase in ingestion incidence of a specific caustic substance, the button battery cell. There are four main types of button cell: mercury, silver, alkaline manganese, and lithium. Although these cells are sealed, they contain corrosive and toxic chemicals. The most serious injuries are usually associated with 20-mm-diameter batteries, about the size of a nickel, as they are likely to get lodged in a small child's esophagus. Lodgment in the esophagus can lead to tissue injury, with mucosal damage and necrosis within hours and with exposure to gastric acid there is a remote risk of leakage of the cell contents leading to perforation or death (Litovitz, Whitaker, Clark, White, & Marsolek, 2010).

1. *Sources*

a. Acids, such as sulfuric acid, hydrochloric acid, and muriatic acid (dilute hydrochloric acid), are found in toilet bowl cleaners, swimming pool chemicals, metal cleaners, and concrete and masonry cleaners. These products tend to be liquids and after ingestion are usually associated with greater injury to the stomach than to the esophagus.

b. Alkaline substances are liquids or solids found in wet cement, drain openers, oven cleaners, laundry detergent packets/pods, and automatic dishwasher detergent. Examples include sodium hydroxide, potassium hydroxide, calcium hydroxide, sodium carbonate, and some phosphates. Children who bite into ammonia capsules are likely to develop an alkaline burn on the tip of the tongue.

2. *Mechanism of Injury*

   a. Acids precipitate proteins and dehydrate tissues; exposure causes vascular thrombosis and the rapid formation of eschar. This hard crust helps to limit further penetration of acid into tissue. In general, serious injury is associated with exposure to products with a pH less than 2.

   b. Alkaline substances cause vascular thrombosis and liquefaction necrosis. They disrupt cell walls and combine with lipids, which accounts for the soapy appearance of tissue and provides no protection whatsoever from further penetration of the chemical into tissue. In general, serious injury is associated with products with a pH higher than 12.

3. The degree of injury is determined by several factors. In addition to pH, the physical form of the substance may influence toxicity: liquid products transit the oropharynx and esophagus quickly and may cause the greatest injury to the stomach. However, a very viscous liquid may cause significantly greater injury. Solids and crystals are associated with injury to the lips, mouth, oropharynx, and esophagus. Duration of contact with tissue also influences the extent of injury. The presence of food and liquid in the stomach minimizes the amount and duration of contact between the caustic substance and the gastric mucosa.

4. Ocular and dermal exposure to caustic substances requires copious irrigation with saline or water. If there are any symptoms after irrigation, ocular exposures to caustic substances require ophthalmologic consultation. After initial irrigation, dermal exposures to caustic substances are treated as thermal burns.

5. After ingestion of a caustic product, there is no strict correlation between the presence or absence of symptoms (including pain) and presence, location, or degree of injury.

   a. Mild effects of inflammation and irritation without blistering require only symptomatic and supportive care.

   b. Partial- or full-thickness injuries occur when the substance burns through the epidermis with partial thickness and down through the dermis with full thickness. With ingestion of an acid (typically a liquid), there is risk of gastric perforation within about 3 days of ingestion.

Otherwise, the risk of perforation is greatest during the granulation phase, perhaps up to 2 weeks. Then the development of scar tissue and esophageal stricture commences.

   c. Initial pain may be oral, substernal, or epigastric.

6. Assessment of the patient during the initial exposure includes visual inspection of exposed tissue, evaluation of acid–base and fluid and electrolyte status, determination of hemoglobin and hematocrit, and perhaps radiographic examinations to determine the presence or absence of free air.

7. *Treatment*

   a. Dilution is not recommended due to the risk of aspiration as well as lack of efficacy. Neutralizing or buffering agents are contraindicated due to the risk of vomiting, causing esophageal reinjury, and the possibility of aspiration. In addition, the risk of heat injury associated with the neutralization process prohibits the use of these agents.

   b. *Observe for respiratory distress*. Soft-tissue swelling and aspiration of caustic material can contribute to respiratory difficulty. If significant edema is present, oral or nasotracheal intubation is dangerous, and a tracheotomy or cricothyrotomy is needed.

   c. Observe for signs of fluid and electrolyte imbalance to evaluate loss of fluids or third-spacing of fluids.

   d. Observe for acidosis if the patient has ingested a large quantity of an acid, as may occur in a suicide attempt. Although direct injury is generally confined to points of contact with the chemical, acidosis is one possible systemic manifestation associated with acid ingestion.

   e. Esophagoscopy and endoscopy may be indicated. If the initial injury is thought to be severe or if circumferential burns are found on esophagoscopy, additional surgical procedures may be indicated. The surgical procedures that may be indicated include gastrectomy to remove necrotic tissue, insertion of a string or stent in the esophogus, or insertion of a gastric feeding tube. Esophagectomy and colonic interposition (removing the esophagus and replacing it with a length of the patient's own colon) may also be performed.

   f. The use of steroids is controversial and depends upon the severity of injury and may be utilized based on the preference and experience of individual treating physicians. Steroids may decrease the formation of restrictive scar tissue after circumferential burns but may also weaken tissue and predispose the patient to infection.

g. Antibiotics are prescribed for patients taking steroids and for patients with specific indications.

h. Observe the patient for signs of perforation and sepsis. Perforation may be accompanied by abdominal distention and a change in the amount or character of the patient's pain.

i. Analgesics are indicated.

j. Patients must remain NPO (taking nothing by mouth) until esophagoscopy is performed.

8. *Special Considerations*

a. Until the patient is decontaminated, healthcare providers must protect themselves with appropriate personal protective equipment to avoid contact with caustic materials.

b. If the patient has sustained a serious injury, psychosocial considerations for the patient and the family come to the forefront. Ocular and dermal exposures may cause significant disfigurement, and ocular exposures may result in permanent blindness. Poisoning with significant injury means that the patient may require permanent tracheostomy or gastrostomy or both, major surgery and follow-up for esophagectomy and colonic interposition, or regular esophageal dilation, for many years to come. Also, the risk of developing cancer at the site of the injury, although delayed for decades, is greater than in the general population.

9. Hydrofluoric acid is different from other caustic agents in that it is absorbed dermally, even through intact skin, and can cause both local and systemic effects. It is used industrially to etch glass and computer chips, as a cleaning agent for metals and air-conditioning units, and as a rust remover. Products with low, but potentially dangerous concentrations of hydrofluoric acid, are sold for home use as rust removers and metal brighteners. Hydrofluoric acid is toxic by all routes of exposure, but dermal exposure is the most common.

a. In concentrations above 50%, hydrofluoric acid causes immediate local tissue injury along with significant pain. In concentrations between 20% and 50%, the onset of local injury and pain

can be delayed for 8 hours or longer. In concentrations lower than 20%, the effects of exposure may not be evident for 24 hours.

b. Hydrofluoric acid is absorbed through the skin and precipitates both calcium and magnesium with resulting intense pain at the exposure site. With significant exposure, systemic hypocalcemia, hypomagnesemia, hyperkalemia, and possibly fatal ventricular dysrhythmias are present.

c. Initial treatment is copious irrigation with running water, even in the absence of local effects. With exposure to the hands, subungual concentrations of hydrofluoric acid may be difficult to remove and often necessitate removal or splitting of the nails or injection of calcium.

d. Local pain is treated with a calcium gluconate gel, prepared by mixing 3.5 g of calcium gluconate powder in 5 oz of water-soluble gel (Taketomo et al., 2015), and is applied to painful areas until the pain subsides. When pain recurs, additional gel is applied. The patient should apply the gel liberally at home if pain recurs and return for further care if the gel ceases to be effective.

e. More serious exposures may be treated with subcutaneous, IV, or intra-arterial infusions of calcium gluconate. Even minimal dermal exposure to high concentrations of hydrofluoric acid may cause systemic hypocalcemia. These patients must be admitted to monitored beds, and serial calcium levels must be closely monitored until adverse effects are corrected.

C. Cyanide

Cyanide is thought of as a fast-acting lethal poison, but in some circumstances a slower onset of symptoms is possible. Treatment involves aggressive supportive care and the rapid administration of amyl nitrite, sodium nitrite, and sodium thiosulfate, packaged as a cyanide antidote kit or hydroxocobalamin.

1. There are many potential sources of cyanide poisoning. Victims of fires may develop cyanide poisoning along with carbon monoxide poisoning. A number of plant seeds (apples, peaches, plums, pears, nectarines, and cherries) contain amygdalin, which generates hydrogen cyanide after ingestion. Laetrile, an ineffective treatment for cancer, is derived from apricot kernels and has caused death from cyanide poisoning. Cyanide is a metabolite of nitroprusside; rapid or prolonged treatment can cause symptoms of cyanide poisoning. Nonoccupational cyanide poisoning in adults and teenagers is likely to result from suicidal ingestion of laboratory or photographic chemicals. Children have died rapidly after swallowing professional jewelry-cleaning solutions containing cyanide. Acetonitrile, which is metabolized to cyanide, is found in liquids used to dissolve artificial fingernail glue; delayed onset of symptoms and death have occurred when this was swallowed.

2. Cyanide binds with ferric iron contained within cytochrome oxidase, impairing adenosine triphosphate (ATP) production and thereby aerobic metabolism and cellular utilization of oxygen results in anoxic tissue injury. Other metalloenzyme systems are affected as well.

3. The toxic dose depends on the form of the chemical and route of administration, but toxic effects are usually severe. Small amounts of cyanide salts can cause rapid loss of consciousness and death. Toxicity develops more slowly with cyanide ingestion than inhalation because absorption takes longer. Substances that are metabolized to cyanide (e.g., amygdalin glycosides, acetonitrile, nitroprusside) have a delayed onset of action, and the toxic dose is variable.

4. Clinical effects are related to hypoxia and typically progress within minutes from dizziness and headache to coma and death. Severe lactic acidosis from tissue hypoxia and hypotension are prominent. The high anion gap metabolic acidosis, high lactate, and elevated mixed venous saturation suggest cyanide toxicity in patients who are at risk. Patients with lesser exposures and those exposed to substances that must be metabolized have a less precipitous onset of symptoms.

5. ABGs must be followed closely in addition to serum electrolytes and lactate. If possible, measuring mixed venous saturation may be helpful. Depending upon the exposure route, co-oximetry to measure carboxyhemoglobin and methemoglobin may be beneficial to determine whether there is a concomitant exposure. Cyanide can be measured in serum, but levels cannot be returned in time to be useful for acutely poisoned patients.

6. Antidote treatment is initiated for patients with known cyanide poisoning and serious clinical effects. In the United States, there are now several types of cyanide antidotes available. The Cyanide Antidote Kit, a three-part cyanide antidote kit, contains amyl nitrite, sodium nitrite, and sodium thiosulfate. This combination of agents is now available as the branded Cyanide Antidote Package or as the generic cyanide antidote kit. Nithiodote, recently approved by FDA, contains sodium nitrite and sodium thiosulfate and is only used in situations deemed life-threatening. In 2006, FDA approved hydroxocobalamin, a novel cyanide antidote, available as the branded Cyanokit.

   a. *Hydroxocobalamin or vitamin B_{12a},* detoxifies cyanide and forms cyanocobalamin, which is renally excreted. Hydroxocobalamin is an appealing cyanide antidote because it is relatively safe, does not compromise the blood's oxygen-carrying capacity, and, unlike the nitrites or sodium thiosulfate, does not produce hypotension. The empiric adult dose of hydroxocobalamin is 5 g, which can be infused over a period of 15 minutes, with the infusion repeated if necessary; the pediatric dose is 70 mg/kg, up to a maximum of the adult dose, administered at the same infusion rate (Taketomo et al., 2015). Hydroxocobalamin is known to cause a reddish discoloration of the urine that typically resolves within 48 hours.

The mechanism of action of amyl nitrite and sodium nitrite as antidotes for cyanide poisoning is to produce methemoglobinemia and vasodilation. Vasodilation may contribute to their therapeutic and adverse effects. If the Cyanide Antidote Kit is used: methemoglobin is first induced with nitrites; cyanmethemoglobin is formed as cyanide and is thus removed from cytochrome oxidase. Rhodanese, an endogenous enzyme, then facilitates the formation of thiocyanate, a much less toxic metabolite, which is renally excreted. Administration of sodium thiosulfate results in the formation of relatively nontoxic thiocyanate.

   b. *Amyl nitrite ampules* are broken, placed in a cloth, and held in front of the patient's mouth for 15 of 30 seconds, then repeated until vascular access is obtained. This permits the formation of about 5% methemoglobin. This step may be skipped in favor of immediate administration of IV sodium nitrite.

   c. *Sodium nitrite* induces the formation of additional methemoglobin. Clinical response to sodium nitrate administration has been seen with methemoglobin levels of less than 10%. Methemoglobin concentrations should be closely monitored and maintained less than 30% and generally discontinued when levels exceed 30%. In children, the amount of sodium nitrite is calculated according to body weight and titrated to actual hemoglobin levels. Doses must be carefully calculated because inducing too high a level of methemoglobinemia worsens hypoxia. High levels cannot be treated with methylene blue because to do so would liberate free cyanide.

d. Administration of *sodium thiosulfate* results in the formation of thiocyanate, which is eliminated renally.

e. Treatment also includes respiratory support and symptomatic and supportive care.

f. Patients with a known cyanide exposure but without clinical effects are treated with sodium thiosulfate component alone if not using hydroxocobalamin.

7. *Special Considerations*

a. Too high a level of *methemoglobin* can itself be fatal. Neither carboxyhemoglobin nor methemoglobin is capable of carrying oxygen, so such patients can develop functional hypoxia. Pediatric doses of nitrites must be carefully calculated, and methemoglobin levels must be monitored.

b. If neurologic criteria for death is met by a patient with cyanide poisoning he or she may be considered a potential organ donor.

D. Envenomations

Envenomations by snakes and spiders will not be considered in depth. Always consult the poison center when treating a patient with a snake or spider bite. All venoms are extremely complex mixtures; any bite resulting in symptoms indicates a poisoning with the potential for serious multisystem effects. Children are at greater risk than adults because of their small body size in relationship to the amount of venom injected.

1. The venom of the Crotalinae (rattlesnakes, copperheads, and cottonmouths [water moccasins]) can cause the rapid onset of life-threatening effects, although this is not expected with bites of copperheads and cottonmouths. Action at numerous venom receptors results in hypotension, increased capillary permeability resulting in local ecchymosis and edema, pulmonary edema, local tissue injury, myocardial injury, and bleeding and clotting disorders. Local wound care and intensive supportive care are both essential. Definitive antidotal treatment is the administration of antivenin; Crotalidae Polyvalent Immune Fab (Ovine [CroFab]) is an antigen-binding fragment antivenin derived from sheep and has superseded equine polyvalent crotalid antivenin as the treatment for

crotalid envenomations. Patients are eligible for therapy with Crotalidae Polyvalent Immune Fab (Ovine) if they have moderate envenomation, severe envenomation, or any degree of envenomation with progression of the envenomation syndrome. As the antivenin dose reflects venom size, not patient size, the FDA recommends the same initial and subsequent doses for pediatric patients. There is no substitute for administration of sufficient quantities of antivenin in a patient poisoned by a rattlesnake. With the reduced side effect profile of antigen-binding fragment antivenin and the improvement in tissue injury with antivenin administration, the threshold for dosing is lower. Common treatment errors include withholding antivenin in a patient with a life- or limb-threatening envenomation for fear of allergic reactions and performing fasciotomy in lieu of administering sufficient antivenin in patients with peripheral edema. The patient should be monitored for signs of an allergic reaction (hives, urticaria, erythema; wheezing, respiratory distress; edema of face, lips, tongue, or throat) to the antivenin during administration. Late coagulopathy has been reported after using Crotalidae Polyvalent Immune Fab (Ovine).

2. The venom of the Elapidae (the coral snakes) tends to have significant neurotoxicity, inducing neuromuscular dysfunction and can cause fatal poisoning specifically by respiratory muscle paralysis. Onset of symptoms may be delayed for 10 to 12 hours after envenomation. Fortunately, such fatalities are extremely rare. Treatment is directed at stabilization and respiratory support. In the United States, production of coral snake antivenin has ceased. The FDA had extended the expiration date for North American Coral Snake Antivenin through April 30, 2017. After this time, unless stock remains and the expiration date is further extended, there will be no commercially available coral snake antivenin.

3. The venom of the black widow spider (*Latrodectus mactans*) produces protein venom that affects the victim's nervous system. This neurotoxic protein is one of the most potent venoms secreted by an animal. Some people are slightly affected by the venom, but others may have a severe response. The first symptom is acute pain at the site of the bite, although there may only be a minimal local reaction. Symptoms usually start within 20 minutes to 1 hour after the bite and can cause paralysis of respiratory muscles, although this is not usual. The most common symptoms are immediate, intense local pain at the site of the bite (which can be identified by two tiny fang marks, about 0.5 cm [¼ in] apart); muscle weakness, ataxia, and ptosis, especially in children; and intensely painful muscle contractions and diaphoresis in the affected limb, across the abdomen for lower-extremity bites and across the back and shoulders for upper-extremity bites. Treatment includes administration of narcotic analgesics and a benzodiazepine. Antivenin is available, but its use is usually required only for severe systemic effects.

E. Ethanol

Ethanol is found in alcoholic beverages, mouthwash, and cosmetics such as perfumes, tonics, and hair spray. It is used therapeutically as the antidote for ethylene glycol and methanol poisoning when fomepizole is not available. Isopropyl alcohol is a low-molecular-weight hydrocarbon commonly found as both a solvent as well as a disinfectant and is commonly used as an ethanol substitute and ingested by individuals. It can be found in many mouthwashes, skin lotions, rubbing alcohol, and hand sanitizers. Young children are poisoned unintentionally or by adults who give them alcoholic beverages. Preteens and adolescents may indulge in binge drinking and may be alcohol dependent. Young adults are devising ways to use ethanol without actually drinking it. They are still becoming intoxicated, since the delicate tissues of the vagina, anus, and eyeball absorb alcohol readily, but without the knowledge that these routes may result in injury or overdose. The addition of energy drinks, typically containing caffeine and other energy-producing supplements, either ingested alone or in combination with alcohol, has created another circumstance in which people do not comprehend the risks. In these cases, they are as vulnerable as adults to atrial dysrhythmias following binges and to medical and behavioral consequences of alcoholism.

1. Ethanol is rapidly absorbed and widely distributed. The primary route of absorption is oral, although it can be absorbed by inhalation and other routes. It is well known as a CNS depressant. The concomitant use of ethanol and other drugs is common, and combinations of ethanol with other sedative-hypnotics or opioids may potentiate the sedative effects. In children, ethanol's hypoglycemic effects are significant; the immature liver does not maintain sufficient glycogen stores to counteract ethanol-induced hypoglycemia.

2. Symptoms related to ethanol-induced CNS depression are lethargy, ataxia, respiratory depression, hypothermia, and coma. These effects may begin within an hour of ingestion, followed within a few hours by hypoglycemic seizures, coma, and death. These signs usually occur when the ethanol level in the blood exceeds 50 to 100 mg/dL. However, hypoglycemia can be seen with serum ethanol levels as low as 50 mg/dL. Metabolic acidosis may be present in large ingestions. Following isopropanol ingestion, the patient may simply appear intoxicated, as with ethanol intoxication and may have a history of abdominal pain, nausea, and sometimes hematemesis.

3. Toxicity may occur with an ethanol ingestion of 1 g/kg. Using the formula: amount of alcoholic product ingested (mL/kg) multiplied by the percentage of ethanol in the product (%) divided by the body weight of the patient (in kilograms), will provide a rough estimate of blood ethanol concentration. A 4 mL/kg ingestion of 100% ethanol is life threatening. A fatal dose in children is approximately 3 g/kg; the fatal dose in adolescents and adults is widely variable, from 5 to 8 g/kg.

4. Physical assessment is straightforward. Laboratory studies required include serum ethanol and methanol levels, electrolytes, glucose, and ABG analysis. It is necessary to evaluate for salicylate and acetaminophen since coingestion is highly probable with ethanol ingestion.

5. *Treatment.* Gastric emptying is not useful greater than 1 hour after ingestion. Activated charcoal does not adsorb ethanol. Careful monitoring and correction of serum glucose are essential. Other treatment is symptomatic and supportive. Ethanol is removed by hemodialysis, which may be indicated for serious or potentially fatal ingestions.

6. *Special Consideration.* Even preteens and young adolescents may be alcohol dependent. Be alert for signs of impending withdrawal: tremors, agitation, hallucinations, and seizures. Benzodiazepines are usually indicated for initial management of alcohol withdrawal.

F. Ethylene Glycol

Ethylene glycol is an ingredient in antifreeze, deicing products, detergents, paints, and cosmetics. The most common source of ethylene glycol poisoning in the pediatric population is from antifreeze. Unintentional ingestions are the norm in young children, whereas adolescents drink antifreeze in suicide attempts or as an ethanol surrogate. This is a dangerous poisoning because ethylene glycol is sweet but extremely toxic in small amounts. Effects are due to metabolites and are therefore delayed. Parents or victims mistakenly may believe that absence of early symptoms indicates absence of toxicity.

1. Ethylene glycol is rapidly absorbed from the GI tract and is widely distributed. During the several steps in its metabolism, glycolic acid, lactic acid, and a number of other organic acids are generated, leading to the metabolic acidosis characteristic of this poisoning. Oxalic acid precipitates with calcium, leading to the deposition of calcium oxalate crystals in soft tissue (including the kidney) and renal failure.

2. The toxic dose is variable but small; a dose requiring medical treatment varies but is considered more than 0.1 mL/kg body weight of pure substance. Poison control centers often use more than a lick or taste in a child or more than a mouthful in an adult as a dose requiring hospital assessment (Caravati et al., 2005). The orally lethal dose in humans is approximately 1.4 mL/kg of pure ethylene glycol (Brent, 2001).

3. Toxic effects are delayed for as long as 12 to 24 hours; early effects resemble alcoholic intoxication. As the poisoning progresses, nonspecific symptoms of lethargy and GI tract complaints, such as nausea and vomiting, evolve into ataxia, seizures, stupor, coma, and renal failure. In the absence of specific history, ethylene glycol poisoning should be suspected in any patient who presents with or develops both coma and metabolic acidosis.

4. A serum ethylene glycol level is most useful but is not always easily obtained. The presence of an anion gap metabolic acidosis is more readily ascertained and is extremely useful. ABG analysis is required. Other laboratory tests that should be performed include screening for coingestions such as acetaminophen and salicylates; CBC, blood glucose, serum electrolytes, magnesium, calcium, BUN, creatinine, lactate, osmolar and anion gap, and urinalysis. A few hours after ingestion, the urine can be examined for the presence of calcium oxalate crystals. A serum ethanol level should be drawn in anticipation of antidotal therapy with ethanol if fomepizole is not available.

5. Treatment includes prevention of absorption (if possible), prevention of metabolism to toxic metabolites, and enhanced elimination.

    a. *Gastric emptying* is useful only within 1 hour of ingestion.

    b. *Specific antidotes* to ethylene glycol poisoning are the alcohol dehydrogenase inhibitors fomepizole and ethanol. The goal of antidotal treatment with fomepizole or ethanol is to prevent metabolism of ethylene glycol into toxic components until ethylene glycol can be eliminated renally or

by hemodialysis. Either antidote is administered until the serum ethylene glycol level is less than 20 mg/dL. Dosing of both is altered by concurrent hemodialysis.

    i. Fomepizole is administered IV every 12 hours. The loading dose is 15 mg/kg; maintenance dose is 10 mg/kg for four doses, followed by 15 mg/kg until therapy is no longer needed.

    ii. The initial dose of ethanol is calculated according to age, whether ethanol is already present, and whether the patient is habituated to ethanol. Subsequent doses are titrated to the serum ethanol level, which should be maintained at 100 mg/dL. To prevent ethanol-induced hypoglycemia, serum glucose must be carefully monitored and corrected if necessary.

    c. *Hemodialysis* is indicated if the ethylene glycol level is greater than 50 mg/dL or with severe acidosis or evidence of end-organ damage irrespective of level.

    d. *Serial ethylene glycol levels* should be measured until they are less than 20 mg/dL. Metabolism of ethylene glycol to nontoxic metabolites is enhanced by administration of pyridoxine and thiamine.

    e. *Renal function and acidosis* must be aggressively monitored and corrected.

6. *Special Considerations.* A high index of suspicion is necessary as ethylene glycol is toxic in extremely small quantities and the most effective time to initiate treatment is before metabolism and symptoms occur. Aggressive treatment is necessary, not only to prevent renal damage and death but to minimize the risks of peripheral nervous system damage in survivors.

G. Methanol

Methanol, also known as *wood alcohol*, is a commonly used organic solvent that, because of its toxicity, can cause metabolic acidosis, neurologic sequelae, and even death, when ingested. Methanol is the ingredient in windshield washer solution. It also is found in antifreeze, perfumes, paint solvents, photocopying fluid, gas-line additives, fuel for chafing dishes and model airplanes, and deicing compounds. It is extremely toxic in small amounts, has a sweet taste, and, in the case of windshield washer solutions, resembles blue soft drinks, especially when transferred to beverage containers. It is also used as an ethanol surrogate and in suicides. The metabolites of methanol are responsible for its toxicity.

1. Methanol is rapidly absorbed from the GI tract. It is metabolized briefly to formaldehyde, then to formic acid. Generation of organic acids accounts for metabolic acidosis, and generation of formic acid accounts for optic nerve damage.

2. The toxic dose is variable but small, with ocular injury associated with serum methanol levels greater than 20 mg/dL and peak methanol concentrations over 50 mg/dL (500 mg/L) indicate serious poisoning, particularly if an anion gap metabolic acidosis is present. Clinical symptoms and mortality correlate more closely with metabolic acidosis rather than with serum methanol concentrations (Barceloux, Bond, Krenzelok, Cooper, & Vale, 2002) with the minimal lethal dose of methanol in adults believed to be 1 mg/kg of body weight.

3. Because toxicity is due to metabolites, there may be no symptoms for 10 to 24 hours. Initially, the symptoms of methanol intoxication are similar to those of ethanol intoxication, often with disinhibition and ataxia. Following a latent period, patients may develop headache, nausea, vomiting, or epigastric pain. As formic acid is generated, ocular complaints begin. They have been described variously as double vision, dim vision like being in a snowstorm, and actual blindness. In later stages, drowsiness may rapidly progress to obtundation, seizures, and coma.

4. Physical assessment requires specific attention to the optic disc for hyperemia and the retina for edema, so ophthalmologic consultation should occur promptly. Determination of methanol levels is ideal but often difficult to obtain and the osmolar gap can be used to estimate serum methanol levels. Presence or absence of an anion gap metabolic acidosis is the critical information, as is the measurement of ABGs. A methanol level should be determined in anticipation of antidotal therapy with ethanol.

5. Treatment includes prevention of absorption (if possible), prevention of metabolism to toxic metabolites, and enhanced elimination.

    a. *Gastric emptying* is useful only within 1 hour of ingestion.

    b. Specific antidotes to methanol poisoning are the alcohol dehydrogenase inhibitors *fomepizole and ethanol*. The goal of antidotal treatment with fomepizole or ethanol is to prevent metabolism of methanol into toxic components of formic

acid, until methanol can be eliminated renally or by hemodialysis. Either antidote is administered until the serum methanol level is less than 20 mg/dL. Dosing of both is altered by concurrent hemodialysis.

    i. Fomepizole is administered via IV every 12 hours. The loading dose is 15 mg/kg; maintenance dose is 10 mg/kg for four doses, followed by 15 mg/kg until therapy is no longer needed.

    ii. The initial dose of ethanol is calculated according to age, whether ethanol is already present, and whether the patient is habituated to ethanol. Subsequent doses are titrated to the serum ethanol level, which should be maintained at 100 mg/dL. To prevent ethanol-induced hypoglycemia, serum glucose must be carefully monitored and corrected if necessary.

    c. *Hemodialysis* is indicated if the methanol level is greater than 50 mg/dL.

    d. *Serial methanol levels* should be measured until they are less than 20 mg/dL. Eventual metabolism of methanol to carbon dioxide and water is enhanced by the administration of folate if the patient is already symptomatic. If the patient is still asymptomatic, leucovorin may be given instead.

    e. *Ocular status* must be monitored. Acidosis must be aggressively monitored and corrected. Other treatment is symptomatic and supportive.

6. *Special Considerations.* A high index of suspicion is necessary because methanol is toxic in extremely small quantities and because the most effective time to initiate treatment is before metabolism occurs. Aggressive treatment is necessary, not only to prevent blindness and death but to minimize the risks of polyneuropathy in survivors.

H. Hydrocarbons

Hydrocarbons may be categorized in many ways: by chemical composition, intended purpose, volatility, and toxic effects. The types of hydrocarbons are aliphatic ([straight-chain] methane, ethane, propane, and butane) and cyclic (gasoline, kerosene, motor oil, mineral oil, creosotes, solvents, and other products with mixtures of hydrocarbons). Some hydrocarbons are of particular danger to the pulmonary tract if aspirated, although not usually damaging to the GI tract if ingested. These less viscous compounds include gasoline, kerosene, lamp oil, mineral spirits, mineral seal oil, and other substances used as fuels, lighter fluids, lubricants, and polishes.

1. When ingested, these less viscous hydrocarbons may be irritating and cause nausea, diarrhea, and eructation. However, they are not absorbed well from the GI tract and are not expected to cause systemic effects unless large quantities are ingested or the hydrocarbon product contains other toxins.

2. Aspiration of any amount of hydrocarbon is dangerous; and just a few drops may cause pneumonitis. Depending on the exact substance and its viscosity, expected effects include airway irritation, pulmonary edema, disruption of surfactant, and impaired oxygen exchange. Less viscous compounds, which include gasoline, mineral oil seal, and kerosene, are much easier to aspirate than more viscous compounds. With less viscous compound aspirations the victim experiences hypoxia, cyanosis, and potentially alveolar collapse. Chest radiographic findings may range from isolated basilar infiltrates to "whiting out," especially after aspiration of such low-viscosity hydrocarbons as charcoal lighter fluid. Bacterial pneumonia may follow.

3. Relevant history includes a history of coughing or choking after ingestion of a hydrocarbon; in these cases, aspiration is likely, and the victim must be assessed in a healthcare facility. Physical assessment should focus on pulmonary findings and CNS abnormalities secondary to hypoxia. The potential for cardiac dysrhythmias also exists with acute exposure, but is more commonly associated with an inhaled hydrocarbon. Laboratory studies are necessary to determine the status of oxygenation, electrolytes for renal injury, ECG, and CBC. A chest radiograph should be taken quickly if the patient is severely symptomatic on arrival at the healthcare facility; otherwise, it should be deferred until 2 hours after exposure to permit detection of changes.

4. Treatment of patients with hydrocarbon aspiration may need to be aggressive but is symptomatic and supportive, primarily of the respiratory system. There is no specific antidote. In general, steroids are not indicated, and antibiotics are indicated only if bacterial pneumonia develops.

I. Mushrooms

Mushrooms of many varieties can be poisonous and even fatal when ingested. Children may eat wild mushrooms unintentionally, as they do many other things.

More dangerous is the situation in which an adult identifies wild mushrooms incorrectly and then cooks and serves them. In these cases, much more of the material is ingested; also, there could be multiple victims. Mycologists divide mushrooms into species; toxicologists divide them into groups based on symptoms. The poison center can help you narrow the group of mushroom and guide treatment on the basis of symptoms and can identify a mycologist for positive identification of wild mushrooms and their spores. (Any available mushroom specimen must be wrapped in waxed paper or a dry paper bag and stored safely until it can be transported for identification or until it can be determined that specific identification is not necessary.) There are a few specific situations in which mushroom ingestion precipitates an ICU admission. The focus is then on decontamination, identification of the mushroom if possible, and aggressive supportive care.

1. In the United States, there are two types of mushrooms that are inherently sufficiently toxic to cause fatalities. Both are differentiated by the delayed onset of GI tract symptoms. Sometimes people do not associate nausea, vomiting, and diarrhea with mushrooms eaten hours or even the day before.

a. The cyclopeptide group of toxins present in *Amanita phalloides*, *Amanita verna*, and *Amanita virosa* are hepatotoxic and are associated with a high fatality rate. The onset of significant GI tract symptoms occurs after a latent period of 6 to 12 hours after ingestion. Death from hepatic and renal failure may occur in about 5 days. There are no antidotes and no universally effective treatments. If ingestion is recognized early enough, GI tract decontamination is necessary. Hemodialysis may remove hepatotoxic metabolites.

b. *Gyromitra esculenta* is sometimes mistaken for the edible morel, with the development of seizures, hepatotoxic consequences, and occasionally is fatal. Vigorous GI tract decontamination is required if the ingestion is recognized early enough. Ingestion of *Gyromitra* species results in monomethylhydrazine poisoning, similar to INH with the development of mild GI symptoms and with delirium, seizures, and coma in severe cases. Methemoglobinemia and hemolysis may be life threatening. Treatment is as for INH poisoning, including pyridoxine 25 mg/kg; repeat as necessary to a maximum dose of 15 to 20 g.

2. Other toxic mushrooms in the United States cause the rapid onset of predominately GI tract and perhaps other symptoms, typically within

30 minutes to 2 hours. Numerous types of mushrooms can cause cholinergic, anticholinergic, or hallucinogenic effects. Treatment includes GI tract decontamination and then symptomatic and supportive care. Numerous mushroom types can cause the rapid onset of GI tract symptoms with associated fluid and electrolyte imbalances. Treatment may include GI tract decontamination and then symptomatic and supportive care with an emphasis on monitoring and replacing fluids and electrolytes.

J. Organophosphate Insecticides

Organophosphate insecticides, which include chemicals used in both domestic and industrial settings, are absorbed via ingestion, inhalation, and dermal contact. They are classified by their relative toxicity; toxicity varies by potency. Several swallows are needed to produce toxicity from low-potency compounds and only a few milliliters may be needed for high-potency compounds. Highly toxic organophosphates, such as sarin, tabun, and soman, were developed as nerve gas agents for warfare and terrorist events; less toxic organophosphates include malathion, dursban, and diazinon, which are used in household settings. Children can be exposed by household exterminations (e.g., for fleas and termites), garden applications, and exposure to agricultural sprays and adolescents by occupational exposure and in suicide attempts.

1. Organophosphate insecticides are acetylcholinesterase inhibitors. By binding to acetylcholinesterase, organophosphate insecticides prevent acetylcholine from being hydrolyzed to choline and acetic acid. There is continued excessive stimulation of acetylcholine receptors in the CNS and at muscarinic and nicotinic sites in the autonomic nervous system. The binding may "mature" and the inhibition over time becomes irreversible. Expected effects of exposure thus are referable to the CNS and to the autonomic nervous system. Onset of symptoms is variable: rapid for nerve gas agents and "typical" household pesticides, delayed and prolonged for extremely fat-soluble agents and for those that must first be metabolized to toxic agents (e.g., fenthion).

   a. *Muscarinic symptoms* can be remembered by the mnemonic *dumbells syndrome*: *d*iaphoresis and *d*iarrhea, *u*rination, *m*iosis, *b*radycardia, *b*ronchospasm and *b*ronchorrhea, *e*mesis and excess of *l*acrimation, and *s*alivation and *s*eizures.

   b. *Nicotinic effects* can be remembered by the mnemonic *mtwthf*: *m*ydriasis, muscle *t*witching, and cramps; *t*achycardia; *w*eakness; *(t)*hypertension; and *f*asciculations.

   c. *CNS effects* include tremor, agitation, confusion, ataxia, lethargy, muscle weakness, paralysis, seizures, and coma.

2. The greatest threat to the patient is respiratory distress from bronchorrhea, bronchospasm, and from weakness or paralysis of the respiratory muscles. The greatest threat to the healthcare provider is poisoning by being exposed to a patient who has not been appropriately decontaminated.

3. Physical assessment of the patient must be thorough as acetylcholinesterase inhibition has broad and diverse systemic effects. The specific laboratory study required is measurement of RBC cholinesterase level. (Often the more easily measured plasma cholinesterase level is measured, but this test is not as useful because it can be affected by many things other than organophosphate insecticide poisoning.) The range of normal varies, but a significant decrease from the expected normal is indicative of cholinesterase inhibition and organophosphate insecticide poisoning.

4. A patient with dermal exposure must be decontaminated. Protect staff with impermeable gowns and gloves to minimize or prevent dermal exposure, remove and isolate contaminated clothing, and wash the patient with copious amounts of soap and water and then repeat the decontamination wash a second time. Even the vomitus of patients who have ingested these compounds can be hazardous to staff members.

5. Atropine is administered to occupy muscarinic receptors and alleviate muscarinic effects. The necessary dose is titrated to symptoms, especially bronchorrhea. The initial pediatric dose is 0.05 to 0.1 mg/kg, repeat every 5 to 10 minutes as needed, doubling the dose if previous dose did not induce atropinization, continue administering repeat dosing every 2 to 12 hours to maintain atropinization, until pulmonary secretions are controlled. In severe cases, atropine by IV infusion may be required for hours or days, depending on the amount of insecticide absorbed and resolution of effects.

6. Pralidoxime (2-PAM) is administered to treat the neuromuscular dysfunction by cleaving the organophosphate–acetylcholinesterase bond before it "matures," or becomes permanent within 24 hours after exposure. It is used in severe organophosphate

insecticide poisoning and may be administered concurrently with atropine. Pediatric dose is 25 to 50 mg/kg (max. dose 2 g) IV based on severity over 30 minutes, followed by 10 to 20 mg/kg/hr. Like atropine, it is administered until the patient remains asymptomatic.

7. Otherwise, care is symptomatic and supportive, with aggressive respiratory nursing.

8. *Special Considerations.* Patients are often undertreated because healthcare providers are reluctant to administer the necessarily high and prolonged doses of atropine or pralidoxime. Permanent neurologic effects have been associated with exposure to some organophosphate insecticides. Young children are especially susceptible to the effects of these insecticides.

9. Carbamate insecticides have the same acute toxic effects as organophosphate insecticides. However, pralidoxime is not indicated for poisoning by carbamate insecticides, since it does not form permanent bonds with acetylcholinesterase but may be given to hasten reversal.

PSYCHOSOCIAL CONSIDERATIONS

Parents often feel guilty about a poisoning episode. Although it is objectively true that most incidents can be anticipated and avoided, the reality is that young children are extremely curious, very mobile, and many times their abilities are underestimated by adults. Even the most vigilant parents and caregivers need to attend to other things, turn their backs, tend to another child, or experience a momentary lapse in concentration. Most parents realize what they could have done differently to prevent the poisoning event from occurring. It is more productive for healthcare providers to focus on what parents did right: recognized a dangerous situation; sought emergency assistance; cooperated with healthcare providers who attempted to elicit a history, identify the drug or product, and reconstruct the scenario; and provided support to the poisoned child and other family members during recovery. This can be followed by specific poison prevention information, which can be obtained from the poison center, to ensure that the child returns to a safe environment.

For older children or adolescents whose poisoning represented impulsive, intentional, or self-destructive behavior, psychiatric or social service consults are required.

If there is any suspicion of child abuse or factitious disorder by proxy, there may be legal requirements to be fulfilled in addition to the need for psychiatric and social services referrals for the caregivers.

CASE STUDIES WITH QUESTIONS, ANSWERS, AND RATIONALES

Toxicology Case Studies

Case Study 9.3

A 15-year-old girl was found unconscious; a bottle of her mother's amitriptyline was found next to her. She had a grand mal seizure in the ambulance en route to the emergency department.

1. Toxicity of tricyclic antidepressants significantly contributes to which effects?
   A. Drooling and respiratory distress
   B. Agitation and restlessness
   C. Prolonged, accelerated hypertension
   D. Dysrhythmias

2. The single most important drug in the management of tricyclic antidepressant overdose is:
   A. Dopamine
   B. Glucagon
   C. Lidocaine
   D. Phenytoin
   E. Sodium bicarbonate

3. In cases of intentional drug overdose, it is especially important to obtain laboratory evaluation of which potential coingestant?
   A. Acetaminophen
   B. Ethanol
   C. Heroin

4. Following a tricyclic antidepressant overdose, death is usually due to:
   A. Cardiac dysrhythmias
   B. Disrupted neurotransmission in the central nervous system
   C. Hepatotoxicity
   D. Profound hypotension
   E. Refractory seizures

Case Study 9.4

A 3-year-old boy was found with an open bottle of his mother's prenatal vitamins with iron. The color of the tablet coating is seen inside the child's mouth. Twenty-five tablets are unaccounted for.

1. Following ingestion of iron, gastrointestinal (GI) decontamination may include all of the following, *except:*
   A. Ipecac syrup
   B. Gastric lavage
   C. Activated charcoal
   D. Whole-bowel irrigation

2. For the next several hours, it is important to observe this child for the development of any of the following, *except:*
   A. GI bleeding
   B. Coma
   C. Acute tubular necrosis
   D. Metabolic acidosis
   E. Coagulopathies

3. The child experienced vomiting, diarrhea, and abdominal pain for about 3 hours and then gradually fell into an undisturbed sleep. The most likely explanation is:
   A. The iron tablets have been eliminated from the GI tract and the child is out of danger.
   B. The child is now in the asymptomatic latent phase, during which iron is being absorbed and metabolized.
   C. Because the child's symptoms are not characteristic of iron poisoning, he probably has a GI virus or food poisoning.
   D. These symptoms are characteristic of an allergic reaction to vitamin supplements and were precipitated by the large amount of vitamins in these adult-strength supplements.

4. The most effective definitive therapy for acute iron intoxication is:
   A. Deferoxamine
   B. Volume expanders
   C. Hemodialysis
   D. Resin hemoperfusion
   E. Exchange transfusion

Case Study 9.5

A 12-year-old female was admitted to the pediatric intensive care unit after her friends called EMS after a social media posting, stating that she had taken pills and wanted to die. EMS reported several pill bottles were found surrounding the patient. The patient states that she took several ibuprofen and salicylates (aspirin). She is complaining of tinnitus and is very lethargic.

1. In cases of intentional drug overdose, it is especially important to obtain laboratory evaluation of which potential coingestant:
   A. Ethanol
   B. Acetaminophen
   C. Benzodiazepines
   D. Opioids

2. The most appropriate GI decontamination method for salicylate poisoning is:
   A. Whole-bowel irrigation
   B. Forced diuresis
   C. Gastric lavage
   D. Activated charcoal

3. After salicylate poisoning, death is usually related to:
   A. Pulmonary edema
   B. Seizures
   C. Arrhythmia
   D. GI bleed

Case Study 9.6

A 17-year-old male with history of depression and multiple suicide attempts who was started on a new dose of tranylcypromine (Parnate; monoamine oxidase [MAO] inhibitor) yesterday, was found agitated, diaphoretic, and shaking and admitted to taking DMX to "feel good." En route to the emergency department, he has a seizure. Vital signs upon presentation:

T: 106.1°F, heart rate: 195 beats/min; respiratory rate: 32 breaths/min; room air: $SaO_2 + 95\%$

1. Hyperthermia is not part of which toxidrome?
   A. Anticholinergic
   B. Cholinergic
   C. Opiate
   D. Serotonin
   E. Neuroleptic malignant

2. What helps you distinguish between serotonin syndrome and anticholinergic syndrome?
   A. Bowel sounds
   B. Mydriasis
   C. Hyperkenesis
   D. Agitation
   E. Rapid onset (<12 hours)

3. What is the relationship between MAO inhibitors and DMX?
   A. MAO inhibitors directly block serotonin reuptake, whereas DMX increases reuptake
   B. MAO inhibitors and DMX both block serotonin reuptake

C. MAO inhibitors reduce breakdown of serotonin and DMX promotes serotonin release

4. The most definitive effective therapy for serotonin syndrome is:
   A. Cyproheptadine
   B. Benzodiazepines
   C. Haloperidol
   D. Naloxone

Case Study 9.7

A 14-year-old female came to her parents with the complaint of nausea and vomiting. She stated that she had taken a "handful of pills." Upon investigation in her room, an empty bottle of extra-strength (500 mg) tablets of acetaminophen was found. EMS was called and transported her to the emergency department.

1. The single most important drug in the management of acetaminophen overdose is:
   A. Sodium bicarbonate
   B. N-acetylcysteine
   C. Naloxone
   D. Dextrose

2. What is the optimal timing to obtain a serum acetaminophen level?
   A. 2 hours postingestion
   B. 4 hours postingestion
   C. 8 hours postingestion
   D. 24 hours postingestion

3. After acetaminophen overdose, death is usually related to:
   A. Respiratory failure
   B. Cardiovascular collapse
   C. Intractable seizures
   D. Hepatic failure

Case Study 9.8

A 16-year-old female presented to the emergency room with her parents. The patient was found by her parents incoherent, ataxic, and complaining of visual disturbances. Laboratory testing reveals metabolic acidosis which is concerning for methanol intoxication. The patient rapidly progresses to coma.

1. If the patient survives the poisoning, what long-term complication is anticipated?
   A. Renal failure
   B. Seizures
   C. Blindness
   D. Cardiomyopathy

2. The antidote for methanol intoxication is:
   A. Renal replacement therapy
   B. Forced diuresis
   C. Fomepizole
   D. Dextrose

3. What is the optimal level to discontinue antidote administration for methanol intoxication?
   A. Less than 100 mg/dL
   B. Less than 40 mg/dL
   C. Less than 20 mg/dL
   D. Less than 10 mg/dL

Toxicology Answers and Rationales

Case Study 9.3

1. **D.** Tricyclic antidepressants have the following effects: anticholinergic, resulting in dry mouth, early hypertension, and hallucinations; delayed uptake of norepinephrine, resulting in some central nervous system (CNS) and cardiac effects; membrane depressant effects on the heart, resulting in numerous dysrhythmias, especially ventricular dysrhythmias and conduction delays; and a-adrenergic blockade, resulting in the hypotension characteristic of this poisoning.

2. **E.** Symptomatic patients are likely to develop acidosis that is resistant to correction. Although hyperventilation is sometimes used to induce respiratory alkalosis, sodium bicarbonate is more effective m treating acidosis and cardiac dysrhythmias.

3. **A.** Acetaminophen is readily available in the home and is contained in more than 100 products.

4. **A.** Cardiac dysrhythmias can occur following antidepressant overdose. The toxic dose cannot be predicted with certainty. Any amount is potentially dangerous in children. At least 6 hours of emergency department evaluation is required for all ingestions in young children and for ingestions larger than the therapeutic dose in older children. Patients who become symptomatic in the 6-hour observation period require admission to a monitored bed until they have been asymptomatic for 24 hours. With intentional overdoses, psych consults are warranted.

Case Study 9.4

1. **C.** Activated charcoal does not bind iron. Gastric lavage is helpful in removing pills and pill fragments

if performed soon after ingestion. Whole-bowel irrigation is the standard of care to remove large amounts of ingested iron.

2. **C.** In overdose, iron causes significant corrosive injury to the GI tract. Circulating free iron injures blood vessels and damages hepatocytes and can cause GI bleeding. As iron is metabolized, free hydrogen is released and in concert with other events produces metabolic acidosis. Symptoms of severe toxicity include coma, cardiovascular collapse, seizures, hepatic failure, and coagulopathies.

3. **B.** The asymptomatic latent phase occurs between 2 and 12 hours after ingestion. Systemic insults occur during this phase; then the child abruptly enters the third phase with a rapid onset of cardiovascular collapse.

4. **A.** Deferoxamine is an iron-chelating agent (it binds iron) and is administered as an intravenous infusion.

Case Study 9.5

1. **B.** Acetaminophen is primarily metabolized in conjugation with sulfate and glucuronide. Patients are typically asymptomatic for up to 24 hours, and during that time hepatic injury can develop if the patient does not receive proper treatment.

2. **D.** Treatment includes GI decontamination with activated charcoal followed by multiple doses of activated charcoal administered every 4 hours with consideration of a cathartic once per 24 hours if salicylate levels continue to rise.

3. **A.** Severe poisoning may have significant neurotoxicity (agitation, coma, convulsions); kidney failure, pulmonary edema, or cardiovascular instability. Treatment must be aggressive but primarily is symptomatic and supportive. Hydration is essential but must be controlled to avoid precipitating pulmonary edema.

Case Study 9.6

1. **C.** Hyperthermia is a symptom in the sympathomimetic and anticholinergic toxidromes, whereas opiates are actually associated with hypothermia.

2. **C.** Serotonin syndrome is a potentially life-threatening condition associated with increased serotonergic activity in the CNS. Neuromuscular hyperactivity can manifest as tremor, muscle rigidity, myoclonus, hyperreflexia, and bilateral Babinski sign. Hyperreflexia and clonus are particularly common; these findings, as well as rigidity, are more often pronounced in the lower extremities. The majority of cases of serotonin syndrome present within 24 hours, and most within 6 hours, of a change or initiation of a drug.

3. **C.** This combination of medications is incredibly dangerous and likely results in serotonin syndrome with seizures, hyperthermia, and hyperkenesis.

4. **A.** Cyproheptadine is a serotonin and histamine antagonist with anticholinergic and sedative effects. Antiserotonin and antihistamine drugs appear to compete with serotonin and histamine, respectively, for receptor sites.

Case Study 9.7

1. **B.** Acetaminophen is primarily metabolized by conjugation with sulfate and glucuronide. Approximately 5% of drug is oxidized by CYP450-dependent pathways to a toxic metabolite, N-acetyl-p-benzoquinoneimine (NAPQI), which is detoxified by glutathione and eliminated in urine or bile. In toxic doses, excessive NAPQI is produced and glutathione stores are depleted. N-acetylcysteine (NAC) increases their synthesis and availability of glutathione, being converted to cysteine and then to glutathione NAC (via reduced sulfur group) can substitute for glutathione and directly bind and thus detoxify highly reactive metabolite, NAPQI.

2. **B.** The Rumack–Matthew nomogram is used to interpret plasma acetaminophen values to assess hepatotoxicity risk after a single, acute ingestion. Nomogram tracking begins 4 hours after ingestion (time when acetaminophen absorption is likely to be complete) and ends 24 hours after ingestion. About 60% of patients with values above the "probable" line develop hepatotoxicity.

3. **D.** Acetaminophen is primarily metabolized by conjugation with sulfate and glucuronide. Approximately 5% of drug is oxidized by CYP450-dependent pathways to a toxic metabolite, NAPQI, which is detoxified by glutathione and eliminated in urine or bile. In toxic doses, excessive NAPQI is produced and glutathione stores are depleted resulting in liver toxicity and necrosis. Patients are typically asymptomatic for up to 24 hours, and during that time coagulopathies can develop if the patient does not receive proper treatment.

Case Study 9.8

1. C. Methanol is rapidly absorbed from the GI tract. It is metabolized briefly to formaldehyde, then to formic acid. Generation of organic acids accounts for metabolic acidosis, and generation of formic acid accounts for optic nerve damage.

2. C. Specific antidotes to methanol poisoning are the alcohol dehydrogenase inhibitors fomepizole and ethanol. The goal of antidotal treatment with fomepizole or ethanol is to prevent meta-bolism of methanol into toxic components of formic acid.

3. C. It is appropriate to discontinue the administration of either antidote, fomepizole, or ethanol when the serum methanol level is less than 20 mg/dL. At this level, the risk associated with the continued metabolism of methanol into toxic components of formic acid is minimized.

TOXICOLOGY REFERENCES

Barceloux, D. G., Bond, R. G., Krenzelok, E. P., Cooper, H., & Vale, J. A. (2002). American Academy of Clinical Toxicology practice guidelines on the treatment of methanol poisoning. *Clinical Toxicology, 40*, 415–446.

Benson, B., Hoppu, K., Troutman, W. G., Bedry, R., Erdman, A., Höjer, J., . . . Caravati, E. (2013). Position paper update: Gastric lavage for gastrointestinal decontamination. *Clinical Toxicology, 51*, 140–146.

Brent, J. (2001). Current management of ethylene glycol poisoning. *Drugs, 61*, 979–988.

Calello, D. P., & Henretig, F. M. (2014). Pediatric toxicology: Specialized approach to the poisoned child. *Emergency Medicine Clinics of North America, 32*, 29–52.

Caravati, E. M., Erdman, A. R., Christianson, G., Manoguerra, A. S., Booze, L. L., Woolf, A. D., . . . Troutman, W. G. (2005). Ethylene glycol exposure: An evidence-based consensus guideline for out-of-hospital management. *Clinical Toxicology, 43*, 327–345.

Gosselin, S., Morris, M., Miller-Nesbitt, A., Hoffman, R. S., Hayes, B. D., Turgeon, A. F., . . . Lavergne, V. (2015). Methodology for AACT evidence-based recommendations on the use of intravenous lipid emulsion therapy in poisoning. *Clinical Toxicology, 53*, 557–564. doi:10.3109/15563650.2015.1052498

Green, S., Harris, C., & Singer, J. (2008). Gastrointestinal decontamination of the poisoned patient. *Pediatric Emergency Care, 24*, 176–186.

Juurlink, D. N. (2016). Activated charcoal for acute overdose: A reappraisal. *British Journal of Clinical Pharmacology, 81*, 482–487.

Litovitz, T., Whitaker, N., Clark, L., White, N. C., & Marsolek, M. (2010). Emerging battery-ingestion hazard: Clinical implications. *Pediatrics, 125*, 1168.

Madden, M. A. (2015). Pediatric toxicology: Emerging trends. *Journal of Pediatric Intensive Care, 4*, 103–110.

Michael, J. B., & Sztajnkrycer, M. D. (2004). Deadly pediatric poisons: Nine common agents that kill at low doses. *Emergency Medicine Clinic North America, 22*, 1019–1050.

Mowry, J. B., Spyker, D. A., Brooks, D. E., McMillan, N., & Schauben, J. L. (2015). 2014 Annual Report of the American Association of Poison Control Centers' National Poison Data System (NPDS): 32nd annual report. *Clinical Toxicology, 53*, 962–1147. doi:10.3109/15563650.2015.1102927

Taketomo, C. K., Hodding, J. H., & Kraus, D. M. (2015). *Pediatric and neonatal dosage handbook* (22nd ed.). Hudson, OH: Lexicomp.

Thanacoody, R., Caravati, E. M., Troutman, B., Höjer, J., Benson, B., Hoppu, K., Erdman, A., . . . Mégarbane, B. (2010). Position paper update: Whole bowel irrigation for gastrointestinal decontamination of overdose patients. *Clinical Toxicology, 53*, 5–12.

Wang, R. Z., Vashistha, V., Kaur, S., & Houchens, N. W. (2016). Serotonin syndrome: Preventing, recognizing, and treating it. *Cleveland Clinic Journal of Medicine, 83*, 810–817.

Weaver, L. K. (2009). Clinical practice: Carbon monoxide poisoning. *New England Journal of Medicine, 360*, 1217–1225.

TOXICOLOGY ADDITIONAL RESOURCES

Bond, G. R., Woodward, R. W., & Ho, M. (2012). The growing impact of pediatric pharmaceutical poisoning. *Journal of Pediatrics, 160*, 265–270.

Beuhler, M. C., Gala, P. K., Wolfe, H. A., Meaney, P. A., & Henretig, F. M. (2013). Laundry detergent "pod" ingestions: A case series and discussion of recent literature. *Pediatric Emergency Care, 29*, 743–747.

Burghardt, L. C., Ayers, J. W., Brownstein, J. S., Bronstein, A. C., Ewald, M. B., & Bourgeois, F. T. (2013). Adult prescription drug use and pediatric medication exposures and poisonings. *Pediatrics, 132*, 18–27.

Chang, T. P., & Rangan, C. (2011). Iron poisoning: A literature-based review of epidemiology, diagnosis, and management. *Pediatric Emergency Care, 27*, 978–985.

Litovitz, T., Whitaker, N., Clark, L., White, N. C., & Marsolek, M. (2010). Emerging battery ingestion hazard: Clinical implications. *Pediatrics, 125*, 1168–1177.

Ong, G. Y. (2011). A simple modified bicarbonate regimen for urine alkalinization in moderate pediatric salicylate poisoning in the emergency department. *Pediatric Emergency Care, 27*, 306–308.

Rosenbaum, C. D., Carreiro, S. P., & Babu, K. M. (2012). Here today, gone tomorrow . . . and back again? A review of herbal marijuana alternatives (K2, Spice), synthetic cathinones (bath salts), kratom, *Salvia divinorum*, methoxetamine, and piperazines. *Journal of Medical Toxicology, 8*, 15–32.

Spiller, H. A., Beuhler, M. C., Ryan, M. L., Borys, D. J., Aleguas, A., & Bosse, G. M. (2013). Evaluation of changes in poisoning in young children: 2000 to 2010. *Pediatric Emergency Care, 29*, 635–640.

Woo, T. M., & Hanley, J. R. (2013). "How high do they look?": Identification and treatment of common ingestions in adolescents. *Journal of Pediatric Health Care, 27*, 135–144.

Wolk, B. J., Ganetsky, M., & Babu, K. M. (2012). Toxicity of energy drinks. *Current Opinion in Pediatrics, 24*, 243–251.

SECTION III. SEPSIS AND SEPTIC SHOCK

Larissa Hutchins and Megan D. Snyder

DEFINITIONS

A. *Infection* is a microbial phenomenon characterized by an inflammatory response to the presence of microorganisms or the invasion of normally sterile host tissue by those organisms.

B. *Bacteremia* is the presence of viable bacteria in the blood.

C. *Systemic inflammatory response syndrome (SIRS)* is a pathophysiologic state of inflammation characterized by acute development of two or more of the following, one of which must be abnormal temperature or leukocyte count (Goldstein, Giroir, & Randolph, 2005):

   1. Fever (>38.5°C) or hypothermia (<36°C)

   2. Tachycardia (age related) or for children younger than 1 year bradycardia

   3. Tachypnea (age related)

   4. Leukocytosis or leukopenia (age related and not caused by chemotherapy), or greater than 10% bands

D. *Sepsis* is the systemic response to infection. It is diagnosed by the presence of SIRS associated with a suspected or proven infectious process and characterized by two or more of the aforementioned findings for SIRS. Documented bacteremia is not necessary for the diagnosis of sepsis.

E. *Severe sepsis* is defined as sepsis with the presence of one of the following—cardiovascular dysfunction, ARDS, or two or more other organ dysfunctions (Goldstein et al., 2005).

F. *Septic shock* is defined as sepsis in the presence of cardiovascular dysfunction (Goldstein et al., 2005). Septic shock is "infection with hypothermia or hyperthermia, tachycardia (may be absent with hypothermia), and altered mental status with of at least one, but usually more than one, of the following: decreased peripheral pulses compared with central pulses, capillary refill prolonged for more than 2 seconds (cold shock) or flash capillary refill (warm shock), mottled or cool extremities (cold shock), and decreased urine output" (Carcillo & Fields, 2003, p. 1370).

G. *Multi organ dysfunction syndrome (MODS)* is defined as the failure of more than one organ (Carcillo & Fields, 2003).

In 2016, the Sepsis-3 consensus definitions for adult sepsis and septic shock were published (Singer et al., 2016), and describe two entities: sepsis and septic shock. The new Sepsis-3 criteria for adult sepsis define sepsis as "life-threatening organ dysfunction caused by a dysregulated host response to infection" (Singer et al., 2016, p. 805). In the adult population, organ dysfunction is classified using the Sequential Organ Failure Assessment (SOFA) score (Vincent et al., 1998). Sepsis-3 defined septic shock as a "subset of sepsis in which underlying circulatory and cellular/metabolic abnormalities are profound enough to substantially increase mortality" (Singer et al., 2016, p. 805). This is operationalized as having a vasopressor requirement to maintain goals for blood pressure and lactate level, in addition to organ dysfunction according to the SOFA score criteria. Furthermore, the Sepsis-3 consensus definitions created a new bedside clinical score, the quickSOFA, consisting of tachypnea, altered mentation, and hypotension. The presence of at least two of these three clinical elements can help rapidly identify adult patients with suspected infection at higher risk of poor outcome. At this time, updated consensus definitions for the pediatric population have not yet been formalized, and pediatric practitioners continue to rely on the pediatric definitions previously described.

ETIOLOGY

A. Children have a predisposition to sepsis and septic shock as a result of environmental, immune maturity, and genetic factors.

B. All microorganisms potentially can lead to septic shock, including bacteria, viruses, fungi, rickettsia, spirochetes, protozoa, mycoplasmas, *Chlamydia* organisms, and parasites. The *Staphylococcus* species was the most common causative infecting organism for sepsis, followed by fungal infections in 1995, 2000, and 2005 (Hartman, Linde-Zwirble, Angus, & Watson, 2013).

C. Causative microorganisms often vary with the following factors:

1. *Patient's age.* Watson and colleagues (2003) have shown that age is the most significant influence in the epidemiology of severe sepsis. Pediatric severe sepsis mortality was highest in children younger than 1 year (19.2%), and children 1 to 4 years old had the second highest mortality (13.8%; Ruth et al., 2014). Immaturity of the infant and child's immune system cause them to be more susceptible to severe infections (Randolph & McCulloh, 2013).

2. *Immunocompetence.* In immunocompromised patients, the usual source of sepsis is the patient's endogenous flora. Alternatively, in immunocompetent patients, the usual source is exogenous flora, with some evidence that patients may benefit from protective isolation against ICU-acquired microorganisms (Maki, 1995). Immune system function also impacts susceptibility to fungal infections: children with cancer are twice as likely to develop fungal infections compared to children with other or no comorbidities (Hartman et al., 2013).

3. *Location.* In healthcare-associated infections (HAIs), the etiologic organism is usually specific to the individual unit, institution, and geographic region. Based on a recent point-prevalence survey, one in 25 hospitalized patients in the United States has an HAI (Magill et al., 2014). Community-acquired infection causes a significant proportion of infections in the pediatric intensive care unit (PICU). Recent studies suggest that there may be an increased risk of mortality with hospital-onset versus community-onset sepsis (Levy et al., 2012; Weiss et al., 2015).

4. *Site of Infection.* Patients with invasive monitoring devices, mechanical ventilation, and invasive catheters are more likely to acquire HAIs (Urrea, Pons, & Serra, 2003). According to Hartman et al. (2013), when a site of infection was identified nearly half of all infections were attributed to respiratory infections followed by bacteremia. In a pediatric point prevalence sepsis study (Sepsis Prevalence Outcomes and Therapies [SPROUT]), the most common site of infection of the 569 children was the lungs (40%). The bloodstream was the second most frequent site at 19%, followed by the abdomen (8%) and central nervous system (4%; Weiss et al., 2015).

EPIDEMIOLOGY

A. *Incidence*

1. According to recent estimates by the Centers for Disease Control and Prevention, the rate of hospitalization for sepsis has more than doubled between 2000 and 2008 (from 11.6 to 24 per 10,000) and now accounts for over 720,000 hospitalizations annually in the United States. Over 75,000 pediatric hospitalizations involved severe sepsis in the United States in 2005, with an estimated mortality of 8% to 10% (Hartman et al., 2013). Sepsis remains among the top 10 leading causes of death in children 0 to 9 years (National Vital Statistics System, National Center for Health Statistics, Centers for Disease Control and Prevention, 2016).

2. The burden of sepsis continues despite advances in medical care (Watson et al., 2003). In 2008, the United States spent an estimated $14.6 billion in healthcare expenditures for septicemia (National Vital Statistics System, National Center for Health Statistics, Centers for Disease Control and Prevention, 2014). Chronic illness is a major predisposing factor for sepsis (Watson et al., 2003). Watson and colleagues (2003) showed that infants have more underlying comorbidities related to neurologic and cardiovascular disease, whereas children usually have comorbidities of cancer and immunodeficiency disorders (Watson et al., 2003). The most common comorbidities for pediatric sepsis patients are neuromuscular, cardiovascular, and respiratory (Hartman et al., 2013).

B. *Risk Factors*

1. Susceptible patients are those with extremes in age (neonates and children younger than 3 years of age), noncompliance with immunization schedules, malnourishment or failure to thrive, chronic illness, malignancy, immunosuppressive therapy (e.g., malignancy, transplant recipient), primary immunodeficiency, asplenia, AIDS, and congenital heart disease.

2. Aggressive microorganisms have changing resistance patterns.

3. Several factors increase the risk of infection in children who are in the PICU. These include invasive procedures, immunosuppression, and the physiologic immunodeficiency related to the age of the child (Urrea et al., 2003). A recent study of 254 long-stay PICU patients without known baseline immunocompromise found several admission characteristics associated with increased HAI risk (increasing age, higher Pediatric Risk of Mortality Score [PRISM] III scores, diagnoses of trauma or cardiac arrest, and lymphopenia; Carcillo et al., 2016). According to Carcillo et al. (2016), up to 40% of children in the PICU for 14 days or longer will acquire an HAI and/or sepsis. It is also important to note that the risk of secondary infections and HAIs is increased in patients with MODS and immunoparalysis (Hall, Knatz, et al., 2011).

DEVELOPMENTAL ANATOMY AND PHYSIOLOGY

A. Immunity of the young child is not equal to that of the developmentally mature host. Several aspects of the infant and young child's first, second, and third lines of defense are immature. The healthy infant and young child are not immunocompromised; rather, they are immunologically *inexperienced*. The immune system is not fully mature until adolescence (Randolph & McCulloh, 2014). See Chapter 8.

B. Relationship of shock to developmental physiology: Shock is present when metabolic demand needs are not met by or are uncoupled from oxygen and energy supply. Metabolic supply and demand are impacted by cardiac output (CO) and oxygen consumption.

> **1.** *CO regulation.* See "Embryonic, Neonatal, and Pediatric Cardiovascular Physiology" section in Chapter 3. Changes in the child's CO accompany the child's growth and development. CO is greatest at birth (200 mL/kg/min) and then decreases throughout childhood to adolescence (100 mL/kg/min; Hazinski, 2013). This decrease is related to two events (Alyn & Baker, 1992): (a) a decrease in fetal hemoglobin and an increase in adult hemoglobin and (b) lower oxygen requirements secondary to a changing surface area. In the young child, CO is directly proportional to heart rate (Hazinski, 2013).

> **2.** *Oxygen consumption.* Oxygen consumption is the volume of oxygen consumed by the tissues per unit of time. Oxygen consumption is the product of the CO and the amount of oxygen extracted from each milliliter of blood, expressed as mL/kg/min. Changes in the child's oxygen consumption accompany the child's growth and development. As with CO, oxygen consumption decreases throughout childhood. Normal values in the fetus are 8 mL/kg/min (Alyn & Baker, 1992); in the infant, 10 to 14 mL/kg/min; and in the child, 5 to 8 mL/kg/min (Hazinski, 2013).

PATHOPHYSIOLOGY

A. All surfaces of the body exposed in any way to the external environment serve as the first line of defense.

When the microorganism breeches any of these barriers, it gains access to the body's internal environment.

B. The inflammatory immune response, the second line of defense, is then triggered in an effort to eliminate or neutralize the microorganism and its toxins, contain the microorganism invasion, prevent access to the body's systemic environment (i.e., bloodstream), and promote rapid healing of involved tissues.

> **1.** SIRS. With systemic release of the microorganism and its toxins, there is an activation and release of various mediators and cytokines, resulting in SIRS. SIRS can occur both in the presence of infections and in a noninfectious state. The SIRS response can also be triggered by a state of hypoperfusion, leading to hypoxic–ischemic injury commonly seen in septic shock. Septic shock includes a component of SIRS, but is triggered by the presence of infection. A local infection may progress into a systemic infection, triggering SIRS in a patient. Left uncontrolled, SIRS in addition to microbiologic toxins may lead to multiple organ system failure and death (Figure 9.7).

> **2.** Mechanisms within the inflammatory response and SIRS are the same, the differences being in the extent and magnitude of the response. Events or mechanisms of the inflammatory response serve protective functions, whereas SIRS can cause deleterious outcomes.

> **3.** The activation and release of various mediators result from two sources: exogenous and endogenous.

>> **a.** *Exogenous mediators* are released by the invading microorganism. Microorganism mediators include, but are not limited to endotoxin (released from gram-negative bacteria), exotoxin (released from gram-positive bacteria), and mannan (released from fungal cell walls). *Endotoxin*, a lipopolysaccharide that is an integral part of the outer membrane of all gram-negative bacteria, is the most commonly studied toxin in sepsis. Endotoxin is shed as bacteria multiply or die. The body's response to infection and presence of endotoxins is seen in inflammation, activation of coagulation, fever, tachypnea, lactic acidosis, and shock (Schoenmakers, Reitsma, & Spek, 2005).

>> **b.** *Endogenous mediators* are synthesized or activated by the host in response to an insult or invading microorganism (*exogenous mediators*).

> **4.** *Proinflammatory mediators.* Cytokines are a group of proteins responsible for the inflammatory

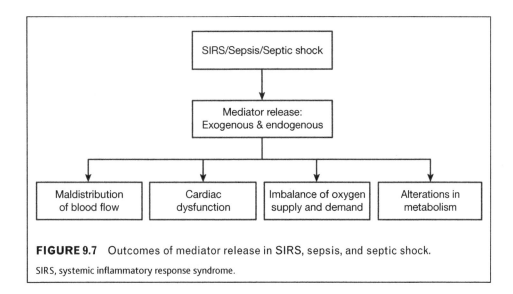

FIGURE 9.7 Outcomes of mediator release in SIRS, sepsis, and septic shock.

SIRS, systemic inflammatory response syndrome.

response. In large-enough concentrations they can cause damage to tissue. Animal studies have demonstrated that the infusion of cytokines (tumor necrosis factor alpha [TNF-α]) in large-enough quantities triggered the inflammatory response as seen in severe infection (Gotts & Matthay, 2016). Proinflammatory cytokines also include interferon gamma, interleukins (IL1 and IL8), histamine, and platelet activating factor.

The initial response of the host to bacteria is the monocyte–macrophage cell response. Neutrophils attempt to manage the infection at a local level to prevent systemic spread by bringing immune cells to the site (Schulte, Bernhagen, & Bucala, 2013). The monocyte cells phagocytose bacteria and release proinflammatory mediators (cytokines) such as TNF and IL-1 (de Pablo, Monserrat, Aprieto, & Alvarez-Mon, 2014).

5. *Anti-inflammatory mediators.* The proinflammatory response of the body is also balanced by an anti-inflammatory response mediated by such cytokines as IL-6, IL-10, transforming growth factor (TGF), and IL-4. The anti-inflammatory response attempts to decrease the inflammatory response, which, if high enough, can cause tissue damage (Schulte et al., 2013). Vagal nerve stimulation also plays a role in managing cytokine signaling and response (Gotts & Matthay, 2016).

C. In septic shock, the mechanisms of each of the mediators vary, but the overall result of the exaggerated release of exogenous and endogenous mediators includes a distributive, a cardiogenic, and a hypovolemic state. Distributive shock is caused by

vascular tone changes and maldistribution of blood flow. Cardiogenic shock is caused by myocardial depression. A hypovolemic shock state is relative to vasodilation and actual dehydration. The patient experiencing septic shock will develop endothelial damage, clotting abnormalities, and metabolic alterations (Figure 9.7).

1. *Distributive Shock*

a. Vasodilation (vascular tone changes). Acute vasodilation caused by inflammatory mediators, nitric oxide release, and presence of endotoxins results in a relative hypovolemia. The vasodilation results in a decrease in systemic vascular resistance (SVR) and decreased preload. Injury of the endothelium also causes the release of nitric oxide by the activation of nitric oxide synthases from the endothelium to the connecting cells. The presence of nitric oxide synthase acts on the vascular smooth muscle by increasing cyclic guanylate monophosphate (C-GMP), which causes smooth muscle relaxation. This relaxation of the vasculature, or vasodilation, can contribute to a state of hypovolemia and hypoperfusion.

b. Maldistribution of blood flow. Maldistribution of blood flow leading to decreased oxygen delivery and tissue hypoxia is seen in septic shock. Endothelial cells stimulated by proinflammatory mediators and endotoxin cause activation of the coagulation cascade, and creation of microvascular plugs. Endothelin, released from the endothelium, and TNF cause vasoconstriction of arterioles, whereas vasodilation occurs in other vessels.

2. *Cardiogenic Shock. Myocardial depression* may be caused by endotoxin release, the presence of cytokines in high concentrations, release of nitric oxide, and alterations in the sympathetic nervous system response. Myocardial depressant factor is thought to be released by the pancreas during hypoperfusion and ischemia.

3. *Hypovolemia.* Hypovolemia is caused by distributive shock and dehydration.

4. *Endothelial Damage.* Damage to the endothelium is caused by the effects of the inflammatory response mediators as well as endotoxin/exotoxin exposure. When damage occurs to the endothelium, small openings on the wall of the endothelium lead to intervascular fluids leaking out of the vasculature and into the interstitial tissues. This capillary leak and shift of fluid from the intravascular space, paired with massive vasodilation, can result in hypovolemia leading to hypoperfusion. Changes to the endothelium may have a direct result on the function of organs, such as the lung, leading to interstitial edema and changes to the alveolar epithelial barrier, leading to impairment in oxygenation, ventilation, and lung compliance (Gotts & Matthay, 2016). In the gut, changes to the endothelial lining may increase the possibility of bacterial translocation and injury to the gut. The liver, kidneys, and nervous systems are all susceptible to injury and malfunction due to the effects of endotheliopathy seen in sepsis (Gotts & Matthay, 2016; Figure 9.8).

5. *Alterations in Coagulation.* DIC may be triggered during the inflammatory response seen with septic

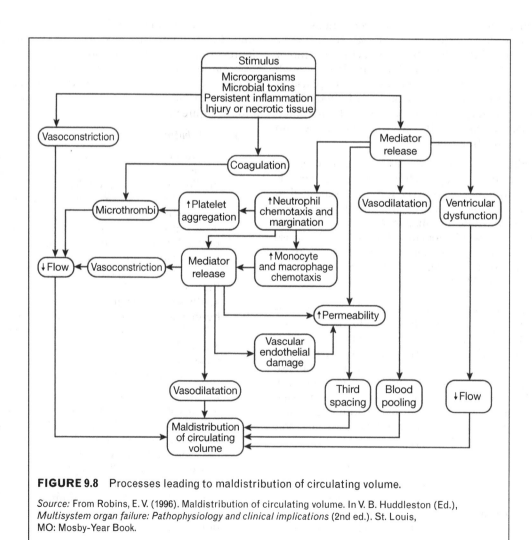

FIGURE 9.8 Processes leading to maldistribution of circulating volume.

Source: From Robins, E. V. (1996). Maldistribution of circulating volume. In V. B. Huddleston (Ed.), *Multisystem organ failure: Pathophysiology and clinical implications* (2nd ed.). St. Louis, MO: Mosby-Year Book.

shock. DIC is an inappropriate accelerated systemic activation of the coagulation system. DIC is triggered by injury to tissue by the release of proinflammatory cytokines, causing a release of tissue factor, which triggers the initiation of the coagulation cascade. As the coagulation cascade is initiated, clotting is occurring with microvascular plugs in small vessels. As the clotting factors and platelets are being consumed, the antithrombotic mechanisms are stimulated and eventually also used up. DIC and the associated ischemia and hemorrhage cause organ dysfunction, and can lead to uncontrolled bleeding (Gotts & Matthay, 2016).

6. *Imbalance of Oxygen Supply and Demand*

a. Maldistribution of blood flow exacerbates hypoxemia and may lead to ventilation perfusion abnormalities and intrapulmonary shunting. Imbalance of oxygen supply and demand with SIRS and septic shock are due to the decrease in the oxygen delivery secondary to myocardial dysfunction and the decrease in the tissue's ability to extract the oxygen.

b. In normal circumstances, with oxygen present the cells produce energy through cellular respiration. In times of stress, such as fever, seizure, or pain, the consumption of oxygen will increase. Oxygen consumption is dependent on oxygen transport. If oxygen delivery does not increase enough to meet the demand, the cells will resort to the use of anaerobic metabolism. This will produce lactic acidosis, quickly using available glucose and is a short-term measure. In order to increase the supply of available oxygen, the body will attempt to compensate by increasing the CO by increasing the heart rate. The presence of low CO more than low SVR, as seen in adults, is associated with mortality in pediatric septic shock (Brierley et al., 2009).

7. Compensatory responses to shock are mechanisms to increase tissue perfusion and prevent cellular, tissue, and vital organ injury in the presence of all shock states. Most compensatory mechanisms are dependent on various "sensing" mechanisms to recognize changes in the CO or arterial blood pressure.

8. *Compensatory mechanisms* are sequentially stimulated in an effort to maintain perfusion.

a. *Stretch receptors* (in the right atrium and pulmonary artery) sense volume changes, either from decreased circulating volume or, in the case of septic shock, from increased venous capacitance. Stimulation of these receptors results in an increase in sympathetic discharge to the medullary vasomotor center.

b. *Baroreceptors* within the renal juxtaglomerular apparatus are stimulated by reduced renal afferent arteriolar pressure. The reduction in pressure causes activation of the renin–angiotensin–aldosterone system, which results in vasoconstriction of arterioles (and, to a lesser extent, veins), increased renal tubular reabsorption of sodium and water, increased water absorption, and increased thirst. A drop in MAP or pulse pressure close to physiologic range results in the decreased stretching of arterial baroreceptors (in aortic arch, carotid bodies, and splanchnic vessels) and loss of their inhibitory effect on the vasomotor center (*baroreceptor reflex*). Sympathetic vasomotor stimulation causes norepinephrine release from nerve endings and widespread vasoconstriction.

c. *Norepinephrine–epinephrine vasoconstrictor reflex.* Sympathetic vasomotor stimulation causes stimulation of the adrenal medulla and the release of epinephrine and norepinephrine. This causes vasoconstriction and increased CO.

d. *Vascular chemoreceptors* are located in tissue beds and are sensitive to changes in PO_2, PCO_2, and decreased pH (increased hydrogen ion concentration) related to low blood pressure. On activation, sympathetic tone increases and respiratory stimulation is triggered to help compensate for the acidosis.

CLINICAL PRESENTATION

A. History

1. *Chief Complaint.* The history is guided by the child's chief complaint. The chief complaint is noted in the patient's or the primary caretaker's own words.

2. History of the present illness includes the date and mode of onset, course, duration, influencing factors, and exposure to infectious agents, including contact with infectious persons, animal (domestic or wild) bites, ingestion of contaminated food or water, and foreign travel. Signs and symptoms to be noted include the following:

a. *General.* Fatigue, change in level of activity, chills, fever, weight loss, change in feeding, night sweats, malaise

b. *Mental status.* Confusion, restlessness, syncope, irritability, somnolence

c. *Skin.* Rash, petechiae, pallor, mottling, lesions, ulcers, rhinitis, temperature

d. *Lymph nodes.* Enlargement (adenopathy), tenderness

e. *Respiratory status.* Tachypnea, respiratory tract infection, respiratory distress, dyspnea, orthopnea, cough, hemoptysis, sputum, chest pain

f. *Cardiovascular status.* Tachycardia, flushed skin

g. *Abdomen.* Anorexia, altered bowel sounds, diarrhea, constipation, melena, vomiting, hematemesis, protuberant abdomen (not age appropriate), abdominal pain, masses, hepatosplenomegaly

h. *Genitourinary tract.* Hematuria, number of voids or diapers per day

3. *Medical History*

a. Aspects that *alter* the child's resistance to infection include recent injury, diet and nutrition, immunization history, and birth history.

b. Aspects that *increase* the child's risk of infection include prolonged antibiotic therapy, previous surgeries (e.g., thymectomy, splenectomy), liver or spleen disorders (functional splenectomy), metabolic and immune disorders (diabetes mellitus, renal disease, primary immunodeficiency, and allergies or hypersensitivities), malignancy, and transplantation.

c. *Previous infections*, including childhood infectious diseases, should be noted.

4. Family history should note familial diseases that may increase the child's risk of infection.

5. Medication history should include those that increase the child's risk of infection. Also consider any dietary supplements the child is taking.

6. Social–cultural history and habits include psychosocial history, environmental exposures such as radiation (either inadvertent exposure or radiation therapies [total or localized]) or chemicals (inadvertent exposure to benzene, lead, etc.), as well as recent travel.

B. *Clinical Assessment*

For patients with suspected sepsis, "a rapid assessment of perfusion should focus on heart rate, blood pressure, capillary refill, quality of peripheral and central pulses, and mental status" (Martin

& Weiss, 2015, p. 143). "Nurses are in an advantageous position to recognize critical status changes, indicating a patient experiencing sepsis" (Jeffery, Mutsch, & Knapp, 2014).

1. Inspection includes LOC, level of activity, general appearance, and respiratory rate, rhythm, and effort. Skin and mucous membranes should be examined for color and consistency, the presence of lesions, and the presence of generalized or localized edema, which is usually periorbital or sacral. Pedal edema may occur after the child begins to walk. Characteristics of fontanelles and jugular venous distention are noted to assess hydration status. Precordial activity is noted and is due to hypertrophy of the right ventricle, causing the lower end of the sternum and ribs to project forward. Although the point of maximal intensity (PMI) may be visible in some children, especially those who are thin, a prominent or heaving precordium may be an indication of cardiac dysfunction.

2. Palpation

a. *Skin and mucous membranes* are palpated for moisture, texture, refill, and temperature (note any demarcation in temperature from distal to proximal extremities and extremities versus the trunk). With cardiac dysfunction, blood is circulated at an insufficient rate, and compensatory vasoconstriction occurs in the extremities to shunt blood toward vital organs. Normal capillary refill is less than or equal to 2 seconds. The presence and intensity of peripheral pulses are noted. Also note proximal versus distal pulse quality because it is reflective of perfusion status. The clinical presentation of septic shock in children is more variable than in adults. Pediatric patients more commonly present in "cold shock"—a state of elevated SVR and low CO with delayed capillary refill and cold extremities (Martin & Weiss, 2015).

b. The level at which the normal liver border may be palpable is related to age. In the infant, the liver is normally felt up to 3 cm below the right costal margin; in the 1-year-old child, up to 2 cm below the right costal margin; and in the 4- to 5-year-old child, up to 1 cm below the right costal margin. The presence of hepatomegaly may indicate cardiac dysfunction, tumor, or hepatitis. An enlarged liver may also indicate fluid overload because the liver may act as a sponge and become engorged when central venous pressure (CVP) increases.

3. *Auscultation.* The presence and quality of breath sounds are noted. Respiratory rate and heart rate should be evaluated within the context of the child's age, clinical condition, and other external factors, such as fever. Apical heart rate and rhythm are auscultated. In the infant and young child, CO is directly proportional to heart rate because stroke volume is small. Blood pressure is a late sign of decompensation, but is still obtained. Blood pressure should be evaluated in the context of the child's age, clinical condition, and other parameters reflective of perfusion.

C. *Invasive and Noninvasive Diagnostic Studies*

1. Serum hematologic studies include:

a. CBC (see Chapter 8)

b. White blood cell (WBC) count: Total WBC count is generally considered normal at 5,000 to 10,000/mm³ but is age specific. Leukocytosis occurs in all forms of shock as a result of the demargination of neutrophils (Kumar & Parrillo, 2001). Leukopenia occurs in late septic shock *or* in infants and young children who are less able to replace neutrophils repeatedly in the face of an overwhelming infection. The WBC differential measures the five subcategories of circulating WBCs and is reported as a percentage. Neutropenia may be seen. An increased percentage (more than 10%) of bands (immature neutrophils) is seen when there is an increased demand for or decreased supply of neutrophils in the presence of an overwhelming infection (a shift to the left). A lymphocyte count of less than 1,000 for longer than 7 days may also be seen (Carcillo & Fields, 2003). Absolute granulocyte or neutrophil counts (AGC or ANC) may be low. An ANC lower than 1,000/mm³ carries a moderate risk for infection, and an ANC lower than 500/mm³ carries a high risk for infection.

c. Hemoglobin is variably affected. With the extravasation of intravascular water, erythrocytosis usually occurs.

d. Platelet count increases acutely but may be followed by thrombocytopenia with progressive septic shock.

e. Other serum tests of inflammation that may be helpful include erythrocyte sedimentation rate (ESR) and C-reactive protein, which are elevated secondary to an infectious process.

f. Procalcitonin (PCT) is an amino acid peptide exclusively produced by the neuroendocrine cells in response to endotoxin or mediators released in response to bacterial infections; thus, PCT normally circulates at very low levels (Pierce, Bingham, & Giuliano, 2014; Schuetz, Albrich, & Mueller, 2011). PCT is a reliable serum marker for detecting the presence or absence of invasive bacterial infection and response to antibiotic therapy (Pierce et al., 2014). PCT levels greater than 2 ng/mL may be predictive of bacterial infection in febrile children.

2. *ABG analysis.* Respiratory alkalosis occurs early in the course of septic shock. Initial respiratory alkalosis occurs as a compensatory mechanism to reduce carbon dioxide in the presence of increasing lactic acidosis from decreased perfusion. As septic shock progresses and respiratory reserves fail, respiratory acidosis develops. The body is unable to compensate for the increasing acid buildup. An anion gap metabolic acidosis is present because of the elevated levels of lactic acid.

3. *Routine chemistries.* Sodium, potassium, chloride, and bicarbonate are required to assess an anion gap. BUN and creatinine levels may initially appear normal. Lactate should be followed serially because it is a marker of tissue oxygen debt and supply-dependent oxygen consumption. It is a late marker of tissue hypoperfusion but one of the few available means of estimating tissue oxygenation. Arterial lactate levels greater than 2 mEq/L are associated with increased mortality in the adult population. Pediatric patients with severe sepsis or septic shock should have their blood glucose and calcium levels monitored because they are at risk of hyper/hypoglycemia and hypocalcemia (Brierley et al., 2009). Low glycogen stores of infants and young children in shock states significantly increase their risk of developing hypoglycemia (Brierley et al., 2009). Furthermore, observational studies have identified hyperglycemia as a risk factor for mortality in children with septic shock (Branco et al., 2005). Current guidelines recommend insulin therapy to avoid hyperglycemia (blood sugar ≥180 mg/dL) while also avoiding hypoglycemia (Brierley et al., 2009).

4. *Blood cultures* may identify causative microorganisms. Aerobic and anaerobic cultures are usually obtained. Obtaining blood cultures is a simultaneous priority with administration of broad-spectrum antibiotic coverage. Attempt to obtain blood cultures before the administration of antibiotics, but *never "hold" antibiotic administration to obtain blood cultures.*

a. The timing of culture results will vary. Results from cultures for common microorganisms, such as *streptococci, staphylococci,* and *Enterobacter,* are available in 24 to 48 hours.

b. Results from blood cultures may be negative. Some microorganisms, such as *Mycobacterium tuberculosis,* shed intermittently, causing negative results from cultures. In these instances, serial cultures may be required. Some patients, especially those who have received antibiotics, may also yield negative results from blood cultures. Only 50% of the patients with clinical signs of sepsis will have an organism isolated (Hartman et al., 2013). When an organism or clear source of infection cannot be identified, it is referred to as *culture-negative sepsis.*

5. *Other specimens and cultures*

a. Sputum specimens from the lower respiratory tract versus oropharyngeal secretions may be helpful.

b. Fecal cultures are used to find organisms that are not a part of the normal bowel flora or to determine normal flora that become pathogenic (e.g., *Clostridium difficile, Escherichia coli*).

c. Urine specimens with bacterial counts of less than 10,000 colony-forming units (CFU)/mL of urine are considered free of infection. Bacterial levels between 10,000 and 100,000 CFU/mL in urine cultures are inconclusive and require a second specimen. Bacterial counts greater than 100,000 CFU/mL of urine represent a definitive urinary tract infection.

d. Cerebrospinal fluid. Lumbar puncture may be needed to evaluate spinal fluid. Gram stains are particularly useful with cerebrospinal fluid infections for the purpose of selecting antibiotics.

6. Routine chest radiography is useful for ruling out pneumonia as the source of infection. Radiographic studies of other areas of the body are indicated by the child's history and physical examination.

7. *Invasive hemodynamic monitoring* should be considered with patients who do not respond quickly to initial fluid boluses or who do not demonstrate adequate physiologic reserve (Davis et al., 2017).

a. All patients with suspected shock should have an indwelling arterial catheter to monitor blood pressure serially. Blood pressure assessment via manual sphygmomanometer or automatic noninvasive oscillometric techniques may be inaccurate in patients in shock secondary to marked peripheral vasoconstriction.

b. CVP is often used to manage the child with septic shock to follow trends in intravascular volume status and responses to therapy. CVP is measured through a central venous catheter with the tip of the line located in the SCV–RA junction.

c. A pulmonary artery catheter may be helpful in managing the child in florid septic shock; however, pulmonary artery catheter use is becoming less common and more controversial. It provides continuous monitoring of cardiac filling pressures (CVP and pulmonary artery wedge pressure [PAWP]), an estimate of left ventricular end-diastolic pressure [LVEDP] and volume [LVEDV]), cardiac flow (CO per cardiac index [CO/CI]), cardiac contractility (stroke volume, stroke volume index, stroke work index), and afterload (SVR, systemic vascular resistance index [SVRI]). It also allows the withdrawal of blood from the pulmonary artery catheter to determine oxygen consumption: pulmonary artery oxygen content and mixed venous oxygen saturation (SvO_2).

8. *Echocardiogram* is a noninvasive tool that can be used to evaluate myocardial contractility and assess hemodynamics in patients with fluid refractory shock (Davis et al., 2017).

D. *Phases and Clinical Manifestations of Septic Shock* (Table 9.24). Stages may be identified in the clinical progression of septic shock in *some* children. During the hyperdynamic compensated phase, blood pressure is maintained. In the later hyperdynamic uncompensated phase, blood pressure begins to fall. The hypodynamic state essentially appears congruent to cardiogenic shock.

PATIENT CARE MANAGEMENT

A. Guidelines for the management of children in septic shock were published in 2002, 2007, and in 2014 (Davis et al., 2017). Use of these guidelines has improved the outcomes for children in septic shock. The updated guidelines provide recommendations that each institution develop tools to identify and manage patients experiencing septic shock. Best practice quality-improvement efforts, including recommendations of treatment within the first hour of recognition, establishing IV access, initiation of IV fluids for resuscitation, administration of antibiotics, and initiation of vasoactive medications to support adequate perfusion, are needed. Many institutions have created management bundles and audit the care provided in the management of patients with septic shock based on these recommendations (Davis et al., 2017).

B. Essential treatment of septic shock *must* include both *definitive treatment*, including identification, localization, and eradication of the source of infection with antibiotic administration and source control procedures if necessary, and *advanced life support treatment*, including oxygenation, ventilation, and circulation with fluid and inotropic administration. *Controversial treatments* are those with conflicting results

or undetermined efficacy such as steroids for fluid refractory catecholamine-resistant shock and plasma exchange. *Futuristic treatments* are those currently under investigation or scheduled for investigation in the near future such as passive immunization and monoclonal antibody administration. Controversial and futuristic treatments often fall into one of two approaches, which include either neutralizing microbiologic toxins or modulating host inflammatory immune responses.

C. Identify those patients at risk for the development of sepsis or septic shock. Rapid identification of the patient experiencing sepsis and septic shock is essential in the rapid treatment and effective management of the patient. The adult literature defines shock by hypotension and increased lactate in a normotensive patient (Brierly et al., 2009). Early recognition of sepsis or septic shock can be challenging in pediatrics (because either may be subtle and insidious), especially in younger patients, such as neonates and infants and patients undergoing treatments or interventions that alter inflammatory immune response, including glucocorticoid administration. Hypotension may be a delayed or late response in young children. Although teenagers and adults may first experience warm shock with increased CO and decreased SVR, a young child may experience vasoconstriction with low CO and poor peripheral perfusion. This vasoconstriction seen with a cold shock state causes the hypotension to be seen later (Martin & Weiss, 2015). The current recommendation is for early recognition of shock in pediatrics using clinical examination (Brierly et al., 2009).

TABLE 9.24   Phases and Clinical Manifestations of Septic Shock

Fluid-resistant shock	Shock persists despite 60 mL/kg resuscitation
Catecholamine-resistant shock	Shock persists despite dopamine 10 mcg/kg/min *and* direct acting catecholamines (epinephrine, norepinephrine)
Warm shock	Vasodilation, low SVR, high CO Warm extremities, flash capillary refill <1 sec, bounding pulse Decreased diastolic blood pressure, wide pulse pressure (>40 mmHg)
Cold shock	High SVR, low CO Cold extremities, prolonged capillary refill (>3 sec), faint pulses Normal or increased diastolic blood pressure Narrow pulse pressure (<30 mmHg)

CO, cardiac output; SVR, systemic vascular resistance.

Source: Permission obtained from Scott Weiss, MD.

Shock may be identified by hypothermia or hyperthermia, tachypnea, altered mental status and oliguria, vasodilation (indicative of warm shock), or vasoconstriction with delayed capillary refill (indicative of cold shock; Brierly et al., 2009; Davis et al., 2017). Bradycardia or tachycardia is also seen. Monitor ongoing changes in the patient or the patient's response(s), such as behavior, level of consciousness, temperature patterns (e.g., fever), and WBC count.

D. *Initial Resuscitation* (see Figure 9.9)

1. *Assess ABCs.* Rapid cardiopulmonary assessment, proposed by the American Heart Association PALS program includes a primary survey of life-threatening conditions followed by a secondary survey. Once the ABCs are ensured, the child should receive, as required, antibiotic administration, volume resuscitation, and vasoactive agents. Vascular access will quickly need to be obtained for fluid and IV therapy. Access may be difficult to obtain in a child or infant experiencing septic shock. PALS guidelines provide direction on the placement of peripheral and central access, including the use of umbilical access and intraosseous access (Brierly et al., 2009).

2. *Volume Resuscitation.* In a child with septic shock who is hypovolemic, an aggressive approach is taken as fluid resuscitation can reverse the shock state and increase odds of survival. A 20 mL/kg IV fluid bolus with subsequent boluses of 20 mL/kg over 5 minutes is started soon after presentation. A septic patient may require a large volume of crystalloid NS or lactated Ringers) reaching 60 to 200 mL/kg in the first hour of resuscitation (Brierly et al., 2009). Fluid boluses should be administered and titrated to assessment of the patient clinical state with frequent reassessment for the development of volume overload. Age-specific parameters for blood pressure and heart rate should be considered. The assessment should include heart rate, blood pressure, peripheral pulses, capillary refill, urine output, level of consciousness, and skin temperature for signs of improvement (Brierly et al., 2009). Colloids, such as 5% albumin, may also be used. Fresh frozen plasma may be used to correct PT or partial thromboplastin time (PTT). Packed red blood cells may also be chosen to increase hemoglobin and to act as a volume expander (Brierly et al., 2009; Davis et al., 2017). During fluid resuscitation, patients should also be assessed for signs of fluid overload such as increased rales, cardiac gallop, or hepatomegaly (Brierley et al., 2009). A study by Rivers and colleagues (2001) found that early aggressive volume resuscitation in patients with severe sepsis and septic shock improved the likelihood of survival. Patients who do not respond to fluid boluses may need invasive hemodynamic monitoring. Serial measurements of cardiac filling pressures (CVP, pulmonary capillary wedge pressure [PCWP]) and ventricular performance (CO/CI, SVR) are useful in monitoring CVP and PAWP's trends during treatment. Approximately 50% of patients with septic shock will have reduced mortality and morbidity and lower organ dysfunction rates associated with adequate intravascular fluid resuscitation (Medeiros, Ferranti, Delgado, & Brunow de Carvalho, 2015). However, risk of mortality doubles per hour delay in restoring the blood pressure level to normal and improving perfusion (Han et al., 2003; Vincent et al., 1998). Patients may require increased fluid administration for multiple days due to capillary leak and leakage of the fluid from the vessels into the tissues (Brierly et al., 2009).

3. Antibiotic Administration. Broad spectrum antibiotics are administered with the initial dose ideally given with in the first hour of recognition (Dellinger et al., 2013). In one pediatric study, patients experienced less sepsis-related organ failure and decreased mortality when antibiotics were administered within 3 hours (Weiss et al., 2014). Blood culture specimens should be obtained before the administration of antibiotics, but antibiotics should never be withheld to obtain a culture. With the emergence of many resistant organisms, antibiotics may be given in accordance with regional resistant/sensitivity patterns. Antibiotic choice will also be influenced by the age, medical history, status of immune compromise of the child as well as the suspected source of infection.

4. *Vasoactive Agents* (Table 9.25). If volume resuscitation fails to restore perfusion or severe hypotension is present, vasoactive agents are indicated in order to maintain organ perfusion (Davis et al., 2017). Fluids should continue to be administered with vasoactive agents until clinical parameters are met. Vasoactive agents may be initiated and changed over time as the patient's clinical condition evolves (Davis et al., 2017).

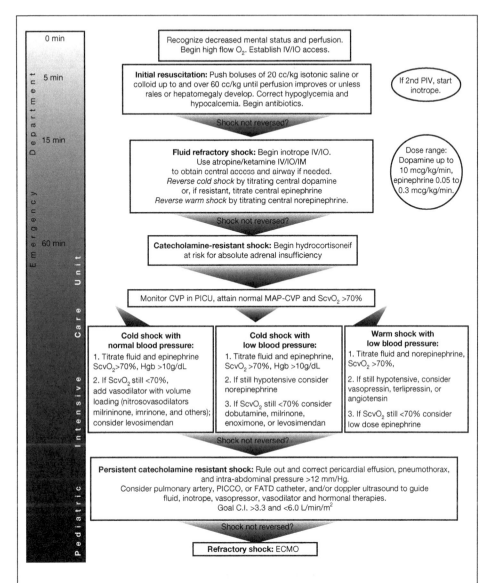

FIGURE 9.9 Algorithm for time-sensitive, goal-directed stepwise management of hemodynamic support in infants and children. Proceed to next step if shock persists. (1) First hour goals—Restore and maintain heart rate thresholds, capillary refill ≤2 sec, and normal blood pressure in the first hour/emergency department. Support oxygenation and ventilation as appropriate. (2) Subsequent intensive care unit goals—If shock is not reversed, intervene to restore and maintain normal perfusion pressure (MAP-CVP) for age, central venous O_2 saturation >70%, and CI >3.3, <6.0 L/min/m² in PICU.

CI, cardiac index; CRRT, continuous renal replacement therapy; CVP, central venous pressure; ECMO, extracorporeal membrane oxygenation; FATD, femoral arterial thermodilution; Hgb, hemoglobin; IM, intramuscular; IO, interosseous; IV, intravenous; MAP, mean arterial pressure, PICU, pediatric intensive care unit; PiCCO, pulse contour cardiac output; PIV, peripheral intravenous line.

Source: From Brierley, J., Carcillo, J. A., Choong, K., Cornell, T., Decaen, A., Deymann, A., . . . Zuckerberg, A. (2009). Clinical practice parameters for hemodynamic support of pediatric and neonatal septic shock: 2007 update from the American College of Critical Care Medicine. *Critical Care Medicine, 37*(2), 677.

TABLE 9.25 Inotropic and Vasoactive Agents Used in the Treatment of Septic Shock

Drug	Site of Action	Dose (mcg/kg/min)	Primary Effect	Secondary Effect
Dopamine	Dopaminergic	2–5	Increase renal perfusion	Dysrhythmias
	Dopaminergic and β_1	2–10	Inotropy Chronotropy Increase renal perfusion	
	α	10–20	Vasoconstriction	
Norepinephrine	$\alpha>\beta$	1–2	Vasoconstriction	>MVO$_2$
			Inotropy	Dysrhythmias
				<Renal BF
Epinephrine	α and β	0.05–1.5	Vasoconstriction	>MVO$_2$
			Inotropy	Dysrhythmias
			Chronotropy	<Renal BF
Dobutamine	β_1	5–20	Inotropy	Tachycardia
				Dysrhythmias
				Vasodilation
				Hypotension
Milrinone	Phosphodiesterase inhibitor	0.25–1	Inotropy	Dysrhythmias
			Vasodilation	<PVR
			Improves diastolic function	

BF, blood flow; ICP, intracranial pressure; MVO$_2$, myocardial oxygen consumption; PVR, pulmonary vascular resistance.

Note: Difficult to predict the dose–response effect. Management requires individual titration at the bedside.

Persistent shock following 40 to 60 mL/kg of fluid administered within the first hour is considered fluid-resistant shock and vasoactive agents are considered (Martin & Weiss, 2015). A mixed α- and β-adrenergic agent, such as epinephrine or dopamine, is considered first-line inotropic support for cold shock in children (Brierly et al., 2009, Martin & Weiss, 2015). If blood pressure continues to be decreased, inotropic agents are added. In the presence of hypotension, the drug of choice is epinephrine due to the preponderance of "cold shock" in children. If a child is in "warm shock," norepinephrine may be more appropriate to increase SVR (Martin & Weiss, 2015). For patients with a normal blood pressure and myocardial dysfunction, dobutamine may be considered a first-line agent to increase contractility when there is a low CO state with high or adequate SVR (Brierly et al., 2009; Martin & Weiss, 2015). Norepinephrine is considered a first-line agent for a patient experiencing warm shock, considered with a high CO state and low SVR. Epinephrine may be initiated in the treatment of cold shock in the lower doses, primarily for its beta-2 adrenergic effects. Higher doses will provide more α-adrenergic effects. Central access is preferred for vasoactive agents, although current recommendations provide support for initial peripheral infusion during resuscitation. Vasopressors can be titrated to clinical parameters, such as CVP or urine output, with the intention to avoid the negative effects of excessive vasoconstriction (Brierly et al., 2009).

Note. Protocols should be used *only* as guides to therapy. Vasoactive support should be evaluated using consistent clinical criteria rather than numeric values only.

E. *Cardiovascular Management*

1. *Support and Optimize CO.* CO may be within the normal range or increased at times in the continuum of septic shock, but it is still inadequate to meet the body's demands. Normal or increased CO is often accompanied by low blood pressure and SVR, thus affecting perfusion and oxygen transport. Recommendations for each of the constituents of CO serve *only* as a guideline. Each patient should be evaluated individually with regard to age, clinical context (including the changing continuum of septic shock), and total hemodynamic profile. Mixed venous saturation ($SCVO_2$) greater than 70%, CI greater than 3.3 L/min/m^2 less than 6.0 L/min/m^2, and a normal perfusion pressure should be the goal of therapy (Brierly et al., 2009).

2. Increase preload with early, aggressive fluid therapy (isotonic crystalloids first and colloids later). Volume administration is used to improve preload and treat hypoperfusion due to increased capillary permeability, vasodilation, and maldistribution of blood flow. Administration and assessment of fluid therapy as discussed previously.

3. *Maximize Contractility.* The left ventricular ejection fraction (LVEF) and overall contractility are significantly lowered in septic shock. Inotropic agents may be indicated for improvement of contractility (see Table 9.25). Dopamine, epinephrine, and norepinephrine all have ionotropic properties. Milrinone and inamrinone, phosphodiesterase inhibitors, may

also be used to increase cardiac contractility and decrease afterload.

4. *Manipulate Afterload (SVR).* Persistent hypotension may occur even in the presence of aggressive volume administration and is often related to mediator release and vasodilation rather than low CO/CI. Vasopressors may be indicated, and larger doses may be required over time because of continuing mediator release, capillary leakage, and decreased responsiveness of α- and β-adrenergic receptors. Sodium nitroprusside or nitroglycerine, short-acting vasodilators may be used in epinephrine-resistant normotensive patients to reduce afterload, increase CO, and improve tissue perfusion (Brierly et al., 2009). Manipulation of afterload most often occurs in combination with an inotropic agent. The inotropic agent maintains the blood pressure and enhances contractility, whereas the vasodilator reduces the afterload and cardiac filling pressures.

F. *Respiratory Management*

1. The patient experiencing septic shock should be monitored and supported. The ability to maintain adequate gas exchange may change quickly. A rapid respiratory rate, hyperventilation, and respiratory alkalosis are seen in early sepsis (Brierley et al., 2009). Due to poor perfusion and decreased oxygen delivery to the cells, a metabolic acidosis develops. As respiratory compromise develops, a child in sepsis may quickly develop a respiratory acidosis and respiratory failure. Supplemental oxygen, adequate positioning of the airway, and preparation for decompensation should be provided to all patients with shock (Davis et al., 2017). A decision to intubate may be necessary to support respirations due to mental status changes causing hypoventilation, worsening lung compliance, and inadequate gas exchange.

2. Assess and maximize tissue oxygenation (see Chapter 2, "Oxygen Transport" section). Support airway and ventilation. Position the child to support maximal airway patency. Provide supplemental oxygen. Anticipate intubation because most children with septic shock require intubation and mechanical ventilation.

3. Assess tissue oxygenation using parameters such as ABG analysis, oxygen saturation, and oxygen content. Normal PaO_2 is 80 to 100 mmHg on room air. With supplemental oxygen, the lower limit of the normal PaO_2 expected for a given FiO_2 is estimated by multiplying the FiO_2 by 5. Hypoxemia is present if the hemoglobin saturation is less than 90%. *Oxygen content* (CaO_2) is the quantity of oxygen in each 100 mL of blood and includes both the amount dissolved in the plasma and carried in the hemoglobin. Normal oxygen content is 18 to 20 mL/dL of blood.

$$CaO_2 = [Hgb\ (g/dL) \times 1.36\ mL\ O_2/g\ Hgb \times SaO_2] + (0.003 \times PaO_2)$$

4. Assess oxygen utilization using the parameters of oxygen delivery and oxygen consumption.

  a. *Mixed venous oxygen saturation (SvO_2)* is a continuous reflection of the balance between oxygen supply and oxygen demand, with the normal range between 70% and 80%.

  b. *Oxygen transport or delivery (DO_2)* is the volume of oxygen delivered to the tissues each minute and reflects the quantity of oxygen available to the tissues.

$$DO_2\ (mL/min)$$

Arterial blood O_2 content (CaO_2) = $(Hgb \times 1.39 \times SaO_2) + (0.0003 \times PaO_2)$

  c. *Oxygen consumption ($\dot{V}O_2$)* is the amount of oxygen consumed by the tissues per minute and reflects an overall index of total body metabolism. VO_2 in infants and children, which ranges from 5 to 14 mL O_2/kg/min, can be measured, estimated, or calculated:

$$\dot{V}O_2 = CO \times [(SaO_2 - S\bar{v}O_2) \times (Hgb\ concentration \times 1.36\ mL/g)] \times 10$$

  d. *Oxygen extraction ratio* is determined by dividing oxygen consumption by oxygen transport or delivery with the normal value, around 20% to 25%. The oxygen extraction ratio (O_2ER) is the percentage of oxygen extracted from the arterial blood by the cells. It is the percentage of difference between the arterial oxygen content and the venous oxygen content.

$$(O_2ER) = (CaO_2 - CvO_2)/CaO_2 \times 100$$

5. *Optimize Oxygen Delivery* (see Chapter 2). Provision of oxygen and mechanical ventilation are key components to increasing oxygen delivery, as well as optimizing carrying capacity through addressing anemia and supporting CO as already described.

6. *Minimize Oxygen Demand.* It is beneficial to limit the patient's metabolic demands, especially patients with little or no metabolic reserve. Interventions include reducing fever, pain, and agitation. It is also important to provide adequate support of ventilation and sedation ± neuromuscular blockade to decrease the patient's work of breathing.

G. *Minimize Iatrogenic Complications*

  1. Barotrauma can be prevented by using the lowest possible peak pressure that will allow for adequate ventilation.

  2. Minimize the risk of and assess for further cardiac dysfunction by monitoring electrolytes and watching for tachyarrhythmias secondary to vasoactive and inotropic agents or electrolyte imbalance. Hypoglycemia, hyperglycemia, or hypocalcemia may require rapid intervention.

  3. Minimize the risk of and assess for aspiration by placing a nasogastric drainage tube, ensuring the tube's patency and function, and elevating the head of the bed 30 degrees if tolerated.

  4. Minimize the risk of and assess for renal toxicity by optimizing tissue perfusion and judiciously using medications that are toxic to the kidneys.

  5. Manage thyroid and adrenal insufficiency. Patients with thyroid or adrenal insufficiency should be monitored closely and may require supplemental pharmaceutical management.

  6. Minimize the risk of VTE formation. VTE prophylaxis should be considered. The presence of a central line increases the risk of development of thrombosis.

H. *Supportive and Investigational Therapies*

  1. Stress-Dose Steroids. Hydrocortisone may be administered to patients who are at risk of adrenal insufficiency. Current guidelines recommend administration of hydrocortisone for patients with fluid-resistant, catecholamine refractory shock and those with absolute adrenal insufficiency (Brierley et al., 2009; Martin & Weiss, 2015). Research has been mixed on the use of steroids as a standard treatment for patients experiencing septic shock (Martin & Weiss, 2015).

2. ECMO may be used to support cardiorespiratory function in the patient with refractory septic shock who has not responded adequately to other therapies (Brierley et al., 2009; Martin & Weiss, 2015). This supportive intervention provides time for other therapies to help the child progress to recovery.

3. Nutritional support should be provided via the enteral route if tolerated. The safety of early nutritional support will need to be considered based on the dose of vasopressors the patient is receiving. The gut mucosa will atrophy quickly in the absence of enteral nutrients. Patients experiencing SIRS are at risk for metabolic alterations. When managed in the ICU, these patients should receive a nutrition consultation for measurement of resting energy expenditure and nutrition enteral nutrition recommendation (Mehta, Comher, & A.S.P.E.N. Board of Directors, 2009).

4. Intravenous immunoglobulin (IVIG). IVIG has been studied for its role in the inflammatory response. It helps balance the inflammatory response and neutralizes endotoxins (Martin & Weiss, 2015). Although some small studies have been favorable and IVIG is mentioned in the guidelines, it is usually considered for specific at-risk patients with immunodeficiency and low immunoglobin levels (Martin & Weiss, 2015). IVIG is also recommended for treatment of toxic shock (Brierley et al., 2009).

5. Continuous renal replacement therapy (CRRT). CRRT should be considered for hemodynamically stable fluid overloaded patients experiencing oliguria or anuria who have been unresponsive to diuretics (Brierly et al., 2009).

I. *Implications for Other Systems.* Given the complexity of the immune system, it is not surprising that SIRS and septic shock influence many body organs and systems. Because many body systems are affected, organ-specific dysfunction may result. Complications of septic shock include ARDS (see Chapter 2), DIC (see Chapter 8), acute renal failure (see Chapter 5), and multiple-organ dysfunction syndrome (MODS).

J. *Multiple-Organ Dysfunction Syndrome.* There are many risk factors that predispose patients to MODS; however, the most common causes are related to shock,

sepsis, and tissue hypoperfusion (Ramirez, 2013). A recent study by Lin et al. (2017) included 567 patients from 128 PICUs in 26 countries, and 384 (68%) patients developed MODS within 7 days of severe sepsis recognition. MODS and new or progressive MODS is a significant risk factor for adverse outcomes in pediatric sepsis (Lin et al., 2017). As compared to adults, pediatric patients have earlier development of MODS and faster multiorgan involvement (Ramirez, 2013). The criteria for pediatric patients with MODS are detailed in Table 9.14.

1. Frequency of specific organ involvement in children experiencing MODS within 7 days of sepsis recognition (Lin et al., 2017):

- Respiratory system (82%)
- Cardiovascular (65%)
- Hematologic (22%)
- Neurologic (15%)
- Renal (12%)

2. The mortality associated with MODS is related to the number of organ systems involved in the dysfunction process. Hospital mortality for patients with progressive MODS was 51% compared to 28% for patients with new MODS and only 10% for patients with single-organ dysfunction without MODS (Lin et al., 2017).

GOALS AND DESIRED PATIENT OUTCOMES

A. Prevention and early recognition of children with sepsis or septic shock

B. Early, accurate, and complete administration of antibiotics

C. Early and aggressive fluid resuscitation until improved perfusion is observed as evidenced by improved mental status, diminished tachycardia, capillary refill of less than 2 seconds, warm extremities, strong pulses, normal urine output, and restoration and maintenance of normal blood pressure (Brierly, 2009)

D. Restoration of optimal balance of oxygen supply and demand and thus tissue perfusion as indicated by arterial oxygen saturation of 92% or higher, hemoglobin concentration of 10 g/dL or greater, CI between 3.3 and 6 L/min/m² body surface area (BSA), oxygen delivery (DO₂) between 500 and 600 mL/min/m², normal oxygen consumption ($\dot{V}O_2$: in infants, oxygen 10 to 14 mL/kg/min; in children, oxygen 7 to 11 mL/kg/min), superior vena cava oxygen saturation (SVC O₂) greater than 70%, and normalization of serum lactate of less than 2 mEq/L

E. Early nutritional support

F. Minimization of the risk and extent of organ dysfunction

CASE STUDIES WITH QUESTIONS, ANSWERS, AND RATIONALES

Sepsis and Septic Shock Case Studies

Case Study 9.9

An 8-year-old male arrives in the ED. He was discharged from the hospital 3 days ago status post two rounds of chemotherapy. At home, he developed watery diarrhea and his mother took him to an outside hospital for dehydration. Vital signs were: temp 39.8°C, heart rate 180 bpm, respiratory rate 30, BP 94/60, SpO₂ 100% on room air. He is ill appearing, mottled with cool extremities, petechia on his chest, and dry mucus membranes. He has a single lumen broviac. Initial labs are: Na 128 mEq/L, k 3.9 mEq/L, Cl 104 mEq/L, CO₂ 19 mEq/L, BUN 23 mg/dL, Creatinine 0.6 mg/dL, glucose 73 mg/dL, lactate 2.9 mmol/L, calcium 6.7 mg/dL, WBC 0.0 per microliter, HgB 9.4 gm/dL, and platelets 12 per microliter. He is given a rapid bolus of 40 ml/kg NSS IV.

1. This child is at highest risk for sepsis due to:
   A. Age, central line, previous hospitalization
   B. Gender, malnourishment
   C. Central line, immunocompromised

As he is waiting to transfer to the ICU, his BP drops to 60/40, heart rate 170 bpm, SpO₂ 97% with weak, thready, peripheral pulses; prolonged capillary refill; and cool extremeties.

2. What type of shock is the patient experiencing?
   A. Cold shock with low blood pressure
   B. Catecholamine-resistant shock
   C. Cold shock with normal blood pressure
   D. Warm shock with low blood pressure

After interventions are provided by the team, he begins to stabilize and is getting prepared to transfer to the ICU. IV antibiotics are administered. Vital signs are: hear rate 180 bpm, respiratory rate 46, SpO₂ 100% with 100% blowby, BP 70/50, venous gas on istat: PH 7.37, PCO₂ 25, PO₂ 24, HCO₃ 4, base deficit -10 Na 137, K 3.9, I cal 0.95, Hgb 6.1, Hct 18.

3. This blood gas reflects:
   A. Respiratory acidosis
   B. Metabolic acidosis
   C. Respiratory alkalosis
   D. Metabolic alkalosis

4. What state of compensation does this blood gas reflect?
   A. Uncompensated
   B. Partially compensated
   C. Fully compensated

On arrival to the PICU, he has had 200 ml urine output and continues to have diarrhea. His mother states that he has had 15 episodes of diarrhea since this started. While getting him settled, you see that his blood pressure has dropped to 50/20. He continues to look mottled, with thready peripheral pulses. His oxygen saturation has dropped to 90% on 100% blowby.

5. Based on the information given here, what is the top priority for this patient?
   A. Administer a unit of packed red blood cells
   B. Place Foley for strict I/O monitoring
   C. Administer a fluid bolus
   D. Prepare for intubation

6. The care team orders multiple STAT interventions (packed red blood cells, antibiotics, fluid bolus, etc.) for this patient, which all need to be completed in a timely manner. The nurse's best course of action would be to:
   A. Independently prioritize interventions
   B. Collaborate with the care team to prioritize and discuss plan of care
   C. Delegate task to neighboring nurse or charge nurse
   D. Update family on plan of care

Sepsis and Septic Shock Answers and Rationales

Case Study 9.9

1. **C.** Pediatric mortality is highest in patients younger than a year and the second highest mortality is seen in patients between the ages of 1 and 4. While the immune system is not fully matured at his age, the presence of an invasive catheter and his immuocompromised status present the greatest risk for this patient.

2. **A.** The patient's physical exam, including weak pulses, and cool extremeties, is consistent with cold shock. His blood pressure is below normal limits and his heart rate remains elevated. A patient in warm shock would present with vasodilation, warm extremeties, and a bounding pulse. Catecholamine-resistant shock would be shock that persists despite dopamine or direct-acting catecholamine administration.

3. **B.** This patient is in metabolic acidosis since the pH is low normal and both the pCO_2 and HCO_3 are low.

4. **C.** For a patient to be fully compensated, the pH will be within normal range. If the pH is less than 7.4 the patient has compensated acidosis; to be metabolic, both the pCO_2 and HCO_3 are less than normal.

5. **C.** According to the Surviving Sepsis Campaign, administration of fluid and antibiotics are the priority interventions for a septic patient. While the Hgb is low, based on initial labs, the likelihood of having a unit readily available to treat the hypotension is unlikely. A Foley would also be helpful, but is not the top priority. Although the patient may need additional respiratory support, the administration of fluid to improve the BP is more concerning at this time.

6. **B.** Collaborating with the care team allows for discussion of priorities and barriers to care. In this example, our patient only has a single lumen Broviac. Discussing limited vascular access would allow the team to decide to obtain more access or other applicable choices to accomplish all interventions in a timely manner. Independently prioritizing the interventions with identified barriers may lengthen the time to complete all interventions. Delegating tasks is important, but in this case will not solve the limited vascular access issue. Updating the family is always important, but the top priority is to stabilize the BP and provide antibiotics to help treat the patient.

SEPSIS AND SEPTIC SHOCK REFERENCES

Alyn, I. B., & Baker, L. K. (1992). Cardiovascular anatomy and physiology of the fetus, neonate, infant, child and adolescent. *Journal of Cardiovascular Nurse, 6*(3), 1–11.

Branco, R. G., Garcia, P. C., Piva, J. P., Casarteli, C. H., Seibel, V., & Tasker, R. C. (2005). Glucose level and risk of mortality in pediatric septic shock. *Pediatric Critical Care Medicine, 6*(4), 470–472.

Brierley, J., Carcillo, J. A., Choong, K., Cornell, T., Decaen, A., Deymann, A., . . . Zuckerberg, A. (2009). Clinical practice parameters for hemodynamic support of pediatric and neonatal septic shock: 2007 update from the American College of Critical Care Medicine. *Critical Care Medicine, 37*(2), 666–688.

Carcillo, J. A., Dean, J. M., Holubkov, R., Berger, J., Meert, K. L., Anand, K. J. S., . . . Webster, A. (2016). Inherent risk factors for nosocomial infection in the long stay critically ill child without known baseline immunocompromised: A post-hoc analysis of the CRISIS Trial. *Pediatric Infectious Disease Journal., 35*(11), 1182-1186 doi:10.1097/INF.0000000000001286

Carcillo, J. A., & Fields, A. I. (2003). Clinical practice meters for hemodynamic support of pediatric and neonatal patients in septic shock. *Critical Care Medicine, 30*(6), 1365–1378.

Davis, A. L., Carcillo, J. A., Aneja, R. K., Deymann, A. J., Lin, J. C., Nguyen, T. C., . . . Zuckerberg, A. L. (2017). American College of Critical Care Medicine clinical practice parameters for hemodynamic support of pediatric and neonatal septic shock. *Critical Care Medicine, 45*(6), 1061–1093. doi:10.1097/CCM.0000000000002425

de Pablo, R., Monserrat, J., Aprieto, A., & Alvarez-Mon, M. (2014). Role of circulating lymphocytes in patients with sepsis. *BioMed Research International, 2014*(2014), 1–11. doi:10.1155/2014/671087

Dellinger, R. P., Levy, M. M., Rhodes, A., Annane, D., Gerlach, H., Opal, S. M., . . . , Moreno, R. (2013). Surviving sepsis campaign: International guidelines for management of severe sepsis and septic shock: 2012. *Critical Care Medicine, 41*(2), 580–637. doi:10.1097/CCM.0b013e31827e83af

Goldstein, B., Giroir, B., & Randolph, A. (2005). International Pediatric Sepsis Consensus Conference: Definitions for sepsis and organ dysfunction in pediatrics. *Pediatric Critical Care Medicine, 6*(1), 2–8. doi:10.1097/01.PCC.0000149131.72248.E6

Gotts, J. E., & Matthay, M. A. (2016). Sepsis: Pathophysiology and clinical management. *BMJ, 353*, i1585. doi:10.1136/bmj.i1585

Hall, M. W., Knatz, N. L., Vetterly, C., Tomarello, S., Wewers, M. D., Volk, H. D., & Carcillo, J. A. (2011). Immunoparalysis and nosocomial infection in children with multiple organ dysfunction syndrome. *Intensive Care Medicine, 37*(3), 525–532. doi:10.1007/s00134-010-2088-x

Han, Y., Carcillo, J. A., Dragotta, M. A., Bills, D. M., Watson, R. S., Westerman. M. E., & Orr, R. A. (2003). Early reversal of pediatric neonatal septic shock by community physicians is associated with improved outcome. *Pediatrics, 112*(4), 793–799.

Hartman, M. E., Linde-Zwirble, W. T., Angus, D. C., & Watson, R. S. (2013). Trends in epidemiology of pediatric severe sepsis. *Pediatric Critical Care Medicine, 14*(7), 686–693. doi:10.1097/PCC.0b013e3182917fad

Hazinski, M. F. (Ed.). (2013). *Nursing care of the critically ill child.* (3rd ed., pp. 101–154). St Louis, MO: Elsevier.

Jeffery, A. D., Mutsch, K. S., & Knapp, L. (2014). Knowledge and recognition of SIRS and sepsis among pediatric nurses. *Pediatric Nursing, 40*(6), 271–278.

Kumar, A., & Parrillo, J. E. (2001). Shock: classification, pathophysiology, and approach to management. In J. E. Parrillo & R. C. Bone (Eds.), *Critical care medicine: Principles of diagnosis and management* (2nd ed., pp. 371-420). St Louis, MO: Mosby.

Levy, M. M., Artigas, A., Phillips, G. S., Rhodes, A., Beale, R., Osborn, T., . . . Dellinger, R. P. (2012). Outcomes of the Surviving Sepsis Campaign in intensive care units in the USA and Europe: A prospective cohort study. *Lancet Infectious Diseases, 12*(12), 919–924.

Lin, J. C., Spinella, P. C., Fitzgerald, J. C., Tucci, M., Bush, J. L., Nadkarni, V. M., . . . Weiss, S. L. (2017). New or progressive multiple organ dysfunction syndrome in pediatric severe sepsis: A sepsis phenotype with higher morbidity and mortality. *Pediatric Critical Care Medicine, 18*(1), 8–16. doi:10.1097/PCC.0000000000000978

Magill, S. S., Edwards, J. R., Bamberg, W., Beldavs, Z. G., Dumyati, G., Kainer, M. A., . . . Fridkin, S. K. (2014). Multistate point-prevalence survey of health care–associated infections. *New England Journal of Medicine, 370*(13), 1198–1208. doi:10.1056/NEJMoa1306801

Maki, D. G. (1995). Nosocomial infection in the intensive care unit. In J. E. Parrillo & R. C. Bone (Eds.), *Critical care medicine: Principles of diagnosis and management* (2nd ed., pp. 371–420). St. Louis, MO: Mosby.

Martin, K., & Weiss, S. L. (2015). Initial resuscitation and management of pediatric septic shock. *Minerva Pediatrica, 67*(2), 141–158.

Medeiros, D. N. M., Ferranti, J. F., Delgado, A. F., & Brunow de Carvalho, W. (2015). Colloids for the initial management of severe sepsis and septic shock in pediatric patients: a systematic review. *Pediatric Emergency Care, 31*(11), e11–e16.

Mehta, N. M., Comher, C., & A. N. Board of Directors. (2009). A.S.P.E.N. clinical guidelines: Nutrition support of the critically ill child. *Journal of Parenteral and Enteral Nutrition, 33*(3), 260–276. doi:10.1177/0148607109333114

National Vital Statistics System, National Center for Health Statistics, Centers for Disease Control and Prevention. (2016). 10 leading *causes of death by age group, United States—2014*. Retrieved from https://www.cdc.gov/injury/images/lc-charts/leading_causes_of_death_age_group_2016_1056w814h.gif

Pierce, R., Bingham, M. T., & Giuliano, J. S. (2014). Use of procalcitonin for the prediction and treatment of acute bacterial infection in children. *Current Opinion in Pediatrics, 26*(3), 292–298. doi:10.1097/MOP.0000000000000092

Ramirez, M. (2013). Multiple organ dysfunction syndrome. *Current Problems in Pediatric and Adolescent Health Care, 43*(10), 273–277. doi:10.1016/j.cppeds.2013.10.003

Randolph, A. G., & McCulloh, R. J. (2014). Pediatric sepsis. *Virulence, 5*(1), 179–189. doi:10.4161/viru.27045

Rivers, E. Nguyen, B, Havstad, S., Ressler, J., Muzzin, A., Knoblich, B., . . . Tomlanovich, M. (2001). Early goal directed therapy in the treatment of severe sepsis and septic shock. *New England Journal of Medicine, 346*, 1368–1377. doi:10.1056/NEJMoa010307

Robins, E. V. (1996). Maldistribution of circulating volume. In V. B. Huddleston (Ed.), *Multisystem organ failure: Pathophysiology and clinical implications* (2nd ed.). St. Louis, MO: Mosby-Year Book.

Ruth, A., McCracken, C. E., Fortenberry, J. D., Hall, M., Simon, H. K., & Hebbar, K. B. (2014). Pediatric severe sepsis: Current trends and outcomes from the pediatric health information systems database. *Pediatric Critical Care Medicine, 15*(9), 828–838. doi:10.1097/PCC.0000000000000254

Schoenmakers, S. H. H. F., Reitsma, P. H., & Spek, C. A. (2005). Blood coagulation factors as inflammatory mediators. *Blood Cells, Molecules & Diseases, 34*(1), 30–37. doi:10.1016/j.bcmd.2004.09.001

Schuetz, P., Albrich, W., & Mueller, B. (2011). Procalcitonin for diagnosis of infection and guide to antibiotic decisions: Past, present and future. *BMC Medicine, 9*, 107. doi:10.1186/1741-7015/9/107/prepub

Schulte, W., Bernhagen, J., & Bucala, R. (2013). Cytokines in sepsis: Potent immunoregulators and potential therapeutic targets— An updated view. *Mediators of Inflammation, 2013*, 165974. doi:10.1155/2013/165974

Singer, M., Deutschman, C. S., Seymour, C. W., Shankar-Hari, M., Annane, D., Bauer, M., . . . Angus, D. C. (2016). The third international consensus definitions for sepsis and septic shock (Sepsis-3). *Journal of the American Medical Association, 315*(8), 801–810. doi:10.1001/jama.2016.0287

Urrea, M., Pons, M., & Serra, M. (2003). Prospective incidence study of nosocomial infections in a pediatric intensive care unit. *Pediatric Infectious Disease Journal, 22*, 490–494.

Vincent, J. L., de Mendonça, A., Cantraine, F., Moreno, R., Takala, J., Suter, P. M., . . . Blecher, S. (1998). Use of the SOFA score to assess the incidence of organ dysfunction/failure in intensive care units: Results of a multicenter, prospective study. *Critical Care Medicine, 26*(11), 1793–8000.

Watson, R. S., Carcillo, J. A., Linde-Zwirble, W. T., Clermont, G., Lidicker, J., & Angus, D. C. (2003). The epidemiology of severe sepsis in children in the United States. *American Journal of Respiratory and Critical Care Medicine, 167*, 695–701.

Weiss, S. L., Fitzgerald, J. C., Balamuth, F., Alpern, E. R., Lavelle, J., Chilutti, M., . . . Thomas, N. J. (2014). Delayed antimicrobial therapy increases mortality and organ dysfunction duration in pediatric sepsis. *Critical Care Medicine, 42*(11), 2409–2417.

Weiss, S. L., Fitzgerald, J. C., Pappachan, J., Wheeler, D., Jaramillo-Bustamante, J. C., Salloo, A., . . . Thomas, N. J. (2015). Global epidemiology of pediatric severe sepsis: The sepsis prevalence, outcomes, and therapies study. *American Journal of Respiratory and Critical Care Medicine, 191*(101), 1147–1157.

SECTION IV. BURNS

Amanda Bettencourt and Melissa Gorman

Caring for a child with a burn injury is challenging; depending on the size and depth of the burn, dramatic alterations in fluid and electrolyte balances, ventilation, and thermoregulation can occur and if not managed properly can result in organ dysfunction and ultimately death. Pediatric burn care has progressed significantly over the past several years, and with proper care and treatment children today can survive burn injuries that involve almost all of their body surface area (BSA). Nursing care of the burned child involves knowledge of the pathophysiology of burn inflammation; management of burn shock; performance of complex wound care; adequate pain and anxiety management; and providing for the psychosocial needs of the child, his or her family, and community. The American Burn Association (ABA) is the interprofessional organization for those who care for patients with burn injuries. In addition to this chapter, nurses who care for burned children on a regular basis are encouraged to familiarize themselves with the ABA and its clinical practice guidelines, which can be found on the organization's website (www.Ameriburn.org).

A. Incidence

1. According to the World Health Organization (2018), an estimated 265,000 deaths are caused worldwide every year by burns. The vast majority of these deaths occur in low- and middle-income countries.

2. According to the ABA (2016), there are approximately 486,000 burn injuries and 40,000 burn-related hospital admissions in the United States annually.

3. Unintentional injury is the leading cause of death for children over the age of 1 year in the United States. Unintentional fire/burn is the fifth leading cause of unintentional injury death in children age 1 to 4 and the third leading cause in children 5 to 9 years of age (CDC, 2016a, 2016b).

4. Children ages 4 and younger are at the greatest risk of suffering burn-related injuries, with an injury rate more than twice that of children aged 5 to 15 years (ABA, 2017).

5. Scald injuries are most prevalent in children younger than 5, whereas fire/flame injuries are the most common in the remaining age categories (ABA, 2017).

B. Types of Burn Injury

Burn types can be classified into four main categories: thermal, electrical, chemical, and radiation. Thermal burns can be further divided into subtypes of scald, flame, contact, and hypothermic. See Table 9.26 for descriptions of each type of burn.

C. Pathophysiology of Burn Injury

1. *Local Inflammation*

  a. The local burn wound is the result of direct damage of skin cells and results in coagulation necrosis of tissue that has both breadth and depth, or more common, a percentage of total body surface area (%TBSA) and degree (i.e., first, second, or third degree) of burn injury. The depth or extent of the burn injury depends on the intensity of the heat, the duration of exposure, and the type of tissue involved.

  b. If the absorption of heat energy exceeds the ability of the tissue to dissipate the absorbed heat, cellular injury occurs at various depths in the skin organ. This phenomenon can best be described by Jackson's functional classification system (Figure 9.10; Lewis, Heimbach, & Gibran, 2012). In this model, the depth of injury is dependent on the relative heat exposure area and the healing process as represented by three distinct zones of injury.

    i. The zone of hyperemia is the most superficial area of viable tissue and will heal itself in a matter of days (i.e., sunburn).

    ii. The zone of stasis is a deeper area inside the zone of hyperemia where vascular damage and inflammation have resulted in some compromise of tissue perfusion but not immediate cell death. This zone is evolving continuously over the first 2 to 3 days postinjury, and may undergo progressive tissue destruction or heal on its own depending on the quality of care the child receives and other physiological factors. Effective resuscitation and immediate postinjury care have been shown to positively affect viability in the zone of stasis (Lewis et al., 2012).

    iii. The third zone is the zone of coagulation, where the heat has damaged the skin most intimately, and cells in the skin have necrosed.

TABLE 9.26 Burn Types

Burn Type	Subtype	Description	Examples
Thermal		Thermal injuries result from direct heat. Extent of injury is dependent on the size or volume and temperature of the thermal agent (surface, steam, or liquid), amount of time the skin was in contact with the heat source, and individual patient characteristics.	
	Scald/steam	Scald burns are caused by contact with hot liquids and are the most common burn type in children younger than 5 years of age.	• A young infant is bathed in water that is too hot. • A toddler reaches and pulls a cup of hot tea off of a table. • A school-age child tries to prepare soup in the microwave.
	Flash and flame	Flash burns are caused by intense heat produced by ignition of flammable liquids for a short period of time. Flame burns are caused by direct contact of the skin with fire and are the most common burn type in children older than 5 years of age.	• A preschooler is playing with a lighter, accidentally igniting his shirt, sustaining a deep flame burn. • An adolescent is burned when gasoline is thrown into a campfire resulting in an explosion and flash burn.
	Contact	Contact burns are caused when hot, solid objects, come in contact with the skin.	• An infant falls against a hot radiator. • A toddler tries to climb on a hot, open oven door.
	Hypothermic	Local cold injury or frostbite occur when the skin is exposed to extreme cold temperatures.	• An adolescent is lost in the woods during a camping trip in extreme cold conditions.
Electrical		Small surface wounds caused by electricity may be associated with larger internal injuries. Electrical injuries are caused by DC or AC, and can be classified as high voltage or low voltage. Electrical injuries may be caused by commercially generated electricity or lightning. Electricity can cause injury via several different mechanisms. These include current flow, arc flash, ignition of clothing, thermal contact burns, and other associated injuries (ABLS Advisory Committee, 2015).	• A toddler places a finger into an electrical outlet. • A school-age child touches a high-tension wire on a dare. • An adolescent is struck by lightning in an open field.

(continued)

TABLE 9.26 Burn Types *(continued)*

Burn Type	Subtype	Description	Examples
Chemical		Chemical burns occur when the skin comes in direct contact with caustic chemicals, such as acids, alkalis, or organic compounds. Severity is related to the agent, its concentration, its volume, and the duration of contact.	• A preschooler spills drain cleaner and slips in the puddle. • An adolescent splashes hydrochloric acid in his eye during chemistry class.
Radiation		Radiation injuries can result from radiation-generating machines and devices, radioactive compounds, and environmental radiation. Ionizing radiation causes tissue damage as energy is transmitted to living tissue (ABLS Advisory Committee, 2015).	• An adolescent falls asleep on the beach without sunblock.

ABLS, Advanced Burn Life Support; AC, alternating current; DC, direct current.

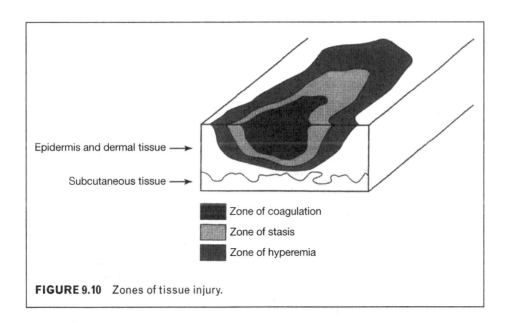

Epidermis and dermal tissue ⟶

Subcutaneous tissue ⟶

■ Zone of coagulation
▨ Zone of stasis
■ Zone of hyperemia

FIGURE 9.10 Zones of tissue injury.

Because this zone is characterized by cellular death, coagulation necrosis is the result of injuries in this zone.

c. At the injury site, the inflammatory response mediated by histamine and prostaglandin causes increased permeability of the cell membrane separating the intravascular and interstitial compartments, resulting in altered exchange of fluid and plasma in the wound bed. When this occurs, it causes all elements of the intravascular space except RBCs to escape, and edema forms, causing a relative intravascular hypovolemia. This is also how a blister forms on the burn wound. As the child's %TBSA and depth of injury increase, the severity of this inflammatory response increases. Thus, children with large burns (>15% TBSA) have local edema formation as well as potential for systemic capillary leak formation, and resultant need for fluid resuscitation to maintain homeostasis. Edema that is the result of increased capillary permeability is at its peak 12 to 24 hours postburn injury. Very large and deep burns can take up to 2 to 3 days to regain capillary cell membrane integrity (Warden, 2014).

2. *Systemic Responses*

   a. A large burn injury (>15% TBSA and deep) affects all organ systems and can cause a phenomenon known as *burn shock*. SIRS is present in burned children to varying degrees after injury. In addition to burn shock, a hypermetabolic and systemic immune response occurs. The events, magnitude, and duration of the systemic manifestations of burn shock are proportional to the extent of burn injury and plateau at approximately 50% to 60% burn surface area. Although the exact etiology of burn shock is not totally understood, characteristic fluid volume shifts and hemodynamic changes that accompany burn shock have been identified. Within several hours of injury, as *edema* forms, the fluid shift and intravascular volume deficit result in hemoconcentration (Kramer, 2014). The hematocrit increases secondary to loss of circulating plasma volume. Blood viscosity also increases.

   b. With increased catecholamine and glucagon production, there is a mobilization of hepatic glycogen stores, coupled with a relative decrease in insulin production that commonly results in high serum glucose levels in the early postburn period. Within 24 to 48 hours after the burn, there is an increase in metabolism directly related to the severity of the injury. This hypermetabolic state is characterized by increases in oxygen consumption and heat production, with an increase in both core and skin temperatures. Both protein synthesis and breakdown are increased. In patients not meeting nutritional goals, breakdown rates exceed synthesis, resulting in a negative nitrogen balance. As capillary integrity is restored, electrolyte replacement therapy becomes an ongoing process and continues until wound closure is achieved. As the wounds heal, either spontaneously or by skin grafting, the metabolic rate gradually returns to normal levels. The decrease in metabolic requirements is a gradual process. In children with large burns, metabolic requirements remain elevated even after the burn wound is fully mature (Jeschke & Herndon, 2014).

3. *Associated Complications*

   a. *General*. Although the exact mechanisms of the immunologic and inflammatory response are not known, characteristic pathophysiologic activities are being recognized as a result of the burn injury. Alteration in the skin's protective function provides opportunity for invasion of microorganisms and primes the defensive mechanisms of the inflammatory and immune systems. It is hypothesized that a massive systemic inflammatory response is caused by the local trauma of a burn. It appears that a burn is a mediator-induced injury; although the local effects occur immediately, the systemic response to the mediators produced within a burn progresses and peaks 5 to 7 days after the injury. It is unclear whether the immunosuppression after a burn injury is the result of biochemical substances (i.e., oxidants, histamine, prostaglandins, arachidonic acid metabolites) liberated from the burn itself, or is produced in response to the burn. In addition, the immunosuppressive effects of anesthetic agents, surgical procedures, multiple transfusions, and the use of systemic antibiotics emphasize postburn immunologic abnormalities during the clinical course of burn therapy (Murphy, Sherwood, & Toliver-Kinsky, 2012).

   b. *Hypothermia*. Children are more prone to the development of hypothermia related to their increased body surface-area-to-mass ratio, resulting in greater evaporative water loss and conductive heat loss. Hypothermia remains a major problem until the wounds have been skin grafted or healed. Hypothermia alone, without any injuries, can cause apnea, progressive metabolic acidosis, and ventricular arrhythmias. Every effort should be made to minimize heat loss in children with burn injuries, including providing care in a heated and humidified hospital room (Lee, Norbury, & Herndon, 2012).

   c. *Compartment syndrome*. Circumferential deep partial-thickness and full-thickness burns of the extremities may impair circulation as a result of rapid edema formation. Thus, it is imperative to maintain continuous elevation of the burned extremities and evaluate skin color, sensation, and capillary refill at frequent intervals during the first 24 to 48 hours after injury. The use of an ultrasonic flow device is indicated if pulses are not palpable or color and sensation assessments are complicated by the burn injury (Advanced Burn Life Support [ABLS] Advisory Committee, 2015). Another assessment strategy is to apply a pulse oximetry probe distal to the circumferential injury and monitor the waveform to assess flow. Because compartment syndrome is associated with loss of life and limb, *escharotomies* should be performed by an experienced clinician provider at the earliest sign of circulatory compromise (i.e., [early] paresthesia, pain with passive stretch, or [later] decreased pulse or complaints of deep aching muscle pain).

    i. Escharotomy/fasciotomy. An escharotomy is performed when the edema from a circumferential deep burn wound is compromising circulation to the deeper tissues. The skin loses elasticity with deep burn injury, and thus cannot expand to accommodate this increased edema, causing circulatory compromise.

    ii. Escharotomies are performed most often at the bedside with a scalpel or electrocautery device, and involve mechanical release of the eschar layer of the skin only on the longitudinal plane. If compartment syndrome becomes severe and escharotomy does not relieve the pressure, a fasciotomy may be required. This procedure is typically performed in the operating room and involves mechanical release of the underlying fascia to alleviate pressure from edema in the muscular compartment. Without prompt intervention, nerve damage and muscle necrosis can result.

d. *Abdominal compartment syndrome.* If the resuscitation volumes are excessive, or the child has suffered from massive (>80%) burns, abdominal compartment syndrome may develop (Lee, Norbury, & Herndon, 2012). In children with abdominal compartment syndrome, mortality risk increases significantly, as multiorgan system failure often results. Careful monitoring and surgical laparotomy intervention or percutaneous peritoneal drainage when abdominal compartment syndrome is suspected/confirmed is key to improving survival and reducing morbidity in children with massive burns.

e. *Electrical injuries.* The complications associated with electrical injuries are related to the type and duration of electrical current that the child has come in contact with. The injuries of most concern for the critical care nurse are high-voltage injuries. According to Ohm's law, electrical current flows through areas that have the least resistance (highest conductivity) to the electrical current flow. When electricity comes in contact with the skin, the skin is injured at the contact points as well as deeper within the skin and underlying tissues where the current has flowed. If electrical current has flowed through the torso, cardiac rhythm disturbances can occur. In addition to cardiac rhythm disturbances, cutaneous injury can occur. Typically, the contact points (or "entrance and exit wounds") appear dry, circumscribed, and depressed.

    i. Electrical injuries are often referred to as "iceberg" injuries, as the true extent of tissue injury is often not visible on the surface of the skin itself. A common complication of high-voltage electrical injury is subfascial edema and tissue necrosis between the contact points. Thus, it is imperative that the nurse measure pulse quality, color, motor function, and sensation in the electrically injured limb closely during the first 24 hours after injury. When a change in color, motor function, sensation, or pulse quality is detected, a provider should be notified and escharotomies or fasciotomies may be performed to relieve the pressure and restore perfusion (ABLS Advisory Committee, 2015). If these symptoms are not recognized and intervened upon, loss of limb can occur.

    ii. Any child who has an electrical injury should have a 12-lead ECG performed to check for arrhythmia. If a loss of consciousness occurred at the scene or any abnormality is detected in the ECG, continuous cardiac monitoring is indicated.

    iii. If the electrical injury is extensive and muscle necrosis has occurred, a common and serious side effect is myoglobinuria due to the hemochromogens present in the bloodstream. If the urine of a child with an electrical injury becomes pigmented, an increase in intravenous fluid rate and addition of bicarbonate or mannitol to the treatment plan is often indicated, as acute tubular necrosis and renal failure can result (ABLS Advisory Committee, 2015).

    iv. Other, less common complications associated with electrical injuries include the following:

        1) Pathologic fractures of long bones due to muscle tetany

        2) Spinal cord injuries due to falling/trauma or spinal fracture

        3) Neurologic complications such as headaches, seizures, diminished memory, difficulty concentrating, and emotional fluctuations that may persist for months to years after injury

f. *Chemical injuries.* The complications associated with chemical injury vary based upon the nature of the chemical. Typical caustic chemicals that can cause injury are acids, alkalis, and petroleum-based products. The most important intervention in the child with a chemical injury is to remove clothing and to brush off all powders, followed by decontamination with tap water. Once the agent has been identified, treatment may be directed at neutralizing the agent, but irrigation should occur continuously from the time of exposure through the evaluation stage in the hospital. Typically, alkalis cause deeper skin damage than acidic compounds due to their high affinity for elements found in the tissue.

   i.   If the chemical has made contact with the eyes, contact lenses should be removed and immediately flushed with copious amounts of water. Irrigation with normal saline or a buffered solution is preferred, but tap water is appropriate if nothing else is readily available (ABLS Advisory Committee, 2015). A prompt consultation to an ophthalmology provider and corneal exam are very important due to the risk of permanent vision loss.

   ii.   The specific treatment modality for each chemical the child has been exposed to can be obtained by contacting a poison control facility, the hazardous materials division of the fire department, or the chemical manufacturer. Prompt treatment with the appropriate antidote is key to minimizing morbidity and mortality in chemically injured children.

D. Initial Assessment and Management

   1. *Assessment and Management at the Scene*

   a. The most important first-aid treatment is *minimizing* the burn wound depth and extent, which is accomplished by eliminating the source of the injury and stopping the burning process (ABLS Advisory Committee, 2015).

   b. After the burning agent is eliminated, *cover* the burns with clean, dry linen. Measures to conserve body heat are essential for all burn survivors, particularly for the infant and young child. Wet compresses may be applied to small wounds but not to large injuries and need only be applied during the first few minutes after injury (Sheridan, 2012). Water increases body heat loss through evaporation and can lead to hypothermia. This is a principal concern in small children, where wet dressings may accentuate the shock state, causing a further decrease in tissue perfusion, cardiac output, and perfusion to vital organs (Lee, Norbury, & Herndon, 2012). Ice or ice water should never be used directly on the skin because of the potential for cold injury or for conversion of a lesser burn to a deeper injury (due to vasoconstriction; ABLS Advisory Committee, 2015).

   c. Rapid primary and secondary assessment

   i.   At the accident scene, the primary and secondary assessments are performed as later described but in a *more rapid manner*. The priority quickly becomes to expediently transport the patient to a hospital.

   ii.   Burn patients are considered multiple trauma victims and must be assessed for other traumatic injuries in addition to the burn, especially if the burn is the result of a motor vehicle crash or an explosion of some kind. Any coexisting trauma must be evaluated and treated during the primary and secondary surveys.

   iii.   Begin fluid resuscitation if the burn appears to be bigger than 15% of the TBSA and deep according to the ABLS prehospital resuscitation rates (Table 9.27). Lactated Ringer's or NS are appropriate choices for resuscitation fluid in the field (ABLS Advisory Committee, 2015).

Example of Calculating Fluid Resuscitation

Parkland Burn Resuscitation Formula
First 24 Hours Postburn 4 mL Ringer's lactate × weight in kg × % burn surface area Give half of the calculated amount in the first 8 hours postburn and the remaining amount over the next 16 hours; *plus daily maintenance volume with dextrose as needed.* Example: 10-kg child with 50% burn surface area: 4 mL × 10 kg × 50% burn surface area = 2,000 mL Ringer's lactate* over 24 hours First 8 hours = 1,000 mL RL = 125 mL/hr Second 8 hours = 500 mL RL = 62.5 mL/hr Third 8 hours = 500 mL RL = 62.5 mL/hr * The fluid is recommended to be lactated Ringer's, but could be normal saline.

   2. *Assessment and Management in the Emergency Department*

   a. Primary assessment. The primary assessment follows the "ABCDE" methodology, beginning with airway and breathing, followed by circulation, disability, and expose/examine.

TABLE 9.27   Burn Resuscitation Fluid Calculation Recommendations

Practice Setting	Age of Patient	Recommended Formula
Prehospital (start if burn looks >15%TBSA and deep)	Infant Child Adolescent/Adult	125 mL/hr of LR or NS 250 mL/hr of LR or NS 500 mL/hr of LR or NS
Emergency department (ABLS consensus formulas)	Adults Children Electrical injury (any age)	2 mL LR × %TBSA × weight (kg) 3 mL LR × %TBSA × weight (kg) 4 mL LR × %TBSA × weight (kg) Take this total and divide by ½. Give the first ½ in the first 8 hours, rest over next 16 hours. Remember to monitor urine output hourly and titrate up/down as needed to meet UOP target of 0.5–1 mL/kg/hr or 2 mL/kg/hr if electrical injury is present.
Inpatient unit/burn center	Adults Children Electrical injury (any age)	Parkland formula Brooke formula Nurse-driven resuscitation All formulas are estimates, careful measurement of clinical endpoints of resuscitation is the key intervention to titrate fluid requirements appropriately.

LR, lactated Ringer's; NS, normal saline, TBSA, total body surface area; UOP, urine output.

b. Assess the airway and breathing. Airway management for the burn patient should be managed as for any trauma victim, including performing basic life-support measures if indicated, providing 100% FiO_2 via face mask, assessing respirations for adequacy of rate and depth, and assessing for bilateral breath sounds.

   i.   Special considerations. The upper airway is susceptible to edema and obstruction as a result of exposure to heat and smoke. Because of relatively small airways in children, upper airway obstruction may occur early and rapidly. Circumferential full-thickness burns to the neck or chest may restrict ventilation.

   ii.   Upper airway obstruction or lower airway compromise should be identified and treated accordingly and may require endotracheal intubation and mechanical ventilation.

c. Assess circulation.

   i.   Determine the exact extent and depth of the burn. Children with deep burns covering 20% or more of their TBSA require circulatory volume support (Sheridan, 2012). See Table 9.27 for appropriate resuscitation formula choices during emergency department stabilization.

   ii.   Establish intravenous (IV) access for fluid resuscitation if indicated. Place two peripheral large-bore IV catheters, appropriate for the size of the child. The peripheral percutaneous route is the method of choice for immediate initial access; if the only accessible veins have overlying burned skin, do not hesitate to use them (ABLS Advisory Committee, 2015). Cannulation of small veins may be difficult in any infant or child but even more so in a child with severe vasoconstriction. Maintaining venous access is a major priority. Adhesive tape is ineffective in securing IV catheters to burned tissue and may compromise blood flow in edematous extremities if applied circumferentially. An intraosseous needle is the vascular access of choice in the child who will need fluids or pain management and peripheral IV access cannot be obtained in a timely fashion (Lee, Norbury, & Herndon, 2012). In the event the child needs continual resuscitation and/or pain management, central venous catheterization is indicated.

   iii.   Evaluate skin color, sensation, and capillary refill. Circumferential deep second- to third-degree burns of the extremities may impair circulation as a result of edema formation. Regardless of circumferential injury, maintain continuous elevation of the burned extremities.

   iv.   Monitor arterial pulses hourly for 24 to 48 hours on all extremities with deep burns, circumferential burns, or electrical burns. Use an ultrasonic flow device or pulse oximetry probe with a pleth waveform if pulses are not palpable. Escharotomies should be performed at the earliest sign of circulatory compromise (i.e., decreased pulse, complaints of deep aching muscle pain) in consultation with an experienced provider.

v. Insert a urinary catheter to monitor the effectiveness of fluid resuscitation.

d. Assess disability/neurologic status. Use the alert, voice, pain, unresponsive (AVPU) method to assess neurologic status (ABLS Advisory Committee, 2015). Typically, the burn survivor is initially alert and oriented. If a decreased level of consciousness is present, consider an associated injury, substance abuse, hypoxia, or preexisting medical condition.

e. Expose and examine

i. Remove all clothing so the extent and severity of injury can be examined. In the case of chemical burns, the clothing could be contaminated and cause further injury and should be immediately removed entirely. Keep any clothing removed from the child in a safe place until it is determined whether it will be needed for law enforcement evidence review.

ii. Remove all jewelry as soon as possible, as jewelry will create a tourniquet effect as systemic and burn wound edema form, restricting blood flow and causing tissue loss (ABLS Advisory Committee, 2015).

f. Secondary assessment

i. Obtain a history of the burn injury. Initial management and definitive care are guided by the mechanism, duration, severity, and time of the injury. As much information as possible should be obtained regarding the incident:

- What was the cause of the burn?
- Did the injury occur in a closed space?
- What was the timing of the injury?
- Were harmful chemicals involved?
- Were others involved?
- Is there suspicion for nonaccidental trauma?

ii. Obtain medical history. Underlying medical conditions frequently complicate burn management and prolong recovery.

Determine the presence of preexisting disease or associated illness; medications, alcohol, or drugs; allergies or sensitivities; recent exposure to communicable diseases (i.e., varicella, tuberculosis); status of tetanus immunization (burn wounds are tetanus-prone wounds and immunizations should be consistent with the recommendations of the American College of Surgeons); and status of other immunizations (ABLS Advisory Committee, 2015). The tetanus status, however, must be documented so as not to be overlooked. As an aid to gaining necessary information, the mnemonic "AMPLET" can be used:

A = Allergy

M = Medications

P = Previous illness

L = Last meal/fluids

E = Events related to the injury

T = Tetanus

iii. Complete physical examination. This includes a complete head-to-toe examination and physical assessment to evaluate more fully any and all injuries or abnormalities, including the burn injury. The severity of a burn injury and its morbidity and mortality are determined by the type of burn; size, depth, and anatomic location of the wound; the patient's age; and any preexisting illness or associated trauma.

iv. Determine burn size.

1) The extent of a burn is calculated as a %TBSA burned. Various methods are available to determine the %TBSA. The exact %TBSA is necessary to calculate definitive resuscitation formulas and ensure adequate volume, but not too much volume, is given to the patient. Superficial first-degree burns with erythema (redness) alone should not be included in %TBSA calculations.

2) In the rule of the palm, the entire palmar aspect of the patient's hand (including the fingers) represents approximately 1% of the TBSA. Therefore, using the child's hand as a visual guide, the extent of a small burn or one with an irregular outline or distribution can easily be estimated by determining how much of that child's palms would cover the injured

area, and multiplying that by 1% to calculate the percentage of TBSA burned.

3) The rule of nines measures the percentage of burn surface area by dividing the body into multiples of nine. In the infant or child, the rule is adjusted because the child's head has a larger proportional percentage of the TBSA and thus is not the most accurate estimation of burn extent in children (ABLS Advisory Committee, 2015).

4) The Berkow formula, or Lund and Browder chart allows for a more accurate assessment in children, as it takes into account differences in BSA related to age and divides the body into smaller areas (e.g., foot, lower leg, thigh).

5) Another method uses a standard height and weight nomogram to calculate the BSA burned in square meters (m^2).

6) Regardless of the calculation method used, accurate communication of the %TBSA calculated upon admission used for resuscitation volume calculations must occur. In most cases, a burn diagram should be completed by a nurse or provider and filed in the child's medical record.

v. Type of burn. Identify the type of burn: Although appropriate initial interventions often occur before arrival at the emergency department, never assume this step has been completed (i.e., chemical burns).

vi. Obtain baseline diagnostic studies. Baseline laboratory studies are essential to evaluate the patient's subsequent progress. Evaluate ABGs and carboxyhemoglobin (if a closed space injury has occurred), hematocrit and hemoglobin, electrolytes, albumin, urinalysis, BUN, chest radiographic examination, and 12-lead ECG with electrical injury, ectopy, or history of underlying cardiovascular disease.

vii. Initial wound care. Wound care is not considered a component of emergency care except in chemical burns, in which immediate removal of the agent is essential. Substantial wound care, such as excessive manual debridement or application of topical antimicrobials (in the field or primary hospital), is not necessary if the patient

will be transferred to a burn care facility in a relatively timely fashion (ABLS Advisory Committee, 2015).

viii. NPO status. Patients must have nothing by mouth (NPO) until they have been seen and evaluated in a hospital and, if necessary, transported to a burn center. A nasogastric tube should be inserted in all patients with a burn size of over 15% BSA, as they are susceptible to gastric dilatation due to a paralytic ileus, and in all patients who are intubated (ABLS Advisory Committee, 2015).

3. *Admission and Transfer Criteria*

a. Children who have suffered deep burns on greater than 15% of their TBSA should be admitted to a pediatric intensive or intermediate level-of-care environment to allow for close monitoring of hydration status and organ perfusion. Criteria established by the ABA exist to guide clinicians in decisions related to transfer of a child to a verified burn center. These criteria are listed in Table 9.28.

b. Additional criteria to consider for a potential admission to a burn critical care environment include the following:

i. Suspected inhalation injury

ii. Concomitant trauma

iii. Circumferential deep burn wounds

iv. Electrical injuries

v. Children who require continuous pain medication infusions

vi. Fluid over-resuscitation in the field/emergency department

vii. Delayed resuscitation

c. Regardless of the care location, priorities of care in the inpatient setting include maintaining intravascular volume to allow for end-organ perfusion, maximizing pain relief, monitoring ventilation, and minimizing wound complications such as compartment syndrome and infection.

E. Ongoing Assessment and Management

1. *Depth of Injury Assessment*

a. It may take up to several days for the burn wound to fully "declare itself" with respect to the depth of injury. Depth of injury is best assessed by visual inspection of the burn wound and palpation of several areas of the burn wound to determine the extent of capillary and tissue injury. As a general rule, a burn wound that is

TABLE 9.28 American Burn Association Burn Center Referral Criteria

Burn injuries that should be referred to a burn center include the following:
1. Partial-thickness burns greater than 10%TBSA
2. Burns that involve the face, hands, feet, genitalia, perineum, or major joints
3. Third-degree burns in any age group
4. Electrical burns, including lightning injury
5. Chemical burns
6. Inhalation injury
7. Burn injury in patients with preexisting medical disorders that could complicate management, prolong recovery, or affect mortality
8. Any patient with burns and concomitant trauma (such as fractures) in which the burn injury poses the greatest risk of morbidity or mortality; in such cases, if the trauma poses the greater immediate risk, the patient may be initially stabilized in a trauma center before being transferred to a burn unit; physician judgment will be necessary in such situations and should be in concert with the regional medical control plan and triage protocols
9. Burned children in hospitals without qualified personnel or equipment for the care of children
10. Burn injury in patients who will require special social, emotional, or rehabilitative intervention

TBSA, total body surface area.

Source: Excerpted from Committee on Trauma American College of Surgeons. (2014). *Resources for optimal care of the injured patient* (p. 101). Chicago, IL: American College of Surgeons.

moist and has blisters is a second-degree (partial-thickness) burn wound. If the skin appears dry and tough, it is most likely a third-degree (full-thickness) burn wound. Skin that appears red and does not have blisters is first degree (superficial) and is not included in %TBSA calculations (ABLS Advisory Committee, 2015).

b. Most burn wounds are a mixture of all three depths of injury, so the nurse must be able to assess depth and healing of the mixed burn wound at the bedside. To assess the depth of a wound that has a mixture of blisters and dry, tough tissue, palpate the tissue with a gloved finger or sterile cotton swab and assess capillary refill, or "blanching" of the wound. A wound with brisk capillary refill when pressed upon is more superficial than one with slower capillary refill when pressed upon. Thus, the part of the wound with slower capillary refill is deeper than the part with the brisk refill. If there is an absence of capillary refill, blood supply to that area is permanently compromised, and that wound is full thickness and will eventually most likely need surgical intervention (see Figure 9.11).

2. Assessment of Systemic Responses to Burn Injury

a. *Burn Shock.* An extensive burn affects all organ systems and is manifested by a biphasic pattern of early hypofunction (i.e., decreased cardiac output, increased capillary permeability) followed by hyperfunction (i.e.,

hypermetabolism). The events, magnitude, and duration of the systemic manifestations of burn shock are proportional to the extent of burn injury and plateau at approximately 50% to 60% burn surface area. Although the exact etiology of burn shock is not totally understood, there are several characteristic fluid volume shifts and hemodynamic changes that accompany burn shock that have been identified.

b. Cardiovascular response

i. The *initial response* to a large burn injury is characterized by a decrease in cardiac output and increased peripheral vascular resistance. An uncharacterized factor present in the circulation following massive burns has been implicated for this characteristic myocardial depression. The increased peripheral vascular resistance develops as an initial physiologic response to hypovolemia, decreased cardiac output, and the release of vasoactive mediators from the stress response following injury (Kramer, 2014).

ii. *Cardiac output* returns to normal 24 to 36 hours after the burn (Kramer, 2014). Peripheral vascular resistance returns to normal as cardiac output improves. As cardiac output improves, it exceeds normal values as the characteristic hyperdynamic state develops. Tachycardia develops as a physiologic response to hypovolemia, decreased cardiac output, and elevated catecholamine levels.

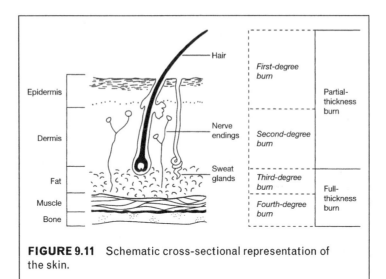

FIGURE 9.11 Schematic cross-sectional representation of the skin.

iii. *Microvasculature changes* in the cell membranes result in the disruption of normal capillary barriers separating the intravascular and interstitial compartments, resulting in free exchange of fluid and plasma. This increased permeability permits essentially all elements of the vascular space, except RBCs and platelets, to escape, creating a relative hypovolemia. The fluid requirement necessary to restore and maintain tissue perfusion is directly related to the burn size. Capillary leak and edema following small burns are localized to the burn wound. Injury greater than 20% burn surface area produces not only a localized burn wound edema but also a systemic capillary permeability and general body edema (Sheridan, 2012). The rate of progression of tissue edema is dependent on the adequacy and volume of fluid resuscitation. The maximal amount of edema occurs 8 to 12 hours after injury in small burns but can last up to 24 hours after injury in large burns. Capillary integrity is restored approximately 18 to 24 hours postburn. Large burns may take up to 30 hours to regain capillary integrity.

c. Pulmonary response

i. In large burns without an inhalation injury, early alterations in pulmonary function occur indirectly through the release of inflammatory mediators (i.e., thromboxane) and intravascular hypoproteinemia resulting in a transient hydrostatic pulmonary edema with a mild derangement in oxygenation.

ii. A decrease in lung compliance may be related to chest-wall edema, circumferential burns to the chest wall, smoke-inhalation injury, preexisting lung disease, or fluid volume overload (Traber, Herndon, Enkhbaatar, Maybauer, & Maybauer, 2012).

d. Hematologic response

i. Within several hours of injury, as *edema* forms, the fluid shift and intravascular volume deficit result in hemoconcentration. The hematocrit increases secondary to loss of circulating plasma volume. Blood viscosity also increases (Kramer, 2014).

ii. The characteristic *anemia* associated with burn injuries has multiple causes. Only about 10% of the RBC mass is lost to hemolysis during the burning process or by the extravasation of RBCs into the wound (Posluszny, Gamelli, & Shankar, 2012). Heat-injured RBCs have a shortened half-life and increased clearance. The ongoing postburn RBC hemolysis has been attributed to the release of inflammatory mediators (i.e., oxygen radicals, lipid peroxides). Although the exact nature is not known, there is an impaired production of new RBCs by the bone marrow with a shortened RBC lifespan (Posluszny et al., 2012). In addition, there is an ongoing effective blood loss related to daily wound care and multiple surgical procedures.

iii. Initially there is a *depression in serum clotting factors* with a concomitant rise in fibrinogen degradation products, followed by a postresuscitation rise in increased levels of coagulation components. Platelet alterations include an increase in adhesiveness and shortened survival time (Posluszny et al., 2012).

e. GI response. Decreased GI tract activity caused by decreased tissue perfusion is the by-product of hypovolemia and the neuroendocrine responses to injury. These responses cause an increased risk for the development of a burn-stress-related ulceration (Curling's ulcer), and the incidence of ulceration has been greatly reduced by the routine use of antacid or histamine (H$_2$) antagonist therapy. With adequate fluid resuscitation, GI tract activity returns to normal within 24 to 48 hours (Chung & Wolf, 2012).

f. Renal response. With decreased intravascular volume there is a decrease in renal plasma flow and glomerular filtration rate (GFR), resulting in low urine output (Chung, & Wolf, 2012). If fluid resuscitation is inadequate or if resuscitation is delayed, oliguria ensues leading to acute renal failure. As the capillary integrity is restored, interstitial fluids are pulled back into the intravascular compartment, and diuresis occurs.

g. Metabolic response

i. With increased catecholamine and glucagon production, there is a mobilization of hepatic glycogen stores, coupled with a relative decrease in insulin production that commonly results in high serum glucose levels in the early postburn period.

ii. Within 24 to 48 hours after the burn, there is an increase in metabolism directly related to the severity of the injury. This hypermetabolic state is characterized by increases in oxygen consumption and heat production, with an increase in both core and skin temperatures. Severe injury accelerates nitrogen flow. Both protein synthesis and breakdown are increased. In patients not meeting nutritional goals, breakdown rates exceed synthesis, resulting in a negative nitrogen balance. As capillary integrity is restored, electrolyte replacement therapy becomes an ongoing process and continues until wound closure is achieved. As the wounds heal, either spontaneously or by skin grafting, the metabolic rate gradually returns to normal levels. The decrease in metabolic requirements is a gradual process. In children with large burns, metabolic requirements remain higher for up to 2 years even after the burn wound is fully mature (Lee, Norbury, & Herndon, 2012).

h. Immune response

i. Although the exact mechanisms of the immunologic and inflammatory response are not known, characteristic pathophysiologic activities are being recognized as a result of the burn injury. Alteration in the skin's protective function provides opportunity for invasion of microorganisms and primes the defensive mechanisms of the inflammatory and immune systems. It is hypothesized that a massive systemic inflammatory response is caused by the local trauma of a burn. It appears that a burn is a mediator-induced injury; although the local effects occur immediately, the systemic response to the mediators produced within a burn progresses and peaks 5 to 7 days after the injury.

ii. It is unclear whether the immunosuppression after a burn injury is the result of biochemical substances (i.e., oxidants, histamine, prostaglandins, arachidonic acid metabolites) liberated from the burn itself, or are produced in response to the burn (Posluszny et al., 2012). In addition, the immunosuppressive effects of anesthetic agents, surgical procedures, multiple transfusions, and the use of systemic antibiotics emphasize postburn immunologic abnormalities during the clinical course of burn therapy. Burn patients are at an increased risk for nosocomial infection and sepsis due to this immune response (Posluszny et al., 2012).

i. Thermoregulation. Children are more prone to the development of hypothermia secondary to their increased BSA-to-mass ratio, and, as a result, children have greater evaporative water loss and greater heat loss from evaporation and convection. Hypothermia remains a major problem until the wounds have been skin grafted or healed. Hypothermia alone, without any injuries, can cause apnea, progressive metabolic acidosis, and ventricular arrhythmias (Lee, Norbury, & Herndon, 2012).

F. Inhalation Injury Assessment and Management

1. *Respiratory Injury.* An *inhalation injury* may be the most important determinant of mortality in burn patients, having a greater effect than either TBSA burn or age. Inhalation injury exists in approximately 30% of hospitalized burn patients

(Traber et al., 2012). Respiratory failure, during the first few hours to days after a burn injury, can be caused by asphyxia, upper airway obstruction, or chemical injury to the airway. The resulting injury can occur alone or in combination with a cutaneous injury.

2. *Classification of injury.* Diagnosis of inhalation injury is typically a subjective decision based on smoke exposure in a closed space. Bronchoscopy during the first 24 hours postinjury can be performed to diagnose inhalation injury formally using a grading scale of 0 to 4 (Dries & Endorf, 2013), but oftentimes the diagnosis of inhalation injury is made based on clinical presentation.

    a. *Acute asphyxia* related to hypoxia and carbon monoxide excess. The process of combustion involves consumption of oxygen; therefore, air inspired by fire victims has considerably lower than normal oxygen concentration, particularly when the fire occurs in a closed space. In a fire, as oxygen is consumed during combustion, carbon monoxide is released because it is a basic by-product of incomplete combustion (Traber et al., 2012).

       i. Carbon monoxide causes toxicity by three mechanisms: the formation of carboxyhemoglobin, shifting the oxygen–hemoglobin dissociation curve to the left, and binding to other heme-containing proteins, namely, cytochrome enzymes and myoglobin. Carbon monoxide is a colorless, tasteless, odorless, nonirritating gas with an affinity for hemoglobin 200 times greater than that of oxygen. As carbon monoxide is transported across the alveolar membrane, it preferentially binds with hemoglobin, in place of oxygen, to form carboxyhemoglobin. Carbon monoxide impedes the dissociation of oxygen from hemoglobin, shifting the oxygen–hemoglobin dissociation curve to the left, thereby impairing oxygen unloading at the tissue level. The result is a major impairment in oxygen delivery. Ninety-seven percent of oxygen is carried to the tissues on hemoglobin. Carboxyhemoglobin also interacts with the myoglobin of cardiac muscle and the cytochrome system, further interfering with oxygen utilization (Traber et al., 2012).

       ii. Tachypnea and cyanosis may be absent because the partial pressure of oxygen in arterial blood (PaO_2) as perceived by the peripheral chemoreceptors (the carotid body and aortic arch) is normal. The peripheral chemoreceptors controlling respiratory drive respond to changes in the PaO_2, and not to changes in the arterial oxygen saturation (SaO_2), even in the presence of high carboxyhemoglobin levels. Standard pulse oximeters are unable to distinguish between hemoglobin molecules saturated with oxygen (oxyhemoglobin) and those saturated with carboxyhemoglobin, producing a false elevation in oxygen saturation in victims with significant carbon monoxide toxicity. Carbon monoxide toxicity is evaluated by measuring the arterial carboxyhemoglobin level. Elevated levels of carboxyhemoglobin serve as indirect evidence for exposure to combustion products. Multiple signs and symptoms have been associated with carboxyhemoglobin levels (Table 9.29). A low carboxyhemoglobin level does not indicate minimal exposure. Administration of 90% to 100% O_2 displaces some, if not all, the carboxyhemoglobin before arrival to the emergency department or before an ABG analysis can be performed (ABLS Advisory Committee, 2015). Carbon monoxide has a constant half-life and is reduced by 50% in 4 hours at room air, and in less than 1 hour if an oxygen concentration of 100% is used. Thus 100% FiO_2 for 6 hours is the treatment of choice for CO inhalation, as hyperbaric oxygen therapy is not typically feasible or available in the first hours following injury (Sheridan, 2012).

b. Airway injury related to edema or obstruction. Heat injury, from inhaling hot air, is limited to the upper airways (above the glottis) and may cause sufficient edema to produce mechanical obstruction (Sheridan, 2012). Direct thermal injury to the lower tracheobronchial tree and alveoli is rare because of the protective reflex closure of the glottis and the heat-dissipating capacity of the upper airway. Mucosal damage may result from both the heat and the chemical components of smoke. Mechanical obstruction of the airway is not limited to those with inhalation injury. The edema that accompanies scalds or even grease burns to the face and neck can be associated with enough edema to cause external airway compromise (Sheridan, 2002).

c. Airway injury related to smoke inhalation. Airway injury due to smoke is essentially a chemical injury caused by inhalation of the by-products of combustion and is related to the composition

TABLE 9.29   Carboxyhemoglobin Level and Associated Signs and Symptoms

Carboxyhemaglobin Level (%)	Symptoms
0–5	Normal value
<15	Often found in smokers
15–20	Headache, mild dyspnea, confusion
20–40	Disorientation, fatigue, nausea, syncope
>50	Coma, seizures, respiratory failure, death

(i.e., benzene from plastics) and duration of the inhaled smoke. When the toxic material is inhaled, it adheres to the mucous membranes, producing a chemical burn to the tracheobronchial mucosa or as far down as the particles descend into the lung. Diagnosing the severity of the injury may be based more on the clinical course of the disease process than on initial physical findings. In general, admission chest radiographic examinations underestimate the severity of lung damage because the injury is usually initially confined to the airways (ABLS Advisory Committee, 2015).

3. *Clinical Assessment*

a. The onset of symptoms is unpredictable, and a patient with possible inhalation injury must be observed closely. Many patients demonstrate minimal symptoms early after injury, and only when airway edema develops over the next 24 to 48 hours after injury do symptoms become evident (Traber et al., 2012).

b. Because of their relatively small airways, upper airway obstruction in the pediatric patient may occur early and rapid. Thus, if edema is expected and any suspicion of inhalation injury is present, the child should have a secure airway placed until they overcome this period of increased airway loss risk (Sheridan, 2002). Securing the ETT is a particular problem in the presence of burn injury. Facial edema—coupled with wounds, secretions, and topical creams—increases the difficulty of securing and maintaining proper tube placement. Tape and commercially available securement devices may not be effective in securing ETTs in the presence of facial burns. Twill tracheostomy ties may be utilized to secure ETTs.

4. *Ventilation Strategies*

a. Ventilator strategies must support oxygenation and ventilation and reflect the experience of the clinical team managing the patient. Limitation of pressure, acceptance of permissive hypercapnia, and strategies to manage secretions, such as aggressive pulmonary toileting and suctioning, are important. Many patients with smoke inhalation will develop pneumonia in association with mechanical ventilation.

b. The nursing care of the child with inhalation injury includes elevation of the head of the bed, frequent position changes and oral care to prevent ventilator-associated events (VAEs). There is no consensus about the most appropriate mode of ventilation, as high-frequency oscillation (HFOV) and airway pressure release ventilation (APRV) have not been shown to improve outcomes in these patients (Dries & Endorf, 2013). Thus, ventilation for the child with inhalation injury includes methods similar to those with ARDS.

G. Fluid Resuscitation Assessment and Management

1. *Fluid Resuscitation.* Ongoing fluid resuscitation is indicated if the child's TBSA burned exceeds 15% second or third degree. If the burn wound is smaller, maintenance IV fluid and encouragement of oral intake is indicated, along with close monitoring of intake and output by the nurse. The goal of resuscitation is to preserve end-organ perfusion in the setting of burn shock, so indicators of good end-organ perfusion should be followed closely during the entire resuscitation phase. It is possible to administer too much or too little fluid to

resuscitate the burned child, and care must be taken in this phase of inpatient admission to ensure that just the amount of fluid the child needs is administered, and not more or less than is necessary to perfuse the child's vital organs. Fluid resuscitation begins at the scene of the injury if possible, and progresses through distinct stages of acute burn care as follows.

2. *Precision Resuscitation.* At the scene of the injury or in the ED upon initial arrival, fluid resuscitation with lactated Ringer's solution is administered using the ABLS prehospital fluid rate based solely on the child's age (see Table 9.27). Once the primary and secondary survey has been completed in the emergency department and precise %TBSA burned has been calculated using one of the methods described earlier, a more prescriptive resuscitation formula is used to guide resuscitation (see Table 9.27). Fluid resuscitation formulas, such as the Parkland, Brooke, Consensus, ABLS, and so forth, are all *estimations* of the total fluids the child will require over the first days of resuscitation. Each child is different, thus close monitoring by the nurse of end-organ perfusion adequacy, such as urine output, vital signs, and mental status, are essential to achieve optimal resuscitation outcomes (Warden, 2014).

3. *Monitoring*

a. Once resuscitation has begun, a urinary catheter should be inserted and used to measure urine output quantity and quality at least hourly. The goal urine output during resuscitation is generally 0.5 to 1.0 mL/kg/hr for children and 2 mL/kg/hr in infants (Lee, Norbury, & Herndon, 2012). Urine output targets may be even higher (1.5–2.0 mL/kg/hr or greater) if electrical injury has occurred (ABLS Advisory Committee, 2015).

b. If the urine output is above this goal, the continuous IV fluid rate should be decreased by 33%, and if it is below the goal the IV fluid rate should be increased by 33% hourly until the child achieves urine output in the goal range (ABLS Advisory Committee, 2015). If the child's urine output is in the goal range and no other signs of decreased end-organ perfusion exist, no adjustments to the IV fluid rates should be necessary, even if the formula initially used to estimate initial resuscitation fluids calls for more to be given.

c. Remember, all resuscitation formulas (i.e., Parkland, Brooke) are estimations; the most accurate guides for resuscitation are end-organ perfusion clinical assessment findings such as urine output, vital signs, and mental status (Sheridan, 2012). The nurse caring for a burned child undergoing resuscitation should be in close communication with the provider directing resuscitation regarding the child's response to fluid therapy.

d. As a general rule, crystalloid boluses are not recommended during the resuscitation phase. Many burn centers include colloid resuscitation as a part of their overall resuscitation plan once certain volumes of crystalloid have been given as colloids have been shown to restore intravascular volume well in the burned child after 24 hours postburn injury have passed (Warden, 2014).

e. Many pediatric burn centers use a *nurse-driven resuscitation* protocol to guide practice. These types of protocols require hourly titrations based on clinical endpoints of resuscitation such as MAP, CVP, and UOP hourly until targets are met. The use of a nurse-driven resuscitation protocol in adults has been shown to improve accuracy and precision in the total volume of resuscitation fluid given as compared with Parkland formula estimations (Fahlstrom, Boyle, & Makic, 2013). See Figure 9.12 for an example of a nurse-driven resuscitation protocol for pediatric patients.

H. Wound Assessment and Management

Wound assessment and care can be one of the most challenging aspects of caring for the burn patient. It takes time and experience to become proficient at wound assessment, interpretation, and dressing application, particularly in the pediatric burn patient. The potential for wound infection is one of the major considerations in patients who sustain a thermal injury. Wound care, daily wound assessment, and documentation are a vital part of the nursing care of a patient following burn injury. Particular attention should be focused on methods and techniques to prevent infection, facilitate wound healing, promote patient comfort, maintain optimal function, and minimize deformities. Any signs of infection, such as odor, drainage, and redness (cellulitis), must be noted and reported, so as to advocate appropriately for the patient. Wound care begins in the emergent phase and continues through the acute and rehabilitative phases.

1. *Initial Debridement and Cleaning: Emergent Phase*

a. Wound care should only be initiated after all potentially life-threatening injuries have been addressed as outlined previously.

b. All clothing and jewelry should be removed from the injured area prior to cleansing wounds, and any decontamination necessary from chemical exposure should occur first.

c. Wound-cleansing methods are somewhat variable, but the underlying principles are the same.

d. Wound cleansing involves using water and a mild soap in a bath basin, or various topical agents, to cleanse the wounds. In some burn care areas, hydrotherapy is utilized; however, immersion hydrotherapy is no longer indicated due to increased risk of bacterial translocation (Tredget et al., 1992; Weber, 2014). Hydrotherapy today typically involves the use of a shower or sprayer to cleanse the wounds. Caution must be taken to prevent hypothermia during wound cleansing. This may include only cleansing one part of the body at a time and keeping parts not being cleaned covered with dressings or a dry sheet or blanket, maintaining a warm room temperature, and using warm water for cleansing. It is best to cleanse areas with known or suspected infection or areas close to the perineum last.

e. Wound debridement involves the removal of necrotic tissue, debris, and foreign material. This can be accomplished by mechanical debridement, chemical debridement, or surgical debridement.

i. *Mechanical debridement* can be accomplished by several different methods. This may involve cleaning the wound with coarse mesh gauze, the application and removal of gauze dressings, irrigation, or the use of scissors and forceps to gently lift and trim loose necrotic tissue. It is recommended that all blisters greater than 2 cm be debrided, as this tissue must be removed to minimize infection risk.

ii. *Chemical or enzymatic debridement* is accomplished by the use of commercially available topical preparations that cause selective lysis of necrotic tissue. Chemical or enzymatic debriding agents are typically used on partial-thickness wounds to minimize the need for or extent of surgical intervention necessary to close the wound. Enzymatic debridement agents should be applied only within the area of eschar or necrotic tissue and should be discontinued once the eschar has been removed and granulation tissue is present.

iii. *Surgical debridement* involves removal of eschar using surgical instruments. This is accomplished via tangential or fascial excision. *Tangential excision* involves removal of thin layers of eschar until viable tissue is reached. *Fascial excision* removes all layers of the skin and subcutaneous tissue. Fascial excisions are infrequently required, but may be indicated in burns that involve subcutaneous fat or large full-thickness burns (Sheridan, 2012).

2. *Dressing Application*

a. In the emergent phase, if the patient is being transferred to a burn center, dry sterile dressings should be applied.

b. Once on the burn unit, wounds should be fully assessed by the nurse with each dressing change and compared to the previous assessment. Assessment findings should be clearly documented and communicated to the patient care team, and any concerning findings escalated to the burn surgeon for evaluation.

c. Infection prevention is the top priority throughout the dressing-change process. Hand hygiene must be performed prior to the dressing-change procedure and appropriate personal protective equipment must be worn throughout. Sterile supplies should always be used for any dressing procedure, including wound cleansing, debridement, or dressing application. The use of sterile gloves should always be considered during dressing changes to prevent the transfer of organisms to the wound site. Sterile gloves should always be worn for a dressing change that involves sharp debridement or during the first 24 hours after surgery (Iwamoto, 2009).

d. The choice of dressing is dependent on the area of the body and the size, depth, and type of burn. Dressings are selected and applied to accomplish several goals. The goals of dressing therapy include the following:

i. Promotion of wound healing

ii. Prevention of infection

iii. Protection of the wound

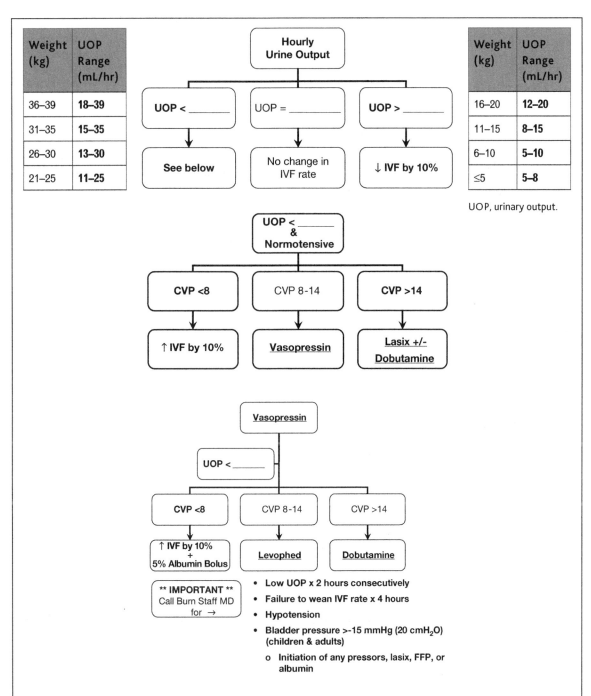

Weight (kg)	UOP Range (mL/hr)
36–39	**18–39**
31–35	**15–35**
26–30	**13–30**
21–25	**11–25**

Weight (kg)	UOP Range (mL/hr)
16–20	**12–20**
11–15	**8–15**
6–10	**5–10**
≤5	**5–8**

UOP, urinary output.

Hourly Urine Output

UOP < _____ → See below

UOP = _____ → No change in IVF rate

UOP > _____ → ↓ IVF by 10%

UOP < _____ & Normotensive

CVP <8 → ↑ IVF by 10%

CVP 8-14 → **Vasopressin**

CVP >14 → **Lasix +/- Dobutamine**

Vasopressin

UOP < _____

CVP <8 → ↑ IVF by 10% + 5% Albumin Bolus

CVP 8-14 → **Levophed**

CVP >14 → **Dobutamine**

** IMPORTANT **
Call Burn Staff MD for →

- Low UOP x 2 hours consecutively
- Failure to wean IVF rate x 4 hours
- Hypotension
- Bladder pressure >-15 mmHg (20 cmH₂O) (children & adults)
  o Initiation of any pressors, lasix, FFP, or albumin

FIGURE 9.12 Nurse-driven resuscitation protocol.

CVP, central venous pressure; FFP, fresh frozen plasma; IVF, in vitro fertilization; UOP, urine output.

Source: Adapted from Regions Hospital Burn Center's Nurse-Driven Resuscitation Protocol, St. Paul, MN. Used with permission.

iv. Promoting comfort

v. Prevention of desiccation

3. *Special Care Areas*

a. *Eyes.* The skin around the eye is delicate and should be gently cleansed. Care must be taken to avoid getting topical preparations and cleansing agents in the eye. Ophthalmic lubricants may be ordered to keep the eyes moist due to decreased lubrication, depressed blink reflex, and/or eyelid injury. An ophthalmology consult is indicated for patients with facial burns to rule out eye injury and foreign-body presence. Though uncommon in the acute stage due to edema, tarsorrhaphy is a procedure in which the eyelids are partially sutured closed that may be indicated for ocular protection when a patient is not able to close the eyes fully (Malholtra, Sheikh, & Dheansa, 2009).

b. *Ears.* Pressure on the ears should be avoided to prevent pressure necrosis and chondritis. If ties are used to secure endotracheal or nasogastric tubes, they should be positioned to prevent contact with the ear. Mafenide cream is an effective antimicrobial cream to prevent infection in the cartilaginous tissue of the ear.

c. *Lips.* The lips are very vascular and sensitive, and should be gently washed with water or normal saline-soaked gauze. Topical antimicrobial ointments such as bacitracin are used, rather than creams, and are reapplied as needed to prevent the lips from drying and cracking.

d. *Perineum.* Due to an increased risk of infection from bacteria commonly found in the perianal area, the perineum should be thoroughly cleaned after urination and defecation and topical agents reapplied to burned areas as ordered. Any diapers or underpads containing stool should be promptly changed, and any contaminated dressings changed after a bowel movement.

e. *Exposed muscle, tendon, or bone.* Dressings over exposed muscle, tendon, or bone must be kept moist to prevent desiccation. This can be accomplished by rewetting the dressing with normal saline or an antimicrobial solution.

f. *Fingers and toes.* Dressings to fingers and toes should allow for frequent assessment of the perfusion to distal digits. Gauze should be placed between fingers and toes to avoid web-space contractures and adherence of digits to

one another. If possible, the child should be able to move his or her hands and fingers to assist with feeding themselves and participate in supervised play with the dressings on, as movement speeds the healing process and minimizes wound edema.

4. *Operative Burn-Wound Management*

a. *Excision and grafting.* Early excision and grafting have been shown to improve morbidity and mortality by decreasing infection and the systemic inflammatory response (Ong, Samuel, & Song, 2006; Sheridan, 2002). *Excision* refers to the surgical removal of eschar via tangential or fascial debridement. The ultimate goal after excision is to provide definitive or permanent wound coverage via grafting. In some cases, such as in the setting of infected wounds or large burns without adequate donor site, temporary wound-closure techniques may be necessary until permanent wound closure can be achieved.

b. *Temporary wound-closure methods*

i. *Homograft* or *allograft* is a biological dressing and is a skin graft from a human donor (i.e., cadaver skin). These grafts provide a temporary wound covering until the area is able to be covered with a permanent wound-closure method. Typically, in 1 to 3 weeks, the grafted site is assessed, the allograft is removed, and the wound is either covered with autograft or left to heal on its own.

ii. *Heterograft* or *xenograft* is a layer of skin from a different species, usually porcine (pig) skin. Xenografts are often used as a temporary wound covering on superficial partial-thickness burns while the underlying wound heals.

iii. Depending on the depth of the burn, it is possible that a temporary coverage method will allow the burned skin to heal well enough that autografts are not needed. Other times, a more permanent wound-closure method is needed.

c. *Permanent wound-closure methods*

i. *Autograft.* An autograft is a skin graft taken from the patient's own unburned or healed skin that is transferred to the injured area after the burn wound has been debrided. The area the autograft is taken from is referred to as the *donor site*. Autografts are utilized for permanent wound coverage, and can be described based on the thickness of the graft as well as the meshing ratio.

ii. *Full-thickness grafts* involve all of the dermis and epidermis. Although they may result in improved cosmetic appearance, the donor site will require primary closure or grafting from another site to heal so they are used selectively.

iii. *Split-thickness grafts* include all of the epidermis and a variable amount of the dermis. Split-thickness grafts are more commonly used in the surgical management of extensive burns as they can cover a relatively large surface area using a smaller graft.

1) Meshed split-thickness skin grafts can be created in a 2:1, 3:1, or even up to a 6:1 meshing ratio depending on the available donor skin and area needing to be covered. Meshing allows the graft to be expanded for greater coverage of large area using a relatively small piece of donor-site skin. Meshed grafts also allow for drainage of fluid and will have a meshed lattice-like appearance once healed. A meshed graft is considered fully healed when the interstices (areas inside the meshed holes) are filled in. This can take up to several weeks to occur.

2) Sheet grafts are applied as a continuous sheet of skin without being meshed. Small holes may be present to allow for fluid drainage. Sheet grafts have improved cosmetic and functional outcomes, but also have greater risk of graft loss or decreased graft take due to accumulation of fluid or blood between the graft and underlying tissue. Any fluid or blood noted under the graft should be reported to the surgeon. In some cases, gentle "rolling" of the graft with a cotton applicator may be indicated to express the fluid and prevent graft loss during the first few days after grafting surgery. Careful monitoring of sheet grafts is essential to prevent clots or fluid pockets from forming between the graft and the wound, causing graft loss.

iv. Artificial dermis. Dermal replacements may be used in conjunction with an autograft to help restore some of the features of the dermis that are lost when a full-thickness burn is excised. Dermal replacements are often placed over the excised wound bed prior to placement of a split-thickness skin graft (Lee, Norbury, & Herndon, 2012) to provide an optimal surface for the autograft to adhere to.

v. Cultured epithelial autograft (CEA). CEA may be necessary in the setting of massive burns when the patient does not have enough suitable (nonburned) donor-site skin available to cover the burned area. CEA is grown in a laboratory from two small full-thickness specimens of the patient's own unburned skin. In approximately 3 weeks after skin samples are taken, sheets of the patient's own keratinocytes have matured in the lab and are available for grafting (Lee, Dibildox, 2012). These types of grafts are expensive and fragile, as they only involve the keratinocyte portion of the skin organ, and are typically only used when absolutely necessary. If applied, the patient will require meticulous wound and nursing care, including specialized antibiotic soak instructions, careful mobility of the patient, and a prescribed "drying time" daily until healed.

d. *Donor site*

i. *Site selection.* An inconspicuous donor site, such as the thigh, is often selected for cosmetic reasons but may be limited by the extent of the burn wound. In children, it is relatively common to harvest donor skin from the scalp and other areas, such as the back or flank, when the burn is extensive. Removal of the donor skin creates a new wound, so care is taken to ensure only what is needed is harvested. Depending on the depth of the graft that was taken, the donor site may heal primarily on its own in about 2 weeks (split-thickness graft) or may require grafting or primary closure to heal using an additional full-thickness autograft.

ii. *Dressings.* There are many options for donor-site dressings. Open donor-site management involves the use of petrolatum-impregnated dressings or fine-mesh gauze over the donor site. The dressing dries and forms a scab-like barrier over the wound and allows the donor site to heal. One disadvantage of this type of dressing is pain is present until the dressing dries and a feeling of tightness occurs once the scab has formed. Closed donor-site dressings involve the use of semipermeable membranes and hydrocolloid dressings. This type of dressing presents challenges in optimal wound healing, as increased drainage and wound colonization can occur (Sheridan, 2012). Regardless of the dressing type used, nursing management of donor sites should include careful assessment for bleeding, drainage, odor, and erythema around the donor site. Pain assessment and management are key until the donor site heals. During the first few days after harvesting donor skin, the donor site typically has sanguineous drainage and is very painful, and toward the end of the healing phase, the donor site can become very itchy and dry.

e. *Graft care.* Postoperatively, grafts are immediately at risk for failure from infection, bleeding, and mechanical forces such as shearing and friction. The postoperative surgical dressing is selected to apply gentle pressure and protect the graft from friction and shear. Often, the initial postoperative dressing is a primary dressing that stays in place for a predetermined number of days. During this time, the dressing must be monitored for bleeding, odor, and drainage. If any of these are present, the surgeon must be notified. The dressing may need to be removed for further inspection because infection or excessive bleeding can disrupt the graft's viability. Negative pressure wound therapy may also be used over grafts to promote adherence. When caring for a patient with a new graft, the prevention of friction and shear must remain a priority, and, in particular, careful repositioning or moving/ambulation of the patient must be performed to avoid disrupting the fragile graft. A new graft typically takes about a week to adhere fully, and become less fragile. In children, care must be given to ensure that the child does not scratch at or disrupt the healing process of the new graft, as graft loss can occur, which requires a new donor site and surgical procedure and is an undesired patient outcome.

5. *Nonoperative Burn-Wound Management*

a. Although full-thickness burns require prompt excision and grafting, more superficial burns may heal on their own. As the wound evolves, in some cases, the true depth may not be determined for several days. If the wound is determined to be able to heal on its own, the wound is often managed expectantly for a period of time. Wounds may be managed with daily dressings or multiday dressings, with close monitoring by the burn team for healing progression and need for grafting surgery over a period of days to weeks. In pediatric scald burns, Cubison, Pape, and Parkhouse (2006) found that burns that healed in fewer than 10 days had a 0% chance of hypertrophic scarring, whereas burns that healed in 10 to 14 days had a 2% chance of hypertrophic scaring and burns that healed in 14 to 21 days had a 20% chance of hypertrophic scarring. As such, surgery should be reserved for pediatric scald burns that are not expected to heal in less than 21 days.

b. *Daily dressing.* Areas of superficial partial-thickness burns will typically heal in 7 to 10 days without surgical intervention. Nursing care of the child with more extensive burns typically includes daily wound assessment and dressing changes. A variety of topical antimicrobial preparations may be used (Table 9.30) for daily dressing changes. Important benefits of daily dressing changes include the ability to assess the wound, daily assessment of healing trajectory, and the ability to change the treatment plan as necessary based on the healing process. The wound must be gently cleansed and all prior topical creams/ointments removed prior to the application of new dressings.

c. *Multiday dressing.* Many dressing products now exist that are intended for long-term wear and infection prevention and can remain in place from 3 to 14 days depending on the product. These dressings may be composed of a hydrofiber or foam-base material, which is often impregnated with silver to provide antimicrobial action as the wound heals. A major advantage to the use of multiday dressings is the less frequent dressing change for the patient, which may translate to decreased pain and stress and trauma for the child. Caution must be used in selection of these dressings as they may not be appropriate in situations where wound depth is unclear. In addition, selection of the product to use must consider factors such as the need to assess the wound, mobility of the area to be dressed, and the stage of healing the wound is in. Each extended-wear dressing has a profile of advantages and disadvantages as compared to others that must

TABLE 9.30 Topical Antimicrobial Agents

Agent	Advantages	Disadvantages
1% silver sulfadiazine Silvadene, SSD, Thermazene	Broad spectrum antimicrobial activity Painless upon application Readily available Minimal sensitivity May be used with open or closed dressing technique Most commonly used topical agent Moderate eschar penetration	Transient leukopenia
Mafenide acetate cream (Sulfamylon)	Penetrates through burn eschar and cartilage Effective gram-negative coverage	Painful upon application May cause metabolic acidosis (alternating Sulfamylon and Silvadene application may diminish this effect)
Bacitracin	Effective against gram-positive organisms Low toxicity	Limited effect against gram-negative organisms Limited ability to penetrate eschar
0.5% silver nitrate solution	Excellent antibacterial spectrum	Requires dressing Messy May cause electrolyte imbalances (hyponatremia and hypochloremia)

SSD, silver sulfadiazine.

be carefully considered by an expert clinician before a dressing therapy is chosen. The decision to move from daily dressing-change therapy to a longer wear dressing should be made in collaboration with the treatment team based on the child's wound appearance and tolerance of the regimen.

d. *Scar management.* As the burn wound heals, scar tissue forms at the injured site. When a scar becomes thick and raised, it is called a *hypertrophic scar*. Deeper burns and burns that take longer to heal are more prone to hypertrophic scarring (Serghiou et al., 2012). Hypertrophic scars can lead to impaired range of motion and a poor cosmetic outcome. Surgical and laser therapies are available to treat hypertrophic scars after they have formed, but interventions to decrease the likelihood of hypertrophic scarring should be instituted as soon as possible in the healing process. See Table 9.31 for scar management techniques.

I. Nonburn Diagnoses With Complex Wound Care: Assessment and Management

1. *Stevens-Johnson Syndrome (SJS) and Toxic Epidermal Necrolysis (TEN)*

a. *SJS and toxic epidermal necrolysis.* Because of their complex wound-care needs and infection risk, children with SJS and TEN are often cared for by nurses with burn-care expertise. SJS and TEN are exfoliative skin diseases that occur from an immunologic reaction in the child's body to a drug or virus, or can be completely idiopathic (Fagan et al., 2012). The principles of infection prevention, pain management, and psychosocial support are similar for children with SJS and TEN to children with burns with a few exceptions.

2. *Medication Therapy.* Treatment of SJS and TENs is mostly supportive; however, IVIG is sometimes given to attempt to slow or halt disease progression because the disease is characterized as an immunologic reaction to a foreign antigen (Fagan et al., 2012). The use of IVIG for SJS and TENs remains controversial (Fagan et al., 2012). The most important first treatment is removal of the causative agent, if known.

3. *Wound Care.* The wound-care goals for SJS and TENs include prevention of infection and protection of sloughed or sloughing skin. Contrary to a burn wound, the blisters that form from these nonburn diagnoses generally should be protected and covered with a biologic or synthetic long-wear dressing rather than forcefully debrided at the bedside frequently by nurses. Depending on the size of the involved skin, wound care, debridement, and

TABLE 9.31 Scar Management Techniques

Scar Management Technique	Description	Nursing Care
Elastic bandages	Ace wraps or tubular elastic bandages may be used on newly healed skin to promote soft, flat, supple scars.	Ace wraps are donned in a figure-8 pattern. Ensure wraps are not too tight to impair circulation or shear fragile skin or grafts. Assess for color changes, cool distal extremities, and decreased sensation. Tubular elastic bandages are available in various sizes. These are typically removed and reapplied one to two times daily.
Pressure garments	Commercially available or custom-made elastic impregnated garments that are worn 23 hr/d and are removed for bathing and skin care.	Patients typically have two pairs of pressure garments to allow one to be worn while the other is being washed. Assess for skin breakdown, signs of circulation compromise, and areas of increasing hypertrophic scarring. Usually worn for 12–18 months. Children may need to be re-measured with pressure garments replaced as they grow and garments wear out.
Inserts	May be used as an adjunct to pressure therapy to provide additional pressure to areas where pressure garments are unable to provide adequate pressure. May consist of various materials, such as silicone gel or foam inserts, and may be custom made or commercially available.	Remove insert to clean and dry. Assess underlying skin for rash, drying, or maceration.
Self-adherent pressure wraps	Often used to apply pressure over the hands, toes, and fingers.	These are typically applied by a burn therapist and should be wrapped around digits in a spiral pattern beginning at the fingertips. The fingertips should always be left exposed to allow for assessment of circulation.
Mask	Transparent plastic face mask is custom made for patient to provide uniform pressure to facial scars. May be lined with silicone.	Assess for rash and signs of skin breakdown. May need to be refined and reformed by a skilled therapist to ensure uniform pressure on scar areas over time.
Massage	Aids in softening and remodeling of scar tissues by freeing adhering fibrous bands and aligning collagen to proper orientation, which allows scars to become more elastic. Often done in combination with a gentle lubricating cream.	Typically performed at least twice daily for 5–10 minutes on each area. Massage with enough pressure to cause skin blanching in a circular motion. Cream and massage techniques may also improve itching.

Source: Serghiou, M. A., Ott, S., Whitehead, C., Cowan, A., McEntire, S., & Suman , O. E. (2012). Comprehensive rehabilitation of the burn patient. In D. N. Herndon (Ed.), *Total burn care* (pp. 517–549). New York, NY: Elsevier.

dressing changes likely will require moderate sedation or an operating room visit under general anesthesia (Fagan et al., 2012). It is important to remove any peeling skin to prevent infection. Careful monitoring of disease progression, including noting and reporting the appearance of new blisters to the healthcare team, is important in the care of a child with SJS or TENs.

4. *Nutritional Requirements.* In SJS and TEN patients, sloughing of the oral mucosa that may make eating and drinking painful. In some cases, this sloughing may compromise the respiratory system and airway (Fagan et al., 2012). The child with SJS and TENs will require high-quality nutrition to heal, and may need a temporary enteral feeding tube or parenteral nutrition while the mouth is healing (Fagan et al., 2012).

5. *Special Care Areas*

a. Care should be taken to ensure the eyes are examined by an ophthalmologist and protected in the child with SJS or TENs to prevent blindness. Most children with SJS and TEN require frequent administration of eye drops and some may require temporary eye membrane placement to protect the cornea (Fagan et al., 2012).

b. Children with SJS or TENs should have a genital and/or gynecologic examination to rule out urethral and/or vaginal sloughing that can cause scarring and strictures (Fagan et al., 2012).

J. Wound Infection Assessment and Management

1. *Etiology.* The use of topical antimicrobial agents and the early excision of deep burn wounds, coupled with early wound closure, have reduced the incidence of serious wound infections that cause mortality (Ludwik, Herndon, Barrow, 2012; Sheridan & Chang, 2014). As such, routine systemic antibiotic prophylaxis is not indicated in the absence of known bacteremia. The moist, protein-rich avascular eschar provides an excellent culture medium for microorganisms. Within a week after the burn injury, bacteria are consistently present on any remaining eschar. In addition, the thermal thrombosis that renders the eschar avascular prevents easy penetration by parenteral antibiotics and impedes delivery of the cellular components of the host defense system to the microorganisms. Consequently, parenteral

antibiotics exert little effect on the rapid colonization of the burn wound itself. Early excision and grafting coupled with strategies to decrease risk of wound infection are the most vital to minimizing infection (Ludwik et al., 2012).

2. *Infection Definitions*

a. *Burn wound bacterial colonization* refers to bacteria present on the wound surface at low concentrations with no invasive infection (Greenhalgh et al., 2007). Treatment is continued: routine burn care with wound cleaning, topical antimicrobials, and surgical intervention (Gallagher, Branski, Williams-Bouyer, Villarreal, & Herndon, 2012). *Burn-wound infection* refers to bacteria present in the wound and wound eschar at high concentrations with no invasive infection (Greenhalgh et al., 2007). Treatment of a burn-wound infection involves continued wound care with cleaning, topical antimicrobials, and the addition of systemic (IV) antimicrobials (Gallagher et al., 2012).

b. *Burn wound invasive infection* refers to the presence of pathogens in a burn wound at concentrations sufficient to cause separation of eschar or graft loss, invasion of adjacent unburned tissue (cellulitis) or systemic bacteremia sufficient enough to produce sepsis pathology (Greenhalgh et al., 2007). Treatment of invasive infection involves surgical elimination of all dead tissue, systemic IV antibiotics, including broad-spectrum medications if the pathogen has not been identified. Careful selection of topical antimicrobial soaks may also be indicated based on the identified organism (Gallagher et al., 2012).

c. *Cellulitis* occurs when bacteria present in the wound and/or eschar are at high concentrations and surrounding tissue demonstrates advancing erythema, induration, warmth, and tenderness (Greenhalgh et al., 2007). Treatment of cellulitis involves continued wound care and systemic IV antibiotics (Gallagher et al., 2012).

d. *Necrotizing infection/fasciitis* is an aggressive, invasive infection with underlying tissue necrosis (Greenhalgh et al., 2007). Treatment includes broad-spectrum antibiotics and aggressive surgical intervention (Fagan et al., 2012). Amputation may be necessary. Careful measurement and assessment of the size of the wound with this type of infection is necessary to identify disease progression and prevent further tissue loss. If the wound size is becoming larger, notify a surgical provider as immediate surgical intervention is most likely indicated.

3. *Assessment*

    a.   Assessment of the burn wounds for signs of infection is the best method for detecting wound infection (Tran & Chin, 2014). The wound should be completely exposed at least daily by the nurse for a clear assessment. Visual assessment findings that may indicate infection include a change in drainage color, increased exudate, increased pain, an unexpected increase in wound depth, or premature separation of burn eschar (Tran & Chin, 2014).

    b.   Nursing care infection-prevention priorities

        i.   Infection-prevention strategies must be in place to decrease the chance of complications associated with sepsis.

        ii.   Hand hygiene is imperative before any contact with the patient, patient environment, or anything that will come in contact with patient environment.

        iii.   The standard precautions that should be maintained for all burn patients to protect against exposure to microorganisms include a gown or apron that is donned before patient care and discarded upon leaving the patient's room, gloves, and a mask. During patient care and dressing changes, soiled gloves should be changed before moving to another site on the same patient (Weber, 2014) and a face mask with shield and hair coverings should be worn.

        iv.   Children with large TBSA burns or multiply drug-resistant organisms should be cared for in a private room.

        v.   Use sterile technique when performing invasive procedures.

        vi.   Strict adherence to institutional guidelines for the frequency of supply and invasive line and tubing changes is necessary to prevent healthcare-associated infections.

        vii.   Clean all equipment around the bedside at least daily with a germicidal solution, according to institutional policy.

        viii.   Restrict flowers, plants, and nonwashable toys at the bedside as they can harbor bacteria and fungi (Weber, 2014).

4. *Monitoring*

    a.   Continually monitor vital signs, including temperature, with a urinary catheter temperature probe or soft rectal probe in patients with large (>15% TBSA) burns, as both hyperthermia and hypothermia are common signs of wound infection (Weber, 2014).

    b.   Wound cultures may be obtained on a routine basis, although practice varies across settings. Some benefits of routine wound cultures include early indication of contaminated wounds, guidance in selecting topical antimicrobials or empiric antimicrobial coverage, and timely detection of cross-colonization (Gallagher et al., 2012; Weber, 2014).

    c.   Ensure all who enter the patient's environment have taken appropriate hand-hygiene measures, including all members of the healthcare team, family, and visitors. Intervene immediately if appropriate hand hygiene was not performed. If the child has a tendency to touch the dressings or invasive lines, the child's hands should be washed frequently as well.

K. Comfort Assessment and Management

1. *Pain Assessment*

    a.   The burn injury itself is the source of continuous (background) pain. Loss of the epidermis and partial loss of the dermis leave nerve endings exposed, creating a painful wound. This type of pain begins from the time of injury until complete wound healing. Wounds that are deeper (deep partial thickness or full thickness) typically have less associated pain initially due to injury of the nerve endings.

    b.   *Acute pain*, or procedural pain, is associated with the multiple procedures required during the clinical course of the burn injury, such as dressing changes, surgical excision and grafting (donor sites, contracture release), daily physical therapy, bed mobility, and ambulation.

2. *Pain Management*

    a.   If pain is not well managed during the initial acute phase, severe anxiety and fear may develop and effective pain management may be more difficult to achieve.

    b.   *Background pain* can be managed by oral or intravenous medications, including acetaminophen, NSAIDs, or opioids. These medications should be administered on a routine basis to maintain a therapeutic blood level while painful stimuli is present, and tolerance should be assessed at regular intervals, with increased dosage given if necessary.

c. *Procedural pain* is generally managed by IV medications, primarily morphine, ketamine, or fentanyl, as they have a relatively short onset and sufficient duration for the procedure. Patients without venous access may receive oral analgesic agents, such as ibuprofen, acetaminophen, and oxycodone, administered 30 to 60 minutes before a painful procedure. Note the onset and duration of the medication given so that the procedure can be timed so that the medication is in full effect as desired. Closely monitor the patient after the administration of opioids, as when the stimulus is removed, as the patient could begin to be oversedated and respiratory distress and failure can occur. Conversely, if pain medication is administered for procedural pain and the child appears uncomfortable, repeated dosing or an adjunct should be administered before proceeding with the painful procedure. Procedures, such as dressing changes, are rarely emergent, so careful attention to pain and anxiety management is a high priority. If pain is not well controlled, it may be best to stop the procedure, administer additional medication, and continue with it at a later time. In the first 48 hours after burn injury, a slower rate of drug distribution and lower renal clearance of drugs is generally observed, then in the days following, clearance of drugs is accelerated and patients may need higher doses of drugs (Bayat, Ramaiah, & Bhananker, 2010). Continuous monitoring of the child's response to any medication given is key to effective pain-management planning.

d. A patient-controlled analgesia (PCA) pump is useful for children who are able to follow directions and may decrease total opioid requirement due to an improved sense of control that the patient may feel over pain management (Bayat et al., 2010). In general, children who are able to play video games can operate a PCA pump. The medication chosen for the PCA should be based on past patient experience and history of tolerance and side effects as well as institutional protocol.

e. Moderate or deep sedation may be required to manage more painful procedures, such as the first bedside debridement (Bayat et al., 2010). Combining opioids and benzodiazepines is useful for moderate and deep sedation; however, meticulous assessment and monitoring of the patient are essential as sedation occurs on a continuum. Medications should be delivered based on the patient's age, weight, and response by a credentialed provider. Continuous vital-sign monitoring, and, if possible, end-tidal carbon dioxide monitoring, are essential; and emergency airway equipment and medication reversal agents must be available at all times. Personnel qualified to monitor sedation and rescue the patient's airway should an unintended level of sedation be achieved must be readily available at all times.

f. When appropriate, collaborate with a child life specialist to develop strategies to give the patient some control over painful encounters. Allow the family to help and be present when appropriate and able.

g. Several nonpharmacologic adjunctive approaches to pain management that work well for the pediatric burn patient include distraction, imagery, relaxation, music, hypnosis, and positive reinforcement. The participation of a child life specialist in routine painful procedures is also a key component of the treatment plan.

3. *Fear and Anxiety Assessment.* The psychological response of fear and anxiety is caused by multiple factors, including fear of the unknown; separation from parents, family, and friends for extended periods; multiple invasive procedures during hospitalization; an inability to communicate with patients receiving mechanical ventilation and chemical paralytics altered sleep patterns and increased activities during the day and night; unfamiliar surroundings, equipment, and people; and pain. Anxiety may also develop as a result of the traumatic nature of the burn injury, thus interventions targeting prevention of the development of fear should routinely be provided.

4. *Anxiety Management.* Anxiolytics are usually a helpful adjunct to opioids to reduce the anxiety associated with a procedure. The most common anxiolytic medication class is the benzodiazepine, but other adjunctive medications, such as nitrous oxide and dexmedetomidine, have been used successfully in the burn-patient population (Bayat et al., 2010). Successful use of anxiolytic medication requires an observational assessment by the treatment team and, if possible, a self-report by the patient to ensure adequate anxiolysis/sedation is achieved. Ongoing monitoring is necessary and adjustments to the plan should be made as needed based on patient response. The most commonly used benzodiazepines include midazolam and lorazepam.

  a. Reduce the patient's anxiety level by explaining procedures and talking to the patient while performing nursing interventions.

  b. Allow frequent visiting for families. Encourage the family to bring items from home to remind the child of family life before the injury. Organize care into routines similar to home (i.e., a time to sleep, eat, play, have dressing changes, see visitors).

  c. Allow the family to participate in the dressing change or painful procedure by distracting or holding their child as tolerated. Ensure parents and caregivers are full partners in their children's care.

5. *Itch Assessment.* The severe itching of burn scars and wounds is another symptom that must be addressed and managed. Many burn survivors report that the itching, not the pain, was the most troublesome aspect of burn recovery. Scratching the wound can lead to breakdown of the fragile newly healing skin and, potentially, infection or the need for further surgery. The nurse may use an assessment tool, such as the Itch Man Scale, to have the child rate the intensity of itching (Meyer et al., 2007), or, if a validated itch assessment tool cannot be used, the nurse can assume itch may be present if the child self-reports itch or appears restless and/or is unable to sleep calmly.

6. *Itch Management*

  a. Dry, scaly, healing skin is more susceptible to itch. Skin-moistening soap should be used daily, followed by moisturizing lotion applied as needed and twice daily to healed skin.

  b. Medications that can be used for treatment include diphenhydramine 1.25 mg/kg every 6 hours and hydroxyzine 0.5 mg/kg every 6 hours. If itch is refractory to treatment with these medications, addition of loratadine (Schneider et al., 2015) may be indicated.

7. *Delirium*

  a. Delirium is often present in the child who has been hospitalized. Factors that increase the burn survivor's risk for delirium include prolonged hospitalization, sleep interruption, fever events, and administration of benzodiazepines for sedation (Silver et al., 2015).

  b. Strategies that can be implemented to reduce the risk for and treat the symptoms of delirium include the implementation of a validated bedside pediatric delirium screening tool such as the Preschool Confusion Assessment Method for the ICU (psCAM-ICU), Pediatric Confusion Assessment Method for the Intensive Care Unit (pCAM-ICU), or Cornell Assessment of Pediatric Delirium (CAPD), and multidisciplinary focused rounding to eliminate as many risk factors as possible (Silver et al., 2015). Normalization of the sleep schedule and minimizing sleep interruptions may also be helpful (Kudchadkar, Sterni, Yaster, & Easley, 2009).

L. Nonaccidental Injury Assessment and Management

1. *Assessment.* When assessing a child with a burn injury, the potential for nonaccidental injury must always be considered. In 2014, an estimated 702,000 children were found to be victims of abuse and neglect in the United States, including 1,580 fatalities (U.S. Department of Health and Human Services, 2016). As many as 20% of pediatric burns are the result of child abuse or neglect (Sheridan, 2012). A thorough history and physical will help the patient care team determine whether additional investigation is warranted. Although none are absolute indicators of nonaccidental injury, some assessment findings that warrant further investigation include (Greenbaum, Donne, Wilson, & Dunn, 2004) the following:

  • Clear lines of demarcation or bilateral symmetrical burns (gloved hand or stocking feet distribution), which may indicate an immersion mechanism

  • The presence of spared areas within areas of burn such as joint flexor surfaces. This may indicate that a child was held in a flexed position at the time of an immersion injury

  • A mechanism of injury that is not compatible with the child's developmental level or injury pattern

  • Unwitnessed or inconsistent accounts of the mechanism of injury

  • Delay in seeking treatment

  • Prior injuries such as burns, bruises, or broken bones

  • Child was in the care of someone other than a parent

2. *Reporting.* Healthcare workers are mandated reporters, which means they are required by law to report cases of suspected child maltreatment or neglect to the appropriate state child welfare agency. The nurse is not required to prove that abuse has occurred, only to report the facts that led him or her to suspect potential abuse or neglect (Child Welfare Information Gateway, 2015). Institutional policies for reporting suspected abuse and neglect often include consultation with a social worker or child protection team.

3. *Nursing Care Interventions*

 a. Ensure safety of the patient at all times, but do not restrict access to the child by any family members unless child protective services have ordered this.

 b. Obtain patient history, including mechanism of injury.

 c. Document all information in a complete, clear, objective manner.

 d. In collaboration with other members of the patient care team, communicate the decision to report suspected abuse or neglect to the appropriate individuals.

 e. Provide support and psychosocial referral as necessary for the child and family.

M. Nursing Priorities During the Acute Phase: Weeks to Months Following Injury

1. *Infection Prevention.* Preventing infection is a priority in both the initial and acute phases of burn injury. Unfortunately, hospital-acquired infections often occur in burn patients as they are exposed to the hospital environment for a long time during hospitalization and have reduced defenses against these types of conditions related to their injury. Careful attention to infection prevention nursing interventions will result in reduced hospital length of stay and morbidity/mortality in this patient population.

 a. Ventilator-associated events (VAE/VAP). Although the definition of VAEs in children at the time of this publication remains controversial, in general, burn survivors of all ages experience a high incidence of VAEs, such as pneumonia, but children experience this condition less frequently than adults due to their relatively healthier lungs (Weber & McManus, 2004). The recommended nursing interventions to prevent pneumonia in ventilated pediatric burn patients are the same as other pediatric patients and include elevation of the head of the bed, meticulous oral care, DVT prophylaxis, and a daily sedation vacation (Resar et al., 2005).

 b. Catheter-associated urinary tract infections (CAUTIs). Burn patients undergoing fluid resuscitation often require a urinary catheter to measure hourly urine output in real time. In addition to needing a catheter during resuscitation, burn patients may need a urinary catheter to promote healing of a burn wound or donor site in the upper thigh, buttocks, or perineum. A daily evaluation of catheter necessity is recommended, and due to the increased risk of infection a burn patient has the catheter should be removed at the earliest possible time. If the burned child requires a urinary catheter, careful attention to preventing a CAUTI is important, and should include strict adherence to hospital and nationally established CAUTI-prevention bundles.

 c. Central line-associated bloodstream infections (CLABSIs). Burn patients often need central venous access to administer fluid resuscitation, antibiotics, and pain management. The current recommendation to prevent central-line infection in burn patients includes placement of the catheter through unburned skin and at a sufficient distance to prevent contamination of the insertion site from the burn wound (Rafla & Tredget, 2011); however, this is not always possible in children with large burns covering common insertion sites. Therefore, changing of the central venous catheter itself at a regular interval may be indicated, but the optimal interval for line changes remains controversial (Sheridan et al., 2012). In addition, the central venous catheter should be coated inside and outside with minocycline and rifampin, as this type of catheter was shown to reduce infection of the central line by about 50% in pediatric burn patients (Weber et al., 2012). If possible, the central-line dressing should be occlusive and be used in conjunction with antiseptic cleansing at the insertion site to prevent infection at routine intervals (Marschall et al., 2014). Occasionally, it is not possible to maintain an occlusive dressing in the burn patient due to moisture or nonintact skin, so in this case, a providone-iodine-containing gauze dressing should be placed and changed every 2 to 4 hours (Rafla & Tredget, 2011). In addition to these strategies, which are specific to burn patients, a daily multidisciplinary assessment of line necessity, including prompt removal when the line is no longer needed, is important (Marschall et al., 2014) as well as is strict adherence to hospital and nationally established CLABSI-prevention bundles.

2. *Metabolic*

   a. Nutritional support

      i. Burn injury is one of the greatest insults the body can sustain and it requires caloric and protein levels exceeding those of any other traumatic injury. Increased metabolic requirements of severe burns make nutritional management a requirement. Energy expenditure in the pediatric patient may reach 2½ times normal, thus early initiation of enteral nutrition is important (Saffle, Graves, & Cochran, 2012).

      ii. Providing aggressive nutritional support to patients with major burns to meet energy requirements, replace protein losses, promote wound healing, and strengthen the immune system is a primary goal of burn therapy. Children normally require greater caloric and protein requirements per kilogram of body weight than adults. For the pediatric burn patient, the nutritional demands required by the hypermetabolic state of the burn injury superimposed on those for growth may result in a compromise in growth with little net weight gain for the duration of the recovery period (Saffle et al., 2012). Determine nutritional goals by using one of the various formulas for estimating the energy requirements in pediatric burn patients such as the Dietary Reference Intake Index (DRI), Galveston, or Curreri Junior formulas (Saffle et al., 2012).

      iii. *Indirect calorimetry* can also be used to calculate the metabolic requirements of the patient. It can also detect significant underfeeding or overfeeding. The respiratory quotient (RQ) is calculated as the ratio of oxygen consumption to CO_2 production (VO_2/VCO_2). Starvation is indicated by an RQ of 0.7 or less, normal metabolism produces an RQ of 0.75 to 0.90, and overfeeding results in an RQ of 1.0 or greater (Saffle et al., 2012).

      iv. For patients with functioning GI tracts, nutrition provided by the enteral route is preferred because it supports the absorptive mechanism of the GI tract and preserves mucosal integrity, which may in turn minimize bacterial translocation from the GI tract. For young children with less than 15% TBSA or older children with less than 25% TBSA, oral intake is generally acceptable. Initiating enteral tube feedings within 24 hours after larger injuries can improve nitrogen balance and nutritional support (Saffle et al., 2012).

Children who are unable to consume the required amount of calories to meet their nutritional goals need enteral tube feedings. Begin tube feedings at a rate of 20 to 40 mL/hr and gradually increase to goal as tolerated. Assess gastric residuals every 1 to 2 hours with enteral tube feedings, and assess GI tract function at least every 4 hours. Note the presence of abdominal distention and diarrhea.

   b. Assess electrolyte status every 8 to 12 hours. Weigh the patient daily and maintain strict input and output. The patient's weight should remain within 10% of the patient's usual preburn weight (dry weight).

   c. Administer antacids or H_2 blockers as ordered. Assess for occult GI tract bleeding and gastric pH every 2 to 4 hours.

   d. Avoid any disruptions of feeding. Enteral feedings can continue preoperatively, intraoperatively, and postoperatively without increased risk of aspiration if given via postpyloric (duodenal) feeding tubes. By avoiding disruptions in feeding, it is easier to meet the patient's nutritional goals (Saffle et al., 2012).

   e. Enteral feeding can oftentimes cause diarrhea. The causes include high glucose loads, medications, infectious causes, and contaminated feeds. Treatment ranges from medications, fiber-containing enteral feedings, altering the formula, reducing the infusion rate, or holding the feeding for a day or 2.

   f. Parenteral nutrition is necessary for those unable to meet nutritional goals through the enteral route. Total parenteral nutrition (TPN) is a safe and effective means of nutritional support in the child who does not tolerate the goal of enteral nutrition (Dylewksi et al., 2013).

3. *Acute Rehabilitation.* The initiation of a rehabilitation program is crucial for the patient sustaining a burn injury. The aim of a rehabilitation program is to restore function and prevent deformities.

   a. Positioning focuses on the prevention of contractures and deformity development. The nurse working with the burn therapist must pay attention to the depth and location of burns and appropriately position the head, extremities, and body so that wound healing is promoted.

   b. Splinting aids in achieving optimal positioning while protecting joints with deep burns and fresh skin grafts. The nurse must be aware of the splints, assess for proper placement, and recognize potential problems associated with the splinting, such as pressure sores.

c. The goals of exercise are to reduce edema, maintain functional joint motion, stretch scar tissue, and return the patient to the optimal level of function (Serghiou, Cowan, & Whitehead, 2009). Initially, postoperative exercise must not be done to grafted areas. However, as soon as possible, the exercises must begin. Active exercises can start on admission and continue throughout the rehabilitation continuum of care. Passive exercises are done with patients who are not able to complete active exercises at that time. Gentle, slow stretching results in blanching of the burn scar.

d. Early ambulation and performance of age-appropriate activities of daily living (ADL) are crucial in the recovery process of the patient with a burn injury and aid in producing optimal functional outcomes.

4. *Psychosocial Care*

a. Several factors complicate the psychosocial sequelae of the burn-injured child. Circumstances surrounding the accident generate feelings of guilt, helplessness, despair, and anger from families. Disfigurement is frequently associated with a burn injury, and severe, lengthy episodes of pain are common. Risks of numerous medical and surgical complications increase during hospitalization. Because of the rollercoaster ride of good days and bad days, progress is made very slowly. Hospitalizations are lengthy, and even longer periods of rehabilitation follow discharge. Burn care may precipitate a financial disaster for the family. Because burn care requires a team approach, there are many people, procedures, and tasks the child must become familiar with each day.

b. Anger, depression, and withdrawal are common sequelae of burn injury and require intervention through education and psychological support. The goal is to assist the child in developing positive coping skills.

c. Changes in appearance and body image are also common concerns of burn patients. Fear of not being accepted by their friends and of being different and wondering how people in general will treat them is common in burn patients. The fear usually occurs as the time for discharge approaches. Planning for discharge begins on admission to the ICU. Encourage burn-injured patients to discuss their concerns. Psychological counseling for patient and family is helpful. School reentry programs facilitate a successful return to school.

d. Financial concerns may be present due to the expense of burn care or missed work. Provide for early social work involvement to facilitate support for the family if needed.

5. *Patient and Family Education and Support*

a. Provide the patient and family with frequent opportunities for education about the burn injury and care regimens required for optimal recovery. Support the family to be involved in ADL, and develop a partnership with the parents. Develop a trusting relationship with the patient and family. Provide honest but positive information.

b. Promote restful periods for the patient during the day and night, and promote a quiet environment.

c. The rehabilitative phase begins on admission to the ICU and comprises prevention of functional deficits and psychosocial support. As wounds heal, correction of functional deficits begins with ongoing psychosocial support.

N. Long-Term Outcomes

1. *Morbidity and Mortality.* Overall, burn mortality has decreased significantly in recent decades. Factors that have contributed to improved burn care and decreased morbidity and mortality include advances in (Sheridan, 2002):

a. Understanding of fluid resuscitation needs

b. Treatment of inhalation injury

c. Support of the hypermetabolic response of burn injury

d. Early excision and grafting of deep burn wounds

e. Pain and anxiety control

f. Rehabilitation and reconstruction

g. Care of patients in pediatric ABA verified burn centers

h. Postburn aftercare programs

i. According to the ABA (2017), the risk of death increases at the extremes of age and increased burn size.

2. *Psychosocial Outcomes*

a. Although burn patients may be at risk for psychosocial sequelae related to their injury, patients can achieve positive outcomes with optimal treatment and follow-up support.

b. Pediatric patients who survived greater than 70% TBSA burns can have outcomes that are comparable to the general population. The involvement of a functional family, early reintegration into preburn activities, and consistent follow-up in a multidisciplinary pediatric burn clinic were found to be predictors of more favorable outcomes (Meyer et al., 2012).

c. Burn patients are at risk for developing PTSD related to the initial injury and/or treatment (Sheridan et al., 2014), and this risk can be mitigated by the use of appropriate pain and anxiety management throughout the healing process. There is a significant impact of early pain management on long-term posttraumatic (PTSD) symptoms. Early and adequate opiate management of burn-wound pain in the first 7 days after injury has been shown to predict the development and resolution rate of PTSD symptoms. The effect is dose related and durable up to 4 years postburn in a large range of burn sizes (Sheridan et al., 2014).

3. *Chronic Issues*

a. Itch. Itch is a common symptom in pediatric burn patients and can have a significant impact on sleep and overall quality of life. Itch is present in up to 93% of pediatric burn patients with greater than 20% TBSA burns at the time of discharge from the hospital. The intensity of itch typically decreases over time, but is still present in 63% of patients 2 years postdischarge (Schneider et al., 2015).

b. Sleep. Following discharge, many patients will have significant sleep disturbances following a burn injury. This may be related to PTSD symptoms, depression, itch, or pain (Low, Meyer, Willebrand, & Thomas, 2012).

The nursing care of the pediatric burn survivor is complex and challenging, but if careful attention is paid throughout the care continuum to key assessment priorities and nursing interventions, the outcome of burn injury in children can be very positive. Nurses are key members of the multidisciplinary team caring for the burned child, and are uniquely positioned to positively influence the child's outcome from the scene of the event through the rehabilitative phase and reintegration of the child to his or her home community.

CASE STUDIES WITH QUESTIONS, ANSWERS, AND RATIONALES

Burns Case Studies

Case Study 9.10

You are the first responder arriving on the scene of a house fire where a child was rescued from the burning home by a firefighter after an unknown amount of time. The child is 10 years old, and her family reports that she was in good health prior to this event. Upon initial evaluation, you notice that she is covered in soot, appears to have singed eyebrows, is gasping for breath, and has burn wounds covering about half of her body.

1. What is your first priority in this situation after you have ensured that the scene is safe?
  A. Stopping the burning process by removing all clothing and placing wet compresses on the patient's skin
  B. Assessing distal extremities for pulses and capillary refill to ensure adequate perfusion
  C. Assessing the airway and establishing a patient airway
  D. Determining the patient's weight and burn size to begin fluid resuscitation

2. Once you have assessed airway, breathing, circulation and neurological status, what is the next priority action you would perform before loading this patient into the transportation vehicle?
  A. Remove all clothing and jewelry and briefly examine the extent of the burn
  B. Insert a foley catheter to assess urine output
  C. Perform escharotomies to the areas of deep burn
  D. Wrap burned areas in sterile dressings

3. You have determined that the burns look deep and are present on about half of the child's body. Does this child need immediate IV access and fluid resuscitation in the field?
  A. Yes
  B. No

4. What fluid would you choose, and at what rate will you run it?
  A. Lactated Ringer's at 50 mL/h
  B. 0.45% NS at 500 mL/hour
  C. Lactated Ringer's at 250 mL/h
  D. D5 at maintenance

The 10-year-old child is now in the trauma room of the pediatric emergency department after being transported by a pediatric EMS team from the field.

The paramedic reports that the child was unresponsive and gasping at the scene, so they intubated the child, placed the child on 100% FiO_2 via Ambu bag, and placed an intraosseous catheter in the left tibia to administer normal saline at a rate of 250 mL/hr. The child's heart rate has been 120 beats per min, BP 120/80 mmHg, respirations have been with assistance only, and temperature is 37°C. The oxygen saturations have been 100% since intubation, and the child has been responsive only to painful stimuli during transport. The paramedic estimates that about 50% of the child is burned.

5. What is your first priority of care in the emergency department for this child?
  A. Airway
  B. Circulation
  C. Neurological status
  D. Pain management

6. You notice that the oxygen saturation on the monitor is consistently reading 100%. Would you advocate for reducing the FiO_2 to 80% at this time?
  A. Yes
  B. No

7. You have completed your primary survey and the child is stable. You wish to turn your attention to fluid resuscitation. What is the first step in calculating the proper fluid resuscitation volume this patient will require per hour?
  A. Calculate the child's maintenance IV fluid rate
  B. Obtain an accurate weight and determine TBSA
  C. Program the pump to run as fast as it can
  D. Obtain a baseline set of labs

8. Let's say that you calculate the %TBSA burned to be 55% deep partial and full-thickness burns and the child weighs 30 kg. What is the rate at which you will set the IV pump to deliver the requisite fluid volume needed for resuscitation?
  A. 206 mL/hour
  B. 250 mL/hour
  C. 70 mL/hour
  D. 309 mL/hour

9. The child has received 2 hours of fluid resuscitation in the ED while a fixed wing transport to a pediatric burn center is arranged. During the 2 hours in the ED, you note urine output of 100 mL with stable vital signs. Is this within the target range for this patient?
  A. Yes
  B. No

10. What is your next step given this urine output value?
  A. No action is necessary, this is an appropriate value
  B. Notify a provider and anticipate an order to decrease the IV fluid rate
  C. Stop fluid resuscitation
  D. Notify a provider and anticipate an order to increase the IV fluid rate

The 10-year-old child rescued from the house fire is now in the PICU of a burn center. From a respiratory standpoint, she has been stable over the first 24 hours postinjury, but is now starting to exhibit desaturations when turned and positioned, and you are beginning to see greyish yellow secretions when you suction her ETT.

11. Is this an expected finding?
  A. Yes
  B. No

12. What are your nursing care priorities for this patient today?
  A. Performing multiple dressing changes throughout the shift to prevent infection
  B. Ensuring range of motion exercises are done frequently to avoid functional impairment
  C. Maintaining a patent airway
  D. Providing age-appropriate stimulation and distraction

13. You are outside of this child's room in the alcove charting, see the child cough, hear the ventilator high-pressure alarm sound, and notice the child's saturations and heart rate are rapidly dropping on the bedside cardiac monitor. What is your first care intervention?
  A. Assess the ventilator closely to determine the cause of the alarm.
  B. Disconnect the patient from the ventilator and attempt to ventilate with an ambu bag.
  C. Page the respiratory therapist.
  D. Administer PRN Albuterol

14. When you attempt to bag the patient, you are unable to squeeze the bag. What could be causing this?
  A. Occlusion of the tube with thick secretions
  B. Swelling around the endotracheal tube
  C. Pulmonary edema
  D. The endotracheal tube is too small

Case Study 9.11

You are the nurse working in the PICU and are receiving report on a 2-year-old child who suffered a scald burn on the lower extremities while in the care of the mother's boyfriend this afternoon. The caregiver reports that he didn't see exactly what happened, but he suspects the child went into the bathroom unsupervised, turned on the hot water, and crawled into the tub. The caregiver reports that he was alerted to this situation when he heard the child crying, and he lifted the child out of the tub and brought the child immediately to the ED. ED personnel did not feel that the child's injuries were worrisome for nonaccidental trauma, so they did not file a report with child services. When you assess the child's burn wounds, you notice that there is flexor sparing behind both knees, and a clear line of demarcation at the child's waist. The caregiver reports the child has been toilet training for a few weeks and was not wearing a diaper. The boyfriend states that the child's mother is out of town this weekend, and left the child in his care a few days ago. You also notice that the wounds are cherry red and dry, with no blistered skin present.

1. Which elements of this child's presentation concern you, and which specific risk factors for nonaccidental trauma are present in this case?
   A. Clear lines of demarcation
   B. Flexor sparing
   C. Unwitnessed injury
   D. All of the above

Burns Answers and Rationales

Case Study 9.10

1. **C.** The first priority of care is the primary survey, so this is the ABCDE assessment of the burned child. Because the child is gasping and you see singed eyebrows, securing the airway with an ETT is the first priority, followed by administration of 100% FiO2 oxygen until a carboxyhemoglobin level can be drawn to rule out CO poisoning. Then ensuring adequate breathing and chest excursion is the next action. A rapid cardiac assessment of pulses and neurologic status prior to intubation is a key finding to report to the hospital team.

2. **A.** The next priority is to expose/examine the patient. So, all clothing and jewelry should be removed in order to stop the burning process, and after quick assessment of the extent of body surface area burned (i.e., is it "big or small"), the child should be wrapped in dry sheets and kept warm.

3. **A.** The best choice of IV fluid for resuscitation is an isotonic crystalloid such as lactated Ringer's or normal saline. The ABLS prehospital resuscitation formula calls for LR to run at 250 mL/hr until arrival at the ED if the burns appear to be greater than 15% to

20% of the TBSA and deep. Insertion of two IVs or an intraosseous catheter is indicated to provide pain management and resuscitation for this patient until central venous access can be established.

4. **C.** This is the ABLS standard for the initial fluid rate as long as a global estimation of the burn size is greater than 15% to 20%. Once precise TBSA is calculated and accurate weight is obtained in a hospital setting, then the precise fluid resuscitation formula is used to continue with resuscitation.

5. **A.** In the ED, the primary and secondary assessment should be repeated and performed in greater detail. The first priority is the child's airway, and the ED nurse should ensure that the ETT is secure and note its size and depth using a standardized landmark. Ensure bilateral breath sounds are audible, and that ventilation is occurring either via Ambu bag or the ventilator. This child is at risk of airway collapse if the ETT is dislodged, so securing it via a commercially available device or twill ties is advised.

6. **B.** This child was involved in a closed-space house fire, and thus is at risk for carbon monoxide poisoning. Remember that children with CO inhalation can demonstrate "normal" oxygen saturations on standard pulse oximetry and a "normal" PaO2 on blood gases and still be hypoxemic. Thus, until a carboxyhemoglobin level is obtained and resulted, the child should remain on 100% oxygen. Typically, this is done for about 4 hours, depending on the child's total CO exposure.

7. **B.** The first step is to obtain an accurate weight and %TBSA burned. This can be accomplished by using the rule of the palm, the rule of nines, or a Lund and Browder chart burn diagram.

8. **D.** ABLS Consensus formula for children calls for 3 mL × %TBSA × wt (kg) over 24 hours, anticipating half of that volume in the first 8 hours, and the rest over the next 16. For this child, that amounts to 3 mL × 55% × 30 kg =4,950 mL total. To get the rate of IV fluid for the pump, divide 4,950 by 2 (=2,475 mL) and divide that total by 8, which equals 309 mL/hr. So, your 4,950 mL will be delivered at approximately 309 mL/hr for the first 8 hours, and 155 mL/hr for the remaining 16 hours. Remember that these formulae are all estimations of what the child will require, close monitoring of urine output and perfusion is the indicator that resuscitation is progressing as planned. Adjustments to the calculated fluid rates and volumes will always need to be made during the first 24 hours.

9. **B.** It is higher than is recommended. This child is in danger of overresuscitation if this trend continues, which can cause compartment syndrome and pulmonary edema.

10. B. Notify a provider that the urine output is higher than the 1 mL/kg/hr target. Most likely, the IV fluid will need to be reduced by one third of the rate hourly until the urine output approaches 1 mL/kg/hr (30 mL/hr) via a urinary catheter.

11. A. This child suffered some degree of inhalation injury and is showing typical signs and symptoms, which occur 24 to 72 hours after injury.

12. C. Maintenance of a patent airway is of utmost importance in this child. Frequent suctioning and pulmonary toileting should be performed, as well as ensuring continued safety of the ETT.

13. B. Take the child off the ventilator and attempt to ventilate with an Ambu bag and 100% oxygen.

14. A. Children with inhalation injury develop thick secretions in the lung that can become viscous and occlude the tube opening. In this case, deep suctioning of the tube is required, and if not successful in clearing the airway, immediate replacement of the ETT is indicated before the child becomes hypoxic. Immediate nursing priorities include immediate provider notification, ensuring equipment for emergent intubation is readily available, and that a bag-mask setup is at the bedside for temporary ventilation. In some circumstances, a surgical airway may need to be emergently placed at the bedside and should be readily available for the provider team.

Case Study 9.11

1. D. You should be most concerned with the injury pattern, as children who are crawling and walking should be able to splash around and attempt to escape from accidental immersion in hot water. There is a clear line of demarcation and flexor sparing, which could indicate that the child was held forcefully in the water for a period of time. Also, the injuries are deep (cherry red) and dry, which indicates severe heat damage either from prolonged immersion or very hot temperatures. Most fresh burn wounds will appear moist and blister, so the lack of blistering and moisture may indicate a delay in seeking treatment, which is an indicator for child neglect. The child's additional risk factors include being in the care of someone other than a parent, and an unwitnessed injury.

BURNS REFERENCES

Advanced Burn Life Support Advisory Committee. (2015). *Advanced burn life support course provider manual*. Chicago, IL: American Burn Association.

American Burn Association. (2016). Burn incidence and treatment in the United States: 2016. Retrieved from http://www.ameriburn.org/resources_factsheet.php

American Burn Association. (2017). *National Burn Repository 2017 update: Report of data from 2008–2017*. Retrieved from http://ameriburn.org/wp-content/uploads/2018/04/2017_aba_nbr_annual_report_summary.pdf

Bayat, A., Ramaiah, R., & Bhananker, S. M. (2010). Analgesia and sedation for children undergoing burn wound care. *Expert Review of Neurotherapeutics*, *10*(11), 1747–1759. doi:10.1586/ern.10.158

Child Welfare Information Gateway (2016). Mandatory reporters of child abuse and neglect. Washington, DC: U.S. Department of Health and Human Services, Children's Bureau.

Chung, K. K., & Wolf, S. E. (2012). Critical care in the severely burned: Organ support and management of complications. In D. N. Herndon (Ed.), *Total burn care* (4th ed., pp. 377–395). Philadelphia, PA: Elsevier.

Centers for Disease Control and Prevention, National Center for Injury Prevention and Control (2016a). 10 leading causes of injury deaths by age group highlighting unintentional injury deaths, United States—2016. Retrieved from https://www.cdc.gov/injury/wisqars/pdf/leading_causes_of_injury_deaths_highlighting_unintentional_injury_2016-508.pdf

Centers for Disease Control and Prevention, National Center for Injury Prevention and Control (2016b). 10 leading causes of death by age group, United States—2016. Retrieved from https://www.cdc.gov/injury/wisqars/pdf/leading_causes_of_death_by_age_group_2016-508.pdf

Committee on Trauma American College of Surgeons. (2014). *Resources for optimal care of the injured patient*. Chicago, IL: American College of Surgeons.

Cubison, T. C. S, Pape, S. A., & Parkhouse, N. (2006). Evidence for the link between healing time and the development of hypertrophic scars (HTS) in paediatric burns due to scalds. *Burns, 32*, 992–999.

Dries, D. J., & Endorf, F. W. (2013). Inhalation injury: Epidemiology, pathology, treatment strategies. *Scandinavian Journal of Trauma, Resuscitation and Emergency Medicine*, *21*(1), 31. doi:10.1186/1757-7241-21-31

Dylewksi, M. L., Baker, M., Prelack, K., Weber, J. M., Hursey, D., Lydon, M., ... Sheridan, R. (2013). The safety and efficacy of parenteral nutrition among pediatric patients with burn injuries. *Pediatric Critical Care Medicine*, *14*(3), e120–e125.

Fagan, S., Chai, J., Spies, M., Hollyoak, M., Muller, M. J., Goodwin, C. W., & Herndon, D. N. (2012). Exfoliative diseases of the integument and soft tissue necrotizing infections. In D. N. Herndon (Ed.), *Total burn care* (4th ed., pp. 471–481). Philadelphia, PA: Saunders.

Fahlstrom, K., Boyle, C., & Makic, M. B. F. (2013). Implementation of a nurse-driven burn resuscitation protocol: A quality improvement project. *Critical Care Nurse*, *33*(1), 25–35. doi:10.4037/ccn2013385

Gallagher, J. J., Branski, L. K., Williams-Bouyer, N., Villarreal, C., & Herndon, D. (2012). Treatment of infection in burns. In D. N. Herndon, *Total burn care* (pp. 138–156). New York, NY: Elsevier.

Greenbaum, A.R., Donne, J., Wilson, D. and Dunn, K.W. (2004). Intentional burn injury: an evidence based, clinical and forensic review. *Burns, 30*, 628–642.

Greenhalgh, D. G., Saffle, J. R., Holmes, J. H., Gamelli, R. L., Palmieri, T. L., Horton, J. W.,...Latenser, B. A. (2007). American Burn Association consensus conference to define sepsis and infection in burns. *Journal of Burn Care and Research, 28*(6), 776–790.

Iwamoto, P. (2009). Aseptic technique. In P. Grota (Ed.), *APIC text of infection control and epidemiology* (pp. 20-1–20-3). Washington, DC: The Association for Professionals in Infection Control and Epidemiology.

Jeschke, M. G., & Herndon, D. N. (2014). Burns in children: Standard and new treatments. *Lancet, 383*(9923), 1168–1178. doi:10.1016/S0140-6736(13)61093-4

Kramer, G. C. (2014). Pathophysiology of burn shock and burn edema. In D. N. Herndon (Ed.), *Total burn care* (4th ed., pp. 103–113). Philadelphia, PA: Saunders.

Kudchadkar, S. R., Sterni, L., Yaster, M., & Easley R. B. (2009). Sleep in the intensive care unit. *Contemporary Critical Care, 7*, 1–12.

Lee, J. O., Dibildox, M., Jimenez, C. J., Gallagher, J. J., Sayeed, S., Sheridan, R. L. and Herndon, D. J. (2012). Operative wound management. In D. N. Herndon (Ed.), *Total burn care* (pp.157-172). New York, NY: Saunders.

Lee, J. O., Norbury, W. B., & Herndon, D. N. (2012). Special considerations of age: The pediatric burned patient. In D. N. Herndon (Ed.), *Total burn care* (4th ed., pp. 405–414). Philadelphia, PA: Saunders.

Lewis, G. M., Heimbach, D. M., & Gibran, N. S. (2012). Evaluation of the burn wound: Management decisions. In N. Herndon (Ed.), *Total burn care* (4th ed.). Philadelphia, PA: Saunders.

Low, J. F. A., Meyer, W., Willebrand, M., & Thomas, C. (2012). Psychiatric disorders associated with burn injury. In D. N. Herndon (Ed.), *Total burn care* (4th ed., pp. 733–741). Philadelphia, PA: Saunders.

Ludwik, K. B., Herndon, D. N., & Barrow, R. E. (2012). A brief history of acute burn care management. In D. N. Herndon (Ed.), *Total burn care* (4th ed., pp. 1–7). Philadelphia, PA: Saunders.

Malholtra, R., Sheikh, I., & Dheansa, B. (2009). The management of eyelid burns. *Survey of Ophthalmology, 54*(3), 356–371.

Marschall, J., Mermel, L. A., Fakih, M., Hadaway, L., Kallen, A., O'Grady, N. P., … Society for Healthcare Epidemiology of America. (2014). Strategies to prevent central line-associated bloodstream infections in acute care hospitals: 2014 update. *Infection Control and Hospital Epidemiology, 35*(Suppl. 2), S89–S107.

Meyer, W., Lee, A. F., Kazis, L. E., Li, N. C., Sheridan, R. L., Herndon, D. N., … Group, M.-C. B. S. W. (2012). Adolescent survivors of burn injuries and their parents' perceptions of recovery outcomes: do they agree or disagree? *Journal of Trauma and Acute Care Surgery, 73*(3 Suppl 2), S213–S220.

Meyer, W., Meyer, W., Wiechman, S., Woodson, L., Jaco, M., & Thomas, C. (n.d.). Management of pain and other discomforts in burned patients. Total burn care (pp. 715–731.e6). [S.l.]: Saunders. doi:10.1016/B978-1-4377-2786-9.00064-3

Murphey, E. D., Sherwood, E. R., & Toliver-Kinsky, T. (2012). The immunological response and strategies for intervention. In D. N. Herndon (Ed.), *Total burn care* (4th ed., pp. 265–276). Philadelphia, PA: Saunders.

Ong, Y. S., Samuel, M., & Song, C. (2006). Meta-analysis of early excision of burns. *Burns, 32*, 145–150.

Posluszny, J. A., Gamelli, R. L., & Shankar, R. (2012). Hematologic and hematopoietic response to burn injury. In D. N. Herndon (Ed.), *Total burn care* (4th ed., pp. 277–288). Philadelphia, PA: Saunders.

Rafla, K., & Tredget, E. E. (2011). Infection control in the burn unit. *Burns, 37*(1), 5–15. doi:10.1016/j.burns.2009.06.198

Resar, R., Pronovost, P., Haraden, C., Simmonds, T., Rainey, T., & Nolan, T. (2005). Using a bundle approach to improve ventilator care processes and reduce ventilator-associated pneumonia. *Joint Commission Journal on Quality and Patient Safety/Joint Commission Resources, 31*(5), 243–248.

Saffle, J., Graves, C., & Cochran, A. (2012). Nutritional support of the burned patient. In D. N. Herndon (Ed.), *Total burn care* (4th ed., pp. 333–353). Philadelphia, PA: Saunders.

Schneider, J. C., Nadler, D. L., Herndon, D. N., Kowalske, K., Matthews, K., Wiechman, S. A., …Ryan, C. M. (2015). Pruritis in pediatric burn survivors: Defining the clinical course. *Journal of Burn Care and Research, 36*(1), 151–158.

Serghiou, M., Cowan, A., & Whitehead, C. (2009). Rehabilitation after a burn injury. *Clinics in Plastic Surgery, 36*(4), 675–686. doi:10.1016/j.cps.2009.05.008

Serghiou, M. A., Ott, S., Whitehead, C., Cowan, A., McEntire, S., & Suman , O. E. (2012). Comprehensive rehabilitation of the burn patient. In D. N. Herndon (Ed.), *Total burn care* (pp. 517–549). New York, NY: Elsevier.

Sheridan, R. L. (2002). Burns. *Critical Care Medicine, 30*(11), S500–S514. Retrieved from https://journals.lww.com/ccmjournal/Abstract/2002/11001/Burns.15.aspx

Sheridan, R. L. (2012). *Burns*. London, UK: Manson.

Sheridan, R. L., & Chang, P. (2014). Acute burn procedures. *Surgical Clinics of North America, 94*(4), 755–764. doi:10.1016/j.suc.2014.05.014

Sheridan, R. L., Neely, A. N., Castillo, M. A., Shankowsky, H. A., Fagan, S. P., Chung, K. K., & Weber, J. M. (2012). A survey of invasive catheter practices in U.S. burn centers. *Journal of Burn Care & Research, 33*(6), 741–746.

Sheridan, R. L., Stoddard, F. J., Kazis, L. E., Lee, A., Li, N.-C., Kagan, R. J.…Tompkins, R. G. (2014). Long-term posttraumatic stress symptoms vary inversely with early opiate dosing in children recovering from serious burns: Effects durable at 4 years. *Journal of Trauma and Acute Care Surgery, 76*(3), 828–832.

Silver, G., Traube, C., Gerber, L. M., Sun, X., Kearney, J., Patel, A., & Greenwald, B. (2015). Pediatric delirium and associated risk factors: A single-center prospective observational study. *Pediatric Critical Care Medicine: A Journal of the Society of Critical Care Medicine and the World Federation of Pediatric Intensive and Critical Care Societies, 16*(4), 303–309.

Traber, D., Herndon, D., Enkhbaatar, P., Maybauer, M., & Maybauer, D. (2012). The pathophysiology of inhalation injury. In D. N. Herndon (Ed.), *Total burn care* (4th ed., pp. 219–228). Philadelphia, PA: Saunders..

Tran, S., & Chin, A. C. (2014). Burn sepsis in children. *Clinical Pediatric Emergency Medicine, 15*(2), 149–157.

Tredget, E. E., Shankowsky, H. A., Joffe, A. M., Inkson, T. I., Vopel, K., Paranchych, W. . . . Burke, J. F. (1992). Epidemiology of infections with Pseudomonas aeruginosa in burn patients: The role of hydrotherapy. *Clinical Infectious Diseases, 15*(6), 941–949.

U.S. Department of Health & Human Services, Administration for Children and Families, Administration on Children, Youth and Families, Children's Bureau (2016). Child maltreatment 2014. Retrieved from http://www.acf.hhs.gov/programs/cb/research-data-technology/statistics-research/child-maltreatment

Warden, G. (2014). Fluid resuscitation and early management. In In D. N. Herndon (Ed.), *Total Burn Care* (4th ed., pp. 115–124). Philadelphia, PA: Saunders.

Weber, J. M. (2014). Burns. In P. Grota (Ed.), *APIC text on infection control and applied epidemiology (pp. 38.1–38.12)*. Washington, DC: The Association for Professionals in Infection Control and Epidemiology.

Weber, J. M., & McManus, A. (2004). Infection control in burn patients. *Burns, 30*(8), 16–24. doi:10.1016/j.burns.2004.08.003

Weber, J. M., Sheridan, R. L., Fagan, S., Ryan, C. M., Pasternack, M. S., & Tompkins, R. (2012). Incidence of catheter-associated bloodstream infection after introduction of minocycline and rifampin antimicrobial-coated catheters in a pediatric burn population. *Journal of Burn Care & Research, 33*(4), 539–543.

World Health Organization (2018, March 6). Burns fact sheet. Retrieved from http://www.who.int/mediacentre/factsheets/fs365/en

SECTION V. DISASTER PREPAREDNESS AND RESPONSE

Nancy Blake

Natural and man-made disasters occur around the world on a frequent basis. The Department of Homeland Security (2016) and the Centers for Disease Control and Prevention (CDC; 2016a) provide current and valuable resources for a wide variety of diseases, emergencies, and disasters that impact patient care, including outbreaks, incidents, natural disasters and severe weather, chemical and radiation emergencies, and bioterrorism. Although beyond the scope of this text to address all aspects of both natural and man-made disasters, this section focuses on content that is more challenging to locate, such as pediatric preparedness for mass casualty incidents (MCIs) and specific information on terrorism, including violent incidents, nuclear or radiologic attacks, chemical attacks, biological attacks, and the psychological impact. More information regarding patient management of pediatric victims of multiple trauma is located in the "Multiple Trauma" section in this chapter.

In the past 15 years, terrorism has unfortunately become an increasingly real threat to the citizens of the United States. During 2016, numerous terrorist acts in various states impacted several hospitals because of the number of victims brought to these hospitals. *Terrorism* by definition is the unlawful use of force or violence against persons or property to intimidate civilians or to coerce a government or a civilian population in the furtherance of political and social objectives and to effect the conduct of a government by mass destruction, assassination, or kidnapping (Federal Bureau of Investigation [FBI], 1992). Because the scale of a terrorist attack can be often widespread, this type of disaster can be overwhelming to a nation's healthcare system.

A report to the Congressional Committee from the U.S. General Accounting Office (GAO) regarding hospital preparedness for a bioterrorist incident was published in August 2003. This report stated that although most urban hospitals nationwide reported participating in basic planning and coordination of activities for bioterrorism response, they did not have the medical equipment, especially ventilators, needed to handle the number of patients who would likely require medical attention as the result of a bioterrorism incident. Four of five hospitals reported having a written emergency response plan that addresses bioterrorism; however, many hospitals lacked key resources, such

as laboratories. Many reported being involved in state or local planning and had conducted some training of staff members; however, few had actually conducted drills to prepare for a bioterrorist attack. Most hospitals admitted a lack of preparedness, particularly in terms of having adequate resources to handle a large influx of patients (GAO, 2003). A similar governmental study has not been done to address the overall hospital preparedness since then, but in 2002 the Hospital Preparedness Program (HPP) was established through the Office of Assistant Secretary for Preparedness and Response (ASPR), which has given funding to 62 awardees, including all states and several major cities and counties to strengthen hospital preparedness (ASPR, 2016). This program took a few years to develop fully and some of this funding still exists. The goal of this program was to improve patient outcomes, minimize the need for supplemental state and federal resources, and enable rapid disaster response recovery. The hospitals that receive funding have several deliverables to sustain their operation in a real disaster, including supplies, equipment, education, pharmaceuticals, and personnel to address whatever disaster they may have. Numerous groups have looked at the needs of pediatric patients and make suggestions to identify their needs specifically, including the report by the National Advisory Committee on Children and Disasters (NACCD; 2015) and the Pediatric Mass Critical Care Task Force (Kissoon, 2011). In addition, numerous resources have been published specific to pediatric response (Foltin, Schonfeld, & Shannon, 2006; Bradley et al., 2014; Hamele, Poss, & Sweeney, 2014). The following website has an archived list of many of the studies and reports regarding pediatric disaster preparedness: https://ncdp.columbia.edu/library/publications.

PEDIATRIC PREPAREDNESS

A. Besides being generally unprepared to deal with a large-scale attack, most hospitals are specifically unprepared to care for pediatric patients. State and federal plans historically have not included provisions for pediatric patients, although that is changing. Children have unique needs for which adult models cannot be adapted easily, because these models were based around military models that did not include children. In February 2003, a National Consensus Conference was convened to address pediatric preparedness for disasters and terrorism. The conference was funded by grants from the Agency for Healthcare Research and Quality (AHRQ) and the Emergency Medical Services for Children (EMSC) program of the Maternal and Child Health Bureau and sponsored by the Program for Pediatric Preparedness of the National Center for Disaster Preparedness, Mailman School of Public Health, Columbia University, the Children's Health Fund, and the Children's Hospital at Montefiore (Markenson & Redlener, 2003). Since that time, several other groups have been convened and resources have been developed specifically for pediatric patients.

B. Several special pediatric considerations in terrorism and disaster preparedness have been identified:

  1. Children are more vulnerable to chemical agents that are absorbed through the skin or inhaled.

  2. Children are especially susceptible to dehydration and shock from a biological attack.

  3. Children cannot be decontaminated in adult decontamination units because of their unique needs.

  4. Children require different dosages, antibiotics, and antidotes to many agents.

  5. Children are more susceptible to the effects of radiation exposure and require responses that are different from those required by adults.

  6. Because they have unique psychosocial vulnerabilities, children require special management plans in the event of mass casualties and evacuation.

  7. Emergency responders, medical professionals, and children's healthcare institutions require special expertise and training to ensure optimal care of those exposed to chemical, biological, or nuclear agents.

  8. Children's developmental ability and cognitive levels may impede their ability to escape danger.

  9. EMS and medical and hospital staff may not have pediatric training, equipment, or facilities (Markenson & Redlener, 2003).

C. Since that conference, several groups have developed resources, but the one most relevant to the pediatric critical care nurses is the Pediatric Mass Critical Care

Task Force project that implemented recommendations that were specific to pediatric patients:

  1. Treatment and triage recommendations

  2. Supplies and equipment

  3. Neonatal and pediatric regionalized recommendations

  4. Education

  5. The role of community preparedness in conserving critical care resources

  6. Legal considerations

  7. Focus on family-centered care

  8. Ethical issues (Kissoon, 2011)

D. The following recommendations were made by the National Advisory Committee on Children and Terrorism:

  1. All planning and training mechanisms must specifically include elements that focus on the needs of infants, children, and adolescents.

  2. Direct attention will be addressed to settings where children normally gather.

  3. Coordination and integration response efforts must be made at all levels of government.

  4. In the event of an incident, priority will be given to returning children to their normal routine (National Advisory Committee on Children and Terrorism, 2003).

E. In 2006, a group was convened to address pediatric terrorism and disaster preparedness that was sponsored by the AAP and the AHRQ. The resource that was developed by this workgroup is very extensive and addresses not only the physical differences between children and adults, but also addresses all of the recommendations for treating nuclear, biological, and chemical terrorism (Foltin et al., 2006).

TYPES OF TERRORISM

Terrorism exists in a variety of forms:

- Violence, explosions, and hijackings

- Nuclear or radiologic attacks

- Chemical attacks

- Biological attacks

A. Violence (Including Active Shooters), Explosions, and Hijackings

1. The United States has an organized trauma system to deal with small-scale violence or explosions, but is not prepared for large-scale attacks. It is important that we become better prepared to deal with large-scale emergencies. In the past, attacks within the United States, including the Oklahoma City bombing, the Columbine High School shootings, and the shootings at the Jewish Community Center in Granada Hills, California, have overwhelmed EDs and pediatric critical care centers. The Sandy Hook Elementary School shooting could have also overwhelmed the system, but unfortunately there were few survivors.

2. MCIs require that patients be assessed and triaged quickly but comprehensively. An MCI is characterized by an influx of large numbers of casualties that exceed the capabilities of local emergency and medical personnel. Nurses perform the primary and secondary survey, as with any other trauma patient. Tables 9.32 and 9.33 list the assessment components of the pediatric trauma patient.

3. As patients go through triage, they are sent to the appropriate level of care. The **JumpSTART triage model** is a model that can be used to triage pediatric patients during mass casualty events. (More information about this triage model can be obtained by visiting www.jumpstarttriage. com.) This differs from the START model, which is adult based, that is traditionally used in an MCI event.

4. In preparing for MCIs, it is important to have the appropriate size and amount of emergency medication, supplies, and equipment. Many new documents related to MCIs in pediatrics have been published, but much more work needs to be done to handle large-scale disasters involving pediatric patients. One crucial step is to ensure that pediatric patients can be placed in a PICU that can take care of pediatric trauma patients as quickly as possible and that the PICU nurses know how to treat victims of weapons of mass destruction. The Pediatric Mass Critical Care Task Force recommended that hospitals prepare to care for patients for at least 10 days and have equipment such as ventilators and ventilation equipment; intravenous fluids; and equipment, sedation, and items to reduce cold stress (Bohn, Kanter, Burns, Barfield, & Kissoon, 2011).

TABLE 9.32   Primary Survey of the Pediatric Trauma Patient

Component	Actions
Airway	Assess for patency; look for loose teeth, vomitus, or other obstruction; note position of head. Suspect cervical spine injury with multiple trauma; maintain neutral alignment during assessment; evaluate effectiveness of cervical collar, cervical immobilization device, or other equipment used to immobilize the spine. Open cervical collar to evaluate neck for jugular vein distention and tracheal deviation.
Breathing	Auscultate breath sounds in the axillae for presence and equality. Assess chest for contusions, penetrating wounds, abrasions, or paradoxic movement.
Circulation	Assess apical pulse for rate, rhythm, and quality; compare apical and peripheral pulses for quality and equality. Evaluate capillary refill; normal is less than 2 seconds. Check skin color and temperature. Assess level of consciousness; check for orientation to person, place, and time in the older child.
Disability	In a younger child, assess alertness, ability to interact with environment, and ability to follow commands. Is the child easily consoled and interested in the environment? Does the child recognize a familiar object and respond when you speak to him or her? Check pupils for size, shape, reactivity, and equality. Note open wounds or uncontrolled bleeding.
Expose	Remove clothing to allow visual inspection of entire body.

TABLE 9.33   Secondary Survey of the Pediatric Trauma Patient

Component	Actions
Head, eye, ear, nose	Assess scalp for lacerations or open wounds; palpate for step-off defects, depressions, hematomas, and pain. Reassess pupils for size, reactivity, equality, and extraocular movements; ask the child whether he or she can see. Assess ears and nose for rhinorrhea or otorrhea. Observe for raccoon eyes (bruising around the eyes) or Battle's sign (bruising over the mastoid process). Palpate forehead, orbits, maxilla, and mandible for crepitus, deformities, step-off defect, pain, and stability; evaluate malocclusion by asking child to open and close mouth; note open wounds. Inspect for loose, broken, or chipped teeth as well as oral lacerations. Check orthodontic appliances for stability. Evaluate facial symmetry by asking child to smile, grimace, and open and close mouth. Do not remove impaled objects or foreign objects.
Neck	Open cervical collar and reassess anterior neck for jugular vein distention and tracheal deviation; note bruising, edema, open wounds, pain, and crepitus. Check for hoarseness or changes in voice by asking child to speak.
Chest	Obtain respiratory rate; reassess breath sounds in anterior lobes for equality. Palpate chest wall and sternum for pain, tenderness, and crepitus. Observe inspiration and expiration for symmetry or paradoxic movement; note use of accessory muscles. Reassess apical heart rate for rate, rhythm, and clarity.
Abdomen/pelvis/genitourinary	Observe abdomen for bruising and distention; auscultate bowel sounds briefly in all four quadrants; palpate abdomen gently for tenderness; assess pelvis for tenderness and stability. Palpate bladder for distention and tenderness; check urinary meatus for signs of injury or bleeding; note priapism and genital trauma such as lacerations or foreign body. Have rectal sphincter tone assessed, usually by physician.
Musculoskeletal	Assess extremities for deformities, swelling, lacerations, or other injuries. Palpate distal pulses for equality, rate, and rhythm; compare to central pulses. Ask child to wiggle toes and fingers; evaluate strength through hand grips and foot flexion/extension.
Back	Logroll as a unit to inspect back; maintain spinal alignment during examination; observe for bruising and open wounds; palpate each vertebral body for tenderness, pain, deformity, and stability; assess flank area for bruising and tenderness.

5. Trauma injuries would result from some type of blast injury, given that explosions and bombings are often the weapons of choice for terrorists. Such injuries can result from either primary, secondary, and tertiary blasts. These were the types of injuries seen in the children during the Boston marathon bombing (Biddinger et al., 2013).

a. *Primary blast injuries* are the result of sudden changes in atmospheric pressure caused by an explosion. The following are examples of primary blast injuries:

   i.   Ear injuries (e.g., perforated eardrums)

   ii. Pulmonary injuries, including hemorrhagic contusion and hemopneumothorax

   iii. Gastrointestinal hemorrhage, bowel perforation, or rupture

b. *Secondary blast injury* occurs when victims are struck by flying objects and debris.

c. *Tertiary blast injuries* occur when the body is hurled through the air and struck by another object.

B. Nuclear/Radiologic Attacks

1. The threat of nuclear attack was more of an issue before the end of the Cold War. Radiation accidents/attacks can arise from problems with nuclear reactors, industrial sources, and medical sources.

It is important that clinicians understand how such an attack can occur and how to treat patients affected by it. Medical consequences depend on the type of device used. A radiologic or nuclear attack occurs in one of five ways:

a. *Simple radiological device (SRD)*. Use of an SRD is a deliberate act of spreading radioactive material without the use of an explosive device, such as putting a high-activity radioactive isotope in a public place, exposing numerous individuals to various levels of radiation.

b. *Radiologic dispersal device (RDD)*. This type of device is formed by combining an explosive agent with radioactive materials that might have been stolen. The initial explosion kills or injures those closest to the bomb, and radioactive substances remain to expose and contaminate survivors and possibly emergency responders. This is also known as a *dirty bomb*. This material is common to labs, medical centers, and used in industry. This is the most common type of exposure (CDC, 2014).

c. *Nuclear reactor sabotage*. This type of incident is uncommon because of sophisticated shielding but could occur with an attack on a nuclear reactor. In addition, no one is known to survive whole-body doses of radiation exceeding about 8 Gy. Acute radiation system results from this type of exposure and care is general supportive care. Because the body retains radioactive materials after death, cremation should be avoided in these patients to avoid vaporizing the radioactive material (CDC, 2014). These patients may receive a bone marrow transplant that may prolong their life for a few months.

d. *Improvised nuclear device (IND)*. An IND is a device designed to cause a nuclear detonation; it is an RDD. Because it is difficult to detonate such a weapon correctly, this type of incident is uncommon; a high level of sophistication is required to engineer it, but a stolen device would generate high levels of radiation.

e. *Nuclear weapon* (American College of Radiology [ACR], 2002; Foltin et al., 2006).

2. There are two categories of radiation incidents:

a. *External exposure*, which is irradiation from a source that is either distant or close to the body. External irradiation can be divided into *whole-body* exposure or *local* exposure.

b. *Contamination*, which is defined as unwanted radioactive material in or on the body (ACR, 2002).

3. Response is based on the type of incident. Most external exposures result in irradiation of the victim. A person exposed to external radiation does not become radioactive and poses no hazard to nearby individuals. Once the victim is removed from the source of radiation, the irradiation ceases.

4. Contamination incidents require a different approach. Caregivers and support personnel must be careful not to spread the contamination to uncontaminated parts of the victim's body, to themselves, or to the surrounding area. Internal contamination can result from inhalation, ingestion, direct absorption through the skin, or penetration of radioactive materials through open wounds (Yu, 2003). Treatment of serious or significant medical conditions should always take precedence over radiologic assessment or decontamination of the patient.

5. Treatment of patients of a radiologic attack involves the following priorities:

a. Treat and stabilize life-threatening injuries. A radiologic assessment should be performed by an individual with radiologic health training. Radiologic measurements can be done using a Geiger counter and swabs containing blood fluid can be sent to the lab for measurement.

b. Prevent and minimize internal contamination. Time is critical to prevent radioactive uptake. Potassium iodide (KI) is administered to prevent radioiodine from accumulating in the thyroid gland. The pediatric dose of KI is listed in Table 9.34. KI should be given within 2 hours of contamination.

c. Assess internal contamination and decontamination. Patients who are contaminated but not seriously injured should be decontaminated before they are treated.

d. Contain contamination and decontamination.

e. Minimize external contamination to medical personnel. Staff should wear personal protective clothing and, if the area is highly contaminated, respirators should be worn.

f. Assess internal contamination (concurrent with the preceding).

g. Assess local radiation injuries and burns and flush if they are contaminated.

h. Follow up on patients with significant whole-body irradiation or internal contamination.

TABLE 9.34   Guidelines for KI Dose Administration

Patient/Age	Exposure, Gy (rad)	KI Dose[a] (mg)
>40 years	>5 (500)	130
18–40 years	0.1 (10)	130
12–17 years	0.05 (5)	65
4–11 years	0.05 (5)	65
1 month–3 years	0.05 (5)	32
Birth–1 month	0.05 (5)	16
Pregnant or lactating women	0.05 (5)	130

KI, potassium iodide.

[a]Children/adolescents weighing more than 70 kg should receive the adult dose (130 mg).

Note: This table was created from recommendations developed at the Consensus Conference and in part is based on reviewed reference materials from the American Academy of Pediatrics, Centers for Disease Control, and U.S. Food and Drug Administration.

Source: American Academy of Pediatrics. (2003). AAP policy statement: Radiation disasters and children. *Pediatrics*, *111*(6), 1455–1466. Retrieved from http://pediatrics.aappublications.org/content/pediatrics/111/6/1455.full.pdf

i. Counsel the patient and his or her family about the potential for long-term risks and effects (Foltin et al., 2006; Linnemann, 2001).

C. Chemical Attacks

1. Chemical warfare agents are hazardous chemicals that have been designed for use by the military to irritate, incapacitate, injure, or kill during wartime (Foltin et al., 2006; Los Angeles County EMSA and Public Health, 2012). The sarin gas attacks in Japan in the mid-1990 resulted in few deaths, but the influx of contaminated patients to medical facilities was overwhelming to the medical system. Chemical attacks may be combined with explosions and blast attacks to make dirty bombs. To have chemical contamination associated with explosions, victims will be in close proximity to the explosion or blast attack. In these situations, casualties occur almost immediately and the attack is recognized right away. First responders need to be cautious as to not expose themselves (Foltin et al., 2006). Children are more vulnerable in these types of attacks because of their physiologic, developmental, and psychological differences.

2. Many nerve agents are transported on a daily basis by truck or rail cars in the United States. Potentially, tear gas, which is sold in stores, could be used in an attack. Chemicals can be absorbed through the eyes, skin, airways, or a combination of these routes.

3. The following are types of chemical agents:

a. *Nerve agents* are the most toxic of all weaponized military agents. They can cause sudden loss of consciousness, seizures, apnea, and death. The diagnosis is usually made on clinical signs and symptoms. Nerve agents inhibit cholinesterase. Examples of these agents are tabun, sarin, saman, and VX, a man-made chemical warfare agent that is very fast acting and very serious.

b. *Vesicants* cause blistering. The most common vesicants are sulfur, mustard, and lewisite. Mustard and lewisite cause injury to the eyes, skin, airways, and some internal organs.

c. *Cyanide* is a chemical agent that is widely used in the United States. Terrorists may use it in confined spaces such as subway cars, shopping centers, convention centers, and small buildings. Shortly after inhalation, victims often become anxious and start to hyperventilate. Convulsions, asystole, and death also can occur. Antidotes should be administered immediately.

d. *Pulmonary intoxicants* can cause severe life-threatening lung injury after inhalation. The effects are generally delayed for several hours. Examples are phosgene and chlorine. An example of this type of accident occurred at the Union Carbide plant in 1984 in Bhopal, India, which was due to an industrial accident (not to a terrorist attack). These intoxicants are irritating to the eyes and respiratory tract and can cause severe pulmonary edema of a noncardiac nature.

e. *Riot-control agents* stimulate the lacrimal glands to produce tears and cause irritation to eyes, nose, mouth, skin, and respiratory tract. These are routinely used by police to control an out-of-control crowd or individual. The effect is immediate and lasts about 30 minutes. Examples of these agents are chloroacetophenone (Mace 7), OC (oleoresin capsicum or pepper spray), and adamsite or chlorobenzylidene malinonitrile (tear gas; Los Angeles County EMSA and Public Health, 2012; CDC, 2016a).

f. *Antidotes* for the aforementioned agents are listed in Table 9.35.

4. *Decontamination Standards*

a. Staff needs to be trained to decontaminate patients appropriately and the staff should have the appropriate personal protective equipment (PPE). Hospitals should have the equipment required to decontaminate victims.

TABLE 9.35 Antidote Therapy for Chemical Weapons Attacks

Chemical	Antidote	Decontamination (Including Removal of Clothing)	Other
Nerve agent	Atropine, 2-PAM	Soap and water	Diazepam (Valium)
Sulfur mustard	None, supportive	Soap and water	Delayed onset, delayed bullae, pulmonary care
Lewisite	BAL, supportive	Soap and water	Acute onset, treat acidosis, volume depletion, pseudomembranes
Cyanide	Methemoglobin, amyl nitrite, sodium nitrite, sodium thiosulfate	Soap and water	Bicarbonate, O_2, fluids, treat acidosis, sudden loss of consciousness
Phosgene	None, supportive	Soap and water	IVF, monitor volume, O_2, early intubation, steroids, watch for pulmonary edema
PFIB	None, supportive	Soap and water	Monitor O_2, watch for pulmonary edema
Ammonia	None, supportive	Irrigate eyes—water only Soap and water	Milk, bronchodilators, Silvadene, GI endoscopy, watch for mediastinitis, liquefaction necrosis
Chlorine	None, supportive	Irrigate eyes—water only Soap and water	Bronchodilators, steroids, intubation, bronchoscopy
CN (mace)	None	Irrigate eyes—water only Soap and water	Remove foreign body from eye, watch for bronchospasm
CS (tear gas)	None	Irrigate eyes—water only Soap and water	
Oleoresin capsicum	None	Irrigate eyes—water only Soap and water	From chili pepper, dermatitis, eye injury

BAL, British anti-Lewisite; CN, chloroacetophenone; CS, chlorobenzylidene malinonitrile; GI, gastrointestinal; IVF, in vitro fertilization; PFIB, perfluoroisobutene.

b. Decontamination shelters should have the following:

    i. A water connection compatible with the facility's water lines

    ii. The ability to collect and contain large quantities of water

    iii. Something to mix with the water to remove the chemicals

    iv. Adequate lighting

    v. Connection to electricity, whether plugged into the hospital or into a generator

    vi. A conveyor system for nonambulatory patients

    vii. Allowance for patient privacy

    viii. Room for two or three personnel, preferably nonhealthcare providers

    ix. Room for families in pediatric facilities. Parents may also require decontamination. Parents can also help with decontaminating their children (Hudson, Reilly, & Dulagh, 2003).

c. Special considerations must be made when decontaminating children. Because children might not be at a developmental level to understand what is going on, they may be uncooperative, even combative. Children are lower to the ground and so might be exposed to more of the contaminant; in addition, their large surface-to-volume ratio places them at higher risk of absorption and exposure to the contaminant. Removing clothing will help with decreasing exposure. Because of their size, a smaller dose may be lethal, so it is important to get them decontaminated as quickly as possible. Children are at a higher risk of thermoregulation and must be placed in a neutral thermal environment and out of the extreme heat or cold. It is important to keep the family unit together if possible so that parents can keep smaller children safe. If parents are not available, appropriate arrangements for supervision must be made.

d. A diagram of a decontamination trailer with all the preceding requirements is illustrated in Figure 9.13.

D. Biological Attacks

Biological warfare is a very real threat. In 1999, the Association of Professionals in Infection Control developed a template for hospitals to adopt when dealing with bioterrorism; this template is entitled the "Bioterrorism Readiness Plan: A Template for Healthcare Facilities" (Association for Professionals in Infection Control [APIC], 1999). A biological attack is called *bioterrorism*. Since this document was developed, there has been a strong focus on preparedness for this type of attack. In 2002, the Public Health Security and Bioterrorism Preparedness and Response Act of 2002 was signed into law. This required facilities to register if they had selected agents. The most recent guidance on this Act can be found at http://www.fda.gov/Food/GuidanceRegulation/GuidanceDocumentsRegulatoryInformation/FoodDefense/ucm331957.htm.

Bioterrorism is defined as the deliberate release of microorganisms (bacteria, viruses, fungi, or toxins) into a community to produce death or disease or to poison humans, animals, or plants (Los Angeles County EMSA and Public Health, 2012). Biological weapons are often called the *poor man's bomb* because they are relatively inexpensive to produce and disseminate. A bioterrorist attack is a real threat, as evidenced by the anthrax attacks in 2001, which resulted in 22 cases of anthrax exposure, five deaths, and a nation on high alert.

    1. *Anthrax*

        a. Etiology

            i. An acute infectious disease caused by *Bacillus anthracis*

            ii. Some spores viable and infectious in soil for up to 50 years

            iii. Found most frequently in sheep, goats, and cattle, but has been used as a biological weapon with serious consequences; considered a national security threat by the U.S. government and guidelines have been developed for pediatric clinical management (Bradley et al., 2014)

            iv. Three types. Cutaneous, gastrointestinal, and pulmonary (usually based on the route of exposure); another new concern is injection anthrax, which has been described for drug abusers, but it is not something that is a real threat at this time; if left untreated, any form of anthrax can lead to serious complications, including hemorrhage, edema, necrosis, or even meningoencephalitis (Bradley et al., 2014)

        b. Clinical features

            i. Cutaneous effects

                1) Local skin involvement if there is direct contact with spores or bacilli

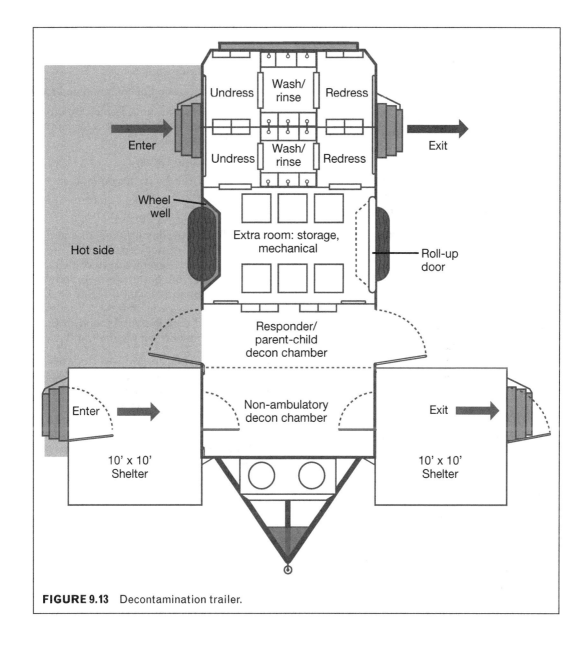

FIGURE 9.13 Decontamination trailer.

2) Most often found on head, chest, and forearms and accounts for 95% of the naturally acquired cases of anthrax

3) Incubation period is about 1 to 12 days until itchy, papular lesion that turns into a vesicle and within 2 to 6 days is black eschar

4) Usually not fatal if treated, but may progress if untreated

ii. Pulmonary effects

1) Nonspecific flu-like symptoms; has the highest case-fatality ratio of this disease; there were five cases of inhalation anthrax reported in pediatrics from 1900 to 2005 (Bradley et al., 2014).

2) 2 to 4 days after initial symptoms, abrupt onset of respiratory failure

3) Hemodynamic collapse

4) Widened mediastinum

5) Dormant in early prodomal stage; high mortality rate after respiratory symptoms

iii. Gastrointestinal effects

1) Abdominal pain, nausea, vomiting, and fever following ingestion of contaminated food, usually meat

2) Bloody diarrhea, hematemesis

3) Positive culture after 2 to 3 days

4) Usually fatal after progression to sepsis

5) Less common form

iv. Meningeal anthrax

1) Bacillus anthracis causes a hemorrhagic meningoencephalitis that involves both deep-brain parenchymal hemorrhagic lesions and an infection in the CSF in the subarachnoid space (Bradley et al., 2014)

2) Signs and symptoms consist of fever, headache, delirium, seizures, emesis, and diarrhea

3) This is such a rare occurrence, there is little known about it.

c. Mode of transmission (route of exposure)

i. Inhalation of spores

ii. Cutaneous contact

iii. Ingestion of contaminated food

iv. Not communicable person to person, but it is believed it can be transmitted through needle sharing

d. Incubation period

i. 2 to 60 days for pulmonary

ii. 1 to 7 days for cutaneous, gastrointestinal, and meningeal modes

e. Treatment/therapy. Pediatric anthrax guidelines have been developed for the care of children and there are several stages of therapy in these guidelines from postexposure prophylaxis to care of the premature infant (Bradley et al., 2014); the therapy for systemic anthrax is listed in Table 9.36; doses and details can be found in Bradley et al. (2014) guidelines for pediatric anthrax

2. *Smallpox.* This disease was declared eradicated by the World Health Organization (WHO) in 1980 (Los Angeles County EMSA and Public Health, 2012). A smallpox vaccine was available in 2003 for healthcare workers, but it was not widely used because of issues related to the exclusion criteria and some issues with cardiac problems after receipt of the vaccine. Smallpox is a strong bioterrorism threat because it has a high morbidity in an otherwise normal population.

a. Etiology

i. Acute viral illness caused by the variola virus

ii. Airborne transmission

iii. One case is a public emergency

TABLE 9.36   Triple Therapy for Systemic Anthrax

1. Administer ciprofloxacin or levofloxacin or moxifloxacin
2. Administer a bacterial antimicrobial
   a. For all strains, regardless of whether penicillin susceptibility is known—meropenem or imipenem/cilastatin or doripenem or vancomycin
   b. Alternatives for penicillin-susceptible strains—Penicillin or ampicillin *plus*
3. Administer a protein synthesis inhibitor—linezolid or clindamycin or rifampin or chloramphenicol
4. Duration of therapy: 2–3 weeks or longer, until clinical criteria for stability are met; will require prophylaxis to complete an antimicrobial course of up to 60 days from onset of illness.

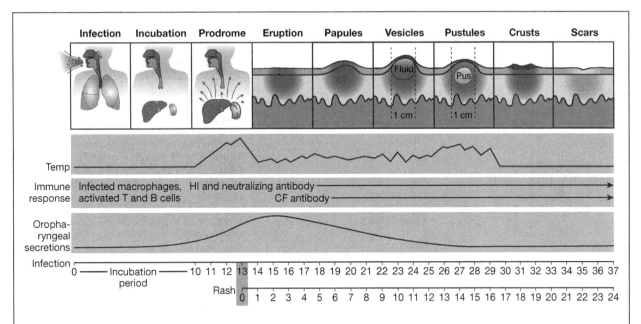

FIGURE 9.14 Clinical manifestations and pathogenesis of smallpox and the immune response.

CF, complement fixation; HI, hemagglutination inhibition.

b. Clinical features (Figure 9.14)

    i. Acute viral symptoms, such as influenza, usually 7 to 19 days after exposure

    ii. Skin lesions appear quickly, progressing from macules to papules to vesicles

    iii. By day 2 to 4, nonspecific flu-like symptoms, high fever, myalgias

    iv. Rash with scabs that begin in the mouth and eventually appear on the skin in 1 to 2 weeks

c. Mode of transmission (route of exposure)

    i. Large and small respiratory droplets

    ii. Patient-to-patient transmission is likely

    iii. Patients are more infectious if they are coughing

    iv. Infectious at the onset of rash until scabs separate (approximately 3 weeks)

d. Incubation period

    i. 7 to 17 days

    ii. Average, 12 days

e. Treatment (Table 9.37)

    i. Vaccine is available

    ii. Vaccine can be given up to 3 days after exposure and still be effective

    iii. Three days after exposure can try the vaccine that can likely decrease the illness; once you have the illness, the vaccine is no longer effective; further treatment with antibiotics that can be tried can be found at the CDC website under smallpox prevention and treatment (CDC, 2016b)

    iv. Negative pressure isolation is required and anyone entering the room must wear an N95 mask (CDC, 2016b; Foltin et al., 2006; Los Angeles County EMSA and Public Health, 2012)

3. *Plague*

  a. Etiology

    i. Acute bacterial disease caused by the gram-negative bacillus *Yersinia pestis*

    ii. Usually transmitted by infected fleas and rodents

    iii. Can be airborne, causing pneumonic plague

    iv. Naturally occurring in rodents

  b. Clinical features of pneumonic plague

    i. Fever, cough, chest pain

    ii. Hemoptysis

TABLE 9.37 Recommended Therapy and Prophylaxis in Children for Additional Select Diseases Associated With Bioterrorism

Disease	Therapy or Prophylaxis	Treatment, Agent, and Dosage[a]
Smallpox	Therapy Prophylaxis	Supportive care Vaccination may be effective if given within the first several days after exposure
Plague	Therapy	Gentamicin 2.5 mg/kg IV every 8 hours *or* Streptomycin[b] 15 mg/kg IM every 12 hours (max. 2 gm/d, although only available for compassionate usage and in limited supply, is a preferred agent) *or*
	Prophylaxis	Doxycyline 2.2 mg/kg PO every 12 hr (if older than 8 years of age or the benefits outweigh the risks) *or* Ciprofloxacin[c] 20 mg/kg PO every 12 hours
Tularemia	Therapy	Same as for plague
Botulism	Therapy	Supportive care, antitoxin may halt progression of symptoms but is unlikely to reverse them
Viral hemorrhagic fevers (including Ebola)	Therapy	Supportive care, ribavirin may be beneficial in select cases for yellow fever[d] For Ebola: Oxygen, IV fluids, and supportive care—Vaccine has been used during the outbreak of 2015/2016, but further research is still being completed
Brucellosis	Therapy[e]	TMP/SMX 30 mg/kg PO every 12 hours and rifampin 15 mg/kg every 24 hours *or* gentamicin 7.5 mg/kg IM for the first 5 days

IM, intramuscular; IV, intravenous; PO, by mouth; TMP, trimethoprim; SMX, sulfamethoxazole.

[a]In a mass casualty setting, parenteral therapy might not be possible. In such cases, oral therapy (with analogous agents) may need to be used.
[b]Concentration should be maintained between 5 and 20 mcg/mL; some experts have recommended that chloramphenicol be used to treat patients with plague meningitis because chloramphenicol penetrates the blood–brain barrier. Use in children younger than 2 years may be associated with adverse reactions but might be warranted for serious infections.
[c]Other fluoroquinolones (levofloxacin, ofloxacin) may be acceptable substitutes for ciprofloxacin; however, they are not approved for use in children.
[d]Ribavirin is recommended for arenavirus, bunyavirus, and may be indicated for a viral hemorrhagic fever of an unknown etiology, although not FDA approved for these indications. For intravenous therapy, use a loading dose of 30 kg IV once (maximum dose, 2 g), then 16 mg/kg IV every 6 hours for 4 days (maximum dose, 1 g), and then 8 mg/kg IV every 8 hours for 6 days (maximum dose, 500 mg). In a mass casualty setting, it may be necessary to use oral therapy. For oral therapy, use a loading dose of 30 mg/kg PO once, then 15 mg/kg/d PO in two divided doses for 10 days.
[e]For children younger than 8 years. For children older than 8 years, adult regimens are recommended. Oral drugs should be given for 6 weeks. Gentamicin, if used, should be given for the first 5 days of a 6-week course of TMP/SMX.

Note: This table was created from recommendations developed at the Consensus Conference and in part is based on reviewed reference materials from the AAP, CDC, and Infectious Disease Society of America.

    iii. Mucopurulent or watery sputum with gram-negative rods on Gram stain

    iv. Bronchopneumonia on x-ray

  c. Mode of transmission (route of exposure)

    i. Infected rodent to humans by infected fleas

    ii. Bioterrorism-related outbreaks likely in the event of aerosol dispersion

    iii. Person-to-person spread is possible via large aerosol droplets

  d. Incubation period

    i. 2 to 8 days if due to flea-borne transmission

    ii. 1 to 2 days if pulmonary exposure has occurred

    iii. Droplet precautions until the patient has completed 72 hours of antimicrobial therapy

iv.   Special air handling is not necessary

v.   Mandatory reporting to public health (Foltin et al., 2006)

e.   Treatment (see Table 9.37)

4. *Tularemia*

a.   Etiology

i.   Caused by the bacteria *Francisella tularensis*, which typically is the cause in animals (rabbit, deer)

ii.   Almost all exposed will be infected

b.   Clinical features

i.   2 to 10 days after exposure: fever, chills, headache, muscle pain, nonproductive cough, pneumonia

ii.   If ingested, regional lymphadenopathy will occur

c.   Mode of transmission (route of exposure)

i.   Humans can be infected from handling infected animals or from diseased fleas, ticks, or mosquitoes

ii.   Can also be spread by aerosol

iii.   Not transmitted person to person

d.   Incubation period is 2 to 14 days after exposure

e.   Treatment (see Table 9.37)

5. *Botulism*

a.   Etiology

i.   Caused by *Clostridium botulinum*

ii.   Food-borne cause is most common, but can come via a wound and infant (intestinal)

iii.   Can be airborne if aerosolized botulinum toxin were used in a bioterrorism incident

b.   Clinical features

i.   Gastrointestinal symptoms are most common but when in a wound it resembles tetanus

ii.   Eyelids drooping, jaw clenching, difficulty swallowing or speaking

iii.   Descending paralysis

iv.   Blurred vision

v.   No sensory deficits

c.   Mode of transmission (route of exposure)

i.   Usually in food

ii.   Can be aerosolized

iii.   Not transmitted from person to person

d.   Incubation period

i.   Ingestion. 12 to 36 hours

ii.   Aerosolized. 24 to 72 hours

e.   Treatment (see Table 9.37)

6. *Viral Hemorrhagic Fever (Ebola)*

a.   Etiology

i.   Diverse group of organisms, such as Ebola virus and yellow fever; the focus of this section will be primarily about Ebola

ii.   Animal or insect hosts (yellow fever)

iii.   Ebola transmission

1) When an infection occurs in humans, the virus can be spread to others through direct contact (through broken skin or mucous membranes, e.g., the eyes, nose, or mouth) with blood or body fluids (including but not limited to urine, saliva, sweat, feces, vomit, breast milk, and semen) of a person who is sick with or has died from Ebola, objects (such as needles and syringes) that have been contaminated with body fluids from a person who is sick with Ebola or the body of a person who has died from Ebola, infected fruit bats or primates (apes and monkeys), and possibly from contact with semen from a man who has recovered from Ebola (e.g., by having oral, vaginal, or anal sex; CDC, 2017)

iv.   Can be released from an aerosol

b.   Clinical manifestations

i.   Vary according to virus

ii.   Usually a nonspecific illness, lasting less than a week, with high fever, headache, and systematic illness followed by flushing, maculopapular rash, and conjunctival infection, progressing to diffuse hemorrhagic disease and multi-organ system failure

iii.   Severe illness may lead to DIC, shock, seizures, and even death

iv.   Mortality varies from 10% to 90%

c.   Mode of transmission (route of exposure)

i.   Ebola is highly infectious and can be transmitted person to person through blood and body fluids

ii.   Infected flea or animal bite for yellow fever

iii. Can be aerosolized

1) CDC has listed the following information for Ebola transmission:

- There is no FDA-approved vaccine available for Ebola.

- If you travel to or are in an area affected by an Ebola outbreak, make sure to do the following:

  – Practice careful hygiene. For example, wash your hands with soap and water or an alcohol-based hand sanitizer and avoid contact with blood and body fluids (such as urine, feces, saliva, sweat, urine, vomit, breast milk, semen, and vaginal fluids).

  – Do not handle items that may have come in contact with an infected person's blood or body fluids (such as clothes, bedding, needles, and medical equipment).

  – Avoid funeral or burial rituals that require handling the body of someone who has died from Ebola.

  – Avoid contact with bats or fruit from the trees that they have eaten from, and nonhuman primates or blood, fluids, and raw meat prepared from these animals.

  – Avoid facilities in West Africa where Ebola patients are being treated. The U.S. embassy or consulate is often able to provide advice on facilities.

  – Avoid contact with semen from a man who has had Ebola until you know Ebola is gone from his semen.

  – After you return, monitor your health for 21 days and seek medical care immediately if you develop symptoms of Ebola.

- Healthcare workers who may be exposed to people with Ebola should follow these steps:

  – Wear appropriate PPE.

  – Practice proper infection control and sterilization measures.

  – Isolate patients with Ebola from other patients.

  – Avoid direct, unprotected contact with the bodies of people who have died from Ebola.

  – Notify health officials if you have had direct contact with the blood or body fluids, such as, but not limited to, feces, saliva, urine, vomit, and semen of a person who is sick with Ebola. The virus can enter the body through broken skin or unprotected mucous membranes in, for example, the eyes, nose, or mouth (CDC, 2017).

d. Incubation period is 2 to 22 days

e. Treatment (see Table 9.37)

7. *Emerging Infectious Diseases—Zika.* As there are more and more diseases that are developing that have not been the focus of a widespread disaster issue, it is important that hospital are prepared to deal with these issues. The 2016 Zika outbreak spread to the United States, creating a public health emergency, as there were birth defects that were the result of infections in pregnant women. This became a serious issue in south Florida in the summer of 2016.

a. Etiology

i. Zika is mostly spread by a bite from a mosquito infected with the virus (*Aedes aegypti* and *Aedes albopictus*)

ii. There have been a few cases spread from human to human by sex or blood transmission

iii. Can be spread from a pregnant woman to her fetus

iv. There have also been cases known to be spread in the laboratory

b. Clinical manifestations

i. Most people will have no symptoms

ii. Those who have symptoms will have fever, rash, joint pain, and possibly conjunctivitis

c. Mode of transmission

i. Mosquito bite from an infected mosquito

ii. Sex

iii. Blood transmission from an infected human

    d. Incubation period

        i. There are no clear dates listed as to when someone can be infected after exposure, but there are recommendations that the virus can stay in a man's semen for as long as 6 months and there are recommendations for women to refrain from getting pregnant for up to 6 weeks after having the virus so as not to expose the baby

    e. Prevention

        i. There is no vaccine

        ii. Avoid mosquito bites or sex and sharing of body fluids with an infected person

        iii. Pregnant women are encouraged to stay away from areas where the infected mosquito is known to be

    f. Birth defects

    g. Microcephaly and other fatal brain defects have been linked to the Zika virus in addition to eye and ear deficits and growth retardation

    h. Treatment

        i. No medicines are available to treat the virus

        ii. Acetaminophen and fluids should be used to treat the symptoms of the virus (CDC, 2016b)

PSYCHOLOGICAL EFFECTS

A. Since the disasters of September 11, 2001, much research has been done related to the psychological effects of children resulting from such events. Blaschke, Palfrey, and Lynch (2003) identify three specific mental health factors unique to pediatrics:

1. Response is dependent on cognitive, physical, emotional, or social development.

2. Response is influenced by the emotional state of the caregivers.

3. Fear or discomfort may cause children to struggle against their providers.

B. Reactions and symptoms of these events vary in children. If they are directly affected by the events, they will experience more obvious symptoms. Some initial symptoms may be hyperventilation, tachycardia, and other symptoms related to fear and paranoia. If left untreated, these symptoms can lead to depression, poor appetite, and weight loss, and children sometimes regress into an earlier stage of growth and development. For example,

children who are potty trained may start to wet the bed. They may also have nightmares.

C. After a major disaster, children are more fearful of what comes next, that the event will recur, that someone they love will be killed or injured, or that they will be left alone. Nurses can help to alleviate these fears by intervening as they do with other traumatic events. They can answer questions and encourage family-centered care. Nurses need to assess the children's growth and developmental levels and treat them accordingly. Nurses also need to assess the psychological symptoms and determine whether the symptoms are severe or out of the ordinary; in the latter situation, social workers or the appropriate mental health members should be notified and allowed to intervene. The Red Cross has numerous resources for healthcare team members called "Helping Children Cope with Disaster."

D. Because children are vulnerable in times of disaster, it is important that they are placed in a safe environment until they can get reunited with their family. There is a lot of research and guidance about reunification to ensure that they are being released to their parents who have legal custody or, in the event of their parent's death in a disaster, to a legal guardian. During these times, there may be individuals who try to take advantage of these vulnerable children. There have been several guidance documents published on this topic (Blake & Stevenson, 2009; Chung & Blake, 2014).

CONCLUSIONS

When mass casualties occur, the impact will be overwhelming to the healthcare system. The potential impact of large numbers of critically ill patients is a real concern, but the overwhelming impact of the additional "worried well" patients can shut down a healthcare system. It is important that all healthcare workers have some understanding of the potential of a larger scale disaster and how to care for themselves and others during this type of disaster. It is also important that hospitals be prepared to deal with MCIs and that they are aware of their need for "surge capacity," specifically, the ability to increase the census and care for more patients in a disaster.

The need for psychological treatment for the effects of bioterrorism cannot be minimized. Even patients with no physical effects may go the hospital to be checked for illness or injury. Initial triage of psychological symptoms is important in the elimination or minimization of long-term psychological effects.

Depending on the environment and area of the world where nurses are practicing, they may experience terrorist incidents more frequently; all nurses, however, need to be knowledgeable about dealing effectively with these issues. They also need to be aware of how care needs differ for adult patients and pediatric patients.

CASE STUDIES WITH QUESTIONS, ANSWERS, AND RATIONALES

Disaster Preparedness and Response Case Studies

Case Study 9.12

A 12-year-old female was at a movie theater with her friends when there was an explosion of unknown origin. She was brought to the ED by paramedics, who reported suspicion of terrorism. She is the first to arrive and you have been informed that there are a total of 15 victims that will be triaged to several different local trauma centers. She is conscious but complaining of a headache and earache and she is tachypneic. Her mother states that she has no previous medical issues. Other than cuts and small bruises, there are no obvious deformities seen on her extremities.

1. What are three components of the primary survey that you would perform first?
   A. Assess airway for patency and obstruction; assess breath sounds for presence and equality; assess heart rate and rhythm
   B. Open cervical collar to evaluate neck for jugular vein extension; assess airway for patency; assess scalp for laceration or open wounds
   C. Assess breathing by listening to breath sounds; log roll to inspect the back for open wounds or injuries; remove clothing to inspect the entire body
   D. Assess airway for patency; assess heart rate and rhythm; palpate bladder for tenderness

2. Primary blast injuries that could be causing her symptoms are:
   A. Exposure to radiation or some type of chemical weapon
   B. A change in atmospheric pressure resulting in a perforated eardrum and hemopneumothorax
   C. Flying debris hitting her in the head and chest
   D. Referred pain from an injury somewhere else in the body

3. If a dirty bomb was expected and the patient needed to be decontaminated, what is the most common form of decontamination after the clothing is removed?
   A. A chlorhexidine bath wipe
   B. An alcohol-based solution
   C. Water alone
   D. Soap and water

Case Study 9.13

A 6-year-old girl presents to your hospital with a high fever and a history of flu-like symptoms for the past 5 days. When her mother is asked screening questions about the patient history, she shares that they just came back from a trip to Africa in an area that has recently had a few new Ebola cases. You are aware of the recent outbreak through a public health alert. No one else is sick in the family. With further questioning, her mother notes that her daughter did play with other children in the village that the family did not know, so they have no information about whether she was exposed to anyone who was sick.

1. What would you do first?
   A. Take a full set of vital signs
   B. Place the patient in isolation and don your PPE
   C. Ask the MD for an order for antibiotics
   D. Perform a full assessment on the child's skin looking for rashes

2. Care for the Ebola patient includes:
   A. Oxygen, IV fluids, and supportive care
   B. The Ebola vaccine
   C. Rifampin 15 mg/kg every 24 hours
   D. Doxycycline 2.2 mg/kg orally every 12 hours

3. As a healthcare worker taking care of this patient until she can be moved to an Ebola treatment center, what you know about Ebola is:
   A. The clinical manifestations are very specific and it is easy to diagnose because the patient presents with a high fever and a headache.
   B. Putting the patient in Universal Precautions is acceptable to protect the healthcare worker.
   C. Insects can spread Ebola so you will ask about insect bites while she was out of the country.
   D. Ebola is a highly infectious disease usually spread from human to human contact with blood or bodily fluids and is usually diagnosed with a history of travel or exposure to a person or area where the Ebola virus is known or suspected.

Disaster Preparedness and Response Answers and Rationales

Case Study 9.12

1. **A.** This is the only answer that includes three items from the primary survey. In a blast injury, airway, breathing, and circulation take priority over items from the secondary assessment. While there are no outward signs of injuries, blast injuries often present with internal injuries, which are not visible.

2. **B.** Blast injuries result in a change in atmospheric pressure caused by the explosion. Frequently, perforated eardrums and chest injuries result from the change

in atmospheric pressure. While the other injuries are common in trauma, they usually result from blunt trauma versus a change in atmospheric pressure.

3. D. Most patients that require decontamination from a possible chemical attack can be decontaminated with soap and water.

Case Study 9.13

1. B. Ebola is highly infectious and your first priority is to isolate the child from other patients and put on your PPE to protect yourself.

2. A. There is currently no vaccine for Ebola and the only available care is supportive care with oxygen and IV fluids.

3. D. There is still a lot of research being done on the Ebola virus but it is known that it is highly infectious, so there are treatment guidelines that include strict PPE and proper infection control measures. While Yellow Fever, which is also a viral hemorrhagic fever, is known to be spread by insects, Ebola is currently viewed as being infectious by direct contact of blood and bodily fluids of an infected person.

DISASTER PREPAREDNESS AND RESPONSE REFERENCES

American Academy of Pediatrics. (2003). AAP policy statement: Radiation disasters and children. *Pediatrics, 111*(6), 1455–1466. Retrieved from http://pediatrics.aappublications.org/content/pediatrics/111/6/1455.full.pdf

American Academy of Pediatrics. (2018). Disaster preparedness to meet children's needs. Retrieved from www.aap.org/terrorism

American College of Radiology. (2002). *ACR disaster planning task force—2002: Disaster preparedness for radiology: Professional response to radiological terrorism, Version 2.0.* Reston, VA: Author.

Assistant Secretary for Preparedness and Response. (2016). Hospital preparedness program: An introduction. Retrieved from http://www.phe.gov/Preparedness/planning/hpp/Documents/hpp-intro-508.pdf

Association for Professionals in Infection Control. Bioterrorism Taskforce and CDC Hospital Infectious Program Bioterrorism Working Group. (1999). *Bioterrorism readiness plan: A template for healthcare facilities.* Washington, DC: Author.

Biddinger, P., Baddish, A., Herrington, L., d'Hemecourt, P., Hooley, J., Jones, J., . . . Dyer, K. S. (2013). Be prepared—The Boston Marathon and mass-casualty events. *New England Journal of Medicine, 368*(21), 158–160.

Blake, N., & Stevenson, K. (2009). Reunification: Keeping families together in crisis. *Journal of Trauma, 67*(Suppl. 2), S147–S151.

Blaschke, G., Palfrey, J., & Lynch, J. (2003). Advocating for children during uncertain times. *Pediatric Annals, 32*(4), 271–274.

Bohn, D., Kanter, R. K., Burns, J., Barfield, W. D., & Kissoon, N. (2011). Supplies and equipment for emergency mass critical care. *Pediatric Critical Care Medicine, 12*(Suppl. 6), S120–S127.

Bradley, J., Peacock, G., Krug, S., Bower, W, Cohn, A. C., Meaney-Delman, D., . . . AAP Committee on Infectious Diseases and Disaster Preparedness Advisory Council. (2014). Pediatric anthrax clinical management: Executive summary. *Pediatrics, 133*(5), 940–942.

Centers for Disease Control and Prevention. (2014). Frequently asked questions about dirty bombs. Retrieved from https://emergency.cdc.gov/radiation/dirtybombs.asp

Centers for Disease Control and Prevention. (2016a). Emergency preparedness and response: Chemical agents. Retrieved from https://emergency.cdc.gov/Agent/AgentlistChem.asp

Centers for Disease Control and Prevention. (2017). Ebola. Retrieved from https://www.cdc.gov/vhf/ebola/treatment/index.html

Centers for Disease Control and Prevention. (2016b). Smallpox prevention and treatment. Retrieved from https://www.cdc.gov/smallpox/prevention-treatment

Chung, S., & Blake, N. (2014, December). Family reunification after disasters. *Clinical Pediatric Emergency Medicine, 15*(4), 334–342.

Department of Homeland Security. (2016). Disasters. Retrieved from https://www.dhs.gov/topic/disasters

Federal Bureau of Investigation. (1992). FBI: Terrorism. Retrieved from https://www.fbi.gov/about-us/investigate/terrorism/terrorism-definition

Foltin, G. L., Schonfeld, D. J., & Shannon M. W. (Eds.). (2006). Pediatric terrorism and disaster preparedness: A resource for pediatricians (AHRQ Publication No: 06(07)-0056). Rockville, MD: Agency for Healthcare Research and Quality.

Government Accounting Office. (2003). *Report to the congressional committees. Hospital preparedness: Most urban hospitals have emergency plans, but lack certain capacities for bioterrorism response.* Washington, DC: Author.

Hamele, M., Poss, W., & Sweeney, J. (2014, February). Disaster preparedness, pediatric considerations in primary blast injury, chemical, and biological terrorism. *World Journal of Critical Care Medicine, 3*(1), 15–23.

Hudson, T., Reilly, K., & Dulagh, J. (2003). Considerations for chemical decontamination shelters. *Disaster Management Response, 1*(4),110–113.

Kissoon, N. (2011). Deliberations and recommendations of the Pediatric Emergency Mass Critical Care Task Force: Executive summary. *Pediatric Critical Care Medicine, 12*(Suppl. 6): S103–S108.

Linnemann, R. E. (2001). *Managing radiation medical emergencies.* Philadelphia, PA: Radiation Management Consultants.

Los Angeles County EMSA and Public Health. (2012). *Terrorism agent information and treatment guidelines for clinicians and hospitals.* Retrieved from http://publichealth.lacounty.gov/acd/Bioterrorism/TerrorismAgentInformation.pdf

Markenson, D., & Redlener, I. E. (2003). *Pediatric preparedness for disasters and terrorism: A national consensus conferenc: Executive summary.* New York, NY: National Center for Disaster Preparedness.

National Advisory Committee on Children and Terrorism. (2015). Recommendations to the Secretary, June 2003.

Yu, C. (2003). Medical response to radiation-related terrorism. *Pediatric Annals, 32*(3), 169–176.

SECTION VI. INITIAL STABILIZATION AND TRANSPORT

Bradley A. Kuch and Michael McSteen

Pediatric critical care transport is a highly specialized area of medicine in which a critically ill infant or child is stabilized and transported to a facility specializing in his or her care. The need for patient transport is indicated by the specific elements of care that cannot be provided by the referring institution. These may include diagnostic procedures, airway management, mechanical ventilation, or ECMO. Transferring patients to a facility specializing in this type of care is often complicated by the severity of illness of pediatric patients and the increased risk of mortality found in the transport setting. These children require more interventions (e.g., endotracheal intubation, inotropic support) and continuous cardiovascular monitoring (both invasive and noninvasive), which warrants a crew with an in-depth understanding of pediatric disease pathology and care. It has been demonstrated that identification and rapid stabilization of the pediatric patients with septic shock decrease morbidity and morbidity rates in the transport setting (Carcillo et al., 2009; Han et al., 2003). In an effort to provide the same level of care found in the PICU, the pediatric critical care specialty transport team was created and continues to grow nationwide.

In 1991, Pollack et al. set the precedent for specialized care by establishing evidence showing an associated decrease in morbidity and mortality in patients who were treated for respiratory failure and head trauma in tertiary care centers versus nontertiary centers (Pollack et al., 1991). A later investigation found that nonspecialized EMS personnel underutilized basic therapies, such as oxygen administration, during the transport of pediatric patients with respiratory illness (Scribano, Baker, Holmes, & Shaw, 2000). More recent, Orr and colleagues demonstrated improved outcomes in patients who were transported by pediatric critical care specialty teams when compared with adult teams (Orr et al., 2009). These findings were validated in a large study of children transferred to a European PICU. They reported an increased survival was associated with the use of a specialized team (Ramnarayan et al., 2010).

In 1990, the AAP recognized this area of medicine as an integral part of the pediatric emergency care system and ultimately creating the section on Transport Medicine (Woodward et al., 2002). As the support for pediatric specialty care teams grows, so does the need for education and a complete understanding of the principles associated with the safe effective transport of the critically ill child (Stroud et al., 2013).

A. Principles and Philosophy of Pediatric Interfacility Transport

1. *Goals of the Critical Care Transport Team*

    a. To provide an *extension of the critical care unit* (i.e., skills, equipment) to the referring facilities

    b. To provide *timely and safe transportation* to a pediatric critical care center without an increase in morbidity or mortality

    c. To provide the *highest quality of care* for critically ill infants and children who require interfacility transport

2. *Trauma Versus Critical Care*

    a. *Scoop and run* is the term given to the concept of transport in which a patient is taken to a facility within the "golden hour," described as the period immediately following a traumatic injury, if surgical intervention is needed or the patient is at risk of physiologic deterioration and needs to be moved quickly to a tertiary center for a higher level of care. The philosophy has never been validated, being developed in an era when prehospital personnel did not provide advanced airway management. Therefore, patients were at increased risk for adverse events, including death, during transport.

        i. Nonspeciality care teams have adopted the "scoop and run" philosophy of patient transport as the standard of practice in the trauma setting. One reason is that there is little triage by a coordinating physician at the time of a trauma call. Most calls received are from local EMS personnel at the scene; thus all calls are considered critical and deserve immediate transport to a trauma care center.

        ii. A clinical situation in which scoop and run would be appropriate would be, for example, a patient who had uncontrollable bleeding, significant head injury for which the immediate lifesaving intervention for a surgical emergency would be an emergent trip to the operating room.

iii. Time is critical in regard to the time of arrival to the scene or referral to a facility by a team that can provide critical care interventions.

b. *Stay and play* suggests that certain aspects of resuscitation must be delivered as quickly as possible (McCloskey & Orr, 1995). The initial trauma resuscitation of any patient starts with the ABCs and must be delivered at either the accident scene or the referring institution.

i. Increased survival rates have been documented in infants and children with shock who received early resuscitative interventions by community hospital physicians leading to shock reversal (Carcillo et al., 2009; Han et al., 2003).

ii. This goal-directed approach to transport care is supported by the American Heart Association PALS concept for treating shock and respiratory failure (Stroud et al., 2015).

3. *Legal Issues*

a. Consolidated Omnibus Budget Reconciliation Act (COBRA)/Emergency Medical Treatment and Active Labor Act (EMTALA). The COBRA passed in 1986 was intended to prevent patients with unstable medical conditions from being transferred without treatment from the initial hospital (Stroud et al., 2013). The statute is also known as *EMTALA* and more accurately describes the statute. Under EMTALA, physicians are obligated to stabilize patients with identified emergency conditions. EMTALA defines *stabilized*—a prerequisite for transport to mean no deterioration is likely to result from or occur during transfer (Stroud et al., 2013). Responsibilities of the referring physicians and hospitals include, but are not limited to, the following:

i. Provide all medical treatment within its capacity.

ii. Stabilize the patient prior to transfer.

iii. Identify a receiving hospital that will accept and provide qualified personnel to treat the patient's clinical needs.

iv. Qualified personnel, with appropriate equipment, must accompany the patient.

b. The decision of who is best qualified to assist the referring hospital in the safe *transport* of the neonatal or pediatric patient is most often made by the common consent of the referring doctor and the receiving hospital physician.

4. *Patient Family Issues.* The transport team's role in the area of family support has continued to undergo many changes (American Association of Critical-Care Nurses [AACN], 2016). Previously, most teams rarely allowed family members to travel with the patient and team. The psychological impact on families in acute or worsening medical conditions (see Chapter 1) has been considered in several studies. These studies support the value of parental presence in decreasing stress in both the patient as well as the parent (AACN, 2016). Woodward has stated that "allowing the presence of family members helps minimize the family's fear of being left to wonder what is happening to their child" (AACN, 2016; Woodward & Flaegler, 2000). The concept of parental presence is becoming incorporated into many transport systems.

a. Woodward and colleagues conducted a survey of parents whose children were transported via ambulance to a large regional children's hospital. They found that allowing the parent to accompany the child during transport was a positive experience that did not hinder intratransport medical care (Woodward & Flaegler, 2000).

b. In the incidence of neonatal transports, the possibility of parental presence is impacted by the inpatient status of the mother. Some programs address the issue of bonding while decreasing parental stress by using various plush bonding tools. Safe sleep standards should be considered in this process.

c. The transport team is the first specialized group of caretakers involved in the child's care. Transport team members are the key participants in a child's definitive medical care. Involving parents in the process benefits the family, patient, and transport system (AACN, 2016; Woodward & Flaegler, 2000).

B. Transport Physiology

The care of critically ill or injured patients during air medical transport is a complex, ever-changing situation that requires a firm knowledge of flight physiology and an understanding of fundamental laws of physics. These include atmospheric composition, basic gas laws, and transport-related stresses that affect both the patient and transport team.

1. Atmospheric composition is an important physical property of which an understanding is essential for building the foundation of the flight physiology. The atmosphere is composed of seven basic gases: nitrogen (78%), oxygen (21%), argon (0.94%), carbon dioxide (0.03%), hydrogen (0.01%), neon (0.0018%), helium (0.0005%), and trace amounts of methane, neon, and krypton. The percentage of each gas in the atmosphere remains constant up to approximately 70,000 feet above sea level. Each gas is responsible for a percentage of the total atmosphere that corresponds to its partial pressure.

2. *Gas Laws.* A complete understanding of gas laws as they relate to temperature, pressure, and volume is crucial for the safe, effective transport of a patient via either a helicopter or fixed-wing aircraft (Blumen & Rinnert, 1995; Nehrenz, 1997; Orsborn, Graham, Moss, Melguizo, & Stroud, 2016).

    a. *Boyle's law* states that "at a constant temperature, the volume of a given gas is inversely proportional to the pressure" (McCloskey & Orr, 1995, p. 144).

$$P_1 V_1 = P_2 V_2$$

In other words, a known volume of gas will expand as the pressure that surrounds it decreases. Boyle's gas law affects any enclosed gas-filled space whether inside or outside the body cavity.

Example: An intubated 17-year-old trauma patient is being transported via a fixed-wing aircraft to a Level 1 trauma center. As the aircraft lifts off and climbs to 12,000 feet above sea level, the ETT cuff will increase in size, causing more pressure on the trachea walls. When the aircraft starts to descend for landing, the cuff will decrease to its size prior to landing, thus decreasing the pressure that was previously on the tracheal walls.

    b. *Dalton's law* describes the partial pressure of various gases, the effect that altitude has on them, which states "the total pressure of a gas mixture equals the sum of the individual (partial) pressures of all the gases in the mixtures" (McCloskey & Orr, 1995, p. 144).

$$P_{total} = P_1 + P_2 + P_3 + P_4 + P_n$$

Another illustration of Dalton's law is as follows: Each gas present in a gas mixture exerts a partial pressure that equals the fractional volume of gas multiplied by the total pressure (Table 9.38).

TABLE 9.38 Level of Inspired Oxygen Related to Altitude

Altitude (ft)	Barometric Pressure (mmHg)	Inspired Oxygen Tension (mmHg)
0	760	149
1,000	733	143
2,000	707	138
3,000	681	133
4,000	656	127
5,000	632	122
6,000	609	117
8,000	564	108
10,000	523	99

Example: What is the partial pressure of oxygen being delivered to a patient being mechanically ventilated at 2,000 feet above sea level (706 torr) with 50% oxygen?

Partial pressure = barometric pressure × gas concentration

Partial pressure = 706 torr × 0.5 oxygen

Partial pressure = 353 torr

    c. *Charles's law* states, "when pressure is constant, the volume of a gas is very nearly proportional to its absolute temperature" (McCloskey & Orr, 1995, p. 114).

$$\frac{V_1}{T_1} = \frac{V_2}{T_2}$$

Charles's law explains the direct relationship between volume and temperature; as the temperature of a gas increases, so does the volume of that gas.

Example: You are transporting a 50-kg patient who is septic and receiving a 1 L bolus of fluid using large-bore tubing and a pressure bag. As you leave the building and assess your patient during the frigid 15°F winter day, you notice a drop in pressure on the manometer (pressure bag) and the volume stops running. Promptly add more air to the bag to ensure that the bolus continues to run. Adding gaseous volume to the pressure bag puts Charles's law to work.

The decrease in temperature causes a direct decrease in gaseous volume in the bag.

d. *Gay-Lussac's Law* states that when a volume of gas is constant, the pressure of this gas is directly proportional to the absolute temperature for a constant volume of gas.

$$\frac{P_1}{T_1} = \frac{P_2}{T_2}$$

In simpler words, Gay-Lussac's law illustrates the direct relationship between pressure and temperature.

Example: While completing the morning checks when the aircraft was in the heated hanger (74°F), the pressure of oxygen was 1,800 psi. Later that morning, the pilot moves the aircraft outside (32°F) so that the maintenance crew can clean the hanger. Before the first flight, the oxygen level is checked once more discovering a pressure of 1,550 psi. The change in pressure is explained by Gay-Lussac's law of temperature and pressure. As the temperature decreases, so will the pressure.

e. *Henry's law* states that "a quantity of gas dissolved in a liquid is proportional to the partial pressure of the gas in contact with that liquid" (McCloskey & Orr, 1995, p. 145). In other words, the partial pressure of a gas above the liquid equals the quantity of gas dissolved in the liquid.

Example: A 15-year-old scuba diver suffering from decompression sickness after a rapid ascent from a depth of 90 feet is being transported. The cause of this illness is the rapid ascent from an environment with a high pressure (i.e., a depth of 90 feet) to an area of relatively low pressure (sea level), causing a release of gas bubbles from the blood. If the teen would have slowly ascended from the depth allowing time for the gas–liquid interface to equilibrate, the situation could have been completely avoided.

3. Transport-related stresses can be placed into two distinct but related categories: environmental and self-imposed. Temperature, hypoxia, dehydration, noise, and vibration are stresses imposed by the environment. Self-imposed stresses can easily be remembered by the acronym DEATH; the components include *d*rugs, *e*xhaustion (fatigue), *a*lcohol, *t*obacco, and *h*ypoglycemia (Holleran, 2010).

In combination with the environmental factors, the self-imposed stresses can magnify the physical and mental fatigue, leading to errors in judgment and decreasing the level of performance. To limit these factors, the transport team must have a solid understanding of the principles of transport-related stresses and the physiologic effects they have on both the patient and crew.

a. *Hypoxia* is described as the relative state of oxygen deficiency that tissues experience from a decreased oxygen supply. Hypoxia is one of the most important stresses that may be encountered during the air medical transport and is found within four physiologic categories (Table 9.39).

   i. *Hypoxic hypoxia* is the oxygen deficiency that is present at the alveolar level. The transfer of gas from the alveolus to the arterial system is compromised, resulting in a low partial pressure of oxygen in the blood.

   ii. *Hyperemic hypoxia* or *anemic hypoxia* occur when the oxygen-carrying capacity of the blood is decreased, resulting in a limited oxygen delivery to the tissues.

   iii. *Stagnant hypoxia* is defined as the lack of adequate blood flow to the body or a specific area of the body. Stagnant hypoxia results from clinical situations with low cardiac output as a component of its pathophysiology.

   iv. *Histotoxic hypoxia (cellular/tissue poisoning)* refers to the clinical situations that affect the cell's ability to metabolize molecular oxygen. A patient may have a normal arterial partial pressure of oxygen (PaO_2), but the tissue is unable to use it because of the cellular metabolic dysfunction.

b. *Changing barometric pressure* is the primary cause for many physical symptoms experienced by the flight crew. As an aircraft ascends, the barometric pressure decreases, in turn, gases within the body cavity expand. The expansion may cause complications such as *barotitis media, barosinusitis, and barodontalgia. The GI system* can hold a significant amount of gas *(methane)*, which is a by-product of normal digestion. As the aircraft ascends, the volume of the gas in the GI tract expands (Boyle's law of volume and pressure), resulting in discomfort and pain. The patient may release the expanded gas by either belching

TABLE 9.39   Clinical Effects and Treatment of Hypoxia

Systems	Signs and Symptoms	Treatment
Cardiovascular	Tachycardia Arrhythmias Hypertension Hypotension (*late*) Bradycardia	**1.** Identify which type of hypoxia is present • Hypoxic • Hyperemic • Stagnant • Histotoxic
Pulmonary	Hyperventilation Dyspnea Tachypnea Cyanosis (*late*)	**2.** Deliver supplemental oxygen • Depending on the severity, an FiO_2 of 1.0 may be required • An increase may be needed in spontaneously breathing and mechanically ventilated patients alike
		3. Patient monitoring • Heart rate/rhythm • Respiratory rate • Blood pressure • End-tidal CO_2 • Ventilator parameters
Neurologic	Seizures Restlessness Euphoria Belligerence Unconsciousness	**4.** Monitor equipment • Indwelling catheters and tubes • Mechanical ventilator • Invasive pressure monitoring equipment
		5. Descend • Increase the partial pressure of oxygen by descending to a lower altitude

or flatus (Holleran, 2010). Nasogastric tubes should be vented, allowing excess gas to escape.

c. *Thermal regulation.* The transport environment exposes both the patient and crew to a wide range of temperatures. Prolonged exposure to this environment has been found to have negative physiologic effects. These effects include increased oxygen consumption, vasoconstriction or vasodilation, an increased susceptibility of motion sickness, disorientation, and an increased metabolic rate (Blumen & Rinnert, 1995; Holleran, 2010).

d. *Humidity.* As altitude increases, humidity in the ambient atmosphere decreases. The crew must be cognizant of the effects that this environmental change will have on both the patient and fellow team members. Effects include dry eyes, chapped lips, thickening of pulmonary secretions, and sore throat. Increasing fluid intake via the oral (crew) or IV routes (patient) will aid in replenishing the fluid lost during flight (Holleran, 2010; McCloskey & Orr, 1995).

e. *Noise and vibration* are common occurrences in the transport setting, dependent on the mode of transportation: ambulance, fixed-wing aircraft (airplane), or rotor-wing aircraft (helicopter; Sittig, Nesbitt, Krageschimidt, Sobczak, & Johnson, 2011). Noise and vibration may or may not affect patients. Some might experience anxiety, which can be exhibited by an increase in heart rate, blood pressure, or combativeness. Noise presents the crew with the added difficulty of patient assessment. It makes the use of a stethoscope for auscultation of breath sound virtually impossible (Tourtier et al., 2014).

f. *Fatigue* is the end product of all contributing stresses on transport personnel, which has been linked to judgment errors, narrowed attention span, limited response, and possibly the cause of several fatal accidents (Blumen & Rinnert, 1995; Holleran, 2010).

C. Transport Equipment

The equipment routinely carried by the transport team should be able to provide ongoing intensive care until the team safely arrives at the receiving institution. The AAP Task Force on Interhospital Transport recommends the following guidelines for transport equipment (MacDonald & Ginzburg, 1999). The equipment will do the following:

1. Provide the capability for life support in the transport setting.

2. Be lightweight (*loadable by two persons*), portable, and self-contained, with a battery life twice the expected transport duration.

3. Be durable enough to withstand altitude and thermal changes, acute decompression vibration (*20-g decelerative forces, both ground and air vehicles*), and repeated use.

4. Have alternating current (AC)/direct current (DC) capabilities.

5. Have no electromagnetic field interference.

6. Be able to fit through standard hospital doors and into transport vehicles and be easily secured to prevent shifting while en route.

7. Supplies and medications carried should be sufficient to maintain ongoing critical care during the transport.

D. Team Configuration

The composition of a critical care transport team varies from institution to institution. Presently, the guidelines for training transport team personnel are designed and implemented by the program director. The goal is for team members to have the clinical skills and expertise needed to deliver the level of care found in the critical care area of the receiving hospital (Stroud et al., 2013).

1. Configuration models that currently exist include RN/respiratory care practitioner (RCP), RN/RN, RN/paramedic, RN/MD, RN/RCP/MD, certified registered nurse practitioner (CRNP)/RN, and CRNP/RCP. A program may choose a constant configuration or change based on patient acuity (Table 9.40).

2. The Transport Section of the AAP recommends that an RN be a member (most likely the team leader) of the team during every transport (MacDonald & Ginzburg, 1999). The task force's rationale behind this is that an RN offers the needed education, versatility, and license requirements needed to perform as the team leader.

E. Advanced Skills Training

It has become common practice in pediatric transport systems to use an RN/RT or RN/RN team without the addition of a physician after a period of specialized training. These individuals are expected to identify and manage problems that might and often do occur during transport. Frequently, the team is expected to intervene on arrival to a referring hospital where staff either is uncomfortable or lacks the skill to perform a specific procedure. The AAP Section on Transport medicine has published specific guidelines that address appropriate training procedures and other team-related issues (Stroud et al., 2013).

TABLE 9.40   Examples of RN/RCP Configuration as Related to Clinical Situation

Type of Patient	Staff to Accompany and Remain With Patient
Stable with one IV	RN/RCP team
Stable with arterial line	RN/RCP team
On mechanical ventilator	RN/RCP team
Vasoactive drips/MV	RN/RCP team
ECMO referral	RN/RCP/transport MD
Sepsis shock w/o access	RN/RCP/transport MD

ECMO, extracorporeal membrane oxygenation; IV, intravenous; MV, mechanical ventilation; RCP, respiratory care practitioner.

Note: Application of this specific triage strategy to other pediatric referral centers may be limited.

1. Many programs require experience in the ED or critical care areas, which serve as a foundation for the development of advanced skills.

2. Many, if not most, programs require staff to have successfully completed one or more advanced life support courses (Advanced Cardiac Life Support [ACLS], PALS, Neonatal Resuscitation Program [NRP]). In general, advanced skill training focuses on (but is not limited to) interventional skills, such as advanced airway management, needle thoracotomy, chest tube placement, cannulation of umbilical vessels, and placing intraosseous (I/O) catheters.

3. Individual programs develop training sessions that not only address technical skills, but a didactic component, including core topics such as pathophysiology, diagnosis, assessment, therapy, and complications for each disease entity. The use of simulation is increasingly common to provide training for low-volume/high-risk procedures, and improve team dynamics and communication.

4. Following initial training, credentialing may occur within the medical structure of the institution. Ongoing competency assessment programs are expected by the AAP (MacDonald & Ginzburg, 1999).

5. Commission on Accreditation of Medical Transport Systems (CAMTSs) is a voluntary accreditation service focused around patient care, safety, and quality in the transport environment. CAMTS certification verifies that a transport program meets current standards, which are based on medical research, ground transport, and aviation developments.

INITIAL STABILIZATION OF THE NEONATAL OR PEDIATRIC PATIENT

A. Principles and Practice

Initial stabilization of any infant or child begins at the referring facility prior to the transfer request. This responsibility is federally mandated by EMTALA and COBRA laws. Patient assessment and therapeutic intervention should be focused on procurement of a patent airway, ensuring effective ventilation, stabilizing circulation, and assessing blood glucose status. These assessments and interventions are outlined in the American Heart Association's PALS course (American Heart Association [AHA], 2016).

1. The transport team's resuscitative efforts are focused on stabilizing the patient before transport, bringing ICU level of care to the patient. The "routine" delivery of intensive care to the critically ill child is complicated by numerous environmental factors during transport, including the following:

    a. *Cramped surroundings* cause restricted access to the patient due to seatbelts of both the patient and the team members.

    b. *Limited access* to all equipment and limited ability to carry anything but essential equipment are issues.

    c. *Low-light conditions, constant vibration, and/or noise* produced by engines may decrease the ability to hear alarms and assess the patient. The low-light conditions may also affect readings of various monitoring devices. Combination of vibration, electronic distortion, and background sound challenges even the most technically advanced equipment.

    d. *Constant movement* of the vehicle increases the risk of accidental extubation.

    e. *Low temperatures* present a significant challenge to team members as they deliver care and also attempt to maintain adequate body temperatures.

B. Transport Population

The pediatric transport patient population differs greatly from that of the adult patient population. Figure 9.15 shows the diagnostic categories of 4,905 patients transported by five pediatric specialty care teams from different regions around the United States.

C. Initial Call and Triage

The initial call may be triaged by a command physician who collects patient information and gives recommendations for stabilization. Stabilization begins at the time of the call. An outline of the components for effective information gathering and therapeutic considerations are presented in Table 9.41.

D. Patient Assessment

1. *Airway.* Assessment of the pediatric airway includes airway patency and airway protection. Rapid assessment of these areas will determine the next intervention. It may be as simple as repositioning the child's head (not recommended in patients with questionable cervical spine injury) or as complex

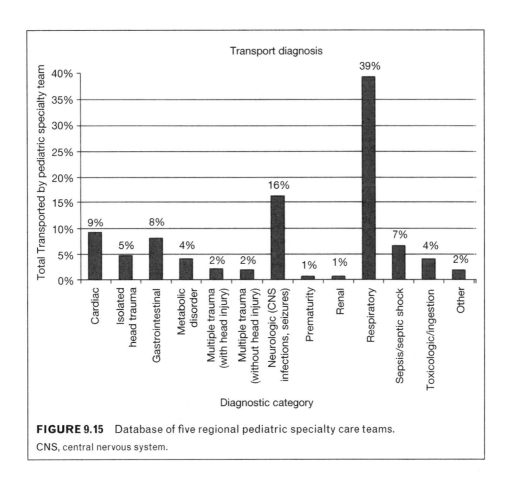

FIGURE 9.15   Database of five regional pediatric specialty care teams.

CNS, central nervous system.

TABLE 9.41   **Information Outline for Initial Transport Triage Call**

Initial Call
(Stabilization Begins at the Time of Call)

I. Report should include a brief but concise past medical history as well as a history of the present illness:
Present condition
     Vital signs (ABCs)
     Patent airway
     Respiratory rate
     Heart rate
     Blood pressure
     Perfusion
Neurologic assessment
     LOC
     GCS
     Presence of seizure activity
Lab data
     Blood glucose level
     CBC
     Electrolytes
     Cultures
Radiologic interpretations

(continued)

TABLE 9.41 Information Outline for Initial Transport Triage Call *(continued)*

Initial Call
(Stabilization Begins at the Time of Call)
II. Treatment recommendations from the transport physician may include, but are not limited to, the following: Fluid resuscitation Inotropic support Aerosolized medication recommendation Anticonvulsant therapy Antibiotics **III.** Decision regarding mode of transportation and team composition: Patient condition Safety Distance Accordance with the referring physician recommendation on the patient's medical necessity EMTALA laws

ABCs, airway, breathing, and circulation; CBC, complete blood count; EMTALA, Emergency Medical Treatment and Active Labor Act; GCS, Glasgow Coma Scale; LOC, level of consciousness.

Note: Ultimately responsibility falls on the referring physician.

as endotracheal intubation. The decision can be made based on the presence or absence of the following:

a. *Patent airway (ventilation/CO_2).* Obstruction of the upper airway can be easily identified by the absence of audible or palpable airflow, upper airway stridor, or asynchronous chest and abdominal motion. If any of the aforementioned symptoms are present, the upper airway should be visually inspected. In this situation, the patient may require repositioning of the head, suctioning of the oral pharynx, or placement of a nasal pharyngeal airway (NPA) to ensure a patent pathway for respiration to occur.

b. *Maintaining an airway.* Patients with an altered level of consciousness or neuromuscular weakness may be unable to maintain their own airway. Presentation can include limited airflow (decreased breath sounds), "snoring respirations," an inability to control secretions, or obstructive apneas. These patients are at risk for pulmonary insufficiency, leading to hypoxia, hypercarbia, respiratory acidosis, and ultimately respiratory insufficiency or failure.

c. *Protective airway reflexes (cough and gag).* Assessment of the upper airway reflexes are performed by using a soft-suction catheter to elicit a cough or gag. The presence of this protective reflex will illustrate whether the infant or child can protect his or her own airway in case of emesis during transport.

2. *Breathing (oxygenation/O_2).* The initial step in the assessment of breathing is a visual inspection of the patient. Identifying the patient's position (i.e., tripod position in epiglottitis); respiratory pattern; and rate, level of distress, and behavior (obtunded or anxiousness) will provide an immediate assessment of the severity of the situation.

a. *Respiratory rate.* An accurate respiratory rate should be obtained before interacting with the patient; interaction with a stranger often causes anxiety in the young child, leading to an elevated respiratory rate.

i. *Tachypnea* in a child can be a caused by pain, anxiety, shock, respiratory distress, metabolic acidosis (i.e., diabetic ketoacidosis), and increased body temperature. Identifying the exact cause is often difficult but may be assisted by the use of pulse oximetry, blood gas analysis, or measurement of the patient's temperature.

ii. *Bradypnea or gasping* is uncommon; it may be caused by a head injury, hypothermia, medications such as narcotics, or impending respiratory failure.

iii. *Apnea* is relatively common in the premature infant population and can lead to cyanosis and bradycardia. It can be an ominous sign in an older infant and should be closely monitored. If apnea continues, treatment is recommended to ensure a positive neurologic outcome. The causes of apnea may be serious in nature and have been implicated as the first sign in the progression of life-threatening critical illness.

b. *Pattern.* Respiratory pattern should be assessed along with the respiratory rate. Assessment should include the depth of each breath, the inspiratory and expiratory time (i.e., prolonged expiratory phase), and the presence of an increased work of breathing (WOB).

    i.   Increased WOB (respiratory distress) is explained with greater detail in Chapter 2.

    ii.   The following clinical findings are signs and symptoms of respiratory distress: grunting, nasal flaring, retractions, paradoxical respiration, and tachypnea. Oxygen is the drug of choice in most cases involving patients who present with signs of an increased WOB. Always obtain the patient's normal pulse oximetry saturation (SpO_2) level, especially with a history of cardiac disease (see Chapter 3, "Congenital Heart Disease" section for more information).

    iii.   Breathing patterns can aid in distinguishing the underlying cause of the clinical manifestations with which a particular patient presents:

        1) *Periodic breathing* is defined by spurts of respiratory activity of 20 seconds or less separated by periodic pauses in the respiratory cycle lasting less than 10 seconds without associated cyanosis or bradycardia. This pattern is common in premature infants (Walsh, 2015).

        2) *Kussmaul breathing* is a deep, continuous breathing pattern commonly observed in patients with diabetic ketoacidosis (DKA). This breathing pattern causes hyperventilation to partially compensate for profound metabolic acidosis.

        3) *Cheyne–Stokes breathing* is a periodic breathing pattern characterized by periods of tachypnea and hyperpnea with periods of apnea, which occurs most often in patients with neurologic injury. It also has been associated with congestive heart failure (CHF) in the adult population.

c. *Breath sounds.* Auscultation of the chest in all lobular regions should be performed to determine whether any adventitious breath sounds are present. Proper breath sound assessment should include documentation of the amplitude of the sound produced, timing of the sound (i.e., early, late), and the quality of air movement. Some commonly used terms to describe adventitious breath sounds include *wheezes, crackles* or *rales, rhonchi,* and *stridor.* Chapter 2 describes the clinical assessment of pulmonary function in more detail.

d. *Skin color.* Assessment of skin color should focus on identifying the presence of cyanosis that may be found either centrally (lips) or peripherally (nail beds). The first line of treatment should be the administration of supplemental oxygen. Causes of cyanosis can be pulmonary and non-pulmonary (see Chapter 2).

3. *Circulation/Peripheral Perfusion.* Assessment of circulation and peripheral perfusion can be done simultaneously during the initial patient survey. The assessment should include heart rate, central versus peripheral pulses, capillary refill time, LOC, and urine output. Early identification and reversal of children with decreased or poor perfusion limits the adverse outcomes associated with uncompensated shock and multiorgan dysfunction syndrome (MODS; Scott, Donoghue, Gaieski, Marchese, & Mistry, 2014). The clinician must be mindful that the presence of one of these signs has been associated with increased risk of MODS, with the presence at least two signs having almost a fivefold increase in organ dysfunction (Kleinman et al., 2010; Scott et al., 2014).

a. *Heart rate* is evaluated for rate, rhythm, strength, and the presence of a murmur. Chapter 3 covers the clinical assessment of cardiovascular function in more detail.

b. *Central and peripheral pulses* are compared by evaluating the pressure differences and the quality between the central (i.e., femoral, carotid, axillary) and the peripheral pulses (i.e., radial, dorsalis pedis, posterior tibial):

- Narrowed pulse pressure is indicative of circulatory compromise.

- "Thready" pulse can occur as a result of a narrowing pulse pressure.

- "Wide pulse" pressures or "bounding pulses" are commonly found in early septic shock.

c. *Capillary refill* is assessed by applying pressure to an extremity and observing the time it takes for the blanched area to reperfuse. Less than 2 seconds is considered normal, whereas a capillary refill time longer than 2 seconds may indicate poor perfusion and may require medical intervention.

    i.   *Flash* or *brisk capillary refill* is present when the blanched area reperfuses in less than 1 second and is considered "warm shock" (Carcillo, 2003; Kleinman et al., 2010; Scott et al., 2014).

ii. Other indicators of poor skin perfusion include pallor, mottling, peripheral cyanosis, and cold extremities (Carcillo, 2003; Kleinman et al., 2010; Scott et al., 2014).

d. *Altered level of consciousness* is often found as an early sign of shock because of inadequate cerebral perfusion (Carcillo, 2003; Kleinman et al., 2010; Scott et al., 2014). See Chapter 4 for a detailed review of age-specific neurologic assessments.

e. *Urine output* is an indicator of renal perfusion and is considered inadequate when it is less than 1 mL/kg/hr (Carcillo, 2003; Kleinman et al., 2010; Scott et al., 2014). Low urine output may be present before any other sign of decreased perfusion. It may be helpful to ask the caregiver the number of diaper changes the patient had today. This will help discern whether the child is experiencing decreased urine output while in the care of the family.

f. *Liver size* should be assessed in any patient with signs of decreased cardiac output or respiratory distress of unknown etiology. The liver edge in a healthy child should be palpated less than 3 cm below the right costal margin. If the liver is enlarged, the patient may be in cardiogenic shock (Carcillo & Fields, 2002; McCloskey & Orr, 1995).

4. *Neurologic.* A brief neurologic evaluation should be part of the ongoing assessment, together with the ABCs. Focus should be directed to several areas:

a. LOC

i. Age-appropriate behavior. One can expect a child to be crying or frightened; however, irritability may be an early sign of neurologic deterioration.

ii. Alertness, level of activity, and quality of cry are all easily assessed at the time of transport.

iii. Ominous signs of neurodeterioration include a child's failure to respond to parents or not crying during a noxious stimulus, such as starting an IV. Urgent medical intervention and support are warranted.

iv. Use of the GCS (see Chapter 4) or AVPU (awake, voice response, pain response, unresponsive) scale provides a brief ongoing method of evaluation of LOC.

b. Pupillary response

i. Observe for size, equality, and reactivity.

ii. Responses may indicate increased ICP, inadequate oxygenation, hypothermia, or ischemic encephalopathy.

iii. Pupillary changes may be a result of pharmacologic intervention.

c. Seizure activity

i. Seizures are a common occurrence in transport.

ii. Woodward and colleagues stated that "the etiologies of seizures and treatments required can be varied and complex. Familiarity with seizure etiologies and treatment options will allow one to manage the event effectively in the short run, while safely transporting the patient for definitive evaluation and therapy" (Woodward, Chun, & Miles, 1999, p. 155).

iii. Comprehensive review of seizures, classification, and defining characteristics are covered in Chapter 4.

d. Signs of increased ICP

i. Irritability progressing to lethargy

ii. Decreased ability to follow commands

iii. Changes in response to painful stimuli

iv. Pupillary changes, decreasing response to light

v. LOC and GCS can be used to evaluate neurologic changes

e. Pain assessment

i. Children with trauma or agitation should be assessed and treated for pain during transport.

ii. Ongoing evaluation and intervention can avert later signs of increased ICP (Figure 9.16).

5. *GI Assessment.* Clinical assessment should be focused on four main areas (see Chapter 7):

a. *Inspection* for abdominal distention, masses, and obvious loops of bowel

b. *Auscultation* for the presence or absence of bowel sounds

c. *Palpation* to note presence of guarding or pain

d. *Percussion*

e. *Review* of recent GI insensible losses

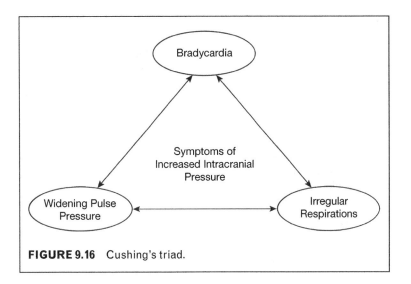

FIGURE 9.16 Cushing's triad.

6. *Head-to-Toe Assessment*

a. *Brief* head-to-toe assessment should be conducted in all patients.

b. *Special areas of focus* may be included based on the reason for transfer as well as team's initial assessment. This may include abdominal survey or observing the skin for rashes or bruises.

E. Airway Management

The single most important intervention during the initial stabilization of any patient is the establishment of a functional patent airway. Understanding the clinical indications and techniques used during the stabilization of the pediatric airway is focused around the basic anatomic difference found between the pediatric and adult patient (see Chapter 2). Some of the more common airway interventions used in the pediatric population include NPAs, oropharyngeal airways (OPAs), laryngeal mask airways (LMAs), and endotracheal intubation. Each of these techniques has relative indications and contraindications that provide the practitioner with a useful means of deciding which maneuver is needed to ensure a safe, effective airway (Table 9.42).

1. NPAs (nasal trumpet) are used in the semiconscious patient with intact airway reflexes (*cough and gag*) to relieve the obstruction created by posterior pharynx. The appropriate-sized NPA is found by measuring the distance from the nares to the tragus for length and using the largest diameter that passes through the nasal passage without traumatizing the mucosa. The NPA should not be used with patients who have suspected head trauma or skull fractures. Always remember the following:

a. *Lubricate* the exterior of the tube with a water-soluble lubricant.

b. If the *airway adjunct is too large*, it may cause blanching of the exterior nares.

c. Placement may cause *laryngospasm, nasal ulceration, or bleeding*.

2. OPAs (oral airway) are used to relieve the obstruction created by the base of the tongue and the posterior portion of the oropharynx, thus providing a patent pathway for ventilation to occur. The devices are useful in unconscious patients with respiratory drive or to facilitate bag–mask ventilation prior to intubation. Sizing of the oral airway is done by aligning the selected airway on the corner of the mouth and the tip at the angle of the mandible. Use of the OPA provides no protection against aspiration of blood, stomach contents, or other material in a patient with an altered LOC. In the pediatric transport setting, patients who tolerate an oral airway may require endotracheal intubation before transfer to protect against aspiration. OPAs should not be used with patients who have oral trauma. Important issues to remember when caring for a patient with an OPA include the following:

a. A *tongue depressor* should be used to displace the tongue downward, which facilitates placement of the oral airway.

b. If the *oral airway is too small*, it may "push" the tongue into the posterior pharynx, exacerbating the airway obstruction.

c. If the *oral airway is too large*, the distal end may force the epiglottis into the entrance of the airway, causing obstruction.

TABLE 9.42 The Indications and Contraindications of Various Airway Adjuncts

Airway Adjuncts	Indications	Contraindications	Clinical Limitations
Nasopharyngeal	Upper-airway obstruction in the semiconscious patient Airway obstruction caused by a clinched jaw (*clonus*)	Coagulopathies Cerebral spinal fluid leaks Basilar skull fractures	No protection against aspiration Risk of laryngospasm Difficult to find pediatric sizes
Oropharyngeal	Upper-airway obstruction caused by the posterior displacement of the tongue against the pharyngeal wall As an adjunct until endotracheal intubation	Coagulopathies Functional gag reflex Consciousness	No protection against aspiration Trauma to lips and teeth Risk of laryngospasm
LMA	Airway in an unconscious patient without protective airway reflexes Difficult airway situation Respiratory failure	High pressures required to effectively ventilate Full stomach Intact airway reflexes	Limited use in patients requiring high ventilatory pressures No protection against aspiration Correct placement of the LMA is difficult to maintain when moving a patient
Endotracheal intubation	Respiratory failure Upper airway obstruction Hemodynamic instability (*shock*) Loss of protective airway reflexes (*cough and gag*) Suspected increase in intracranial pressure	Intubation is often indicated by the failure or limitations of the prementioned adjuncts; therefore the need for endotracheal intubation has only technical contraindications	Requires highly trained clinicians to perform Demands an advanced knowledge of the pediatric airway and the pharmacologic agents used during intubation

LMA, laryngeal mask airway.

d. This type of airway is not well tolerated in patients with *intact airway reflexes.*

e. Oral airway does not protect against *aspiration.*

3. LMA is an airway adjunct often used in the operating room as the primary method of securing an artificial airway. The device consists of a tube with a large balloon or mask at the end that seals the hypopharynx. Placement of the LMA is relatively simple and is accomplished by blindly advancing it into the pharynx until resistance is met. The balloon is then inflated and ventilation is assessed. The AHA recognizes the device as an acceptable alternative to endotracheal intubation in unresponsive patients when performed by healthcare providers trained in its use. Important facts about the LMA include the following:

a. A *relative ease of placement* (Guyette, Roth, Lacovey, & Rittenberger, 2007; Pennant & Walker, 1992).

b. It is *contraindicated* in conscious patients with intact gag reflex (Chameides, Samson, Schexnayder, & Hazinski, 2011).

c. *Sedation or neuromuscular blockade* may be required to prevent coughing or gagging during placement (Martin, Ochsner, & Jarman, 1999; Tung, 2005).

d. Does not protect against *aspiration* (Chameides et al., 2011; Martin et al., 1999; Tung, 2005.

e. Limited use in patients who require *high ventilatory pressures* as leaks at higher pressures are common (Guyette et al., 2007; Martin et al., 1999).

f. *Correct placement* of the LMA is difficult to maintain when moving a patient.

g. An LMA is an acceptable method of *initial airway stabilization*; an ETT is the recommended method of airway management during transport (Warren, Fromm, Orr, Rotello, & Horst; American College of Critical Care Medicine, 2004).

4. *Oral Endotracheal Intubation (OETI)*, when performed by the skilled practitioner, is considered the gold standard in the patient with respiratory failure. Endotracheal intubation can be complicated by a number of undesirable factors, potentially leading to catastrophic pulmonary and neurologic complications. These factors include prolonged hypoventilation resulting in decreased cardiopulmonary reserve, increased ICP, hemodynamic instability (shock), and the potential of a full stomach. Successful endotracheal intubation is defined by the limitation of the adverse effects that may occur as a result of airway manipulation in the critically ill patient. To limit these effects, many pediatric emergency care systems have adopted the technique of rapid sequence intubation (RSI) for all patients requiring OETI (Algie et al., 2015; Goto et al., 2016; Sagarin et al., 2002). RSI is a systematic approach to OETI, which has a 3- to 5-minute period of breathing 100% oxygen, the simultaneous administration of an induction agent and neuromuscular blockade, and when intubating conditions are present, a proper-sized ETT is passed into the trachea (Figure 9.17). It has been associated with a higher success rate and lower rate of serious adverse effects (Goto et al., 2016; Sagarin et al., 2002; Smith et al., 2015). When assisting with the endotracheal intubation of the pediatric patient, the practitioner should remember a few important points:

a. Always gather the equipment first. Intubation equipment includes a high FiO_2 delivery appliance, functional proper-sized resuscitation bag (bag–valve–mask [BVM]), proper-sized laryngoscope blades with functional bulbs and handle, ETTs (one proper size and one size smaller) and a stylet, monitoring equipment, suction and suction equipment, clinically indicated drugs for induction and paralysis, a device to secure the ETT, and an end-tidal carbon dioxide detection device (for secondary confirmation).

b. Complete a team pause. This is final verification that the correct patient, procedure, staff, equipment, and medications are present.

c. Use sedation first, neuromuscular blockade second.

d. Always confirm ETT placement by multiple methods. Equal bilateral breath sounds, no air entry into the stomach (epigastric region), end-tidal carbon dioxide detection, effective chest rise, oxygen saturation (SpO_2), condensation in the ETT tube, and CXR (especially in neonates) are effective ways to identify an appropriately placed ETT. Confirmation should be used as a quality-improvement measure, which is discussed later in the chapter.

F. Vascular Access

1. Establishing peripheral vascular access via a peripheral intravenous line (PIV) before transport is essential.

2. In the presence of cardiovascular collapse, PIV access may be difficult. PALS guidelines advocate that peripheral access be obtained rapidly. The term *rapidly* is defined by the patient's acuity rather than by a 90-second time frame as previously published.

3. If PIV access cannot be obtained, I/O vascular access in the proximal tibia or distal femur should be initiated. Updated 2016 guidelines state the I/O access is acceptable for

a. Delivery of all IV medications, including epinephrine, adenosine, fluids, blood products, and catecholamines (Kleinman et al., 2010). Each medication should be followed by saline flush to promote entry to the central circulation (Kleinman et al., 2010). To maintain patency, consider a continuous infusion to keep the line open.

b. Onset of action is comparable to venous administration (Kleinman et al., 2010).

c. Can be used to obtain blood samples for analysis, including type and crossmatch and blood gases during CPR (Kleinman et al., 2010). Acid–base analysis is inaccurate after sodium bicarbonate administration via an I/O cannula (Kleinman et al., 2010).

4. Central venous access is not advocated as a first choice. However, it may be attempted by qualified personnel after initial access is obtained.

5. In the neonatal population, umbilical venous access is the preferred means of access, and it is easily located and cannulated by trained healthcare practitioners.

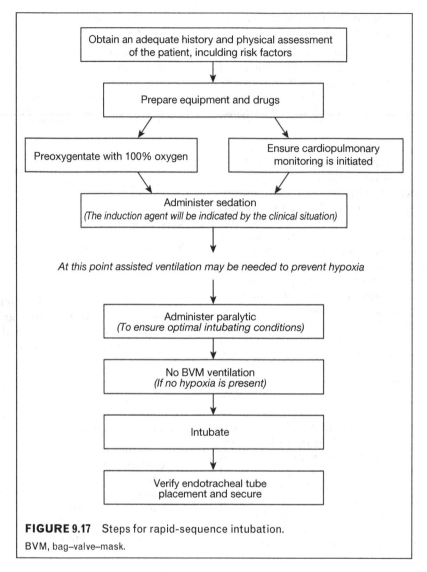

FIGURE 9.17 Steps for rapid-sequence intubation.

BVM, bag–valve–mask.

G. Fluid Resuscitation

The rapid administration of isotonic fluid is imperative for the reversal of dehydration and the treatment of low cardiac output states such as shock. The recommended crystalloid solutions are normal saline (0.9% NS), and lactated Ringer's (Carcillo 2003; Carcillo & Fields, 2002; Dellinger et al., 2013). Colloids (5% albumin) may also be used as an initial resuscitation fluid; the evidence is inconclusive, however (Carcillo, 2002; Dellinger et al., 2013; Lighthall & Pearl, 2003).

1. Fluid administration should be given as a rapid IV bolus of either 10 mL/kg in the neonatal population or 20 mL/kg in the pediatric population within 10 minutes (Figure 9.18) and repeated as needed.

2. After each bolus, the patient should be reassessed. The assessment must include heart rate, blood pressure, urine output, capillary refill, and LOC (Carcillo & Fields, 2002; Dellinger et al., 2013). Assess for pulmonary edema and hepatomegaly in children with cardiac or renal disease or if obstructive shock or myocardial dysfunction is suspected (AHA, 2016).

3. Initial fluid resuscitation may require up to or over 60 mL/kg. Recent guidelines recommend the initiation of vasopressor support in the patient with septic shock who does not respond to total 60 mL/kg of volume (Dellinger et al., 2013). Consider starting a second peripheral IV if severity and time permits. A second IV will allow for the simultaneous administration of fluid and inotropes (Dellinger et al., 2013).

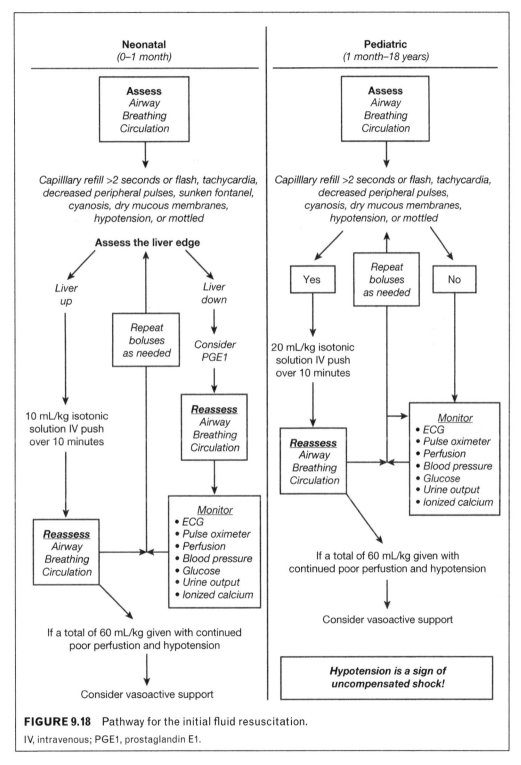

FIGURE 9.18 Pathway for the initial fluid resuscitation.

IV, intravenous; PGE1, prostaglandin E1.

a. Indications for the administration of isotonic IV fluids in the neonatal population include a capillary refill time longer than 2 seconds, sustained tachycardia, tachypnea, hypotension, mottled or cyanotic appearance, cool skin temperature, dehydration, weak or thready pulses, or narrowed pulse pressure (High & Yeatman, 2000).

b. Pediatric patients who require fluid resuscitation may present with delayed capillary refill longer than 2 seconds, sustained tachycardia, tachypnea, hypotension, mottled or cyanotic appearance, cool skin temperature, dehydration, or narrowed pulse pressure (High & Yeatman, 2000).

H. Vasoactive Drug Support

Inotropic agents are useful in the treatment of shock (cardiogenic or distributive) or in any condition in which myocardial function is impaired. The International Guidelines for Management of Serve Sepsis and Septic Shock call for rapid, stepwise execution of therapeutic interventions with the goal to restore normal blood pressure and perfusion within 1 hour of patient presentation (Dellinger et al., 2013). Institution of these guidelines should be recommended by the command physician (Figure 9.19). Han and colleagues demonstrated that the early reversal of shock using therapeutic interventions consistent with the established guidelines is associated with improved outcome when initiated by the community physician (Han et al., 2003).

1. Inotropic agents work through α- and β-adrenergic receptors. The hemodynamic impact of catecholamine infusions may be blunted by inadequate fluid resuscitation in shock states (Dellinger et al., 2013; Han et al., 2003). For this reason, less than 60 mL/kg maybe indicated, which requires ongoing cardiovascular and liver position assessment.

2. Dobutamine may be administered to improve capillary refill in normotensive patients by improving cardiac output.

3. Hypotensive patients commonly require epinephrine, norepinephrine, or dopamine. Epinephrine may be more effective because children and infants commonly have an age-specific insensibility to dopamine (Han et al., 2003). First-line agents and threshold doses include (Dellinger et al., 2013):

a. Epinephrine up to 0.05 to 0.3 mcg/kg/min continuous infusion as first-line treatment for cold shock.

b. Dopamine up to 10 mcg/kg/min—For patients in shock, intrinsic norepinephrine stores are often depleted, making dopamine an ineffective agent.

4. In warm shock, norepinephrine is commonly used (Dellinger et al., 2013). Norepinephrine dosing is 0.1 to 2 mcg/kg/min IV/IO continuous infusion.

5. Detailed review of agents, along with dosages, is found in Chapter 3 and in the "Sepsis and Septic Shock" section of this chapter.

6. In the transport setting, inotropes may be administered through a peripheral vein or I/O in the absence of central venous access (Turner & Kleinman, 2010). Turner and Kleinman demonstrated that peripheral administration of vasoactive agents was safe; however, 15% developed IV infiltration (Turner & Kleinman, 2010). For this reason, IV sites should be assessed every 15 minutes during transport. The greatest effects and safety are attained via central access and should be obtained as soon as possible (Turner & Kleinman, 2010).

I. Glucose

Hypoglycemia can result quickly as the critically ill child depletes his or her glycogen stores. Losek demonstrated that 18% of children requiring resuscitative interventions were found to be hypoglycemic with an associated increase in mortality (Losek, 2000). Both hyper- and hypoglycemia have been associated with mortality in critically ill children (Li et al., 2015). Early identification of hyperglycemia or hypoglycemia can easily be accomplished with a bedside rapid glucose testing system.

1. *Hypoglycemia.* The presentation of hypoglycemia in the neonate may include seizures, altered LOC, jitteriness, apnea, irregular respirations, hypothermia, and hypotonia. In the infant or child, it may present as palpitations, tremors, anxiety, sweating, hunger, paresthesias, confusion, coma, headache, weakness, abdominal pain, and seizures (Thornton et al., 2015). If a patient presents with a history of poor feeding or any of the associated symptoms mentioned herein, a serum or whole-blood sample is used to rule out hypoglycemia as an underlying cause. If hypoglycemia is present, a 0.5 to 1 g/kg IV/IO bolus (5–10 mL/kg D10W bolus in children [AHA, 2016] or 2–3 mL/kg D10W bolus in neonates) should be administered (Figure 9.20).

a. Causes of hypoglycemia include the following:

i. Ingestions. Salicylates, alcohol, hypoglycemic agents, β-adrenergic blocking agents, and propranolol

ii. Infection. Gram-negative sepsis, septic shock

iii. Endocrine disorders. Genetic or metabolic etiology such as insulin-dependent diabetes mellitus (IDDM), growth hormone deficiencies, hypothyroidism, and Addison disease; rare genetic causes include

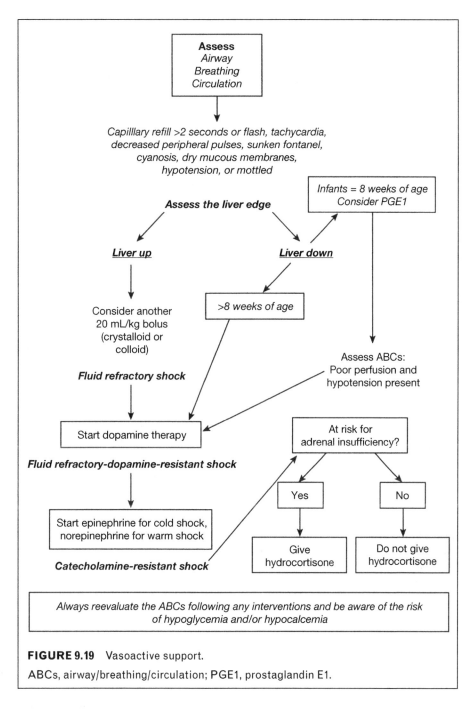

FIGURE 9.19 Vasoactive support.

ABCs, airway/breathing/circulation; PGE1, prostaglandin E1.

congenital hyperinsulinism or hypopituitarism; more common in neonates is prolonged neonatal hyperinsulinism (Thornton et al., 2015); the most common complication in children with IDDM is hypoglycemia (Bhatia & Wolfsdorf, 1991)

iv. Other. CHF, respiratory failure, and idiopathic ketotic hypoglycemia

b. Complications of hypoglycemia include coma, seizures, aspiration pneumonia, and hypoxia due to the patient's inability to maintain his or her own airway (Jaimovich & Vidyasagar, 2002). Rapid identification and management of a patient with neurologic compromise will limit risk of these untoward events.

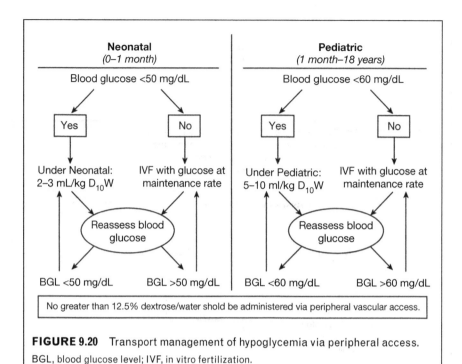

Neonatal
(0–1 month)

Blood glucose <50 mg/dL

Yes   No

Under Neonatal: IVF with glucose at
2–3 mL/kg D$_{10}$W   maintenance rate

Reassess blood
glucose

BGL <50 mg/dL   BGL >50 mg/dL

Pediatric
(1 month–18 years)

Blood glucose <60 mg/dL

Yes   No

Under Pediatric: IVF with glucose at
5–10 ml/kg D$_{10}$W   maintenance rate

Reassess blood
glucose

BGL <60 mg/dL   BGL >60 mg/dL

No greater than 12.5% dextrose/water shold be administered via peripheral vascular access.

FIGURE 9.20 Transport management of hypoglycemia via peripheral access.
BGL, blood glucose level; IVF, in vitro fertilization.

2. *Hyperglycemia/Diabetic Ketoacidosis.* See Chapter 6 for etiology, pathophysiology, and definitive treatment of DKA, the leading cause of morbidity and mortality in children with insulin-dependent diabetes mellitus (type 1). Death is most commonly associated (57%–87%) with the occurrence of cerebral edema (Dunger et al., 2004). A child who presents with a long duration of symptoms, signs of circulatory compromise, altered LOC, who is younger than 5 years, or who is a patient with "new-onset" DKA is associated with the highest risk of cerebral edema and should be managed in a PICU (White, 2003). In the transport setting, the initial treatment is focus on the reversal of hypovolemic shock secondary to the severe dehydration, which is a major component of this disease process (Wolfsdorf et al., 2014; Figure 9.21).

    a. Type 1 IDDM is an autoimmune disease that is most commonly found in infants and children. Type 1 is associated with DKA. Goals of DKA therapy include:

        i) Correct dehydration and shock.

        ii) Normalize acid–base balance and reverse ketosis.

        iii) Restore blood glucose to near normal.

        iv) Monitor for complications of DKA and its treatment.

        v) Identify and treat any precipitating events.

    b. Type 2 non–insulin-dependent diabetes mellitus (NIDDM) is most often found in adults and is related to insulin resistance. Hyperglycemic hyperosmolar state (HHS) occurs frequently in children but can occur with type 1 diabetes, type 2 diabetes, as well as in infants. HHS is characterized by extreme hyperglycemia and hyperosmolality without significant ketosis. When HHS does occur, the treatment differs from DKA. Children with HHS are less acidotic but more severely dehydrated with hyperglycemia as well as serum osmolality greater than 320 mOsm/kg. Goals of therapy include:

        i) Expand intravascular and extravascular volume.

        ii) Restore renal perfusion.

        iii) Promote a gradual decline in osmolality.

    c. Associated complications of hyperglycemia/DKA include cerebral edema (*most common*), other CNS complications such as dural sinus thrombosis, intracranial hemorrhage, cerebral infarction, as well as heart disease, myocardial

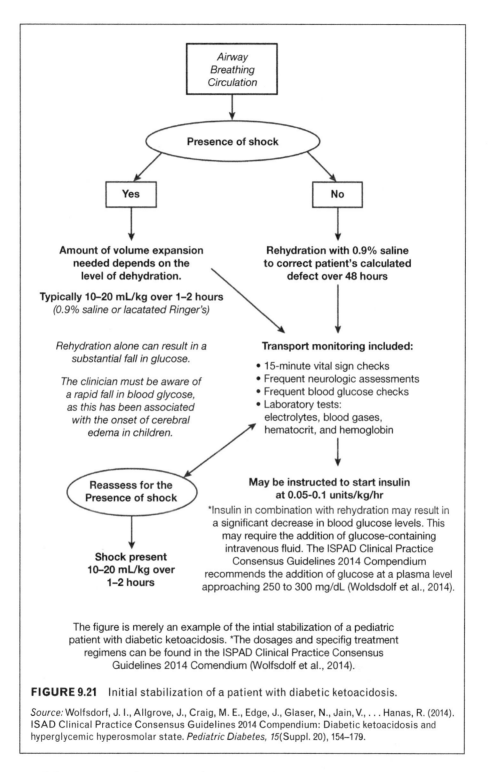

FIGURE 9.21   Initial stabilization of a patient with diabetic ketoacidosis.

Source: Wolfsdorf, J. I., Allgrove, J., Craig, M. E., Edge, J., Glaser, N., Jain, V., . . . Hanas, R. (2014). ISAD Clinical Practice Consensus Guidelines 2014 Compendium: Diabetic ketoacidosis and hyperglycemic hyperosmolar state. *Pediatric Diabetes, 15*(Suppl. 20), 154–179.

infarction, adult respiratory distress syndrome, thrombosis, aspiration pneumonia, pulmonary embolism, and rhabdomyolysis (Wolfsdorf et al., 2014).

J. Respiratory Care

Respiratory distress may be caused by a variety of pulmonary and nonpulmonary pathologies (see Chapter 2). Nonpulmonary causes include sepsis, congenital cardiac disease, and shock. Pulmonary pathophysiology can be divided into two distinct areas of origin:

1. Upper airway, including croup, epiglottitis, foreign-body aspiration, tracheal malacia, subglottic stenosis (*acquired and congenital*), and vocal cord paralysis

2. Lower airway and the lung parenchyma, including asthma, bronchiolitis, bronchomalacia, pneumonia, pediatric acute respiratory distress syndrome (PARDS), hyaline membrane disease (*neonatal RDS*), and aspiration

3. Patient assessment should be aimed at identifying the origin of respiratory distress

4. Supplemental oxygen delivery in the pediatric transport setting requires knowledge of the basic principles of oxygen therapy as well as the baseline peripheral pulse oximetry (SpO_2) for patients with congenital heart disease (Walsh, 2015). A concise report of the patient's medical history should reveal the presence of any underlying cyanotic heart disease.

a. The previously healthy child who demonstrates signs of respiratory distress, hypoxia, cyanosis, and shock should have supplemental oxygen administered as the first step.

b. The proper device for oxygen delivery is based on the patient's age, size, fraction of inspired oxygen (FiO_2) needed, and inspiratory flow rate.

5. Aerosolized medications have become the treatment of choice in the pediatric patient presenting with an increased WOB secondary to acute reversible airway obstruction.

a. Medications are indicated, depending on the origin of the airway obstruction (i.e., upper versus lower airway). Table 9.43 includes a synopsis of commonly used pharmacologic agents for the acute treatment of airway obstruction. Clinicians must assess known drug allergies or past adverse drug reactions.

b. Selection of a delivery method is based on the severity of illness and the duration of treatment needed to electively reverse acute airway obstruction. Both small-volume (*intermittent*)

TABLE 9.43 Medications for the Acute Treatment of Airway Obstruction

Pharmacologic Agent	Mode of Action	Indications	Contraindications	Complications
Racemic epinephrine (*Vaponephrine*)	Equal α and β adrenergic stimulation Causes both vasoconstriction and bronchodilation	Bronchospasm Upper airway inflammation	Hypersensitivity to epinephrine or of the drug suspension Cardiac arrhythmias	Bronchospasm Palpitations Cough Muscle tremors Nervousness Tachycardia
Albuterol sulfate (*Ventolin, Proventil*)	β_2-adrenergic stimulation Little β_1 receptor activity	Bronchospasm	Hypersensitivity to albuterol or other components of the drug suspension Congestive heart failure Hypertension	Bronchospasm Palpitations Cough Muscle tremors Nervousness Tachycardia
Levalbuterol (*Xopenex*)	Single isomer β_2-agonist	Bronchospasm	Hypersensitivity to albuterol or other components of the drug suspension	Tachycardia Hypertension Anxiety Headache Chest Pain Nausea
Ipratropium bromide (*Atrovent*)	Anticholinergic agent that causes bronchodilation by parasympathetic pathways	Used in conjunction with β_2-agonist for the treatment of bronchospasm	Hypersensitivity to ipratropium or other components of the drug suspension	Dry mouth Blurred vision Nausea Palpitations Cough Bronchospasm

and large-volume (*continuous*) nebulizers can be used to administer medications via a mask, oxyhood (*infant*), or an artificial airway (Bower et al., 1995; Walsh, 2015).

i. Small-volume nebulizers are used to deliver intermittent drug aerosol treatments for either acute exacerbations or the daily therapeutic delivery of maintenance medications. In the emergency treatment of bronchospasm, this type of nebulizer can be used to deliver multiple single-dose treatments as needed.

ii. The National Heart, Lung, and Blood Institute recommends multiple nebulized low-dose albuterol at 0.15 mg/kg (minimum dose 2.5 mg) every 20 minutes for three doses, then 0.15 to 0.3 mg/kg up to 10 mg every 1 to 4 hours as needed, or 0.5 mg/kg/hr via continuous nebulization treatments in pediatric patients with acute asthma (National Asthma Education and Prevention Program, Third Expert Panel on the Diagnosis and Management of Asthma, 2007).

iii. Multiple doses of ipratropium bromide (Atrovent) added to frequent high doses of nebulized albuterol might aid in the treatment of severe bronchospasm (Kline-Krammes, Patel, & Robinson, 2013; Schuh et al., 1995).

iv. Nebulized racemic epinephrine (Vaponephrine) has become a common treatment for children with upper-airway obstruction secondary to croup (Petrocheilou et al., 2014). It also has been found to be effective in the treatment of bronchiolitis. The positive effect in infants with bronchiolitis has been demonstrated by improvement in clinical scores and a decrease in airway resistance (Bertrand, Araníbar, Castro, & Sánchez, 2001; Numa, Williams, & Dakin, 2001). However, large randomized studies failed to demonstrate any differences between groups (Anil et al., 2010)

v. Large-volume nebulizers are used to deliver aerosolized medications continuously over an extended period. The delivery method has been associated with a more rapid clinical improvement in children with severe status asthmaticus compared with intermittent delivery of the same drug concentration in and outside the PICU (Kenyon, Fieldston, Luan, Keren, & Zorc, 2014; Papo, Frank, & Thompson, 1995).

6. *Adjunctive Therapies*

a. Glucocorticoids in conjunction with aerosolized medication have been found to be beneficial in the treatment of acute upper-airway and lower-airway obstruction. Administration can be by either by mouth (PO), IM, IV, or by nebulization (Klassen, 1999; Volovitz & Nussinovitch, 2002). The effect of glucocorticoids is not immediate; thus the initial treatment of these patients should focus on stabilizing ABCs.

i. Dexamethasone (Decadron) is most commonly used to treat upper-airway inflammation. Strong evidence has been published that demonstrates a more rapid clinical improvement, shortened hospital stays, and a significant reduction in the rate of endotracheal intubation in patients who receive dexamethasone versus those who do not (Klassen, 1999).

ii. Methylprednisolone (Solu-Medrol), when given as an initial bolus of 2 mg/kg followed by 1 to 2 mg/kg in two divided doses (maximum 60 mg/d), shows no documented advantage with higher doses of corticosteroids (National Asthma Education and Prevention Program, Third Expert Panel on the Diagnosis and Management of Asthma, 2007).

iii. Budesonide (Pulmicort) has been proven an effective alternative to oral steroids as maintenance therapy in asthma. Nebulization of budesonide results in a high percent of the drug being deposited in the upper airway. Budesonide for the treatment of croup has been associated with more rapid clinical improvement, a lower rate of hospitalization, and shorter stays in the ED compared with use of a placebo (Petrocheilou et al., 2014).

b. IV medications may be indicated in the patient with refractory bronchospasm and impending respiratory failure. Administration must include continuous cardiopulmonary monitoring and frequent clinical assessments to monitor respiratory and neurologic status.

i. Terbutaline is the IV β-agonist of choice in the United States, which is most commonly used in patients who do not respond to continuous nebulized treatment and is initiated as an initial loading dose of 5 to 10 mcg/kg over 5 minutes. Recommended dosages for continuous infusion of terbutaline are 0.1 to 6.0 mcg/kg/min

(Stephanopoulos, Monge, Schell, Wyckoff, & Peterson, 1998; Werner, 2001). Adverse reactions to terbutaline include arrhythmias, tachycardia, hypertension, hypotension, nausea, and palpitations (Doymaz & Schneider, 2018).

ii. Magnesium sulfate administration via either a single bolus or continuous infusion may be beneficial in the treatment of refractory bronchospasm (Bloch et al., 1995; Ciarallo , Sauer, & Shannon, 1996; Okayama et al., 1987; Singhi, Grover, Bansal, & Chopra, 2014). Boluses are most commonly given in doses between 25 and 75 mg/kg over 20 minutes (Singhi et al., 2014; Werner, 2001). Singhi and colleagues describe the safety of continuous infusions at a rate of 50 mg/kg/hr in children (Singhi et al., 2014). Adverse reactions to IV magnesium sulfate include nausea, flushing, somnolence, vision changes, and muscle weakness (Glover, Machado, & Totapally, 2002). The most severe effects occur at a concentration of greater than 12 mg/dL and include respiratory depression and arrhythmias (DeNicola, Monem, Gayle, & Kissoon, 1994).

7. *Mechanical Ventilation*

a. *Indications.* The noise, vibration, poor lighting, and lack of assistive personnel make advanced airway procedures extremely difficult while in the transport vehicle. For this reason, the indications for the initiation of mechanical ventilation in the transport setting tend to be more aggressive and include, but are not limited to, cardiac or respiratory arrest, combativeness (safety), airway obstruction, impaired control of ventilation, impending respiratory failure, inadequate gas exchange, fluid refractory shock, or circulatory failure (McCloskey & Orr, 1995).

b. *Ensuring effective ventilation* in the mechanically ventilated patient is an essential skill in the transport setting. The movement associated with transport as well as multiple patient transfers add to the increased risk of ETT displacement.

   i. A rapid visual inspection of the child's chest should be completed. Unilateral rise of a patient's chest may be the first sign of either a mainstem intubation or a pneumothorax. If this occurs, the clinician should perform a physical assessment of the patient. A radiograph or illumination of the chest may also aid in the identification of a pneumothorax.

   ii. Auscultation of the patient's chest and abdomen should be done postintubation as part of initial airway assessment. If the patient has already been intubated by the referring hospital the team should assess the patient's breath sounds immediately upon arrival.

   iii. A disposable end-tidal carbon dioxide (CO_2) detector is a useful tool for identifying whether the ETT is in the trachea. The CO_2 detector is placed on the 15-mm flange of the ETT while it is in the trachea, and then the patient is given a manual breath. The presence of exhaled CO_2 will result in a color change inside the CO_2 detector. Giving six artificial breaths before assessing color change on the CO_2 detector is recommended (Chameides et al., 2011). If there is no color change when the CO_2 detector is in place, the ETT is in the esophagus, the patient has little or no pulmonary perfusion, or the ETT is completely occluded.

   iv. Continuous end-tidal CO_2 monitoring is useful in identifying esophageal intubation, displaced artificial airways, and adjunctive in monitoring mechanical ventilation in an environment with excessive noise (Bhende, Karr, Wiltsie, & Orr, 1995; Price, Wilson, & Fee, 2007). The use of end-tidal CO_2 monitors should not replace the use of blood gas analysis.

c. *Trouble shooting.* Use of the DOPE algorithm (Table 9.44) may aid in identifying situations that might cause acute patient decompensation during mechanical ventilation.

d. *Humidity.* Inadequate humidification in the patient with an artificial airway can cause damage to tracheal epithelium, reduce motility of cilia, and result in excessive mucus production and plugging (Walsh, 2015). A heat and moisture exchanger (HME) is a lightweight hygroscopic condenser that adds humidity by retaining moisture from patient's exhaled gas.

   i. HME may add resistance to the airway, thus increasing the WOB in the spontaneously breathing patient.

   ii. HME should be used with caution in patients with excessive pulmonary

TABLE 9.44 Algorithm for Troubleshooting a Mechanically Ventilated Patient in Respiratory Distress

DOPE
D = Displacement of the airway
O = Obstruction of the airway
P = Pneumothorax
E = Equipment failure

Source: Data from American Heart Association (AHA). 2016. *Pediatric advanced life support: Provider manual.* Dallas, TX: Author.

TABLE 9.45 Normal Neonatal and Infant Temperature Values

Temperature Site	Celsius (°C)	Fahrenheit (°F)
Skin	36–36.5	96.8–97.7
Axillary	36.5–37.5	97.7–98.6
Rectal	36.5–37.0	97.7–98.8

Source: Adapted from McCloskey, K. A., & Orr, R. A. (Eds.). (1995). *Pediatric transport medicine.* St Louis, MO: Mosby.

secretions because there have been reports of ETTs becoming completely obstructed with thickened mucus (Walsh, 2015).

iii. One must ensure the proper-sized HME for the patient because this may add a significant amount of dead space to the ventilation circuit, elevating the patient's $PaCO_2$. If the HME is too small, it will add resistance to the ventilation system.

K. Thermoregulation

The maintenance of normothermia in the transport setting is complex because of the constant changing physical environment and the increased risk of ineffective thermoregulation of the critically ill child.

1. *Hypothermia*

a. The neonatal or infant population is at a greater risk for hypothermia because it has a limited nutritional reserve, a large surface area-to-body ratio, extremely low birth weight, and increased metabolic demands (McCloskey & Orr, 1995). These risks are especially elevated in the infant who is unconscious, sedated, or immobilized (Hazinski, 2013). The following should be considered in the stabilization of the hypothermic infants:

i. Ensure that the infant is completely dry and remove any wet clothing or linen.

ii. Place a stocking cap on the infant's head or swaddle the infant in a blanket.

iii. Transport the infant (i.e., one who weighs <10 lb) in a double-walled incubator. A heat shield, insulated incubator cover, or a heating mattress/pack may be needed to maintain a stable thermal environment within the incubator.

iv. Monitor both skin and axillary temperatures throughout transport (Table 9.45).

Skin temperature is monitored by placing a skin-temperature probe directly onto the infant's abdomen (McCloskey & Orr, 1995).

b. Pediatric hypothermia may be caused by environmental exposure, infection, shock, surgery, traumatic brain injury, congenital nervous system malformation, and medications such as vasopressors, sedatives, or anesthetics (Curley & Moloney-Harmon, 2001; Hazinski, 2013). The following will aid in the reversal of hypothermia in the pediatric patient:

i. Remove all wet clothing and linens.

ii. Cover the patient in warm blankets, and use a radiant insulated blanket to prevent continued heat loss during transport.

iii. Resuscitation of a patient in cardiopulmonary arrest should continue until the patient's core temperature reaches 30°C.

c. Hypothermia impairs both myocardial function and vascular tone, which may lead to profound hemodynamic collapse. Profound hypotension may occur from the rewarming process secondary to the peripheral vasodilation (Curley & Moloney-Harmon, 2001; Hazinski, 2013).

2. *Hyperthermia*

a. Clinical hyperthermia is a state of sustained elevated body temperature greater than 37.8°C orally or 38.8°C rectally. As in hypothermia, the causes of hyperthermia are either internal or environmental in nature. Internal causes include fever (*most common*), malignant hyperthermia, traumatic brain injury, CNS malformation medications (*phenytoin, histamine blockers, and antibiotics*), or heat-related illnesses (Curley & Moloney-Harmon, 2001; Hazinski, 2013). Environmental causes include exposure to extreme elevated ambient temperatures and accidental overheating. Treatment of hyperthermia may include, but is not limited, to the following:

    i. Antipyretic therapy, such as aspirin, acetaminophen, and ibuprofen, effectively resets the hypothalamic set-point to normal limits (Curley & Moloney-Harmon, 2001; Hazinski, 2013).

    ii. Aspirin has been associated with gastritis, GI bleeding, diminished platelet function, and Reye syndrome.

    iii. The use of external cooling may aid in controlling elevated body temperature in the transport setting.

    iv. When fever is associated with suspected bacteremia, treatment will include antibiotics (Curley & Moloney-Harmon, 2001; Hazinski, 2013).

SPECIAL CONSIDERATIONS IN TRANSPORT

A. Cardiac Patient Population

Medical advances in cardiology, intensive care, and surgical intervention have led to the increased survival of infants and children with previous untreatable congenital and acquired cardiac disease. The referral-based nature of neonatal and pediatric cardiac care results in a large number of these children presenting to community-based hospital's nurseries, and EDs for initial care prior to being transferred to regional tertiary care centers for definitive diagnostic, surgical, and/or critical care. Some estimate that approximately 10% of children undergoing interfacility transport have a final diagnosis of cardiac disease (Kuch, Munoz, & Orr, 2006). Primary reason for transfer in this multicenter study included cyanotic heart disease (43%), arrhythmia (15%), CHF (12%), need for critical care monitoring (6.8%), cardiogenic shock (5.8%), respiratory distress/failure (5.7%), congenital abnormalities (1.8%), sepsis syndrome (1.1%), and other (4.2%; Kuch et al., 2006).

1. *Defects With Increased Pulmonary Blood Flow* are characterized by pulmonary overcirculation, which may present with symptoms of CHF around 3 months of age. Those infants less than 8 weeks of age presenting with CHF should be evaluated for left outflow tract obstruction, as the symptoms may be associated with the closure of the patent ductus arteriosus (PDA). Defects with pulmonary overcirculation include:

- Atrial septal and ventricular defects
- PDA
- Truncus arteriosus
- Anomalous pulmonary venous return

a. *Clinical presentation.* Children with cardiac lesion resulting in pulmonary overcirculation most commonly present with respiratory symptomatology, resulting from pulmonary edema or complicating infectious pneumonitis (Munoz, Morell, da Cruz, & Vetterly, 2010). Parental history and physical exam may also reveal (Munoz et al., 2010):

    i. Progressive increased WOB

    ii. Poor feeding tolerance and weight gain

    iii. Pale, thin appearance with normal length and normal head circumference

    iv. Tachycardia

    v. Tachypnea and varying degrees of respiratory distress

    vi. Hepatomegaly

b. *Chest radiography.* Radiologic evaluation may demonstrate cardiomegaly with or without increased pulmonary vascular markings (Munoz et al., 2010). Atelectatic or hyperinflated lung fields may be found as well.

c. *Stabilizing intervention.* Initial stabilization of patients with defects resulting in pulmonary overcirculation should focus on reversing hypoxemia, respiratory distress, and preventing the need for advanced airway management (Munoz et al., 2010). Interventions may include:

    i. Use the lowest concentration required to increase SpO_2 to a clinically acceptable level, as oxygen is a potent pulmonary vasodilator that may worsen left-to-right shunting.

    ii. Administration of diuretics may improve respiratory workload and gas exchange via decreasing pulmonary venous and intrapulmonary shunting.

    iii. Patients with poor cardiac function should be considered. Epinephrine and/or dopamine are considered first-line treatment during the initial resuscitation; however, amrinone or milrinone (phosphodiesterase III inhibitors) may also be indicated (Munoz et al., 2010).

2. *Defects With Left Heart Outflow Tract Obstruction.* Left heart outflow tract obstruction is the most common cause of cardiogenic shock in infants under 1 month of age and frequently presents with CHF before closure of the ductus (Munoz et al., 2010). Often these infants appear "septic" as a result of low cardiac output and resulting metabolic acidosis. Infants under 8 weeks of age should be treated for both conditions until definitive diagnosis is made. These infants may become symptomatic over hours or as late as 8 weeks of age (Munoz et al., 2010). Defects with left heart outflow tract obstruction include the following:

- Aortic stenosis
- Coarctation of the aorta
- Hypoplastic left heart syndrome

a. *Clinical presentation.* Infants with left heart outflow tract obstruction present with varying degrees of tachycardia, irritability, and shock (Munoz et al., 2010). Additional laboratory and physical findings may include the following:

  i.   Respiratory distress or apnea
  ii.   Altered mental status
  iii. Prolonged capillary refill
  iv.   Hepatomegaly
  v.   Absent or weak thready pulses
  vi.   Blood gas analysis will demonstrate severe metabolic acidosis, low $PaCO_2$, and mild to moderate hypoxemia.

b. *Chest radiography.* Will demonstrate cardiomegaly (cardiothoracic ratio > 60%) with pulmonary edema and thickening of the perihilar regions of the lungs fields.

c. *Stabilizing intervention.* The focus of intervention in left heart outflow tract obstruction is to reestablish systemic blood flow via a PDA (Munoz et al., 2010). Establishing adequate systemic blood flow can be identified by return of peripheral pulses, urine output, and correction of metabolic acidosis. See Figure 9.19 for suggested resuscitation guidelines. The following interventions may be indicated during early stabilization of cardiogenic shock secondary to left heart outflow tract obstruction.

  i.   Prostaglandins E1 (PGE1). Initial dose of 0.05 to 0.1 mcg/kg/min up to doses of 0.4 mcg/kg/min may improve ductal flow to restore systemic blood flow, and improve perfusion (Huang et al., 2013). PGE1 at the doses previously mentioned has been

associated with apnea requiring intubation (Huang et al., 2013).

  ii.   Sodium bicarbonate ($NaHCO_3^-$). Metabolic acidosis will decrease heart function and $NaHCO_3^-$ will help correct a low pH thus improving response to inotropes and function.

  iii. Inotropic and vasopressor support. Clinical situations with decreased cardiac function may indicate administration of IV inotropic support. Agent may include dopamine and/or dobutamine. As previously mentioned, amrinone or milrinone may be effective in increasing inotropy, lusitropy, and peripheral vasodilatation (Wessel, 2001).

  iv.   Advanced airway management/intubation. Any patient meeting intubation criterion and/or whose cardiopulmonary status presents a risk of decompensation while en route should have an advanced airway placed prior to transport.

3. *Defects with decreased pulmonary blood flow* are characterized by central cyanosis and are often difficult to diagnosis as etiologies for cyanosis may include pulmonary, cardiac, or a combination of both (Munoz et al., 2010). The correct cause of cyanosis is determined with a concise accurate familial and prenatal history, conducting a physical exam, and reviewing lab data. These defects include the following:

- Tetralogy of Fallot
- Critical pulmonary stenosis
- Pulmonary atresia with intact ventricular septum
- Transposition of the great arteries

a. Transport crews should quickly assess the *family and prenatal history* for congenital heart or birth defects, syndromes, or early deaths (Munoz et al., 2010). Maternal history should be evaluated for diabetes or for any exposure to rubella, Coxsackie, or radiation. Onset of cyanosis and/or respiratory distress should also be documented, as it will provide important clues to the closure of the ductus arteriosus or development of sepsis (Munoz et al., 2010).

b. *Clinical presentation.* Assessment should begin with the appearance and severity of respiratory distress. Irritability, tachypnea, nasal flaring, grunting, and retractions suggest pulmonary pathophysiology (Munoz et al., 2010). Central cyanosis with a comfortable appearance or "quiet tachypnea" is associated with cyanotic heart disease. In the presence of central cyanosis, application of pre- and postductal pulse oximetry is extremely useful in identifying shunting at the ductal level. The presence of "differential cyanosis" is also helpful as blue upper extremities and pink lower extremities are highly suggestive of cyanotic heart disease (Munoz et al., 2010).

c. *Chest radiography and laboratory data.* Chest radiographs and ABG analysis are helpful in identifying cyanotic heart disease.

    i. Chest radiograph demonstrating clear lung fields, decreased pulmonary vascular markings, and cardiomegaly is suggestive of cardiac defects with decreased pulmonary blood flow (Munoz et al., 2010).

    ii. If cyanotic heart disease is suspected, a hyperoxia test may be useful in identifying the etiology of the hypoxia. If the PaO_2 is less than 200 mmHg in 100% oxygen ($FiO_2 = 1.0$), right to left shut is likely.

d. *Stabilizing intervention.* Focus of stabilization should be on the restoration of pulmonary blood flow in infant with suspected cyanotic heart disease.

    i. *PGE1* should be initiated to promote ductal patency and improve oxygenation. Intubation maybe required, as PGE1 has been associated with clinically significant apnea. Control of respiratory status may require the use of sedation and/or neuromuscular blockade (Munoz et al., 2010).

    ii. Supplemental oxygen for ductal-dependent defects should be managed with a goal of maintaining arterial saturations between 80% and 85%, and a PaO_2 in the range of 35 to 45 mmHg (Munoz et al., 2010). This will minimize the risk of PDA closure while en route.

4. *Arrhythmias.* Management of arrhythmias during transport should be aimed at those that may or are resulting in hemodynamic instability. Frequently, the cause of the arrhythmia is related to compromised ABCs, hypoglycemia, or electrolyte imbalances. Management should follow the most recent AHA PALS arrhythmia-specific guidelines (Kleinman et al., 2010). Arrhythmias can be separated into tachyarrhythmias and bradycardiac arrhythmias.

a. *Tachyarrhythmias*

    i. Supraventricular tachycardia (SVT). Commonly occurring in infants younger than 4 months, which can present as poor feeding, inconsolability, tachypnea, and poor perfusion (Munoz et al., 2010). The presence of SVT should be considered as follows (AHA, 2016):

- Infants: QRS duration less than or equal to 0.09 seconds and heart rate greater than or equal to 220/min

- Pediatrics: QRS duration less than or equal to 0.09 seconds and heart rate greater than or equal to 180/min

- Absent or abnormal *P*-waves

- Lack of heart rate variability

    ii. Ventricular tachycardia (VT). Differs from SVT by a wide complex QRS complex (≥ 0.09) with poor perfusion. Frequently, children presenting with VT have a past medical history of congenital or acquired heart disease (Munoz et al., 2010).

b. *Bradycardiac arrhythmias.* Primary etiology of bradycardia in infants and children is hypoxemia with or without hypoventilation (Munoz et al., 2010). Additional causes include hypothermia, hypoglycemia, hypothyroidism, elevated ICP, seizures, and vagal stimulation (Munoz et al., 2010; Table 9.46). Treatment should follow the AHA PALS pediatric bradycardia algorithm unless otherwise indicated (AHA, 2016).

    i. *First-degree AV block.* Rarely symptomatic and is defined as a prolonged PR interval greater than 0.20 in any age group.

    ii. *Second-degree Mobitz type I (Wenckebach block).* May be caused by digoxin toxicity and is defined as growing prolongation of the PR interval leading to a nonconducted P wave.

    iii. *Mobitz type II second-degree block and third-degree heart block* is associated with congenital complete heart block and complex heart disease—may indicate more serious cardiac disease. The arrhythmia(s) is defined as P waves "marching through" the ECG tracing with no association with QRS complexes (Munoz et al., 2010).

TABLE 9.46   Hs and Ts of Treatable Causes of Arrhythmias

"Hs"	"Ts"
Hypovolemia	Toxins
Hypoxia	Tamponade, cardiac
Hydrogen ion (*acidosis*)	Tension pneumothorax
Hypo- or hyperkalemia	Thrombosis (*coronary or pulmonary*)
Hypoglycemia	Trauma (*hypovolemia*)
Hypothermia	
Heart block	

Source: Adapted from American Heart Association. 2016. *Pediatric advanced life support: Provider manual.* Dallas, TX: Author; Munoz, R. A., Morell, V. O., da Cruz, E. M., & Vetterly, C. G. (2010). *Critical care of children with heart disease: Basic medical and surgical concepts.* London, UK: Springer Verlag.

B. Neonatal Hypoxic Ischemic Encephalopathy

1. *Definition.* "Hypoxic ischemic encephalopathy (HIE) in newborns is caused by an injury to the brain following a hypoxic or an ischemic event during the peripartum, intrapartum, or postpartum period. HIE may result in death or cause serious impairment in survivors, and remains a significant cause of morbidity and mortality among neonates" (Merrill, 2012, p. 127). Therapeutic hypothermia is recognized as the standard in the treatment of infants with hypoxic ischemic encephalopathy (HIE; Schierholz, 2014; Thoresen et al., 2013). The therapy is an effective but time-critical treatment for moderate to severe HIE in term infants (Mitchell & Johnston, 2011).

2. *Etiology.* The cause of HIE in infants can be a result of several factors, including maternal or uteroplacental complications, or fetal complications and in some instances, is never fully explained. "A variety of conditions decrease placental perfusion or disrupt the delivery of oxygen and glucose in the umbilical cord, including placental abruption, prolapse of the umbilical cord, and uterine rupture" (Douglas-Escobar & Weiss, 2015, p. 397). Infants born in a medical center with therapeutic hypothermia capabilities are ideally started on the therapy as soon as it is determined that the infant meets the criteria. Recent literature has shown that outcomes correlate with the time of initiation of therapeutic hypothermia. Neonates undergoing earlier cooling therapy (within 180 minutes of birth) had better outcomes compared with those who

underwent the therapy later (180–360 minutes after birth) as cited by Douglas-Escobar and Weiss (2015).

3. *Clinical Presentation.* The following criteria are provided by the Children's Hospital of Pittsburgh of UPMC. Patient must meet *all* of the following criteria:

   a. Older than 36 0/7 weeks

   b. Birth weight greater than 1.8 kg

   c. Infant younger than 6 hours old

   d. No major congenital or known chromosomal anomalies

   e. No immediate plan to redirect care

   f. Either of the following criteria:

   i. Blood gas less than 1 hour of life (cord gas/ABG/VBG [venous blood gas]): pH less than 7.01 and base deficit greater than 16

   ii. If gas is not available *or* if pH less than 7.10 *or* if base deficit greater than 12, then *all* of the following need to be met:

   • 10-minute Apgar score less than 5

   • Continued resuscitation/ventilation greater than 10 minutes

   • Identified acute perinatal event, including but not limited to severe late/variable decelerations, umbilical cord prolapse, umbilical cord rupture, placental abruption, uterine rupture, maternal trauma, maternal arrest, maternal seizure.

   g. Either of the following criteria

   i. Seizure (clinical seizures or documented by EEG)

   ii. Moderate or severe encephalopathy as defined in Table 9.47:

   (*Must identify at least one finding in three of six separate categories.*)

4. *Transport Management of Cooling.* Infants who are born at facilities without the capacity to care for infants with HIE will require a higher level of care and transport to a neonatal ICU by either ground or air.

   a. Even if the referring hospital does not have the equipment to begin active cooling, the accepting neonatologist will instruct the referring physician to turn off the radiant warmer and allow the infant rectal temperature to fall between 33°C and 34°C.

   b. The rectal temperature should be obtained every 15 minutes, so that if the temperature falls below 33°C the radiant warmer can be

TABLE 9.47   Categories to Measure Severity of Hypoxic Encephalopathy

Category	Moderate Encephalopathy	Severe Encephalopathy
Level of consciousness	• Lethargic *or* obtunded • *Lethargic*: Delayed but complete response to stimuli • *Obtunded*: Delayed and incomplete response to stimuli	• Stupor *or* coma • *Stupor*: Response only to strong or noxious stimuli, absent gag, shallow breathing or apnea • *Coma*: No response
Spontaneous activity	• Decreased activity	• No activity
Posture	• Distal flexion with complete extension (posturing of arms with flexion at wrists and extension at elbows, usually enhanced by stimulation)	• Decerebrate posturing (rigid posturing with flexion at wrists, extension of arms and legs, toes pointing, and opisthotonos)
Tone	• Hypotonic	• Flaccid
Primitive reflexes	• Weak suck *or* incomplete Moro *or* strong ATNR	• Absent suck *or* Moro
Autonomic system	• Miosis (constricted pupils) *or* bradycardia *or* irregular breathing pattern	• Variable/unequal/absent Light reflexes *or* apnea

ATNR, asymmetric tone neck reflex.

Note: Goal should be to initiate cooling of eligible infants as rapidly as possible, and ideally every effort should be made to initiate cooling within 6 hours of life. However, if infant is younger than 6 hours of age, an attending physician can initiate cooling per their discretion.

Source: Amended from Children's Hospital of Pittsburgh of UPMC therapeutic hypothermia criteria; Rodriguez Perez, J. M., GolomBek, S., & Sola, A. (2017). Clinical hypoxic-ischemic encephalopathy score of the Iberoamerican Society of Neonatology (Siben): A new proposal for diagnosis and management. *Revista da Associação Médica Brasileira, 63*(1), 64–69.

turned back on at 0.5°C above the current infant temperature.

c. The specialized neonatal team will have the necessary equipment to begin the active-cooling phase. At present, the two types of treatment used include whole-body hypothermia and selective head cooling. Although the two cooling methods are equally effective, clinicians predominantly use whole-body cooling owing to its reduced cost and ease of use (Douglas-Escobar & Weiss, 2015).

  i. The infant's head, torso, and limbs will be wrapped in a water bath-filled blanket that will be connected to a machine that will circulate the water through the blanket in order to keep the infant at the target set point between 33°C and 34°C.

  ii. The infant's temperature will be continuously monitored with a combination of two of the following, esophageal temperature probe, axillary skin probe, or a rectal probe. The two temperature readings will allow the machine to accurately maintain the infant temperature by circulating the water through the therapeutic hypothermia blanket.

d. During the transport phase to the accepting hospital, the equipment will be properly secured to maintain the safety of the transport. The infant will have constant monitoring and assessment performed by the neonatal transport team. When the team arrives at the receiving facility, a proper handoff will be performed with records and details about the transport provided. The receiving facility may have the same equipment as the transport team and this will allow for an easy transition to the bedside.

C. ECMO Transport

A fast-growing area of neonatal pediatric specialty care transport is ECMO transport or "mobile ECMO." Mobile ECMO has been used for close to two decades for interfacility transport (Bryner et al., 2014). Bryner et al. reported a 61% survival rate in patients transported on ECMO, which is comparable to age and treatment matched ECMO patients who were not transported (Bryner et al., 2014). Broman and colleagues evaluated the safety of mobile ECMO during both long- and short-distance transfers (Broman, Holzgraefe, Palmer, & Frenckner, 2015). The group reported 27.3% of transport experienced an adverse event, with 22% being patient related and 5.3% being equipment related (Broman et al., 2015). It was concluded that mobile ECMO can be performed safely with low mortality risk by highly competent staff (Broman et al., 2015).

Safe successful transport of patients on ECMO requires a team highly competent in pediatric critical care, ECMO physiology, cannulation, transport medicine, and air medical physiology. A team developing an ECMO program should develop training and competency prior to their first transport. These programs should meet the Extracorporeal Life Support Organization Guidelines for training (Annich, Lynch, MacLaren, Wilson, & Bartlett, 2012).

1. *Transport ECMO Equipment.* Specialized ECMO transport equipment is required and often developed by the receiving center, as few commercially available systems currently exist. ECMO transport systems/carts must have pumps (primary and backup), monitors, medical-grade gas tanks, IV pumps, and the capability to be safely secured and operated in ambulances, helicopters, and fixed-wing platforms (Annich et al., 2012). These platforms must have a high-capacity inverter and medical gas systems able to support the additional oxygen/air needs. In addition, the following equipment should be carried:

a. *ECMO pumps.* Increased use of centrifugal pumps has allowed for the miniaturization of transport systems and increased the ability to bring a second pump as backup.

b. *Backup ECMO circuit* should include extra cannulas, connectors, tubing, and an oxygenator. Custom circuit packs can be developed, helping to ensure sterility during transport. Bio-coated circuits are recommended as the coatings will decrease the inflammatory response to the foreign surface if or when a circuit change is indicated (Wendel & Ziemer, 1999).

c. *Laboratory devices.* Activated clotting time (ACT) and blood gas monitoring devices should be included during transport. These devices will help monitor anticoagulation and blood gas changes during transport, ensuring hemostasis and ensuring quick identification of respiratory compromise during transport.

d. *Standard transport equipment.* The team should carry a patient monitor, additional IV pump, transport ventilator, and indicated medications. These may need to be augmented as clinically indicated prior to transport. Discussion should occur prior to transport to ensure the team is prepared for patient care needs.

2. *Referring Institution Responsibility.* Often mobile ECMO is used to transfer patients from centers

unable to support long-term patients to centers with transplant or ventricular assist device capabilities. Following the formal request for transfer and acceptance, the following information must be obtained:

a. *Past medical history.* Information regarding the patient's past medical history, reason for cannulation, duration of support, and procedures should be obtained.

b. *ECMO information.* The ECMO team should be included during information gathering as specific support data is required for successful transport. Information must include pump type and size; cannula location and size; and oxygenator type, including last oxygenator gas, which identifies the functional status of the devices. The information will help the ECMO team prepare for the transfer.

c. *Hemostatic information.* Transport physician must obtain the most recent hemostatic information, which includes ACT, PTT, platelet count, hemoglobin and hematocrit, Xa (antithrombin factor 10a), and fibrinogen values. The data will help stabilize the patient prior to transport.

d. *Medications.* Detailed information regarding medication currently being delivered and the site(s) of administration must be obtained. In some circumstances, the team will need to acquire medications from the pharmacy prior to departing on transport.

e. *Respiratory status.* Ventilator support information must be obtained to ensure the correct device is available for transport. Most transport ventilators are capable of supporting the ECMO patient during transport.

3. *At the Referring Facility.* At the referring institution, the team should conduct a thorough bedside assessment, including review of laboratory and radiographic studies (Annich et al., 2012). In addition, any physiologic changes or trend in ECMO parameters must be identified. Stabilizing intervention should follow institutional transport and ECMO protocols.

4. *During Transport.* Following stabilization, the most critical components of the transport is patient movement to and from the transport vehicle, the effect of altitude on the oxygenator, and recognition and management of in-transport events (Annich et al., 2012). It is recommended that "time-outs" are included prior to each move, ensuring all crew members are prepared. A team leader should manage each move using good situational awareness techniques.

a. *Effect of altitude of the oxygenator.* Gas exchange capacity of the oxygenator declines with decreasing barometric pressure (Annich et al., 2012). See section on transport physiology, in this chapter, for detail regarding the effect of altitude on oxygen delivery. This aspect along with temperature change must be considered. Extreme cold will make plastic components brittle; thus, care must be taken to ensure the circuit and its components are protected. Breakage of any circuit component can be catastrophic.

b. ECMO transport is complex and requires an in-depth knowledge of all aspects of ECMO as well as critical and transport medicine. The section offers a brief introduction to mobile ECMO. Additional information can be found in the Extracorporeal Life Support Organization's *ECMO: Extracorporeal Cardiopulmonary Support in Critical Care*, 4th edition (Annich et al., 2012).

D. Nonaccidental Trauma

1. Identification and care of a child who is a victim of NAT is challenging, as the etiology of the illness, mechanism of the injury, and the history of the event is not always clear at the time of referral request. The CDC defines *pediatric abusive head trauma (AHT)* "as an injury to the skull or intracranial contents of an infant or young child (<5 years of age) due to inflicted blunt impact and/or violent shaking" (Parks, Annest, Hill, & Karch, 2012, p. 10). The definition excludes gunshot wounds, stab wounds, or penetrating trauma (Parks et al., 2012). It also excludes unintentional injuries resulting from neglectful supervision. NAT is a leading cause of childhood traumatic injury and death in the United States.

a. An estimated 1,400 children died from maltreatment in the United States in 2002 and AHT accounted for 80% of these deaths (Paul & Adamo, 2014).

b. AHT is a leading cause of physical child abuse deaths in children younger than 5 years in the United States (Klevens & Leeb, 2010).

c. AHT accounts for approximately one third of all child maltreatment deaths (Palusci & Covington, 2014).

2. Transport teams may be dispatched for an infant or child with a history of "not acting himself or herself," lethargy with unclear etiology, presence of bruising, and/or bone fractures or a fall with a history that is inconsistent with the events leading to the child presenting to the referring ED. History of the present illness and onset of current symptoms with a proper assessment, intervention, evaluation, and documentation are important aspects in the care of these infants and children. Children who present with evidence of respiratory compromise, seizures, or coma are more likely to be accurately diagnosed with AHT.

a. During initial contact, careful attention should be given to the emergency management of ABCs and neurological disability. Early communication with pediatric intensive care specialists, neurosurgeons, and radiologists is advised for more severely injured children in order to expedite transfer to a Level 1 trauma facility (Colbourne, 2004).

b. A thorough assessment using the PALS primary survey for initial care of the infant and child would also include a rapid trauma assessment. Stabilization of the child is the priority if the child is compromised, followed by transport to a Level 1 trauma center for further intervention and treatment. An organized approach to this stabilization should include, but is not limited to, airway, breathing, circulation, and bedside blood sugar assessment. The process should include the following:

i. Cervical spine should be maintained in the neutral position and an appropriate-sized cervical collar placed. Cervical spine should be immobilized in the following situations:

1) All patients with decreased or ALOC in which an adequate history of trauma cannot be ruled out (NAT, AHT).

2) All patients with physical findings suggesting neck or back injury.

ii. Assess, secure, and maintain a patent airway. If an airway adjunct is needed on suspected C-spine injury, consider endotracheal intubation ensuring in line mobilization and no movement of the neck, using rapid sequence induction as needed with brain-protective drugs for the intubation. Intubation should be considered for signs of increasing ICP and GCS less than 9 or decreasing by 2.

iii. Assess the breathing and expose the chest and assess the rate, pattern, and depth of respirations. Auscultate breath sounds, administer oxygen to maintain SaO_2 greater than 95%.

iv. Assess circulation, including the quality, rate, and regularity of the pulses. Assess the color, temperature, moisture of skin, and capillary refill time. Place the child on a cardiac monitor with pulse oximetry. If the blood pressure is normal and there are no other signs of shock or respiratory distress, administer 0.9% normal saline solution for fluid maintenance. If the child is or is becoming hypotensive, exhibits signs of shock or respiratory distress, volume resuscitation with isotonic saline and/ or packed red blood cells may be indicated. Be cautious of compensatory mechanisms that may mask signs of shock.

v. Ventilate the child to a $PaCO_2$ goal of 30 to 35 (Vavilala et al., 2014).

vi. Obtain imaging at the referring hospital if the child is stable and it does not delay the transfer. CT of the head is the mainstay of the diagnosis of AHT. Interpretation of these scans should be carried out by a radiologist familiar with pediatric imaging techniques. CT findings may include subdural hemorrhage (both acute and chronic), interhemispheric falx hemorrhage, diffuse axonal injury, and cerebral edema (Colbourne, 2004).

vii. Labwork includes a blood gas that will assist with stabilization and ventilator management. End-tidal CO_2 monitoring is the standard of care in children with an advanced airway during transport.

viii. Rapid transfer to a Level 1 trauma center is the goal once the child is stable for travel.

c. In children with less severe injuries, more time can be given to completing a full head-to-toe assessment at the referring hospital, paying attention to the abdomen, back, and any other bruising inconsistent with the history provided. Concise documentation is critical, as records are required if it has been confirmed that the child has been abused by a caregiver.

d. During transport, continuous serial assessment (every 15 minutes), planning, intervention, and evaluation are indicated. A concise handoff should be given with patient records, imaging, history of the events, and interventions provided by the team and referring facility upon arrival to the receiving facility.

E. Infectious Disease

1. The transport environment is unique, however, this does not abdicate the use of appropriate infection-control techniques, such as proper handwashing and the use of PPE such as masks, gloves,

and gowns. Safety of the crew and the patient, however, remains the primary focus of air and ground medical transport. It is recommended that all air operations are performed cold (no engines turning, blades have stopped) in order to prevent the hazard of foreign-object debris on the helipad.

2. Care of a neonatal or pediatric patient with an unknown illness requires the transport team to protect themselves and the crew of the ambulance or aircraft by alerting them of the potential illness. The uniform of the transport team does not take the place of using PPE and preventing the spread of infections does not stop during transport. The CDC has recommendations for disease prevention with the most obvious being proper and frequent hand washing before and after patient contact (CDC, 2017a). Handwashing with soap and water and use of alcohol-based hand sanitizers has been shown to prevent the spread of infection and help to prevent viral illnesses, including influenza and respiratory syncytial virus (RSV; CDC, 2017b). Influenza and RSV are the two viral illnesses that commonly affect the neonatal and pediatric transport population.

a. RSV is the most common cause of lower respiratory tract infections among young children worldwide. Most infants are infected before 1 year of age, and virtually everyone gets an RSV infection by 2 years of age. Each year, on average, in the United States, RSV leads to (Hall et al., 2009):

i. 57,527 hospitalizations among children younger than 5 years

ii. 2.1 million outpatient visits among children younger than 5 years

b. Influenza (flu) is a contagious respiratory illness caused by influenza viruses that infects the nose, throat, and lungs. It can cause mild to severe illness, which can lead to death (CDC, 2018). During the 2015 to 2016 influenza season, the CDC reported 70 deaths from influenza infection. Flu season generally starts in October and may last until May of the following year in certain areas of the country. When a transport team is dispatched for an infant or child with a suspected viral illness, the team should protect themselves with the appropriate PPE. Information gathered from the referring provider may alert the team that the infant or child being referred may have a viral illness and may consider RSV or the flu as an etiology. EDs, urgent care centers, and pediatricians have the ability to send rapid tests to determine whether the infant or child has RSV or the flu. Knowing this information prior to departure, the crew can protect themselves by wearing

PPE when caring for the patient. However, this does not mean that the team should not wear PPE if there are no definitive test results. If an infant presents with a history of difficulty breathing, poor feeding, nasal drainage, cough, and fever, the transport team should treat the patient as infectious and don PPE.

F. Telemedicine

1. Teleconferencing or videoconferencing has been used in the business world since the 1960s, allowing people from various locations to communicate—accomplishing tasks remotely and allowing coworkers to visualize presented items. Teleconferencing in medicine, or telemedicine, has been used since 1950 with the transmission of radiology images over telephone lines (Field, 1996). The technology allows a referring physician to discuss patients with an accepting/consulting physician and make decisions based on assessment by both parties.

2. Telemedicine successfully crossed over to the transport environment providing emergency medicine physicians in remote locations the ability to consult with a physician with greater pediatric expertise. Visualizing a child via video allows the accepting physician to consult with the referring physician to provide recommendations until the transport team arrives. In addition, the technology can improve remote diagnostic, therapeutic, and transport decisions among children receiving care in nonpediatric institutions (Ellenby & Marcin, 2015). Some tertiary care centers have developed networks for their referral area to use a telemedicine cart prior to the transfer to the accepting tertiary care center. A single center study demonstrated a pediatric critical care telemedicine program used for consultations for seriously ill children in rural and community EDs was feasible, sustainable, and used relatively infrequently, typically for the more critical ill patients (Hernandez et al., 2016). Most common reasons for consultation were respiratory illnesses, acute injury, and neurological conditions (Hernandez et al., 2016). Telemedicine is not restricted to ED transfers. Referring hospitals may use telemedicine for consultation of patients with non–life-threatening conditions, as well. For example, physicians may use telemedicine to consult a subspeciality service line, such as dermatology, for evaluation of rashes or skin conditions considered uncommon.

3. Other subspecialities, such as neonatology and cardiology, have set up telemedicine systems with referring hospitals to aid pediatricians when assistance is needed. The referring physician can bring the telemedicine cart, which includes a computer with videoconferencing software, video screen, and a camera, to the bedside—focusing the camera on the infant or child. The referring provider and accepting physician discuss the situation in real time with the accepting physician providing additional recommendations prior to transport team arrival. In some instances, the transport team is able to participate in the telemedicine call, promoting clinical awareness. Telemedicine is certainly not limited to local or rural referral hospitals. Some servicelines have developed relationships with hospitals abroad allowing them to add expertise internationally.

G. Transport Metrics

1. In 2001, the Institute of Medicine released a report titled, *Crossing the Quality Chasm: A New Health Care System for the 21st Century*. The report stated that the American healthcare system was broken and requires sweeping overhauls in order to fix the many problems that exist (Institute of Medicine [IOM], 2001). It outlined six aims for improvement, including 10 steps for the redesign of the healthcare system. One of the steps for healthcare redesign is a focus on safety as a system property and by focusing on safety, patients should be free from injury caused by the system.

2. Safety of the patient and crew is the number one priority for a transport service (IOM, 2001). Quality-improvement indicators are tracked with the expectation that the team will use the measures to advance the system process. Benchmarking of these measures is essential for a critical care transport service to improve patient outcomes, advance quality of care, and correct known deficiencies. Neonatal and pediatric transport teams consist of highly skilled practitioners who strive to consistently improve the care resulting in improved patient outcomes. For example, teams may track the number of successful intubations on the first attempt or mobilization time, the time from the call to the team departure. In the past, neonatal and pediatric teams tracked multiple measures, however, no systematically defined metrics were benchmarked to improve patient outcomes. During the 2012 American Academy of Pediatrics, Section on Transport Medicine Meeting, a group of experts developed 12 quality metrics to improve the care delivered by pediatric specialty care teams (Schwartz et al., 2015). Table 9.48 lists these metrics (Schwartz et al., 2015).

3. Use of these standardized metrics allows neonatal and pediatric transport teams to benchmark their system against nationally accepted benchmarks. The Ground and Air Medical Quality in Transport (GAMUT; http://gamutqi.org) is a free resource for

TABLE 9.48   AAP Consensus Neonatal and Pediatric Transport Quality Metrics, Including Metrics Definition and Reporting Nomenclature

Metric	Definition and Reported Nomenclature
Unplanned dislodgement of therapeutic devices	Number of documented dislodgement (may be >1 per transport while under the care of the team of the following devices (I/O lines, IVs, UAC/UVC, central venous lines, arterial catheters, ETTs, chest tubes and tracheostomy tubes) divided by the number of transports during the calendar month. Reported as *"dislodgement of therapeutic devices/1,000 transports."*
Verification of tracheal tube placement	Number of ETTs on transport (regardless of whether or not the team placed them) for which there is documentation confirming placement using a minimum of two of the following confirmatory techniques: radiograph, direct visualization through the cords, continuous capnometry or colorimetric capnometer, and assessment of symmetric breath sounds divided by the number of intubated patients transported during the calendar month. Reported as *"percentage of intubated patients with documented ETT verification."*
Average mobilization time of the transport team	Average time (including all transports in the calendar month, excluding transport scheduled in advance and patient transports out of the originating facility) in minutes (rounded up to nearest minute) from the start of the referring phone call to the transport team to the time the team is en route to the referring facility. "Stacked" trips or transports done right after the last during which the team never returns to base should be included in this count. Reported as *"average mobilization time for an unscheduled transport."*
First attempt tracheal tube placement	Total number of intubations successful on the first attempt divided by the number of patients on whom intubation was attempted by the transport team during the calendar month. *Intubation attempt* is defined as laryngoscopy by any member of the team regardless of whether there is an attempt to pass a tracheal tube. This number should be reported separately for patients younger than 28 days (neonates) and those 28 days and older (nonneonatal). Reported as *"percentage of neonatal intubations with a successful first attempt"* and *"percentage of nonneonatal intubations with a successful first attempt."*
Rate of transport-related patient injuries	Number of documented transport-related injuries or deaths divided by the number of transports during the calendar month. Excluded are injuries and deaths related to medical care itself or the omission of medical care. Reported as *"rolling 12-month transport-related patient injury rate per 10,000 transports."*
Rate of medication administration errors	Number of documented medication administration errors during a calendar month divided by the number of transports during the calendar month. Medication administration errors are further defined as drug administrations violating any of the "five rights"—right patient, right medication, right dose, right route, and right time. Reported as *"medication administration errors per 1,000 transports."*
Rate of patient medical equipment failure during transport	Number of documented medical equipment failures (may be >1 per transport) while under the care of the team divided by the number of transports during the calendar month. Reported as *"medical equipment failure per 1,000 transports."*
Rate of CPR performed during transport	Number of transports during which chest compressions are performed from the time the team assumes care ("hands on") until the patient handoff is completed at the destination facility divided by the number of transports during the calendar month. Multiple episodes of chest compressions in a single transport should only be counted as one episode. If CPR is in progress when the team arrives, this should not be included in this count. Reported as a *"rolling 12-month CPR rate per 10,000 transports."*

(continued)

TABLE 9.48 AAP Consensus Neonatal and Pediatric Transport Quality Metrics, Including Metrics Definition and Reporting Nomenclature *(continued)*

Metric	Definition and Reported Nomenclature
Rate of SREs	Number of SREs during the calendar month divided by the number of transports during the calendar month. An *SRE* is defined as any unanticipated and largely preventable event involving death, life-threatening consequences, or serious physical or psychological harm. Reported as "*rolling 12-month SRE rate per 10,000 transports.*"
Unintentional neonatal hypothermia upon arrival to destination	Number of neonates (infants < 28 d) with admission temperatures at the destination facility less than 36.5°C axillary (excluding those being actively cooled) divided by the number of neonates transported during the calendar month. Reported as "*percentage of transported neonates found hypothermic at admission.*"
Rate of transport-related crew injury	Number of transport-related crew injuries or deaths reported to the institution's employee health department or equivalent during the calendar month divided by the number of transports during the calendar month. Reported as "*rolling 12-month transport-related crew injury rate per 10,000 transports.*"
Use of standardized patient care handoff	Number of transports for which there is documented use of a standardized handoff procedure for turning over patient care at the destination hospital divided by the number of transports during the calendar month. Reported as "*percentage of transports involving a standardized patient care handoff.*"

AAP, American Academy of Pediatrics; CPR, cardiopulmonary resuscitation; ETT, endotracheal tube; I/O, intraosseous; IV, intravenous; SRE, serious reportable event; UAC, umbilical artery catheter; UVC, umbilical venous catheter.

Source: Adopted from Schwartz, H. P., Bigham, M. T., Schoettker, P. J., Meyer, K., Trautman, M. S., & Insoft, R. M. (2015). Quality metrics in neonatal and pediatric critical care transport: A national Delphi project. *Pediatric Critical Care Medicine, 16*(8), 711–717. Retrieved from https://journals.lww.com/pccmjournal/Abstract/2015/10000/Quality_Metrics_in_Neonatal_and_Pediatric_Critical.3.aspx

transport teams to track, report, and analyze their performance on transport-specific quality metrics by comparing it to other programs. It is recommended that pediatric speciality teams utilize measures mentioned earlier as part of a quality-improvement program to ensure the highest quality of care.

CONCLUSIONS

The goal of any pediatric transport system is to provide an extension of the critical care unit to the referring facilities, ensure a timely and safe transport to a pediatric critical care center without an increase in morbidity or mortality, and to provide the highest quality of care for critically ill infants and children who require interfacility transport. The first step in this process is the initial stabilization, which must begin at the referring facility before the request for transfer. Stabilization begins with a thorough assessment of the child's ABCs. Once identified, airway compromise, ineffective respiration, stabilization of circulation, and correction of hypoglycemia must be treated without delay. Using the American Heart Association's PALS course guidelines may be beneficial in both assessing and treating the critically ill child. The second step is the transfer to a facility specializing in pediatric care. This transfer is often complicated by the severity of illness and the innate increased risk of mortality found in the transport setting. Children needing medical transport often require more advanced procedures, such as endotracheal intubation, inotropic support, and continuous cardiovascular monitoring (invasive and noninvasive), which warrants a crew with an in-depth understanding of pediatric disease pathology and advanced care.

CASE STUDIES WITH QUESTIONS, ANSWERS, AND RATIONALES

Initial Stabilization and Transport Case Studies

Case Study 9.14

A 14-month-old male presented to a local community hospital with tachypnea, increased work of breathing, and arterial saturations (SpO$_2$) ranging from 86% to 90% on room air (FiO$_2$ 0.21). At the time of the call, the following information was conveyed: patient weight of 12 kg, heart rate of 186 bpm, blood pressure of 98/60 (mean pressure 76), capillary refill time of approximately 4 seconds, patent airway, respiratory rate of 68 with intercostal retractions, and SpO_2 of 92% on 8 lpm blow-by oxygen. The referring hospital was attempting to gain peripheral access to administer a bolus of fluids. The transport team was dispatched and is in route to the referring hospital.

Upon arrival, the team finds the patient alert and interactive in mild respiratory distress, receiving oxygen via 8 lpm blow with SpO_2 of 90%. Care included suctioning of the nasal and oral airway, administration of a 20 cc/kg bolus of NS, and a drug aerosol treatment of 2.5 mg albuterol with no improvement. Vital signs upon the team's arrival are as follows: heart rate 172 bpm, blood pressure 88/64 (mean pressure 74), capillary refill time greater than 2 seconds, and alert and crying.

1. What additional information would you like to gather regarding the metabolic state of the patient at the time of initial referral request?
   A. Blood glucose level
   B. Date of birth
   C. Anion gap
   D. Carbon monoxide level

2. In preparation for transport, which is the best device for oxygen delivery for this patient?
   A. 100% nonrebreather mask
   B. Blow-by oxygen
   C. 2 lpm nasal cannula
   D. None of the above is acceptable

3. Given the hemodynamic and perfusion status of the child, another 20 cc/kg bolus of NSS is indicated.
   A. True
   B. False

Case Study 9.15

While transporting a 6-year-old female for liver transplant by fixed-wing aircraft, you observed an increase in heart rate from 80 to 120 bpm during ascent to cruising altitude. The patient is now crying and trying to roll on her side, at times holding her abdomen. When you assess her level of pain, she states "my belly hurts." There is a nasal gastric tube in place and you noticed on her abdomen radiograph that she had an increased amount of gas in her stomach and gastrointestinal tract. Further assessment revealed that the nasal gastric tube is capped, not allowing excess gas to vent to the atmosphere.

1. What is the cause of the onset of abdominal pain during ascent?
   A. Expansion of abdominal gas secondary to decreased atmospheric pressure associated with altitude
   B. Narcotic withdrawal

C. Peripheral IV infiltration
D. Anxiety associated with flight

2. Which gas law is the cause for the abdominal pain?
   A. Dalton's Law
   B. Charles's Law
   C. Boyle's Law
   D. Gay-Lussac's Law

3. Venting the nasal gastric tube to either suction or atmosphere will allow the expanded volume to vent to the atmosphere and help relieve the increased abdominal pressure.
   A. True
   B. False

Initial Stabilization and Transport Answers and Rationales

Case Study 9.14

1. **A.** Young children and infants are at increased risk of hypoglycemia during illness as increased metabolic demands quickly deplete glycogen stores and often they have poor oral intake. Clinicians should obtain and record a serum glucose level at the time of the request for transfer and upon the team's arrival.

2. **C.** The best method for oxygen administration is a nasal cannula for this patient. The transport environment exposes the patient to temperature changes and external air flow. The nasal cannula will ensure a stable increased concentration of oxygen that is easily maintained during transport. The liter flow can be increased and decreased as required to maintain a SpO_2 greater than 92% during transport.

3. **A.** The patient continues to have increased heart rate and prolonged capillary refill greater than 2 seconds. Another 20 cc/kg bolus of NSS is indicated, as increased respiratory rate and decreased oral intake result in greater insensible losses via the respiratory tract. This leads to volume loss and hypovolemia.

Case Study 9.15

1. **A.** At a constant temperature, the volume of a given gas is inversely proportional to the pressure, therefore as barometric pressure decreases with ascent—a volume of gas will increase. This may cause abdominal pain and discomfort.

2. **C.** Boyle's law states that a known volume of gas will expand as the pressure that surrounds it decreases, affecting any enclosed gas-filled space inside or outside the body cavity.

3. A. Venting the nasal gastric tube will decrease the pressure in the stomach alleviating the abdominal discomfort.

INITIAL STABILIZATION AND TRANSPORT REFERENCES

American Association of Critical-Care Nursing. (2016). AACN practice alert: Family presence during resuscitation and invasive procedures. *Critical Care Nurse*, 36(1), e11–e14.

Algie, C. M., Mahar, R. K., Tan, H. B., Wilson, G., Mahar, P. D., & Wasiak, J. (2015). Effectiveness and risks of cricoid pressure during rapid sequence induction for endotracheal intubation. *Cochrane Database of Systematic Reviews*, 2015(11), CD011656. doi:10.1002/14651858.CD011656.pub2

American Heart Association. (2016). *Pediatric Advanced Life Support: Provider manual*. Dallas, TX: Author.

Anil, A. B., Anil, M., Saqlam, A. B., Cetin, N., Bal, A., & Aksu, N. (2010). High volume normal saline alone is as effective as nebulized salbutamol-normal saline, epinephrine-normal saline, and 3% saline in mild bronchiolitis. *Pediatric Pulmonology*, 45(1), 41–47.

Annich, G. M., Lynch, W. R., MacLaren, G., Wilson, J. M., & Bartlett, R. H. (2012). *ECMO: Extracoporeal cardiopulmonary support in critical care* (4th ed.). Ann Arbor, MI: Extracorpeal Life Support Organization.

Bertrand, P., Araníbar, H., Castro, E., & Sánchez, I. (2001). Efficacy of nebulized epinephrine versus salbutamol in hospitalized infants with bronchiolitis. *Pediatric Pulmonology*, 31(4), 284–288.

Bhatia, V., & Wolfsdorf, J. L. (1991). Severe hypoglycemia in youth with insulin-dependant diabetes mellitus: Frequency and causative factors. *Pediatrics*, 88(6), 1187–1193.

Bhende, M. S., Karr, V. A., Wiltsie, D. C., & Orr, R. A. (1995). Evaluation of a portable infrared end-tidal carbon dioxide monitor during pediatric interhospital transport. *Pediatrics*, 95(6), 875–878.

Bloch, H., Silverman, R., Mancherje, N., Grant, S., Jagminas, L., & Scharf, S. M.. (1995). Intravenous magnesium sulfate as an adjunct in the treatment of acute asthma. *Chest*, 107(6), 1578–1581.

Blumen, I. J., & Rinnert, K. J. (1995) Altitude physiology and the stresses of flight. *Air Medical Journal*, 14(2), 87–100.

Bower, L. K., Barnhart, S. L., Betit, P., Czervinske, M. P., Masi-Lynch, J., & Wilson, B. G. (1995). Selection of an aerosol delivery device for neonatal and pediatric patients. *Respiratory Care*, 40(12), 1325–1335.

Broman, L. M., Holzgraefe, B, Palmer, K., & Frenckner, B. (2015). The Stockholm experience: Interhospital transports on extracorporeal membrane oxygenation. *Critical Care*, 19, 278–284.

Bryner, B., Cooley, E., Copenhaver, W., Brierley, K., Teman, N., Landis, D., . . . Bartlett, R. H. (2014). Two decades' experience with interfacility transport on extracorporeal membrane oxygenation. *Annals of Thoracic Surgery*, 98(4), 1363–1670.

Carcillo, J. A. (2003). Pediatric septic shock and multiple organ failure. *Critical Care Clinics*, 19(3), 413–440.

Carcillo, J. A., & Fields, A. I. (2002). Clinical practice parameters for hemodynamic support of pediatric and neonatal patients in septic shock. *Critical Care Medicine*, 30(6), 1365–1378.

Carcillo, J. A., Kuch, B. A., Han, Y. Y., Day, S., Greenwald, B. M., McCloskey, K. A., . . . Orr, R. A. (2009). Mortality and functional morbidity after the use of PALS/APLS by community physicians. *Pediatrics*, 124(2), 500–508.

Centers for Disease Control and Prevention. (2017a). Handwashing: Clean hands save lives. Retrieved from http://www.cdc.gov/handwashing

Centers for Disease Control and Prevention. (2017b). Respiratory syncytial virus. Retrieved from http://www.cdc.gov/rsv

Centers for Disease Control and Prevention. (2018). Influenza (Flu). Retrieved from http://www.cdc.gov/flu

Chameides, L., Samson, R. A., Schexnayder, S. M., & Hazinski, M.F. (Eds). (2011) *Pediatric advanced life support provider manual*. Dallas, TX: American Heart Association.

Ciarallo, L., Sauer, A. H., & Shannon, M. W. (1996). Intravenous magnesium therapy for moderate to severe pediatric asthma: results of a randomized, placebo-controlled trial. *Journal of Pediatrics*, 129(6), 809–814.

Colbourne, M. (2004). Abusive head trauma. *British Columbia Medical Journal*, 46(2), 72–76.

Curley, M. A. Q., & Moloney-Harmon, P. (2001). *Critical care nursing of infants and children* (2nd ed.). Philadelphia, PA: Saunders.

Dellinger, R. P., Levy, M. M., Rhodes, A., Annane, D., Gerlach, H., Opal, S. M., . . . Moreno, R. (2013). Surviving sepsis campaign: International guidelines for management of severe sepsis and septic shock: 2012. *Critical Care Medicine*, 41(2), 580–637.

DeNicola, L. K., Monem, G. F., Gayle, M. O., & Kissoon, N. (1994). Treatment of critical severe status asthmaticus in children. *Pediatric Clinics of North America*, 41(6), 1293–1324.

Douglas-Escobar, M., & Weiss, M. D. (2015). Hypoxic-ischemic encephalopathy: A review for the clinician. *JAMA Pediatrics*, 169(4), 397–403. doi:10.1001/jamapediatrics.2014.3269

Doymaz, S., & Schneider, J. (2018). Safety of terbutaline for treatment of acute severe pediatric asthma. *Pediatric Emergency Care*, 34(5), 299–302.

Dunger, D. B., Sperling, M. A., Acerini, C. L., Bohn, D. J., Daneman, D., Danne, T. P., ... LWPES. (2004). ESPE/LWPES consensus statement on diabetic ketoacidosis in children and adolescents. *Archives of Disease in Childhood*, 89(2), 188–194.

Ellenby, M. S., & Marccin, J. P. (2015). The role of telemedicine in pediatric critical care. *Critical Care Clinics*, 31(2), 275-290.

Field, M. J. (Ed.). (1996). *Telemedicine: A guide to assessing telecommunications in health care*. Washington, DC: National Academies Press.

Glover, M. L., Machado, C., & Totapally, B. R. (2002). Magnesium sulfate administered via continuous intravenous infusion in pediatric patients with refractory wheezing. *Journal of Critical Care*, 17(4), 255–258.

Goto, T., Gibo, K., Hagiwara, Y., Okubo, M., Brown, D. F., Brown, C. A. 3rd., & Hasegawa, K. (2016). Factors associated with first-pass success in pediatric intubation in the emergency department. *Western Journal of Emergency Medicine*, 17(2), 129–134.

Guyette, F. X., Roth, K. R., Lacovey, D. C., & Rittenberger, J. C. (2007). Feasibility of laryngeal mask airway use by prehospital personnel in simulated pediatric respiratory arrest. *Prehospital Emergency Care*, 11(2), 245–249.

Hall, C. B., Weinberg, G. A., Iwane, M. K., Blumkin, A. K., Edwards, K. M., Staat, M. A., . . . Szilagyi, P. (2009). The burden of respiratory syncytial virus infection in young children. *New England Journal of Medicine*, 360(6), 588–598.

Han, Y. Y., Carcillo, J. A., Dragotta, M. A., Bills, D. M., Watson, R. S., Westerman, M. E., & Orr, R. A. (2003). Early reversal of pediatric-neonatal septic shock by community physicians is associated with improved outcome. *Pediatrics*, 112(4), 793–799.

Hazinski, M. F. (2013). *Nursing care of the critically ill child* (3rd ed.). St. Louis, MO: Elsevier Mosby.

Hernandez, M., Hojman N., Sadorra C., Dharmar, M., Nesbitt, T. S., Litman, R., & Marcin, J. P. (2016). Pediatric Critical Care Telemedicine Program: A single institution review. *Telemedicine and e-Health, 22*(1), 51–55

High, K., & Yeatman, J. (2000). Transport considerations for the pediatric trauma patient. *Journal of Emergency Nursing, 26*(4), 346–351.

Holleran, R. S. (2010). *ASTNA patient transport: Principle and practice* (4th ed.). St Louis, MO: Mosby.

Huang, F. K., Lin, C. C., Huang, T. C., Weng, K. P., Liu, P. Y., Chen, Y. Y., . . . Hsieh, K. S. (2013). Reappraisal of the prog-taglandin E1 dose for early newborns with patent ductus arteriosus-dependent pulmonary circulation. *Pediatrics and Neonatology, 54*(2), 102–106.

Institute of Medicine. (2001). *Crossing the quality chasm: A new health system for the 21st century*. Washington, DC: National Academies Press.

Jaimovich, D. G., & Vidyasagar, D. (2002). *Handbook of pediatric and neonatal transport medicine* (2nd ed.). Philadelphia, PA: Hanley & Belfus.

Kenyon, C. C., Fieldston, E. S., Luan, X., Keren, R., & Zorc, J. J. (2014). Safety and effectiveness of continuous aerosolized albuterol in the non-intensive care setting. *Pediatrics, 134*(4), 976–982.

Klassen, T. P. (1999). Croup, a current perspective. *Pediatric Clinics of North America, 46*(6), 1167–1178.

Kleinman, M. E., Chameides, L., Schexnayder, S. M., Samson, R. A., Hazinski, M. F., Atkins, D. L., . . . Zaritsky, A. L. (2010). Part 14: Pediatric Advanced Life Support: 2010 American Heart Association guidelines for cardiopulmonary resuscitation and emergency cardiovascular care. *Circulation, 122*(Suppl. 3), S876–S908.

Klevens, J., & Leeb, R. (2010). Child maltreatment fatalities in children under five: Findings from the national violent death reporting system. *Child Abuse & Neglect, 34*(4), 262–266.

Kline-Krammes, S., Patel, N. H., & Robinson, S. (2013). Childhood asthma: A guide for pediatric emergency medicine providers. *Emergency Medicine Clinics of North America, 31*(3), 705–732.

Kuch, B. A., Munoz, R., & Orr, R. A. (2006). Interfacility transport of infants and children with congenital heart disease: A multi-center analysis. *Cardiology in the Young, 16*, S91.

Li, Y., Bai, Z., Li, M., Wang, X., Pan, J., Wang, J., & Feng, X. (2015). U-shaped relationship between early blood glucose and mortality in critically ill children. *BMC Pediatrics, 15*, 88–97.

Lighthall, G. K., & Pearl, R. G. (2003). Volume resuscitation in the critically ill: Choosing the best solution. *Journal of Critical Illness, 18*, 252–260.

Losek, J. D. (2000). Hypoglycemia and the ABC's (sugar) of pediatric resuscitation. *Annals of Emergency Medicine, 35*(1), 43–46.

Martin, S. E., Ochsner, M. G., & Jarman, R. H. (1999). The LMA: Available alternative for securing the airway. *Air Medical Journal, 18*(2), 89–92.

MacDonald, M. G., & Ginzburg, H. M. (Eds.). (1999). *Guidelines for air and ground transport of neonatal and pediatric patients* (2nd ed.). Elk Grove Village, IL: American Academy of Pediatrics.

McCloskey, K. A., & Orr, R. A. (Eds.). (1995). *Pediatric transport medicine*. St Louis, MO: Mosby.

Merrill, L. (2012). Therapeutic hypothermia to treat hypoxic ischemic encephalopathy in newborns. *Nursing for Women's Health, 16*(2), 126–134. doi:10.1111/j.1751-486X.2012.01718.x

Mitchell, A. P., & Johnston, E. D. (2011). Provision of therapeutic hypothermia during neonatal transport. *Infant, 7*(3), 79–82.

Munoz, R. A., Morell, V. O., da Cruz, E. M., & Vetterly, C. G. (2010). *Critical care of children with heart disease: Basic medical and surgical concepts*. London, UK: Springer Verlag.

National Asthma Education and Prevention Program, Third Expert Panel on the Diagnosis and Management of Asthma. (2007). *Expert panel report 3: Guidelines for the diagnosis and management of asthma*. Bethesda, MD: National Heart, Lung, and Blood Institute. Retrieved from https://www.ncbi .nlm.nih.gov/books/NBK7232/

Nehrenz, G. (1997). Motion interpretation. *Internet Journal of Aeromedical Transportation, 1*(1), 1–4. Retrieved from http:// www.ispub.com/journals/IJAMT/VOL1N1/altox.htm

Numa, A. H., Williams, G. D., & Dakin, C. J. (2001). The effect of nebulized epinephrine on respiratory mechanics and gas exchange in bronchiolitis. *American Journal of Respiratory and Critical Care Medicine, 164*(1), 86–91.

Okayama, H., Aikawa, T., Okayama, M., Sasaki, H., Mue, S., & Takishima, T. (1987). Bronchodilating effect of intravenous magnesium sulfate in bronchial asthma. *Journal of the American Medical Association, 257*(8), 1076–1078.

Orr, R. A., Felmet, K. A., Han, Y., McCloskey, K. A., Dragotta, M. A., Bills, D. M., . . . Watson, R. S. (2009). Pediatric specialized teams are associated with improved outcomes. *Pediatrics, 124*(1), 40–48.

Orsborn, J., Graham, J., Moss, M., Melguizo, M., & Stroud, M. (2016). Pediatric endotracheal tube cuff pressures during aeromedical transport. *Pediatric Emergency Care, 32*(1), 20–22.

Palusci, V. J., & Covington, T. M. (2014). Child maltreatment deaths in the U.S. national Child Death Review Case Reporting System. *Child Abuse & Neglect, 38*(1), 25–36.

Papo, M. C., Frank, J., & Thompson, A. E. (1995). A prospective, randomized study of continuous versus intermittent nebulized albuterol for severe status asthmaticus in children. *Critical Care Medicine, 21*(10), 1479–1486.

Parks, S. E., Annest, J. L., Hill, H. A., & Karch, D. L. (2012). *Pediatric abusive head trauma: Recommended definitions for public health surveillance and research*. Atlanta, GA: Centers for Disease Control and Prevention. Retrieved from http://www.cdc .gov/ViolencePrevention/pdf/PedHeadTrauma-a.pdf

Paul, A. R., & Adamo, M. A. (2014). Non-accidental trauma in pediatric patients: Review of epidemiology, pathophysiology, diagnosis and treatment. *Translational pediatrics, 3*(3), 195–207.

Pennant, J. H., & Walker, M. B. (1992). Comparison of the endotracheal tube and laryngeal mask in airway management by paramedical personnel. *Anesthesia and Analgesia, 74*(4), 531–534.

Petrocheilou, A., Tanou, K., Kalampouka, E., Malakasioti, G., Giannios, C., & Kaditis, A. G. (2014). Viral croup: Diagnosis and a treatment algorithm. *Pediatric Pulmonology, 49*(5), 421–429.

Pollack, M. M., Alexander, S. R., Clarke, N., Ruttimann, U. E., Tesselaar, H. M., & Bachulis, A. C. (1991). Improving outcomes from tertiary pediatric intensive care: A statewide comparison of tertiary and nontertiary care facilities. *Critical Care Medicine, 19*(2), 150–159.

Price, D. D., Wilson, S. R., & Fee, M. E. (2007). Sidestream end-tidal carbon dioxide monitoring during helicopter transport. *Air Medical Journal, 26*(1), 55–59.

Ramnarayan, P., Thiru, K., Parslow, R. C., Harrison, D. A., Draper, E. S., & Rowan, K. M. (2010). Effect of a specialized retrieval teams on outcomes in children admitted to paediatric intensive care units in England and Wales: A retrospective study. *Lancet, 376*(9742), 698–704.

Rodriguez Perez, J. M., Golombek, S., & Sola, A. (2017). Clinical hypoxic-ischemic encephalopathy score of the Iberoamerican Society of Neonatology (Siben): A new proposal for diagnosis and management. *Revista da Associação Médica Brasileira, 63*(1), 64-69.

Sagarin, M. J., Chiang, V., Sakles, J. C., Barton, E. D., Wolfe, R. E., Vissers, R. J., & Walls, R. M. (2002). Rapid sequence intubation for pediatric emergency airway management. *Pediatric Emergency Care, 18*(6), 417–422.

Schierholz, E. (2014). Therapeutic hypothermia on transport: Providing safe and effective cooling therapy as the link between birth hospital and the neonatal intensive care unit. *Advances in Neonatal Care, 14*(Suppl. 5), 24–31. doi:10.1097/ANC.0000000000000121

Schuh, S., Johnson, D. W., Callahan, S., Canny, G., & Levison, H. (1995). Efficacy of frequent nebulized ipratropium bromide added to frequent high-dose albuterol therapy in severe childhood asthma. *Journal of Pediatrics, 126*(4), 636–645.

Schwartz, H. P., Bigham, M. T., Schoettker, P. J., Meyer, K., Trautman, M. S., & Insoft, R. M. (2015). Quality metrics in neonatal and pediatric critical care transport: A national Delphi project. *Pediatric Critical Care Medicine, 16*(8), 711–717.

Scott, H. F., Donoghue, A. J., Gaieski, D. F., Marchese, R. F., & Mistry, R. D. (2014). Effectiveness of physical exam signs for early detection of critical illness in pediatric systemic inflammatory response syndrome. *BMC Emergency Medicine, 14*, 24–30.

Scribano, P. V., Baker, M. D., Holmes, J., & Shaw, K. N. (2000). Use of out-of-hospital intervention for the pediatric patient in an urban emergency medical service system. *Academic Emergency Medicine, 7*(7), 745–750, 2000.

Singhi, S., Grover, S., Bansal, A., & Chopra, K. (2014). Randomized comparison of intravenous magnesium sulphate, terbutaline and aminophylline for children with severe asthma. *Acta Paediatrica, 103*(12), 1301–1306.

Sittig, S. E., Nesbitt, J. C., Krageschimidt, D. A., Sobczak, S. C., & Johnson, R. V. (2011). Noise levels in a neonatal transport incubator in medically configured aircraft. *International Journal of Pediatric Otorhinolaryngology, 75*(1), 74–77.

Smith, K. A., Gothard, M. D., Schwartz, H. P., Giuliano, J. S. Jr., Forbes, M., & Bigham, M. T. (2015). Risk factors for failed tracheal intubation in pediatric and neonatal critical care speciality transport. *Prehospital Emergency Care, 19*(1), 17–22.

Stephanopoulos, D. E., Monge, R., Schell, K. H., Wyckoff, P., & Peterson, B. M. (1998). Continuous intravenous terbutaline for pediatric status asthmaticus. *Critical Care Medicine, 26*(10), 1744–1748.

Stroud, M. H., Sanders, R. C. Jr., Moss, M. M., Sullivan, J. E., Prodhan, P., Melguizo-Castro, M., & Nick, T. (2015). Goal-directed resuscitative interventions during pediatric interfacility transport. *Critical Care Medicine, 43*(8), 1692–1698.

Stroud, M. H., Trautman, M. S., Meyer, K., Moss, M. M., Schwartz, H. P., Bigham, M. T., . . . Insoft, R. (2013). Pediatric and neonatal interfacility transport: Results from a national consensus conference. *Pediatrics, 132*(2), 359–366.

Thoresen, M., Tooley, J., Liu, X., Jary, S., Fleming, P., Luyt, K., . . . Sabir, H. (2013). Time is brain: Starting therapeutic hypothermia within three hours after birth improves motor outcome in asphyxiated newborns. *Neonatology, 104*(3), 228–233. doi:10.1159/000353948

Thornton, P. S., Stanley, C. A., De Leon, D. D., Haris, D., Haymond, M. W., Hussain, K., . . . Wolfsdorf, J. I. (2015). Recommendations from the Pediatric Endocrine Society for evaluation and management of persistent hypoglycemia in neonates, infants, and children. *Journal of Pediatrics, 167*(2), 238–245.

Tourtier, J. P., Libert, N., Clapson, P., Dubourdieu, S., Jost, D., Tazarourte, K., . . . Auroy, Y. (2014). A simulation-based study of in-flight auscultation. *Simulation in Healthcare, 9*(2), 81–84.

Tung, B. J. (2005). The pediatric rescue airway. *Air Medical Journal, 24*(2), 55–58.

Turner, D. A., & Kleinman, M. E. (2010). The use of vasoactive agents via peripheral intravenous access during transport of critically ill infants and children. *Pediatric Emergency Care, 26*(8), 563–566.

Vavilala, M. S., Kernic, M. A., Wang, J., Kannan, N., Mink, R. B., Wainwright, M. S., . . . Rivara, F. P. (2014). Acute care clinical indicators associated with discharge outcomes in children with severe traumatic brain injury. *Critical Care Medicine, 42*(10), 2258–2286.

Volovitz, B., & Nussinovitch, M. (2002). Management of children with severe asthma exacerbation in the emergency department. *Pediatric Drugs, 4*(3), 141–148.

Walsh, B. K. (2015). *Neonatal and pediatric respiratory care* (4th ed.). St. Louis, MO: Elsevier Saunders.

Warren, J., Fromm, R. E. Jr., Orr, R. A., Rotello, L. C., & Horst, H. M. (2004). Guidelines for the inter- and intrahospital transport of the critically ill patient. *Critical Care Medicine, 32*(1), 256–262.

Wendel, H. P., & Ziemer, G. (1999). Coating-techniques to improve the hemocompatibility of artificial devices used for extracorporeal circulation. *European Journal of Cardio-thoracic Surgery, 16*(3), 342–350.

Werner, H. A. (2001). Status asthmaticus in children. *Chest, 119*, 1913–1929.

Wessel, D. L. (2001) Managing low cardiac output syndrome after congenital heart surgery. *Critical Care Medicine, 29*(Suppl. 10), S220–S230.

White, N. H. (2003). Management of diabetic ketoacidosis. *Reviews in Endocrine and Metabolic Disorders, 4*(4), 343–353.

Woodward, G. A., Chun, T. H., & Miles, D. K. (1999). It's not just a seizure: Etiology, management, and transport of the seizure patient. *Pediatric Emergency Care, 15*(2), 147–155.

Woodward, G. A., & Fleegler, E. W. (2000). Should parents accompany pediatric interfacility ground ambulance transport? The parent's perspective. *Pediatric Emergency Care, 16*(6), 383–390.

Woodward, G. A., Insoft, R. M., Pearson-Shaver, A. L., Jaimovich, D., Orr, R. A., Chambliss, R., . . . Westergaard, F. (2002). The state of pediatric interfacility transport: Consensus of the second National Pediatric and Neonatal Interfacility Transport Medicine Leadership Conference. *Pediatric Emergency Care, 18*(1), 38–43.

Wolfsdorf, J. I., Allgrove, J., Craig, M. E., Edge, J., Glaser, N., Jain, V., . . . Hanas, R. (2014). ISAD Clinical Practice Consensus Guidelines 2014 Compendium: Diabetic ketoacidosis and hyperglycemic hyperosmolar state. *Pediatric Diabetes, 15*(Suppl. 20), 154–179.

10 PROFESSIONAL ISSUES—QUALITY, SAFETY, WORK ENVIRONMENT, AND WELLNESS

Brandis Thornton and Jaime Manley

The foundation of nursing is rooted in the "protection, promotion, and restoration of health and well-being; the prevention of illness and injury; and the alleviation of suffering" (American Nurses Association, 2015). Nurses are the frontline health professionals who provide safe, effective, and timely care in sometimes under resourced and chaotic settings, such as the ICU. As such, nurses are obligated to participate in establishing and sustaining a culture that values and promotes quality and safety for staff and patients. The purpose of this chapter is to provide critical care nursing with an introduction to the history of the patient safety movement (including how patient safety techniques evolved out of knowledge from other industries outside of healthcare), strategies to promote a culture of patient safety, and how to implement quality-improvement (QI) methodologies in clinical care. In addition, this chapter addresses the issue of a healthy work environment (HWE) because meeting the needs of nursing staff is paramount to ensuring safe and effective patient care.

KEY STAKEHOLDERS IN THE HISTORY OF THE PATIENT SAFETY MOVEMENT

Patient safety is a relatively "young" field, with most work being done in the past 20 to 25 years (Figure 10.1).

A. Institute of Medicine

In 2000, the Institute of Medicine (IOM) published *To Err Is Human: Building a Safer Health System* (Kohn, Corrigan, & Donaldson, 2000). This report estimated that between 44,000 and 98,000 patients annually are harmed by medical errors. As such, its authors called for a ≥50% *reduction in medical errors over a 5-year time period* by:

1. Establishing a national focus on patient safety

2. Identifying and learning from errors via mandatory and voluntary reporting systems (VRS)

3. Raising standards and expectations of healthcare organizations by professional groups, payers, and oversight organizations

4. Helping healthcare organizations implement systems and culture change to improve patient safety (IOM, 2000)

B. The Joint Commission

1. The National Patient Safety Goals® (NPSG) program was established by The Joint Commission (TJC) in 2002 and represents the highest priorities for patient safety across the nation. NPSG are used as part of TJC's accreditation process for healthcare organizations. Table 10.1 outlines 2017's NPSG for hospitals; each healthcare setting (hospitals, long-term care, ambulatory, laboratory services, etc.) has its own set of goals. TJC also issues Elements of Performance, which further provide guidance for of standards related to each NPSG (TJC, 2018).

2. In 2008, the Joint Commission Center for Transforming Healthcare was created to assist providers to transform patient care into a higher quality healthcare delivery system "by developing highly effective, durable solutions to healthcare's most critical safety and quality problems" (Joint Commission Center for Transforming Healthcare, n.d., "Mission Statement"). The Center works collaboratively with healthcare organizations, providing support in dissemination and adoption of best practices (Joint Commission Center for Transforming Healthcare, n.d.).

C. Agency on Healthcare Research and Quality

The Agency on Healthcare Research and Quality (AHRQ) was created in 1989 as a part of the U.S. Department of Health and Human Services and was originally known as the Agency for Health Care Policy and Research. It was founded with the goal of making "health care safer, higher quality, more accessible, equitable, and affordable"

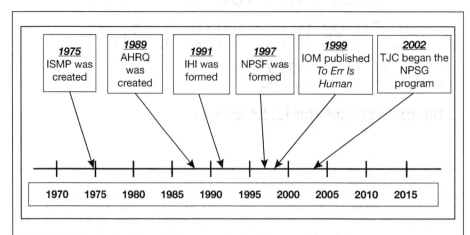

FIGURE 10.1   A timeline of milestones in the patient safety movement.

AHRQ, Agency for Healthcare Research and Quality; IHI, Institute for Healthcare Improvement; IOM, Institute of Medicine; ISMP, Institute for Safe Medication Practices; NPSF, National Patient Safety Foundation; NPSG, National Patient Safety Goals; TJC, The Joint Commission.

TABLE 10.1   2018 National Patient Safety Goals for Hospitals

General Goal	Specific Goal
Goal 1: Improve the accuracy of patient identification.	Use at least two patient identifiers when providing care, treatment, and services.
	Eliminate transfusion errors related to patient misidentification.
Goal 2: Improve the effectiveness of communication among caregivers.	Report critical results of tests and diagnostic procedures on a timely basis.
Goal 3: Improve the safety of using medications.	Label all medications, medication containers, and other solutions on and off the sterile field in perioperative and other procedural settings.
	Reduce the likelihood of patient harm associated with the use of anticoagulant therapy.
	Maintain and communicate accurate patient medication information.
Goal 6: Reduce the harm associated with clinical alarm systems.	Improve the safety of clinical alarm systems.
Goal 7: Reduce the risk of health care-associated infections.	Comply with either current Centers for Disease Control and Prevention hand-hygiene guidelines or the current World Health Organization hand-hygiene guidelines.
	Implement evidence-based practices to prevent healthcare-associated infections due to multidrug-resistant organisms in acute care hospitals.
	Implement evidence-based practices to prevent central line-associated bloodstream infections.

(continued)

TABLE 10.1 2018 National Patient Safety Goals for Hospitals *(continued)*

General Goal	Specific Goal
	Implement evidence-based practices for preventing surgical site infections.
	Implement evidence-based practices to prevent indwelling catheter-associated urinary tract infections.
Goal 15: The hospital identifies safety risks inherent in its patient population.	Identify patients at risk for suicide.
Universal Protocol: Prevent mistakes in surgery.	Conduct a preprocedure verification process.
	Mark the procedure site.
	A time-out is performed before the procedure.

Source: From The Joint Commission. (2018). 2018 National Patient Safety Goals®. Retrieved from https://www.jointcommission.org/standards_information/npsgs.aspx

(AHRQ, n.d.-a, "AHRQ Profile") by working with the U.S. government and other partners. AHRQ contributes the following to the field:

1. Publication of AHRQ Quality Indicators, which are measures that hospitals and healthcare organizations can use to benchmark themselves against other organizations in a variety of care contexts, including prevention, inpatient care, patient safety, and pediatric care

2. Development of the Consumer Assessment of Healthcare Providers and Systems (CAHPS), a patient and family experience survey tool

3. Regulation of patient safety organizations (PSOs), which are entities that "have expertise in identifying the causes of, and interventions to reduce the risk of, threats to the quality and safety of patient care" (AHRQ, n.d.-b). Healthcare organizations contract with PSOs to engage in patient safety activities, including development of protocols and recommendations, encouraging a culture of safety, and the collection and analysis of patient safety work product. By working with PSOs, organizations are protected by the a Patient Safety Act from legal liability for issues that are uncovered as part of patient safety activities.

D. National Patient Safety Foundation

The National Patient Safety Foundation (NPSF) was formed to promote "patient safety by using a systems approach to analyze human or organizational errors that may lead to patient injuries and thereby discover and eliminate their root cause" (Goldsmith, 1997, p. 1561). NPSF's contributions include:

1. Sponsorship of the annual Patient Safety Awareness Week

2. Creation of the Lucian Leape Institute, a strategic think tank

3. Establishment of the American Society of Professionals in Patient Safety (ASPPS), which provides educational resources and certification examinations in the area of patient safety (National Patient Safety Foundation, n.d.)

E. Institute for Safe Medication Practices

The Institute for Safe Medication Practices (ISMP) began medication safety efforts in 1975 and is the "nation's only ... nonprofit organization devoted entirely to medication error prevention and safe medication use" (ISMP, n.d.). ISMP's contributions include:

1. The Medication Errors Reporting Program (MERP), which is a voluntary medication error reporting program that allows identification of trends in errors and sharing of lessons learned

2. Medication safety alert newsletters for healthcare professionals and consumers

3. Production of patient and healthcare provider education materials (ISMP, n.d.)

F. Institute for Healthcare Improvement

The Institute for Healthcare Improvement (IHI) was founded in 1991 with the mission to "improve health and health care worldwide." IHI utilizes "the science of improvement" to drive change in healthcare systems; this science draws on principles from multiple disciplines, including systems theory, psychology, statistics, human factors, and clinical science. IHI's commitment to improvement is evidenced in its multiple contributions to the fields of quality and safety:

1. The Breakthrough Series, which is IHI's model to achieve rapid and dramatic change by forming learning collaboratives involves multiple healthcare organizations that can learn best practices from each other (Institute for Healthcare Improvement, 2003)

2. Open School, which offers web-based training on quality and safety topics for healthcare professionals and trainees (courses are free for IHI member institutions, and nurses can receive continuing education credit)

3. Working to achieve the Triple Aim, which improves the experience of individual patients, improves the health of the population, and reduces the cost of healthcare per capita (Berwick, Nolan, & Whittington, 2008; IHI, n.d.-b)

CREATING A CULTURE OF SAFETY IN HEALTHCARE

Singer, Lin, Falwell, Gaba, and Baker (2009) defined the safety culture of an organization as "the values shared among organization members about what is important, their beliefs about how things operate in the organization, and the interaction of these with work unit and organizational structures and systems, which together produce behavioral norms in the organization that promote safety" (p. 400). A strong safety culture has been associated with desired outcomes, including improved patient and family satisfaction and reduced patient mortality, readmissions, medication errors, and hospital-acquired pressure ulcers (PUs; DiCuccio, 2015). Table 10.2 outlines dimensions of a culture of safety in the healthcare setting. The first part of the unfolding Case Study 10.1 illustrates key points of a safety culture.

A. Person Approach Versus System Approach

Historically, "safety" in healthcare has been the responsibility of the individual practitioner, that is, with enough training and motivation, errors will not happen (Chera et al., 2016). This is known as the "person approach" to error management (Reason, 2000). However, it is unrealistic to expect humans functioning in high-risk environments like healthcare settings to do so error-free. Organizations that have adopted a

TABLE 10.2 Dimensions of a Culture of Safety in Healthcare

Safety Culture Element	Basic Tenets
Communication	Staff are encouraged to respectfully question each other (including those in positions of authority) and speak up when there is a safety concern.
Feedback	After an event is reported, staff receive communication on process and policy changes in response to the error, and how to prevent it from happening again.
Just culture	Staff feel that mistakes are not held against them, and that there is a system approach to patient safety.
Organizational learning	The organization strives to continuously improve and learn from event reports.
Staffing	There is adequate staffing to prevent errors and safety events.
Leadership expectations	Leadership at the unit and hospital levels promotes a culture of safety by prioritizing safe work, providing adequate resources, and supporting staff in managing issues.
Teamwork	Staff within and between units support one another, cooperate and coordinate, and treat each other with respect.
Handoffs	Thorough and adequate handoffs are a part of every patient transfer, shift change, and provider sign-out.

Sources: Adams-Pizarro, I., Walker, Z., Robinson, J., Kelly, S., & Toth, M. (2008). Using the AHRQ Hospital Survey on Patient Safety Culture as an intervention tool for regional clinical improvement collaboratives. In K. Henriksen, J. B. Battles, M. A. Keyes, & M. L. Grady (Eds.), *Advances in patient safety: New directions and alternative approaches* (Vol. 2: Culture and Redesign). Rockville, MD: Agency for Healthcare Research and Quality. Retrieved from https://www.ncbi.nlm.nih.gov/books/NBK43728; Burlison, J. D., Quillivan, R. R., Kath, L. M., Zhou, Y., Courtney, S. C., Cheng, C., & Hoffman, J. M. (2016). A multilevel analysis of U.S. hospital patient safety culture relationships with perceptions of voluntary event reporting. *Journal of Patient Safety.* doi:10.1097/PTS.0000000000000336

CASE STUDY 10.1   Patient Safety Introduction

Joe is a nurse orientee in a pediatric cardiac intensive care unit and is caring for a 13-year-old male in heart failure. The patient is on a ventricular assist device, and requires multiple continuous medications, including analgesia. Today is a particularly busy day, because the patient had a bronchoscopy this morning, has required multiple ventilation setting adjustments, and is being switched to a bed that will allow him to lie prone. The patient is receiving significant pain control and due to the syringe concentration is requiring syringe and line replacement every 2 hours. Prior to sending up a new syringe of hydromorphone (0.2 mg/mL) when the old one runs out, the clinical pharmacist contacts the bedside nurse (Joe's preceptor, Liz) to ask whether the medication can be switched to a higher concentration (4 mg/mL) to allow for less frequent changes. The bedside nurse agrees that the change would be appropriate, and the pharmacist collaborates with the ordering practitioner to change the order in the electronic medical record. Around 18:00, the patient begins to decompensate, and the attending physician and multiple other staff enter the room to assist with patient management and transition to the new bed. Meanwhile, the old hydromorphone syringe runs out, and Joe goes down to pharmacy to pick up the new hydromorphone. While Liz and the physician are managing the patient, Joe and a second nurse double-check the new hydromorphone and verify that the syringe matches the concentration ordered in the electronic medical record (4 mg/mL). However, they are unable to reach the medication pump to hook up the new syringe because of space constraints in the room (multiple staff and a large rotating bed). Instead, they leave the medication at the bedside for the night shift nurse, Amy, to hang. Liz provides shift change handoff to Amy, but they aren't able to do a typical double check of infusing medications and lines due to the patient status. When the patient is stabilized around 19:30, Amy hangs the syringe and restarts the pump at the previously programmed rate of 8.25 mL/hr. Amy doesn't notice the "Note Dosage Strength" sticker on the syringe. Around 20:50, Amy performs her medication double checks with a second nurse, and they realize that the hydromorphone is being infused at a higher rate than intended.

---

culture of safety have done so by moving beyond individual blame and instead focusing on system failures (Chera et al., 2016). The "system approach" to error management is rooted in the belief that errors will happen when humans are involved, and "though we cannot change the human condition, we can change the conditions under which humans work" (Reason, 2000). The second part of Case Study 10.1 outlines some system issues that contributed to the harm event.

B. Promoting a Just Culture

Although system failures often contribute to adverse events, caregivers must be held accountable for individual failures, when appropriate. A just culture is one that considers system failures as root causes for errors, yet also recognizes the need for individual accountability (Boysen, 2013; Petschonek et al., 2013). It is a balance between blamelessness and punitive action, and although this seems straightforward, it is often a fine line (Brink, 2017). Multiple approaches (Frankel, Leonard, & Denham, 2006; Marx, 2007) exist for application of just-culture principles in the wake of an adverse event or near miss. Figure 10.2 presents some key questions and considerations that can be useful in determining event response, and the third part of Case Study 10.1 shows how just-culture principles can be used in the case of patient harm.

CASE STUDY 10.1   System Issues Contributing to Harm Event (Part 2)

In this scenario, there are multiple system issues that contributed to this adverse drug event:

- Multiple hydromorphone concentrations are available.

- The patient environment was chaotic due to multiple staff present and patient deterioration.

- A new, unfamiliar bed type was being utilized, and staff required just-in-time training for use, adding to the chaotic nature of the day.

- The "Note Dosage Strength" sticker on the syringe was inadequate to alert the nurse that a concentration change had occurred.

- Barcode scanning and other technology was inadequate to prevent the new hydromorphone from being infused at the rate intended for the old concentration.

- The intensive care unit culture allowed for nurses to skip or delay bedside handoff and double check of high-risk infusions.

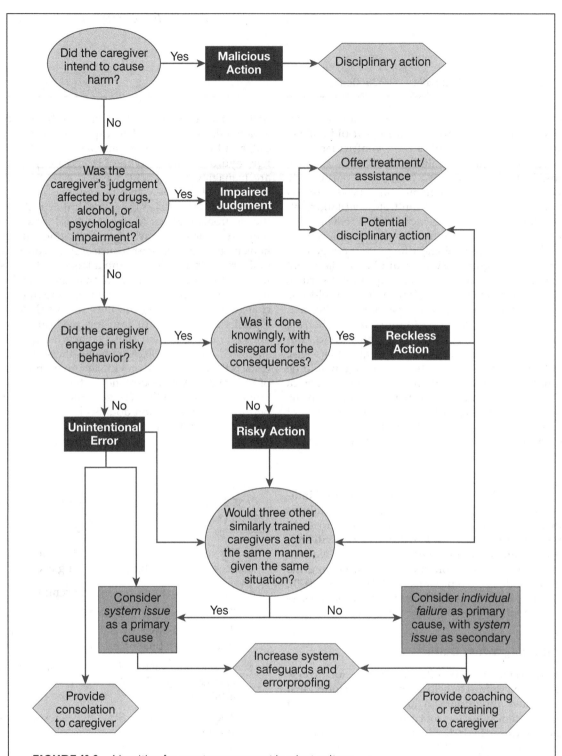

FIGURE 10.2 Algorithm for event management in a just culture.

Sources: Boysen, P. G., II. (2013). Just culture: A foundation for balanced accountability and patients safety. *Oschner Journal, 13,* 400–406 . Retrieved from https://www.ncbi.nlm.nih.gov/pmc/articles/PMC3776518; Frankel, A. S., Leonard, M. W., & Denham, C. R. (2006). Fair and just culture, team behavior, and leadership engagement: The tools to achieve high reliability. *Health Services Research, 41*(4, Pt. 2), 1690–1709. doi:10.1111/j.1475-6773.2006.00572.x

> **CASE STUDY 10.1   Application of "Just-Culture" Principles (Part 3)**
>
> This scenario lends itself to application of just culture principles. Although there were multiple system failures that contributed to this event, nursing staff, particularly trainees and orientees, can be coached to improve safety practices in the future. None of the nurses involved were acting maliciously or recklessly or were under the influence of a substance. However, Joe's manager can help him learn to assert himself by asking staff to move so he can reach the head of the bed and perform a thorough double check of the medication at the pump, and not just at the computer.

C. Understanding the Swiss Cheese Model

Indeed, the root cause of many errors in healthcare can be attributed to inadequate system design and functioning. Furthermore, it is often *several* system failures that occur (or system failures in conjunction with individual failures), allowing an adverse event to happen. This is known as the "Swiss cheese model." Each line of defense in the healthcare system (training, policies/procedures, alarms, physical barriers, etc.) is akin to a slice of cheese in a stack. Holes in one slice are inconsequential because the other slices prevent the adverse event from reaching the patient. However, on occasion, the holes of the slices align such that an error finds a path through the stack of slices and affects a patient (Reason, 2000).

1. *Latent Errors.* These are system issues that lie dormant until they are combined with an active, individual error to cause an adverse event. Examples include inadequate policies and procedures, suboptimal staffing, an unsafe work environment, or a lack of safety culture in the organization (S. J. Collins, Newhouse, Porter, & Talsma, 2014).

2. *Active Errors.* There are individual failures that, when combined with latent errors, have the potential to produce harm to a patient. Factors that contribute to active errors include fatigue, stress, inexperience, inadequate training, distractions, and disregard for policies and procedures (S. J. Collins et al., 2014).

D. Strategies to Reduce Errors

Some errors are inevitable, but many are preventable. There are some specific strategies that can be used on the front lines of healthcare to reduce the "holes in the Swiss cheese."

1. Implement clear, evidence-based policies and procedures.

2. Develop and use checklists, especially in procedural areas (S. J. Collins et al., 2014).

3. Identify situations in which staff commonly use workarounds; adjust workflow to optimize patient safety and system capability, while reducing staff frustration and workflow burden (Seaman & Erlen, 2015).

4. Reduce practice variation and consistently implement evidence-based practice (EBP) by implementing protocols, algorithms, guidelines, clinical pathways and bundles (Buchert & Butler, 2016; Institute for Healthcare Improvement, 2017).

5. Provide distraction-free work zones, particularly in those areas in which high-risk activities occur, such as in medication preparation areas (Connor et al., 2016).

6. Provide simulation training for high-stakes, chaotic, and dynamic situations that have the potential to produce patient harm (Deutsch et al., 2016)

7. Utilize *Failure and Mode Effects Analysis (FMEA)*, which is a tool that proactively assesses processes to determine risk and prevent errors or harm from occurring. FMEA is most often used for new processes or those being significantly revamped. IHI includes a more detailed FMEA template in its QI Essentials Toolkit (available to member institutions at www.ihi.org), but the basic steps are as follows (Institute for Healthcare Improvement, 2017a):

    a. Convene a multidisciplinary team.

    b. List all of the steps in the process of interest.

    c. For each step, determine potential failure modes (how things could go wrong).

    d. For each failure mode, determine causes and consequences (why things could go wrong and what would happen if they did).

    e. Utilize a scoring scale to determine how likely the event is to happen, how detrimental the consequences would be if it did happen, and how likely current systems would be to detect the failure if it did happen.

    f. Assign a summary "risk priority number" based on scores from the scoring scale (likelihood score × severity score × detection score).

    g. Prioritize and implement action plans based on those failure modes with the highest risk priority number.

E. Learning From Event Reporting and Huddles

According to James Reason, creator of the Swiss cheese model, "effective risk management depends crucially on establishing a reporting culture" (Reason, 2000, p. 768). That is, system issues can only be identified when frontline staff report adverse events, near misses, or situations that have the potential to produce patient harm. VRS are commonly used in healthcare organizations to capture these safety events. However, there are multiple barriers to staff use of VRS, including (N. Miller et al., 2017):

1. Fear of the consequences, which can include disciplinary action and negative reactions from patients or colleagues: "I don't want to be blamed for something that wasn't my fault."

2. Lack of feedback about the root cause of the event and how it can be prevented in the future: "No one ever keeps staff in the loop of what's being done to prevent events like this from happening again."

3. Lack of understanding about what types of events (i.e., near misses) should be reported: "The patient wasn't actually harmed, so I don't need to report it."

4. Doubt that action will be taken in response to the event report: "Those event reports go into a black hole and no one ever looks at them or does anything about them."

Hospitals can overcome lack of VRS use by enhancing elements of their safety culture (Table 10.2). Literature suggests that increased voluntary reporting is associated with staff perceptions of feedback about errors, management support for patient safety, organizational learning, a just culture, and teamwork within a given unit (Burlison et al., 2016; N. Miller et al., 2017).

"Huddles" or debriefings may be a useful way to follow up with staff after event reports. This opportunity can allow for event investigation and brainstorming of prevention strategies, and/or can instill a sense of closure after a particularly traumatic event (McQuaid-Hanson & Pian-Smith, 2017). Although debriefing is most often used in simulation training, adverse events can be reduced after inception of a standardized huddle process (Blankenship Harrison, Brandt, Joy, & Simsic, 2016; Morvay et al., 2014).

F. Safety II: The New Frontier

"Safety I" is an umbrella term for the historical approach of patient safety and is characterized by a focus on failures. Safety I seeks to eliminate adverse events through identification of potential or actual adverse events, determination of root cause of the event, and development of plans to mitigate future risk (which often involves training, work standardization, or development of policies and procedures; Braithwaite, Wears, & Hollnagel, 2015; McNab, Bowie, Morrison, & Ross, 2016; Patterson & Deutsch, 2015). However, multiple experts in the patient safety field have begun to question whether the Safety I approach is adequate for healthcare because of the following reasons:

1. Patient safety is not just the absence of adverse events. Without minimizing the seriousness of adverse events, it is clear that most interactions between a patient and the healthcare system actually end in a safe outcome. Patient safety must also be the study of how and when things go right (Braithwaite et al., 2015; McNab et al., 2016; Patterson & Deutsch, 2015).

2. In traditional safety thinking, it is assumed that if the system inputs function correctly (technology, caregivers, protocols, etc.), the system will yield outputs without defect (i.e., patient encounters without adverse events). In fact, there is evidence to the contrary. Even in systems in which components function as intended, adverse events can happen, "due to the way that goals and context change" (McNab et al., 2016, p. 446).

3. Policies, procedures, and standardization of work (via protocols, guidelines, algorithms, etc.) are not fool-proof methods of ensuring patient safety.

a. These tools can rarely account for all context variations and individual patient scenarios. As such, humans will always be looked upon to be agile and innovative in healthcare settings where there is no guidance, or where traditional guidance is not relevant because of the setting or context (i.e., resource limitations, dramatic changes in patient volume, etc.; McNab et al., 2016).

b. In some cases, work standardization (i.e., checklists) can prevent optimal patient outcome, because the checklist is completed without critical thinking and situational awareness. That is, the caregiver's attention is on the checklist and not the patient. The caregiver may miss subtle clinical signs and may have a false sense of security in the checklist (Patterson & Deutsch, 2015).

c. If protocols are blindly followed for the sake of compliance, the system may miss an opportunity to implement an adaptation that would actually result in an improved patient outcome (McNab et al., 2016).

4. Methodologies used in Safety I were conceived in industries that are less complex and operate in a more linear fashion than healthcare.

a. Healthcare is an increasingly complex environment with multiple stakeholders, including providers, patients, regulatory organizations, and payers. There are multiple external influences, including the media, the season, and even the weather (McNab et al., 2016).

b. Events in healthcare occur in a nonlinear fashion (Patterson & Deutsch, 2015) versus a car manufacturing plant where A always happens before B, which always occurs before C, and so on.

c. It is generally not possible to break down a healthcare system into its individual components in order to understand the how each part and unit work together (McNab et al., 2016); the whole is more (complex) than the sum of its parts.

d. The industry's substrates (patients) are unique and may react in different ways to standard work (for instance, a patient may refuse the standard of care or may react different than another patient to a commonly used medication).

e. In healthcare, functioning is usually compared with "work-as-imagined" rather than "work-as-done" (McNab et al., 2016). "Work-as-imagined" often fails to consider the real-world situations that caregivers face, such as staffing shortages, medication and resource shortages, equipment malfunction, patient treatment adherence, and so on (Braithwaite et al., 2015).

f. Because of some of the limitations of Safety I, patient safety experts have begun to advocate for a balanced approach between traditional tenets of Safety I and the more contemporary thinking of "Safety II." Safety II is the study of why and how things go right in healthcare (Braithwaite et al., 2015; McNab et al., 2016; Patterson & Deutsch, 2015). Safety II was borne of "resilience engineering," a field that purports that "things usually go right because people adjust their performance to the everyday conditions they face" (McNab et al., 2016, p. 444). Those everyday conditions are "work-as-done." Some key principles of Safety II include (Braithwaite et al., 2015; McNab et al., 2016; Patterson & Deutsch, 2015):

i. Maximizing the number of events that end successfully

ii. Identifying determinants of success (workarounds, tradeoffs, etc.) that are difficult to pinpoint in complex systems like healthcare

iii. Promoting resilience, which is the ability to react and adjust to changes and "thereby sustain required operations under both expected and unexpected conditions" (Patterson & Deutsch, 2015, p. 387)

iv. Understanding how variations in care may be warranted and should not be seen simply as blatant, unwarranted deviations from the standard of care

g. Safety II is not meant to replace Safety I; rather, the two are meant to exist in a complementary fashion to achieve desired outcomes. It is undoubtedly necessary to understand why adverse events occur and to try to prevent them from happening in the future; however, this approach does not tell the whole story of patient safety. Focusing only on principles of Safety I may cause us to miss the opportunity to learn how caregivers in the healthcare system can adapt in dynamic, unexpected, and resource-constrained situations to achieve optimal outcomes. McNab et al. (2016) and Patterson and Deutsch (2015) suggested the following strategies to introduce Safety II into healthcare:

i. While investigating adverse events, also consider cases that yielded a successful outcome.

ii. Do not automatically assume that standardization is the best way to react to an adverse event. We should "prioritize managing variability rather than simply eliminating it. Flexible ways of working that are beneficial can be encouraged (as long as people are mindful of risks and responsibilities)" (McNab et al., 2016, p. 447).

iii. Incorporate resilience engineering activities into adverse event prevention efforts by practicing skills and critical thinking (i.e., simulation and real-time feedback) and debriefing after events (part four of Case Study 10.1).

CASE STUDY 10.1 Event Response and Follow-Up (Part 4)

As soon as the error was realized, management reports the event in the hospital's event reporting system. Medication safety leadership begins to investigate the event by reviewing the infusion pump memory and the electronic medical record. A huddle is convened within a week of the incident, and relevant parties work together to discover elements of the event's context that led to the adverse event (system failures) as well as opportunities in which individuals could have prevented the error. The team also considers other high-risk situations in which staff naturally adapt to prevent an error like this from happening (they attempt to learn from successes). An action plan is developed and staff will be educated about the incident and prevention strategies.

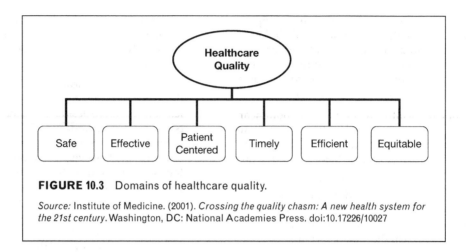

FIGURE 10.3 Domains of healthcare quality.

Source: Institute of Medicine. (2001). *Crossing the quality chasm: A new health system for the 21st century.* Washington, DC: National Academies Press. doi:10.17226/10027

G. Safety as a Domain of Quality

Quality and *safety* are terms often used together, and indeed the concepts are closely intertwined. Many, including the IOM (2001), consider safety to be an element of quality (Figure 10.3). The World Health Organization [WHO] (2009) defines *quality* as "the degree to which health services for individuals and populations increase the likelihood of desired health outcomes and are consistent with current professional knowledge." Although WHO (2009) uses a Safety I-minded definition of patient safety ("the reduction of risk of unnecessary harm associated with healthcare to an acceptable minimum"), we know that an emerging definition of patient safety (in accordance with Safety II) is centered around maximizing the number of healthcare occurrences that end successfully. Patient safety's new focus on increasing desirable outcomes rather than minimizing failures further aligns healthcare safety with healthcare quality.

As presented in Figure 10.3, the five other quality domains according to IOM (2001) are:

1. *Effective.* Providing evidence-based care to those patient populations that would benefit

2. *Patient Centered.* Providing care that takes into consideration the patient's wants, needs, values, and beliefs and involving the patient as a key decision maker in all treatment decisions

3. *Timely.* Reducing delays in care provision

4. *Efficient.* Reducing waste (including equipment, supplies, manpower, time, etc.)

5. *Equitable.* Providing care to all patients, regardless of gender, socioeconomic status, race, ethnicity, or location

LEARNING FROM ULTRA-SAFE, HIGH-RELIABILITY INDUSTRIES

Certain industries, including nuclear power, commercial aviation, and railway transportation, are considered "ultra-safe," with less than one death per million exposures (Amalberti, Auroy, Berwick, & Barach, 2005). These industries are also considered to be high-reliability organizations (HROs), because they are characterized by operations that are high risk, yet have very few adverse events (Amalberti et al., 2005; Lekka, 2011; Yip & Farmer, 2015). However, this has not always been the case. For instance, in 1959, U.S. airline passengers experienced 40 fatal crashes per 1 million flights. By 1970, this reduced to less than two per 1 million flights, and today is at 0.1 per 1 million flights (S. Collins, 2015). Undoubtedly, improvements in aviation technology have contributed to this drastic improvement in passenger safety, but work done in the area of human factors deserves equal attention, particularly when considering applications of aviation safety work in the field of healthcare.

In the 1970s, the National Aeronautics and Space Administration (NASA) determined that 70% of aviation safety events were due to human errors, more specificly, to failures in teamwork, decision making, and leadership (American Psychological Association, 2014). As such, multiple strategies and tools have emerged to establish a culture of safety in the aviation industry (MacDonald, 2016; Rutherford, 2003).

A. Strategies to Achieve a Culture of Safety in the Aviation Industry

1. An understanding that errors *will* happen when humans are involved; HROs have a preoccupation with failure (Reason, 2000) and don't just accept

that failures are part of doing business (Chassin & Loeb, 2013)

2. Increase in transparency and establishment of the expectation that events and "near misses" be reported (Rutherford, 2003)

3. Increase in standardization of work and processes (reduction in autonomy of the pilot) (Rutherford, 2003) coupled with deference to expertise (usually at the front line and not at the top of the organizational hierarchy), when appropriate (Chassin & Loeb, 2013)

4. Leveraging the power of the team, rather than an individual, to optimize safety and prevent errors

5. "Sensitivity to operations," which means the organization is in tune to even small anomalies that can evolve into major issues (Chassin & Loeb, 2013)

6. Introduction of *crew resource management (CRM)*, which encompasses use of all available resources (human, data, technology, equipment, etc.) to optimize safety (Rutherford, 2003); rather than focusing on the technical skills of the pilot, CRM teaches the crew how to leverage cognitive (decision making and situational awareness) and interpersonal skills (communication and teamwork) to prevent errors; key principles of CRM include (Crew Resource Management, n.d.-a, n.d.-b):

   a. Leadership and teamwork

   b. Effective and standardized communication

   c. Situational awareness

   d. Informed decision making

   e. Team briefings and debriefings

   f. Conflict resolution

   g. Use of critical language

   h. Threat and error management

   i. Recognition of stress and fatigue

B. Translation to Healthcare

There are many similarities between aviation and healthcare (Table 10.3). As such, patient safety experts have sought to translate aviation tools and processes into the healthcare setting (Table 10.4). However, there are also important differences between the two industries. There is a fundamental tradeoff between productivity and safety (sometimes referred to as the *efficiency–thoroughness tradeoff* [McNab et al., 2016]), and in healthcare, the pendulum does not always swing in the direction of safety. If an airline crew has exceeded work time limits, flights can be delayed or canceled, but if a surgeon has been operating all night or there are staffing shortages, emergency surgeries and care of the ICU patient cannot be delayed because of concerns for patient safety.

The Joint Commission Center for Transforming Healthcare, by working with experts in high-reliability science, suggests the following as key elements for healthcare organizations seeking to become HROs:

   1. The leadership of the organization must commit to prioritizing elimination of patient harm. This fulfills one of the characteristics of an HRO—preoccupation with failure and an unrelenting desire to improve performance and safety (Chassin & Loeb, 2013).

   2. The organization must embrace and perpetuate a culture of safety. This likely involves assessing the current state using a safety culture survey, but should not stop there. Instead, leaders should use survey results to determine opportunities for improvement in the areas of teamwork, communication, respect, training, and stress recognition (Chassin & Loeb, 2013).

   3. The organization must adopt and disseminate effective methods for quality and process improvement. TJC calls this "robust process improvement," and asserts that a blend of Lean, Six Sigma, and change management methodologies are most effective (Chassin & Loeb, 2013).

TABLE 10.3   Similarities Between Aviation and Healthcare

- The stakes are high
- Life-and-death decisions must be made quickly
- Technology is heavily relied upon, but can be lethal when misused
- Operators are highly skilled, independent, and assertive
- Embodies a traditionally hierarchical nature, with deference to the team leader (physician or pilot)
- Overcrowding and service delays

Sources: McKeon, L. M., Cunningham, P. D., & Detty Oswaks, J. S. (2009). Improving patient safety: Patient-focused, high-reliability team training. *Journal of Nursing Care Quality, 24*(1), 76–82. doi:10.1097/NCQ.0b013e31818f5595; Rutherford, W. (2003). Aviation safety: A model for health care? *BMJ Quality and Safety in Health Care, 12*, 162–163. doi:10.1136/qhc.12.3.162

TABLE 10.4   The Use of Aviation Safety Tools in Healthcare

Domain	Example	Barriers to Implementation in Healthcare
Transparency and event reporting	• Event reporting systems that facilitate identification of system issues • Safety records are publicly available • Event reporting is mandatory, not optional	• Providers are hesitant to self-report due to fear of consequences, i.e., litigation, patient reaction, or judgment by peers
Standardization of work	• Use of checklists • Use of algorithms, decision trees, and protocols • Idea that the success of the event (flight, surgical procedure, etc.) is not dependent on the players; i.e., one pediatric surgeon is as good as another	• Providers are resistant to a reduction in professional autonomy • Patients have a relationship with a particular physician and would not willingly accept a substitution
Leveraging the team	• Airline crew members are expected to "speak up" if there is a safety concern; any crew member can halt operations	• Healthcare has a hierarchical nature

Source: Chera, B. S., Mazur, L., Adams, R. D., Kim, H. J., Milowsky, M. I., & Marks, L. B. (2016). Creating a culture of safety within an institution: Walking the walk. *Journal of Oncology Practice, 12*(10), 880–883. doi:10.1200/jop.2016.012864

APPLYING QI METHODOLOGY TO IMPROVE PATIENT SAFETY

Multiple models exist to facilitate QI efforts (Table 10.5). Six Sigma and Lean are the most recognized and were both developed for manufacturing settings (electronics and automotive, respectively). The Model for Improvement (MFI) was developed more recently for a variety of settings, including healthcare (Langley et al., 2009), and it is the model that has been adopted by IHI. This section focuses on utilization of the MFI to drive change in hospitals, although, in reality, most healthcare organizations actually blend tools and approaches from more than one model.

A. Assemble a Project Team

Prior to beginning QI efforts, it is critical to assemble a project team of relevant stakeholders, subject matter experts, and frontline staff who understand work-as-done. Including the individuals increases buy-in and enhances the project's likelihood of success (Crowl Sharma, Sorge, & Sorensen, 2015; Dixon & Pearce, 2011). Case Study 10.2 introduces a project to reduce pressure injuries in the ICU setting.

B. Scope and Plan the Project

The MFI is shown in Figure 10.4. The first part of the model involves answering three questions to scope and plan the project, and the second part utilizes multiple, iterative Plan–Do–Study–Act (PDSA) cycles to attempt small tests of change before changes are implemented system-wide.

1. What are we trying to accomplish?

By answering this question, the project team determines the project aim statement (Langley et al., 2009). An effective aim statement should be SMART—specific, measurable, attainable, realistic, and time-bound. Aim statements should identify the population of interest for the project, as well as the baseline and goal levels. The second part of Case Study 10.2 provides an example of an appropriate aim statement.

2. How will we know that a change is an improvement?

The second step involves development of measures for the project. Measurement is a critical part of any QI project, and informs the team if changes are producing the desired result. There are three types of measures commonly used in QI work (Langley et al., 2009):

a. *Outcome measures.* These quantify how the system impacts patients (i.e., average cholesterol levels, percentage of patients readmitted to the hospital within 7 days of discharge, adverse event rates, and mortality rates).

b. *Process measures.* These measure whether the components of a system are performing as intended or if processes are completed as intended (i.e., percentage of patients who receive nutrition counseling, percentage of patients who receive standardized medication reconciliation upon discharge, and adherence to medication barcode scanning procedures).

TABLE 10.5 Methodologies Used in Quality Improvement

Improvement Methodology	Basic Principles
Model for Improvement	Part 1: Addresses three basic questions: 　a. What are we trying to improve? 　b. What can we measure so we know that we're making an improvement? 　c. What changes can we make to drive improvement? Part 2: Uses PDSA cycles as small tests of change to rapidly pilot potential interventions in real-world situations
Six Sigma	Focuses on reducing process variation to less than 3.4 defects per million opportunities
Lean	Focuses on culture and behavior change to identify and eliminate waste in a process

PDSA, plan, do, study, act.

CASE STUDY 10.2 An Example of Quality-Improvement Project to Reduce Pressure Injuries

In the pediatric ICU (PICU) at a Children's Hospital, the pressure injury rate is two injuries per 100 patient days, which is almost twice the benchmark rate for other children's hospitals. The nursing leadership of the PICU determines this to be a focus area for QI efforts. To begin the project, the PICU manager assembles a team of bedside nurses, attending physicians, advanced practice nurses (APNs), respiratory therapists, and wound/ostomy care nurses, all of whom are passionate about reducing preventable harm.

CASE STUDY 10.2 Sample Aim Statement for a Pressure Injury Reduction Project (Part 2)

The PICU pressure injury team develops the following aim statement for their project:

Reduce pressure injury (stage II–IV, unstageable, and deep tissue injury) rates in the pediatric ICU population from a baseline of two injuries per 100 patient days to a goal of one injury per 100 patient days in the next 12 months and sustain this change for 12 months.

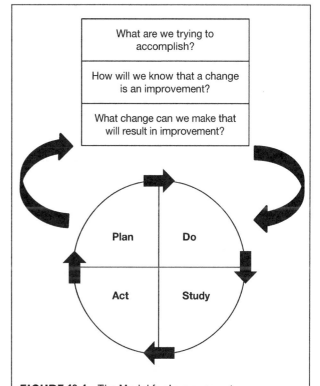

FIGURE 10.4   The Model for Improvement.

Source: Langley, G. L., Moen, R., Nolan, K. M., Nolan, T. W., Norman, C. L., & Provost, L. P. (2009). *The improvement guide: A practical approach to enhancing organizational performance* (2nd ed.). San Francisco, CA: John Wiley and Sons.

3. What changes can we make that will result in improvement?

Teams can determine potential interventions by first exploring why the system isn't currently performing at desired levels. Multiple tools can be employed; three of the most commonly used are presented here (Langley et al., 2009):

c. *Balancing measures.* These measure whether changes to one part of the system inadvertently and negatively affect another part of the system (i.e., by decreasing hospital readmission rates, we inadvertently increase hospital length of stay).

a. *Fishbone (Ishikawa or cause-and-effect) diagrams* (Figure 10.5). This type of diagram categories potential reasons for suboptimal performance into like categories. Not all individual reasons or whole categories are modifiable or can have associated interventions, but it is useful to put them on the diagram in order to understand all of the factors that affect the system.

b. *Process-flow map.* This is a flow chart that depicts the steps in a process and is useful in determining waste or inefficient processes.

c. *Pareto charts* (Figure 10.6). This type of chart quantitatively depicts characteristics of a given system, such as reasons for pressure injuries, and can help a project team determine where to target initial interventions. The

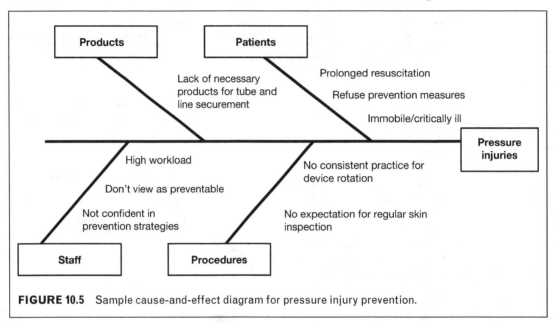

FIGURE 10.5 Sample cause-and-effect diagram for pressure injury prevention.

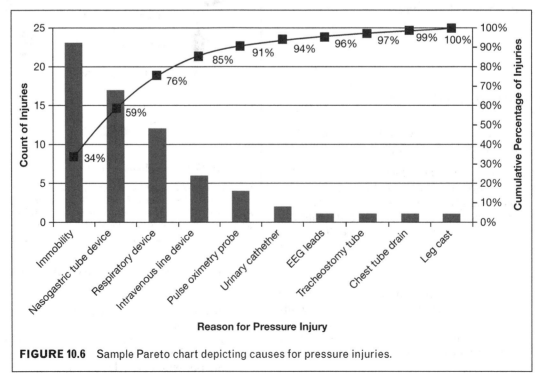

FIGURE 10.6 Sample Pareto chart depicting causes for pressure injuries.

Pareto rule states that 80% of problems (or variations) are due to 20% of reasons (part 3 of Case Study 10.2).

Dixon and Pearce (2011) provide additional tools that can be used in healthcare QI, as well as a matrix that will help the reader decide which tools are helpful in which improvement situations. For member institutions, IHI offers a QI Essentials Tooklit, which contains templates for common QI tools, on their website (www.ihi.org).

The results borne of these tools can help the group determine the project's key drivers, which are the main leverage points that, when optimized, should result in aim achievement. Key drivers are the "whats." Once key drivers are determined, interventions (the "hows") relating to each driver can be determined and prioritized. All of these elements can be depicted on a key driver diagram (KDD; Figure 10.7), which serves as an ever-evolving, dynamic project roadmap (fourth part of Case Study 10.2).

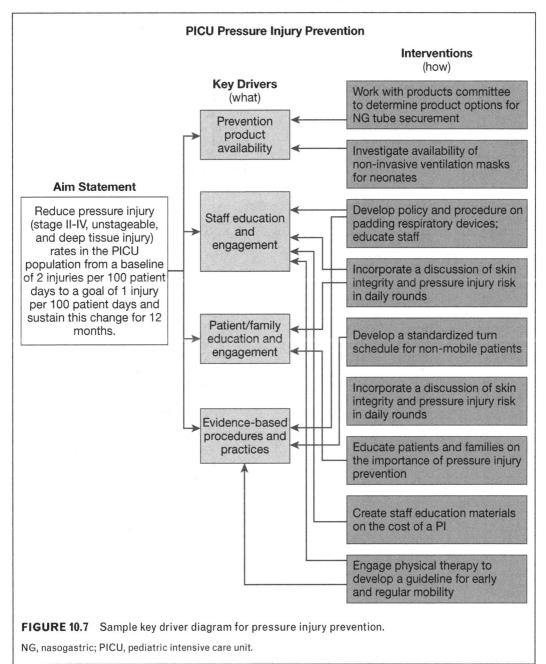

FIGURE 10.7 Sample key driver diagram for pressure injury prevention.

NG, nasogastric; PICU, pediatric intensive care unit.

C. Begin Small Tests of Change

A PDSA cycle is a powerful tool used to rapidly test potential process changes and interventions and to obtain knowledge to answer any of the three questions that are part of the MFI. Of note, some interventions will not require PDSA cycles, but many will, especially those that are complex and affect many stakeholders. PDSA cycles are particularly useful in understanding whether a particular intervention has the capability to produce desired improvement in a certain context and

---

CASE STUDY 10.2   Measures for a Pressure Injury Reduction Project (Part 3)

The PICU pressure injury team chooses the following measures for their project:

Outcome measure: Pressure injury rate per 100 PICU patient days

Process measure: Percentage of patients following the evidence-based practice prevention bundle

Balancing measure: Unplanned extubation rate associated with increased frequency of patient turning and repositioning

---

CASE STUDY 10.2   Intervention Planning for the Pressure Injury Reduction Project (Part 4)

The PICU pressure injury team brainstorms potential reasons for events in their population and they develop the cause-and-effect diagram seen in Figure 10.6. The Pareto chart (Figure 10.7) is created based on the baseline data and shows that about 80% of the injuries are caused by three reasons: immobility, nasogastric tubes, and respiratory devices. Using the categories in the cause-and-effect diagram, key drivers are identified and a KDD (Figure 10.8) is created. Based on the most common causes of pressure injuries, the group brainstorms and prioritizes interventions in order to begin its first PDSA cycle.

CASE STUDY 10.2   A Plan–Do–Study–Act Cycle for Pressure Injury Reduction (Part 5)

Because most of the pressure injuries in the PICU are due to immobility, the PICU pressure injury team decides to design and test an intervention that would affect immobility-related pressure injuries. More specific, they decide to test a turning schedule, which relates both to their key drivers of staff engagement and education and evidence-based procedures and practices. Their PDSA cycle happens as follows:

1. *Plan*
   a. Objective: Test the implementation of a turning schedule on PICU patients
   b. Who: Sarah Smith, RN
   c. What: Turn one PICU patient every 2 hours
   d. When: During her 12-hour shift on February 1
   e. Hypothesis: We hypothesize that Sarah will be successful in turning her dayshift patient every 2 hours

2. *Do*
   a. On February 1, Sarah completed the test of change with a 1-month-old infant with increased work of breathing due to respiratory syncytial virus.

3. *Study*
   a. At first, Sarah found it hard to remember to turn the patient every 2 hours. This became easier once she added it to her to-do list.

The patient's mother was hesitant for Sarah to disturb the baby while he was sleeping.

4. *Act*
   a. Modify the turning protocol to every 3 to 4 hours for infants, so that turning can be aligned with other cares, like feedings and diaper changes.
   b. Sarah will try the new schedule with her next infant patient and will enlist another bedside nurse to implement the turning schedule with one of her patients.

The PDSA cycles continue until the new turning schedule (every 2 hours for older kids and every 3 to 4 hours for infants) is spread throughout the PICU. Over time, the PICU finds stage I pressure injuries earlier than before, and can implement interventions to prevent progression to stage II and higher. Over time, their rate of pressure injury due to immobility decreases, and other critical care units in the hospital become interested in implementing a similar turning schedule. The PICU moves on to PDSA other interventions that could prevent injuries due to nasogastric tube and respiratory device securement. The team tracks the outcome measure (pressure injury rate), the process measure (adherence to the turning schedule protocol), and balancing measures (rate of unplanned extubations due to patient repositioning).

to evaluate the unintended consequences and costs of a process change. Cycles can begin with an "n of 1," and ramp up in an iterative fashion, affecting more patients and broader contexts (Langley et al., 2009). Unlike traditional research methodology, PDSA cycles do not require one large, controlled, randomized intervention. Rather, the interventions evolve over time after collecting data and learning from prior cycles (IHI, n.d.-a).

The steps of a PDSA cycle are outlined as follows and are exemplified in the fifth part of Case Study 10.2 (Langley et al., 2009):

1. *Plan*
   a. Determine the purpose of the test.
   b. Generate a hypothesis about what will happen and why.
   c. Develop a plan (who, what, where, and when) to implement the test of change.

2. *Do*
   a. Try out the test on a small scale (i.e., one patient, one clinic session, one provider, one set of morning rounds, etc.).
   b. Document the outcome.

3. *Study*
   a. Compare the data with the prediction.
   b. Summarize the findings.

4. *Act*
   a. Adjust the change based on the results of the "study."
   b. Plan for the next test, which could involve:
      i. Retooling the intervention and trying again on the same scale
      ii. Refining the intervention and trying again on a slightly larger scale
      iii. Spreading the intervention in varied contexts

D. Measure Changes Over Time

The most widely used method of tracking changes in data over time is the run chart (sixth part of Case Study 10.2; see Figure 10.8). A run chart is a graphical display of data organized in sequence, with the x-axis representing a unit of measure (months, quarters, days, or consecutive patients) and the y-axis representing the measure being tracked (infection rate, percentage of patients adherent to a treatment bundle, or satisfaction scores, etc.). Run charts are powerful because data are plotted over time, so QI teams can see changes in measures in relation to PDSA cycles and intervention implementation.

CASE STUDY 10.2 Measuring Change in the Pressure Injury Reduction Project (Part 6)

The team tracks the outcome measure (pressure injury rate), the process measure (adherence to the turning schedule protocol), and balancing measure (rate of unplanned extubations due to patient repositioning) using a run chart. An example is provided in Figure 10.8. The team identifies that a change has happened in the system, resulting in first a downward trend and then a downward shift in the pressure injury rate. They postulate that these nonrandom changes in the rate are due to their QI efforts.

In addition, established rules of run chart interpretation allow project teams to distinguish between random and nonrandom variation in their data. Identification of nonrandom variation signals a true change in the system, which could be related to intended changes as part of a QI project or to confounding variables. Two of the most common signals of nonrandom variation include the shift and the trend (Perla, Provost, & Murray, 2011).

1. A *shift* is characterized by multiple (6–8) consecutive data points either above or below the run chart's median value.

2. A *trend* is characterized by five consecutive data points all going up or all going down.

Statistical process control refers to a set of statistical tools and principles used to aid in improvement work, but a full discussion is out of the scope of this chapter. *The Healthcare Data Guide* by Provost and Murray (2011) is an excellent reference on this topic.

RECENT PEDIATRIC QUALITY AND SAFETY INITIATIVES

Multiple pediatric-focused collaboratives have found success in improving clinical outcomes through the use of QI methodology (i.e., the MFI and the IHI Breakthrough Series) and high-reliability practices (Billett et al., 2013). These networks pool data from multiple institutions and accelerate learning and improvement by sharing ideas and information. Each collaborative is founded on transparency of outcomes and a commitment to learning from each other (an "all teach, all learn" mentality). Most have regular webinars or conference calls with periodic in-person learning sessions to facilitate information-sharing. Member hospitals routinely report outcome and process data to a

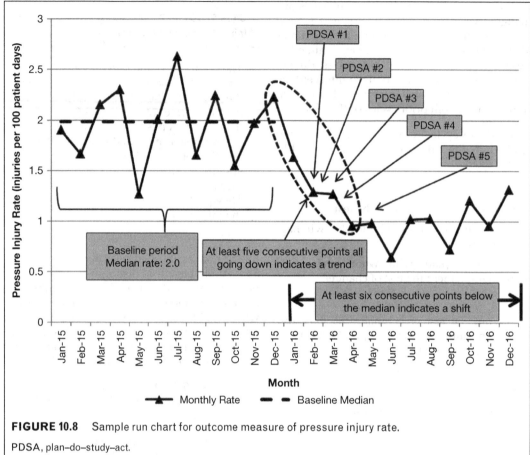

FIGURE 10.8   Sample run chart for outcome measure of pressure injury rate.

PDSA, plan–do–study–act.

Source: Perla, R. J., Provost, L. P., & Murray, S. K. (2011). The run chart: A simple analytical tool for learning from variation in healthcare processes. *BMJ Quality & Safety, 20*(1), 46–51. doi:10.1136/bmjqs.2009.037895. With permission from BMJ Publishing Group Ltd.

central registry, which allows examination of data for the entire population, but also facilitates stratification of data into high performers and low performers. With this approach, low performers can seek out and learn from those centers that are performing well. Presented here are a few examples of successful pediatric-focused quality collaboratives.

A. Solutions for Patient Safety

In 2009, eight pediatric referral centers formed the Ohio Children's Hospitals Solutions for Patient Safety (OCHSPS), an organization focused on reducing harm in pediatric patients. Initially, prevention bundles were created and implemented for surgical site infections (SSIs) and adverse drug events (ADEs). In 2010, OCHSPS began efforts to reduce serious safety events (SSE) as a third harm domain; SSEs are those that result in serious patient harm as a result of a deviation from the standard of care or recognized best practice (Lyren, Brilli, Bird,

Lashutka, & Muething, 2016). In 2012, the OCHSPS spread to a national forum by adding 25 hospitals from outside the state of Ohio, forming Solutions for Patient Safety (SPS; n.d.-a). SPS now has membership in over 100 children's hospitals across the United States and Canada and, as shown in Table 10.6, works to reduce the incidence of multiple hospital-acquired conditions (SPS, n.d.-a, n.d.-b).

B. ImproveCareNow

The ImproveCareNow Network (www.improvecarenow .org) focuses on the care of children with inflammatory bowel disease (IBD), including Crohn's disease and ulcerative colitis. Initially, the network focused on standardization of diagnostic criteria, disease severity definitions, and evaluation of nutrition status. Later, the network developed standardized recommendations for medication and nutrition management. By reducing variation and implementing EBP in a consistent

TABLE 10.6   Patient Harm Reduction in the Solutions for Patient Safety Collaborative

Harm Domain	Data as of December 2017
Overall harm	Savings of over $162 million Prevented harm in 9,677 children
Adverse drug events	64% reduction
Catheter-associated urinary tract infections	59% reduction
Falls with moderate or greater injury	81% reduction
Pressure injuries	26% reduction
Surgical site infections	31% reduction

Source: Solutions for Patient Safety. (n.d.-b). Our results. Retrieved from http://www.solutionsforpatientsafety.org

manner, the network observed an increase in the proportion of patients with IBD who were in remission (Crandall et al., 2012). At present, there are more than 100 centers across the globe participating in the network (ImproveCareNow, n.d.).

C. National Pediatric Cardiology Quality Improvement Collaborative

The National Pediatric Cardiology Quality Improvement Collaborative (NPC-QIC; https://npcqic.org) began in 2009 to improve the care of infants with hypoplastic left heart syndrome (HLHS) and similar single ventricle physiology. The collaborative has a three-part goal to (1) reduce mortality between the first and second operations in the first year of life (the "interstage"), (2) reduce interstage growth failure, and (3) reduce interstage hospitalizations for major medical events. Because HLHS is a rare heart defect, it is difficult for any one center to make conclusions about how improvements may affect clinical outcomes; as such, in this population, the data-pooling element of the collaborative is particularly helpful. NPC-QIC is unique in that it involves parents as a fundamental part of the collaborative. They feel that parents are crucial in motivating teams to achieve breakthrough levels of improvement. NPC-QIC has been successful in reducing interstage mortality by a relative 44% from baseline (Anderson et al., 2015) in its approximately 60 sites (National Pediatric Cardiology Quality Improvement Collaborative, n.d.).

D. California Perinatal Quality of Care Collaborative

The California Perinatal Quality of Care Collaborative (CPQCC) was formed in 1997 to improve health outcomes

for mothers and infants in California. Stakeholders include neonatal intensive care units (NICUs), birthing hospitals, obstetricians, private organizations (i.e., March of Dimes), public health organizations, and professional groups (i.e., California Association of Neonatologists; Gould, 2010). Using the IHI model, CPQCC has been successful in reducing overall NICU nosocomial infection rates (Wirtschafter et al., 2011) and more specific, central line-associated bloodstream infections (Wirtschafter et al., 2009), as well as improving breast milk use in very-low-birthweight infants (Lee et al., 2012). CPQCC currently has a membership of 137 hospitals and affects the care of over 90% of all neonates in California (California Perinatal Quality Care Collaborative, n.d.).

E. Pediatric Trauma Quality Improvement Program

The Pediatric Trauma Quality Improvement Program (Pediatric TQIP) is an initiative of the American College of Surgeons. The purpose of the program is to provide risk-adjusted benchmarking for pediatric and adult trauma centers that treat pediatric trauma patients in order to evaluate outcomes and improve the quality of patient care. Valid and reliable data associated with improved outcomes from the National Trauma Data Bank is provided to participating Level I and II designated trauma centers (American College of Surgeons, n.d.).

PROFESSIONAL COMMUNICATIONS THAT ENHANCE PATIENT SAFETY

A. Effective Communication

Effective communication only occurs when communication is complete, concise, accurate, timely, and relevant. The recipient must be ready to receive and potentially act on the information, and the sender must communicate in a way that respectfully yet fully shares the information.

  1. Communication in a healthcare environment must be treated differently than that which occurs during normal social interactions. It involves very private, intimate, difficult, and sometimes life-changing or even life-ending conversations.

  2. Pediatric critical care is a particularly high-stress environment in which clear communication can be key to ensuring optimal patient outcome (Blake, Searle, Robbins, Pike, & Needleman, 2013).

B. Potential Outcomes of Poor Communication

  1. According to TJC's sentinel event (defined as a catastrophic event in healthcare that should not have occurred) database, communication failures were the root cause of 70% of the sentinel events that occurred between 1994 and 2005 (Kear, 2016; Pettit & Duffy, 2015).

2. Literature has established that poor communication or lack of communication lead to a decrease in patient safety. Outcomes can include loss of critical patient information, misrepresentation of information, and delay in treatment or recognition of deterioration (Pettit & Duffy, 2015).

3. Communication errors in healthcare occur most frequently during some type of handoff or care transition.

C. Barriers to Effective Communication

Barriers are multifaceted and can be related to cultural, personality, hierarchical, behavioral, or knowledge differences. They are typically related to varying perceptions of roles, goals, and responsibilities. Breakdown in communications can also occur related to (Gordon, Deland, & Kelly, 2015):

1. Systematic complexity

2. Poor health literacy

3. Poor or incorrect recall

4. Interruption during communication

Fear of confrontation can lead many healthcare providers to hesitate to speak up when they identify a concern. They may have previously experienced intimidating or inappropriate behaviors from others after recognizing or communicating a concern, even in the face of deteriorating patient status.

In addition, situations that are not conducive to clear communication occur frequently in healthcare (Weller, Boyd, & Cumin, 2017):

1. *Geography*: The patient being discussed may be in another ICU or area, such as radiology or the operation room, and is being cared for by another employee.

2. Information shared via technology (email, emergency medical records [EMR] notes, text pages) are open to misinterpretation and minimizes the ability to ask for clarification.

3. Key players are missing during conversations, such as the bedside nurse missing rounds or a consult service being unavailable to discuss plans.

4. Cultural differences (beliefs, language, behavior, social norms) exist.

D. MD to RN Communication Barriers

Physicians and RNs experience the most frequent challenges and breakdowns in communication (Petit & Duffy, 2015). Literature demonstrates that nurses' and physicians' prelicensure education on communication styles are very different from each other (Beckett & Kipnis, 2009).

1. *Nursing Communication Style*

   a. Detailed

   b. Descriptive

   c. Emphasis placed on nursing diagnosis

   d. Focused on next " task" (i.e., drawing blood, giving medication)

2. *Physician Communication Style*

   a. Brief

   b. Factual

   c. Emphasis placed on medical diagnosis

Vertical hierarchies can impede appropriate communication channels by closing off opportunities for clarification. Individuals who are in traditionally "higher" positions of power may be concerned with appearing incompetent or unsure of their knowledge or decisions, perceive that the "subordinate" is less competent, or use silence as a way to retain their power. The subordinate in the relationship may fear appearing incompetent, disrespectful, inexperienced, or fear retaliation as a result of questioning an order or directive (Pettit & Duffy, 2015). Studies show that RNs in general are less satisfied with team communication than physicians (Blake et al., 2013).

E. Methods and Models to Improve Communications

Standardized handoffs: A 2007 TJC patient safety goal required that hospitals "implement a standardized approach to hand-off communications and provide an opportunity for staff to ask and respond to questions about a patient's care" (Pettit & Duffy, 2015, p. 24). In 2014, TJC further defined *successful handoffs* as those including:

1. Transfer from one caregiver to another with acceptance of responsibility for the patient and care

2. Handoff in real time

3. Passing of specific patient information

4. Limited interruptions

5. A process in place to verify information received

6. Ability to review historical data when needed

F. Handoff Tools

Handoffs should occur at *any point* when the patient is cared for by a different healthcare provider, even if for a very short time (i.e., lunches or during testing). Frequently utilized hand-off tools include:

1. *SBAR.* A structured communication tool that stands for "situation, background, assessment, and recommendation." This tool helps to structure information in a clear and concise format, while also allowing for the most pertinent information to be shared quickly. It can be utilized for any situation or for any communication, patient related or otherwise, and by any discipline, and still be a recognizable communication technique. In addition, it allows nurses to make communicate concerns in a respectful and collaborative manner, and to make suggestions for next steps (Beckett & Kipnis, 2009; Figure 10.9)

2. *Five Ps.* The five Ps stand for *patient, plan, precautions, problem, and precaution* (Kear, 2016)

3. *I PASS the BATON.* Introduction, patients, assessment, situation, safety concerns, background, actions, timing, ownership, next (Kear, 2016)

4. *I-PASS* (frequently taught in graduate medical education). Illness, patient summary, action list, situation awareness and contingency plans, synthesis (opportunity to ask questions; AHRQ, 2017b)

G. Additional Tools That Aid in Communication

1. *Teach-Back Method (typically utilized for families, can be effective for anyone).* Asks the other person to explain back, in his or her own words, the

S	**Situation:** What is the situation you are calling about? • Identify self, unit, patient, room number. • Briefly state the problem, what is it, when it happened or started, and how severe.	
B	**Background:** Pertinent background information related to the situation could include the following: • The admitting diagnosis and date of admission • List of current medications, allergies, IV fluids, and labs • Most recent vital signs • Lab results: provide the date and time test was done and results of previous tests for comparison • Other clinical information • Code status	
A	**Assessment:** What is the nurse's assessment of the situation?	
R	**Recommendation:** What is the nurse's recommendation or what does he/she want? Examples: • Notification that patient has been admitted • Patient needs to be seen now • Order change	

FIGURE 10.9 SBAR report to physician about a critical situation.

Source: Institute for Healthcare Improvement. (2017). SBAR: Situation-Background-Assessment- Recommendation. Retrieved from http://www.ihi.org/resources/Pages/Tools/SBARToolkit.aspx

information they have just been provided. Achieves improved retention and comprehension, and identification of incorrect understanding of the original information.

2. *Institutional Procedures and Policies.* Created to help standardize care across the institution and to decrease variation and questionable practices that are not evidenced based. Minimizes questions and can clarify communication regarding care standards and practices (Stein & Heiss, 2015).

3. *Interdisciplinary Rounding.* The rounding process allows all members of the care team to discuss progress, concerns, and care planning in a controlled environment where each team member's input is respected. For the best outcome, rounds should be done at the bedside and the patient and family should be invited to participate.

4. *Creation of Distraction-Free Zones for Communication.* Certain communications and tasks should take place in areas where staff is less likely to be interrupted, and those situations (such as report hand-off and medication administration) should be respected and untouchable.

5. *Implementation of a just culture* by senior or unit leadership of the institution/area can aid in effective communication by encouraging all employees to speak up regarding either their own actions or others' actions without fear of retaliation or reprisal, with the end goal being safe patient care. This aids the recognition of errors or improper communications (Gordon et al., 2015; Stein & Heiss, 2015). The environment created should be nonpunitive, while also encouraging individual or system-level accountability when indicated.

6. *Debriefing.* "Debriefing is defined as a dialogue between two or more people" (AHRQ, 2017a, para. 2) to review and reflect on the rationale for actions taken during specific patient care events. Clinical event debriefing has been identified by the AHRQ as a useful strategy to improve team performance, especially in emergency events, and has included debriefing in the TeamSTEPPS training program. Debriefing is an effective strategy for recognizing actions that were effective and opportunities for improvement, at individual, team, and systems levels (AHRQ, 2017a). Although real-time debriefing can be difficult to operationalize, it is a valuable educational tool for QI.

TEAMWORK—LEVERAGING MULTIDISCIPLINARY TEAMS AND GROUPS

Teamwork is defined as the way in which a team's members are able to coordinate effort in order produce a "synchronized" output (Reader, Flin, Mearns, & Cuthbertson, 2009). The increased complexity of healthcare over the past 20 years has led the industry to realize the value of teamwork in quality and patient safety. Healthcare has moved from a traditionally hierarchical model to one that requires knowledge, skills, and input from all members of the healthcare team to achieve optimal patient outcomes. Each member must be accountable for his and her own actions and participate equally in the team to succeed (Lighter, 2011).

1. Communication failure between team members is the number one reason for poor collaboration (Weller, Boyd, & Cumin, 2014).

2. Poor collaboration between team members increases patient morbidity and mortality (Blake et al., 2013; Weller et al., 2014).

3. Poor collaboration among caregivers in ICUs is associated with significantly lower nurse turnover and intention to leave (Blake et al., 2013).

A. Identified Barriers to Effective Teamwork in an ICU Environment:

1. Shiftwork

2. Educational rotations (particularly of physicians)

3. Staff attrition

4. Inappropriate power dynamics

5. Poor or ineffective communication

6. Poor understanding of roles and responsibilities

7. Emotional exhaustion/moral distress

8. Constraints of resources or time

9. Increasing patient complexity and acuity

10. Discipline-specific backgrounds (can lead to differing goals/processes)

The list identifies a few barriers that can be outside of the control of team members regardless of effectiveness. Strategies to improve collaboration may need to be adjusted to accommodate those barriers (Rose, 2011).

B. Successful ICU Specific Frameworks

Literature demonstrates four specific teamwork *processes* that are crucial for predicting optimal team functioning: team communication, team leadership, team coordination, and team decision making (Reader et al., 2009).

1. *Team Communication.* Relies on the clear and concise transfer of ideas, opinions, and knowledge among team members. Requires closed-loop communication, direct requests, honest feedback, appropriate urgency of problems, and agreement and understanding of the patient plan. Communication is at the greatest risk of failure during patient handoffs and under reluctance by any member to report concerns or errors. Includes both verbal and nonverbal communications.

2. *Team Leadership.* Refers to the guidance the team receives in setting expectations for everyone; organizing resources, coordinating activities, and defining goals. Leaders can be clinical (attending physicians, charge nurse), operational (unit leadership, departmental managers), and strategic (vice-presidents, chief executive officer, chief nursing officer).

3. *Team Coordination.* Refers to the synchronicity of the team within assigned work activities, how well each member is aware of the others' role and function. Coordination can suffer when team members are overworked, lack delegation skills, have poor prioritization abilities, and communicate needs poorly.

4. *Team Decision Making.* Includes decisions made as a whole or by a recognized team leader. Poor decision-making processes can include inappropriate resource utilization or incorrect care planning. Decision-making behaviors must be adapted to the situation accordingly, a high-stress situation (i.e., code blue) may have more formal leadership framework, with one person (most senior physician) making decisions. Lower stress situations with less risk encourage leadership behaviors from all members of the team, including autonomous decision making and coordination.

C. TeamSTEPPS Model

The *Team Strategies and Tools to Enhance Performance and Patient Safety* (TeamSTEPPS) system was developed by the AHRQ. It was created as a result of 20 years of team training knowledge from not only healthcare, but from high-reliable institutions such as the military and aviation research (Pettit & Duffy, 2015). It emphasizes team skills that include:

1. *Communication.* How information should be exchanged between team members.

2. *Leadership.* How are activities coordinated, and by whom? Are they clearly understood and shared, and are resources available when needed?

3. *Situation Monitoring.* The team is actively monitoring the situation, gaining understanding for what steps are needed next and how they can best support team function.

4. *Mutual Support.* Team has knowledge and provides support by understanding all members' needs, responsibilities, and workloads.

The model's triangle holds the knowledge and competencies (inside the triangle) needed for all team members (at the circle), and identifies the skills (inside the circle) the team needs to use to achieve optimal outcomes and details the knowledge, skills, and attitudes needed. This model can be particularly effective when used during simulation and role-playing activities (Figure 10.10).

LEVERAGING FAMILY INVOLVEMENT IN SAFETY AND QUALITY

In recent years, patient and family experiences during inpatient encounters have been scrutinized and considered by many as a pillar of quality to be measured. This is supported by the American Academy of Critical-Care Nurses (AACN) synergy model: "dimensions of a nurse's practice are driven by the needs of a patient and family" (The AACN Synergy Model for Patient Care, n.d., para. 2). See Chapter 1 for additional information on the AACN Synergy Model.

A. Pillars of Patient- and Family-Centered Care

1. Patient- and family-centered healthcare have been associated with several positive patient and family outcomes, which can include not only improved clinical outcomes, but increased receipt of patient preventative care, adherence to prescribed treatments and self-care, and ultimate decrease of healthcare utilization overall (Toomey et al., 2017).

2. In 2001, the IOM stated that ensuring healthcare workers provide patient- and family-centered care (FCC; respectful, responsive, and indicative of the patient/family values and beliefs) is one of the pillars of assuring high-quality health care (IOM, 2001).

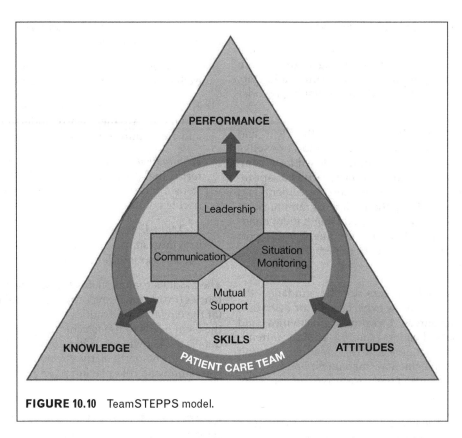

FIGURE 10.10 TeamSTEPPS model.

3. The Patient Protection and Affordable Care Act (ACA) of 2010 mandates that public reporting of patient experience (in adult inpatient institutions) be made available to the Centers for Medicare & Medicaid Services (CMS). Although not yet mandatory, many healthcare economists believe that the CMS will ask for this information from pediatric institutions in the near future.

4. The availability of this public reporting means that families have a transparent way of determining which providers and institutions they feel will provide the best quality outcomes for their child.

B. Leveraging FCC to Improve Quality

1. The FCC healthcare movement did not begin in America until the 1970s, and, in 1993, it was formally introduced through the Institute for Patient- and Family-Centered Care (Williams, 2016).

2. There are general FCC principles that are the same among groups such as Family Voices, the American Academy of Pediatrics (AAP), the Institute for Patient- and Family-Centered Care, and the Maternal and Child Health Bureau (MCHB; Kuo et al. 2011).

a. *Sharing of information.* Transparent, objective, and honest

b. *Showing respect and honoring differences.* Respect for diverse cultures, religious and spiritual beliefs, linguistic differences, and care preferences

c. *Collaboration and partnership.* When medically suitable decisions can be made together that fulfill the needs, wishes, strengths, abilities, and values of the patient and family; the family will participate at the level of involvement that they choose and can handle

d. *Care that is provided within the context of the family and its community.* Decision making and medical care that aligns with their home and community needs and acceptable quality of life

C. Applications of FCC in Pediatric Critical Care

Given the many challenges pediatric critical care areas face to provide care to just the patient, it can be daunting to determine how best to incorporate these FCC principles to serve the patient, family, and care team as well as improve quality outcomes. Examples of implementing FCC on a unit level, at the bedside:

1. Family-centered rounding processes (recent research proves this is one of the easiest and most effective ways to improve and implement FCC; Butler, Copnell, & Willetts, 2013; Blankenship, Harrison, Brandt, Joy, & Simsic, 2015)

2. Allowing families to stay at the bedside during procedures when medically possible

3. Preparing families for what they may see, hear, and experience during their child's stay—prior to admission when possible

4. Scheduling regular-care conferences with the multidisciplinary care team and family, particularly during long inpatient stays

5. Encouraging families to provide additional "normal" child care when the child is medically ready

6. Personalizing the patient's space with pictures, items from home, and the child's own clothing when possible

7. Shifting nursing handoff out of conference rooms and to the bedside, including the family in the discussions and welcoming questions

8. Providing families with multiple resources to learn about their child's diagnosis, treatments, and care—including handouts, books, electronic resources, and classes

There are several proven methods to improve staff understanding of FCC on a formal and larger institutional basis:

1. Formation of family advisory boards

2. Family peer/mentor support groups

3. Family presentations for staff regarding personal experiences

4. Asking family members to serve on hospital committees

Consideration should be given to evaluating FCC interventions as part of QI projects, setting measurable goals and metrics to objectively identify outcomes.

D. Identified Barriers to FCC Practice

There are barriers to implementing FCC on an institutional or unit level—these include lack of resources (time, money, staff), lack of leadership support, additional research on FCC (particularly in pediatric critical care areas) that can help to support and guide

best practices (Kuo et al., 2012). It is also important to consider that families themselves may have barriers (time, money, resources) that prevent them from being at the bedside as much as they would wish; therefore, the team must be creative in making sure they are able to update these families on their child's progress. The team should welcome inquiries that may require frequent medical updates as well as reassurance that the child is receiving high-quality care and support, despite absence of the parent/support person.

Many institutions continue to exercise outdated practices that decrease parental engagement in FCC and detract from care of their child (Butler et al., 2013; Williams, 2016).

1. Restricted visiting hours for family members (including no visiting surrounding shift changes)

2. Denial of sibling/young family member visitation

3. Being forced to leave their child during medical procedures (when they could safely stay)

4. Limiting holding, comforting, singing, or talking to their child despite medical stability to do so

5. Withholding information, particularly during care conferences or medical rounding

6. Not inviting parents and social support persons to be present at the bedside, despite being present in the room

E. Future Assessment of Patient/Family Needs and FCC

1. Most adult inpatient institutions utilize psychometrically sound survey tools such as the Consumer Assessments of Healthcare Providers and Systems Hospital Survey (HCAHPS).

2. Poor scores gathered by these tools are used in the Hospital Value-Based Purchasing Program and can affect the reimbursement that a hospital receives for the care they provide to patients covered under governmental assisted care (Angang Price et al., 2014).

3. CAHPS (Child HCAHPS) was developed by Boston Children's Hospital (AHRQ, 2017b), mirroring the adult tool to capture patient/family needs in the pediatric realm. Institutions are able to benchmark their scores against other pediatric institutions.

4. These surveys focus on the patient care experience that can help patients and families reflect on the *quality of the care* provided to them as a whole (Angang Price et al., 2014), beyond just the physiological outcome of the patient.

5. This is a relatively new method of assessing patient experience in pediatrics, and additional research is needed to understand how the data on FCC corresponds to both perceived and actual patient quality outcomes (Toomey et al., 2017).

UNDERSTANDING RISK RELATED TO QI

QI activities are about *advancing practice.* Determining the effectiveness of processes and disseminating solutions to practices are the crucial part of nursing's contribution to patient care. QI is about improving the care we currently provide, through "systematic, data-guided activities" (Hicks, 2016). These change activities should demonstrate measured improvement. QI is different than traditional formal research or EBP, in which the goal is generating new knowledge about a previously little-known (or unknown), subject or problem. EBP is also different than QI, as EBP seeks to have the best available evidence at the bedside to direct care.

A. Differences Among QI, Research, and EBP

1. *Research.* Research is utilized to generate new knowledge about a currently known, little-known, or unknown subject. It is meant to be generalizable, and uses experimental methods that may be yet unproven, rather than currently accepted standards of care. Research follows protocols and procedures that are strictly regulated and help to protect human subjects from any exposed risk as a result of participating (Stausmire, 2014). Institutional review board (IRB) approval is required and has to be obtained prior to any implementation of the project.

2. *EBP.* EBP guides implementation of evidence that is already available to answer pressing questions. Evidence must be systematically reviewed and critically appraised to produce the most recent and relevant answers. Done correctly, it should be a rigorous process. EBP aids in translating new knowledge to help address an administrative, educational, or clinical problem. IRB approval is not normally required, unless projects can potentially cause patient harm or are intended for eventual publication.

3. *QI.* QI is data driven and systematic. QI can provide the most rapid solution to concerns, whether they be workflow-process, clinical outcomes, or administrative or educational issues. IRB approval is not required for projects determined to not be human subject research; QI data collection may be in that category. Some organizations have developed an alternative review process for QI projects. Projects that may be eventually intended for publication, go beyond individual institutional improvements, or may result in patient risk should be reviewed. Although important to disseminate, QI activities are done at a local level. Therefore, it is important to consider that a project may not be generalizable to a particular region or other patient population.

B. Understanding and Minimizing Risk

Regardless of activity—research, EBP, and QI should be able to demonstrate that certain ethical standards were upheld during the project and process. The standards and oversight that are necessary to uphold and provide via documentation vary based on the activity. The oversight needed should be determined at the beginning stages of creation to reduce possible risk to patients and save time for the team members involved in obtaining appropriate permissions (Morris & Dracup, 2007). The key difference in determining what oversight is necessary for a project involves the discussion of potential patient exposure to risk.

The Office for Human Research Protection falls under federal government oversight and defines the research process as a "systematic investigation ... designed to develop or contribute to generalizable knowledge" (Morris & Dracup, 2007, p. 425). QI, EBP, and research activities can be confused with one another as they share common characteristics. Risk is what separates the oversight needed for each. A primary nursing care goal is based on patient benefit, what can we do, (or not do), to best benefit the patient? Research conducted does not always relate to patient benefit. Therefore, ethical caution must be used when planning or conducting research to also protect human subjects' well-being and welfare and prevent abuse. To be certain research conforms to those federal standards set to minimize risk, the investigators must seek approval by the IRB.

IRBs were established in the 1970s to provide protection to individual human subjects under federally funded research (Graham et al., n.d.). IRBs provide the following oversight: Review and approve protocols that involve human subjects, monitor ongoing research, approve forms for consent, and investigate allegations of wrong-doing or adverse events in research.

C. Risk as It Relates to QI and Safety Initiatives

One approach used to distinguish activities that are exempt from IRB oversight versus those that require it is to examine the generalizability of the project, the degree of risk to human subjects involved, the design used and features of the project, and desired potential publication goals (Olsen & Smania, 2016).

1. *Generalizability.* Knowledge that is generalizable expands the knowledge base of a field. This knowledge can generally be expanded to populations outside of a local setting. The limitation of generalizability is considered a weakness in research, but is not uncommon. In contrast, a QI project goal is changing the delivery of healthcare in a particular setting, and although the project can and should be shared with others, it should not be recreated exactly in another setting with the expectation of similar results.

2. *Risk.* EBP and QI activities should not pose any risk to patients, such as withholding a treatment from patients that may provide a potential benefit. This extends to the collection of information, even retroactively, that is not required for clinical treatment or the improvement of clinical treatment interventions. If any question regarding risk arises, the project proposal can be submitted to the IRB for review and determination.

3. *Design.* Control of variables, widespread additions of new information to the discipline, randomization, blinding, using placebos, and comparison of interventions (especially when withheld from one group and given to another) are all frequent characteristics of research designs. Improvement of local problems with little control of variables and flexibility regarding data collection are associated with QI.

4. *Publication.* Both QI and research projects can and should be published to expand the knowledge of nursing and improve the profession. Understanding that many nurses may read the publication with the intent of applying the findings to their own situations suggests that they may feel there may be some generalizability. The distinction between QI and a research study should be made clear to the reader (Table 10.7).

COMPETENCIES FOR QUALITY AND SAFETY IN NURSING

A. QSEN Competencies

In 2003, the IOM challenged educators of medicine, nursing, and other health professions to implement a new era of quality and safety into their programs. The *Quality and Safety Education for Nurses (QSEN)* project was borne of the need for educators of undergraduate nursing programs to implement learning that prepared prelicensure nursing students to deliver care through its' core competencies. QSEN was funded by the Robert Wood Johnson Foundation and was created with an expert advisory board using nursing literature and existing IOM nursing competencies to form a curriculum that would serve not only academic programs, but transition to practice (residency) and continuing-education programs for existing nurses as well. Six competencies, along with the knowledge, skills, and attitudes needed for success, were formed

TABLE 10.7 Differentiation of Quality Improvement Versus Research Activities

Measured Criteria	Quality Improvement	Research
Purpose	Improve current processes and outcomes— guide actions	Create new knowledge where more is needed or none exists
Risk	No risk to humans	Potential risk, even when slight or mitigated
Consent	Typically not required	Required when human subjects are involved
Intended audience	Organization where QI conducted	Scientific community
Scope	Internal organizational processes—one site	Potentially generalizable to other sites, patients, or situations
Results	Used primarily by originating institution— although publishing processes and results is becoming common	Published with recommendations for usage
Subjects	Institutional patients or subpopulation of patients	Based on study design and purpose

QI, quality improvement.

with the goal of being applicable to all registered nurses (Cronenwett et al., 2007):

1. *Patient-Centered Care.* Care based on the patient/family being a full partner with the nurse, providing care that is compassionate and respects patient/family values, preferences, and needs

2. *Teamwork and Collaboration.* To function within interdisciplinary teams in an effective manner, fostering respect and open communication, and achieving quality care by practicing shared decision making

3. *EBP.* To follow and integrate best evidenced-based nursing evidence into clinical practice

4. *Quality Improvement.* To continuously improve outcomes by gathering and tracking data utilizing established improvement methods

5. *Safety.* To recognize and minimize the risk of harm to patients and families through improvement of both individual and system performance

6. *Informatics.* To utilize information technology to improve communications, minimize errors, house knowledge, and support shared decision making

B. Validating QSEN Across Agencies

The American Nurses Credentialing Center (ANCC) Magnet® recognition is a prestigious award that signifies the institution achieves the highest quality of nursing practice. Accreditation by TJC and/or ANCC maximizes third-party reimbursement to the institution through the Hospital Value-Based Purchasing program led by the CMS. Following recommendations from both agencies can be crucial to the welfare of institutions. In 2016, Lyle-Edrosolo and Waxman (2016) recognized that both schools of nursing and healthcare institutions may find that there are varying definitions and recommendations regarding quality and safety found across these agencies compared to QSEN competencies. A crosswalk document demonstrates both TJC and ANCC standards do align with QSEN competencies, further validating the value of QSEN centered education.

STARTING WITH SMALL STEPS AND MOVING TO HIGHER GOALS

Exposure to QI's history, tools, and models gives us base knowledge regarding its importance; implementing it into everyday practice can seem overwhelming. Creating a practical approach with topics already familiar to the ICU nurse can help with implementation. An

easy-to-understand model involves three components: *structure, process, and outcome* (Curtis et al., 2006).

1. *Structure* refers to those ways in which we organize care. These features can include items such as the geographical setup, patient population, technology utilized, and various clinician roles and responsibilities.

2. *Process* is considered to be the things we do, or fail to do, for patients and families. Bedside nurses are most familiar with processes; medication administration, dressing changes, care planning, and so on.

3. *Outcomes* are the results that are achieved as a result of the processes and structure. Although most ICU nurses are familiar with the goal of achieving results by following their processes (i.e., decreased blood sugars with the administration of insulin, improvement in lung sounds following treatments), QI challenges RNs to consider the larger picture of care provided. Based on the quality of our central-line care, have we prevented infections? Have we implemented enough successful interventions to prevent PUs in the critically ill intubated patient?

Changing the structure of a unit is the most challenging, expensive, and resource-rich component. A bedside RN, unit, or institution who is new to QI may wish to start with changing *processes* to achieve improved *results*. Although not examined in-depth here, an RN will want to involve a project manager (and team) familiar with QI to aid in the creation of initiatives.

A. Power of Nursing to Improve Care

There are hundreds of quality indicators to consider for improvement in the pediatric ICU environment. Nurses at the bedside have the most power to change the safety of the care they provide; therefore, it makes sense to start with safety metrics. Scanon, Mistry, and Howard (2007) translated three qualitative patient safety concepts into quantitative metrics for pediatric ICUs:

1. *Injury-Based Metrics.* Many nurses are familiar with these metrics, which include harm-based events that are largely believed to be preventative, including:

   a. Central line-associated blood stream infections (CLABSIs)

   b. Catheter-associated urinary tract infections (CAUTI)

   c. Ventilator-associated pneumonia (VAP)

   d. PU or PI

   e. ADE

2. *Error-Based Metrics.* Achieving the best clinical outcome is reliant on successfully delivering the *correct* plan of care. In order to do so, actual errors that do and do not reach the patient (also known as *near misses*) need to be captured and measured (see "The Importance of Nurses Reporting"). Recognizing errors that occur with frequency can point teams in the direction of determining which metrics need first action.

3. *Risk-Based Metrics.* What are hazards that increase the likelihood of errors at the point of care? Examples include depending on verbal versus written orders and administering high-risk medications without double checks. Risk-based metrics depend not only on identifying past errors, but proactively considering which behaviors contributed to them.

Once metrics have been identified for QI, nurses need not start from scratch to create interventions and implement process changes. The IHI, AHRQ, and SPS all have ready-made care *bundles* (a group of proven EBP interventions that direct caregivers on how to deliver care for optimal outcomes) available on a wide variety of pediatric ICU specific initiatives, including frequently utilized indicators such as reducing CLABSIs, CAUTIs, and VAPs.

B. The Importance of Nurse Reporting

Nurses have an ethical responsibility to ensure that patient care maintains high standards and to report it when they do not (Attree, 2007). By reporting errors and near misses, risk-based metrics can be developed that can help prevent the event from occurring again, thus increasing patient safety. Literature agrees that there is still widespread under-reporting of errors in healthcare, although how much occurs is still unknown. There have been studies that recognize which factors may lead nurses to raise concerns or report errors regarding quality of care (Attree, 2007):

1. *Punitive Environment.* Nurses who speak up regarding lapses in care are "written-up" or punished and fear retribution or retaliation by others or the institution.

2. *Poor System Reception to Concerns.* Nurses are encouraged to keep quiet by peers or superiors. Concerns that are raised are ignored or minimized.

3. *Little Support.* The nurse who reports or experiences the error is unsupported following the report. The nurses receive little guidance or advice for improvement. No recognition exists regarding the emotional stress of being involved in an incident.

Organizations that recognize the importance of reporting patient safety concerns will implement a "just-" culture environment of nonpunitive error reporting. A just culture identifies human fallibility and engages a system-level approach to errors. In other words, unless an event is caused by deliberate intention to harm or a failure to adhere to policies and procedures that have been shown to keep patient care safe, it must be investigated as a systems-level failure, and the institution, not the *nurse*, takes the blame (M. R. Miller, Takata, Stucky, & Neuspiel, 2011).

There are numerous ways to facilitate and support nurses to encourage error and near-miss reporting in a just-culture environment:

1. *Open Environment.* Nurses should be emboldened to report concerns. The objective should be to create a shame- and blame-free system that proves the system is trustworthy and wants to hear about errors and near-misses that can comprise patient safety.

2. *Approach.* The environment should approach reporting as writing up the incident, not writing up the person. Leaders and peers should take notice of the concern and respond to it in a timely manner. Concerns should be investigated and discussed in a safe and supportive setting. All parties should be professional and avoid "you" statements that suggest errors were the result of incompetence or inattention.

3. *Support.* Advice given should be reliable and depersonalized. All parties should feel respected and accepted for reporting. Interventions should be implemented to help prevent incidents from occurring again.

C. Striving for Systems-Level Thinking

The ultimate goal for nursing is to achieve *systems-level thinking* when assessing QI (Dolansky & Moore, 2013). The strategy encourages recognizing patterns of behavior, and how actions can strengthen or counteract each other. Systems-level thinking is how nurses understand their behavior can be linked to their environment. Ultimately, we strive to appreciate how individual patient care can be linked to a larger, more complex health system, and vice-versa. Figure 10.11 shows an example of bedside care that demonstrates systems-level thinking.

D. What Does This Mean to Your Practice?

There is no question that QI activities and initiatives require the gift of time. There must be support from leadership and administration to give that time to bedside nurses who are engaged in improving processes and

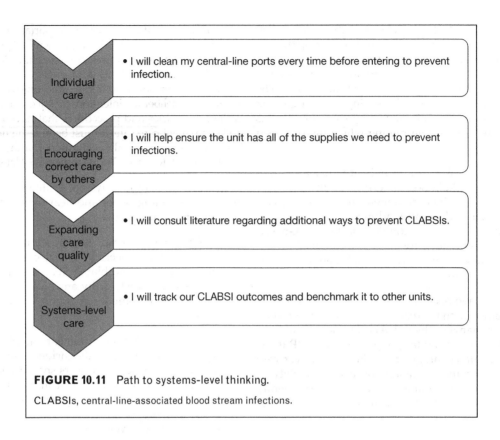

FIGURE 10.11 Path to systems-level thinking.

CLABSIs, central-line-associated blood stream infections.

outcomes. This time may come in administrative "off-unit" time during which the nurse is asked to complete audits, compile data, or evaluate outcomes. However, when patient needs exceed current nurse availability, the nurse will be asked to resume bedside duties. How can we encourage participation while acknowledging that QI is resource intensive?

1. *Focus on QI Activities That Improve Workflow.* Is there a way to streamline auditing by inserting it into everyday tasks? Example: A nurse utilizes a checklist to complete a central-line dressing, following it during the change and checking it off when completed. He or she notes any difficulties he or she had during the procedure and anything that could have been done differently to improve it (i.e., needed additional supplies, required help from additional staff member). After several feedback forms, the nurse manager realizes that current supply availability is not adequate for needs. The manager requests to increase the par levels delivered by central supply and future procedures are not delayed by nurses looking for additional supplies.

2. *Buy-In.* QI initiatives can only be successful if nurses are engaged in the creation of a new process or intervention. At a minimum, understanding the value of the change aids in acceptance. Nurses are encouraged to ask, "Why are we doing this? And where is the evidence that it is effective?"

3. *Encourage a Time to Adapt.* Numerous theories exist on the best way to implement lasting change in healthcare. One of the most simplistic, by Kurt Lewin (Mitchell, 2013), emphasizes that after a change is implemented, there must be a period of *refreezing*. Refreezing allows new interventions to become embedded in everyday practice. Once it has been established that the intervention is effective, nurses will need a period of time to adapt their workflow to the change. This is a time to discourage additional initiatives; multiple new interventions during this time can cause confusion and distress (Mitchell, 2013).

4. *Tracking Data.* Nurses need to know that the work they're doing at the bedside produces improved outcomes. It is vitally important to not only track this data, but to be transparent in sharing it with staff. If a QI measure is not producing the desired effects, new interventions should be considered, or the project should be abandoned.

5. *Rewarding Outcomes.* Once projects have measured success, they should be celebrated! Publicly thanking those involved and sharing success stories (including patient details where pertinent) will help nurses feel their work in the project is valued and will encourage future projects.

CREATING AN HWE FOR NURSING PRACTICE TO ENSURE PATIENT SAFETY

A. AACN's Healthy Workplace Initiative

In 2005, the AACN set forth six standards for organizations to follow to help create an HWE that fosters the spirit of quality care and ensures patient safety. Based on the increasing body of literature published surrounding nursing care quality and safety, these guidelines were reviewed and validated in 2016. The AACN document believes that the nursing profession is uniquely positioned to be a front-runner in QI, and encourages healthcare organizations to consider abiding by their recommendations to provide an environment that allows nurses to fulfill the call (AACN, 2016).

1. *Skilled Communication.* Communicating clearly and concisely must be considered as important as having clinical competence.

2. *True Collaboration.* Support and coaching must be provided for all members of the care team to participate in care equally.

3. *Effective Decision Making.* Nursing should be a valued part of the team for its contributions and decisions as patient advocates.

4. *Appropriate Staffing.* Far from the simple process of having a certain number of nurses for a set number of patients, at its most basic, patient needs must match nurse competencies.

5. *Meaningful Recognition.* Nurses should be recognized in an ongoing manner for their contributions, recognition should be specific and sincere.

6. *Authentic Leadership.* Leaders, too, must hold competence in implementing truthful practices that demonstrate trust, effective communication, strategic thinking, and continuing support of the nurses they lead.

The AACN urges each nurse, leader, and organization to embrace these values and follow through on them to create an HWE. The six standards are interdependent on each other to fulfill the goal of creating an environment that interconnects and helps lead to clinical excellence and optimal patient outcomes (Figure 10.12).

The AACN website provides an HWE assessment tool for free at www.aacn.org/nursing-excellence/healthy-work-environments/aacn-healthy-work-environment-assessment-tool (Case Study 10.3).

B. Challenges to Creating an HWE

1. Breakdowns in communication

2. Lack of collaboration

3. Effective decision making

4. Appropriate staffing

5. Meaningful recognition

6. Authentic leadership

SELF-CARE AND WELLNESS PROMOTION

A. Health-Promoting Behaviors

Nurses must engage in healthy behaviors, both personally and professionally. They should make attempts to partner with institutions that support and foster wellness and self-care in order to be best prepared to provide the safe and quality care that the complex healthcare climate demands. Despite previous knowledge regarding best self-care and wellness practices, research demonstrates that many nurses do not fulfill the duty to care for themselves so that they can care for others. Common health-promoting behaviors nurses should both personally practice as well as educate patients and families on include eating a proper diet, getting adequate exercise, proper sleep hygiene, and stress-reduction activities.

1. *Diet.* The American Heart Association (AHA) recommends eating a varied diet high in fruits, vegetables, and whole grains, with limited amounts of trans-fats and sugars.

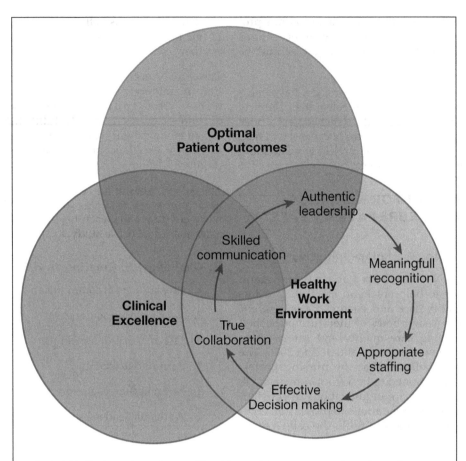

FIGURE 10.12 Interdependence of healthy work environment, clinical excellence, and optimal patient outcomes.

Source: AACN. (2016). Interdependence of healthy work environment, clinical excellence, and optimal patient outcomes. In *AACN standards for establishing and sustaining healthy work environments; A journey to excellence* (2nd ed., p. 11. Aliso Viejo, CA: Author.

CASE STUDY 10.3   Healthy Work Environment

Our busy cardiothoracic ICU has frequent and significant census changes, which can lead to difficulty staffing appropriately while also ensuring too many nurses aren't cancelled or floated to other units. One day we kept getting admission after admission, to the point that our previously "good" staffing was simply not enough to keep up! As the charge nurse, I knew that the nightshift was going to be in trouble if we couldn't receive adequate help. We immediately huddled with our physicians, APNs, and manager to devise a plan for that night. The physicians knew they needed to help us monitor our patients more than usual for signs and symptoms of issues, the APNs aided us in getting routine lab work and even completed some treatments, and the manager set off to make phone calls and adjust future schedules to encourage other staff to come in and help for that night. We ended up making it through the night with adequate help and no adverse outcomes in patient safety (or quality!) occurred. What could have been a disaster waiting to happen was thwarted by communication, collaboration, and a dedication to creating an environment in which everyone is valued for what she or he adds to the team.

Monica, RN, CTICU

(M. G., personal communication, February 13, 2017)

2. The Centers for Disease Control and Prevention (CDC) recommendations include 150 minutes of moderate exercise or 75 minutes of intense physical exercise per week.

3. *Sleep.* Although the exact amount of sleep needed for healthy adults has not yet been established, the American Nurses Association (ANA) states 7 to 8 hours of sleep per each 24-hour period is recommended (V. Hughes, 2016).

4. *Stress Reduction.* Techniques are tailored to what is most effective for the person, and can include exercise, meditation, prayer, mindfulness activities, engaging in hobbies, counseling, employee assistance programs, support groups, and socializing with friends and family.

In 2010, Tucker et al. found that of 3,132 nurses, only 50% participated in the CDC-recommended amount of physical activity weekly, with 62% consuming fast-food meals twice weekly. Geiger-Brown et al. (2012) reported that of both day- and night-shift nurses who work 12-hour shifts, the average amount of sleep reported was 5.5 hours in a 24-hour period, with increasing amounts of daytime/nighttime drowsiness reported for each consecutive shift worked.

B. Barriers to Health-Promoting Activities

Both intrinsic (personal) and extrinsic factors (external or professional) can create barriers to practicing adequate self-care. Intrinsic factors can include fatigue, depression, anxiety, and obtaining ongoing inadequate amounts of sleep can prevent self-wellness. Poor sleep or lack of sleep alone is linked to an increased risk of causing medication errors. Prolonged periods of wakefulness (20–25 hours) can produce impairments similar to a blood alcohol level of 0.01% (R. G. Hughes, 2008). Extrinsic factors can be social, interpersonal, or professional. Related to the work environment, long shifts, high acuity, poor communication, and competing personal and professional demands can interfere with an individual desire to care for one's self. In 2008, 55% of a nationally represented sample of 33,549 RNs reported having an adult or child dependent (or both) in their household to care for, in addition to the care they provide to patients at work (Ross, Bevans, Brooks, Gibbons, & Wallen, 2016). This leaves little time nor inclination for nurses to focus on themselves.

C. Workplace Stress and Wellness

In addition to long hours, physical and emotional challenges, staffing shortages, and increasing patient acuity, nurses report other significant workplace stressors.

In 2015, the ANA published the primary findings of their "Health Risk Appraisal" with responses from 3,765 RNs, completed between October of 2013 and October of 2014 (Carpenter, 2015):

1. Eight-two percent replied they were at significant risk of experiencing workplace stress.

2. More than 50% reported experiencing some type of musculoskeletal pain at work.

3. Almost 60% reported they work through breaks and come in early or stay late to complete work-related tasks.

4. Thirty-three percent reported they had cared for a greater number of patients than they were comfortable with.

McElligott, Siemers, Thomas, and Kohn (2009) found that critical care nurses in particular scored lower than medical-surgical nurses on the Health Promoting Lifestyle Profile II, which examines personal wellness activities, including seeking professional assistance when experiencing ongoing stress.

D. Creating Workplace Wellness

Despite the presence of workplace stress, many nurses reported positive examples of workplaces supporting personal wellness.

1. Ninety percent reported their workplace as tobacco free.

2. Seventy percent had access to health-promotion activities and programs.

3. Fifty-nine percent had ready access to health foods at work, including fruits, vegetables, and whole grains.

Ways for nurses and leaders to increase employee health-promotion in their institution:

1. Support employee participation in existing health-promotion activities, ask whether employees would like to be involved in creating programs for peers.

2. Create a culture of healthy eating. Instead of cake on birthdays, donuts for morning meetings or pizza at lunch, provide fruits and vegetables for snacks or provide healthy wraps or salads.

3. Encourage nurses to take breaks and to eat uninterrupted lunches whenever possible.

4. Build an environment where nurses can feel supported when experiencing stress and feel their suggestions for improvement are taken seriously. Provide feedback regardless of whether the suggestions can be implemented or not.

5. Discourage staff from working many (more than three) shifts in a row without at least a 24-hour break in between.

6. Create an area where nurses can feel safe to engage in quiet reflection or meditation.

E. Self-Care and the Night Shift

In addition to the potential increase of health risks, such as obesity, cancers, irritable bowel syndrome, and cardiovascular disease, nurses who work steady night shifts also suffer from sleep-related disturbances and threat of drowsy driving (V. Hughes, 2016). Professionally, some literature has shown a higher percentage of errors occur at night, including drug and equipment mistakes; needle-stick injuries are also higher during the nighttime hours (V. Hughes, 2016).

Regardless of risk, patient care still must occur 24 hours a day, 7 days a week, with no holidays! Many nurses begin their careers on nights shift (with dayshift being a "seniority" perk), or choose to work the night shift for the increased pay, to fulfill family obligations during the day, or prefer the differing pace and culture that may occur in their institution at night. However, there is no doubt that consistently working at night brings challenges separate from those of their dayshift colleagues (Case Study 10.4).

Institutions are increasingly realizing that to avoid turnover, to increase productivity, and to help create a safe environment at night, these nurses need additional attention. In 2015, Nationwide Children's Hospital, in Columbus, Ohio, started a "night-shift friendly committee." A small group of managers met to discuss how the institution could recognize and address the challenges faced by night-shift staff. A needs assessment identified the institution's night-shift needs, including more learning opportunities offered between 7 p.m. and 7 a.m., an increase in healthy foods offered by the cafeteria, and additional leadership recognition. They've since implemented evening and night-shift educational breaks, celebrate each year's "lag night" (daylight savings night, during which night-shift nurses work 13 hours), partnered with nutrition services to increase both coffee availability and healthy cafeteria offerings, offer TB shots and test-reading during nighttime hours, and increased senior leadership recognition of the night-shift staff. A list of "night-shift tips" acknowledges

> **CASE STUDY 10.4   Night Shift Challenges**
>
> I worked night shift for 11 years. Originally, it was the only shift offered. Eventually, I grew to love the teamwork and camaraderie of those of us dedicated to providing care during this difficult shift, and it worked well with my young and growing family. It's not without its challenges. Resources are fewer at night. Departments we count on during the day would never stay open 24 hours. We have less staff at night, there is less access to leadership for questions, educational opportunities rarely occurred during my shifts, mandatory meetings were held during the day, the cafeteria was only open for a few hours and served only leftovers or fried food, and we frequently were unable to access all of the supplies we needed. There was a lot that could have been done to improve the experiences of nurses working at night.
>
> Michelle, RN
>
> (M. M., personal communication, March 16, 2017)

the difficulties of working at night while also implementing self-care and wellness practices (P. Creech, personal communication, April 4, 2017). Examples of some helpful tips:

1. To optimize the sleep cycle, wear sunglasses when leaving and until you get to your dark bedroom. Refrain from using any device with a "blue light" (TV, cell phone) before sleep.

2. If you think you're too tired to drive home, call a friend, taxi, or take a nap before going home.

3. Avoid rotating shifts frequently or working every other night.

4. Build a community of friends and coworkers who also work the night shift. Talk with others who understand your lifestyle.

5. Consider creating a "business card" with your name and describing your sleep hours, asking friends/families/contacts not to call you during the day.

6. Be *patient* with yourself as you adjust to your new schedule. You will not discover the best way to handle your "new normal" until you give it some time.

NURSING AND MORAL DISTRESS

The concept of moral distress was first introduced to medical bioethics circles in 1984 by Andrew Jameton; "when nurses know the right thing to do; but institutional constraints make it nearly impossible to pursue the right course of action" (Jameton, 1984, p. 6). The nurse experiencing moral distress feels that she or he can no longer be an adequate advocate for the patient, which is an inherent and core tenet of the nursing profession. Moral distress can also occur when a nurse does not necessarily know what is ethically correct, but is forced to make a decision (af Sandeberg, Wenemark, Barthodson, Lützén, & Pergert, 2017). A specificity exists between *moral distress* and a *moral dilemma*, in that dilemmas suggest that there may be more than one course of action (Dyo, Kalowes, & Devries, 2016; Prentice, Janvier, Gillam, & Davis, 2016). Moral distress can make a nurse (correctly or incorrectly) believe that the path she or he may wish to take with or for a patient is not the one she or he is to practice. Short-term responses to experiencing moral distress include sadness, fear, anguish, guilt, anger, frustration, powerlessness, and loneliness (Thomas, Thammasitboon, Balmer, Roy, & McCullough, 2016). Long-term consequences can include significant workplace stress, avoidance of professional interactions, low-job satisfaction, burnout, and intention to leave a nursing position (af Sandeberg et al., 2017; Dyo et al., 2016; Trotochaud, Ramsey Coleman, Krawiecki, & McCracken, 2015).

Moral distress exists across nursing specialties, but is particularly common among those practicing in critical care (Browning, 2013; Leggett, Wasson, Sinacore, & Gamelli, 2013; Ulrich, Lavandero, Woods, & Early, 2014). Several studies have validated higher levels of distress in pediatric critical care areas versus other pediatric specialty care areas as well (Prentice et al., 2016; Trotochaud et al., 2015).

A. Root Causes of Moral Distress

Root causes can be internal (specific to the caregiver), or external (constraints created by the institution or situation).

1. *Internal Causes*

    a. *Feelings of powerlessness.* The nurse may feel that she or he has no control over the care provided to the patient, even if she or he feels the care provided is ethically or morally wrong.

    b. *Lack of knowledge.* The nurse may not know what the correct ethical action should be, but is uncomfortable with the identified plan and intervention.

    c. *Increased moral sensitivity.* The nurse (through personal experience or personality type) feels particular sympathy, empathy, or depression toward the patient, family, or situation.

2. *External Causes*

    a. Work overload related to staffing or poor care provided by others

    b. Inaction of others to intervene appropriately when providing care

    c. Difference in perception of truth-telling and communication

    d. Differing interprofessional (RN to MD) opinions

    e. Provider-specific and dramatic changes in plans of care

    f. Witnessing or giving false hope

    g. Performing painful treatments against a child's will

    h. Futility of care or prolonging the dying process

    i. Treatments that the nurse may fear will hasten death

Nurses who feel they practice in a more ethical climate may experience less moral distress (af Sandeberg et al., 2017; Prentice et al., 2016). Tenured professionals may encounter a "crescendo effect" due to multiple negative experiences over time (Epstein & Hamric, 2009).

B. Moral Distress Related to Resuscitation and End-of-Life Care Challenges

Moral distress in pediatric critical care can occur as a result of disproportionate treatment of the child compared to a likely positive outcome (Case Study 10.5). With the increasing availability of new life-saving technology, nurses may more often encounter instances in which families and practitioners, or even patients themselves, disagree on whether continuing treatment is futile.

End-of-life care and resuscitation in pediatrics may represent the "ultimate moral endeavor" (Thomas et al., 2016, p. e304) with the goal of restoring health and life to the most innocent and vulnerable of patients. Results of a qualitative study asking for caregiver feelings surrounding pediatric resuscitation (Thomas et al., 2016) found four common themes of moral distress triggers:

1. *Misunderstanding and Disagreement of the "Big Picture."* When nurses and physicians fundamentally

> **CASE STUDY 10.5   Morally Distressing Situations**
>
> Samantha is an 8-year-old patient with a congenital heart defect who has been placed on the transplant list for a new heart after multiple failed surgeries. She is clinically deteriorating and requiring escalating care for heart failure. Despite enduring painful procedures and ongoing treatment, Samantha's parents refuse to let staff either tell her or speak of the need for transplant around her. Samantha asks her nurse why she is continuing to be so sick and still in the hospital. The nurse is frustrated and not sure how to respond.
>
> Makil is a 4-year-old end-stage neuroblastoma patient in the PICU. He is mechanically ventilated and the oncology team has decided there are no further treatment options available. The palliative care team has met with Makil's parents and collectively decided not to pursue additional lifesaving measures should he deteriorate further. His night-shift nurse responds to a bradycardia alarm that she knows requires the start of compressions, but steps back to allow natural death (AND) because of his AND status. His mother is at the bedside and starts screaming at the nurse to "do everything possible" to save her child despite the earlier decision.

3. *Ineffective Leadership.* The team leader's ability to direct a resuscitation effort can negatively affect patient outcomes. Team leaders who make poor decisions or ineffectually communicate create ambiguity regarding the process and lead the team to question what is right. Leaders should demonstrate skillful execution of resuscitation while also seeking input and feedback from the team. Being at the mercy of another's opinions and judgments, particularly when they are medically or morally unsound, produces distress and doubt in the efficacy of future situations.

4. *Ambiguity of Role Responsibilities.* Similar to ineffective leaders, nurses who are unfamiliar with or confused about their role in the event risk losing their ability to critically think about tasks and interventions. A perceived knowledge gap can lead a nurse to avoid speaking up and giving feedback, allowing mistakes to occur or omitting what could be valuable information. Even in more seasoned nurses, second-guessing themselves can lead to distress if they later felt that their input could have changed the patient outcome.

COMPASSION FATIGUE AND BURNOUT

Nurses, particularly those who care for acuity ill patients and families facing suffering, pain, and possible death, face difficult emotional challenges and potentially, moral distress, on a daily basis. Confronting additional trials such as staffing issues, complex workflows, constant change, lack of management support, and a shortage of resources means that at any point, available coping mechanisms used to handle these challenges may exceed what the nurse can offer. Repeated exposure to these challenges leads to a depletion of empathy, which can also be considered *compassion fatigue*. Compassion fatigue has also been called the "cost of caring," and is especially prevalent in healthcare providers (Branch & Klinkenberg, 2015). Compassion is a feeling of sympathy that leads to a desire to alleviate a patient's suffering and is the core of nursing and most healthcare professions. However, humans do not have an endless supply of compassion; mismanagement or ignorance of repeated emotional stress and its' resulting negative cumulative effects can lead to devastating consequences for the nurse and potential patients as well.

Although used interchangeably with the term *burnout* in a significant amount of research on the subject, there is also research that demonstrates that compassion fatigue is actually one phenomenon with two components. One is burnout, and

disagree on the child's overall condition and prognosis, it challenges individual integrity and can produce moral distress. This is particularly evident when various services and care teams with multiple stakeholders interpret results differently, creating primary caregiver and family misperceptions of the overall picture.

2. *Variations on Resuscitation.* Caregivers and families often perceive the definition of resuscitation differently. Caregivers may feel morally obligated to do everything possible for a child when the family wishes to do so, despite a professional medical opinion that further care will be futile. One nurse in the study described participating in events such as "slow codes" (delayed response times), "chemical codes" (meds only), and "long codes" (past the point of a reasonably good clinical outcome even if successful). She also vocalized that she believed viewing the resuscitation process may help the family feel that both they and the medical team did everything medically possible to save their child, and ultimately aids in the grieving and healing process.

is not specific to healthcare, (having been demonstrated in other professions), but is common in occupations with frequent emotional interactions with other people (Jennings, 2008; Meyer, Li, Klaristenfeld, & Gold, 2015). The other component of compassion fatigue is *secondary trauma syndrome (STS)* and can occur as a result of repeated contact with others suffering traumatic events. The resulting traumatic emotions transfer from the patient to the nurse, leaving him or her with feelings of empathy (internalizing the same feelings) with the patient versus sympathizing and providing compassion (Sacco, Ciurzynski, Harvey, & Ingersoll, 2015).

A. Symptoms Specific to Compassion Fatigue, Burnout, and STS

1. *Compassion Fatigue*

    a. Emotional distancing from one's job

    b. Helplessness and anger

    c. Anxiety and depression

    d. Health issues, including hypertension, coronary artery disease, diabetes, obesity, and gastrointestinal disorders (Berger, Polivka, Smoot, & Owens, 2015)

    e. Poor coping mechanisms and self-destructive behaviors, including abuse of drugs, alcohol, and food (Slatten, David Carson, & Carson, 2008)

2. *Burnout*

    a. Exhaustion

    b. Cynicism and frustration

    c. Decreased engagement in work

    d. Inefficacy

    e. Inability to meet goals

    f. Desire to quit

    g. Intention to leave

3. *STS*

    a. Having intrusive thoughts or images of traumatic events

    b. Decreased tolerance with frustration

    c. Outburst of anger or rage

    d. Depression

    e. Self-destructive behaviors

    f. Difficulty separating work and personal-life issues

    g. Diminished sense of purpose or enjoyment

    h. Loss of hope

4. Individual characteristics of nurses with increased levels of compassion fatigue and burnout include younger age with fewer years in nursing, working shifts longer than full time per week, weak or few support systems, negative colleague relationships (Hinderer et al., 2014), self-medicating or self-destructive behaviors, poor coping mechanisms for normal life events, and increased moral sensitivity.

5. Institutions with higher rates of nurses experiencing compassion fatigue typically have poor work environments. They do not embrace the AACN's six standards of HWEs, and also suffer from inconsiderate or distant leadership, abusive work relationships, excessive patient workloads, very limited resources and staffing, low salaries, and unclear work and role expectations.

B. Increasing Compassion Satisfaction to Reduce Compassion Fatigue

What allows some nurses to continue practicing for years without experiencing compassion fatigue, whereas in the same unit other nurses suffer from it? One answer may be an increase in *compassion satisfaction. Compassion satisfaction* refers to the positive feelings and sentiment one feels when he or she has the ability to feel empathy and connect with patients. These individuals also feel a great sense of achievement and believe their actions have a positive impact on outcomes. In nursing, experiencing compassion satisfaction is a vital part of staying satisfied and fulfilled (Slatten et al., 2011).

Psychological capital consists of preexisting resilience, optimism, and feelings of worth and efficacy (Slatten et al., 2011). The amount available is not endless, and existing amounts vary greatly among nurses. Psychological strength training can be effective in increasing psychological capital, and therefore can increase compassion satisfaction. In addition, the trait of hardiness has been found in those nurses who have high compassion satisfaction. Hardiness consists of three individual components and includes an understanding and acceptance of the meaning of life, personal belief in the ability to control one's basic course of life, and expectations of change (acceptance that change is inevitable throughout life).

Compassion satisfaction has also been considered an important element in determining overall professional quality of life (ProQOL), first conceptualized by Stamm in 2002. *ProQOL* is defined as "the quality one feels in relation to their work as a helper" (Stamm, 2010, p. 6). A balance between compassion satisfaction and compassion fatigue can achieve a sustainable ProQOL. The ProQOL model encourages this balance to exist in both professional and home settings, emphasizing the importance of positive work–life balance standards (Sacco et al., 2015). The ProQOL Scale was created to help assess ProQOL for individuals in helping professions to measure and track both compassion satisfaction and compassion fatigue levels (Stamm, 2010).

C. Personal Strategies to Reduce Compassion Fatigue

By increasing compassion satisfaction and creating an HWE, institutions can decrease the incidence of compassion fatigue. There are additional individual actions a nurse can take as well:

1. *Limit or Diversify Patient Acuity or Caseload Mix.* Often the most dependable, compassionate, and competent nurses are assigned the sickest patients. The balance between available psychological resources and the ability to care for these acutely ill patients needs readjustment and time for the nurse to recover. Caring for less ill patients and experiencing positive outcomes can allow nurses time to reset their compassion levels.

2. *Encourage Participation in or Creation of Self-Care Initiatives.* These activities should include education on how to recognize STS, burnout, and compassion fatigue in self and others.

3. *Create Strict Structured Time Between Work and Home Life.* Decrease overtime work if possible, take mini-vacations, and do not take work home or check email often.

4. *Maintain Appropriate Professional Boundaries With Patients and Families.* During the care of acutely ill or dying children, bonds of trust can form quickly among caregivers, patients, and families. If a nurse finds herself or himself thinking about patients frequently outside of work, dreaming about them, speaking or meeting with families during nonwork time, or consistently requesting to be their caregivers during a shift, there is potential that the relationships have violated professional boundaries. The nurse should immediately create emotional and physical distance.

D. The Second-Victim Phenomenon

First described by Wu in 2000, second victims are healthcare providers who experience profound trauma as a result of involvement in a patient safety event, particularly when they occur as a result of a medical error (Case Study 10.6). Second victims can experience symptoms similar to STS, with the addition of guilt, isolation, and concerns

> **CASE STUDY 10.6   Second-Victim Kim Hiatt**
>
> Kim Hiatt was a well-respected pediatric ICU nurse who worked over 24 years in the same hospital. In September 2010, she mistakenly gave a tenfold overdose of calcium chloride to an 8-month-old critically ill infant. Five days later, the infant died. Although a state investigation found no proof that the overdose led to the infant's death, a cardiologist stated that he believed the overdose exacerbated the child's already tenuous cardiac dysfunction. Kim was suspended following the incident, and her employment involuntarily terminated several weeks later. Her state nursing commission placed her on a 4-year probationary period, which included supervision during any medication administration to patients. She was unable to obtain other employment. Distraught, guilt-ridden, and devastated over the loss of the profession she loved and dedicated her life to, she committed suicide 7 months after the incident. Kim's experience as a *second victim*, although an extreme example, is indicative of the importance of understanding this relatively newly defined phenomenon (Saavedra, 2015).

of job loss and litigation (Quillivan, Burlison, Browne, Scott, & Hoffman, 2016). The second-victim phenomenon can even occur with a near-miss event, creating feelings of paranoia (of making the mistake again), decreased self-confidence, and low self-esteem, leading to anxiety and depression if feelings continue.

Undoubtedly, increased focus on creating safe environments and reviewing medical errors and mistakes closely is the right thing to do. However, there is increasing evidence that it also leads nurses involved in adverse events to feel cumulative amounts of personal responsibility and failure. Although adverse events can result from an individual failure to follow accepted procedures, system-level failures often frequently contribute to events. Transparent discussion of emotional stress experienced by caregivers involved in adverse events encourage reporting and personal responsibility or error. Root-cause analyses by a dedicated group of safety experts, plus those caregivers involved, encourage dialog of how to improve individual performance and address system-level failures. A just-culture philosophy and nonpunitive environments in which individuals do not shoulder blame alone creates HWEs (Joeston, Cipparrone, Okuno-Jones, & DuBose, 2015). Caregivers in these environments can feel comfortable sharing errors with others to promote learning and contribute to constructive system changes to prevent future events. Institutions that provide emotional support following events can decrease probable incidents of compassion fatigue, burnout, and STS. Recent literature discussing the phenomenon encourages the creation of formal programs to provide support, including a tutorial toolkit endorsed by TJC (Pratt, Kenney, Scott, & Wu, 2012).

CONCLUSIONS

Nurses are the frontline providers of patient care in the ICU setting. As such, they must be able to articulate and implement elements of safe, quality care. By understanding the Swiss cheese model and how latent and active errors can interact to produce patient harm events, nurses can proactively identify system issues that contribute to patient safety events, while holding each other accountable for individual performance using principles of a just culture. Critical care nurses can be leaders in establishing and sustaining a culture of safety in their units by maintaining competencies outlined in the IOM's QSEN program. Some examples include practicing and promoting effective communication, involving families and patients in bedside care, and engaging in QI and EBP activities. In addition, to ensure safe and quality patient care at all times, nurses should ensure there is "care for the caregiver." That is, fatigue and burnout should be reduced by implementing strategies to promote an HWE.

REFERENCES

AACN. (2016). Interdependence of healthy work environment, clinical excellence, and optimal patient outcomes. In *AACN standards for establishing and sustaining healthy work environments; A journey to excellence* (2nd ed., p. 11. Aliso Viejo, CA: Author.

Adams-Pizarro, I., Walker, Z., Robinson, J., Kelly, S., & Toth, M. (2008). Using the AHRQ Hospital Survey on Patient Safety Culture as an intervention tool for regional clinical improvement collaboratives. In K. Henriksen, J. B. Battles, M. A. Keyes, & M. L. Grady (Eds.), Advances in patient safety: New directions and alternative approaches (Vol. 2: Culture and Redesign). Rockville, MD: Agency for Healthcare Research and Quality. Retrieved from https://www.ncbi.nlm.nih.gov/books/NBK43728

af Sandeberg, M., Wenemark, M., Bartholdson, C., Lützén, K., & Pergert, P. (2017). To change or not to change—Translating and culturally adapting the paediatric version of the Moral Distress Scale-Revised (MDS-R). *BMC Medical Ethics, 18,* 14. doi:10.1186/s12910-017-0176-y

Agency for Healthcare Research and Quality. (n.d.-a). About AHRQ. Retrieved from https://www.ahrq.gov/cpi/about/index.html

Agency for Healthcare Research and Quality. (n.d.-b). Frequently asked questions. Retrieved from https://info.ahrq.gov/app/answers/detail/a_id/426/~/where-can-i-find-out-about-ahrqs-history%3F

Agency for Healthcare Research and Quality. (2017a). Debriefing for clinical learning. Retrieved from https://psnet.ahrq.gov/primers/primer/36/learning-through-debriefing

Agency for Healthcare Research and Quality. (2017b). Handoffs and signouts. Retrieved from https://psnet.ahrq.gov/primers/primer/9

Amalberti, R., Auroy, Y., Berwick, D., & Barach, P. (2005). Five system barriers to achieving ultrasafe health care. *Annals of Internal Medicine, 142*(9), 756–764. doi:10.7326/0003-4819-142-9-200505030-00012

American Association of Critical-Care Nurses. (n.d.) Synergy Model. Retrieved from https://www.aacn.org/nursing-excellence/aacn-standards/synergy-model

American Association of Critical-Care Nurses. (2016). *AACN standards for establishing and sustaining healthy work environments: A journey to excellence (2nd ed.).* Retrieved from https://www.aacn.org/WD/HWE/Docs/HWEStandards.pdf

American College of Surgeons. (n.d.). Pediatric trauma quality improvement program. Retrieved from https://www.facs.org/quality-programs/trauma/tqip/pediatric-tqip

American Nurses Association. (2015). *Code of ethics for nurses with interpretive statements.* Silver Spring, MD: Author Retrieved from http://nursingworld.org/DocumentVault/Ethics-1/Code-of-Ethics-for-Nurses.html

American Psychological Association. (2014, February). Safer air travel through crew resource management. Retrieved from http://www.apa.org/action/resources/research-in-action/crew.aspx

Anderson, J. B., Beekman, R. H., Kugler, J. D., Rosenthal, G. L., Jenkins, K. J., Klitzner, T. S., ... Lannon, C. (2015). Improvement in interstage survival in a national pediatric cardiology learning network. *Circulation: Cardiovascular Quality and Outcomes, 8*(4), 428–436. doi:10.1161/circoutcomes.115.001956

Angang Price, R., Elliott, M. N., Zaslavsky, A. M, Hays, R. D., Lehrman, W. G., Rybowski, L., ... Cleary, P. D. (2014). Examining the role of patient experience surveys in measuring health care quality. *Medical Care Research and Review, 71*(5), 522–554. doi:10.1177/1077558714541480

Attree, M. (2007). Factors influencing nurses' decisions to raise concerns about care quality. *Journal of Nursing Management, 15,* 392–402. doi:10.1111/j.1365-2834.2007.00679.x

Beckett, C. D., & Kipnis, G. (2009). Collaborative communication: Integrating SBAR to improve quality/patient safety outcomes. *Journal for Healthcare Quality, 31*(5), 19–28. doi:10.1111/j.1945-1474.2009.00043.x

Berger, J., Polivka, B., Smoot, E. A., & Owens, H. (2015). Compassion fatigue in pediatric nurses. *Journal of Pediatric Nursing, 30,* e11–e17. doi:10.1016/j.pedn.2015.02.005

Berwick, D. M., Nolan, T. W., & Whittington, J. (2008). The Triple Aim: Care, health, and cost. *Health Affairs, 27*(3), 759–769. doi:10.1377/hlthaff.27.3.759

Billett, A. L., Colletti, R. B., Mandel, K. E., Miller, M., Muething, S. E., Sharek, P. J., & Lannon, C. M. (2013). Exemplar pediatric collaborative improvement networks: Achieving results. *Pediatrics, 131*(Suppl. 4), S196–S203. doi:10.1542/peds.2012-3786f

Blake, N., Searle, L. S., Robbins, W., Pike, N., & Needleman, J. (2013). Healthy work environments and staff nurse retention. *Nursing Administration Quarterly, 37*(4), 356–270. doi:10.1097/NAQ.0b013e3182a2fa47

Blankenship, A. C., Fernandez, R. P., Joy, B. F., Miller, J. C., Naguib, A., Cassidy, S. C., ... Yates, A. R. (2016). Multidisciplinary review of code events in a heart center. *American Journal of Critical Care, 25*(4), e90–e97. doi:10.4037/ajcc2016302

Blankenship, A. C., Harrison, S., Brandt, S., Joy, B. & Simsic, J. (2015). Increasing parental participation during rounds in a pediatric cardiac intensive care unit. *American Journal of Critical Care, 24*(6), 532–538. doi:10.4037/ajcc2015153

Boysen, P. G., II. (2013). Just culture: A foundation for balanced accountability and patients safety. *Oschner Journal*, *13*, 400–406. Retrieved from https://www.ncbi.nlm.nih.gov/pmc/articles/PMC3776518

Braithwaite, J., Wears, R. L., & Hollnagel, E. (2015). Resilient health care: Turning patient safety on its head. *International Journal for Quality in Health Care*, *27*(5), 418–420. doi:10.1093/intqhc/mzv063

Branch, C., & Klinkenberg, D. (2015). Compassion fatigue among pediatric healthcare providers. *American Journal of Maternal/Child Nursing*, *40*(3), 160–166. doi:10.1097/NMC.0000000000000133

Brink, J. A. (2017). Is achieving "just culture" just culture, or something more? *Journal of the American College of Radiology*, *14*(2), 143–144. doi:10.1016/j.jacr.2016.12.018

Browning, A. M. (2013). Moral distress and psychological empowerment in critical care nurses caring for adults at end of life. *American Journal of Critical Care*, *22*(2), 143–151. doi:10.4037/ajcc2013437

Buchert, A. R., & Butler, G. A. (2016). Clinical pathways: Driving high-reliability and high-value care. *Pediatric Clinics of North America*, *63*(2), 317–328. doi:10.1016/j.pcl.2015.12.005

Burlison, J. D., Quillivan, R. R., Kath, L. M., Zhou, Y., Courtney, S. C., Cheng, C., & Hoffman, J. M. (2016). A multilevel analysis of U.S. hospital patient safety culture relationships with perceptions of voluntary event reporting. *Journal of Patient Safety*. Advance online publication. doi:10.1097/PTS.0000000000000336

Butler, A., Copnell, B., & Willetts, G. (2013). Family-centred care in the paediatric intensive care unit: An integrative review of the literature. *Journal of Clinical Nursing*, *23*(15-16), 2086–2100. doi:10.1111/jocn.12498

California Perinatal Quality Care Collaborative. (n.d.). Membership. Retrieved from https://www.cpqcc.org/about-us/membership

Carpenter, H. (2015). ANA releases preliminary findings from health risk appraisal. *American Nurse*. Retrieved from http://www.theamericannurse.org/2015/03/01/preliminary-data-released-from-anas-hra

Chassin, M. R., & Loeb, J. M. (2013). High-reliability health care: Getting there from here. *Milbank Quarterly*, *91*(30), 459–490. http://doi.org/10.1111/1468-0009.12023

Chera, B. S., Mazur, L., Adams, R. D., Kim, H. J., Milowsky, M. I., & Marks, L. B. (2016). Creating a culture of safety within an institution: Walking the walk. *Journal of Oncology Practice*, *12*(10), 880–883. doi:10.1200/jop.2016.012864

Collins, S. (2015). *Safer skies: How aviation safety has improved.* Retrieved from http://www.agcs.allianz.com/assets/PDFs/GRD/GRD%20individual%20articles/012015/GRD2015-1-AviationSafety.pdf

Collins, S. J., Newhouse, R., Porter, J., & Talsma, A. (2014). Effectiveness of the surgical safety checklist in correcting errors: A literature review applying Reason's Swiss Cheese Model. *AORN Journal*, *100*(1), 65–79.e5. doi:10.1016/j.aorn.2013.07.024

Connor, J. A., Ahern, J. P., Cuccovia, B., Porter, C. L., Arnold, A., Dionne, R. E., & Hickey, P. A. (2016). Implementing a distraction-free practice with the red zone medication safety initiative. *Dimensions of Critical Care Nursing*, *35*(3), 116–124. doi:10.1097/dcc.0000000000000179

Crandall, W. V., Margolis, P. A., Kappelman, M. D., King, E. C., Pratt, J. M., Boyle, B. M., … Colletti, R. B. (2012). Improved outcomes in a quality improvement collaborative for pediatric inflammatory bowel disease. *Pediatrics*, *129*(4), E1030–E1041. doi:10.1542/peds.2011-1700

Crew Resource Management. (n.d.-a). Introduction. Retrieved from http://www.crewresourcemanagement.net/introduction

Crew Resource Management. (n.d.-b). Human factors for pilots. Retrieved from http://www.crewresourcemanagement.net

Cronenwett, L., Sherwood, G., Barnsteiner, J., Disch, J., Johnson, J., Mitchell, P., … Warren, J. (2007). Quality and safety education for nurses. *Nursing Outlook*, *55*(3), 122–131. doi:10.1016/j.outlook.2007.02.006

Crowl, A., Sharma, A., Sorge, L., & Sorensen, T. (2015). Accelerating quality improvement within your organization: Applying the Model for Improvement. *Journal of the American Pharmacists Association*, *55*(4), e364–e376. doi:10.1331/japha.2015.15533

Curtis, J. R., Cook, D. J., Wall, R. J., Angus, D. C., Bion, J., Kacmarek, R., … Puntillo, K. (2006). Intensive care unit quality improvement: A "how-to" guide for the interdisciplinary team. *Critical Care Medicine*, *34*(1), 211–218. doi:10.1097/01.CCM.0000190617.76104.AC

Deutsch, E. S., Dong, Y., Halamek, L. P., Rosen, M. A., Taekman, J. M., & Rice, J. (2016). Leveraging health care simulation technology for human factors research. *Human Factors*, *58*(7), 1082–1095. doi:10.1177/0018720816650781

DiCuccio, M. H. (2015). The relationship between patient safety culture and patient outcomes. *Journal of Patient Safety*, *11*(3), 135–142. doi:10.1097/pts.0000000000000058

Dixon, N., & Pearce, M. (2011, October). *Guide to using quality improvement tools to drive clinical audits.* Retrieved from https://www.hqip.org.uk/resource/hqip-guide-to-using-quality-improvement-tools-to-drive-clinical-audit

Dolansky, M. A. & Moore, S. M. (2013). Quality and safety education for nurses (QSEN): The key is systems thinking. *The Online Journal of Issues in Nursing*, *18*(3), 1. doi:10.3912/OJIN.Vol18No03Man01

Dyo, M., Kalowes, P., & Devries, J. (2016). Moral distress and intention to leave: A comparison of adult and paediatric nurses by hospital setting. *Intensive and Critical Care Nursing*, *36*, 42–48. doi:10.1016/j.iccn.2016.04.003

Epstein, E. G., & Hamric, A. B. (2009). Moral distress, moral residue, and the crescendo effect. *Journal of Clinical Ethics*, *20*(4), 330–342. Retrieved from https://www.ncbi.nlm.nih.gov/pmc/articles/PMC3612701

Frankel, A. S., Leonard, M. W., & Denham, C. R. (2006). Fair and just culture, team behavior, and leadership engagement: The tools to achieve high reliability. *Health Services Research*, *41*(4, Pt. 2), 1690–1709. doi:10.1111/j.1475-6773.2006.00572.x

Geiger-Brown, J., Rogers, V. E., Trinkoff, A. M., Kane, R. L., Bausell R. B., & Scharf, S. M. (2012). Sleep, sleepiness, fatigue, and performance of 12-hour-shift nurses. *Chronobiology International*, *29*(2), 211–219. doi:10.3109/07420528.2011.645752

Goldsmith, M. F. (1997). National patient safety foundation studies systems. *Journal of the American Medical Association*, *278*(19), 1561. doi:10.1001/jama.1997.03550190025014

Gordon, J. E., Deland, E., & Kelly, R. E. (2015). Let's talk about improving communication in healthcare. *Columbia Medical Review*, *1*(1), 23–27. doi:10.7916/D8RF5T5D

Gould, J. B. (2010). The role of regional collaboratives: The California Perinatal Quality Care Collaborative Model. *Clinics in Perinatology*, *37*, 71–86. doi:10.1016/j.clp.2010.01.004

Graham, D. G., Pace, W., Kappus, J., Holcomb, S., Galliger, J. M., Duclos, C. W., & Bonham, A. J. (n.d.). *Institutional review board approval of practice-based research network patient safety studies.* Retrieved from https://www.ahrq.gov/sites/default/files/wysiwyg/professionals/quality-patient-safety/patient-safety-resources/resources/advances-in-patient-safety/vol3/Graham.pdf

Hicks, R.W. (2016). Maintaining ethics in quality improvement. *AORN, Journal 103*(2), 139–141. doi:10.1016/j.aorn.2015.12.014 doi:10.1016/j.aorn.2015.12.014

Hinderer, K. A., VonRueden, K. T., Friedmann, E., McQuillan, K. A., Gilmore, R., Kramer, B. & Murray, M. (2014). Burnout, compassion fatigue, compassion satisfaction, and secondary traumatic stress in trauma nurses. *Journal of Trauma Nursing, 21*(4), 160–169. doi:10.1097/JTN.0000000000000055

Hughes, R. G. (Ed.). (2008, March). *Patient safety and quality: An evidence-based handbook for nurses.* (AHRQ Publication No. 08-0043). Rockville, MD: Agency for Healthcare Research and Quality.

Hughes, V. (2016). Safe night-shift work. *Nursing Management, 47*(8), 30–36. doi:10.1097/01.NUMA.0000488857.54323.64

ImproveCareNow. (n.d.). Purpose & success. Retrieved from https://www.improvecarenow.org/purpose-success

Institute for Healthcare Improvement. (n.d.-a). How to improve. Retrieved from http://www.ihi.org/resources/Pages/HowtoImprove/default.aspx

Institute for Healthcare Improvement. (n.d.-b). Triple Aim for populations. Retrieved from http://www.ihi.org/Topics/TripleAim/Pages/Overview.aspx

Institute for Healthcare Improvement. (2003). *The breakthrough series: IHI's collaborative model for achieving breakthrough improvement.* Boston, MA: Author.

Institute for Healthcare Improvement. (2017a). SBAR tool: Situation-background-assessment-recommendation. Retrieved from http://www.ihi.org/resources/Pages/Tools/SBARToolkit.aspx

Institute for Healthcare Improvement. (2017b). *QI essentials toolkit: Failure modes and effects analysis (FMEA).* Retrieved from www.ihi.org

Institute for Safe Medication Practices. (n.d.). *Historical timeline.* Retrieved from http://www.ismp.org/about/timeline.aspx

Institute of Medicine. (2001). *Crossing the quality chasm: A new health system for the 21st century.* Washington, DC: National Academies Press. doi:10.17226/10027

Jameton, A. (1984). *Nursing practice: The ethical issues.* Englewood Cliffs, NJ: Prentice Hall.

Jennings, B. (2008). Work stress and burnout among nurses: role of the work environment and working conditions. In R. Hughes (Ed.), *Patient safety and quality: An evidence-based handbook for nurses* (chap. 26, pp. 1–22). Rockville, MD: Agency for Healthcare Research and Quality.

Joeston, L., Cipparrone, N., Okuno-Jones, S., & DuBose, E. R. (2015). Assessing the perceived level of institutional support for the second victim after a patient safety event. *Journal of Patient Safety, 11*(2), 73–78. doi:10.1097/PTS.0000000000000060

Joint Commission Center for Transforming Healthcare. (n.d.). About us. Retrieved from https://www.centerfortransforminghealthcare.org

The Joint Commission. (2018). 2018 National Patient Safety Goals®. Retrieved from https://www.jointcommission.org/standards_information/npsgs.aspx

Kohn, L. T., Corrigan, J. M., & Donaldson, M. S. (Eds.). (2000). *To err is human: Building a safer health system.* Washington, DC: National Academies Press. doi:10.17226/9728

Kuo, D. Z., Houtrow, A. J., Arango, P., Kuhlthau, K. A., Simmons, J. M. & Neff, J. M. (2011). Family-centered care: Current applications and future directions in pediatric health care. *Maternal and Child Health Journal, 16*, 297–305. doi:10.1007/s10995-011-0751-7

Langley, G. J., Moen, R. D., Nolan, K. M., Nolan, T. W., Norman, C. L., & Provost, L. P. (2009). *The improvement guide: A practical approach to enhancing organizational performance* (2nd ed.). San Francisco, CA: Jossey-Bass.

Lee, H. C., Kurtin, P. S., Wight, N. E., Chance, K., Cucinotta-Fobes, T., Hanson-Timpson, T. A., ... Sharek, P. J. (2012). A quality improvement project to increase breast milk use in very low birth weight infants. *Pediatrics, 130*(6), e1679–e1687. doi:10.1542/peds.2012-0547

Leggett, J. M., Wasson, K., Sinacore, J. M., & Gamelli, R. L. (2013). A pilot study examining moral distress in nurses working in one United States burn center. *Journal of Burn Care and Research, 34*(5), 521–528. doi:10.1097/BCR.0b013e31828c7397

Lekka, C. (2011). *High reliability organisations: A review of the literature.* Retrieved from http://www.hse.gov.uk/research/rrpdf/rr899.pdf

Lighter, D. E. (2011). *Advanced performance improvement in health care: Principles and methods.* Sudbury, MA: Jones & Bartlett.

Lyle-Edrosolo, G. & Waxman, K. T. (2016). Aligning healthcare safety and quality competencies: Quality and Safety Education for Nurses (QSEN), the Joint Commission, and American Nurses Credentialing Center (ANCC) Magnet® standards crosswalk. *Nurse Leader, 14*(1), 70–75. doi:10.1016/j.mnl.2015.08.005

Lyren, A., Brilli, R., Bird, M., Lashutka, N., & Muething, S. (2016). Ohio children's hospitals solutions for patient safety: A framework for pediatric patient safety improvement. *Journal for Healthcare Quality, 38*(4), 213–222. doi:10.1111/jhq.12058

MacDonald, R. D. (2016). Articles that may change your practice: Crew resource management. *Air Medical Journal, 35*(2), 65–66. doi:10.1016/j.amj.2015.12.010

Marx, D. (2007). *Patient safety and the "just culture"* [Lecture]. Retrieved from https://www.unmc.edu/patient-safety/_documents/patient-safety-and-the-just-culture.pdf

McElligott, D., Siemers, S., Thomas, L., & Kohn, N. (2009). Health promotion in nurses: Is there a healthy nurse in the house? *Applied Nursing Research, 22*(3), 211–215. doi:10.1016/j.apnr.2007.07.005

McKeon, L. M., Cunningham, P. D., & Detty Oswaks, J. S. (2009). Improving patient safety: Patient-focused, high-reliability team training. *Journal of Nursing Care Quality, 24*(1), 76–82. doi:10.1097/NCQ.0b013e31818f5595

McNab, D., Bowie, P., Morrison, J., & Ross, A. (2016). Understanding patient safety performance and educational needs using the "Safety-II" approach for complex systems. *Education for Primary Care, 27*(6), 443–450. doi:10.1080/14739879.2016.1246068

McQuaid-Hanson, E., & Pian-Smith, M. C. (2017). Huddles and debriefings: Improving communication on labor and delivery. *Anesthesiology Clinics, 35*(1), 59–67. doi:10.1016/j.anclin.2016.09.006

Meyer, R., Li, A., Klaristenfeld, J., & Gold, J. I. (2015). Pediatric novice nurses: Examining compassion fatigue as a mediator between stress exposure and compassion satisfaction, burnout, and job satisfaction. *Journal of Pediatric Nursing, 30*, 174–183. doi:10.1016/j.pedn.2013.12.008

Miller, M. R., Takata, G., Stucky, E. R., & Neuspiel, D. R. (2011). Principles of pediatric patient safety: Reducing harm due to medical care [Policy statement]. *Pediatrics, 127*(6), 1199–1210. doi:10.1542/peds.2011-0967

Miller, N., Bhowmik, S., Ezinwa, M., Yang, T., Schrock, S., Bitzel, D., & McGuire, M. J. (2017). The relationship between safety culture and voluntary event reporting in a large regional ambulatory care group. *Journal of Patient Safety.* doi:10.1097/PTS.0000000000000337

Mitchell, G. (2013). Selecting the best theory to implement planned change. *Nursing Management, 20*(1), 32–37. doi:10.7748/nm2013.04.20.1.32.e1013

Morris, P. E., & Dracup, K. (2007). Quality improvement or research? The ethics of hospital project oversight. *American Journal of Critical Care, 16*(5), 424–426. Retrieved from http://ajcc.aacnjournals.org/content/16/5/424.full

Morvay, S., Lewe, D., Stewart, B., Catt, C., McClead, R. E., & Brilli, R. J. (2014). Medication event huddles: A tool for reducing adverse drug events. *The Joint Commission Journal on Quality and Patient Safety, 40*(1), 39–45. doi:10.1016/s1553-7250(14)40005-9

National Patient Safety Foundation. (n.d.). History and timeline Retrieved from http://www.npsf.org/?page=historyandtimeline

National Pediatric Cardiology Quality Improvement Collaborative. (n.d.). Retrieved from https://npcqic.org/

Olsen, D. P. , & Smania, M. A. (2016). Determining when an activity is or is not research. *American Journal of Nursing, 116*(10), 55–60. doi:10.1097/01.NAJ.0000503304.52756.9a

Patterson, M., & Deutsch, E. S. (2015). Safety-I, Safety-II, and resilience engineering. *Current Problems in Pediatric and Adolescent Health Care, 45,* 382–389. doi:10.1016/j.cppeds.2015.10.001

Perla, R. J., Provost, L. P., & Murray, S. K. (2011). The run chart: A simple analytical tool for learning from variation in healthcare processes. *BMJ Quality & Safety, 20*(1), 46–51. doi:10.1136/bmjqs.2009.037895

Petschonek, S., Burlison, J., Cross, C., Martin, K., Laver, J., Landis, R. S., & Hoffman, J. M. (2013). Development of the just culture assessment tool: Measuring the perceptions of health-care professionals in hospitals. *Journal of Patient Safety, 9,* 190–197. doi:10.1097/PTS.0b013e31828fff34

Pettit, A. M. & Duffy, J. J. (2015). Patient safety: Creating a culture change to support communication and teamwork. *The Journal of Legal Nurse Consulting, 26*(4), 23–26. Retrieved from http://www.aalnc.org/page/journal-v2.0

Pratt, S., Kenney, L., Scott, S. D., & Wu, A. W. (2012). How to develop a second victim support program: A toolkit for health care organizations. *The Joint Commission Journal on Quality and Patient Safety, 38*(5), 235–240. doi:10.1016/S1553-7250(12)38030-6

Prentice, T., Janvier, A., Gillam, L., & Davis, P. G. (2016). Moral distress within neonatal and paediatric intensive care units: A systematic review. *Archives of Disease in Childhood, 101,* 701–708. doi:10.1136/archdischild-2015-309410

Provost, L. P., Murray, S. K., (2011). *The healthcare data guide.* San Francisco, CA: Jossey-Bass.

Quillivan, R. R., Burlison, J. D., Browne, E. K., Scott, S. D., & Hoffman, J. M. (2016). Patient safety culture and the second victim phenomenon: Connecting culture to staff distress in nurses. *The Joint Commission Journal on Quality and Patient Safety, 42,* 377–384, AP1–AP2. doi:10.1016/S1553-7250(16)42053-2

Reader, T. W., Flin, R., Mearns, K. & Cuthbertson, B. H. (2009). Developing a team performance framework for the intensive care unit. *Critical Care Medicine, 37*(5), 1787–1793. doi:10.1097/CCM.0b013e31819f0451

Reason, J. (2000). Human error: Models and management. *British Medical Journal, 320,* 768–770. doi:10.1136/bmj.320.7237.768

Rose, L. (2011). Interprofessional collaboration in the ICU: How to define? *BACN Nursing in Critical Care, 16*(1), 5–10. doi:10.1111/j.1478-5153.2010.00398.x

Ross, A., Bevans, M., Brooks, A. T., Gibbons, S., & Wallen, G. R. (2016). Nurses and health-promoting behaviors: Knowledge may not translate into self-care. *AORN Journal, 105,* 267–275. doi:10.1016/j.aorn.2016.12.018

Rutherford, W. (2003). Aviation safety: A model for health care? *BMJ Quality and Safety in Health Care, 12,* 162–163. doi:10.1136/qhc.12.3.162

Saavedra, S. M. (2015, November 25). Remembering Kimberly Hiatt: A casualty of second victim syndrome. Retrieved from https://nurseslabs.com/remembering-kimberly-hiatt-casualty-second-victim-syndrome

Sacco, T. L., Ciurzynski, S. M., Harvey, M. E., & Ingersoll, G. L. (2015). Compassion satisfaction and compassion fatigue among critical care nurses. *Critical Care Nurse, 35*(4), 32–43. Retrieved from http://ccn.aacnjournals.org/content/35/4/32.full

Scanon, M. C., Mistry, K. P., & Jeffries, H. E. (2007). Determining pediatric intensive care unit quality indicators for measuring pediatric intensive care unit safety. *Pediatric Critical Care Medicine, 8*(2 Suppl.), S3–S10. doi:10.1097/01.PCC.0000257485.67821.77

Seaman, J. B., & Erlen, J. A. (2015). Workarounds in the workplace: A second look. *Orthopaedic Nursing, 34*(4), 235–240. doi:10.1097/nor.0000000000000161

Singer, S., Lin, S., Falwell, A., Gaba, D., & Baker, L. (2009). Relationship of safety climate and safety performance in hospitals. *Health Services Research, 44,* 399–421. doi:10.1111/j.1475-6773.2008.00918.x

Slatten, L. A., David Carson, K., & Carson, P. P. (2011). Compassion fatigue and burnout: What managers should know. *Health Care Manager, 30*(4), 325–333. doi:10.1097/HCM.0b013e31823511f7

Solutions for Patient Safety. (n.d.-a). How it all got started. Retrieved from http://www.solutionsforpatientsafety.org

Solutions for Patient Safety. (n.d.-b.). Our results. Retrieved from http://www.solutionsforpatientsafety.org

Stamm, B. H. (2002). Measuring compassion satisfaction as well as fatigue: Development and history of the compassion fatigue test. In C. R. Figley (Ed.), *Treating compassion fatigue* (pp. 107–122). New York, NY: Brunner-Routledge.

Stamm, B. H. (2010). *The concise ProQOL manual* (2nd ed.). Pocatello, ID: ProQOL.org.

Stausmire, J. M. (2014). Quality improvement or research—Deciding which road to take. *American Association of Critical-Care Nurses, 34*(6), 58–63. doi:10.4037/ccn2014177

Stein, J. E. & Heiss, K. (2015). The swiss cheese model of adverse event occurrence—Closing the holes. *Seminars in Pediatric Surgery, 24,* 272–282. doi:10.1053/j.sempedsurg.2015.08.003

The Joint Commission. (2018). *National patient safety goals.* Retrieved from https://www.jointcommission.org/standards_information/npsgs.aspx

Thomas, T. A., Thammasitboon, S., Balmer, D. F., Roy, K., & McCullough, L. B. (2016). A qualitative study exploring moral distress among pediatric resuscitation team clinicians: Challenges to professional integrity. *Pediatric Critical Care Medicine, 17*(7), e303–e308. doi:10.1097/PCC.0000000000000773

Toomey, S. L., Elliott, M. N., Zaslavsky, A. M., Klein, D. J., Ndon, S., Hardy, S., … Schuster, M. A. (2017). Variation in family experience of pediatric inpatient care as measured by child HCAHPS. *Pediatrics, 139*(4). doi:10.1542/peds.2016-3372

Trotochaud, K., Ramsey Coleman, J. Krawiecki, N., & McCracken, C. (2015). Moral distress in pediatric healthcare providers. *Journal of Pediatric Nursing, 30,* 908–914. doi:10.1016/j.pedn.2015.03.001

Tucker, S. J., Harris, M. R., Pipe T. B., & Stevens, S. R. (2010). Nurses' ratings of their health and professional work environments. *Workplace Health & Safety*, *58*(6), 253–267. doi:10.1177/216507991005800605

Ulrich, B. T., Lavandero, R., Woods, F., & Early, S. (2014). Critical care nurse work environments 2013: A status report. *Critical Care Nurse*, *34*(4), 64–79. doi:10.4037/ccn2014731

Weller, J., Boyd, M. & Cumin, D. (2014). Teams, tribes and patient safety: Overcoming barriers to effective teamwork in healthcare. *Postgraduate Medical Journal*, *90*, 149–154. doi:10.1136/postgradmedj-2012-131168

Williams, L. (2016). Impact of family-centered care on pediatric and neonatal intensive care outcomes. *AACN Advanced Critical Care*, *27*(2), 158–161. doi:10.4037/aacnacc2016579

Wirtschafter, D. D., Pettit, J., Kurtin, P., Dalsey, M., Chance, K., Morrow, H. W., … Kloman, S. (2009). A statewide quality improvement collaborative to reduce neonatal central line-associated blood stream infections. *Journal of Perinatology*, *30*(3), 170–181. doi:10.1038/jp.2009.172

Wirtschafter, D. D., Powers, R. J., Pettit, J. S., Lee, H. C., Boscardin, W. J., Subeh, M. A., & Gould, J. B. (2011). Nosocomial infection reduction in VLBW infants with a statewide quality-improvement model. *Pediatrics*, *127*(3), 419–426. doi:10.1542/peds.2010-1449

World Health Organization. (2009). Conceptual framework for the international classification for patient safety (Rep. No. V1.1). Retrieved from http://www.who.int/patientsafety/taxonomy/icps_full_report.pdf?ua=1

Wu, A. W. (2000). Medical error: The second victim: The doctor who makes the mistake needs help too. *British Medical Journal*, *18*(320), 726. doi:10.1136/bmj.320.7237.726.

Yip, L., & Farmer, B. (2015). High reliability organizations—Medication safety. *Journal of Medical Toxicology*, *11*(2), 257–261. doi:10.1007/s13181-015-0471-2

INDEX

Note: Page numbers followed by f indicate figures and t indicate tables.

A waves, 390, 391f
AACN. *See* American Association of Critical-Care Nurses
AAP. *See* American Academy of Pediatrics
AAPCC. *See* American Association of Poison Control Centers
ABA. *See* American Burn Association
ABGs. *See* arterial blood gases
abdomen
  assessments of, 533–534
  child abuse-related injuries, 723
  distention of, 533
  pediatric assessments, 830t
  post-traumatic assessment of, 687
  stab wounds to, 706
  traumatic injuries to, 706, 723
abdominal compartment syndrome, 797
abdominal computed tomography, 536t, 549
abdominal radiography, 544
abdominal reflex, 372
abdominal ultrasound, 536t, 549
abdominal wall, 534
abdominal wound care, 546
abdominal x-rays, 536t, 549
abducens nerve
  in children, 377t
  function of, 364t
  in infants, 374t
ABO blood groups, 607
absence seizures, 404
absolute neutrophil count, 604
absolute refractory period, 160
absorption, 353
abuse
  child. *See* child maltreatment
  emotional, 719, 727
  sexual, 719–720
abusive head trauma (AHT), 874
acceleration-deceleration injury, 674
accidental injury, 668
acetaminophen
  pain management using, 14, 16t
  poisoning, 743t, 744–746
acetazolamide, 464
acetylcholine, 365
acetylcholinesterase inhibitors, 768

acid–base balance
  description of, 452–453
  renal responses to changes in, 463t
acidosis
  acute kidney injury and, 458t, 460, 462
  caustic substance poisoning and, 759–761
  description of, 463t
  hyponatremic, 452
  respiratory, 463t
acids, 759–761
acoustic nerve
  in children, 378t
  function of, 364t
  in infants, 375t
acquired immunity, 593t, 594
acquired immunodeficiency syndrome (AIDS). *See also* human immunodeficiency virus
  in children, 639
  definition of, 638–639
  etiology of, 638–639
  incidence of, 639
acquired myopathy, 309
acrocyanosis, 162, 166
ACT. *See* activated clotting time
ACTH. *See* adrenocorticotropic hormone
action potential, 159, 159f, 360
activated charcoal, 742, 756
activated clotting time (ACT), 607, 873
activated partial thromboplastin time, 606
activation gate, 160
active errors, 889
active immunity, 593t
active transport, 446
activities of daily living (ADL), 821
acute abdomen, 580
acute abdominal trauma
  blunt, 548
  clinical presentation of, 548–549
  definition and etiology of, 548
  diagnostic studies of, 550
  management of, 550
  mechanisms of, 548
  pathophysiology of, 548
  patient care management, 549–553
  signs and symptoms of, 550
  spleen, 550–551, 551t
acute chest syndrome, 633–634
acute glomerulonephritis, 466
acute hemolytic reactions, 620

acute hypoglycemia, 515–518
  complications, 518
  diagnostic studies, 517
  etiology, 516
  management, 517–518
  pathophysiology, 515–516
  risk factors, 516
  sign and symptoms, 516–517
acute idiopathic pulmonary hemorrhage of infancy, 104
acute ischemic stroke (AIS)
  characteristics, 408–409
  definition of, 408
  diagnostic tests, 409
  etiology, 408
  management of, 409–410
  neuroimaging, 409
  outcomes for pediatric, 410
  pathophysiology, 408
  symptoms, 409
acute kidney injury (AKI)
  acetazolamide for, 464
  acute glomerulonephritis and, 466
  cardiac failure and, 467
  causes of, 457–459
  in children, 457
  complications of, 458, 458t, 464, 465
  definition of, 456
  diuretics for, 464
  fenoldopam for, 464
  hematologic changes, 462
  hemolytic uremic syndrome and, 465
  hepatorenal syndrome and, 466–467
  hyperkalemia, 458t, 460–461
  hypermagnesemia, 458t, 461
  hyperphosphatemia, 458t, 461
  hypocalcemia, 458t, 461
  intrinsic. *See* acute tubular necrosis
  laboratory findings in, 459–463, 459t, 463t
  management of, 463–464
  metabolic acidosis in, 462, 463t
  multisystem complications secondary to, 463, 463t
  nephrotic syndrome and, 465–466
  postrenal, 459
  prerenal, 457, 457t
  renal diseases or conditions that cause, 466–468
  replacement therapy, 464
  rhabdomyolysis and, 467–468, 468t
  tumor lysis syndrome and, 467
acute lung injury (ALI), 68, 92, 132
acute pulmonary embolism, 90–91

acute renal failure, 456. *See also* acute
kidney injury
acute respiratory distress syndrome
(ARDS), 68. *See also* pediatric
acute respiratory distress
syndrome
acute spasmodic laryngitis, 76t, 78
acute surgical abdomen
clinical presentation of, 556, 562
definition of, 556
etiology of, 556
intervention for, 562
management, 562
pathophysiology of, 556
acute tubular necrosis (ATN), 454,
455, 571
clinical course of
diuretic phase, 459
oliguric phase, 458, 459
onset/initiating phase, 458
recovery phase, 459
description of, 457
ischemic, 458
nephrotoxic, 457
true intrinsic, 464
acyclovir, 398
adaptive pressure ventilation, 121
adaptive support ventilation, 121
Addison disease, 501
additional labs, 517
adenohypophysis, 486–487
adenosine (Adenocard), 197
adenosine triphosphate, 446, 762
ADH. *See* antidiuretic hormone
adhesiveness, 590–591
adjunctive therapies, chest trauma, 110
adolescent idiopathic scoliosis
(AIS), 434
adolescents. *See also* children
cerebral blood flow in, 360
cognitive development, 5
communication by, 17
cough in, 50t
death, concept of, 5
fear responses by, 8
hospitalization response of, 7–8
noninsulin-dependent diabetes, 508
pain assessment and management,
12t, 13t
as parents, 6
personality development, 5
play with, 20
poisoning of, 737
principles for working with, 6
psychosocial development, 4–5
scoliosis in, 433
stress response of, 7–8
traumatic injuries in, 672t
adrenal crisis, 502
adrenal glands
adrenal cortex, 481t, 499
adrenal medulla, 482t
cell types, 499–500
embryology of, 499

location of, 499
structure of, 499
zones of, 499
adrenal insufficiency, 507, 788–789
adrenocorticotropic hormone
(ACTH), 501
characteristics of, 489–490
cortisol secretion and, 501
embryologic production of, 484
functions of, 480t
stimulation test, 505
adult-onset diabetes, 508
adult respiratory distress syndrome,
123t, 644, 863
advanced cardiac life support
airway management, 210
cardiopulmonary assessments, 784
cardiopulmonary failure, 209–210
circulatory support, 210–212
fluid resuscitation, 213
initiation of, 210
neonatal resuscitation, 214
parental presence during, 216–217
pharmacologic support, 213, 214
postresuscitation care, 214–216, 215f
septic shock management, 784
vascular access, 212, 213, 213f, 214f
ventilation, 210
Advanced Trauma Life Support
(ATLS), 668
adventitious sounds, 47
adverse drug event, 887
AED. *See* automatic electrical
defibrillation
afferent fibers, 362
afterload, 156, 230, 253, 787
Agency for Health Care Policy and
Research, 883
Agency on Healthcare Research and
Quality (AHRQ), 883, 885
agglutination, 594
aggregation, 590
aggressive therapy, 107
AHRQ. *See* Agency on Healthcare
Research and Quality
AHT. *See* abusive head trauma
AIDS. *See* acquired immunodeficiency
syndrome
airflow resistance, 37
airway. *See also* asthma
and acute laryngotracheobronchitis,
77f
assessment of, 680, 799, 829t, 850–851
chemical burns, 96
conducting, 37–38
contraindications, 856t
description of, 855
edema, 97
endotracheal, 210, 211f, 212f
foreign material in, 688
head-tilt/chin-lift method for,
114, 688
hyperresponsiveness, 97
indications for, 856t

inflammation, 97–98
during initial stabilization of patient,
855–857
injury, 799, 805–806
intrapulmonary, 37
jaw thrust maneuver for, 688
limitations of, 856t
maintenance of, 210, 852
management of
during initial stabilization of
patient, 855–857
in mechanical ventilation, 126, 127
nasopharyngeal, 689, 856t
oropharyngeal, 689, 856t
patent, 210, 214, 852
pediatric, 829t
post-trauma assessments, 681
postnatal development of, 35
remodeling, 97
airway-clearance therapies, 69
diagnosis and implementation of, 69
types of, 69t–70t
airway obstruction, 98, 114
description of, 864t
foreign-body aspiration-related, 88
airway pressure release ventilation
(APRV), 121, 807
airway reflexes, 852
airway resistance, 39
AIS. *See* acute ischemic stroke;
adolescent idiopathic scoliosis
AKI. *See* acute kidney injury
alagille syndrome, 163t, 574
alanine aminotransferase, 534t
albumin, 535t, 619t
albuterol
airway obstruction treated with, 864t
hyperkalemia managed using, 460
aldosterone
characteristics of, 450–451, 500–501
functions of, 481t, 501
regulation of, 500–501, 500f
ALI. *See* acute lung injury
alkaline phosphatase, 534t
alkaline substances, 759–760
alkalosis
metabolic, 463t
respiratory, 463t, 781
Allen test, 182, 213
allergen control, asthma, 98
allergy testing, 98
allograft, 811
alloimmunization, 622
alpha-1 antitrypsin deficiency, 574
alpha cells, 482t, 497
alpha-fetoprotein, 420, 437
Alprostadil. *See* prostaglandin E1 (PGE1)
alteplase, 615
alveolar-arterial gradient (A-a gradient),
187–188
alveolar ischemia, 234
alveolar overdistention, 132
alveolar pores of Kohn, 38
alveolar ventilation, 118t, 119

alveoli
 anatomy of, 38
 epithelial cells of, 38
 postnatal development of, 35
Amanita spp., 767
ambrisentan, 206
American Academy of Critical-Care
  Nurses (AACN)
 healthy work environment, 913,
  914, 914f
 synergy model, 905
American Academy of Pediatrics
  (AAP), 668, 832, 839, 876
American Association of Critical-Care
  Nurses (AACN)
 Essentials of Pediatric Critical Care
  Orientation, 8
 Synergy Model for Patient Care, 1–3
American Association of Poison Control
  Centers (AAPCC), 746
American Board of Surgery, 667
American Burn Association (ABA), 793
 burn center referral criteria, 802t
American College of Emergency
  Physicians, 668
American Heart Association (AHA), 878
 CPR guidelines, 113
 diet recommendations, 913
American Nurses Association (ANA)
 "Health Risk Appraisal," 915
 sleep recommendations, 915
American Nurses Credentialing Center
  (ANCC), 910
American Society of Professionals in
  Patient Safety (ASPPS), 885
amiodarone hydrochloride
  (Cordarone), 196
ammonia, 535t, 833t
amoxapine, 748
amphetamines, 739t, 755
Amplatzer device, for atrial septal
  defect, 255, 256f
amputations, 691, 710, 715–716
amygdalin, 761–762
amyl nitrite, 761–762
amylase, 531, 552
amylin, 499
anal examination, 687
analgesia
 in children, 395, 396t
 management of, 221, 223
 patient-controlled, 631, 635, 817
 remedial agents for, 65–67, 65t–66t
analgesics, 59t–62t
anaphylactic shock, 232
anaphylaxis
 management of, 627
 transfusion-related, 620t
anaplastic astrocytoma and
  glioblastoma, 419
anemia
 assessment of, 623–624
 burn-related, 803
 chronic kidney disease and, 454

definition of, 587, 623
 iatrogenic, 624
 interventions for, 626
 renal failure and, 462
 sickle cell, 631t
 signs and symptoms of, 623
anemic hypoxia, 847
anencephaly, 437
anesthetics, 746
aneurysm
 characteristics of, 410–411
 definition of, 410–411
 types of, 411
angiography
 cardiovascular system
  evaluations, 180
 cerebral, 384
 coronary, 179
 magnetic resonance, 179, 180
 pulmonary function evaluations
  using, 53
 thoracic trauma, 112
angiotensin I, 157
angiotensin II, 157, 454, 492
angiotensin-converting enzyme
  inhibitors, 229
animal bites, 673t, 674
anisocoria, 426
ANP. *See* atrial natriuretic peptide
anterior cord syndrome, 429, 701
anterior fontanelle
 anatomy of, 352, 352f
 auscultation of, 369
 external fiber-optic transducer
  attached to, 388
anterior pituitary gland, 487
 cells of, 486
 characteristics of, 486
 embryology of, 484
 hormones produced by, 480t,
  489–490
anthrax, 834, 836t
anthropometrics, 542
anti-inflammatory drugs, 68, 99
anti-inflammatory mediators, 777
antiarrhythmic agents, 314
 class I agents, 193
 class II agents, 194–196
 class IV agents, 196–197
 miscellaneous medications, 197–198
antiarrhythmic therapies, 230
antiarrhythmics, 237. *See also* specific
  drugs
 class I, 193–194
 class II, 194–196
antibiotics
 asthma treated with, 99
 septic shock treated with,
  783, 784, 819
antibleeding agents, 537
antibodies
 detection of, 606
 monoclonal, 606, 613–614
antibody-dependent cytotoxicity, 594

anticholinergics, 743t
 asthma treated with, 99
 characteristics of, 65
anticipatory guidance, 27
anticoagulants, 743t
 description of, 590, 599
 heparin, 614–615
 warfarin, 615
anticoagulation
 description of, 471–472
 in pulmonary hypertension, 107
anticonvulsant medications
 long-term effects of, 407–408
 for seizures, 398, 399t, 407
 status epilepticus treated with, 407
antidepressant poisoning, 743t, 746–749
antidiuretic hormone (ADH), 527
 abnormalities of, 492
 characteristics of, 491–492
 description of, 450
 diabetes insipidus testing, 522
 functions of, 481t
 in newborns, 484
 receptors, 492
 regulation of, 492f
 secretion, 492f
antidotes
 for cyanide poisoning, 762
 for ethylene glycol poisoning, 765
 for poison exposures, 742–743
antidromic pathway, 235
antigen-antibody interaction, 594
antigens
 definition of, 591
 detection of, 606
 human leukocyte, 591, 605
 processing, 594
antihistamines, 736t
antihypertensives, 198–203. *See also*
  specific drugs
antimicrobials
 bacterial meningitis treated with, 418
 burn wounds treated with, 813t
 therapy for central nervous system
  infections, 396, 397t, 398
antipyretic administration, 107
antipyretic therapy, 868
antiretroviral medications, 641
antithrombin III, 590, 614
antithrombin system, 590, 600
antithymocyte globulin, 613
anuria, 458
anxiety
 assessment, 818
 hospitalization-related, 8, 9
 management, 818–819
 pain versus, 11
 parental, 25
anxiolytics, 817
aortic arch
 coarctation of the aorta and, 275
 segments of, 276f
aortic area, 167f, 168, 171
aortic atresia, 301

aortic injuries, 110, 111
aortic stenosis
    congenital, 272
    definition of, 271
    discrete subaortic, 274
    interventions for, 277, 278f
    subaortic, 274–275, 275f, 292f
    supravalvular, 274–275, 276f, 284f, 285
    valvular, 271–274
aortoplasty, for coarctation of the aorta,
    277, 278f
apical area, 167f, 168, 171
apixaban, 204–205
aplasia
    bone marrow, 610
    definition of, 585
aplastic anemia, 623
aplastic crisis, 631t, 633
apnea, 112, 690, 852
apneustic breathing, 46f
apneustic respiratory pattern, 380
APRV. *See* airway pressure release
    ventilation
AquaMEPHYTON. *See* vitamin K
aqueduct of sylvius, 352
arachnoid, 357
arachnoid villi, 353
argatroban, 203
arginine vasopressin (AVP), 491–492
arrhythmias, 210, 226–227
    atrial fibrillation, 240, 240f
    atrial flutter, 239–240, 240f
    causes of, 871t
    definition of, 235
    etiology of, 235
    junctional tachycardia, 239, 239f
    management of, 870
    pathophysiology, 235
    sick sinus syndrome, 237
    sinus arrhythmia, 235, 236, 236f
    sinus bradycardia, 236f, 237
    sinus tachycardia, 236, 236f
    supraventricular, 235–240, 236f
    supraventricular tachycardia,
        237–238, 238f
    therapy, 213
    ventricular, 240–242
arrhythmogenic right ventricular
    myopathy (ARVM)
    complications, 318
    diagnostic evaluation, 318
    etiology of, 317
    pathophysiology of, 317
    phenotypic expression, 317–318
    treatment for, 318
arterial blood, 356
arterial blood gases (ABGs), 100
    description of, 554
    during mechanical ventilation, 128
    septic shock evaluations using, 781
arterial occlusion, 716
arterial oxygen
    content, 42
    saturation, 43t

arterial partial pressure of oxygen,
    calculation of, 43t
arterial pressure
    description of, 157
    monitoring of, 182–183
arterial switch operation, for
    transposition of the great arteries,
    297, 298f
arterial vascular access, 213, 214f
arterial waveforms, 183, 185f
arteries, 150
arteriohepatic dysplasia, 574
arterioles, 150
arteriovenous malformations (AVMs),
    410–411
arteriovenous oxygen difference, 43t
artificial dermis, 811
ASA. *See* aspirin
ascending spinal tract, 358t
ascites, 572–573
ASD. *See* atrial septal defect
aspartate aminotransferase, 534t
asphyxia, 805
aspiration pneumonia
    causes of, 89t
    clinical presentation of, 89
    definition of, 88
    outcomes of, 90
    pathophysiology of, 88–89
    patient care management, 90
aspirin, 205, 614, 754, 755, 868
ASPPS. *See* American Society of
    Professionals in Patient Safety
assist/control ventilation, 120
asterixis, 573
asthma
    acute episodes of
        management of, 98–101
        prognosis for, 101
    airflow limitation in, 97
    allergen control, 98
    breathing exercises, 99
    bronchoconstriction in, 97
    categories, 97
    clinical presentation of, 98
    complications, 101
    critical care management, 99–100
    definition, 97
    diagnostic evaluation, 98
    differential diagnosis, 98
    drug therapy, 98–99
    hyposensitization, 99
    inflammation, 97–98
    laboratory testing, 98
    long-term care, 100–101
    nursing care management,
        99–101
    outcome of, 101
    pathophysiology of, 97–98
    risk factors, 101
    tobacco smoke exposure, 96
astrocytes, 352
astrocytoma, 419
asymmetric tonic neck response, 372

asynchronous mode, of pacemaker,
    245, 246t
ataxia-telangiectasia syndrome, 637
ataxic breathing, 46f
ataxic respirations, 380
atelectasis, 132
atenolol (Tenormin), 195
ATLS. *See* Advanced Trauma Life
    Support
atracurium, 58t
atria
    autonomic nerve stimulation effects
        on, 367t
    depolarization of, 160
atrial asynchronous mode, of
    pacemaker, 246t
atrial demand mode, of pacemaker, 246t
atrial fibrillation, 240, 240f
atrial flutter, 239–240, 240f
atrial kick, 239
atrial myocytes, 479
atrial natriuretic peptide (ANP), 155,
    451, 479
atrial septal defect (ASD)
    Amplatzer device, 255, 256f
    anatomy of, 254
    atrial septal defect, 255, 256f
    in atrioventricular septal defect,
        258, 258f
    classification of, 256–257
    closure of, 255, 255f
    complications, 256
    definition of, 256
    diagnostic evaluation, 254
    familial, 163t
    incidence of, 254
    intervention for, 257
    management, 254–256
    patent foramen ovale and, 255
    pathophysiology of, 256
    signs and symptoms, 254
atrioventricular block
    complete, 243
    first-degree, 242, 242f
    Mobitz type I, 242–243, 242f
    Mobitz type II, 242f, 243
    second-degree, 242f, 243
atrioventricular node, 157–158, 367t
atrioventricular septal defect,
    258–259, 258f
atrioventricular sequential mode, of
    pacemaker, 246t
atrioventricular valves
    anatomy of, 147
    embryologic development of, 147
atropine sulfate
    characteristics of, 65t, 198
    diphenoxylate and, 752
    organophosphate insecticide
        poisoning treated with, 768–769
Atrovent. *See* ipratropium
auscultation
    of abdomen, 533
    of blood pressure, 169

auscultation (*cont.*)
    of diaphragm, 47
    heart, 602
    during mechanical ventilation, 128
    pulmonary function assessments,
        47–48
    in septic shock assessments, 780–781
    of skull, 369
auto positive end-expiratory pressure, 129
autoantibodies, 628
autoantigens, 628
autogenic drainage, 69t
autografts, 811
autoimmune diseases, 628
autoimmune-mediated disease, 508
automatic electrical defibrillation
        (AED), 211–212
automaticity
    in arrhythmias, 235
    description of, 158
autonomic dysreflexia, 430
autonomic nervous system
    components of, 363
    heart regulation by, 155
    innervation of, 366, 367t–368t
    neural transmission in, 365–366
    parasympathetic division of, 364–365
    sympathetic division of, 363–364
autonomic testing, 177
autoregulation, 153, 448
aviation industry, 892–893
    safety tools in healthcare, 893,
        893t, 894t
AVP. *See* arginine vasopressin
axillary temperature, 867t
AZA. *See* azathioprine
azathioprine (AZA), 542, 612
azidothymidine, 610
azotemia, 462

β-adrenergic receptors, 226
β-agonists, 68
β-blockers, 229, 313–314, 743t
    discontinuation of, 231
B cells
    congenital disorders of, 636–637
    description of, 585, 589, 594
B lymphocytes, 589, 594
    disorders, 636
B-type natriuretic peptide (BNP), 107
B waves, 390, 391f
Babinski's reflex, 372
Bachmann's bundle, 157
bacitracin, 813t
back blows, 114
backup extracorporeal membrane
        oxygenation circuit, 873
bacteremia, 774, 775
bacterial meningitis, 397t, 415–419
bacterial tracheitis
    clinical presentation of, 78–79
    definition of, 78
    differential diagnosis, 76t

outcomes of, 79
    pathophysiology of, 78
    patient care management, 79
Bacteroides fragilis, 533
BAER. *See* brainstem auditory evoked
        response
bag-valve-mask device, 114, 210, 690
Bainbridge reflex, 155
balancing measures, 895, 898
balloon angioplasty, 278f
balloon valvuloplasty, 285, 285f
band, 587
barbiturates
    coma induced using, 403, 407
    description of, 64
    indications for, 64
    overdose of, 739t
    pain management using, 15
barcode scanning, 887
barium swallow, 536t
barometric pressure, 847
baroreceptor reflex, 779
baroreceptors, 154, 491, 492, 779
barotrauma, 132
barrel chest, 98
Barth syndrome, 163t
basal ganglia, 354
basilar cistern, 381
basilar fractures, 424–426
basophil, 588
basophilia, 588
basophilopenia, 588
Battle's sign, 425, 687, 699
behavioral pain assessment scale, 693
benzodiazepines, 743t
    description of, 58, 749–750
    indications for, 58
    nursing considerations for, 64
    overdose of, 749–750
    pain management using, 14–15
    seizure control using, 398
    types of, 59t–60t
bereaved families, 28–30
Berkow formula burn record, 801
    description of, 801
    fear assessments, 822
berry aneurysm, 411
beta-adrenergic agonists, 99
beta cells, 482t, 497
Betapace. *See* sotalol
bicarbonate, 509
bidirectional cavopulmonary shunt,
        305, 305f–306f
bilevel positive airway pressure
        (BiPAP), 103
biliary atresia, 537, 574
biliary tree, 533
bilirubin, 535t, 563
biochemical mediators, 592
biological attacks. *See also* bioterrorism
    blast injuries, 830
    chemical attacks, 832–834, 833t
    definition of, 827
    explosions, 829

mass casualty incidents, 827
    nuclear attacks, 830–832
    psychological effects of, 841
    radiologic attacks, 830–832
    trauma injuries from, 830
    types of, 828–841
    violence, 829–830
biomarkers, 91, 106
biopsy
    bone marrow, 608
    central nervous system tumors
        diagnosed using, 420–421
    encephalitis diagnosed using, 418
    liver, 536t
    lymph node, 608
    percutaneous liver, 536t
    renal, 456
bioterrorism, 834
    anthrax, 834
    botulism, 838t, 839
    definition of, 834
    hospital preparedness for, 827
    plague, 837–839, 838t
    psychological effects of, 841
    smallpox, 836–837, 837f, 838t
    tularemia, 838t, 839
    viral hemorrhagic fevers, 838t
bite injuries
    dog, 674
    snake, 763
    spiders, 763
        black widow, 763–764
bladder
    autonomic nerve stimulation effects
        on, 367t–368t
    description of, 709
    traumatic injuries to, 708–709
bladder catheter, 691
blast injuries, 830
bleeding
    gastrointestinal tract. *See* upper
        gastrointestinal tract bleeding
    management of, 221, 224
    time, 607
blood-brain barrier, 355
blood chemistries, 505
blood component therapy
    blood products, 616, 617t–619t
    complications of, 620–623
    cross-matching, 616
    disseminated intravascular
        coagulation treated with, 618t, 620t
    donors, 616
    hemophilia treated with, 618t–619t
    infectious disease transmission, 622
    reactions to, 620–622, 621t
    red blood cells
        administration of, 616, 620
        packed, 617t
blood-cerebrospinal fluid barrier
    characteristics of, 356
    circulation of, 353f, 356
    description of, 40–41
    external ventricular, 394

blood-cerebrospinal fluid barrier
(*cont.*)
  methods for promoting, 402
  production of, 352–353
blood cultures, in septic shock, 782
blood flow
  cerebral
    description of, 361
    hyperventilation effects on, 402
    redistribution of, 227
    xenon computed tomography
      scan of, 385
  renal
    glomerular filtration rate and, 448
    regulation of, 454
blood gas, 871
blood pressure
  arterial, 453–454
  assessment of, 380, 784
  auscultation of, 169
  measurement of, 169–170
blood products
  administration of, 616, 620
  bedside filtration of, 616
  description of, 616
  irradiation effects on, 616
  modification of, 616
  types of, 617t–619t
blood typing, 607–608
blood urea nitrogen (BUN), 454, 456
blood vessels, 367t
blood warmer, 616, 620
blunt trauma
  child abuse–related, 722
  description of, 548, 669, 673
  example of, 669
  head injuries caused by, 669, 696
  renal, 473–474
  thoracic, 110–111
BNP. *See* brain natriuretic peptide
body temperature, 380, 867. *See also*
  hyperthermia; hypothermia
bone
  burns of, 810
bone marrow
  aplasia of, 610
  biopsy of, 608
  erythrocyte production by, 454
  necrosis of, 635
  neutrophils in, 604
  suppressive agents, 609–611
bone marrow transplantation, 609, 654
bosentan, 206
botulism, 743t, 838t, 839
bowel infarction, 556
bowel obstruction, 556
bowel perforation, 556
Bowman's capsule, 445
Boyle's law, 846
bradycardia, 689
  cardiopulmonary failure, 210
  respiratory support for, 214
  sinus, 236f, 237
bradycardia-tachycardia syndrome, 237

bradycardiac arrhythmias, 870–871
bradypnea, 852
  respiratory failure caused by, 209, 210
brain. *See also* central nervous system
  development of, 350
  divisions of, 354–356
  glucose metabolism by, 361
  metabolism by, 361
  myelination of, 350
  oxygen metabolism by, 361
  traumatic injury of, 424–427
brain biopsy
  central nervous system tumors
    diagnosed using, 420–421
  encephalitis diagnosed using, 418
brain death, 27, 380–381
brain natriuretic peptide (BNP), 155, 479
  heart failure, 228
brain tissue oxygen monitoring, 392
brainstem
  description of, 355, 355f
  gliomas of, 419, 421
  tumors, 420
brainstem auditory evoked response
  (BAER), 387
Breakthrough Series, 886
breast milk, 543
breath sounds, 47–48, 209, 853
breathing
  assessment of, 829t, 852–853
  chemical control of, 40–41, 41f
  control of, 40
  disordered control of, 209
  exercises, 99
  Kussmaul, 853
  management of, after traumatic
    injuries, 690
  mechanics of, 41
  nasal, 36
  patterns, 46f, 853
  rescue, 211
Brevibloc. *See* esmolol hydrochloride
Broca's motor speech area, 354
bronchi, 37
bronchial breath sounds, 47
bronchial rupture, management of, 110
bronchiectasis, 102
bronchioles, 37–38
bronchiolitis
  clinical presentation of, 80
  definition of, 79
  etiology of, 80
  outcomes of, 80
  pathophysiology of, 79–80
  patient care management, 80
bronchitis
  clinical presentation of, 79
  definition of, 79
  pathophysiology of, 79
  patient care management, 79
bronchoconstriction, 97
bronchodilators
  anti-inflammatory agents, 68
  β–agonists, 68

bronchopulmonary dysplasia treated
  with, 117
  definition of, 68
bronchopulmonary dysplasia
  clinical presentation of, 115
  complications of, 117–118
  definition of, 114
  diagnostic tests for, 115–116
  etiology of, 115
  management of
    growth and development
      promotion, 116
    infection prevention, 117
    from mechanical ventilation, 116
    oxygen therapy, 116
    pharmacologic, 117
  neurodevelopmental problems
    associated with, 117–118
  outcomes of, 117–118
  pathophysiology of, 115
  respiratory distress syndrome
    and, 114
  viral respiratory illness risks in, 117
bronchoscopy, thoracic trauma, 112
bronchospasm, 865
bronchovesicular breath sounds, 47
Brown–Sequard syndrome, 702
bruises, 721–722, 724
bruit, 267
budesonide, 865
bullet wounding mechanisms, 675
bumetanide, 464
Bumex, 207, 464
BUN. *See* blood urea nitrogen
bundle-branch block, 243
bundle-branch system, 158
bundle of His, 158
burns
  acute phase management, 819–821
  American Burn Association burn
    center referral criteria, 802t
  anxiety reductions after, 817–818
  assessments after, 806
    airway, 799
    Berkow formula burn
      record, 801
    breathing, 799
    circulation, 799–800
    history-taking, 800
    medical history, 800
    neurologic status, 800
    physical examination, 800
    rule of nines, 801
  body image changes after, 821
  burn-center referral criteria, 802t
  cardiovascular response to,
    802–803
  chemical, 795t, 797–798
  child abuse-related
    assessment for, 818
    treatment of, 818
  chronic issues, 822
  delirium, 818
  to ears, 810

burns (*cont.*)
electrical, 794t, 797
complications associated with, 796
flash-flame type, 794t
in emergency room, 798–801
enteral feedings, 820
eschar removal, 808
escharotomy/fasciotomy, 797
extent, 800
to eyes, 810
family education about, 821, 827
fasciotomy, 797
fear assessments, 817
first aid for, 798
fluid management after, 807–808
fluid resuscitation for
formulas for, 807–808
goals of, 807
inadequate, 804
initiation of, 808
monitoring of, 807–808
Parkland formula, 808
fourth-degree, 803f
gastrointestinal response to, 804
gunshot, 667
hematologic response to, 803–804
hypothermia risks after, 804
immune response to, 804
incidence of, 793
inflammatory response to, 804
inhalational injury associated with
classification of, 793, 805–806
smoke inhalation, 805
initial care of, 800, 801
itch, 822
to lips, 810
long-term outcomes, 821–822
management of
assessments. *See* burns,
assessments after
enteral feedings, 820
metabolic support, 820
nutritional support, 820
metabolic response to, 804
metabolic support, 820
morbidity and mortality, 821
multiday dressing, 813
nonaccidental injury, 818–819
nutritional support, 820
occupational therapy after, 713, 716
pain assessment and management
after, 816–817, 822
parenteral nutrition, 820
pathophysiology of, 793–798
patient education about, 821, 827
pediatric patients, 822
physical therapy after, 713, 716, 816
pressure sores after, 820
psychosocial care, 821
psychosocial outcomes, 821–822
psychosocial sequelae, 821
pulmonary response to, 803
radiant, 676
radiation, 795t

rehabilitation, 820–821
renal response to, 804
reporting of, 818–819
at scene of accident, 798
second-degree, 803f
shock, 796, 802
size, 800–801
sleep, 822
sociocultural assessment and care, 821
stab, 680, 874
Stevens–Johnson syndrome, 813, 815
systemic responses to, 802–804
thermal, 793
third-degree, 803f
toxic epidermal necrolysis, 813, 815
transport, 801
types of, 793, 794t–795t, 801
ventilator strategies, 807
World Health Organization, 793
burn wound
autograft for, 811
bacterial colonization, 815
cleansing of, 808
closure methods, 811–812
debridement of, 808
dressings for, 810
eschar removal, 808
excision of, 808, 810
hydrotherapy of, 808
infection in, 808, 815, 819, 822
invasive infection, 815
itching, 818
itching of, 820
nonoperative management, 812–813
sepsis of, 816
special care areas, 810
surgical debridement of, 808
temporary closure of, 811
topical preparations for, 808, 813t
burnout, 918–919
butemadine (Bumex), 207

C-reactive protein, 605
lymphocyte, 585
C-type natriuretic peptide, 155
C waves, 388, 390, 391f
caffeine, 758t
CAH. *See* congenital adrenal
hyperplasia
CAHPS. *See* Consumer Assessment
of Healthcare Providers and
Systems
CAHPS Child Hospital Survey (Child
HCAHPS), 907
calcarine sulcus, 350
calcitonin, 495
calcium
blood levels of, 195, 452, 495
clinical manifestations of, 461
description of, 452
disorders of, 455, 465
hypercalcemia, 452, 496
hypocalcemia. *See* hypocalcemia

calcium carbonate, 539
calcium channel blockers, 313–314
overdose of, 743t, 750–751
pulmonary hypertension treated
with, 107–108
calcium chloride, 750
calcium elevations, 226
California Perinatal Quality of Care
Collaborative (CPQCC), 901
cAMP release, 226
canals of Lambert, 38
CAPD. *See* continuous ambulatory PD
capillaries, 150
capillary blood gases, 52t
capillary filling time, 168
capillary filtration, 150
capillary refill, 780, 853–854
captopril (Capoten), 201–202
caput succedaneum, 369
carbamate insecticides, 769
carbamazepine, 408
carbohydrates
digestion of, 533
metabolism of
glycogen stores in, 781
insulin's role in, 498
carbon dioxide
diffusion of, 42
monitoring of, 54–55
carbon monoxide, 96
after burns, 805
characteristics of, 805
poisoning, 743t, 758–759
toxicity, 805
carbonic acid, 41, 42
carboxyhemoglobin, 758, 805, 806t
cardiac catheterization, 106–107, 220, 228
aortic stenosis, 272
atrioventricular septal defect
findings, 257
cardiac transplantation, 328
coarctation of the aorta
findings, 277
complications of, 181, 182
contrast agents, 181, 182
D-transposition of the great
arteries, 296
diagnostic uses of, 180–181
dilated cardiomyopathy
findings, 311
double-outlet right ventricle
findings, 260
Ebstein anomaly findings, 263–264
endocarditis findings, 322
hypertrophic cardiomyopathy
findings, 313
hypoplastic left heart syndrome
findings, 302
Kawasaki disease findings, 327
L-transposition of the great
arteries, 300
mitral insufficiency findings, 280
mitral stenosis findings, 283
myocarditis findings, 319

cardiac catheterization (*cont.*)
  pericarditis findings, 323
  pulmonary atresia intact ventricular
    septum, 291
  pulmonary atresia with ventricular
    septal defect, 289
  pulmonary stenosis, 285
  restrictive cardiomyopathy
    findings, 315
  supravalvular aortic stenosis,
    274, 285
  tetralogy of Fallot, 287
  tricuspid atresia findings, 292
  ventricular septal defect
    findings, 257
cardiac center, 154
cardiac glycosides, 192–193
cardiac index, 155, 181
cardiac magnetic resonance imaging
    (cMRI), 228
  dilated cardiomyopathy, 311
  hypertrophic cardiomyopathy, 313
  left ventricular noncompaction
    cardiomyopathy, 317
  restrictive cardiomyopathy, 315
cardiac monitoring, 182, 183f
cardiac muscle. *See also* heart
  excitation-contractile process of,
    159–160
  hypertrophy of, 226
  refractoriness of, 160
cardiac output (CO)
  after burn, 802
  calculation of, 155, 181, 187–188
  low
    extracorporeal life support
      for, 217
    heart failure, 224, 225
    obstructive shock, 233
    postcardiotomy, 217
    in septic shock, 787
  measurement of, 181
  regulation of, 776
  in septic shock, 787
cardiac patient population, 868–871
cardiac reserve, mechanism of, 225, 225f
cardiac resynchronization therapy
    (CRT), 229
cardiac septa, 147
  embryologic development of, 148t
cardiac tamponade, 332
cardiac transplantation
  definition of, 327
  diagnostic evaluation, 328, 329t
  goals for, 327
  indications for, 327–328
  management of, 328, 330–331
  signs and symptoms, 328
  transplant evaluation, 328, 330f
cardiac trauma, 110, 332–334
cardiac valves, 147
  embryologic development of, 148t
cardinal signs, respiratory failure, 112
cardinal veins, 148t

cardioaccelerator center, 154
cardiogenic pulmonary edema, 91
cardiogenic shock, 232, 234, 777, 778
cardiomyopathy, 225, 226
  dilated, 310–312
  human immunodeficiency virus
    and, 642
  hypertrophic, 312–314
  left ventricular noncompaction,
    316–317
  pediatric, 308–310
  restrictive, 314–316
cardiopulmonary bypass, 467
cardiopulmonary exercise testing, 107
cardiopulmonary failure, 209–210
cardiopulmonary resuscitation (CPR),
    113–114, 210
cardiovascular disorders, 368
cardiovascular function assessments,
    209, 234
  history-taking, 161–162
  physical examination
    auscultation, 168–171
    inspection, 162, 166–167
    palpation, 167–168
cardiovascular system
  burn-related response by, 802–803
  diagnostic studies
    autonomic testing, 177
    cardiac catheterization,
      180–182
    chest radiography, 172–173
    echocardiography, 177–178, 177f
    electrocardiogram, 173–175
    electrophysiologic studies, 182
    exercise stress testing, 176–177
    Holter monitoring, 175–176
    laboratory studies, 172
    pulse oximetry, 171–172
  embryologic development of heart,
    147, 148f–149f, 148t
  genetic signals to embryonic
    development, 147
  heart. *See* heart
  human immunodeficiency virus
    effects on, 642
  multiple-organ dysfunction
    syndrome findings, 726t
  symptoms of concern, 601t
cardioversion
  atrial flutter treated with, 240
  ventricular tachycardia treated
    with, 241
Cardizem. *See* diltiazem
care-and-comfort-only policy, 26
caregivers, 19, 24, 29
carvedilol (coreg), 208
cat eye syndrome, 164t
catastrophic syndrome, 414
CATCH-22 syndrome, 164t
catecholamine-resistant
    shock, 783t
catecholamines, 189–193, 492
cathartics, 742

catheter-associated urinary tract
    infections (CAUTIs), 475,
    475t–476t, 476, 819
catheter-tipped transducers, 389
catheters
  catheter-tip strain-gauge, 388
  epidural, 389
  for external ventricular drainage, 393
  fiber-optic, 388
  intraparenchymal fiber-optic
    transduced tipped, 389
  subdural, 389
cauda equina, 362
cause-and-effect diagram, for pressure
    injuries, 896, 896f
caustic substance poisoning, 759–761
CAUTIs. *See* catheter-associated urinary
    tract infections
cavopulmonary shunt, bidirectional,
    305, 305f–306f
CD4 cells, 589, 604
CD8 cells, 589, 604
CD4:CD8 lymphocyte ratio, 604
CEA. *See* cultured epithelial autograft
CECT. *See* contrast-enhanced CT
cell-mediated immunity (CMI)
  description of, 589, 594, 639
  human immunodeficiency virus
    effects on, 639
cellular edema, 400
cellular immunity, 585
cellular respiration, 42–43
cellulitis, 815
Centers for Disease Control and
    Prevention (CDC), 475, 668, 695,
    726, 837, 840, 874, 875, 915
Centers for Medicare & Medicaid
    Services (CMS), 906, 910
central cord syndrome, 429, 702
central diabetes insipidus, 520, 521, 522
central herniation, 401
central line-associated bloodstream
    infections (CLABSIs), 819
central nervous system. *See also* brain;
    spinal cord
  congenital abnormalities of, 436–439
  developmental anatomy of,
    349–359
  developmental physiology of,
    359–362
  embryogenesis of, 349–351
  human immunodeficiency virus
    effects on, 642
  impulse conduction in, 359–360
  infections of, 415–419
  ischemia, 778
  sensory components of, 351
  tumors of, 419–422
central neurogenic hyperventilation,
    46f, 380
central pontine demyelination, 526
central pontine myelinolysis, 520
central pulse, 853
central sulcus, 350, 354f

central venous pressure (CVP), 782
  monitoring of, 183, 184
  waveform, components of, 185f
central venous vascular access, 212
centrifugal pumps, 218f, 873
cephalhematoma, 369
Cephulac. *See* lactulose
cerebellar tumors, 420
cerebellum
  anatomy of, 356
  function testing of, 373
cerebral angiogram, 384
cerebral blood flow
  description of, 361–362
  hyperventilation effects on, 402
  xenon computed tomography scan
    of, 385
cerebral contusions, 425
cerebral edema, 400, 513t, 527
  diabetic ketoacidosis for, 513t
cerebral hemispheres, 354
cerebral hypoxia, 678
cerebral lacerations, 425
cerebral metabolic rate of oxygen, 361
cerebral perfusion pressure (CPP), 188,
    361–362, 526, 527, 697
  monitoring of, 188–189
cerebral salt wasting syndrome (CSWS),
    403, 527
  complications, 526
  conditions associated with, 523–524
  diagnostic studies, 525
  differential diagnosis for, 524t, 525
  hypertonic saline in treatment of, 525
  management, 525–526
  mechanism for production of, 523f
  pathophysiology, 523
  signs and symptoms, 524
  urine sodium levels, 525–526
cerebrospinal fluid (CSF) analysis,
    384–385
cerebral swelling, hyperosmolar
    therapy for, 398
cerebral veins, 356
cerebral venous drainage, 402
cerebral venous sinus thrombosis
    (CVST), 408
cerebrospinal fluid (CSF), 353, 353f
  analysis of
    bacterial meningitis diagnosed
      by, 415–416
    hydrocephalus diagnosed by, 423
    septic shock diagnosed by, 782
  blood-cerebrospinal fluid barrier, 356
  characteristics of, 354
  circulation of, 353
  description of, 40–41
  function of, 353
cerebrovascular accident (CVA), 635
cerebrum
  circulation in, 356
  diffuse generalized swelling of, 425
  hemispheres of, 354, 354f
cervical nerves, 362–363

cervical spine
  immobilization of, 689
  post-trauma assessments, 681,
    689–690
CF. *See* cystic fibrosis
CFTR. *See* cystic fibrosis transmembrane
    regulation gene
Char syndrome, 163t
Charles's law, 846
CHD. *See* congenital heart disease
chelation, 753
chemical debridement, of burn
    wounds, 808
chemical injuries, 95, 676, 795t, 797–798
chemical warfare attacks, 832–834
chemoreceptors, 155, 779, 805
chemotaxis, 592
chemotherapeutic agents, 609
chemotherapy
  agents used in, 421, 610
  central nervous system tumors
    treated with, 421
chest
  asthma, 98
  asymmetric movement, 209
  compression, 113
  contours of, 44
  imaging, 93t, 94, 104
  in infants, 35
  pediatric assessments, 830t
  percussion of, 46
  post-traumatic assessment of, 686
  thrusts, 114
chest compressions, 210, 214. *See also*
    compressions (cardiac)
chest pain, 43
chest physiotherapy, 69t
chest radiographs
  aortic stenosis findings, 272
  atrial septal defect findings, 257
  atrioventricular septal defect
    findings, 257
  bronchopulmonary dysplasia
    findings, 115–116
  cardiovascular system evaluations,
    172–173
  chronic lung disease, 115–116
  coarctation of the aorta findings, 277
  D-transposition of the great
    arteries, 296
  double-outlet right ventricle
    findings, 260
  Ebstein anomaly findings, 263, 265f
  endocarditis findings, 322
  hypoplastic left heart syndrome
    findings, 302
  L-transposition of the great arteries,
    299–300
  left heart outflow tract
    obstruction, 869
  mitral insufficiency findings, 280
  mitral stenosis findings, 283
  myocarditis findings, 319
  pediatric cardiomyopathy, 310

pericarditis findings, 323
  post-traumatic uses of, 692
  pulmonary atresia intact ventricular
    septum, 291
  pulmonary atresia with ventricular
    septal defect, 289
  pulmonary blood flow, 868
  pulmonary stenosis, 284–285
  pulmonary vascularity, 172f
  tetralogy of Fallot, 287
  total anomalous pulmonary venous
    return findings, 294
  tricuspid atresia findings, 292
chest wall
  anatomy of, 38
  in children, 683t
  compliance of, 119
  violence to, 109
chest x-ray, 227
Cheyne-Stokes breathing, 853
Cheyne-Stokes respirations, 46f, 380
chief cells, 532
chief complaint, 161
Child Abuse Prevention and Treatment
    Act, 719, 725
child maltreatment
  abuse, 719
    bite marks, 722
    bruises, 721–722
    burns, 722, 819
    cutaneous injuries, 721
    emotional, 727
    head trauma, 723–724
    history of, 721
    internal organ injuries, 722
    long-bone fractures, 722–723
    physical, 721–725
    sexual, 669, 725–726
    treatment for, 725
  definition of, 719
  diagnostic tests associated with, 724t
  indicators of, 728t
  Munchausen syndrome by proxy. *See*
    factitious disorder
  neglect
    definition of, 719
    description of, 726
    prevalence of, 669
  organ donation in victims of, 27
childhood development, 3–5
childhood hypoglycemia, 516
childhood injuries, 668
children. *See also* adolescents; infants;
    neonates; preschoolers; school-
    age children; toddlers
  abdomen in, 533
  acquired immunodeficiency
    syndrome in, 639
  acute ischemic stroke in, 408
  acute kidney injury in, 457
  assessment of, 5–6
  cerebral blood flow in, 361
  circulation in, 151–152
  with cognitive impairment, 12t

children (*cont.*)
  cranial nerves in, 376t–379t
  decontamination of, 833
  developmental stages for, 3–5
  disaster preparedness for,
    827–843, 829t
  emotional, 725, 727
  gallbladder disease in, 567–568
  hematologic values in, 603t
  with iatrogenic withdrawal
    syndrome, 17
  intracranial hypertension in, 401
  intracranial pressure in, 360
  leading causes of injury, 669, 669t
  limited understanding by, 9
  misconceptions about pain in, 8t–9t
  nephrotic syndrome in, 465
  principles for working with, 5–6
  sexual abuse, 725–726
chloral hydrate, 15
chloramphenicol, 610
chlorhexidine gluconate, 676
chloride, 451
  reabsorption, 450, 453
chlorine, 833
Chloromycetin. *See* chloramphenicol
chloroquine, 751
chlorothiazide, 207–208
choanal atresia
  clinical presentation of, 72
  definition of, 72
  outcomes of, 73
  pathophysiology of, 72
  patient care management, 73
choking infant, 114
cholestatic jaundice, 565
cholinergic, 743t
cholinesterase, 366
choroid plexus, 353
Christmas disease, 647
chromaffin cells, 500
chronic diarrhea, 638
chronic lung disease, 93t
  clinical presentation of, 115
  definition of, 114
  diagnostic tests for, 115–116
  management of
    growth and development
      promotion, 116
    infection prevention, 117
    oxygen therapy, 116
    pathophysiology of, 115
    pharmacologic, 117
    tracheomalacia and, 116
    viral respiratory illness risks
      in, 117
chronically ill children, 24
chyme, 532
cimetidine, 537
cingulate herniation, 400f
ciprofloxacin, 836t, 838t
circadian rhythms, 19, 19t
CIRCI. *See* critical illness–related
  corticosteroid insufficiency

circulation
  after burns, 799–800
  assessment of, 210, 799–800, 829t,
    853–854
  cerebral, 356
  cerebrospinal fluid, 353, 353f
  fetal, 151, 152f
  neonatal, 153
  pediatric, 153, 829t
  post trauma
    assessments of, 686
    management of, 690
  spinal column, 359
  transitional, 151–152
circulatory failure, 210
circulatory overload, 622
circumflex artery, 150
citrate lock, 472
citrate regional anticoagulation, 471–472
citrate toxicity, 622
CLABSIs. *See* central line-associated
  bloodstream infections
clearance, 448, 471
clindamycin, 836t
clonidine, 200–201, 540, 739t, 752
clopidogrel, 205
closed pneumothorax, 705t
clotting factors, 642–643, 647–649
  agents that affect, 614–616
  description of, 590
clouding of consciousness, 369
clubbing, 162, 166, 166f
cluster breathing, 46f
clusters of differentiation, 589
CMI. *See* cell-mediated immunity
CN, 833, 833t
CO. *See* cardiac output
co-trimoxazole. *See* trimethoprim–
  sulfamethoxazole (TMP–SMX)
coagulation
  alterations in, 778–779
  assessment of, 606–607
  description of, 590
  disseminated intravascular, 554,
    642–644
coagulation cascade, 599
coagulopathy, 571, 573, 623
coarctation of the aorta
  balloon angioplasty of, 278f
  classification of, 275
  complications, 280f
  definition of, 275
  diagnostic tests, 277
  incidence of, 275
  interrupted aortic arch, 277–278
  interventions for, 277, 278f
  pathophysiology of, 275–276
  signs and symptoms, 276–277
  surgical approach, 279f
cocaine, 739t, 755
cognitive development, 4, 5
cold exposure injuries, 676–677
cold-reactive autoantibodies, 608
cold shock, 783t

collaboration
  and partnership, 906
  poor, 904
  teamwork and, 910
  true, 913
colon, 533
colonoscopy, 536t
colony-stimulating factors, 586f, 596t
coma
  barbiturate-induced, 403, 407
  definition of, 370
coma scales, 370, 371t
combined B- and T-lymphocyte
  disorders, 637
combined variable immunodeficiency
  (CVID), 636
comminuted fracture, 711f
Commission on Accreditation of
  Medical Transport Systems, 850
committed stem cells, 585
common carotid arteries, 356
common pathway, 599
communicating hydrocephalus, 422
communication
  age-appropriate methods of, 17
  barriers, 902
  debriefing, 904
  distraction-free zones for, 904
  effective, 901
  failure, 904
  handoffs, 903, 903f
  in healthcare environment, 901
  implementation of just culture, 904
  institutional procedures and
    policies, 904
  with intubated children, 17–18
  with parents, 23
  patient safety. *See* patient safety,
    communication and
  poor, 901–902
  rounding process, 904
  skilled, 913
  strategies for, 18
  teach-back method, 903, 904
  team, 905
  TeamSTEPPS model, 904, 905, 906f
  tools, 903, 904
compartment syndrome, 717, 796–797
compassion fatigue, 918
  strategies to reduce, 920
  symptoms, 919
compassion satisfaction, 919
compensated shock, 231
complement assays, 605
complement disorders, 637
complement system
  description of, 592–593
  disorders of, 637
complete atrioventricular block, 243
complete blood count (CBC)
  absolute cell counts, 604
  absolute lymphocyte counts, 604
  absolute neutrophil count, 604
  assessment, 456

complete blood count (CBC) (*cont.*)
    hematocrit, 602
    hemoglobin, 602
    peripheral smear, 602
    red blood cell count, 602
    reticulocyte count, 602
    sickle cell disease findings, 630
    white blood cell count, 602, 604
compliance
    chest-wall, 119
    definition of, 39, 39f, 119
    dynamic, 55
    equation for, 118
    lung, 119
    measurement of, 55–56
compressed fracture, 711f
compressions (cardiac), 211
computed tomography (CT), 178–179
    advantages/disadvantages of, 179
    cardiac level imaging, 179f
    clinical uses of, 381–382
    contrast-enhanced, 382
    description of, 381
    endocrine system evaluations, 505
    interpretation of, 381, 382f
    magnetic resonance imaging versus, 381–382, 383
    meningitis evaluations, 417
    neurologic system evaluations, 381–383, 382f
    nursing implications for, 382–383
    pulmonary function evaluations using, 53
    renal diagnosis using, 455, 474
    for renal trauma evaluation, 474
    restrictive cardiomyopathy, 315
    thoracic trauma, 112
    traumatic brain injury evaluations, 426
    xenon, for cerebral blood flow assessments, 385
concrete operational stage, 4
concussion, 698-699
    brain, 424–425
    spinal cord, 430
conducting airways, 37–38
conductivity, 159
congenital adrenal hyperplasia (CAH), 501
congenital bleeding disorders, 600
congenital diaphragmatic hernia
    definition of, 70
    diagnosis of, 71
    outcomes of, 71
    pathophysiology of, 70–71
    patient care management, 71
    prognosis for, 71
congenital disorders, 368
congenital heart disease (CHD). *See also* specific diseases
    acyanotic lesions
        description of, 251
        physiology of, 251–252
    children with, 178

chromosomal defects associated with, 164t
classification of, 250–251, 256–257
cyanotic, 285–295
environmental factors, 165t, 250
etiology of, 250
gene defects associated with, 163t, 250
infection risks in, 250
maternal and paternal, 161
multifactorial inheritance syndromes associated with, 165t
nursing diagnoses for, 253
persistent ductus arteriosus, 251
systemic exposures associated with, 165t
congenital hydrocephalus, 422
congenital mitral insufficiency, 280
congenital neurologic abnormalities
    anencephaly, 437
    clinical presentation of, 437–438
    etiology of, 436–437
    outcomes of, 438–439
    pathophysiology of, 437
    patient care management, 438
congenital scoliosis, 433
congestive heart failure. *See* heart failure
conivaptan, 520
conotruncal cushions, 148t
consciousness
    clouding of, 369
    level of, 369–370, 854
Consolidated Omnibus Budget Reconciliation Act, 845
Consumer Assessment of Healthcare Providers and Systems (CAHPS), 885
contact burns
    description of, 722
    intentional versus unintentional, 722
contamination injuries, 831, 832
continuous ambulatory PD (CAPD), 469
continuous flow VAD, 222
continuous positive airway pressure
    in bronchiolitis patients, 92
    definition of, 103, 121
    description of, 126
    nasal, 81
continuous renal replacement therapy (CRRT), 789
    anticoagulation during, 471–472
    filtration capability measurements, 471
    fluid balance during, 472
    hemodynamic stability during, 472
    indications for, 470
    nursing implications, 471–472
    process used in, 470–471
continuous venovenous hemodiafiltration (CVVH-DF), 470
continuous venovenous hemofiltration with dialysis (CVVH-D), 470

contractility
    description of, 156, 252
    in septic shock, 787
contrast agents, 178
contrast echocardiography, 178
contrast-enhanced CT (CECT), 382
contusions
    cardiac, 705t
    cerebral, 425
    pulmonary, 705t
    renal, 473
    spinal cord, 430
conus medullaris, 429
convection, 468
convective transport, 468
Coombs' test, 605
coordination, team, 905
Cordarone. *See* amiodarone hydrochloride
Coreg. *See* carvedilol
coronal suture, 352f
coronary angiography, 180
coronary arteries
    anatomy of, 150, 151f
    anomalous, 287
coronary, autonomic nerve stimulation effects on, 367t
coronary sinus (CS), 833, 833t
corpus callosum, 354
cortical nephrons, 445
corticosteroids, 499
    asthma treated with, 99, 100
    bronchopulmonary dysplasia, 117
    definition of, 68
    description of, 611
    indications for, 611
    lung development in premature infants, 35
    mechanism of action, 611
    pulmonary disorders, 68
    secretion of, 499
    sickle cell disease, 627
    side effects of, 611
corticotropin-stimulation tests, 507
corticotrophs, 486
corticotropin-releasing hormone (CRH), 487
cortisol
    characteristics of, 481t, 501
    fetal, 499
    gluconeogenesis affected by, 501
    random levels, 507
cortisol-binding globulin (CBG), 501
corticosterone, 481t
cough
    age-related causes of, 50t
    asthma and, 98
    causes of, 50t
    definition of, 50
cough reflex, 852
Coumadin. *See* warfarin
counterregulatory hormones, 509
CPK. *See* creatine phosphokinase
CPP. *See* cerebral perfusion pressure

CPQCC. *See* California Perinatal
  Quality of Care Collaborative
CPR. *See* cardiopulmonary resuscitation
crackles, 47–48
cranial nerves
  description of, 363, 364t
  function assessments, 373, 373t–379t
cranial sutures, 352, 352f
craniopharyngiomas, 419
craniotomy, postoperative, 422
creatine kinase (CK), 467
creatine phosphokinase (CPK), 467
creatinine, 454
  age, variation with, 456, 456t
creatinine clearance, 448, 449
cremasteric reflex, 372
"crescendo effect," 917
crew resource management (CRM), 893
CRH. *See* corticotropin-releasing
  hormone
cricoid cartilage, 682t
cricoid cartilage ring, 37
critical-care transport
  advanced skills training for, 849–850
  atmospheric considerations, 846
  barometric pressure changes, 847
  clinical effects of, 848t
  configuration of, 849
  equipment, 849
  family issues, 845
  humidity considerations, 848
  hyperthermia during, 867–868
  hypothermia during, 852, 854, 867
  legal issues for, 845
  overview of, 844
  physiology of, 845–848
  population utilizing, 850, 851t
  principles of, 844–845
  stabilization of patient during. *See*
    stabilization of patient
  stress caused by, 847
  thermal regulation during, 847–848
  thermoregulation during, 867–868
  treatment of, 848t
critical illness-related corticosteroid
  insufficiency (CIRCI), 501, 506
  complications, 508
  conditions associated with, 506
  diagnostic studies, 507
  differential diagnoses, 507
  etiology, 506
  lab data, 507
  management, 507–508
  pathophysiology, 506
  signs and symptoms, 506
  treatment goals, 507
critical labs, 517
CRM. *See* crew resource management
crossmatching, 605
croup
  definition of, 74–75
  diagnostic features of, 76t
  management of, 75–76
  postextubation, 68

CRRT. *See* continuous renal replacement
  therapy
CRT. *See* cardiac resynchronization
  therapy
crush injuries, 673–674
cryoprecipitate, 618t, 643
CS. *See* coronary sinus
CSA. *See* cyclosporine A
CSF. *See* cerebrospinal fluid
CSF analysis. *See* cerebrospinal fluid
  (CSF) analysis
CSWS. *See* cerebral salt wasting syndrome
CT. *See* computed tomography
culture, 23
cultured epithelial autograft (CEA),
  811–812
Curling's ulcer, 804
Cushing syndrome, 502
Cushing's reflex, 380
Cushing's triad, 855f
CVA. *See* cerebrovascular accident
CVID. *See* combined variable
  immunodeficiency
CVP. *See* central venous pressure
CVST. *See* cerebral venous sinus
  thrombosis
CVVH-D. *See* continuous
  venovenous hemofiltration with
  dialysis
CVVH-DF. *See* continuous venovenous
  hemodiafiltration
cyanide, 743t
  poisoning from, 761–763
  terrorist uses of, 830
cyanosis, 209, 210, 805
  chronic, 166
  definition of, 49
  differential diagnosis, 45
  etiology of, 49f
  evaluation of, 49, 162, 166
  peripheral, 166
  respiratory, 166
cyanotic heart disease, 93t
  chest radiography, 870
  clinical presentation, 869–870
  intervention, 870
  laboratory data, 870
cyclic antidepressant poisoning, 739t,
  746–748
cyclosporine, 541
cyclosporine A (CSA), 611–612
cyproheptadine, 749
cysteinyl leukotriene, 69
cystic fibrosis (CF), 101–102
  description of, 136
  diabetes mellitus and, 504
  lung transplantation for, 137
cystic fibrosis transmembrane
  regulation gene (CFTR),
  101–102
cystitis, hemorrhagic, 660
cytokines, 595, 597t, 776–777
cytotoxic T cells, 589, 604
Cytovene. *See* ganciclovir

D-dimer, 607
d-Hand, 147
D-transposition of the great arteries
  (D-TGA)
  definition of, 295
  diagnostic tests for, 296
  incidence of, 295
  intervention of, 297
  pathophysiology of, 295–296
  patient management, 297–298
  signs and symptoms, 296
dactylitis, 631t
daily dressing, burns, 812–813
Dalton's law, 846
Damus–Kaye–Stancel operation, 293
Darvon. *See* propoxyphene
day-night cycle, 19, 19t
DCDD. *See* donation after circulatory
  determination of death
DCM. *See* dilated cardiomyopathy
ddl. *See* didanosine
deactivation gate, 160
dead-space ventilation, 55, 119
death
  age-appropriate reactions to, 4, 5
  family interventions, 29–30
debridement, burn wounds, 808
debriefing, 890, 904
Decadron. *See* dexamethasone
decannulation, extracorporeal
  membrane oxygenation, 221
decerebrate posturing, 372
decision making
  effective, 913
  team, 905
decompensated shock, 231
decontamination, from chemical
  warfare attacks, 833–834, 833t
decorticate posturing, 372
deep tendon reflexes, 372
defibrillation
  automatic electrical, 211–212
  electrical, 212
dehydration, 509
delirium, 18–19, 369, 818
delta cells, 482t, 497
demand pacing, 245
Demerol. *See* meperidine
dental injuries, 700
denticulate ligaments, 357
depolarization, 159, 160, 360
dermatomes, 362, 363f
descending spinal tract, 358t
desmopressin, 648
dexamethasone, 68, 418, 865
dexmedetomidine, 15, 16, 62–65
  in children, 396t
dextromethorphan, 755, 757t
DI. *See* diabetes insipidus
diabetes insipidus (DI), 503, 527
  antidiuresis, 522
  central, 520, 521, 522
  complications of, 522–523
  diagnoses associated with, 522

diabetes insipidus (DI) (*cont.*)
  diagnostic studies for, 521–522
  laboratory findings, 519t
  management of, 522
  nephrogenic, 520, 521, 522
  pathophysiology, 520
  risk factors for, 521
  signs and symptoms of, 521
  syndrome of inappropriate
    antidiuretic hormone versus, 519t
  water-deprivation test for, 505,
    521–522
diabetes mellitus (DM)
  cystic fibrosis and, 504
  definition of, 508
  insulin-dependent, 508, 862
  non-insulin-dependent, 508, 862
  type 1a, 508
  type 1b, 508
  type 2, 508
diabetic ketoacidosis (DKA), 527
  categories of, 509
  for cerebral edema, 513t
  complications, 512–513
  definition, 508–509
  description of, 862–863
  diagnoses associated with, 510–511
  electrolyte therapy for, 511
  etiology of, 509
  fluid therapy for, 511
  hyperglycemia and, 509
  hyperglycemic hyperosmolar
    syndrome and, 514t
  insulin infusion, 512
  management of, 511–512
  pathophysiology of, 509
  risk factors for, 509, 513t
  signs and symptoms of, 509, 510t
  stabilization of patient with, 863f
  treatment goals, 511
diagnostic peritoneal lavage (DPL),
  549, 692
dialysis
  continuous venovenous
    hemofiltration with, 470
  hemodialysis, 469–470
  peritoneal, 468–469
Diamox. *See* acetazolamide
diaphragm
  anatomy of, 38
  auscultation of, 47–48
  traumatic blunt rupture of, 110–111
diaphragmatic hernia, 561t
diastasis, 424
diastolic heart failure, 225
diastolic murmurs, 170, 171f
diazepam
  contraindications, 60t
  dosing of, 60t
  pain management using, 16t
  seizure control using, 398, 399t
DIC. *See* disseminated intravascular
  coagulation
didanosine, 610

dideoxynucleosides, 610
diencephalon, 350, 350f, 355
diet, 107, 913
differential white blood cell
  count, 604
differentiation, 585
diffusion, 41–42, 446, 447, 468
DiGeorge syndrome, 164t
digestive tract, 531, 531f. *See also*
  gastrointestinal tract
digitalis, 751–752
digoxin, 229, 314, 743t
  characteristics of, 192–193
  contractility affected by, 229
  overdose of, 751–752
Dilantin. *See* phenytoin
dilated cardiomyopathy (DCM), 311f
  complications of, 312
  definition of, 310
  diagnostic evaluation, 311
  etiology of, 310
  pathophysiology of, 310
  phenotypic expression, 310–311
  treatment for, 311–312
diltiazem, 197
dimercaptosuccinic acid scanning
  (DMSA), 455
diphenoxylate–atropine
  combination, 752
dipyridamole, 205
direct antiglobulin test (DAT), 605
direct Coomb's test, 605
disaster preparedness
  overview of, 827
  pediatric, 827–828, 829t
  terrorism. *See* terrorism
discrete subaortic stenosis, 274
disopyramide, 314
disseminated intravascular coagulation,
  554, 643–644
  symptoms, 643
distributive shock, 232, 234, 777
diuretic agents
  loop, 207
  potassium sparing, 208
  thiazide, 207–208
diuretic management, 229
diuretics, 314
  acute kidney injury with, 464
  bronchopulmonary dysplasia treated
    with, 117
  fluid status controlled using, 229
  loop, 464
  mannitol and, 403
  osmotic, 464
  potassium-sparing, 464
  thiazide, 464
dive reflex, 678
DKA. *See* diabetic ketoacidosis
DM. *See* diabetes mellitus
DMSA. *See* dimercaptosuccinic acid
  scanning
DNR. *See* do-not-resuscitate (DNR) order
do-not-resuscitate (DNR) order, 26

dobutamine, 189, 860
  septic shock treated with, 786t
Dobutrex. *See* dobutamine
dog bites, 674
donation after circulatory determination
  of death (DCDD), 27
donors
  blood component therapy, 616
  potential, caring for, 27–28
dopamine, 213, 487
  description of, 189–190
  hypotension treated with, 860
  septic shock treated with, 786
Doppler, 178
Doppler echocardiography, 178
Doppler ultrasound, transcranial, 385
dorsal root, of spinal nerves, 362
double-outlet right ventricle, 259–261, 261f
Down syndrome, 164t
doxycycline, 842
DPL. *See* diagnostic peritoneal lavage
dressings, burn wounds, 810, 812–813
droperidol, 66t
drowning, 677–679
drug(s). *See also* specific drugs
  dosing of, 56
  protein binding, 57
drug therapy, asthma, 98
dual chambered pacing, 246t
Duchenne's syndrome, 163t
ductus arteriosus
  closure of, 152, 252
  patent, 251–253, 290
  surgical closure of, 258
duodenum, 532
dura mater, 357
dying child
  caring for conscious, 28
  interventions for, 25–30
  remembrance packet of, 30
  sibling of, 29
  staff support, 30
dynamic compliance, 55
dysmetria, 373

E-CPR (ECMO cannulation during
  CPR), 214
ears
  burns of, 810
  infection, 96
  trauma-related evaluation of, 687
EBP. *See* evidence-based practice
Ebstein anomaly
  anatomy of, 264f
  assessment of, 263–265
  definition of, 261
  diagnostic findings for, 263
  etiology of, 263
  incidence, 262
  interventions for, 264
  pathophysiology of, 262–263
  prognosis for, 264
  surgical repair of, 264–265, 266f

ECG. *See* echocardiography
echocardiogram, 782
echocardiography
  cardiac transplantation, 328
  tetralogy of Fallot findings, 285
  three-dimensional, 178
  transesophageal, 178
  two-dimensional, 177, 178
echocardiography (ECG), 106
  aortic stenosis findings, 271,
    272, 274
  atrioventricular septal defect
    findings, 259
  coarctation of the aorta findings, 277
  contrast, 178
  D-transposition of the great
    arteries, 296
  dilated cardiomyopathy, 311
  Doppler, 178
  double-outlet right ventricle
    findings, 259–261
  endocarditis findings, 322
  fetal, 178
  heterotaxy syndromes, 308
  hypertrophic cardiomyopathy, 313
  hypoplastic left heart syndrome
    findings, 302
  interrupted aortic arch, 278
  Kawasaki disease findings, 327
  L-transposition of the great
    arteries, 300
  left ventricular noncompaction
    cardiomyopathy, 317
  M-mode, 177
  mitral insufficiency findings, 280
  mitral stenosis findings, 283
  myocarditis findings, 319
  patient management, 285
  pediatric cardiomyopathy, 310
  pericarditis findings, 323
  pulmonary atresia intact ventricular
    septum, 291
  pulmonary atresia with ventricular
    septal defect, 290
  pulmonary stenosis findings, 285
  purpose of, 178
  restrictive cardiomyopathy, 315
  single ventricular variants, 307
  technique for, 177–178, 177f
  tetralogy of Fallot findings, 287
  three-dimensional, 178
  total anomalous pulmonary venous
    return findings, 294
  transesophageal, 178
  tricuspid atresia findings, 292
  two-dimensional, 177–178
  ventricular septal defect
    findings, 243
ECMO. *See* extracorporeal membrane
    oxygenation
ECMO pumps, 873
ectoderm, 349
ectopic area, 167f
Edecrin. *See* ethacrynic acid

edema
  cellular (cytotoxic), 400
  cerebral, 400, 513t, 527
  interstitial, 400
  mechanical ventilation requirements
    for, 123t
  vasogenic, 400
Edwards syndrome, 164t
EES. *See* erythromycin
efficiency–thoroughness tradeoff, 893
EIB. *See* exercise-induced
    bronchospasm
Eisenmenger syndrome, 253, 257
elastance, 360
elastase inhibitors, 108
elbow fractures, 712–713
electrical burn
  complications associated with, 797
  mechanism of injury, 797
electrical defibrillation, 212
electrical injury, 676, 794t, 797
electrical stimulation, 70t
electrical synapse, 352
electrocardiogram, 173–175
electrocardiography
  arrhythmogenic right ventricular
    myopathy, 318
  cardiac transplantation, 328
  D-transposition of the great
    arteries, 296
  dilated cardiomyopathy, 311
  double-outlet right ventricle
    findings, 259–261
  Ebstein anomaly findings, 263–264
  endocarditis findings, 322
  hemodynamic measurements, 181
  heterotaxy syndromes findings, 308
  hypertrophic cardiomyopathy
    findings, 313
  interrupted aortic arch, 278
  Kawasaki disease findings, 327
  L-transposition of the great
    arteries, 299
  mitral insufficiency, 280
  myocarditis findings, 319
  pediatric cardiomyopathy, 310
  pericarditis findings, 323
  persistent ductus arteriosus findings,
    261–265
  pulmonary atresia intact ventricular
    septum, 290
  pulmonary atresia with ventricular
    septal defect, 289–290
  pulmonary stenosis, 284
  restrictive cardiomyopathy, 315
  single ventricular variants, 307
  total anomalous pulmonary venous
    return findings, 294
  tricuspid atresia findings, 292
  ventricular septal defect
    findings, 256
electroencephalograms, 385–386, 386f
  description of, 385–386
  nursing implications, 386

electrolytes
  calcium. *See* calcium
  diabetic ketoacidosis treated
    with, 511
  disturbances, 510
  hyperglycemic hyperosmolar
    syndrome treated with, 515
  magnesium, 452
  phosphate, 452
  potassium, 451-452, 511
  sodium, 452
electrophysiologic studies, 182
electrophysiology, 158–161
embryonal tumors, 419
emergence/agitation delirium, 369
Emergency Medical Treatment and
    Active Labor Act, 845
Emergency Nursing Pediatric Course
    (ENPC), 668
emotional abuse, 727
emotional support
  after traumatic injuries, 693–695
  description of, 20–21
emotions
  grief-related, 29
  range of, 20
empiric antimicrobial therapy, 396, 398
empty heart syndrome, 691
enalapril maleate, 202
enalaprilat, 199–200
encephalitis, 397t, 416–418
encephalopathy, 427–429, 573
  clinical presentation of, 427–428
  definition and etiology of, 427
  outcomes of, 429
  pathophysiology of, 427
  patient care management, 428–429
end-of-life care
  and moral distress, 917–918
end-stage liver disease, 575
end-stage renal disease (ESRD), 465, 473
end-tidal carbon dioxide detector
    (ETCO$_2$), 866
end-tidal carbon dioxide monitors,
    54–55, 128
end-to-end anastomosis, for coarctation
    of the aorta, 279f
endocardial cushions, 148t
endocardial fibroelastosis, 226
endocarditis
  etiology of, 320–321
  management of, 322
  pathophysiology of, 320
  signs and symptoms of, 321
  terminology, 321t
endocardium, 147
endocrine disorders, 368
endocrine glands
  description of, 479
  pituitary gland. *See* pituitary gland
endocrine system
  developmental anatomy and
    physiology, 484–503
  diagnostic studies, 505–506

endocrine system (*cont.*)
　family history, 504
　functions of, 479
　growth and development factors, 503
　history of, 503–504
　hypothalamic–pituitary complex. *See*
　　hypothalamic–pituitary complex
　laboratory studies, 505
　medication history, 503–504
　neonatal history, 504
　physical assessment, 504–505
　prenatal history, 503
　radiologic tests, 505–506
　role of, 479
　summary of, 479t–483t
endoderm, 349
endogenous mediators, 776–777
endoscopic retrograde
　　cholangiopancreatography, 536t
endoscopy
　diagnostic uses of, 536t
　upper gastrointestinal tract bleeding
　　evaluations, 555
endothelial cell dysfunction, 105
endothelial damage, 778
endothelial dysfunction, 105
endothelin-1, 206
endothelin receptor antagonists, 108
endotoxin, 776
endotracheal intubation, 210, 211f, 212f
　complication of, 689
　for initial stabilization of
　　patient, 855
　post-traumatic indications for, 689
endotracheal tube (ETT)
　description of, 689
　displacement of, 866
　indications for, 37
　with mechanical ventilation, 127
　size of, 131
　suctioning of, 127
　in ventilator-associated pneumonia, 131
energy drinks, 758t
enoxaparin, 203–204, 229
ENPC. *See* Emergency Nursing
　　Pediatric Course
enteral feeding, 820
enteral nutrition, 95
　in bronchopulmonary dysplasia, 116
　in burn patients, 820
　enteral feedings, 820
　in septic shock, 789
enterocytes, 532
envenomations, 763–764
environmental tobacco smoke
　　exposure, 96
enzymatic debridement, burn
　　wounds, 808
enzyme-linked immunosorbent
　　assay, 606
enzyme-replacement therapy, 638
eosinopenia, 588
eosinophil(s), 588
　in children, 603t

eosinophilia, 588
EPCCO. *See* Essentials of Pediatric
　　Critical Care Orientation
ependyma, 352
ependymomas, 419
epicardial leads, 244
epicardium, 147
epidural catheters, 389
epidural hematoma, 425–426
epidural space, 357
epigastric area, 167f
epiglottis, 37, 37f, 682t
epiglottitis, acute
　clinical presentation of, 75
　complications of, 76
　definition of, 74–75
　diagnostic tests of, 75
　differential diagnosis, 76t
　outcome of, 76
　pathophysiology of, 75
　patient care management, 75, 76
　physical examination, 75
　swollen epiglottis in, 74f
epilepsy, definition of, 404
epinephrine, 483
　advanced life support use of, 213
　airway obstruction treated with, 864t
　biosynthesis of, 502
　characteristics of, 190, 502
　dopamine versus, 860
　endogenous, 482t
　exogenous, 67
　regulation of, 502
　septic shock treated with, 786t
epiphyseal growth plate, 710
epithalamus, 355
epithelial cells of alveoli, 38
epitopes, 591
epitrochlear lymph nodes, 587f
eplerenone, 208
epoprostenol, 205–206
Epstein–Barr virus, 571, 576
ER. *See* evoked response
*Err Is Human: Building a Safer Health
　　System*, 883
error-based QI metrics, 911
error management, 886
errors reduce strategies, 889
erythrocyte(s), 454, 587
erythrocyte enzymes, 638
erythrocyte sedimentation rate, 604–605
erythromycin, 540
erythropoietin, 454, 585, 608–609
eschar, 808
escharotomies, 796–797, 800
Escherichia coli, 533
Escherichia coli 0157:H7, 465
esmolol hydrochloride, 195
esophageal atresia, 71
esophageal varices, 556, 573
esophagus
　embryologic development of, 531
　functions of, 531
　injuries to, 110

ESRD. *See* end-stage renal disease
Essentials of Pediatric Critical Care
　　Orientation (EPCCO), 8
estrogen, 482t
ETCO$_2$. *See* end-tidal carbon dioxide
　　detector
ethacrynic acid, 207
ethanol poisoning, 743t, 757t, 764
ethyl alcohol, 757t
ethylene glycol, 764–765
etomidate
　in children, 396t
ETT. *See* endotracheal tube
EVD. *See* external ventricular drainage
event management algorithm, in just
　　culture, 888f
evidence-based practice (EBP), 910
　quality improvement versus,
　　908, 909
evoked potential studies, 387
evoked response (ER), 387
excision, 810
excitability, description of, 159
exercise
　for asthma patients, 99
　CDC recommendations, 915
exercise-induced bronchospasm
　　(EIB), 99
exercise stress testing, 176–177
exocrine glands, 479
exogenous mediators, 776
expiratory positive airway
　　pressure, 126
expiratory stridor, 49
expiratory wheezing, 48
explosions, 829
exposed muscle, burns of, 810
exposure injuries, 676–677,
　　684t, 691
external carotid arteries, 356
external fiber-optic transducer, 388
external ventricular drainage (EVD),
　　393–394, 393f
extracorporeal circuit
　continuous renal replacement
　　therapy, 472
extracorporeal membrane oxygenation
　　(ECMO), 125, 219t, 789
　bleeding management, 221
　cardiac catheterization, 220
　circuit, 220f
　complications, 222
　continuous monitoring, 220–221
　continuous renal replacement
　　therapy, 472
　contraindications, 217–218
　decannulation, 221
　hemodynamic function, optimization
　　of, 219
　indications for, 217
　initiation of, 218
　neurologic assessment and sedation,
　　218, 219
　nursing care for, 221–222

extracorporeal membrane oxygenation (ECMO) (*cont.*)
  nutrition/electrolyte optimization, 222
  respiratory support, 218
  sedation and analgesia, 221
  ventricular assist device, 217
extracorporeal membrane oxygenation (EMCO) transport, 872–874
extradural hematomas, 425, 426
extremities, 688
extrinsic pathway, 599
eyes
  autonomic nerve stimulation effects on, 367t
  burns near, 810
  poison exposure, 740
  symptoms of concern, 601t
  trauma-related evaluation of, 687

fab antivenin, 763
face mask, 690
faces, legs, activity, cry, and consolability (FLACC) scale, 693
facial nerve
  in children, 378t
  function of, 364t
  in infants, 375t
factitious disorder, 727–729
factor IX assay, 647–649
factor VIII assay, 647–649
factor VIII concentrate, 618t
failure and mode effects analysis (FMEA), 889
falls, 669, 670t–672t
familial hypertrophic syndrome, 164t
familial inherited cardiomyopathy, 309
family. *See also* parents
  anticipatory guidance for, 27
  assessment of, 21–23
  bereaved, 28–30
  cultural considerations, 22
  interventions with, 23–25
  psychosocial needs of, 21–25
  separation from, 9
  spiritual considerations, 22–23
  stress on, 21–22
  support systems for, 22
family-centered care (FCC), 905, 906
  barriers to, 907
  patient/family needs assessment, 907–908
  in pediatric critical care, 906–907
  quality improvement, 906
  staff understanding of, 907
family-centered rounding processes, 907
family education, 231
family smoking, 96
famotidine, 538
fascial excision, 808
fasciotomy, 797
fat embolism, 635
fat embolism syndrome, 717–718

fat metabolism, 498
fat-soluble bilirubin, 564
FCC. *See* family-centered care
fear
  adolescent's response to, 8
  assessment of, 817
  of confrontation, 902
  hospitalization-related, 8
  infant's response to, 8
  preschooler's response to, 8
  school-age child's response to, 8
  toddler's response to, 8
febrile seizure, 404
feelings of powerlessness, 917
femoral fractures, 713–714
fenoldopam, 200, 464
fentanyl
  in children, 396t
  contraindications, 60t
  dosing of, 60t
  overdose of, 754
  pain management using, 15t
ferritin, 455t
fetal circulation, 151, 152f
fetal echocardiography, 178
fetal hemoglobin, 42, 361
fetal posterior pituitary, 485
fever, 91
  hyperthermia versus, 626
  interventions for, 626
  signs and symptoms of, 626
FF. *See* filtration factor
FFP. *See* fresh frozen plasma
fiber-optic catheters, 388
fibrin clot, 590
fibrin degradation products, 600
fibrin split products, 600
fibrinogen, 607
fibrinolytic agents, 615–616
fibrinolytic system, 590, 599–600
fick method, 181
fight-or-flight reaction, 500f
filtration factor (FF), 471
filum terminale, 357
finger-to-nose test, 373
fingers, burns of, 810
firearm injuries, 674–675
first-degree atrioventricular block, 242, 242f
first-degree AV block, 870
first-degree burns, 803f
first-line therapy, 642
Fishbone diagram, 896
five Ps, hand-off communications, 903
flaccidity, 372
flexible colonoscopy, 536t
flexible upper endoscopy, 536t
Florinef. *See* fludrocortisone
flow sensors, 122
flow spirometers, 55
fludrocortisone, 508, 525
fluid(s)
  diabetic ketoacidosis, 511
  regulation of, 533

fluid balance, 472
fluid-coupled ICP transducer, 389
fluid-coupled systems, 388
fluid-filled systems, zeroing and calibrating, 389
fluid management, pulmonary hypertension, 107
fluid-resistant shock, 783t
fluid resuscitation, 213
  algorithm for, 859f
  description of, 798
  fluid management after, 807
  fluid volume for, 860
  formulas for, 807–808
  goals of, 807
  inadequate, 804
  initiation of, 807
  monitoring of, 807
  Parkland formula, 808
  for stabilization of patient, 860
fluid therapy
  diabetic ketoacidosis treated with, 511
  hyperglycemic hyperosmolar syndrome treated with, 515
  septic shock treated with, 787
fluid-volume excess, 253
flumazenil, 65–66, 65t, 750
fluoroscopy, 53, 536t
FMEA. *See* failure and mode effects analysis
focal epileptiform patterns, 406t
focal seizures, 404
focused abdominal sonography for trauma, 549
follicle-stimulating hormone, 480t, 490
fomepizole
  for ethylene glycol poisoning, 765
  for methanol poisoning, 766
fondaparinux, 204
Fontan procedure, 306, 306f
  complications, 307
  fenestration in, 307
  hypoplastic left heart syndrome treated by, 306, 306f
  tricuspid atresia treated by, 293, 293f
fontanelles
  anatomy of, 352
  anterior, 352, 352f, 369
  palpation of, 369
  posterior, 352, 352f, 369
Food and Drug Administration (FDA), 745
foramen of Magendie, 353
foramen of Monro, 352, 413
foramen ovale, 152
foramina of Luschka, 352
forced expiratory technique, 69t
foregut, 531
foreign-body aspiration
  clinical course, 88
  clinical presentation of, 87–88

foreign-body aspiration (*cont.*)
  definition of, 86–87
  outcomes of, 88
  pathophysiology of, 87
  patient care management, 88
forgoing life-sustaining medical
    treatment, 26–27
forkhead transcription factor
    Mfh 1, 147
formal operational stage, 5
fosphenytoin, 398, 399t
fourth-degree burns, 803f
fractional excretion of sodium
    (FENa), 456
fractures
  child abuse-related, 727
  compression plating of, 714
  description of, 710
  displaced, 711
  elbow, 712–713
  external fixation of, 714
  femoral, 714
  immobilization of, 691
  internal fixation of, 714
  LeFort, 687, 701
  mandibular, 700
  midfacial, 701
  nondisplaced, 711
  open, 711–712
  pelvic, 714–715
  physeal, 712, 712t
  rib
    clinical presentation of, 705t
    management of, 705t
  Salter–Harris classification of, 712,
      712f
Frank–Starling law, 156, 156t
fremitus, 45
fresh frozen plasma (FFP), 618t, 643–644
friction rubs, 168
Friedreich's ataxia, 166t
friends, separation from, 9
frontal bone, 352f
frontal lobe
  description of, 354
  tumors of, 420
frontal sinus, 36
frostbite, 676
FSH. *See* follicle-stimulating hormone
full-thickness grafts, 811
fulminant hepatic failure, 569
functional residual capacity
  definition of, 119
  description of, 35, 41
  equation for, 118t
  positive end-expiratory pressure
      effects on, 120f
funduscopic examination, 373, 379
furosemide, 464
  bronchopulmonary dysplasia treated
      with, 117
furosemide (lasix), 207
fusiform aneurysm, 411
fusion/entry inhibitors, 641

gag reflex, 852
gait, 373
gallbladder, 533
gallbladder disease
  clinical presentation of, 567–568
  definition and etiology of, 567
  description of, 533
  pathophysiology of, 567
  patient care management, 568
γ –aminobutyric acid, 749, 754
γ –glutamyl transpeptidase, 535t
ganciclovir, 576
gap junctions, 352
gas exchange
  anatomy involved in, 38
  pediatric acute respiratory distress
      syndrome, 94
  physiology of, 41–42
gas laws, 846–847
gastric acid secretion, 57
gastric emptying, 57, 532
gastric lavage, 740–741
gastroesophageal reflux
  clinical presentation of, 547–548
  definition and etiology of, 547
  medications for, 537–539
  in newborns, 531
  pathophysiology of, 547
  patient care management, 548
gastrointestinal system
  abdominal assessments, 533–534
  abnormalities of, 557t–561t
  anatomy and physiology of, 531–533
  assessment of, 854
  burn-related response by, 804
  case studies of, 580
  development of, 531
  diagnostic studies, 536t
  gastrointestinal disorders evaluated
      using, 536t
  gastrostomy tube, 545
  infection of, 568–569
  liver function tests, 534t–535t
  nasogastric tube, 544–545, 545t
  nasojejunal tube, 545–546
  nutrition assessment, 542
  pharmacologic agents, 537–542
  postresuscitation care, 216
  schematic diagram of, 532
  structures of, 532f
  surgical drains, 546
gastrointestinal tract
  bleeding from. *See* lower
      gastrointestinal tract bleeding;
      upper gastrointestinal tract
      bleeding
  decontamination of, after poison
      exposure, 741
  dysfunction of, after stem cell
      transplantation, 657–658
gastrointestinal tract ischemia, 234
gastroschisis, 558t
gastrostomy tube, 545
GCS. *See* Glasgow Coma Score

gene therapy, 638
general somatic afferent fibers, 362
general somatic efferent fibers, 362
general visceral afferent fibers, 362
general visceral efferent fibers, 362
generalized epileptiform patterns, 406t
generalized seizures, 404
generalized tonic–clonic (GTC) status
    epilepticus, 405
genetic disorders, 368
genetic epilepsy, 404
genetic testing, 107
genitourinary system
  pediatric assessments, 830t
  post-traumatic management
      of, 691
  symptoms of concern, 601t
genitourinary tract injuries, 780
germ cell layers, 349
germ cell tumors, 420
GFR. *See* glomerular filtration rate
GH stimulation, 505
GHRH. *See* growth hormone-releasing
    hormone
giant aneurysm, 411
"giant cell" hepatitis, 571
Glasgow Coma Score (GCS), 370,
    371t, 667
glipizide, 752
glomerular filtrate, 447
glomerular filtration rate (GFR), 448,
    448t, 449f, 804
glomerulonephritis, acute, 466
glomerulus, 445
glossopharyngeal nerve
  in children, 379t
  function of, 364t
  in infants, 375t
glucagon, 482t, 498
glucocorticoids, 495
  airway obstruction treated
      with, 865
  definition of, 68
  endogenous, 481t
  pulmonary disorders treated
      with, 68
gluconeogenesis, 497, 501
glucose
  assessment, 456
  brain metabolism of, 361
  hypoglycemia treated with,
      515–516, 860
glucose homeostasis, 497
glucose intolerance, 461
glucose tolerance test, 510
glyburide, 752
glycogenolysis, 498
glycosuria, 509, 510
glycosylated hemoglobin, 505, 510
GnRH. *See* gonadotropin-releasing
    hormone
GoLYTELY. *See* polyethylene glycol-
    electrolyte solution
gonadotrophs, 486

gonadotropin-releasing hormone (GnRH), 487, 490
gonadotropins, 480t
GORE-TEX patch, 287
graft-versus-host disease (GVHD), 578
    acute, 660–662
    after stem cell transplantation, 661
    chronic, 661–662
    description of, 606
    gastrointestinal manifestations of, 660–661
    hepatic manifestations of, 662
    prophylaxis for, 661
    risk factors for, 638
    skin manifestations of, 660
    stages of, 660–661
    transfusion-associated, 616, 623
    treatment of, 661–662
granulocyte colony-stimulating factor, 585, 597t, 609
granulocyte monocyte-colony stimulating factor, 597t, 609
gray matter, of spinal cord, 357, 358f
great veins, 147
    embryologic development of, 148t
great vessel injuries, 111
grief
    definition of, 28
    emotions associated with, 29
    phases of, 29
Group A β-hemolytic streptococci pharyngitis, 325
growth factors, 608
growth hormone
    characteristics of, 480t, 488–489
    deficiency of, 489, 505
growth hormone-releasing hormone (GHRH), 487, 488
grunting, 209
GSWs. *See* gunshot wounds
Guillain-Barré syndrome, 123t
gunshot wounds (GSWs), 667
Guy-Lussac's law, 847
GVHD. *See* graft-versus-host disease
gyromitra esculenta, 767

haemophilus influenzae type b
    bacterial meningitis caused by, 415–416
    in sickle cell disease, 633
HALF-PINT. *See* Heart and Lung Failure–Pediatric Insulin Titration
hallucinogenic amphetamines, 756
handoff
    successful, 902
    tools, 903, 903f
handwashing, 624–625
hashimoto thyroiditis, 494
HbSS. *See* hemoglobin SS (HbSS) disease
head, eyes, ears, nose, and throat (HEENT) survey, 504, 829t–830t
head tilt–chin lift maneuver, 114

head trauma
    child abuse-related, 723–724
    description of, 696
health-promoting behaviors, 913, 915
    barriers to, 915
Health Promoting Lifestyle Profile II, 915
"Health Risk Appraisal," ANA, 915
Healthcare Data Guide, 899
healthcare quality domains, 892, 892f
healthy eating, 915
healthy work environment (HWE), 883, 913, 914, 914f
heart
    automaticity of, 158
    autonomic nerve stimulation effects on, 367t
    borders of, 172–173, 172f
    conduction system of, 157–158, 158f
    contusions, 705t
    coronary vasculature in, 150
    electrophysiology of, 158–160, 158–161
    embryologic development of, 147–149
    function assessments. *See* cardiovascular function assessments
    human immunodeficiency virus effects on, 642
    neurohormonal control of, 155
    size of, 172
    stem cell transplantation-related complications, 659
    transplantation, 224, 231
    vasculature in, 150
    ventricles of, 147
Heart and Lung Failure–Pediatric Insulin Titration (HALF-PINT), 498
heart failure (HF)
    classification of, 225
    definition of, 224
    diagnostic studies, 227–228
    etiology of, 226–227
    management, 228–231
    pathophysiology, 224–226
    signs and symptoms, 224, 227
heart loop, 147
    embryologic development of, 148t
heart rate (HR), 230, 853
    and rhythm, 156–157
heart sounds, 169–170
heart transplantation. *See* cardiac transplantation
heart tube, 147
    embryologic development of, 148t
heart valves
    anatomy of, 147
    embryologic development of, 147
heat and moisture exchanger, 866–867
heat cramps, 677
heat exhaustion, 677
heat exposure injuries, 676–677, 684t

heat injury, 95
heat stroke, 677
heated plastics, 95–96
heel-shin test, 373
helical CT, renal diagnosis using, 455
helium-oxygen gas, reactive airway disease treated with, 132
helper T cells, 589, 604
helper T lymphocyte, 639
hemarthrosis, 647, 649
hematemesis, 554
hematochezia, 554
hematocrit
    in children, 603t
    in complete blood count, 602
    description of, 575
    in infants, 603t
hematologic system
    anatomy and physiology, 585–590
    assessment of, 600–602
    burn-related response by, 803–804
    diagnostic tests of, 602–608
    function of, 591–600
    pharmacologic agents that affect, 608–616
    physical examination, 602
    postresuscitation care, 216
    white blood cells. *See* white blood cells
hematoma
    epidural, 425–426
    extradural, 425, 426
    periorbital, 721
    renal, 474
    subdural, 426
hematopoiesis, 585
hematopoietic stem cell transplantation (HSCT)
    allogeneic, 654
    autologous, 654
    complications of cardiac, 659
    gastrointestinal tract dysfunction, 657–658
    graft-versus-host disease, 659–663
    hemorrhagic cystitis, 660
    hepatic dysfunction, 656–657
    infection, 656
    interstitial pneumonitis, 659
    pulmonary, 658–659
    renal dysfunction, 658
    veno-occlusive disease, 656–657
        conditioning regimens before, 654
        definition of, 656
        indications for, 654–655
        management after, 656–657
        severe combined immunodeficiency treated with, 654
        supportive care after, 656
        syngeneic, 654
        types of, 654
hematopoietic stem cells. *See* stem cell(s)
hematotympanum, 687

hemodialysis, 469–470
hemodynamic function, optimization of, 219
hemodynamic monitoring
    arterial pressure, 182, 183, 185f
    calculations, 187–188
    central venous pressure, 183, 184, 186f
    left atrial monitoring, 185f, 186–187
    pulmonary artery, 184, 186
    pulmonary artery wedge pressure, 184, 186
hemofiltration, 470
hemoglobin
    A, 587
    carbon monoxide binding to, 758–759
    in children, 603t
    in complete blood count, 602
    definition of, 587
    F, 587
    fetal, 42, 361
    glycosylated, 505
    in infants, 603t
    oxygen transport by, 42
    pulse oximetry evaluations, 53
hemoglobin F, 587
hemoglobin SS (HbSS) disease, 629, 635
hemolytic reactions, 620–621
hemolytic-uremic syndrome (HUS), 465, 645
hemophilia
    A, 647–648
    B, 647–648
    complications of, 648–649
    diagnostic studies, 647–648, 649
    etiology of, 647
    management of, 648
    pathophysiology of, 647
    patient outcomes, 649
    risk factors for, 647–648
    signs and symptoms of, 647
hemoptysis, 103
hemorrhage
    clinical presentation of, 554–555, 555t
    definition, 553
    esophageal varices, 556
    etiology of, 553, 554t
    heparin administration, 91
    hypovolemia related to, 629
    intraventricular, 413–415
    liver, 551
    outcomes of, 556
    pathophysiology of, 553, 554
    patient care management, 555–556
    periventricular, 413, 415
    pulmonary, 103–104
    signs and symptoms of, 554
hemorrhagic component, 643
hemorrhagic cystitis, 660
hemorrhagic stroke, 408, 410
    etiologies for, 410
    mortality range for, 413

hemostasis
    assessment of, 606
    description of, 598, 598f
hemothorax, 110, 111, 111t
    clinical presentation of, 705t
    management of, 705t
hemotympanum, 425
Henry's law, 847
heparin, 203
    description of, 614–615
    disseminated intravascular coagulation treated with, 644
heparin administration, 91
heparin-induced thrombocytopenia, 615, 646–647
heparinization, 471
hepatic failure
    acute
        definition of, 569–570
        drug-induced, 571
        etiology of, 570
        pathophysiology of, 571
        signs and symptoms of, 572
    chronic
        definition of, 572
        diagnosis of, 572
        diagnostic tests, 573
        etiology of, 572
        fulminant, 569
        outcomes of, 574
        pathophysiology of, 572–573
        patient care management, 573–574
        signs and symptoms of, 573
hepatitis A virus, 570
hepatitis B virus, 570, 622
hepatitis C virus, 570, 622
hepatobiliary excretion scan, 536t
hepatoblastoma, 574–575
hepatocellular carcinoma, 575
hepatorenal syndrome, 466–467, 571, 573
hepatosplenomegaly, 572, 602
herbal products, 756–758
hernia, diaphragmatic, 561t
herniation, 401
heterograft, 811
heterotaxy syndromes, 165t, 308
    definition of, 308
    diagnostic evaluation, 308
    incidence of, 308
    interventions of, 308
    pathophysiology of, 308
    patient management, 308
    signs and symptoms, 308
HF. *See* heart failure
HFJV. *See* high-frequency jet ventilation
HFOV. *See* high-frequency oscillation ventilation
HFPV. *See* high-frequency percussive ventilation
HHS. *See* hyperglycemic hyperosmolar syndrome
HI. *See* humoral immunity

HIE. *See* hypoxic ischemic encephalopathy
high-frequency jet ventilation (HFJV), 94, 124–125
high-frequency oscillation ventilation (HFOV), 124–125, 807
high-frequency percussive ventilation (HFPV), 94, 96
high-frequency ventilation, 123–125
high-reliability organizations (HROs), 892–894
hindgut, 531
hip spica casts, 714
Hirschsprung's disease, 561t
histamine-2 receptor antagonists, 538
histocompatibility testing, 605
histotoxic hypoxia, 847
HIV. *See* human immunodeficiency virus
HLHS. *See* hypoplastic left heart syndrome
holosystolic murmurs, 170
Holt-Oram syndrome, 163t
Holter monitoring, 175–176
    nuclear medicine studies, 180
homeostasis, 591
homograft, 811
hormones. *See also* specific hormones
    characteristics of, 479, 480t
    chemical structures of, 483
    definition of, 479
    feedback mechanism for, 483, 485
    target cells for, 479, 485f
hospital tours, 20, 25
Hospital Value-Based Purchasing Program, 907, 910
hospitalization
    adolescent's response to, 8
    anxiety associated with, 8
    fear associated with, 8
    infant's response to, 8
    preschooler's response to, 8
    responses to, 7–8
    school-age child's response to, 8
HROs. *See* high-reliability organizations
HSCT. *See* hematopoietic stem cell transplantation
huddles, 890
huff-coughing, 69t
human chorionic gonadotropin, 420
human immunodeficiency virus (HIV). *See also* acquired immunodeficiency syndrome
    antiretroviral medications, 641
    blood transfusion-related transmission of, 623
    classification of, 639
    course of, 640
    definition of, 638–639
    diagnosis of, 641
    latency stage of, 639
    management of, 640–642
    needlestick injuries and, 641
    occupational risks, 641

human immunodeficiency virus (HIV)
(*cont.*)
on other organ systems, impact
of, 642
pathophysiology of, 639
perinatal transmission, 640
Pneumocystis carinii pneumonia
characteristics of, 641
diagnostic findings, 640
pentamidine isethionate for, 642
postexposure prophylaxis, 641
prophylaxis, 641–642
signs and symptoms of, 641
transmission of, 641
treatment of, 642
trimethoprim-sulfamethoxazole
for, 641
zidovudine for, 610
postexposure prophylaxis for, 641
transmission of, 639
human immunoglobulins, 596t
human leukocyte antigens, 591, 605
humoral disorder, 636
humoral immunity
description of, 585, 594, 639
human immunodeficiency virus
effects on, 639
HUS. *See* hemolytic-uremic syndrome
HWE. *See* healthy work environment
hydralazine (Apresoline), 201
hydrocarbons, 766–767
hydrocephalus
circulation theory, 422–423
clinical presentation of, 423
definition and etiology of, 422
outcomes of, 424
pathophysiology of, 422–423
patient care management, 423–424
hydrochlorothiazide, 464
hydrocortisone, 788
hydrocortisone therapy, 489
HydroDIURIL, 464
hydrofluoric acid, 761
hydromorphone, pain management
using, 15t
hydrotherapy, 808
hydroxocobalamin, 762
hydroxyurea, 632
hyperalgesia, 693
hyperbaric oxygen therapy, 96
hyperbilirubinemia
clinical presentation of, 565
definition and etiology of,
563–564
pathophysiology of, 564–565
patient care management, 565
hypercalcemia, 452
hypercarbia
description of, 45
permissive, 128
hyperdynamic circulation, 466
hyperemic hypoxia, 847
hyperglycemia, 472, 508, 509, 510,
860–862

hyperglycemic hyperosmolar syndrome
(HHS)
complications, 515
diabetic ketoacidosis and, 514t
diagnostic studies, 514–515
differential diagnoses, 514–515
fluid and electrolyte therapy for, 515
incidence of, 513
insulin therapy for, 515
precipitating factors, 513
signs and symptoms, 513–514
hyperkalemia, 458t, 460–461, 501,
651, 658
hyperleukocytosis, 651–652
hyperlipoproteinemia, 250
hypermagnesemia, 458t, 461
hypernatremia, 520–522
hyperosmolality, 509, 511, 514
hyperosmolar therapy, 398, 403
hyperparathyroidism, 496
hyperphosphatemia, 458t, 461
hyperresonance, 47
hypersensitivity reactions, 627, 628t
hypersplenism, 571
hypertension
intracranial. *See* intracranial
hypertension
pulmonary. *See* pulmonary
hypertension
systemic, 226
hyperthermia
causes of, 380, 867
fever versus, 626
during transport, 867–868
treatment of, 402–403, 868
hyperthyroidism, 494, 495
hypertonic saline, 398, 403
hypertrophic cardiomyopathy
(HCM), 313f
complications, 314
diagnostic tests for, 313
etiology of, 312–313
pathophysiology of, 312–313
patient management, 313–314
phenotypic expression, 313
treatment for, 313
hypertrophic scar, 813
hypertrophy of cardiac muscle, 226
hyperuricemia, 458t
hyperventilation, 691
after head injury, 697
cerebral blood flow affected by, 402
intracranial pressure reduced by, 402
hypocalcemia, 472
acute renal failure and, 453,
458t, 461
parathyroid hormone release
and, 496
hypodynamic state, 783
hypogammaglobulinemia, 636
hypoglossal nerve
in children, 379t
function of, 364t
in infants, 376t

hypoglycemia, 512
acute, 515–518
algorithm, 517f
causes of, 860–861
childhood, 516
clinical presentation of, 860–862
complications of, 861
definition, 515
in diabetes, 516
glucose for, 860
neonatal, 516
neurologic responses to, 516
transport mechanism of, 862f
hypoinsulinemia, 498
hypokalemia, 512, 658
hyponatremia, 452, 501
acute renal failure and, 458t
syndrome of inappropriate
antidiuretic hormone as cause of,
403, 518
hypoparathyroidism, 497
hypopharynx, 37, 37f
hypophyseal portal system, 486, 486f
hypophysis, 486. *See also* pituitary
gland
hypoplasia, 585
hypoplastic left heart syndrome
(HLHS), 302f, 901
bidirectional cavopulmonary shunt,
305, 305f–306f
Blalock–Taussig shunt, 304f
complications of, 307
diagnostic findings for, 302
Fontan procedure, 306, 306f
incidence of, 300
Norwood procedure, 293, 302f, 304f
pathophysiology of, 301
postoperative care, 307
preoperative stabilization, 303
surgical reconstruction in, 304f
hyposensitization, for asthma
patients, 99
hypotension, 210, 231, 683t, 697, 748
hypothalamic–pituitary complex,
484–493, 487f. *See also*
hypothalamus; pituitary gland
hypothalamohypophysia tract, 486
hypothalamus
anatomic location of, 486
cell types of, 486–487
description of, 355
embryology of, 484
functions of, 485
hormones produced by, 487
role of, 485
hypothermia
after burns, 796, 804
description of, 676
intracranial hypertension treated
with, 402–403
submersion injuries and, 678–679
during transport, 867
hypothyroidism, 490, 494
hypovolemia, 629, 778

hypovolemic shock, 554, 707
hypoxemia, 90, 100, 102
 causes of, 779
 in septic shock, 779
 ventilation-perfusion mismatch
  and, 116
hypoxia, 104, 697, 805
 after head injury, 698
 during air medical transport,
  845–846
 definition of, 698, 847
 severe, 112
hypoxic hypoxia, 847
hypoxic ischemic encephalopathy
  (HIE), 427–429
 clinical presentation, 871
 definition of, 871
 etiology of, 871
 measure severity of, 872t
 transport management, 871–872
hypoxic-ischemic injury, 679

I-PASS, 903
I PASS the BATON, 903
IADSA. *See* intra-arterial digital
  subtraction angiography
iatrogenic anemia, 624
ibuprofen, 14, 16t
ICP. *See* intracranial pressure
identity, role confusion versus, 4–5
idiopathic cardiomyopathy, 309
idiopathic disease, 508
idiopathic scoliosis, 434
IgA deficiency, 51t, 636
IHI. *See* Institute for Healthcare
  Improvement
ileum, 532
iloprost, 205–206
imidazoline derivatives, 752
imipramine, 746
immobilization
 after spinal cord injury, 432, 702
 cervical spine, 689
 of fractures, 691
immune reconstitution, 638
immune response, 594
immune system
 antiglobulin test, 605–606
 burn-related response, 804
 C-reactive protein, 605
 complement assays, 605
 Coombs' test, 605
 description of, 585–587
 diagnostic testing of, 604–606
 erythrocyte sedimentation rate, 605
 histocompatibility testing, 605
 pharmacologic agents that affect,
  608–616
immune thrombocytopenic purpura
  (ITP), 644–646
immunity
 acquired, 593t, 594
 active, 593t

cell-mediated
 description of, 594, 639
 human immunodeficiency virus
  effects on, 639
 description of, 585, 639
 humoral
 description of, 594, 639
 human immunodeficiency virus
  effects on, 639
 passive, 593t
 specific acquired, 594, 595f
immunocompetence, 775
immunodeficiency
 acquired immunodeficiency
  syndrome. *See* acquired
  immunodeficiency syndrome
 congenital diseases, 636–638
 definition of, 636
 human immunodeficiency virus. *See*
  human immunodeficiency virus
 secondary, 642
 severe combined, 637–638
immunoglobulin(s)
 A, 51t, 594, 596t, 598t
 D, 51t, 594, 596t, 598t
 E
  asthma and, 97–98
  characteristics of, 596t, 598t
  pulmonary function evaluations
   using, 51t
 G, 51t, 466, 594, 596t, 598t, 607
 M, 51t, 594, 596t, 598t
 total level of, 596t
immunosuppression, 636
immunosuppressive therapy
 description of, 541–542
 immune thrombocytopenic purpura
  treated with, 646
Imodium, 540
ImproveCareNow Network, 900, 901
improvised nuclear device, 831
Inapsine. *See* droperidol
Inderal. *See* propranolol
indirect calorimetry, 820
indirect Coombs' test, 605–606
indwelling catheters, uses of, 476t
infants. *See also* children; neonates
 acute idiopathic pulmonary
  hemorrhage of, 104
 airway obstruction, 114
 breast milk, 543
 chest compression, 113
 chest in, 35
 choking, 114
 cognitive development in, 4
 communication by, 17
 cough in, 50t
 cranial nerves in, 373t–379t
 energy needs, assessment of,
  542, 543t
 enteral nutrition, 543
 fear responses by, 8
 fluids, calculation of, 543
 hematologic values in, 603t

homicide, 668
hospitalization response of, 7
intracranial hypertension in, 401
intracranial pressure in, 360
kidneys of, 445
leading causes of injury, 669, 669t
nasal breathing by, 36
nutrition assessment, 542
pacifier for, 14
pain assessment and management,
  11t, 13t
parenteral nutrition, 543–544
personality development in, 4
play with, 20
poisoning of, 735–736
principles for working with, 5
psychosocial development in, 4
separation anxiety in, 8
shaken impact syndrome, 723
stress response of, 7
traumatic injuries in, 670t–671t
infections
 antimicrobial agents for, 625
 assessment and monitoring, 221
 blood transfusion-related
  transmission of, 622–623
 burn wound, 808, 819, 822
 central nervous system, 415–419
 clinical presentation of, 568–569
 definition of, 568, 774
 description of, 117, 625
 etiology of, 568
 human immunodeficiency virus and,
  639–640
 inflammation versus, 627
 interventions for, 626
 during intracranial pressure
  monitoring, 389
 nosocomial, 775
 pathophysiology of, 568
 patient care management, 569
 postresuscitation care, 216
 posttransplant, 576
 in severe combined
  immunodeficiency, 637–638
 in sickle cell disease, 632–633
 signs and symptoms of, 624
 stem cell transplantation, 656
 systemic, 625
 vaccines for, 632
 wound, 808
infectious disease, 875–876
inferior vena cava (IVC), 151
inflammation
 airway, 97–98
 infections versus, 627
 signs and symptoms of, 627
inflammatory cells, 96
inflammatory-immune response, 776
inflammatory mediators, 97
inflammatory response
 to burns, 804
 description of, 592
influenza (flu), 875

influenza vaccination, 107
informatics, 910
infratentorial herniation, 401
infratentorial tumors, 419–420
infundibular stenosis, 284f
infundibulum, 486
inhalational anthrax, 836t
inhalational injury, 95–96, 804–805
    assessment of, 806
    classification of, 805–806
    description of, 804–805
    smoke inhalation, 805
injuries
    adolescent, 672t
    all age groups, 672t–673t
    causes of, 669
    infants, 670t–671t
    kinetic forces, 673–676
    mechanism of, 670
    preschool age, 671t
    school age, 672t
    toddler, 671t
injury-based QI metrics, 910
inotropic agents
    mechanism of action, 189
    septic shock treated with, 786t
    types of, 189–193
insecticides, 768–769
insertion site care, 389
inspiratory flow, 118t, 119–120
inspiratory stridor, 48
inspiratory time, 118t
inspiratory wheezing, 48
inspiratory:expiratory ratio, 123
Institute for Healthcare Improvement
    (IHI), 886
Institute for Safe Medication Practices
    (ISMP), 885
Institute of Medicine (IOM), 876, 883
    quality domains, 892
institutional review board (IRB), 908
insulin
    autoantibodies, 510
    basal, 512
    biosynthesis of, 497–498
    in carbohydrate metabolism, 498
    effects of, 498
    embryologic production of, 497–498
    in fat metabolism, 498
    functions of, 482t
    gluconeogenesis affected by, 498
    hyperglycemic hyperosmolar
        syndrome treated with, 515
    hyperkalemia managed using, 460
    inhibition of, 498
    intermediate-acting, 512
    lack of, 508
    long-acting, 512
    production of, 482t
    in protein metabolism, 498
    rapid-acting, 512
    regulation of, 498
    release of, 498
    secondary effects of, 498

    secretion, 498
    short-acting, 512
insulin-dependent diabetes
    mellitus, 862
insulin replacement therapy, 512
insulin tolerance test, 505
integrase inhibitors, 641
interdisciplinary rounding, 904
interferon alfa, 597t
interferon beta, 597t
interferon gamma, 597t
interleukin-1, 597t, 777
interleukin-2, 597t
interleukin-3, 597t
interleukin-4, 597t
interleukin-6, 597t
intermittent mandatory ventilation, 120
internal cardioverter defibrillators, 231,
    244–250
international normalization ratio, 606
internodal atrial pathways, 157
interrupted aortic arch
    Celoria and Patton
        classification, 281f
    coarctation of the aorta and, 277–278
    definition of, 277–278
    incidence of, 278
    pathophysiology of, 278
    patient management, 278, 280
    signs and symptoms, 278
    surgical correction of, 282f
interstitial edema, 400
interstitial pneumonia, 81
interstitial pneumonitis, 659
intervertebral discs, 356–357
intestinal atresia, 559t
intestine
    anatomy of, 532–533
    atresia of, 559t
    autonomic nerve stimulation effects
        on, 559t
    injuries to, 553
    transplantation, 576–579
        Bianchi procedure, 578
        bowel-lengthening
            procedures, 578
        congenital conditions, 557t–561t
        nursing care of, 579t
        PN-induced cholestasis, 578
        procedures of, 579f
intra-arterial digital subtraction
    angiography (IADSA), 384
intracranial hemorrhage
    aneurysm, 410–411
    arteriovenous malformation,
        410–411
    clinical presentation of, 411–412
    definition of, 410–411
    etiology of, 410–411
    intraventricular hemorrhage,
        413–415
    pathogenesis of, 414
    pathophysiology of, 411
    periventricular hemorrhage, 413–415

intracranial hypertension
    characteristics of, 401
    in children, 401
    clinical course, 402
    description of, 400
    diagnostic tests, 401–402
    etiology of, 400
    herniation symptoms, 401
    in infants, 401
    management of, 402–403
    neuromuscular blockade for, 402
    pathophysiology of, 400–401, 400f
intracranial pressure
    after head injury, 697
    anatomic locations for, 388–389
    carbon dioxide monitoring in, 55
    cerebral edema effects on, 400
    description of, 387
    dynamics of, 360–362
    fiber-optic catheters for, 388
    hypertonic saline, 398
    infection control during, 389
    interventions for, 402
    intraventricular drainage system
        with, 393f
    intraventricular location for, 388
    mannitol for, 398
    nursing considerations for, 389
    signs of, 854
    systems for, 388–389
    transcranial Doppler ultrasound, 385
        after traumatic brain injury, 426
        waveforms, 385, 386f
    waveforms, 389–390, 390f
intrahepatic cholestasis, 574–575
intraosseous vascular access, 212, 213f
intraparenchymal fiber-optic
    transduced tipped catheters, 389
intrapulmonary airways, 37
intravenous cannulation, 690
intravenous immunoglobulin (IVIG),
    619t, 638, 646, 789
intravenous pyelogram (IVP), 474
intraventricular hemorrhage
    clinical presentation of, 414–415
    definition of, 413
    etiology of, 413
    outcomes of, 415
    pathogenesis of, 413–414
    patient care management, 415
    risk factors of, 413
    severity and grading of, 414
    subependymal germinal matrix,
        413–414
intraventricular tunnel repair, of
    double-outlet right ventricle, 262f
intrinsic factor, 532
intrinsic pathway, 599
intrinsic renal failure. *See* acute tubular
    necrosis
Intropin. *See* dopamine
intubation, 94
    of children, 17–18
    complications of, 132, 689

intubation (*cont.*)
  equipment of, 126
  for initial stabilization of patient, 855
  post-traumatic indications for, 689
  procedure of, 127
  rapid sequence, 689, 858f
intussusception, 560t
invasive hemodynamic monitoring, 782
inverse-ratio ventilation, 123
ion trapping, 742
ionized calcium, 452
ipecac syrup, 740
ipratropium, 864t
iron
  overdose, 743t
  overload, 623
  poisoning, 752–754
  replacement therapy, 454, 455t
  supplementation, 454
irradiation, 616
irritant gases, 96
ischemic acute tubular necrosis, 457, 458
ischemic stroke, 222. *See also* acute
  ischemic stroke
Ishikawa diagram, 896
islet cell antibodies, 510
islets of Langerhans, 482t
ISMP. *See* Institute for Safe Medication
  Practices
isometric relaxation, 160
isoniazid overdose, 743t, 754
isoproterenol (Isuprel), 190–191
Isoptin. *See* verapamil
isovolumetric relaxation, 160
ITP. *See* immune thrombocytopenic
  purpura
IVIG. *See* intravenous immunoglobulin

Jackson–Pratt drainage, 546, 575
jaundice, 564
jaw-thrust maneuver, 688
jejunum, 532
Jervell-Lange-Nielsen syndrome, 165t
jugular venous oxygen saturation
  monitoring, 390–392
JUMPStart triage model, 829
junctional tachycardia, 239, 239f
just culture principles, 887, 911
  application of, 889
  event management algorithm in, 888f
  implementation of, 904
juxtaglomerular nephrons, 445
juxtamedullary nephrons, 450

Kawasaki disease, 325–327
Kayexalate. *See* sodium polystyrene
  sulfonate
Kehr's sign, 550
kernicterus, 565
ketamine
  characteristics of, 64
  in children, 396t
  contraindications, 59t

  dosing of, 59t
  pain management using, 15, 16t
ketoacidosis. *See* diabetic ketoacidosis
ketogenesis, 498
ketone bodies, 509
ketonuria, 510
ketorolac, 14, 16t
kidney(s). *See also* acute kidney injury
  acid-base balance regulated by,
    452–453, 463t
  angiogram, 455–456
  arterial blood pressure regulation by,
    453–454
  biopsy of, 456
  capsule, 445
  cortex, 445
  development, 445
  diagnostic studies, 454–456
  dysfunction, 466
    after stem cell
      transplantation, 658
  erythrocyte production by bone
    marrow stimulated by, 454
  failure of. *See* acute renal failure
  filtration by, 448, 449
  location, 445
  medulla, 445
  metabolic wastes, elimination of, 454
  nephron
    anatomy of, 445–446
    collecting ducts, 446
    cortical, 445
    definition of, 445
    juxtaglomerular, 445
    tubular components of, 446, 447f
    vascular components of, 445, 446
  pelvis, 445
  reabsorption in, 449–450
  replacement therapies. *See* renal
    replacement therapies
  response to shock, 448, 449f
  secretion, 450
  solute clearance, 468
  structure, 445–446, 446f
  toxins, elimination of, 454
  transport mechanisms, 446, 447
  trauma to, 473–474
  urine formation by, 447–450
kidney, ureter, and bladder (KUB)
  film, 474
killer T cells, 589
kinetic energy
  blunt-force trauma injuries caused
    by, 673
  definition of, 673
kinetic forces injury, 673
  acceleration–deceleration
    injury, 674
  blunt-force trauma, 673
  bullet wounding mechanisms, 675
  crush injury, 673–674
  GSW characteristics, 675
  penetrating injury, 674–675
  primary survey, 675–676

  risk for injury, 675
  shear injury, 674
knife wounds, 674
Konno procedure, for aortic stenosis,
  272, 273f
Kupffer's cells, 587
Kussmaul breathing, 853

L-transposition of the great arteries
  (L-TGA)
  definition of, 298
  diagnostic test for, 299–300
  incidence of, 298
  pathophysiology of, 298
  patient management, 300
  signs and symptoms, 298–299
LA. *See* left atrial monitoring
labetalol, 199
laceration
  cerebral, 425
  renal, 473
  spinal cord, 430
lack of privacy, 10
lactotrophs, 486
lactulose, 540
laetrile, 761
Lanoxin. *See* digoxin
lansoprazole, 539
Laplace's law, 150
large intestine, injuries to, 553
laryngeal mask airway
  contraindications, 856t
  description of, 855
  indications for, 856t
  limitations of, 856t
laryngotracheobronchitis
  airway edema and, 77f
  clinical presentation of, 77
  definition of, 76–77
  differential diagnosis, 76t
  outcomes of, 78
  pathophysiology of, 77
  patient care management, 77–78
larynx, 687
  anatomy of, 37, 37f
  embryology of, 37
Lasix. *See* furosemide
latent errors, 889
latent tuberculosis infection, 85
lead, 743t
leadership
  authentic, 913
  ineffective, 918
  team, 905
  TeamSTEPPS model, 905, 906f
LeFort fractures, 687, 700–701
left atrial monitoring, 185f, 186–187
left bundle branch (LBB), 158
left bundle branch block, 243
left coronary artery (LCA), 150
left heart outflow tract obstruction, 869
  chest radiography, 869
  clinical presentation, 869
  intervention, 869

left intercostal space (LICS), 167
left-sided heart failure, 225, 226
left-to-right shunts, 253
left ventricular dysfunction, 93t, 642
left ventricular ejection fraction, 787
left ventricular end-diastolic pressure
     (LVEDP), 155
left ventricular end-diastolic volume
     (LVEDV), 155
left ventricular hypertrophy (LVH), 167
left ventricular noncompaction
     cardiomyopathy (LVNC), 317f
  diagnostic evaluation, 316–317
  etiology of, 316
  pathophysiology of, 316
  phenotypic expression, 316
left ventricular outflow tract
     reconstruction, 266f
left ventricular outward tract
     obstruction (LVOTO), 312–314
LET. *See* lipid emulsion therapy
leukocytes
  in children, 603t
  description of, 587
  enzymes, 638
  in infants, 603t
leukocytosis, 602
leukodepletion, 616
leukopenia, 602
leukotriene inhibitors
  asthma treated with, 99
  pulmonary disorders treated with, 69
levalbuterol, 864t
level of consciousness, 369–370, 854
levetiracetam, 398, 399t
levocardia, 302
Levophed. *See* norepinephrine bitartrate
levosimendan, 231
lewisite, 833t
LH. *See* luteinizing hormone
lidocaine, 193
life support
  advanced cardiac
     airway management, 210
     cardiopulmonary failure, 209–210
     circulatory support, 210–212
     fluid resuscitation, 213
     neonatal resuscitation, 214
     parental presence during, 216–217
     pharmacologic support, 213, 214
     postresuscitation care,
        214–216, 215f
     vascular access, 212, 213,
        213f, 214f
     ventilation, 210
  cardiopulmonary assessments, 784
  extracorporeal. *See* extracorporeal
     membrane oxygenation
  septic shock management, 784
  withdrawal of, 27
life-sustaining medical treatment,
     forgoing of, 26–27
lifts, 168
limbic system, 354

lipase, 498, 552
lipid emulsion therapy (LET), 742, 748
lipolysis, 498
lipopolysaccharide, 776
lips, burns of, 810
liver
  assessment of, 854
  border of, 780
  failure of. *See* hepatic failure
  functions of, 533
  hemorrhage of, 551
  injuries to, 551, 552t
  palpation of, 168, 602, 780–781
  size of, 854
  transplantation
     biliary atresia, 574
     complications of, 576
     intrahepatic cholestasis, 574
     malignant disease, 574–575
     metabolic diseases, 574
     nursing care, 575–576
     orthotopic, 575
     pretransplant considerations, 575
liver biopsy, 536t
liver function tests, 534t–535t
liver ischemia, 234
log rolling, 688
long-acting beta agonists, 99
long QT syndrome, 242
loop diuretics, acute kidney injury
     treated with, 464
loop of Henle
  anatomy of, 445, 446
  potassium reabsorption in, 451
lorazepam
  contraindications, 60t
  dosing of, 60t
  pain management using, 16t
  seizure control using, 398, 399t
     in children, 396t
loss of control, 9
low CO syndrome (LCOS), 217
lower airways. *See also* lung
  bronchitis, 79
  development of, 37–38
lower gastrointestinal tract bleeding
  clinical presentation of, 555t
  etiology of, 554t
lumbar puncture, 384–385
Lund and Browder chart, 801
lung
  autonomic nerve stimulation effects
     on, 367t
  burn-related response, 803
  development of, 38, 38f
  embryology of, 35, 36f
  fissures, 37, 38f
  gas exchange in, 37–38
  lobes of, 37, 37f
  perfusion of, 40
  physiologic function of, 40–41
  in premature infants, 35
  vascularization of, 35
lung compliance, 119

lung transplantation
  candidate evaluation, 137–138
  complications of, 139, 140t
  in cystic fibrosis patients, 136
  definition of, 136
  donor evaluation, 138
  indications for, 136, 137t
  mortality rates, 139
  patient care management during,
     138–139
  posttransplantation
     lymphoproliferative disease, 139
  rejection after, 138–139
  survival after, 139
lung volumes, 41, 42f
luteinizing hormone (LH), 480t,
     490, 491f
lymph nodes, 586
  biopsy of, 608
  symptoms of concern, 601t
lymphatic system, 39
lymphoblasts, 585
lymphocyte(s)
  B. *See* B cells
  in children, 603t
  description of, 585, 587f, 589
  in infants, 603t
  T. *See* T cells
lymphocyte immune globulin
     preparations, 612–613
lymphocytic interstitial pneumonitis,
     612–613
lymphocytosis, 589
lymphokines, 595
lymphopenia, 589
lymphoproliferative disease, 578

mace, 833, 833t
Macewen's sign, 423
macitentan, 206
macrophages, 588–589
mafenide acetate cream, 813t
MAG3 renal scan, 455
magical thinking, 9
magnesium, 452
magnesium citrate, 742
magnesium hydroxide, 541
magnesium sulfate
  asthma treated with, 99, 100
  bronchospasm treated with, 866
magnetic expansion control, 436
magnetic resonance angiography
     (MRA), 179, 180
magnetic resonance imaging
  central nervous system tumors
     diagnosed using, 420
  clinical uses of, 381–382, 383
  computed tomography versus,
     381–382, 383
  description of, 179
  endocrine system evaluations, 506
  gastrointestinal disorders evaluated
     using, 536t

magnetic resonance imaging (*cont.*)
  meningitis evaluations, 417
  neurologic system evaluations, 383–384, 383f
  pulmonary function evaluations using, 53
  renal diagnosis using, 455
  for renal trauma evaluation, 474
  traumatic brain injury evaluations, 426
major histocompatibility complex molecules, 591
maldistribution
  of blood flow, 777, 779
  of circulating volume, 778f
malformation syndromes, 309
malnourishment, 139
malnutrition, 572–573
malocclusion, 687
malrotation with volvulus, 559t
mandatory minute ventilation, 121
mandibular fractures, 700
mannitol, 398, 464, 697, 698
MAOIs. *See* monoamine oxidase inhibitors
MAP. *See* mean arterial pressure
Marfan syndrome, 163t
margination, 592
mass casualty incidents, 827
maternal smoking, 96
maturity-onset diabetes of youth (MODY), 508
maxillary sinus, 36
maxillofacial injuries, 700–701
MCL-1. *See* modified chest lead
MDAC. *See* multiple doses of activated charcoal
mean airway pressure, 119, 124
mean arterial pressure (MAP), 40, 156–157, 360, 779
mean corpuscular volume, 603t
mechanical cardiac support (MCS). *See* extracorporeal membrane oxygenation
mechanical debridement, burn wounds, 808
mechanical insufflation–exsufflation, 70t
mechanical ventilation, 224, 230
  airway management in, 127
  assessment of patient during, 128
  barotrauma in, 132
  bronchopulmonary dysplasia caused by, 114
  complications of, 132–133
  extracorporeal membrane oxygenation, 125
  flow delivery, 122
  high-frequency ventilation, 123–125
  after hypoxic-ischemic injury, 679
  inverse-ratio ventilation, 123
  monitoring during, 128
  negative-pressure ventilation, 126
  noninvasive, 126
  nutrition during, 130
  objectives of, 118

pain management during, 130
physiologic interface with child, 119–120
positive-pressure ventilation
  controls, 121–122
  definition of, 120
  flow delivery, 122
  mechanics of, 121f
  modes of, 120–121
  noninvasive, 126
  phase variables for, 122–123
  sensing mechanisms, 122
pressure, flow, and resistance relationships, 119
psychological needs during, 129–130
sedation during, 130
shock managed using, 234
during transport, 866–867
after traumatic injuries, 690
troubleshooting of, 867t
variables for, 123, 123t
weaning from
  dysfunctional, 222
  readiness for, 131
  techniques for, 131–132
mechanoreceptors, 40
Meckel scan, 536t
medication errors reporting program (MERP), 885
medulla
  respiratory control by, 40
  vasomotor center in, 155
medulla oblongata, 355
medulloblastoma, 419
megakaryoblasts, 585
megakaryocytes, 589
melanocyte-stimulating hormone (MSH), 480t
melanotrophs, 487
melena, 554
membrane potentials, 451
memory cells, 589, 594
meninges, 352
meningitis, 415–419
meningocele, 437
meningococcal vaccine, 614
mental status assessments, 370
meperidine, 754
mephedrone, 757t
MERP. *See* medication errors reporting program
mesencephalon, 350, 350f, 355
meshed grafts, 811
mesoderm, 349
metabolic acidosis
  description of, 463t
  hyponatremic, 452
metabolic alkalosis, 463t
metabolic hypothesis, 153
metabolism
  burn-related response, 804
  insulin's role in, 498
metencephalon, 350, 350f, 355

methadone
  contraindications, 60t
  dosing of, 60t
  overdose of, 754
  pain management using, 15t–16t
methanol poisoning, 765–766
methemoglobin, 762–763
methemoglobinemia, 49f, 743t, 746
methylene chloride, 758
methylone, 757t
methylprednisolone, 68, 541–542, 865
methylxanthines, 117
metoclopramide, 66t, 540
metolazone, 464
metrics, for quality improvement, 910–911
MFI. *See* Model for Improvement
microglia, 352
midazolam, 749
  contraindications, 59t
  dosing of, 59t
  pain management using, 16t
  seizure control using, 398, 399t
    in children, 396t
midbrain, 355
midfacial fractures, 701
midgut, 531
Milk of Magnesia. *See* magnesium hydroxide
milrinone, 193
  septic shock treated with, 786t
mineralocorticoids, 481t
minute ventilation, 118t, 121
MiraLax. *See* polyethylene glycol 3350
mistrust, trust versus, 4
mitral insufficiency
  anatomy of, 280
  complications, 281–282
  diagnostic test for, 280
  incidence of, 280
  pathophysiology of, 280
  patient management, 280–281
  signs and symptoms, 280
  surgical correction of, 282f
mitral stenosis
  complications, 284
  definition of, 282
  diagnostic test for, 283
  incidence of, 282
  pathophysiology of, 282–283
  patient management, 283–284
  signs and symptoms, 283
  surgical correction of, 283f
mitral valve, 148t, 301
mixed venous oxygen saturation
  definition of, 788
  monitoring of, 54, 188
mixed venous oxygen saturation (SvO$_2$)
  measurements, 228, 234
MMER. *See* multimodality-evoked response
mobile ECMO, 872
Mobitz type I atrioventricular block, 242–243, 242f

Mobitz type II atrioventricular block, 242f, 243
Mobitz type II second-degree block, 870
Model for Improvement (MFI), 894
modified Blalock-Taussig shunt, 287, 288f
modified chest lead (MCL)-1, 182
modified Monroe-Kellie doctrine, 360
MODS. *See* multiple organ dysfunction syndrome
MODY. *See* maturity-onset diabetes of youth
molecular typing, 605
monoamine oxidase inhibitors (MAOIs), 749
monoblasts, 585
monoclonal antibodies, 99, 606, 613–614
monocyte-colony stimulating factor, 597t
monocytes
    in children, 603t
    description of, 588
    in infants, 603t
monocytopenia, 588
monocytosis, 588
monokines, 595
mononuclear phagocytes, 588–589
moral dilemma, 917
moral distress, 917
    causes of, 917
    end-of-life care and resuscitation, 917–918
moral sensitivity, 917
Moro reflex, 371, 565
morphine
    agitation managed using, 286
    in children, 396t
    contraindications, 60t
    dosing of, 60t
    pain management using, 15t, 635
MOSF. *See* multi-organ system failure
motor function assessments, 371–372
motor vehicle crashes, 429–430
motor vehicle occupant, 679
motor vehicle traffic-related deaths, 668
mouth, 601t
Moyamoya syndrome, 409
MPA. *See* mycophenolic acid
MRA. *See* magnetic resonance angiography
MRI. *See* magnetic resonance imaging
MSH. *See* melanocyte-stimulating hormone
mucosa-associated lymph tissues, 587
mucositis, 627, 656–658
mucous membranes, 162, 166, 780
MUGA scan. *See* multigated acquisition (MUGA) scan
multi-organ system failure (MOSF), 635–636
multiday dressing, wounds, 813
multifactorial inheritance syndromes, 165t

multigated acquisition (MUGA) scan, 180
multimodality-evoked response (MMER), 387
multiple doses of activated charcoal (MDAC), 742, 755
multiple organ dysfunction syndrome (MODS), 776, 789
multiple trauma, 667
Munchausen syndrome by proxy, 727–729. *See* factitious disorder
murmurs
    continuous, 170–171, 171f
    diastolic, 170, 171f
    holosystolic, 170
    systolic, 170, 170f
musculoskeletal injuries, 691, 710–715, 830t
mushrooms, 767–768
mycophenolate mofetil, 542, 612
mycophenolic acid (MPA), 612
Mycostatin. *See* nystatin
mycotic aneurysm, 411
myelencephalon, 350, 350f, 355
myelin sheath, 350
myelination, of brain, 350
myeloblasts, 585
myelodysplasia, 436
myeloid growth factors, 609
myelomeningocele, 437–438
myocardial conduction system, 158–159
myocardial contractility, 226
myocardial contusions, 110
myocardial depressant factor, 778
myocarditis
    etiology of, 319
    management of, 319
    pathophysiology of, 318–319
    signs and symptoms of, 319
myocardium
    contractility of, 156
    fetal, 151
    neonatal, 153
myoclonic seizures, 404
myocyte-enhancing transcription, 147
myogenic response hypothesis, 153
myoglobin, 716
myoglobinuria, 467, 468t, 673–674
myomectomy/myectomy, 314
myxedema coma, 494

N-acetyl-p-benzoquinoneimine, 745
N-acetylcysteine, 745
nalbuphine, 63, 65t
naloxone, 65, 65t
Narcan. *See* naloxone
NASA. *See* National Aeronautics and Space Administration
nasogastric tube, 72, 544–545, 545t, 691
nasojejunal tube, 545–546
nasopharyngeal airway, 210, 689, 856t
nasopharynx, 37, 37f
NAT. *See* nonaccidental trauma

National Aeronautics and Space Administration (NASA), 892
National Patient Safety Foundation (NPSF), 885
National Patient Safety Goals (NPSG) program, 883, 884t–885t
National Pediatric Cardiology Quality Improvement Collaborative (NPC-QIC), 901
National Trauma Data Bank (NTDB), 667, 901
natriuresis, 501
natriuretic peptides, 155
natural killer cells, 589
near drowning, 678
near-infrared spectroscopy (NIRS), 392–393
nebulizers, 864–865
neck
    pediatric assessments, 830t
    trauma-related evaluation of, 687
necrotizing enterocolitis, 562–563
necrotizing infection/fasciitis, 816
negative chronotropy, 155
negative dromotropism, 155
negative feedback, 483
negative-pressure ventilation, 126
Neo-Synephrine. *See* phenylephrine hydrochloride
neonatal hepatitis, 571
neonatal intensive care units (NICUs), 901
neonates. *See also* children; infants
    body fat in, 497
    cerebrospinal fluid production by, 354
    circulation in, 153
    extracorporeal membrane oxygenation in, 125
    gastric emptying in, 57
    high-frequency oscillation ventilation settings in, 124
    hypoglycemia in, 516
    hypoglycemic prevention in, 497
    intracranial pressure in, 360
    myocardium in, 153
    pain assessment in, 11t, 13t, 693
    phagocytosis in, 592
    resuscitation of, 214
nephrogenic diabetes insipidus, 520–522
nephron
    anatomy of, 445–446
    collecting ducts, 446
    cortical, 445
    definition of, 445
    juxtaglomerular, 445
    juxtamedullary, 450
    tubular components of, 446, 447f
    vascular components of, 445, 446
nephrotic syndrome, 465–466
nephrotoxic acute tubular necrosis, 457
nerve agents, 832, 833t
nerve injury, 715

nervous system
central. *See* central nervous system
stress-related response of, 6
nesiritide, 230
neural crest, 349
neural groove, 349
neural plate, 349
neural tissue, 349, 351
neural tube, 349–350
neural tube defects, 437
neuroendocrine system. *See*
hypothalamic–pituitary complex
neurogenic shock, 232–233
neuroglia, 352
neurohormonal control, of heart, 155
neurohypophysis, 486–487
neurologic disorders, 368
neurologic dysfunction, 411
neurologic system
anatomic integrity assessments, 381–384
cerebellar function, 384
cerebral angiogram, 384
computed tomography, 381–383, 382f
magnetic resonance imaging, 383–384, 383f
radiographs, 381
radioisotope scan, 384
brain-death determination, 380–381
brain-tissue oxygen monitoring, 392
central nervous system. *See* central
nervous system
cerebellar function, 373
cranial nerves, 373, 373t–379t
deep tendon reflexes, 372
description of, 854
family history, 368
fiber-optic catheters for, 388
fundoscopic examination, 373, 379
history-taking, 368
intracranial devices, 393
external ventricular shunt, 393–394, 393f
internal ventricular shunt, 394–395, 395f
intracranial pressure, 387–390, 390f
jugular venous oxygen saturation monitoring, 390–392
level of consciousness, 369–370
motor function, 371–372
near-infrared spectroscopy, 392–393
peripheral nervous system. *See*
peripheral nervous system
pharmacology, 395–399, 396t, 397t, 399t
analgesia and sedation, 395–396, 396t
anticonvulsant medications, 398, 399t
antimicrobial therapy, 396, 397t, 398
hyperosmolar therapy, 398
physical examination, 369–380

physiologic alterations, 384–387, 386f
electroencephalograms, 385–386, 386f
evoked potential studies, 387
lumbar puncture and CSF analysis, 384–385
transcranial Doppler ultrasound, 385
video-EEG, 386–387
xenon-enhanced CT scan, 385
post-traumatic, 684t, 686
post-traumatic assessment of, 684t, 686
postresuscitation care, 216
reflexes, 371–372
sensory function, 372–373
vital signs, 379–380
neuromuscular blockade, 95
intracranial hypertension treated with, 402
monitoring of, 128–129
neuromuscular blocking agents
depolarizing, 57
description of, 26, 57
indications for, 57
nondepolarizing, 57
nursing considerations for, 57–58
types of, 58t
neuromuscular disorders, 309
neuromuscular scoliosis, 433–434
neuron, 351, 351f
neuronal processes, 351
neuropilin 1, 147
neurotransmitter, 351
neurulation, 349–350, 349f
neutral protamine Hagedorn (NPH), 512
neutropenia, 588, 609, 637
neutrophil(s)
characteristics of, 587–588
in children, 603t
in infants, 603t
neutrophilia, 588
NICUs. *See* neonatal intensive care units
nidus, 410
nifedipine (Procardia), 202–203
night shift, self-care and, 916
ninhydrin print test, 715
Nipride. *See* nitroprusside
NIRS. *See* near-infrared spectroscopy;
noninvasive infrared spectroscopy
nitric oxide
in septic shock, 777–778
therapy, 206–207
vasodilation caused by, 108
ventilation-perfusion matching affected by, 67
nitroglycerin, 198–199, 787
nitroprusside (Nipride), 199
NKX2.5 transcription factor, 147
NMB. *See* neuromuscular blockade
nodes of Ranvier, 351, 360

noise
description of, 9–10
minimization of, 19
non-insulin-dependent diabetes mellitus, 862
nonaccidental injury
assessment, 818
nursing care interventions, 819
reporting, 818–819
nonaccidental trauma (NAT), 667, 874–875
noncardiogenic pulmonary edema, 91
noncommunicating hydrocephalus, 422
noninsulin-dependent diabetes, 508
noninvasive infrared spectroscopy (NIRS), 188–189
noninvasive positive-pressure ventilation (NPPV), 94
nonpharmaceutical agents. *See*
poisoning
nonpharmacologic therapy
asthma, 98
pulmonary hypertension, 108
nonprescription drugs, 601
nonshivering thermogenesis, 684t
nonsteroidal anti-inflammatory drugs, 68
indications for, 614
pain management using, 16t
nonthiazide diuretics, 464
Noonan's syndrome, 163t, 338
noradrenaline. *See* norepinephrine
norepinephrine, 366, 482t
in critical illness, 502–503
septic shock treated with, 786t
norepinephrine bitartrate (Levophed), 191
norepinephrine-epinephrine vasoconstrictor reflex, 779
normal-pressure hydrocephalus, 422
normal sinus rhythm (NSR), 235, 240
normothermia, 867
normoventilation, 691
Norwood operation, 293, 302f, 303
nose
embryology of, 36
fractures of, 701
symptoms of concern, 601t
trauma-related evaluation of, 687
nosocomial infections, 775
noxious irritants, inhalation of, 96
NPC-QIC. *See* National Pediatric Cardiology Quality Improvement Collaborative
NPH. *See* neutral protamine Hagedorn
NPPV. *See* noninvasive positive-pressure ventilation
NPSF. *See* National Patient Safety Foundation
NPSG program. *See* National Patient Safety Goals (NPSG) program
NSR. *See* normal sinus rhythm
NTDB. *See* National Trauma Data Bank
Nubain. *See* nalbuphine

nuclear attacks, 830–832
nuclear medicine studies, 180
nucleic acid tests (NATs), 640
nurse-driven resuscitation protocol, for pediatric patients, 808, 809f
nursing communication style, 902
nursing competencies, 2
Nursing Mutual Participation Model of Care, 23, 23t
nutritional competency, heart failure and, 231
nystatin, 576

obstruction of forward flow, 226
obstructive respiratory disease, 55
obstructive shock, 233, 234
obstructive sleep apnea syndrome (OSAS), 102–103
obtundation, 370
occipital lobe
    description of, 354
    tumors of, 420
occipital lymph nodes, 587f
occipitofrontal circumference, 44
occult bleeding, 554
OCHSPS. *See* Ohio Children's Hospitals Solutions for Patient Safety
octreotide, 499
octreotide acetate, 537
oculomotor nerve
    in children, 377t
    function of, 364t
    in infants, 374t
Office for Human Research Protection, 908
Ohio Children's Hospitals Solutions for Patient Safety (OCHSPS), 900
oleoresin capsicum, 833t
olfactory nerve
    in children, 376t
    function of, 364t
oligodendrocytes, 352
omalizumab (Xolair), 99
omeprazole, 538
omphalocele, 557t
ondansetron, 66t
open fractures, 711–712, 712t
open pneumothorax, 109, 110, 705t
opiates, 60t–62t
opioid receptors, 63
opioids
    characteristics of, 66t
    overdose of, 739t, 754
    pain management using, 14, 15t–16t, 26
opsonization, 594
optic nerve
    in children, 376t
    function of, 364t
    in infants, 373t
oral candidiasis, 638
oral cavity
    anatomy of, 531
    trauma-related evaluation of, 687

oral glucose tolerance test, 505
oral hypoglycemic agents, 752
organ donor, 28
organophosphate insecticides, 739t, 768–769
orogastric tube, 689
oropharyngeal airway, 210, 688–689, 856t
oropharynx, 37, 37f
orthodromic pathway, 235
OSAS. *See* obstructive sleep apnea syndrome
oscillatory devices, 70t
osmoreceptors, 486, 491
osmosis, 447
osmotic diuretics, 464
ostium primum defect, 256
ostium secundum defect, 254
ostomy care, 546–547
outcomes, 2–3
ovaries, 482t
overdose
    acute, 734
    benzodiazepine, 749–750
    calcium channel blockers, 743t, 750–751
    chloroquine, 751
    chronic, 734
    digoxin, 751–752
    iron, 743t, 752–754
    isoniazid, 743t, 754
    opioids, 754
    poisoning versus, 734
    sympathomimetics, 755–756
overwhelming postsplenectomy infection, 551
oxidative burst, 592
oxygen
    arterial content of, 42
    brain metabolism of, 361
    diffusion of, 41
    supply and demand, imbalance of, 779
    transport of, 42
oxygen consumption, 187
    calculation of, 43t, 187, 788
    definition of, 776, 788
    oxygen transport and, 779, 788
oxygen content, 788
oxygen delivery, 215
oxygen extraction ratio, 788
oxygen monitoring
    pulse oximetry for, 53–54
    transcutaneous, 54
oxygen saturation
    description of, 43t
    mixed venous, 54
oxygen therapy, 116
oxygen toxicity, 132
oxygen transport, 779, 787, 788
oxygenator, 873
oxyhemoglobin dissociation curve, 42, 43f, 43t

oxytocin
    characteristics of, 492–493
    functions of, 481t
    production of, 486

P_1 (percussion wave), 390, 390f
P_2 (rebound or tidal wave), 390, 390f
P_3 (dicrotic wave), 390, 390f
P wave, 173–175
PA. *See* pulmonary artery
PA catheter placement, 228
pacemakers
    capture by, 246
    complications of, 247, 248t
    electrocardiographic evidence of, 246–247
    functions of, 244–246, 245t
    indications for, 244
    modes of, 246t
    nomenclature for, 244–246, 245t
    noncapture by, 247, 248t
    nursing care evaluations, 253
    nursing interventions, 243
    oversensing by, 247, 248t
    permanent, 244, 249
    settings for, 246
    system components, 244
    temporary, 244, 247
    undersensing by, 246, 248t
pacifier, 14
packed red blood cells (PRBCs), 614, 619t
PAH. *See* pulmonary arterial hypertension
pain
    in adolescents, 13t
    anxiety versus, 11
    assessment of, 11–12, 11t–12t, 692–693
    in infants, 13t
    misconceptions about, 8, 8t–9t
    in neonates, 13t, 693
    nursing diagnoses, 250
    in preschoolers, 13t
    reassessment of, 12
    in school-age children, 13t
    in toddlers, 13t
    tolerance to, 250
pain management
    in burn patients, 816–817, 822
    during mechanical ventilation, 130
    morphine sulfate, 635
    nonpharmacologic, 13–14, 13t
    nutritional support during, 820
    patient-controlled analgesia, 14, 631, 635, 817
    pharmacologic, 14–15, 15t–16t
    in sickle cell disease, 635
    in terminally ill, 26
    after traumatic injuries, 692–693
palmar grasp reflex, 371

palpation
    of fontanelles, 369
    of liver, 168, 602, 780
    mucous membranes, 780
    percussion, 45–46
    of peripheral pulses, 168
    of precordium, 167–168
    pulmonary function assessments,
      45–46
    of skin, 780
    of spleen, 602
    of trachea, 45
PALS. *See* Pediatric Advanced Life
    Support
pancreas
    autonomic nerve stimulation effects
      on, 368t
    cell types, 497
    embryology of, 497
    functions of, 533
    injuries to, 551–553, 553t
    insulin, 497–498
    islets of Langerhans, 482t
    location, 497
pancreatic buds, 497
pancreatic injury, 553t
pancreatitis, 508
    acute pancreatitis, 565
    chronic pancreatitis, 565
    clinical presentation of, 566
    definition and etiology of, 565–566
    outcomes of, 567
    pathophysiology of, 566
    patient care management, 566–567
pancuronium, 58t
panda sign, 425
panhypogammaglobulinemia, 636
pantoprazole, 539
PAP. *See* pulmonary artery pressure
papillary muscles, 147
parachute reflex, 371
paralysis
    communication during, 18
    pharmacologic, 15
paraplegia, 429
parasympathetic nervous system
    anatomy of, 364–365
    heart regulation by, 154
    schematic diagram of, 366f
parasympathetic stimulation, 155
parathyroid glands
    cell types, 496
    embryology of, 495–496
    hormones produced by, 481t, 496
    location, 496
parathyroid hormone (PTH), 452, 481t, 497
parathyroid hormone-related protein
    (PTHrP), 495
paraventricular nuclei, 486
parental smoking, 95
parenteral nutrition, 543–544, 820
parents. *See also* family
    adolescents as, 6
    of chronically ill children, 24

communicating with, 23
decision making by, 27
forgoing life-sustaining medical
    treatment by, 26–27
inadequacy feelings by, 21
mutual care planning with, 24
needs of, 21
psychosocial effects of poisoning
    on, 769
stress on, 21–22
support systems for, 22
of terminally ill child, 26
withdrawal of treatment by, 27
Pareto charts, for pressure injuries,
    896, 896f
parietal cells, 532
parietal lobe
    description of, 354
    tumors of, 420
parietooccipital sulcus, 350
Parkland formula, 808
parotid glands, 531
partial spinal cord syndrome, 429
partial thromboplastin time, 554, 599
PASG. *see* pneumatic antishock garment
passive immunity, 593t
passive transport, 446, 447
Patau syndrome, 164t
patch aortoplasty, for coarctation of the
    aorta, 277, 278f
patent ductus arteriosus (PDA), 251–253,
    290, 868
patient-centered care, 905, 906, 910
patient-controlled analgesia (PCA), 14,
    631, 635, 817
Patient Protection and Affordable Care
    Act (ACA), 906
Patient Safety Act, 885
patient safety, communication and
    barriers, 902
    debriefing, 904
    distraction-free zones for, 904
    effective, 901
    handoffs, 902–903, 903f
    implementation of just culture, 904
    institutional procedures and
      policies, 904
    poor, 901–902
    rounding process, 904
    teach-back method, 903, 904
    tools, 903–904
patient safety movement, 883–886
    Agency on Healthcare Research and
      Quality, 883, 885
    historical approach, 890
    Institute for Healthcare
      Improvement, 886
    Institute for Safe Medication
      Practices, 885
    Institute of Medicine, 883
    The Joint Commission, 883
    milestones in, 884f
    National Patient Safety
      Foundation, 885

National Patient Safety Goals
    program, 883, 884t–885t
    outcome measure of, 900f
    quality-improvement methodology,
      894–899
    solutions for, 900
patient safety organizations (PSOs), 885
PAWP monitoring. *See* pulmonary
    artery wedge pressure monitoring
PAX 3, 147
PCA. *See* patient-controlled analgesia
PCAR. *See* pediatric care after
    resuscitation
PCWP. *See* pulmonary capillary wedge
    pressure
PD. *See* peritoneal dialysis
PDA. *See* patent ductus arteriosus
PDSA cycles. *See* plan–do–study–act
    cycles
PE. *See* pulmonary embolism
PEA. *See* pulseless electrical activity
peak inspiratory pressure, 119, 121–122
pectus carinatum, 45
pectus excavatum, 45
Pediatric Acute Lung Injury Consensus
    Conference, 92
pediatric acute respiratory distress
    syndrome (PARDS)
    definition of, 92, 93t
    enteral nutrition, 95
    extracorporeal support, 94
    gas exchange, 94
    long-term outcomes of, 95
    morbidity, 95
    neuromuscular blockade, 95
    noninvasive support, 94
    pathophysiology of, 92
    pulmonary-specific patient care
      management, 94–95
    ventilatory management, 92–94
Pediatric Advanced Life Support
    (PALS), 507, 667
pediatric cardiomyopathy (PCM)
    anticoagulation, 309–310
    definition of, 308
    diagnostic evaluation, 310
    genetic testing, 309
    incidence of, 308
    mechanical ventilation, 309
    medical management, 309
    orthotopic heart transplant, 310
    oxygen demand/consumption, 309
    quality of life, 309
    symptomatic relief, 309
    thrombus formation, 309–310
    transfusion, 309
    treatment goals, 309–310
pediatric cardiomyopathy registry
    (PCMR), 309
pediatric care after resuscitation
    (PCAR), 667–668
pediatric critical care, 542, 906–907
Pediatric Glasgow Coma Score
    (PGCS), 686

pediatric intensive care unit (PICU), 370, 667
pediatric quality and safety initiatives, 899–901
  California Perinatal Quality of Care Collaborative, 901
  ImproveCareNow Network, 900–901
  National Pediatric Cardiology Quality Improvement Collaborative, 901
  Pediatric Trauma Quality Improvement Program, 901
  Solutions for Patient Safety, 900, 901t
pediatric stroke outcome measure (PSOM), 410
Pediatric TQIP. *See* Pediatric Trauma Quality Improvement Program
pediatric trauma
  accidental injury, 668
  age and gender, 668
  care, 667
  centers, 667
  developmental risk factors, 670t–673t
  environment and, 669–670
  firearm incidents, 668
  homicide, 668
  mechanisms of injury, 669, 669t
  mortality, 668
  teams, 667
Pediatric Trauma Quality Improvement Program (Pediatric TQIP), 667, 901
pediatric trauma score (PTS), 688
PEEP levels, pediatric acute respiratory distress syndrome, 93
pelvis
  fractures of, 714–715
  pediatric assessments, 830t
  post-traumatic assessment of, 687
penetrating trauma. *See also* traumatic injuries
  abdominal, 548
  firearm injuries, 674–675
  knife wounds, 674
  renal, 473–474
penicillin G, 836t
pentamidine isethionate, 642
pentobarbital, 396t
Pepcid. *See* famotidine
pepsinogen, 532
percussion
  of abdomen, 534
  definition of, 46
  pulmonary function assessments, 46–47
percutaneous liver biopsy, 536t
pericardial rubs, 602
pericardial tamponade, 705t
pericardiocentesis, 322, 686
pericarditis
  etiology of, 322
  management of, 323

pathophysiology of, 322
  signs and symptoms of, 323
  uremic, 462
pericardium, 147
perikaryon, 351
perimembranous ventricular septal defect, 258
perineum, burns of, 810
periodic breathing, 853
periorbital hematomas, 721
peripheral blood lymphocyte phenotype, 638
peripheral blood vessel physiology, 153–154
peripheral chemoreceptors, 41, 805
peripheral cyanosis, 166
peripheral nervous system
  developmental anatomy of, 362–365
  physiology of, 365–368
peripheral pulse, 168, 853
peripheral vascular resistance, 155–156, 453–454, 453f
peritoneal dialysis (PD), 468–469
peritonitis, 469, 556
periventricular hemorrhage, 413, 415
permissive hypercarbia, 128
person approach versus system approach, 886, 887
personal protective equipment (PPE), 875
personality development, 4, 5
pertussis
  clinical presentation of, 83
  definition of, 83
  outcomes of, 84
  pathophysiology of, 83
  patient care management, 83–84
PFA-100, 607
PFIB, 833t
PFT. *See* pulmonary function testing
PGCS. *See* Pediatric Glasgow Coma Score
PH. *See* pulmonary hypertension
phagocyte dysfunction disorders, 636–637
phagocytosis, 592
pharmacologic paralysis, 15
pharynx
  anatomy of, 37, 37f
  embryology of, 36
phencyclidine, 739t
phenobarbital, 398, 399t, 408
phentolamine, 200
phenylephrine hydrochloride (Neo-Synephrine), 191–192
phenytoin, 398, 403
pheochromocytoma, 503
phlebostatic axis, 182, 184f
phosgene, 833t
phosphate, 452
phosphodiesterase inhibitors, 108, 230
phosphodiesterase type 5 (PDE-5), 68, 206

photic stimulation, during electroencephalography, 386
physeal fractures, 712, 712t
physical restraints, 9
physician communication style, 902
physiologic dead space, 118t
physiologic hypogammaglobulinemia, 598
physostigmine, 748
phytonadione, 537
pia mater, 352, 357
PICU. *See* pediatric intensive care unit
pilocarpine lontophoresis, 52t
pineal-region tumors, 420
Pitressin. *See* vasopressin
pituicytes, 486
pituitary gland, 487f
  cells of, 486
  characteristics of, 486
    embryology of, 484, 485
    hormones produced by, 480t, 481t, 488–489, 488f
  lobes of, 486
  location of, 487f
  posterior
    characteristics of, 486
    embryology of, 484, 485
    hormones produced by, 481t, 491–492
placing reflex, 372
plague, 837–839, 838t
plan–do–study–act (PDSA) cycles, 894, 898–899
plasma clotting factor disorder, 647–649
plasma factors
  description of, 590
  functions of, 599–600
plasma protein factors, 619t
plasmapheresis, 104
plasmin, 615
plasminogen, 590
platelet(s)
  description of, 589
  function of, 598
  hemostatic response of, 598, 598f, 606
  human leukocyte antigen-matched, 616
  indications for, 589
  medications that affect, 599
  physiologic conditions that affect, 598–599
  suppressive agents for, 614
  transfusion of, 617t, 643–644, 646
platelet-activating factor, 430, 777
platelet count, 599, 606
platelet function tests, 607
play facilitation, 19–20
pluripotent hematopoietic stem cells, 585
pneumatic antishock garment (PASG), 691
pneumatic sensor, 388
pneumococcal vaccination, 107

Pneumocystis carinii pneumonia
  characteristics of, 641
  diagnostic findings, 640
  pentamidine isethionate, 642
  prophylaxis, 641–642
  signs and symptoms of, 641
  transmission of, 641
  treatment of, 642
  trimethoprim-sulfamethoxazole
      for, 641
  ventilator-associated, 128, 131
  zidovudine for, 610
pneumonia
  bronchopneumonia, 81
  clinical presentation of, 81–82
  definition and etiology of, 81
  interstitial, 81
  lobar, 81
  outcomes of, 83
  pathophysiology of, 81
  patient care management, 82–83
pneumonitis
  interstitial, 659
  mechanical ventilation requirements
      for, 123t
pneumothorax, 100, 109f
  closed, 705t
  open, 109, 110, 705t
  radiographic evaluation of, 111t
  tension, 109f
      clinical presentation of, 111, 705t
      description of, 109, 110
      management of, 705t
      radiographic evaluation of, 111t
point of maximal impulse (PMI), 106, 167
Poiseuille's law, 39
poison center, 734–735
poison exposures
  acute, 734
  antidotes, 742–743
  chronic, 734
  common types of, 736t
  definition of, 734
  epidemiology of, 735
  eyes, 740
  gastrointestinal tract, 741
  history-taking, 737–738
  in infants, 735–736
  management of
      absorption prevention, 740
      activated charcoal, 742
      assessment, 738–740
      cathartics, 742
      elimination enhancements, 742
      interventions, 740–742
      ipecac syrup, 740
  prevention of, 744
  risk factors for, 735–737
  routes of, 734
  skin, 740
      toxidromes, 739t
poisoning
  acetaminophen, 743t, 744–746
  of adolescents, 737

anesthetics, 746
antidepressants, 746–749
benzodiazepines, 749–750
calcium-channel blockers,
    750–751
carbon monoxide, 743t, 758–759
caustic substances, 759–761
cyanide, 761–763
diphenoxylate-atropine
    combination, 752
envenomations, 763–764
ethanol, 764
ethylene glycol, 764–765
hydrocarbons, 766–767
imidazoline derivatives, 752
of infants, 735–736
iron, 743t, 752–754
methanol, 765–766
mushrooms, 767–768
oral hypoglycemic agents, 752
organophosphate insecticides,
    768–769
overdose versus, 734
psychosocial considerations, 769
salicylate, 754–755
of school-age children, 737
of toddlers, 736–737
topical anesthetics, 746
polyethylene glycol 3350, 541
polyethylene glycol-electrolyte
    solution, 541
polymorphonuclear neutrophils
    (PMNs), 587
polysomnography (PSG), 103
polysynaptic reflex arc, 359
polytrauma, adult and pediatric
    physiologic response, 667, 668t
pons, 40, 355
portal hypertension, 573
portal venous system, 533
portosystemic shunting, 573
positive end-expiratory pressure
  auto-PEEP, 129
      definition of, 120
          functional residual capacity
              affected by, 120f
          mechanical ventilation
              requirements for, 123t
positive expiratoy pressure, 70t
positive-pressure ventilation
  controls, 121–122
  definition of, 120
  flow delivery, 122
  mechanics of, 121f
  modes of, 120–121
  noninvasive, 126
  phase variables for, 122–123
  sensing mechanisms, 122
postcentral gyrus, 354f
posterior cervical chain lymph
    nodes, 587f
posterior cord syndrome, 429
posterior descending artery, 150
posterior fontanelle, 352, 352f, 369

posterior pituitary gland
  characteristics of, 486
  embryology of, 484, 485
  hormones produced by, 481t,
      491–492
posterior pituitary hormones, 491–492
postoperative craniotomy, 422
postrenal failure, 459
postresuscitation care, 214–216, 215f
postsynaptic membrane, 360
posttransplantation lymphoproliferative
    disease, 139
posttraumatic atelectasis, 110
postventricular atrial refractory
    period, 246
potassium, 477
  description of, 451–452
  replacement therapy, 511
potassium iodide, 831, 832t
potassium-sparing diuretics, 464
PPE. *See* personal protective equipment
PR interval, 174–175, 174f
pralidoxime, 768–769
prayer, 22–23
PRBCs. *See* packed red blood cells
preacinar arteries, 38–39
preauricular lymph nodes, 587f
precentral gyrus, 354f
precordium
  inspection of, 166–167
  palpation of, 167–168
prednisone, 541–542
preganglionic fibers, 363–365
preload
  definition of, 155–156
  maintenance of, 254
premature newborns
  lung development in, 35
  persistent ductus arteriosus in, 253
  surfactant therapy for, 67–68
premature ventricular contractions,
    240, 241f
prerenal azotemia, 571
prerenal failure, 463
preschoolers. *See also* children
  cognitive development in, 4
  communication by, 17
  cough in, 50t
  death, concept of, 4
  fear responses by, 8
  hospitalization response of, 7
  pain assessment and management,
      12t, 13t
  personality development in, 4
  play with, 20
  principles for working with, 6
  psychosocial development of, 4
  stress response of, 7
  traumatic injuries in, 671t
prescription agents, 600
preserved ejection fraction HF
    (HFpEF), 229
pressoreceptors, 451
pressure cycle, 122

pressure injury prevention, 898
pressure injury reduction project, 895
  cause-and-effect, 896, 896f
  intervention planning for, 898
  key driver diagram for, 897, 897f
  measure changes over time, 899
  measures for, 894, 895, 898, 899
  Pareto chart for, 896, 896f
  plan–do–study–act cycle for, 898–899
pressure manometers, 55
pressure sensors, 122
pressure sores, 820
pressure support ventilation, 120, 131
presynaptic axon, 351
presynaptic membrane action
        potential, 360
pretransplant management, 638
PRF. *See* prolactin-releasing factor
priapism, 631t, 636
Prilosec. *See* omeprazole
primary lymphocytic tissue, 585
primary myopathy, 309
privacy
  confidentiality and, 27
  lack of, 10
procainamide (Pronestyl), 193–194
Procardia. *See* nifedipine
procedural pain, 817
process-flow map, 896
process measures, 894, 898
procoagulants, 590, 599
proerythroblasts, 585
professional quality of life (ProQOL),
        919–920
progesterone, 482t
progressive familial intrahepatic
        cholestasis, 574
proinflammatory mediators, 776–777
prokinetic agents, 540
prolactin, 480t, 490–491
prolactin inhibitory hormone, 487
prolactin-releasing factor (PRF), 487
Pronestyl. *See* procainamide
propafenone (Rythmol), 194
prophylaxis, 641–642
propofol, 59t, 64–66, 396t
propoxyphene, 754
propranolol, 194–195, 286
proprioception testing, 372–373
ProQOL. *See* professional quality of life
prosencephalon, 350, 350f
prostacyclin, 108, 454
prostaglandin E1 (PGE1), 152, 208, 869
prostaglandin E2 (PGE2), 454
prostaglandins, 108, 454
prostanoids, 205–206
Prostin. *See* prostaglandin E1 (PGE1)
protease inhibitors, 641
protein binding, 57
protein C, 590, 781
protein metabolism, 498
protein S, 590
proteolysis, 498
prothrombin time (PT), 535t, 554, 572, 606

proton-pump inhibitors, 538
Protonix. *See* pantoprazole
proximal tubule
  anatomy of, 446, 447f
  potassium reabsorption in, 451
  tubular reabsorption, 449
pruritus, 573
PS. *See* pulmonary stenosis
PSOM. *See* pediatric stroke outcome
        measure
PSOs. *See* patient safety organizations
psychological capital, 919
psychological stress, 7–8
psychosocial development, 4
psychosocial support, 20–21, 29
PT. *See* prothrombin time
PtcO₂. *See* transcutaneous carbon
        dioxide monitoring
PTH. *See* parathyroid hormone
PTHrP. *See* parathyroid hormone-
        related protein
PTS. *See* pediatric trauma score
Pulmicort. *See* budesonide
pulmonary angiography
  cardiovascular system
        evaluations, 180
  pulmonary function evaluations, 53
pulmonary arterial hypertension
        (PAH), 105t, 186, 186f, 205–207
pulmonary artery (PA), 184, 186
pulmonary artery pressure (PAP), 40,
        105, 181, 337
pulmonary artery wedge pressure
        (PAWP) monitoring, 184, 186
pulmonary atresia
  intact ventricular septum
        complications, 291
    definition of, 290
    diagnostic test for, 290–291
    incidence of, 290
    pathophysiology of, 290
    patient management, 291
    signs and symptoms, 290
  with ventricular septal defect
    anatomy of, 287
    complications, 290
    diagnostic test, 289–290
    incidence of, 287–288
    pathophysiology of, 288–289
    patient management, 290
    signs and symptoms, 289
pulmonary blood flow, 40, 288, 290, 868
pulmonary capillary wedge pressure
        (PCWP), 186, 283
pulmonary circulation
  description of, 38–39
  postnatal changes in, 39–40
pulmonary compliance, 39, 39f
pulmonary contusions, 110, 705t
pulmonary edema, 91–92
  acute respiratory failure caused
        by, 75
  mechanical ventilation requirements
        for, 123t

pulmonary embolism (PE),
        90–91
pulmonary fibrosis, 123t
pulmonary function
  assessment of, 43–50, 118, 209
  diagnostic studies for, 50–53,
        55–56
  history-taking, 43
  laboratory evaluation of,
        51t–52t
  physical examination
    abnormal findings, 48–50
    auscultation, 47–48
    inspection, 44–45
    palpation, 45, 46
    percussion, 46–47, 47f
  radiologic procedures for
        evaluating, 53
pulmonary function testing (PFT),
        55–56, 56f, 98
pulmonary hemorrhage, 103–104
pulmonary hemosiderosis, 103
pulmonary hypertension (PH)
  cardiac catheterization evaluation,
        106–107
  classification of, 105, 105t–106t
  clinical presentation, 105–107
  definition, 105
  endothelial dysfunction in, 105
  etiology of, 104–105
  management of, 107–108
  mortality rates, 104, 108
  outcomes, 108
  pathophysiology of, 105
  primary, 136–137
  prognosis for, 108
  prostacyclin for, 108
  vasoconstriction, 105
  ventilation–perfusion mismatching
        in, 107
pulmonary infarction, 90
pulmonary intoxicants, 832
pulmonary pressure, intravascular, 40
pulmonary stenosis (PS)
  anatomy of, 284f, 285
  balloon valvuloplasty for,
        285, 285f
  complications, 285
  definition of, 284
  diagnostic tests for, 284–285
  double-outlet right ventricle
        and, 260
  incidence of, 284
  interventions for, 285, 285f
  management, 285
  pathophysiology of, 284
  signs and symptoms, 284
  supravalvular, 286f
  types of, 284f
  valvulotomy for, 285, 286f
pulmonary valve, 153f, 284,
        290, 297
pulmonary vascular obstructive disease
        (PVOD), 227

pulmonary vascular resistance (PVR), 151, 186
  definition of, 39–40, 119
  in persistent ductus arteriosus, 251
pulmonary vasoconstriction, 40
pulmonary vasodilators, 230
pulmonary veins, 294, 295
pulmonary venous engorgement, 227
pulmonic area, 167f, 168, 171
pulsatile ventricular assist device, 218, 222
pulse, 380, 853
pulse check, 113, 212
pulse oximetry
  limitations of, 53–54
  oxygen monitoring using, 54
  post-traumatic assessment of, 688
  principles of, 53
pulse pressure, 157
pulseless electrical activity (PEA), 678, 686
pulsus alternans, 168
pulsus paradoxus, 169
pupillary response, 854
Purkinje system, 158
PVOD. *See* pulmonary vascular obstructive disease
PVR. *See* pulmonary vascular resistance

QI. *See* quality improvement
QRS interval, 174–175, 175f
QSEN. *See* Quality and Safety Education for Nurses
QT interval, 174–175
quadriplegia, 429
Quality and Safety Education for Nurses (QSEN), 909–910
quality improvement (QI), 894–899, 895t, 910–913
  balancing measures, 895, 898
  definition of, 908
  EBP versus, 908, 909
  error-based metrics for, 911
  Essentials Toolkit, 889, 898
  family-centered care, 906
  generalizability, 909
  injury-based metrics for, 910
  IRB oversight, 908–909
  model for, 895f
  nurse reporting, importance of, 911
  outcome measures, 894, 898
  plan–do–study–act cycle, 894, 898–899
  process measures, 894, 898
  research versus, 908, 909, 909t
  rewarding outcomes, 913
  risk-based metrics for, 911
  risk minimization, 908
  scope and planning, 894
  structure, process, and outcome model, 910
  systems-level thinking, 911, 912f
  tracking data, 912–913

"raccoon eyes," 425, 687, 699
racemic epinephrine, 864t
radial artery cannulation, 214f
radiant burns, 676
radiation injuries, 795t
radiation therapy, 421
radiofrequency ablation, 182, 241, 318
radiographs, 381
  chest. *See* chest radiographs
  congenital neurologic abnormalities, 437
  skull, 426
radioisotope scan, 384
radiologic attacks, 830–832
radiologic dispersal device, 831
radionucleotide renal scan, 474
radionuclide studies, 555
radionuclide ventriculography, 318
rales, 209
ranitidine, 538
RAP. *See* right atrial pressure
Rapamune. *See* sirolimus
rape, 725
rapid sequence intubation, 689, 857, 858f
Rastelli operation, 298, 299f
Rathke's pouch, 484
RBF. *See* renal blood flow
RCA. *See* right coronary artery
reactive airway disease, 132
recombinant factor VIII concentrate, 648–649
recombinant factor IX concentrate, 648–649
recreational substances, 757t–758t
rectal examination, 687
rectal temperature, 867t
recurrent bacterial infections, 642
red blood cell count, 602
red blood cells (RBCs), 354. *See also* white blood cells; specific cells
  administration of, 620
  burn accident effects on, 803
  description of, 587
  function of, 591
  mature, 587
  packed, 619t
  sickle cell disease. *See* sickle cell disease
  transfusion of, 620, 621–622
red marrow, 585
reduced ejection fraction heart failure (HFrEF), 229–230
reentry, 235, 237
reexpansion pulmonary edema, 91
reflex arc, 359, 359f
reflexes
  deep tendon, 372
  primitive, 371–372
  superficial, 372
refractory status epilepticus (RSE), 403
refreezing, 912
Reglan. *See* metoclopramide
rehabilitation, 820–821

relative refractory period, 160
remedial agents, 65–67, 65t–66t
renal blood flow (RBF)
  glomerular filtration rate and, 448
  regulation of, 454
renal disorders, 368
renal failure, 468
  acute. *See* acute renal failure
  anemia associated with, 462
  prevention of, 468
renal fascia, 445
renal function, 216, 459, 464, 467, 765
renal replacement therapies
  continuous
    anticoagulation during, 471–472
    filtration capability measurements, 471
    fluid balance during, 472
    hemodynamic stability during, 472
    indications for, 470
    nursing implications, 471–472
    process used in, 470–471
  hemodialysis, 469–470
  peritoneal dialysis, 468–469
renal transplantation, 473
renal trauma, 473–474
renal ultrasound with Doppler (RUS), 454, 455
renin–angiotensin–aldosterone system, 225, 227, 453, 453f
  captopril effects on, 201
  description of, 157, 779
reperfusion pulmonary edema, 91
repolarization, 160, 360
rescue breathing, 211
research, quality improvement versus, 908, 909, 909t
residual volume, 41, 42f
respiration. *See also* breathing
  assessment of, 42–43, 379–380
  ataxic, 46f, 380
  Cheyne–Stokes, 380
  patterns, 379–380
respiratory acidosis, 463t
respiratory alkalosis, 463t, 781
respiratory burst, 592
respiratory clearance exercises, 224
respiratory cyanosis, 166
respiratory decompensation, 209
respiratory disease, 72, 102
respiratory distress syndrome (RDS). *See also* pediatric acute respiratory distress syndrome
  adjunctive therapies for, 865–866
  aerosolized medications for, 864
  bronchopulmonary dysplasia and, 114
  mechanical ventilation requirements for, 123t
  oxygen delivery for, 864
respiratory emergency, 112–113

respiratory failure, 112–113
  assessment of, 209
  etiology of, 209
respiratory frequency, 118t
respiratory insufficiency, 48t
respiratory monitoring, 50–51
respiratory muscle, 131, 133
  paralysis of, 763, 768
  strength training, 70t
respiratory pattern, 853
respiratory rate, 125, 852
respiratory reflex, 155
respiratory syncytial virus (RSV), 875
respiratory system, 642. *See also*
    breathing
  anatomy of, 35–39
  human immunodeficiency virus
    effects on, 642
  pharmacologic considerations, 56–69
  physiology of, 39–43
  post-trauma assessments, 686
  postnatal development of, 35, 36t
  symptoms of concern, 601t
resting membrane potential (RMP),
    159, 359
restraints, 9
restrictive airways disease, 55
restrictive cardiomyopathy (RCM)
  complications, 316
  diagnostic evaluation, 315
  etiology of, 314
  pathophysiology of, 314
  phenotypic expression, 314–315
  treatment for, 315–316
resuscitation, 211
  fluid. *See* fluid resuscitation
  and moral distress, 917–918
  neonatal, 214
  postresuscitation care, 214–216, 215f
  in septic shock, 784
  trauma, 679
resynchronization therapy, 314
reticular formation, 355-356
reticulocyte(s)
  in children, 603t
  description of, 587
  in infants, 603t
reticulocyte count, 602
reverse transcriptase inhibitors, 641
revised trauma score (RTS), 688
Rh system, 607
rhabdomyolysis, 467–468, 468t, 716–717
rheumatic fever, 325, 326t
rhinorrhea, 425
Rh$_o$(D), 646
rhombencephalon, 350, 350f
rhythm, 230
  check, 212
  sinus, 236f
rhythmicity, 158–159
rib fractures
  chest injury associated with, 683t
  clinical presentation of, 111, 705t
  description of, 108–109

management of, 705t
  radiographic evaluation of, 111t
rickets, 573
right atrial pressure (RAP), 186
right atrium, 296f
right bundle branch (RBB), 150, 158
right bundle branch block (RBBB), 244
right coronary artery (RCA), 150
right-sided heart failure (right HF), 225,
    226–227
right-to-left shunt, 276, 277
right ventricle, double-outlet,
    259–261, 261f
right ventricular end-diastolic pressure
    (RVEDP), 189
right ventricular hypertrophy
    (RVH), 167
right ventricular outflow tract
    obstruction (RVOTO), 287
Ringer's lactate, 807
risk-based QI metrics, 911
rivaroxaban, 205
robust process improvement, 893
rocuronium, 58t, 689
role confusion, identity versus, 4–5
Romano-Ward syndrome, 165t
Romazicon. *See* flumazenil
rooting reflex, 371–372
Ross–Konno procedure, 272, 273f
rounding processes
  family-centered, 907
  interdisciplinary, 904
RSV. *See* respiratory syncytial virus
RTS. *See* revised trauma score
RUS. *See* renal ultrasound with Doppler
RVEDP. *See* right ventricular end-
    diastolic pressure
RVOTO. *See* right ventricular outflow
    tract obstruction
Rythmol. *See* propafenone

SA node. *See* sinoatrial (SA) node
saccular aneurysm, 411
safety culture, in healthcare, 886–892
  aviation industry, 892–893
  error reduction strategies, 889
  event reporting and huddles, 890
  healthcare quality domains, 892, 892f
  just culture principles, 887, 888f, 889
  new frontier, 890–892
  person approach versus system
    approach, 886, 887
  Swiss cheese model, 889
Safety II approach, 890–892
sagittal suture, 352f
salicylate poisoning, 754–755
saliva, 531, 591
salivary cortisol testing, 507
salivary glands, 531
saltatory syndrome, 414
Salter–Harris classification, 712, 712f
salvia (*Salvia divinorum*), 757t
sano operation, 303

sarcolemma, 147
sarcomeres, 156, 159, 312
SBAR (Situation-Background-
    Assessment-Recommendation),
    903, 903f
scald burns, child abuse and, 722
scalp, 352
scar management techniques, 813, 814t
SCD. *See* sickle cell disease
school-age children. *See also* adolescents;
    children
  cognitive development in, 4
  communication by, 17
  cough in, 50t
  death, concept of, 4
  developmental stages of, 4
  fear responses by, 8
  hospitalization response of, 7
  pain assessment and management,
    12t, 13t
  personality development in, 4
  play with, 20
  poisoning of, 737
  principles for working with, 6
  psychosocial development in, 4
  stress response of, 7, 8
  traumatic injuries in, 672t
SCID. *See* severe combined
    immunodeficiency disorder
scoliosis
  clinical presentation of, 434–435
  etiology of, 433–434
  outcomes of, 436
  pathophysiology of, 434
  patient care management, 435–436
SCUF. *See* slow continuous
    ultrafiltration
SDAC. *See* single doses of activated
    charcoal
second-degree burns, 803f
second-degree Mobitz type I, 870
second-victim phenomenon, 920–921
secondary lymphoid tissue, 585
secondary nephrotic syndrome, 465
secondary trauma syndrome (STS), 919
sedation
  in children, 395, 396t
  communication during, 18
  extracorporeal membrane
    oxygenation, 218, 219
  management of, 221, 223
  for mechanical ventilation, 130
  pain management using, 817
  remedial agents for, 65–67, 65t–66t
sedatives
  description of, 58
  indications for, 58
  nursing considerations for, 63
  overdose of, 739t
  pain management using, 14, 16t
  types of, 59t–62t
seizures
  absence, 404
  alternative therapies, 407

seizures (*cont.*)
  anticonvulsant medications for, 398, 399t
  barbiturate-induced coma for, 403, 407
  benzodiazepines, 398, 399t
  classification of, 404
  definition of, 403
  diagnostic tests, 405–406, 406t
  direct care, 407
  etiology of, 404
  focal, 404
  general anesthesia for, 407
  generalized, 404
  generalized tonic-clonic, 405
  ictal period, 405
  incidence of, 403
  management of, 398, 399t, 406–408
  myoclonic, 404
  outcomes, 408
  pathophysiology of, 404–405
  physical examination, 405
  postictal period, 405
  preventive care, 406–407
  prodromal (preictal) period, 405
  risk factors for, 404
  second phase of therapy, 398, 399t
  supportive care, 407–408
  systemic effects of, 404–405
  third-phase therapy, 398
  tonic, 404
self-care and wellness promotion
  barriers to, 915
  health-promoting behaviors, 913, 915
  night shift challenges, 916
  workplace stress, 915
sella turcica tumors, 420
semilunar valves, 148t
Sengstaken–Blakemore tube, 556
sensorimotor stage, 4
sensory deprivation
  description of, 10
  interventions for, 19
sensory function assessments, 372–373
sensory overload
  description of, 9–10
  interventions for, 19
sentinel events, 901–902
separation anxiety, 8
sepsis
  burn wound, 816, 821
  definition of, 774
  pathogenesis of, 777f
  severe, 774, 781
septic shock, 232
  after burns, 821–822
  afterload in, 787
  arterial blood gases in, 781
  auscultation, 780–781
  blood cultures for, 782
  blood volume maldistribution associated with, 776–777
  cardiac dysfunction in, 780
  cardiac output in, 787

cerebrospinal fluid evaluations, 782
clinical manifestations of, 783, 783t, 821–822
compensatory responses to, 779
complications in iatrogenic, 788
contractility in, 787
defenses against, 776
definition of, 774, 776, 783, 819
developmental anatomy and physiology, 776
diagnoses associated with, 781
diagnostic studies for, 781–782
epidemiology of, 775–776
etiology of, 774–775
factors that affect, 775–776
gram-negative, 776
heart rate in, 787
hemodynamic support, 785f
history-taking, 779–780
incidence of, 775
invasive hemodynamic monitoring, 782
laboratory findings, 781–782
management of
  antibiotics, 784, 819
  cardiovascular, 787
  fluid resuscitation, 784, 822
  nutritional support, 789
  overview of, 783–784, 822
  pediatric advanced life support program, 784
  respiratory, 787–788
  resuscitation, 784, 786-787
  vasoactive agents, 784, 786t
mediators associated with, 776–778
multiple-organ dysfunction syndrome, 789
nursing examination, 780
oxygen extraction in, 42–43
oxygen supply and demand imbalance in, 779
palpations, 780–781
pathophysiology of, 776–779
patient outcomes, 783–784
phases of, 783, 783t
risk factors for, 775–776
stages of, 783
supportive therapies, 788–789
systemic inflammatory response syndrome, 625, 776, 777f
tissue oxygenation in, 787–788
urine specimen evaluations, 782
vasoactive agents, 784, 786–787, 786t
white blood cell count in, 781
Septra. *See* trimethoprim–sulfamethoxazole
sequential compression devices, 718
serious safety events (SSE), 900
serotonin syndrome, 748
serotonin uptake inhibitors, 748–749
serotonin–norepinephrine reuptake inhibitors (SNRIs), 749
serum calcitonin, 495
serum osmolality, 510

"setting-sun" sign, 369, 401, 423
severe combined immunodeficiency disorder (SCID), 637–638
sex hormones, 481t
sexual abuse, 725–726
sexual assault, 725
shaken impact syndrome, 723
shear injury, 674
sheet grafts, 811
shock
  anaphylactic, 232
  cardiogenic, 232, 778
  compensated, 231
  compensatory phase, 233, 233f
  complications, 235
  decompensated, 231
  definition of, 231
  diagnostic evaluation, 234
  distributive, 232–233, 777
  etiology of, 231–233
  goals for, 234–235
  hypodynamic, 783
  hypovolemic, 232, 707
  management of, 215f, 234–235
  mechanical ventilation for, 234
  neurogenic, 232–233
  obstructive, 233
  pathophysiology of, 231–233
  refractory phase, 234
  septic. *See* septic shock
  signs and symptoms, 233–234
  uncompensated phase, 233, 234
short-acting vasodilators, 787
short gut syndrome, 576
shunt
  bidirectional cavopulmonary, 305, 305f–306f
  modified Blalock–Taussig, 287, 288f
  right-to-left, 276, 277
  ventricular, 393–395, 393f, 395f
  ventriculoperitoneal, 395f
SIADH. *See* syndrome of inappropriate antidiuretic hormone
siblings
  of dying child, 29
  working with, 24
sick sinus syndrome (SSS), 237
sickle cell anemia, 631t
sickle cell disease (SCD)
  clinical manifestations of, 630, 631t
  complications of
    acute chest syndrome, 633–634
    aplastic crisis, 633
    bone marrow necrosis, 635
    cerebrovascular accident, 635
    fat embolism, 635
    infections, 632–633
    multi-organ system failure, 635–636
    priapism, 636
    splenic sequestration crisis, 633
    vaso-occlusive crisis, 634–635
  corticosteroids for, 637
  definition, 629
  etiology, 629–630

sickle cell disease (SCD) (*cont.*)
   management of, 633
   pain management in, 634–635
   pathophysiology, 630
   patient-controlled analgesia for, 631
   prevention of, 632
   risk factors for, 630
   transfusion of, 630, 634
   types of, 628t, 630
SIDS. *See* sudden infant death
   syndrome
sieving coefficient, 471
sildenafil, 68, 206
silent syndrome, 414
silver nitrate solution, 813t
silver sulfadiazine, 813t
simple radiological device (SRD), 831
single doses of activated charcoal
   (SDAC), 741–742
single ventricular variants
   complications, 308
   definition of, 307
   diagnostic evaluation, 307
   incidence of, 307
   pathophysiology of, 307
   patient management, 307–308
   signs and symptoms, 307
sinoatrial (SA) node
   autonomic nerve stimulation effects
     on, 367t
   conduction disorders, 236–237
   description of, 157, 158f
sinus arrhythmia, 235, 236, 236f
sinus bradycardia, 236f, 237
sinus pause, 236–237, 236f
sinus tachycardia, 236, 236f
sinus venosum, 254
sirolimus, 612
SIRS. *See* systemic inflammatory
   response syndrome
situation monitoring, TeamSTEPPS
   model, 905, 906f
SJS. *See* Stevens-Johnson syndrome
SjVO₂ monitoring. *See* jugular
   venous oxygen saturation
   monitoring
skin
   anthrax effects on, 834, 836t
   assessment of, 162, 166, 853
   autonomic nerve stimulation effects
     on, 367t
   color of, 162, 853
   hydrofluoric acid absorption, 761
   palpation of, 780
   poison exposure, 740
   symptoms of concern, 601t
   temperature of, 867t
skin-prick testing, 98
skull
   anatomy of, 352
   auscultation of, 369
   examination of, 369
   fractures of, 424
   inspection of, 369

skull radiographs
   description of, 381
   traumatic brain injury
     evaluations, 426
sleep, ANA recommendations for, 915
sleep deprivation
   description of, 10, 10t
   interventions for, 19
sleep study, with PH patients, 107
sleeping habits, 44
slow continuous ultrafiltration
   (SCUF), 471
small intestine
   anatomy of, 532
   injuries to, 553
small-volume nebulizer, 864–865
smallpox, 836–837, 837f, 838t
smoke-inhalation injury, 95–96, 805
snake venom, 763
SNRIs. *See* serotonin–norepinephrine
   reuptake inhibitors
sodium, 447
   active transport of, 450
   aldosterone effects on, 450–451
   balance of, 452
   levels of, 452
   reabsorption, 449, 451
   in syndrome of inappropriate
     antidiuretic hormone, 520
sodium bicarbonate, 107, 213, 511,
   747, 869
sodium nitrite, 762–763
sodium nitroprusside, 787
sodium polystyrene sulfonate, 460
Solu-Medrol. *See* methylprednisolone
Solutions for Patient Safety (SPS),
   900, 901t
somatosensory-evoked response
   (SSER), 387
somatostatin, 482t, 487, 499
somatotrophs, 486, 488
somatotropic hormone, 480t
sorbitol, 742
sotalol, 195–196
space-occupying lesions
   brain tumors, classification of, 419
   chemotherapy, 421
   clinical presentation of, 420–421
   definition and etiology of, 419
   outcomes of, 422
   pathophysiology of, 419
   patient care management, 421–422
   radiation therapy, 421
   targeted therapy, 421
specific acquired immunity, 594, 595f
sphenoidal sinus, 36
spica casting, 714
spider bites, 763
spina bifida cystica, 436–437
spina bifida occulta, 437
spinal accessory nerve
   in children, 379t
   function of, 364t
   in infants, 375t

spinal canal decompression, 432
spinal column
   anatomy of, 356, 357f
   circulation, 359
   vertebrae, 356, 357f
spinal cord. *See also* central nervous
   system
   anatomy, 357
   compression, 653
   concussion of, 430
   contusion of, 430
   coverings of, 357
   cross section, 358f
   development of, 350
   hemorrhage, 430
   transection, 430
spinal cord injury
   autonomic dysreflexia secondary
     to, 430
   complete, 429
   deep vein thrombosis, 433
   defining characteristics of, 429
   description of, 429
   etiology of, 429–430
   immobilization after, 432, 702
   incidence of, 429
   incomplete, 429
   mechanical ventilation requirements
     for, 123t
   neurodiagnostic studies for,
     432–433
   neurological level of injury, 431
   partial, 700, 701–703
   pathophysiology of, 430
   spinal stabilization after, 432
   transection of, 430
   without radiographic abnormality,
     429, 701–702
spinal dysraphism, 436
spinal fusion, 433–436
spinal muscular atrophy, 123t
spinal nerves, 362–363
spinal shock, 430–431
spinal tracts, 357, 358t
spine
   cervical
     immobilization of, 689, 702
     post-trauma assessments, 681, 689
   curvatures of, 433
   radiographs of, 381
spirituality, 22–23
spirometry, 55, 98
spironolactone, 208, 464
splanchnic circulation, 533
spleen
   humoral immunity and, 585
   injuries to, 550–551, 550t, 551t
   palpation of, 602
splenectomy, 550, 646
splenic sequestration, 599, 631t, 633
splenomegaly, 574
splenorrhaphy, 550
split-thickness grafts, 811
SPS. *See* Solutions for Patient Safety

sputum culture, description of, 52t
SSE. *See* serious safety events
SSER. *See* somatosensory-evoked response
SSIs. *See* surgical site infections
SSS. *See* sick sinus syndrome
ST segment, 174
stab wounds, 680, 874
stabilization of patient
  airway
    assessment of, 850, 852
    endotracheal intubation, 856t, 857
    laryngeal mask, 856–857, 856t
    management of, 855–857
    nasopharyngeal, 855, 856t
    oropharyngeal, 689, 855, 856, 856t
  assessments
    airway, 850, 852
    breathing, 852–853
    circulation, 853–854
    gastrointestinal, 854, 855
    neurologic, 854
  cardiac patient population, 868–871
  extracorporeal membrane oxygenation transport, 872–874
  fluid resuscitation, 858–860
  glucose, 860–863
  hypoglycemia, 860–862
  hypoxic ischemic encephalopathy, 871–872
  infectious disease, 875–876
  initial call and triage, 850, 852t
  management of, 855–857
  mechanical ventilation, 866–867
  nonaccidental trauma, 874–875
  principles and practice, 850
  respiratory care, 863–867
  telemedicine, 876
  transport metrics, 876–878, 877t–878t
  transport population, 850
  vascular access, 857
  vasoactive drug support, 860, 861f
stagnant hypoxia, 847
Staphylococcus species, 774–775
static compliance, 56
statistical process control, 899
status asthmaticus, 99–100
status epilepticus, 380, 405
  anticonvulsants for, 407
  definition of, 380, 403
stem cell(s)
  cell differentiation from, 586f
  committed, 585
  pluripotent, 585
  transplantation. *See* hematopoietic stem cell transplantation
sternoclavicular area, 167f
sternotomy, 258
Stevens-Johnson syndrome (SJS), 813
  nutritional requirements, 815
  special care areas, 815
  treatment of, 815
  wound-care goals, 815

stomach
  anatomy of, 532
  injuries to, 553
Streptococcus pneumoniae, 551, 634
streptokinase, 615
stress
  on family, 21–22
  financial, 23
  nervous system response to, 6
  on parents, 21–22
  physiologic response to, 6
  psychological, 7–8
  reduction, 915
  sources of, 21
  transport-related, 847
  workplace, 915
stress-dose steroids, 788–789
stress responses
  by adolescents, 7–8
  by families, 21–23
  by infant, 7
  by parents, 21–23
  by preschooler, 7
  by school-age child, 7
  by toddler, 7
stress testing, 176–177
stretch receptors, 154, 155, 779
stridor
  evaluation of, 48t, 49
  expiratory, 49
  infectious causes of, 76t
  inspiratory, 48
  upper-airway obstruction and, 209
stroke. *See also* acute ischemic stroke; hemorrhagic stroke
  definition of, 408
  heat, 677
  measurement of, 181t
stroke volume (SV), 155
STS. *See* secondary trauma syndrome
stupor, 370
subaortic stenosis, 274–275, 275f, 292f
subarachnoid bolts, 388–389
subdural catheters, 389
subdural hematoma, 425, 426
sublingual glands, 531
submandibular glands, 531
submaxillary lymph nodes, 587f
submental lymph nodes, 587f
submersion injury, 678–679
subthalamus, 355
successful handoffs, 902–903
succinylcholine, 58t, 689
sucralfate, 539
sudden cardiac arrest, 210
sudden infant death syndrome (SIDS), 96, 728
sulfonamide diuretics, 464
sulfonylureas, 743t
sulfur mustard, 833t
superficial cervical lymph nodes, 587f
superior mediastinal syndrome, 652–653
superior vena cava (SVC), 151

suppressor T cells, 589
supraclavicular lymph nodes, 587f
supraoptic nuclei, 486
suprasternal notch, 168
supratentorial herniation, 400
supratentorial tumors, 420
supravalvular aortic stenosis, 274–275, 276f, 285, 286f
supraventricular arrhythmias, 235–240, 236f
supraventricular tachycardia (SVT), 237–238, 238f, 870
surface antigens, 587
surfactant replacement therapy
  for premature newborns, 67–68
  ventilation–perfusion matching affected by, 67
surgical debridement, burn wounds, 808
surgical embolectomy, for pulmonary embolism, 91
surgical site infections (SSIs), 900
sutures
  cranial, 352, 352f
  definition of, 352
SVC. *See* superior vena cava
SvO$_2$ measurements. *See* mixed venous oxygen saturation (SvO$_2$) measurements
SVR. *See* systemic vascular resistance
SVT. *See* supraventricular tachycardia
sweat chloride test, 52t
sweat glands, 591
Swiss cheese model, 889, 890
swollen epiglottis, 74f, 75
sympathetic nervous system
  anatomy of, 363–364
  heart regulation by, 155
  norepinephrine secretion, 154
  schematic diagram of, 365f
sympathetic stimulation, 155, 227
sympathomimetics, overdose of, 755–756
synapse, 351
synaptic cleft, 351
synchronized intermittent mandatory ventilation, 120, 131
syndrome of inappropriate antidiuretic hormone (SIADH), 527
  causes of, 518t
  complications of, 520
  conditions associated with, 518–519
  description of, 132
  diabetes insipidus versus, 519t
  diagnostic studies, 519
  differential diagnosis for, 524t, 525
  etiology of, 518–519
  hyponatremia caused by, 403, 518
  laboratory findings, 519, 519t
  management of, 520
  medications associated with, 519
  pathophysiology of, 518
  risk factors for, 518–519
  serum sodium normalization in, 519
  signs and symptoms, 519

syndromic scoliosis, 433
Synergy Model for Patient Care, 1–3
synthetic cannabinoid receptor agonists, 757t
synthetic cathinone stimulants, 757t
synthetic compounds, 756–758
systemic compensatory response, 225, 226
systemic inflammatory response syndrome (SIRS)
    definition of, 774
    description of, 625, 776
    mediator release in, 778f
    pathogenesis of, 777f
systemic injury, 96
systemic vascular resistance (SVR), 231, 232
    description of, 150, 156, 187
    in septic shock, 777, 787
systemic venous engorgement, 227
systems-level thinking, 911, 912f
systolic heart failure, 225
systolic murmurs, 170, 170f

T3. *See* triiodothyronine
T4. *See* thyroxine
T cells (T lymphocytes)
    description of, 589, 594
    disorders of, 636–637
T tubules, 159
T wave, 174
tachyarrhythmias, 870
tachycardia, 210, 314
    avoidance of, 230
    junctional, 93, 93f
    management of, 690
    pathophysiology of, 231
    sinus, 236
    ventricular, 241, 241f
tachypnea, 805
    definition of, 852
    respiratory failure caused by, 209, 210
tacrolimus, 541, 612
tadalafil, 206
tangential excision, 808
target concentration, 56
target effect, 56
TBI. *See* traumatic brain injury
TCAR Education Programs, 668
TDD. *See* total digitalizing dose
teach-back method, 903, 904
TeamSTEPPS model, 904, 905, 906f
teamwork
    barriers, 904
    and collaboration, 910
    communication, 905
    coordination, 905
    decision making, 905
    definition of, 904
    leadership, 905
    TeamSTEPPS model, 905, 906f
tear gas, 832, 833t

technology-dependent child
    complications of, 136
    definition of, 133
    emergency care, 134
    etiology of, 133
    home medical equipment, 134
    hospital readmission, 134–135
    from liberation, 136
    monitoring of, 135
    noninvasive mechanical ventilation, 133
    supportive care of, 135–136
    tracheostomy, 133, 133t, 135t
technology-dependent patients, 10
TEE. *See* transesophageal echocardiography
teeth, injuries to. *See* dental injuries
telangiectasis, 573
telemedicine, 876
telencephalon, 350, 350f, 354
temporal lobe
    description of, 354
    tumors of, 420
TEN. *See* toxic epidermal necrolysis
tendon
    burns of, 810
    injuries, 716
Tenormin. *See* atenolol
tension pneumothorax, 109f
    clinical presentation of, 111, 705t
    description of, 109, 110
    management of, 705t
    radiographic evaluation of, 111t
terbutaline, 865–866
terrorism. *See also* bioterrorism
    definition of, 827
    pediatric considerations in, 828
testes
    hormones produced by, 483t
    traumatic injuries to, 703, 707
testosterone, 483t
tetraiodothyroxine, 493
tetralogy of Fallot
    anatomy of, 286f
    anomalies associated with, 286
    clinical presentation, 286–287
    complications, 287
    definition of, 285
    diagnostic tests for, 287
    genetic syndromes, 286
    hemodynamics of, 252f
    incidence, 286
    interventions for, 286–287
    modified Blalock–Taussig shunt, 287, 288f
    pathophysiology of, 286
    patient management, 287
    pulmonary atresia with ventricularseptal defect, 287–290
TGA. *See* transposition of the great arteries
thalami, 355
thalidomide, 165t

theophylline, 99
therapeutic holding, 9
thermal injuries, 95, 676, 794t
thermodilution method, 181
thermoregulation. *See also* hyperthermia; hypothermia
    description of, 471
    during transport, 867–868
thiazide diuretics, 464
third-degree burns, 803f
third-degree heart block, 870
thirst receptors, 486
thoracic aorta, rupture of, 110
thoracic cavity, 38
thoracic duct, 586
thoracic excursion, 45
thoracic injuries, 704, 705t
thoracic trauma
    aorta injuries, 110, 111
    blunt, 110–111
    cardiac injuries, 110
    clinical presentation, 111–112
    definition, 108
    diagnostic tests, 111–112, 111t
    esophageal injuries, 110
    etiology of, 108
    great vessel injuries, 111
    hemothorax, 109f, 110
    management of, 112
    outcomes of, 112
    pathophysiology of, 108–111
    physical examination, 111
    rib fractures, 108–109
    supportive care for, 112
    tension pneumothorax, 109–111
    thoracoabdominal injuries, 111
    tracheobronchial injuries, 110
thoracoabdominal injuries, 111
thorax
    age-appropriate contours, 45f
    anatomic landmarks of, 44–45
    contour of, 44, 45f
    percussion of, 46–47, 47f
three-dimensional echocardiography, 178
threshold potential, 159
thrills, 167–168
thrombin time, 606
thrombocytes, 589–590
thrombocytopenia
    description of, 599
    heparin-induced, 615, 646–647
    immune thrombocytopenic purpura, 642–644
    platelet therapy for, 617t
thromboelastography, 607
thromboembolism, 90, 718–719
thrombopoetin, 585
thromboxane A$_2$, 454
thymoglobulin, 613
thyrocalcitonin, 481t
thyroglobulin, 493

thyroid gland
  cell types of, 493
  embryology of, 493
  hormones produced by, 481t, 493
  location, 493
thyroid-stimulating hormone (TSH), 480t, 490
thyroid storm, 495
thyrotrophs, 487, 490
thyrotropin, 480t, 490
thyrotropin-releasing hormone (TRH), 487, 505
thyroxine, 481t, 483, 490, 493–495
TIBC. *See* total iron-binding capacity
tidal volume, 118t, 124
tissue oxygenation, 787–788
tissue perfusion, 252
tissue plasminogen activator, 590, 600
tissue typing, 605
TLS. *See* tumor lysis syndrome
TMP–SMX. *See* trimethoprim–sulfamethoxazole
TNCC. *See* Trauma Nursing Core Course
TNF. *See* tumor necrosis factor
tobacco smoke exposure, 96
toddlers. *See also* children; infants
  cognitive development in, 4
  communication by, 17
  death, concept of, 4
  fear responses by, 8
  hospitalization response of, 7
  pain assessment and management, 11t, 13t
  personality development in, 4
  play with, 20
  poisoning of, 736–737
  principles for working with, 5–6
  psychosocial development of, 4
  stress response of, 7
  traumatic injuries in, 671t
toe-to-heel walking, 373
toes, burns of, 810
tonic neck response, 372
tonic seizures, 404
tonsillar lymph nodes, 587f
total anomalous pulmonary venous return, 169
  anatomy, 293–294
  diagnostic tests for, 294
  pathophysiology of, 294
  from pulmonary venous confluence, 294f
  to right atrium, 296f
total cavopulmonary connection, 292, 294f
total digitalizing dose (TDD), 192
total iron-binding capacity (TIBC), 454, 455t
total lung capacity, 41, 118t
total lung compliance, 118
total parenteral nutrition (TPN), 820
toxic alcohols, 743t
toxic epidermal necrolysis (TEN), 813, 815
  nutritional requirements, 815

special care areas, 815
treatment of, 815
wound-care goals, 815
toxidromes, 739t
TPN. *See* total parenteral nutrition
trachea
  anatomy of, 37, 37f
  embryology of, 37
  palpation of, 45
tracheal aspirate culture, 52t
tracheal stenosis, 74
  clinical presentation of, 74
  definition of, 73–74
  outcomes of, 74
  pathophysiology of, 74
  patient care management, 74
tracheal trauma, 687
tracheobronchial rupture, 705t
tracheobronchial trauma, 110
tracheoesophageal fistula, 560t
  clinical presentation of, 72
  definition of, 70
  outcomes of, 72
  pathophysiology of, 71–72
  patient care management, 72
tracheomalacia
  chronic lung disease and, 116
  definition of, 73
  mechanical ventilation requirements for, 123t
  pathophysiology of, 73
  patient care management, 73
tracheostomy, 103
  for BPD patients, 116
  causal factors for, 133t
  emergency supplies and equipment, 135t
  intubation versus, 76
traditional safety thinking, 890
transcortin, 501
transcranial Doppler ultrasound, 385
  pressure-volume relationships, 360–361, 360f
transcription factors, 147
transcutaneous carbon dioxide monitoring, 54
transcutaneous oxygen monitoring, 54
transducers, for intracranial pressure monitoring, 388
transesophageal echocardiography (TEE), 178
transferrin, 455t
transferrin saturation (Tsat), 455t
transitional circulation, 151–152
transplantation
  heart, 224, 231
  intestine, 576–579
  liver, 574–576
  renal, 473
transport metrics, 876–878, 877t–878t
transport of critically ill patients
  advanced skills training for, 850
  atmospheric considerations, 846
  barometric pressure changes, 847

configuration of, 849
equipment, 849
family issues, 845
humidity considerations, 848
hyperthermia during, 867–868
hypothermia during, 852, 854, 867
legal issues for, 845
overview of, 844
physiology of, 845–848
population utilizing, 850, 851t
principles of, 844–845
stabilization of patient during. *See* stabilization of patient
stress caused by, 847
thermal regulation during, 847–848, 867–868
transposition of the great arteries (TGA), 252f, 295, 296, 298f. *See also* D-transposition of the great arteries; L-transposition of the great arteries
transthoracic pacing, 244
transvenous catheters, 244
Trauma Nursing Core Course (TNCC), 668
trauma scoring, 688
traumatic aneurysm, 411
traumatic arrest, 691
traumatic brain injury (TBI)
  clinical presentation of, 425–426
  definition, 424
  etiology, 424
  management of, 426–427
  outcomes of, 427
  pathophysiology of, 424–425
traumatic injuries. *See also* blunt trauma; penetrating trauma
  abdominal, 704, 706
  acceleration-deceleration injury, 674
  in adolescents, 672t
  airway management
    assessment of, 681
    endotracheal intubation, 689
    foreign material in, 688
    jaw thrust maneuver for, 688
    nasopharyngeal, 689
    oropharyngeal, 688–689
    rapid-sequence intubation, 689
  amputations, 672t, 691, 710, 716
  animal bites, 674
  assessment after, 681–686
    abdomen, 687
    airway, 681
    back, 688
    cervical spine, 681
    chest, 687
    circulatory system, 686
    ears, 687
    exposure, 684t, 686, 687
    extremities, 688
    face, 687
    head, 687
    neck, 687
    neurologic system, 686

traumatic injuries (*cont.*)
  assessment after (*cont.*)
    nose, 687
    oral cavity, 687
    pelvis, 692
    primary, 681–686
    pulse oximetry, 688
    respiration, 686
    respiratory, 686
    secondary, 686–688
    vital signs, 688
  breathing management, 690
  cervical spine management, 681, 688–690
  chemical injury, 676
  circulation management, 690–691
  cold exposure, 676–677, 684t, 686
  complications of
    compartment syndrome, 717
    fat embolism syndrome, 717–718
    rhabdomyolysis, 716–717
    venous thromboembolism, 718–719
  crush injuries, 673–674
  dental, 700
  diagnostic testing, 691–692
  disability assessments after, 691
  drowning, 677–679
  electrical injury, 676
  emotional support after, 693–695
  epidemiology of, 668–670
  exposure injuries, 676–677, 684t, 686, 691
  factors that affect, 669–670
  falls, 669, 670t–672t
  firearm injuries, 674–675
  gastrointestinal management, 691
  genitourinary management, 691
  head, 695–700, 701
  health history, 680
  heat exposure injuries, 676–677, 684t, 686
  history-taking, 679–680
  incidence of, 668–670
  in infants, 670t–671t
  kinetic energy-related, 673–676
  knife wounds, 674
  leading causes of, 669t
  mandibular fractures, 700
  maxillofacial, 700–701
  mechanical ventilation, 690
  mechanisms of injury, 669, 670, 673–679
  midfacial fractures, 701
  motor vehicle traffic-related deaths, 668
  musculoskeletal, 691, 710–715
  nasal fractures, 701
  nerve injuries, 715
  neurologic assessments after, 691
  pain assessments, 692–693
  penetrating, 674–675
  in preschool-age children, 671t
  prevention of, 670, 670t–673t
  radiant burns, 676
  renal, 473–474, 698
  resuscitation after, 679
  in school-age children, 672t
  shear injury, 674
  spinal cord, 701–702
  submersion, 678–679
  tendon injuries, 716
  terrorism, 827
  thermal injury, 676
  in toddlers, 671t
  trauma scoring, 688
traumatic pneumothorax, 109–110, 109f
treatment
  life-sustaining, forgoing of, 26–27
  withdrawal of, 27
treprostinil, 205–206
TRH. *See* thyrotropin-releasing hormone
tricuspid area, 171
tricuspid atresia
  anatomy of, 291
  classification of, 292f
  diagnostic tests for, 292
  etiology of, 291
  incidence of, 291, 294
  interventions for, 293
  pathophysiology of, 291–292
  with transposition of the great arteries, 292f
tricyclic antidepressant poisoning, 743t, 746–747
trigeminal nerve
  in children, 378t
  function of, 364t
  in infants, 374t
triiodothyronine, 481t, 483, 490, 494–495
trimethoprim–sulfamethoxazole (TMP–SMX), 26, 610, 641
Triple Aim, 886
Trisomy 13, 164t
Trisomy 18, 164t
Trisomy 21, 164t
trochlear nerve
  in children, 377t
  function of, 364t
  in infants, 374t
truncus arteriosus (TA), embryologic development of, 147, 148t
trust
  building of, 24
  establishing of, 5
  versus mistrust, 4
TSH. *See* thyroid-stimulating hormone
tuberculosis
  clinical presentation of, 84
  definition of, 84
  outcomes of, 85
  pathophysiology of, 84
  patient care management, 84–85
tularemia, 838t, 839
tumor(s)
  central nervous system, 419–422
  definition of, 419
  infratentorial, 419–420
  supratentorial, 420
tumor lysis syndrome (TLS), 467, 649–651
tumor necrosis factor (TNF), 597t, 777
Turner syndrome, 164t
2,3-diphosphoglycerate, 42
two-dimensional echocardiography, 177–178
two-point discrimination, 717
tympany, 47
type 2 diabetes mellitus (T2DM), 508
type I hypersensitivity reactions, 628t
type II hypersensitivity reactions, 628t
type III hypersensitivity reactions, 628t
type IV hypersensitivity reactions, 628t
tyrosine, 493
tyrosinemia, 574

Ufd1, 147
ultrafiltration
  definition of, 468
  slow continuous, 471
ultrasonography, 423, 474
ultrasound
  abdominal, 536t
  acute abdominal trauma evaluations, 549
  renal diagnosis using, 454, 455
umbilical veins, 148t
uncal herniation, 401
unobstructed veins, 270
upper airways
  in airway resistance, 39
  anatomy of, 36–37, 37f
  development of, 36–37
  diseases, 98
  mechanical ventilation requirements for, 123t
  stridor associated with, 209
upper gastrointestinal tract bleeding
  clinical presentation, 554–555, 555t
  definition of, 554
  esophageal varices, 556
  etiology of, 553, 554t
  in infants and children, 554t
  management of, 574
  pathophysiology of, 553–554
  patient care management, 555–556
  signs and symptoms of, 554
urea, 454
uremia, 454, 458, 462, 599
uremic pericarditis, 462
uric acid, 454
urinalysis, 456
  acute abdominal trauma evaluations, 549
  acute kidney injury findings, 459, 460
  rhabdomyolysis findings, 717
urine
  concentration of, 447, 450
  "dumb," 459
  electrolyte measurement, 456
  formation of, 447–450
urine osmolarity, 450

urine output
monitoring of, during fluid
resuscitation, 807
renal perfusion and, 854
urokinase, 615

v-EEG. *See* video-EEG
V/Q scan. *See* ventilation–perfusion
(V/Q) scan
vaccination, 107
VAD. *See* ventricular assist device
VAE. *See* ventilator-associated events
vagus nerve
in children, 379t
function of, 364t
in infants, 375t
vagus nerve stimulator (VNS), 407
valproic acid, 398, 399t
valvular aortic stenosis, 271–274
valvuloplasty
for aortic stenosis, 272, 272f, 281, 285f
balloon, 285, 285f
valvulotomy, 286f
varices, 556, 573
vascular access, 212, 213, 213f, 214f, 857
vascular bed, 361
vascular chemoreceptors, 779
vascular endothelium, 105
vaso-occlusive crisis, 634–635
vasoactive agents, 231
description of, 784–787, 785t
mechanism of action, 189
septic shock treated with, 786t
types of, 189–193
vasoactive drugs, 860, 861f
vasoconstriction, 231, 492
vasodilation, 107, 108, 592, 777
vasodilators
inhaled, 108
pulmonary, 230
vasogenic edema, 400
vasopressin, 191, 213, 492, 518, 518t, 521.
See also antidiuretic hormone
antibleeding uses of, 537
description of, 191, 213, 450, 481t
Vasotec. *See* enalapril maleate
VCUG. *See* voiding
cystourethorography
vecuronium, 58t
veins, 150, 411, 412
cannulation of, 125, 799
pulmonary, 149f, 269–270, 294
unobstructed, 270
velocardiofacial syndrome, 164t
veno-occlusive disease (VOD), 656–657
venoconstriction, 154
venous blood, 356
venous occlusion, 716
venous oxygen content, 43t
venous oxygen saturation
description of, 43t
jugular, 390–392
monitoring of, 188

venous partial pressure of oxygen, 43t
venous thromboembolism, 718–719
ventilation
in advanced cardiac life support, 210
airway management in, 127
assessment of patient during, 128
barotrauma in, 132
bronchopulmonary dysplasia caused
by, 114
complications of, 132–133
extracorporeal membrane
oxygenation, 125
flow delivery, 122
high-frequency, 94, 123–125
inverse-ratio, 123
monitoring during, 128
negative-pressure, 126, 230
nutrition during, 130
objectives of, 118
pain management during, 130
patient position, 212f
pediatric acute respiratory distress
syndrome, 92–94
physiologic interface with child,
119–120
positive-pressure, 230
controls, 121–122
definition of, 120
flow delivery, 122
mechanics of, 121f
modes of, 120–121
noninvasive, 126
phase variables for, 122–123
sensing mechanisms, 122
pressure, flow, and resistance
relationships, 119
psychological needs during, 130
pulmonary hypertension, 107
sedation during, 130
shock managed using, 234
variables for, 123, 123t
weaning from
dysfunctional, 222
readiness for, 131
techniques for, 131–132
ventilation–perfusion matching
agents that affect, 67–68
description of, 40, 40f
ventilation–perfusion mismatching
hypoxemia caused by, 116
in pulmonary hypertension, 107
ventilation–perfusion (V/Q) scan,
53, 106
ventilator-associated events (VAE), 819
ventilator-associated pneumonia, 128
ventral root, of spinal nerves, 363
ventricles
anatomy of, 352
autonomic nerve stimulation effects
on, 367t
external drainage of, 393–394, 393f
of heart
depolarization of, 160
description of, 147

embryologic formation of, 147, 148t
factors that affect, 155–157
repolarization of, 160
ventricular arrhythmias, 240–242, 241f
ventricular assist device (VAD),
217, 223f
complications, 224
continuous flow, 222
contraindications, 217–218
neurologic evaluation, 222
patient care and management,
222–224
pulsatile, 218, 222
selection, 218f
types of, 222
ventricular asynchronous mode, of
pacemaker, 246t
ventricular compliance, 225, 225f
ventricular demand mode, of
pacemaker, 246t
ventricular failure, 92
ventricular fibrillation, 241, 241f
ventricular septal defect
assessment of, 256
in atrioventricular septal defect,
258–259, 258f
classification of, 256–257, 257f
definition of, 256
etiology of, 256
interventions for, 257
pathophysiology of, 256
perimembranous, 256
pulmonary atresia with, 287–290
subaortic, double-outlet right
ventricle with, 261f
ventricular shunt, 393–395
external, 393–394, 393f
internal, 394–395, 395f
ventricular tachycardia (VT), 241,
241f, 870
ventriculoperitoneal shunt, 395f
venules, 150
VER. *See* visual-evoked response
verapamil, 196–197
vertebrae, 356–357
vertebral arteries, 356
vertebral column, 357f
vesicants, 832
vesicular breath sounds, 47
video-EEG (v-EEG), 386–387
violence, 829–830
viral hemorrhagic fevers, 838t
viral meningitis, 397t, 416, 417
"visiting privileges," 25
visual-evoked response (VER), 387
vital capacity
definition of, 119
description of, 41, 42f
equation for, 118t
vital signs, 379–380, 688
vitamin D, 452
vitamin K
deficiency of, 629
description of, 590, 615, 629

vitamin K1, 537
vitelline veins, 148t
VNS. *See* vagus nerve stimulator
VO$_2$. *See* oxygen consumption
vocal cords, 37
VOD. *See* veno-occlusive disease
voiding cystourethrography
　　(VCUG), 455
volume overload, 226
voluntary reporting systems (VRS), 883
volvulus, 559t
von Hippel-Lindau disease, 419
VRS. *See* voluntary reporting systems
VT. *See* ventricular tachycardia

warfarin, 204, 229, 615
warm-reactive autoantibodies, 608
warm shock, 783t
water
　balance
　　hormonal control of, 450–451
　　measuring of, 450
　reabsorption, 450
water-deprivation test, 505, 521–522
waterhammer pulse, 168, 253
waveforms
　arterial, 183, 185f
　intracranial pressure monitoring,
　　389–390, 390f
WBCs. *See* white blood cells
weaning, from mechanical ventilation
　dysfunctional, 222
　readiness for, 131
　techniques for, 131–132
Wenckebach block, 870
Wenckebach phenomenon,
　242–243, 242f

West's zones of perfusion, 40
wheezing, 48, 81, 209
Whipple's triad, 515
white blood cell count
　description of, 52t, 602, 604
　in septic shock, 781
white blood cell disorders, 636–638
white blood cells (WBCs), 354. *See also*
　　specific cells
　in bone marrow, 588
　cellular response, 592
　description of, 587
　functions of, 591
　homeostasis, 591
　hyperactivity of, 627–628
　hypoactivity of, 624–627
　physiologic mechanisms of, 591–598
　surveillance, 591
　transfusion of, 617t
　vascular response, 592
white matter, of spinal cord, 357
white rami communicants, 363
whole-bowel irrigation, 741
Williams syndrome, 164t
Wilson's disease, 571
Wiskott–Aldrich syndrome, 637
Wolff–Parkinson–White (WPW)
　　syndrome, 163t, 238–239
work of breathing
　in bronchopulmonary dysplasia, 116
　description of, 36, 853
　respiratory mechanics for
　　evaluating, 209
workplace stress, 915
workplace wellness, 915–916
wound(s)
　bullet, 675
　burn. *See* burn wound

cultures, 816
gunshot, 548, 667
knife, 674
stab, 548
wound debridement, 808
　chemical or enzymatic, 808
　mechanical, 808
　surgical, 808
WPW syndrome. *See* Wolff–Parkinson–
　　White syndrome
wrinkle test, 715

X-linked agammaglobulinemia, 636
xanthomas, 573
xenograft, 811
xenon-enhanced CT scan, 385
Xolair (omalizumab), 99
Xopenex. *See* levalbuterol

yaw, 675

Zantac. *See* ranitidine
Zaroxolyn, 464
zidovudine, 610
Zofran. *See* ondansetron
zona fasciculata, 499, 500
zona glomerulosa, 499
zona reticularis, 499, 500
zone of coagulation, 793, 795, 795f
zone of hyperemia, 793, 795f
zone of stasis, 793, 795f
Zovirax. *See* acyclovir